CURRENT
Diagnosis & Treatment in OTOLARYNGOLOGY— HEAD & NECK SURGERY

Edited by

Anil K. Lalwani, MD
Mendik Foundation Professor and Chairman
Department of Otolaryngology
Professor of Pediatrics, and Physiology & Neuroscience
New York University School of Medicine
New York, New York

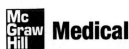

Mc Graw Hill **Medical**

New York Chicago San Francisco Lisbon London Madrid Mexico City
Milan New Delhi San Juan Seoul Singapore Sydney Toronto

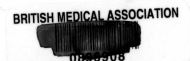

Current Diagnosis & Treatment in Otolaryngology—Head & Neck Surgery

1 2 3 4 5 6 7 8 9 0 DOC/DOC 0 9 8 7

ISBN 978-0-07-146027-9
ISSN 1545-6307
MHID 0-07-146027-6

Notice

Medicine is an ever-changing science. As new research and clinical experience broaden our knowledge, changes in treatment and drug therapy are required. The authors and the publisher of this work have checked with sources believed to be reliable in their efforts to provide information that is complete and generally in accord with the standards accepted at the time of publication. However, in view of the possibility of human error or changes in medical sciences, neither the authors nor the publisher nor any other party who has been involved in the preparation or publication of this work warrants that the information contained herein is in every respect accurate or complete, and they disclaim all responsibility for any errors or omissions or for the results obtained from use of the information contained in this work. Readers are encouraged to confirm the information contained herein with other sources. For example and in particular, readers are advised to check the product information sheet included in the package of each drug they plan to administer to be certain that the information contained in this work is accurate and that changes have not been made in the recommended dose or in the contraindications for administration. This recommendation is of particular importance in connection with new or infrequently used drugs.

The editors were Marsha Loeb and Harriet Lebowitz.
The production supervisor was Phil Galea.
Cover design: Mary McKeon
Cover photos: clockwise from upper left:
Cochlear implant. Illustration of a cochlear implant in a human ear. Credit: John Bavosi/Photo Researchers, Inc.
Sinusitis. Colored computed tomography (CT) scan of a coronal section through the face of a 65 year old woman, showing sinusitis and a nasal polyp. Credit: M. Kulyk/Photo Researchers, Inc.
Cosmetic eyelid surgery. Face of a woman about to undergo cosmetic eyelid surgery. Credit: Coneyl Jay/Photo Researchers, Inc.
The index was prepared by Ann Blum.
The printer was RR Donnelley.

This book is printed on acid-free paper.

ISE 978-0-07-128741-8
ISE MHID 0-07-128741-8

To the *original* NYU Dream Team, Robert M. Glickman, MD, Richard I. Levin, MD, Andrew W. Brotman, MD, Eric C. Rackow, MD, and John M. Deeley for their compassionate leadership and warm friendship.

To my parents, Madan and Gulab, for giving me life;
to my in-laws, Rikhab and Ratan, for greatly adding to my life;
to my wife, Renu, who is my life,
and, to my children, Nikita and Sahil, who show me how to enjoy life.

A special dedication of this second edition to the memory of:
Kelvin C. Lee, MD
1958-2005
A loving father and husband, a compassionate physician, a superb teacher, and a wonderful colleague
and friend who left a positive impact on all of our lives and is deeply missed.

CONTENTS

AUTHORS

Sumit K. Agrawal, MD, FRCSC
Neurotology Fellow, Department of Otolaryngology—
Head and Neck Surgery, Stanford University School of
Medicine
Stanford, California
sagrawal@ohns.stanford.edu
Occupational Hearing Loss

Demetrio J. Aguila, MD
Chief Resident, Department of Otolaryngology—
Head and Neck Surgery, Mount Sinai School of
Medicine
Brooklyn, New York
viperdoc@gmail.com
*Parapharyngeal Space Neoplasms and
Deep Neck Space Infections*

Min S. Ahn, MD
Medical Director, The Anesthetic Wellness Center
Westborough, Massachusetts
minahn@awcenter.com
Hair Restoration—Surgical and Medical Therapy

Milan R. Amin, MD
Assistant Professor of Otolaryngology—Head and Neck
Surgery, Chief, Division of Laryngology, Department of
Otolaryngology—Head and Neck Surgery, NYU School
of Medicine
New York, New York
milan.amin@nyumc.org
Laryngeal Trauma

Shahram Anari, MD, MSc, MRCS
Specialist Registrar in Otolaryngology—Head and Neck
Surgery, Department of Otolaryngology—Head and
Neck Surgery, Freeman Hospital
Newcastle upon Tyne, United Kingdom
sssanari@yahoo.co.uk
Stridor in Children; Otitis Media

Joseph M. Bernstein, MD
Assistant Professor of Otolaryngology and Pediatrics, Direc-
tor, Pediatric Otolaryngology, NYU School of Medicine
New York, New York
joseph.bernstein@med.nyu.edu
Management of Adenotonsillar Disease

Kofi D.O. Boahene, MD
Assistant Professor, Department of Otolaryngology—Head
and Neck Surgery, John Hopkins Medical Institute
Baltimore, Maryland
dboahen1@jhmi.edu
Otosclerosis

William E. Brownell, PhD
Professor and Jake and Nina Kamin Chair of Otorhinolaryngology, Bobby R. Alford Department of Otolaryngology, Baylor College of Medicine
Houston, Texas
brownell@bcm.tmc.edu
Anatomy and Physiology of the Ear

Fidelia Yuan-Shin Butt, MD
Adjunct Clinical Assistant Professor, Department of
Otolaryngology—Head and Neck Surgery, Stanford
University School of Medicine
Staff Physician, The Permanente Medical Group Santa Clara
Santa Clara, California
fidelia.butt@stanfordalumni.org
Benign Diseases of the Salivary Glands

Troy Cascia, AuD
Clinical Audiologist, Audiology Clinic, University of
California, San Francisco Medical Center
San Francisco, California
Troy.cascia@ucsfmedctr.org
Rehabilitation and Hearing Aids

Kelvin Chan, BA
Research Assistant, Department of Radiation Oncology,
Memorial Sloan-Kettering Cancer Center
New York, New York
chank@mskcc.org
*Benign and Malignant Lesions of the Oral Cavity,
Oropharynx, and Nasopharynx*

C.Y. Joseph Chang, MD
Professor and Chairman of the Department of Otolaryn-
gology—Head and Neck Surgery, University of Texas-
Houston Medical School
Houston, Texas
c.y.chang@uth.tmc.edu
Cholesteatoma

Steven W. Cheung, MD
Associate Professor, Department of Otolaryngology—Head and Neck Surgery, University of California, San Francisco
San Francisco, California
aritter@ohns.ucsf.edu
Osseous Dysplasia of the Temporal Bone; Implantable Middle Ear Hearing Devices

Peter V. Chin-Hong, MD
Assistant Professor of Medicine, University of California, San Francisco
San Francisco, California
phong@php.ucsf.edu
Antimicrobial Therapy for Head and Neck Infection

Jeannie H. Chung, MD
Associate Staff, Department of Otolaryngology—Head and Neck Surgery, Massachusetts Eye and Ear Infirmary
Salem, Massachusetts
Microvascular Reconstruction

Adriane P. Concus, MD
Participant Physician, The Permanente Medical Group, Inc., Department of Head and Neck Surgery, Kaiser, South San Francisco
South San Francisco, California
adriane.concus@kp.org
Malignant Diseases of the Salivary Glands; Malignant Laryngeal Lesions

Minas Constantinides, MD
Director, Facial Plastic and Reconstructive Surgery, Department of Otolaryngology, NYU School of Medicine
New York, New York
minas.constantinides@med.nyu.edu
Blepharoplasty; Rhinoplasty; Otoplasty; Facial Fillers and Implants

Allen M. Dekelboum, MD
Clinical Professor, Retired, Department of Otolaryngology—Head and Neck Surgery, University of California, San Francisco
Instructor Trainer, Emeritus, National Association of Underwater Instructors, Tampa, Florida, Divers Alert Network (Duke University), Durham, North Carolina
Novato, California
divedoc@mindspring.com
Diving Medicine

Mark D. DeLacure, MD, FACS
Chief, Division of Head and Neck Surgery and Oncology, Department of Otolaryngology—Head and Neck Surgery, Associate Professor of Plastic Surgery, Institute of Reconstructive Plastic Surgery, Department of Surgery, NYU Clinical Cancer Center, NYU School of Medicine
New York, New York
mark.delacure@nyumc.org
Malignant Diseases of the Salivary Glands; Malignant Laryngeal Lesions

Jaimie DeRosa, MD
Department of Otolaryngology, Geisner Medical Center
Danville, Pennsylvania
jaimie.derosa@bmc.org
Mandible Reconstruction

Daniel G. Deschler, MD, FACS
Associate Professor, Department of Otolaryngology, Harvard Medical School
Director, Division and Head and Neck Surgery, Director, Norman Knight Hyperbaric Medicine Center, Massachusetts Ear and Eye Infirmary
Director, Head and Neck Surgical Oncology, Massachusetts General Hospital
Boston, Massachusetts
daniel_deschler@meei.harvard.edu
Neck Masses; Microvascular Reconstruction

Nripendra Dhillon, MBBS, MS
Lecturer in Anatomy, Department of Anatomy, University of California, San Francisco
San Francisco, California
nripendra.dhillon@itsa.ucsf.edu
Anatomy

Colin L.W. Driscoll, MD
Associate Professor, Mayo Medical School
Consultant, Department of Otolaryngology, Mayo Clinic and Mayo Foundation
Rochester, Minnesota
driscoll.colin@mayo.edu
Otosclerosis; Cochlear Implants

Joseph L. Edmonds, Jr., MD
Clinical Assistant Professor, Division of Otolaryngology and Plastic Surgery, Department of Surgery, Baylor College of Medicine, Weill Cornell Medical College, Attending Physician, Texas Children's Hospital
Houston, Texas
otodoc@edmondsmd.com
Hemangiomas of Infancy and Vascular Malformations

David W. Eisele, MD, FACS
Professor and Chairman, Department of Otolaryngology—Head and Neck Surgery, University of California, San Francisco
San Francisco, California
deisele@ohns.ucsf.edu
Malignant Thyroid Neoplasms; Parathyroid Disorders

Ivor A. Emanuel, MD
Assistant Clinical Professor, Department of Otolaryngology, University of California, San Francisco
Private Practice in Otolaryngology and Allergy
Adjunct Clinical Faculty, Department of Otolaryngology, Stanford University
San Francisco, California
emanuelmd@comcast.net
Nonallergic and Allergic Rhinitis

Nancy J. Fischbein, MD
Associate Professor of Radiology and, by courtesy, of Otolaryngology—Head and Neck Surgery
Chief, Head and Neck Radiology
Stanford University School of Medicine
Stanford, California
fischbein@stanford.edu
Radiology

Steven F. Fowler, MD
Postdoctoral Research Fellow, University of California, San Francisco
San Francisco, California
steven.fowler@cshs.org
Congenital Disorders of the Trachea and Esophagus

Michael B. Gluth, MD
Instructor, Department of Otorhinolaryngology, Mayo Clinic College of Medicine, Rochester, Minnesota, Director of Otology, Ear, Nose, and Throat Center of the Ozarks
Springdale, Arkansas
gluth.michael@mayo.edu
Cochlear Implants

Greg Goddard, DDS
Associate Clinical Professor, Division of Dentistry, Department of Oral and Maxillofacial Surgery, University of California, San Francisco
San Francisco, California
Greg.goddard@ucsf.edu
Temporomandibular Disorders

Andrew N. Goldberg, MD, MSCE, FACS
Professor, Div. of Rhinology and Sinus Surgery, Department Otolaryngology—Head and Neck Surgery, University of California, San Francisco
San Francisco, California
agoldberg@ohns.ucsf.edu
Frontal Sinus Fractures; Sleep Disorders

Eli Grunstein, MD
Assistant Professor of Clinical Otolaryngology—Head and Neck Surgery, Department of Otolaryngology—Head and Neck Surgery, Columbia University Medical Center
eg582@columbia.edu
Diseases of the External Ear

Nicolas Gürtler, MD
Hals-Nasen-Ohren-Universitatsklinik, University Hospital Basel
Basel, Switzerland
nguertler@uhbs.ch
Hereditary Hearing Impairment

Fernando Augusto Mardiros Herbella, MD
Instructor, Attending Surgeon, Department of Surgery
Federal University of Sao Paulo
Sao Paulo, Brazil
Herbella.dcir@epm.br
Benign and Malignant Disorders of the Esophagus

William Y. Hoffman, MD
Professor and Chief, Division of Plastic and Reconstructive Surgery, Department of Surgery, University of California, San Francisco
San Francisco, California
hoffmanw@surgery.ucsf.edu
Cleft Lip and Palate

C.P. Hybarger, MD, FACS
Assistant Clinical Professor, Department of Otolaryngology—Head and Neck Surgery, University of California, San Francisco, Chief of Micrographic Surgery, San Rafael Kaiser Permanente Medical Center
San Rafael, California
pat.hybarger@kp.org
Cutaneous Malignant Neoplasms

Krzysztof Izdebski, FK, MA, PhD, CCC-SLP, FASHA
Assistant Clinical Professor, Department of Otolaryngology—Head and Neck Surgery, Stanford Voice and Swallowing Center, Stanford University School of Medicine
Chairman, Pacific Voice and Speech Foundation
San Francisco, California
kizdebski@ohns.stanford.edu; kizdebski@pvsf.org
Clinical Voice Assessment: The Role and Value of the Phonatory Function Studies

David M. Jablons, MD
ADA Distinguished Professor of Surgery, Chief, Section of General Thoracic Surgery, University of California, San Francisco
San Francisco, California
jablonsd@surgery.ucsf.edu
Benign and Malignant Disorders of the Trachea

Robert K. Jackler, MD
Sewall Professor and Chair, Department of Otolaryngology—Head and Neck Surgery, Professor of Neurosurgery and Surgery, Associate Dean of Continuing Medical Education, Stanford University School of Medicine
Stanford, California
jackler@stanford.edu
Occupational Hearing Loss; Neurotologic Skull Base Surgery

Richard A. Jacobs, MD, PhD
Clinical Professor of Medicine and Clinical Pharmacy, University of California, San Francisco
San Francisco, California
jacobsd@medicine.ucsf.edu
Antimicrobial Therapy for Head and Neck Infection

Jacob Johnson, MD
Assistant Clinical Professor, Department of Otolaryngology—Head and Neck Surgery, University of California, San Francisco
San Francisco, California
jjohnson@ohns.ucsf.edu
Vestibular Disorders; Vestibular Schwannoma (Acoustic Neuroma); Nonacoustic Lesions of the Cerebellopontine Angle

Michael J. Kaplan, MD
Professor, Department of Otolaryngology—Head and Neck Surgery, Stanford University
Stanford, California
mjkaplan@stanford.edu
Lesions of the Anterior Skull Base

Eugene J. Kim, MD
Private Practice in Otolaryngology, Communal Medial Group
Mountain View, California
Rhytidectomy, Browlifts, and Midface Lifts; Blepharoplasty

W. Michael Korn, MD
Assistant Professor of Medicine in Residence, Divisions of Gastroenterology and Hematology/Oncology, University of California, San Francisco
San Francisco, California
mkorn@cc.ucsf.edu
Bening and Malignant Disorders of the Esophagus

Christina J. Laane, MD
Partner, Ear, Nose, and Throat Associates of San Mateo County
San Mateo, California
christina@onebox.com
Congenital Anomalies of the Nose

Anil K. Lalwani, MD, FACS
Mendik Foundation Professor and Chairman, Department of Otolaryngology; Professor of Pediatrics, and Physiology & Neuroscience, New York University School of Medicine
New York, New York
anil.lalwani@nyumc.org
Olfactory Dysfunction; Sensorineural Hearing Loss; The Aging Inner Ear; Vestibular Disorders; Vestibular Schwannoma (Acoustic Neuroma); Nonacoustic Lesions of the Cerebellopontine Angle; Neurofibromatosis Type 2; Cochlear Implants

Hanmin Lee, MD
Associate Professor of Surgery, Pediatrics, Obstetrics, Gynecology, and Reproductive Sciences, Director, Fetal Treatment Center, Department of Surgery, University of California, San Francisco
San Francisco, California
leeh@surgery.ucsf.edu
Congenital Disorders of the Trachea and Esophagus

Grace A. Lee, MD
Clinical Fellow, Department of Endocrinology and Metabolism, University of California, San Francisco
San Francisco, California
galee@itsa.ucsf.edu
Disorders of the Thyroid Gland

Nancy Lee, MD
Assistant Attending, Department of Radiation Oncology, Memorial Sloan-Kettering Cancer Center
New York, New York
leen2@mskcc.org
Management of Adenotonsillar Disease; Benign and Malignant Lesions of the Oral Cavity, Oropharynx, and Nasopharynx

Derrick T. Lin, MD
Assistant Professor, Department of Otology and Laryngology, Harvard Medical School, Massachusetts Eye and Ear Infirmary
Boston, Massachusetts
derrick_lin@meei.harvard.edu
Neck Masses

Errol P. Lobo, MD, PhD
Professor of Anesthesia and Perioperative Care, Department of Anesthesia and Perioperative Care, University of California, San Francisco
San Francisco, California
loboe@anesthesia.ucsf.edu
Anesthesia for Head and Neck Surgery

Lawrence R. Lustig, MD
Associate Professor, Division of Otology, Neurotology, and Skull Base Surgery, Department of Otolaryngology—Head and Neck Surgery, University of California, San Francisco
San Francisco, California
llustig@ohns.ucsf.edu
Anatomy, Physiology, and Testing of the Facial Nerve; Disorders of the Facial Nerve

Corey S. Maas, MD, FACS
Associate Clinical Professor, Division of Facial Plastic Surgery, University of California, San Francisco
San Francisco, California
drmaas@drmaas.com
Rhytidectomy, Browlifts, and Midface Lifts; Blepharoplasty; Rhinoplasty

Aditi H. Mandpe, MD
Assistant Clinical Professor, Department of Otolaryngology—Head and Neck Surgery, University of California, San Francisco
San Francisco, California
Paranasal Sinus Neoplasms; Neck Neoplasms and Neck Dissection

Umesh Masharani, MRCP
Clinical Professor of Medicine, Division of Endocrinology and Metabolism, University of California, San Francisco
San Francisco, California
Umesh.masharani@ucsf.edu
Disorders of the Thyroid Gland

Nathan Monhian, MD, FACS
Director, Monhian Center for Facial Cosmetic Surgery
Great Neck, New York
drmonhian1@verizon.net
Scar Revision; Local and Regional Flaps in Head and Neck Reconstruction

Karsten Munck, MD
Staff Otolaryngologist, Department of Otolaryngology—Head and Neck Surgery, Travis Air Force Base
Travis, California
kmunck@ohns.ucsf.edu
Parathyroid Disorders; Osseous Dysplasia of the Temporal Bone

Andrew H. Murr, MD, FACS
Professor of Clinical Otolaryngology, Department of Otolaryngology—Head and Neck Surgery, University of California, San Francisco, Chief of Service, Department of Otolaryngology—Head and Neck Surgery, San Francisco General Hospital
San Francisco, California
ahmurr@ohns.ucsf.edu
Maxillofacial Trauma; Laryngeal Trauma

John K. Niparko, MD
George T. Nager Professor of Otolaryngology—Head and Neck Surgery, Director, Division of Otology, Neurotology, and Skull Base Surgery, The Johns Hopkins University
Baltimore, Maryland
Anatomy, Physiology, and Testing of the Facial Nerve; Disorders of the Facial Nerve

William A. Numa, MD
Department of Otolaryngology—Head and Neck Surgery, New England Medical Center, Tufts University
Boston, Massachusetts
Nasal Trauma

Rupert J. Obholzer, MD
Specialist Registrar, Department of Otolaryngology—Head and Neck Surgery, St. Bartholomew's and The Royal London Hospitals
London, England
Benign Laryngeal Lesions; Vocal Cord Paralysis

John S. Oghalai, MD
Assistant Professor of Otology, Neurotology, and Skull Base Surgery, Bobby R. Alford Department of Otolaryngology—Head and Neck Surgery, Baylor College of Medicine
Houston, Texas
jso@bcm.tmc.edu
Anatomy and Physiology of the Ear; Temporal Bone Trauma; Neoplasms of the Temporal Bone and Skull Base; Peripetrosal Arachnoid Cysts

Kenneth C. Ong, MD
Chair, Department of Radiology, Good Samaritan Hospital of San Jose
San Jose, California
kennycong@hotmail.com
Radiology

Vicki L. Owczarzak, MD
Resident, Department of Otolaryngology—Head and Neck Surgery, Weill Medical College of Cornell University, New York Presbyterian Hospital
New York, New York
vlo109@gmail.com
Congenital Disorders of the Middle Ear

Marco G. Patti, MD
Professor of Surgery, Division of General Surgery, Department of Surgery, University of California, San Francisco
San Francisco, California
pattim@surgery.ucsf.edu
Benign and Malignant Disorders of the Esophagus

Francesca Pellegrini, MD
Anesthesiologist, Department of Anesthesia, University of Ferrara
Ferrara, Italy
f.pellegrini@ospfe.it
Anesthesia for Head and Neck Surgery

Steven D. Pletcher, MD
Assistant Professor, Department of Otolaryngology—Head and Neck Surgery, University of California, San Francisco
San Francisco, California
spletcher@ohns.ucsf.edu
Frontal Sinus Fractures

Alexander L. Ramirez, MD
Private Practice
Monterey, California
ramirez_alexander@yahoo.com
Rhinoplasty

Scott T. Robinson, MPH, CIH, CSP
Assistant Clinical Professor, Department of Medicine, University of California, San Francisco
San Francisco, California
scorob@comcast.net
Occupational Hearing Loss

Kristina W. Rosbe, MD
Associate Professor, Director of Pediatric Otolaryngology, Department of Otolaryngology—Head and Neck Surgery, University of California, San Francisco
San Francisco, California
krosbe@ohns.ucsf.edu
Foreign Bodies; Airway Reconstruction

John M. Ryzenman, MD
Department of Otolaryngology—Head and Neck Surgery, University of Cincinnati College of Medicine
Cincinnati, Ohio
ryzenshine@doctor.com
Nasal Manifestations of Systemic Disease

Jennifer Henderson Sabes, MA
Research Audiologist, Department of Otolaryngology—Head and Neck Surgery, University of California, San Francisco
San Francisco, California
jennifer.henderson-sabes@ucsfmedctr.org
Audiologic Testing

Frank N. Salamone, MD
Resident, Department of Otolaryngology—Head and Neck Surgery, University of Rochester
Rochester, New York
fns99@yahoo.com
Acute and Chronic Sinusitis

Nicholas Sanfilippo, MD
Assistant Professor, Department of Radiation Oncology, NYU School of Medicine
nicholas.sanfilippo@nyumc.org
Malignant Laryngeal Lesions

Felipe Santos, MD
Resident-Research Fellow, Department of Otolaryngology—Head and Neck Surgery, University of Washington School of Medicine
Seattle, Washington
fsantos@u.washington.edu
Diseases of the External Ear

Bulent Satar, MD
Associate Professor of Otolaryngology—Head and Neck Surgery, Department of Otolaryngology—Head and Neck Surgery, Gulhane Military Medical Academy
Ankara, Turkey
bulentsatar@yahoo.com
Lasers in Head and Neck Surgery; Vestibular Testing

Michael C. Scheuller, MD
Clinical Instructor of Otolaryngology—Head and Neck Surgery, McKay-Dee Hospital
Ogdon, Utah
mscheuller@hotmail.com
Malignant Thyroid Neoplasms

David N. Schindler, MD
Clinical Professor, Department of Otolaryngology—Head and Neck Surgery, University of California, San Francisco
San Francisco, California
ohns2429@sbcglobal.net
Occupational Hearing Loss

Yelizaveta Schnayder, MD
Assistant Professor, Otolaryngic Head and Neck Surgery Foundation, University of Kansas Medical Center
Kansas City, Kansas
yshnayder@kumc.edu
Management of Adenotonsillar Disease

Andrew J. Schreffler, MD
Fellow, Division of General Thoracic Surgery, University of California, San Francisco
San Francisco, California
atschref@mindspring.com
Benign and Malignant Disorders of the Trachea

Samuel H. Selesnick, MD, FACS
Professor and Vice Chairman, Department of Otorhinolaryngology, Weill College of Medicine of Cornell University
New York, New York
shselesn@med.cornell.edu
Diseases of the External Ear; Congenital Disorders of the Middle Ear

Saurabh B. Shah, MD, FAAOA
Attending Surgeon, Granger Medical Clinic
West Valley City, Utah
utahshah@yahoo.com
Nonallergic and Allergic Rhinitis

Ashish Shah, MD
Resident, Department of Otolaryngology—Head and Neck Surgery, University of Cincinnati
Cincinnati, Ohio
shah2400@hotmail.com
Nasal Manifestations of Systemic Disease; Acute and Chronic Sinusitis

Anil R. Shah, MD
Assistant Professor, Division of Facial Plastic Surgery, Department of Otolaryngology—Head and Neck Surgery, NYU School of Medicine
shaha05@med.nyu.edu
Lasers in Head and Neck Surgery; Scar Revision; Rhytidectomy, Browlifts, and Midface Lifts; Otoplasty; Facial Fillers and Implants, Congenital Anomalies of the Nose

Edward J. Shin, MD
Regional Director, Elmhurst Medical Center
Assistant Professor, Mount Sinai School of Medicine
Elmhurst, New York
entshin@yahoo.com
Parapharyngeal Space Neoplasms and Deep Neck Space Infections

Richard A. Smith, DDS
Clinical Professor Emeritus of Oral and Maxillofacial Surgery, Department of Oral and Maxillofacial Surgery, University of California, San Francisco
Kentfield, California
ras144@aol.com
Jaw Cysts

Jeffrey H. Speigel, MD, FACS
Associate Professor, Chief of Facial Plastic and Reconstructive Surgery, Department of Otolaryngology—Head and Neck Surgery, Chief, Facial Plastic and Reconstructive Surgery, Boston University School of Medicine
Boston, Massachusetts
jeffrey.spiegel@bmc.org
Nasal Trauma; Mandible Reconstruction

Robert W. Sweetow, PhD
Director of Audiology, Professor of Otolaryngology, Department of Otolaryngology—Head and Neck Surgery, University of California, San Francisco
San Francisco, California
robert.sweetow@ucsfmedctr.org
Audiologic Testing; Rehabilitation and Hearing Aids

Abtin Tabaee, MD
Assistant Professor, Department of Otolaryngology—Head and Neck Surgery, Albert Einstein College of Medicine
Director of Rhinology and Endoscopic Sinus Surgery, Department of Otolaryngology, Beth Israel Medical Center
New York, New York
atabaee@chpnet.org
Congenital Disorders of the Middle Ear

Thomas A. Tami, MD
Professor, Department Otolaryngology—Head and Neck Surgery, University of Cincinnati College of Medicine
Cincinnati, Ohio
thomas.tami@uc.edu
Nasal Manifestations of Systemic Disease; Acute and Chronic Sinusitis

Tuyet-Phuong N. Tran, MD
Assistant Professor, Division of Head and Neck Surgery and Oncology, Department of Otolaryngology—Head and Neck Surgery, NYU School of Medicine
New York, New York
Theresa.tran@med.nyu.edu
Malignant Diseases of the Salivary Glands; Malignant Laryngeal Lesions

Michael J. Wareing, FRCS(ORL-HNS)
Consultant Otolaryngologist and Associate Clinical Director, Department of Otolaryngology—Head and Neck Surgery, St. Bartholomew's and The Royal London Hospitals
London, England
mjw@orl-hns.co.uk
Benign Laryngeal Lesions; Vocal Cord Paralysis

Kevin C. Welch, MD
Chief Resident, Department of Otorhinolaryngology—Head and Neck Surgery, University of Maryland
Baltimore, Maryland
kwelch@smail.umaryland.edu
Sleep Disorders

Jeffrey B. Wise, MD
Fellow, Facial Plastic and Reconstructive Surgery, Department of Otolaryngology—Head and Neck Surgery, NYU School of Medicine
New York, New York
jeffreywisemd@gmail.com
Local and Regional Flaps in Head and Neck Reconstruction; Otoplasty; Facial Fillers and Implants

Philip D. Yates, MV, MB Chb, FRCS
Consultant Otolaryngologist, Department of Otolaryngology, Freeman Hospital
Newcastle upon Tyne, United Kingdom
philip.yates@nuth.nhs.uk
Stridor in Children; Otitis Media

Kenneth C.Y. Yu, MD
Department of Otolaryngology—Head and Neck Surgery, Travis Air Force Base
Vacaville, California
kenneth.yu@afghan.swa.army.mil
Airway Management and Tracheotomy; Implantable Middle Ear Hearing Devices

PREFACE

Otolaryngology—head and neck surgery is a unique subspecialty in medicine that deals with medical and surgical management of disorders affecting the ear, nose, throat, and the neck; the care of the senses including smell, taste, balance and hearing fall under its domain. As a specialty, it interfaces with other medical and surgical subspecialties including allergy and immunology, endocrinology, gastroenterology, hematology, neurology, neurosurgery, oncology, ophthalmology, pediatrics, plastic and reconstructive surgery, pulmonology, radiation oncology, rehabilitation medicine, rheumatology, thoracic surgery, among others. Further, the specialty encompasses the care of the young and the old, man and woman, as well as benign and malignant diseases.

Symptoms and diseases affecting the ear, nose, throat, and neck are common and commonly lead to patients seeking medical care. These include sinusitis, upper respiratory tract infections, hoarseness, balance disturbance, hearing loss, dysphagia, snoring, tonsillitis, ear infections, thyroid disorders, head and neck cancer and ear wax. In this updated second edition of *Current Diagnosis & Treatment in Otolaryngology—Head & Neck Surgery,* these and many other diseases are covered in crisp and concise manner. Striking just the right balance between comprehensiveness and convenience, it emphasizes the practical features of clinical diagnosis and patient management while providing a comprehensive discussion of pathophysiology and relevant basic and clinical science. With its consistent formatting chapter by chapter, this text makes it simple to locate the practical information you need on diagnosis, testing, disease processes, and up-to-date treatment and management strategies. The book will be of interest to both otolaryngologists as well as all of the medical and surgical specialties and related disciplines that treat patients with head and neck disorders.

OUTSTANDING FEATURES OF THE SECOND EDITION

- Comprehensive review of basic sciences relevant to otolaryngology
- Concise, complete, and accessible clinical information that is up-to-date
- Discussion of both medical and surgical management of otolaryngologic disorders
- Thorough radiology chapter with more than 150 images
- Inclusion of the usual and the unusual diseases of the head and neck
- More than 400 figures to better illustrate and communicate essential points
- Organization by anatomic region to facilitate quick identification of relevant material
- Inclusion of addition Facial Plastic and Reconstructive chapters

INTENDED AUDIENCE

With its comprehensive review of the sciences and the clinical practice of otolaryngology—head and neck surgery, this second edition will be invaluable for medical students, house staff, physicians of all specialties, nurses, physician assistants, audiologists, speech pathologists, and ancillary health care personnel. The book has been designed to meet the clinician's need for an immediate refresher in the clinic as well as to serve as an accessible text for thorough review of the specialty for the boards. The concise presentation is ideally suited for rapid acquisition of information by the busy practitioner.

Anil K. Lalwani
New York

SECTION I

Introduction

Anatomy

1

Nripendra Dhillon, MBBS, MS

■ FACE

Muscles

The muscles of facial expression develop from the second branchial arch and lie within the skin of the scalp, face, and neck.

A. OCCIPITOFRONTALIS MUSCLE

The occipitofrontalis muscle, which lies in the scalp, extends from the superior nuchal line in the back to the skin of the eyebrows in the front. It allows for the movement of the scalp against the periosteum of the skull and also serves to raise the eyebrows.

B. ORBICULARIS OCULI MUSCLE

The orbicularis oculi muscle lies in the eyelids and also encircles the eyes. It helps to close the eye in the gentle movements of blinking or in more forceful movements, such as squinting. These movements help express tears and move them across the conjunctival sac to keep the cornea moist.

C. ORBICULARIS ORIS MUSCLE

The orbicularis oris muscle encircles the opening of the mouth and helps to bring the lips together to keep the mouth closed.

D. BUCCINATOR MUSCLE

The buccinator muscle arises from the pterygomandibular raphe in the back and courses forward in the cheek to blend into the orbicularis oris muscle in the lips. It helps to compress the cheek against the teeth and thus empties food from the vestibule of the mouth during chewing. In addition, it is used while playing musical instruments and other actions that require the controlled expression of air from the mouth.

E. PLATYSMA MUSCLE

The platysma muscle extends from the skin over the mandible through the superficial fascia of the neck into the skin of the upper chest, helping to tighten this skin and also to depress the angles of the mouth. Although lying primarily in the neck, it is grouped with the muscles of facial expression.

Arteries

The blood supply of the face is through branches of the facial artery (Figure 1–1). After arising from the external carotid artery in the neck, the facial artery passes deep to the submandibular gland and crosses the mandible in front of the attachment of the masseter muscle. It takes a tortuous course across the face and travels up to the medial angle of the eye, where it anastomoses with branches of the ophthalmic artery. It gives labial branches to the lips, of which the superior labial artery enters the nostril to supply the vestibule of the nose.

The occipital, posterior auricular, and superficial temporal arteries supply blood to the scalp. They all arise from the external carotid artery.

The superficial temporal artery gives a branch, the transverse facial artery, which courses through the face parallel to the parotid duct.

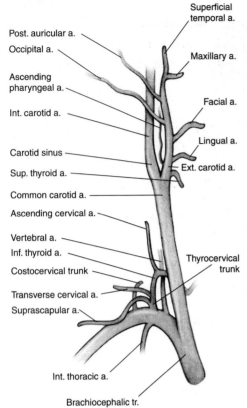

Figure 1–1. Arteries of the neck and face. (Reproduced, with permission, from White JS. *USMLS Road Map: Gross Anatomy*, 2nd edition, McGraw-Hill, 2003.)

Veins

The superficial temporal and maxillary veins join to form the retromandibular vein. The facial vein joins the anterior division of the retromandibular vein to drain into the internal jugular vein. Additional details about the venous drainage pattern of the scalp and face are provided in the discussion of the veins of the neck. The facial vein communicates with the venous plexus in the orbit, which has connections to the cavernous sinus, thus allowing infections to spread from the face into the cranium.

Innervation

A. SENSORY INNERVATION

The sensory innervation of the face is through terminal branches of the trigeminal nerve (CN V) (Figure 1–2). Two imaginary lines that split the eyelids and the lips help to approximately demarcate the sensory distribution of the three divisions of the trigeminal nerve.

In addition to the skin of the face, branches of the trigeminal nerve are also responsible for carrying sensation from deeper structures of the head, including the eye, the paranasal sinuses, the nose, and the mouth. The details of this distribution are discussed with the orbit and the pterygopalatine and infratemporal fossae.

1. Ophthalmic division of the trigeminal nerve— The ophthalmic division of the trigeminal nerve (V1) carries sensation from the upper eyelid, the skin of the forehead, and the skin of the nose through its cutaneous branches, which, from lateral to medial, are the lacrimal, supraorbital, supratrochlear, and nasal nerves.

2. Maxillary division of the trigeminal nerve—The maxillary division of the trigeminal nerve (V2) carries sensation from the lower eyelid, the upper lip, and the face up to the zygomatic prominence of the cheek through its cutaneous branches, which are the infraorbital, zygomaticofacial, and zygomaticotemporal nerves.

3. Mandibular division of the trigeminal nerve— The mandibular division of the trigeminal nerve (V3) carries sensation from the lower lip, the lower part of the face, the auricle, and the scalp in front of and above the auricle through its cutaneous branches, which are the mental, buccal, and auriculotemporal nerves.

B. MOTOR INNERVATION

All the muscles of facial expression are innervated by branches of the facial nerve (CN VII). After emerging from the stylomastoid foramen, the facial nerve lies within the substance of the parotid gland. Here, it gives off its five terminal branches: (1) The temporal branch courses up to the scalp to innervate the occipitofrontalis and orbicularis oculi muscles. (2) The zygomatic branch courses across the cheek to innervate the orbicularis oculi muscle. (3) The buccal branch travels with the parotid duct and innervates the buccinator and orbicularis oris muscles and also muscles that act on the nose and upper lip. (4) The mandibular branch innervates the orbicularis oris muscle and other muscles that act on the lower lip. (5) The cervical branch courses down to the neck and innervates the platysma muscle.

◼ NOSE & SINUSES

THE NASAL CAVITY

The nose is bounded from above by the cribriform plate of the ethmoid bone and from below by the hard palate. It extends back to the choanae, which allow it to communicate with the nasopharynx. The nasal septum is formed by the perpendicular plate of the ethmoid

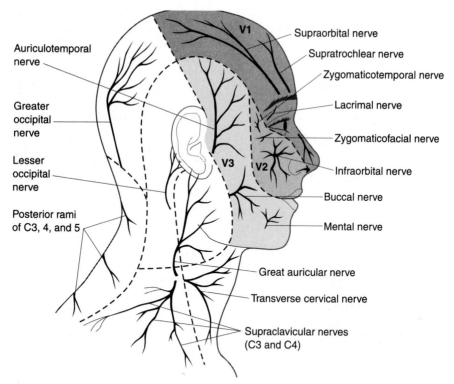

Figure 1–2. Sensory innervation of the head.

bone and by the vomer bone. The lateral wall of the nose has three bony projections, the conchae, which increase the surface area of the nasal mucosa and help to create turbulence in the air flowing through the nose. This allows the nose to humidify and clean the inhaled air and also to change the air to body temperature. The spaces between the conchae and the lateral wall of the nose are called the meatuses. The middle meatus typically has a bulge in its lateral nasal wall, the bulla ethmoidalis, which is created by the presence of ethmoidal air cells. This bulge is bounded from below by a groove, the hiatus semilunaris. The mucous membrane of the nasal cavity is primarily ciliated columnar epithelium and is specialized for olfaction in the roof of the nose and on the upper surface of the superior concha.

THE PARANASAL SINUSES

Several bones that surround the nose are hollow, and the spaces contained within, the paranasal sinuses, are named for the skull bone in which they lie. They are lined by a mucous membrane that is continuous with the nasal mucosa through openings with which the paranasal sinuses communicate with the nose. The presence of the sinuses decreases the weight of the skull and provides resonant chambers for voice. The secretions of the sinuses are carried

into the nose through ciliary action. The frontal sinus drains into the anterior part of the hiatus semilunaris via the infundibulum. The maxillary sinus also drains into the hiatus semilunaris, as do the anterior and middle ethmoidal sinuses. The posterior ethmoidal sinuses drain into the superior meatus. The sphenoid sinus drains into the space above the superior concha called the sphenoethmoidal recess. The inferior end of the nasolacrimal duct opens in the inferior meatus, allowing tears from the conjunctival sac to be carried into the nose. The maxillary sinus lies between the orbit above and the mouth below. The roots of the upper premolar and molar teeth project into the maxillary sinus, often separated from the contents of the sinus only by the mucous membrane that lines the sinus cavity.

Sensory Innervation

The olfactory nerves (CN I) pass through the cribriform plate of the ethmoid bone into the olfactory bulb lying in the anterior cranial fossa, carrying the sensations of smell from the olfactory mucosa in the roof of the nose. General sensory fibers to the nose are provided by the ophthalmic and maxillary divisions of the trigeminal nerve. Specifically, the sensory innervation of the mucosa lining the anterior part of the nasal cavity, as well as that surrounding the olfactory mucosa in the roof of the nose, is by the ethmoidal branches of the ophthalmic division of the trigeminal nerve. Sensation from the lateral wall of the nose is carried by the lateral nasal branches of the maxillary division of the trigeminal nerve. Sensation from the nasal septum is carried by the nasopalatine branch of the maxillary division of the trigeminal nerve. Sensory innervation of the lining of the frontal sinus is by the supraorbital branch of the ophthalmic division of the trigeminal nerve. Sensory innervation of the sphenoid and ethmoid sinuses is by the ethmoidal branches of the ophthalmic division of the trigeminal nerve. Sensory innervation of the maxillary sinus is by the infraorbital branch of the maxillary division of the trigeminal nerve.

Arteries

The rich blood supply of the nasal cavity is primarily from the sphenopalatine branch of the maxillary artery that enters the nose from the pterygopalatine fossa (Figure 1–3). The superior labial branch of the facial artery supplies the vestibule of the nose. In addition, the oph-

thalmic branch of the internal carotid artery supplies the roof of the nose. All of these vessels anastomose with each other.

■ SALIVARY GLANDS

PAROTID GLAND

The parotid gland is wedged into the space between the mandible in front and the temporal bone above and behind. It lies in front of and below the external auditory meatus. It extends as deep as the pharyngeal wall and is enclosed within a sheath formed by the investing fascia of the neck, which is attached to the zygomatic arch above. The parotid duct passes forward over the masseter muscle and can be palpated just in front of the clenched muscle, about half an inch below the zygomatic arch. It passes into the oral cavity by piercing the

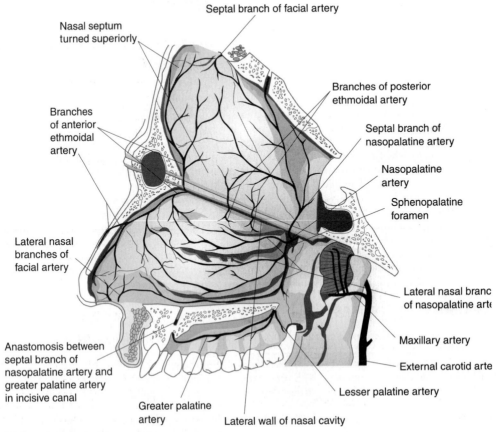

Figure 1–3. Arteries of the nasal cavity.

buccinator muscle and opens in the buccal mucosa opposite the upper second molar tooth.

Several important structures lie within the capsule of the parotid gland. The facial nerve enters the gland after emerging from the stylomastoid foramen and gives off its terminal branches within the substance of the gland. The external carotid artery ascends up the neck, into the gland, and gives off its two terminal branches—the maxillary and superficial temporal arteries—within the gland. The superficial temporal and maxillary veins come together in the substance of the gland to form the retromandibular vein, which divides into its anterior and posterior divisions as it emerges from the gland.

SUBMANDIBULAR GLAND

The submandibular gland lies in the digastric triangle of the neck, below the mylohyoid muscle. Like the parotid gland, it is enclosed within a sheath formed by the investing fascia of the neck that is attached to the mandible above. A part of the gland extends around the posterior, free edge of the mylohyoid muscle to lie above the muscle in the floor of the mouth. The submandibular duct arises from this deep portion of the gland and extends forward, alongside the tongue, to open at the base of the frenulum of the tongue on the submandibular caruncle.

SUBLINGUAL GLAND

The sublingual gland lies below the tongue in the floor of the mouth. It creates a fold of mucous membrane, the sublingual fold, which lies along the base of the tongue, above the mylohyoid muscle. The gland has multiple ducts that open along the sublingual fold.

Innervation

A. SECRETOMOTOR INNERVATION

Although the facial nerve is responsible for almost all the parasympathetic secretomotor innervation of the head, it is interesting to note that the one gland to which it does not provide secretomotor innervation is the very gland in which it is buried. The secretomotor innervation of the parotid gland is by fibers carried on the glossopharyngeal nerve (CN IX). The preganglionic parasympathetic fibers originate in the inferior salivary nucleus and join the glossopharyngeal nerve (Figure 1–4). They course through the lesser superficial petrosal nerve and the foramen ovale to synapse at the otic ganglion. The postganglionic fibers now join the auriculotemporal branch of the mandibular division of the trigeminal nerve to reach the parotid gland.

The secretomotor innervation of the submandibular and sublingual glands is by fibers carried on the facial nerve (CN VII). The preganglionic parasympathetic fibers originate in the superior salivary nucleus and join the facial nerve (Figure 1–5). They course through the chorda tympani nerve and the petrotympanic fissure to join the lingual branch of the mandibular division of the trigeminal nerve in the infratemporal fossa, and they synapse at the submandibular ganglion. Postganglionic fibers coursing to the submandibular gland usually reach the gland directly from this ganglion. Postganglionic fibers coursing to the sublingual gland reach the gland on branches of the lingual nerve.

B. SYMPATHETIC INNERVATION

The sympathetic innervation to the salivary glands controls the viscosity of the glandular secretions. The preganglionic neurons originate in the thoracic spinal cord and ascend in the sympathetic trunk to synapse in the superior cervical ganglion in the neck. From here, postganglionic sympathetic fibers travel as plexuses on the external carotid artery and its branches to reach the salivary glands.

■ CAVITY

The mouth is bounded by the palate above, the mylohyoid muscle below, the buccinator muscles in the cheek on each side, and the palatoglossal arches behind. In addition to the oral cavity proper, the mouth includes the vestibule, which is the space between the cheek and the teeth.

PALATE

The hard palate is formed by the palatal process of the maxilla and the horizontal process of the palatine bone, which are covered by a mucous membrane. The soft palate is formed by contributions from a number of muscles.

Muscles of the Soft Palate

A. TENSOR VELI PALATINI MUSCLE

The tensor veli palatini arises from the scaphoid fossa of the sphenoid bone and descends in the lateral wall of the nose, narrowing to a tendon that turns medially around the pterygoid hamulus. It then fans out to become the palatine aponeurosis and attaches to the muscle of the opposite side. Together, the two

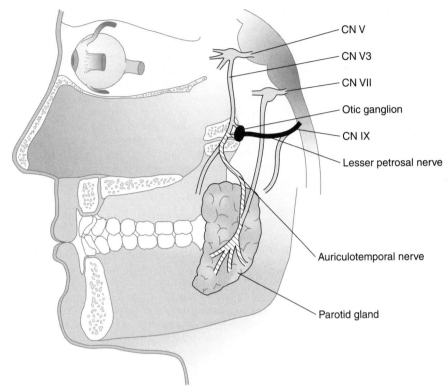

Figure 1–4. Schematic of the innervation of the parotid gland by the glossopharyngeal nerve. **Solid black:** Preganglionic parasympathetic nerves leave the brainstem with the glossopharyngeal nerve (CN IX) and run via the lesser petrosal nerve to the otic ganglion. **Hatched segment:** Postganglionic parasympathetic nerves travel with the auriculotemporal branch of CN V3 and then the facial nerve (CN VII) to reach the parotid gland.

muscles tense the soft palate for other muscles to act upon it.

B. Levator Veli Palatini Muscle

The levator veli palatini arises from the petrous part of the temporal bone near the base of the styloid process and from the cartilage of the eustachian tube. It passes between the lowest fibers of the superior pharyngeal constrictor muscle and the highest fibers of the middle pharyngeal constrictor muscle, attaching to the upper surface of the palatine aponeurosis. It helps to elevate the soft palate and, together with the palatopharyngeus and superior pharyngeal constrictor muscles, it closes off the nose from the oropharynx during swallowing.

C. Palatoglossus Muscle

The palatoglossus muscle arises from the lower surface of the palatine aponeurosis and passes down, in front of the palatine tonsil, to attach to the side of the tongue. It pulls the back of the tongue upward and approximates the soft palate to the tongue, closing off the mouth from the pharynx.

D. Palatopharyngeus Muscle

The palatopharyngeus muscle also arises from the lower surface of the palatine aponeurosis and passes down, behind the palatine tonsil, to blend into the longitudinal muscle layer of the pharynx. It helps to pull the pharyngeal wall upward during swallowing, and, together with the levator veli palatini and superior pharyngeal constrictor muscles, it closes off the nose from the oropharynx.

E. Musculus Uvulae

The musculus uvulae is a small muscle that helps to elevate the uvula.

Arteries

The blood supply of the palate is from the ascending palatine branches of the facial artery as well as from the

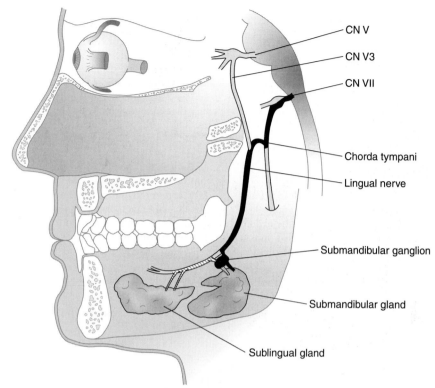

CN V

CN V3

CN VII

Chorda tympani

Lingual nerve

Submandibular ganglion

Submandibular gland

Sublingual gland

Figure 1–5. Schematic of the innervation of the submandibular and sublingual glands by the facial nerve. **Solid black:** Preganglionic parasympathetic nerves leave the brainstem with the facial nerve (CN VII) and run via the chorda tympani and the lingual branch of CN V3 to the submandibular ganglion. **Hatched segment:** Postganglionic parasympathetic nerves travel either directly to the submandibular gland or travel back to the lingual branch of CN V3 to the sublingual gland.

palatine branch of the maxillary artery, both of which drop down to the palate from the pterygopalatine fossa by passing through the palatine canal.

TONGUE

The anterior two thirds of the tongue develop separately from the posterior third, and the two parts come together at the sulcus terminalis. The surface of the anterior two thirds of the tongue is covered by filiform, fungiform, and vallate papillae. The posterior third of the tongue contains collections of lymphoid tissue, the lingual tonsils.

Muscles

The mass of the tongue is made up of intrinsic muscles that are directed longitudinally, vertically, and transversely; these intrinsic muscles help to change the shape of the tongue. The extrinsic muscles help to move the tongue.

A. GENIOGLOSSUS MUSCLE

The genioglossus arises from the genial tubercle on the inside surface of the front of the mandible and passes upward and backward into the tongue. It acts to protrude and depress the tongue.

B. HYOGLOSSUS MUSCLE

The hyoglossus arises from the hyoid bone and passes upward to attach to the side of the posterior part of the tongue. It acts to depress and retract the back of the tongue.

C. STYLOGLOSSUS MUSCLE

The styloglossus arises from the styloid process and passes downward and forward through the middle pharyngeal constrictor muscle to attach to the side of the tongue. It acts to elevate and retract the tongue.

D. PALATOGLOSSUS MUSCLE

The palatoglossus muscle (described previously) acts on the tongue but is considered a muscle of the palate.

Arteries

The blood supply of the tongue is from the lingual branch of the external carotid artery. The lingual artery reaches the tongue by passing behind the posterior edge of the hyoglossus muscle and turning forward into the substance of the tongue, thus coursing medial to the hyoglossus. In contrast, all the other nerves and vessels of the tongue pass lateral to the hyoglossus before entering the tongue.

FLOOR OF THE MOUTH

The floor of the mouth is formed by the mylohyoid muscle upon which lie the geniohyoid muscles (Figure 1–6). The digastric muscle lies immediately below the mylohyoid muscle. Both the geniohyoid and the digastric muscles are discussed with the suprahyoid muscles of the neck. The mylohyoid arises from the similarly named line on the inside surface of the mandible and attaches to the front of the hyoid bone. It is the main support of the structures in the mouth. It helps to elevate the hyoid bone during movements of swallowing and speech. Also, with the infrahyoid muscles holding the hyoid bone in place, the mylohyoid and digastric muscles help to depress the mandible and open the mouth.

The deep part of the submandibular gland and the duct that emerges from it lie above the mylohyoid muscle. The sublingual gland also shares this relationship. The hypoglossal nerve (CN XII) enters the mouth from the neck by passing lateral to the hyoglossus muscle and above the free posterior edge of the mylohyoid muscle. It continues in the mouth, inferior to the submandibular duct, and enters the substance of the tongue at its side. The lingual branch of the mandibular division of the trigeminal nerve enters the mouth from the infratemporal fossa by passing medial to the lower third molar. It initially lies above and lateral to the submandibular duct and then spirals under the duct as it comes to lie above and medial to the duct, where it gives off its terminal

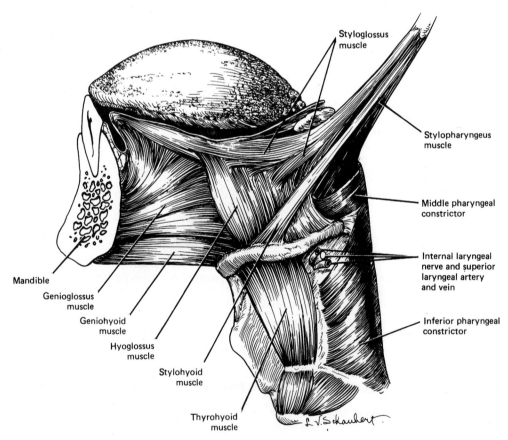

Figure 1–6. Muscles of the tongue and pharynx. (Reproduced, with permission, from Lindner HH. *Clinical Anatomy*, McGraw-Hill, 1989.)

branches to the tongue and the floor of the mouth. The glossopharyngeal nerve passes from the pharynx to the mouth, lies lateral to the bed of the palatine tonsil, and courses into the posterior third of the tongue.

Innervation

A. SENSORY INNERVATION

Sensation from the palate is carried by branches of the maxillary division of the trigeminal nerve (Figure 1–7). From the front of the hard palate, just inside the incisors, sensation is carried by the incisive branch of the nasopalatine nerve. From the rest of the hard palate and the mucosa lining the palatal aspect of the upper alveolar margins, sensation is carried by the greater palatine nerve. From the soft palate, sensation is carried by the lesser palatine nerve.

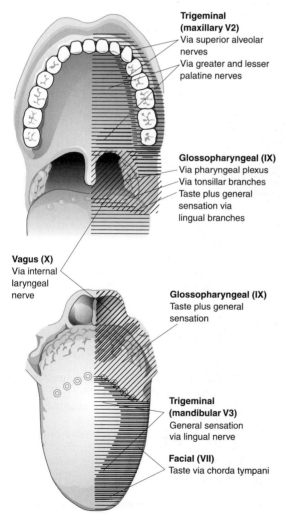

Trigeminal (maxillary V2)
Via superior alveolar nerves
Via greater and lesser palatine nerves

Glossopharyngeal (IX)
Via pharyngeal plexus
Via tonsillar branches
Taste plus general sensation via lingual branches

Vagus (X)
Via internal laryngeal nerve

Glossopharyngeal (IX)
Taste plus general sensation

Trigeminal (mandibular V3)
General sensation via lingual nerve

Facial (VII)
Taste via chorda tympani

Figure 1–7. Sensory innervation of the oral cavity.

Sensation from the tongue is carried by nerves predicated upon the development of the tongue. There are general sensory fibers that carry sensations of touch, pressure, and temperature. In addition, there are special sensory fibers that carry the sensation of taste.

General sensation from the anterior two thirds of the tongue is carried by the lingual branch of the mandibular division of the trigeminal nerve. General sensation from the posterior third of the tongue is carried by the glossopharyngeal nerve. Taste sensation from the anterior two thirds of the tongue is carried by the chorda tympani branch of the facial nerve. Taste sensation from the posterior third of the tongue is carried by the glossopharyngeal nerve.

Sensation from the floor of the mouth and the mucosa lining the lingual aspect of the lower alveolar margins is carried by the lingual branch of the mandibular division of the trigeminal nerve. Sensation from the buccal mucosa and the mucosa lining the buccal aspect of the upper and lower alveolar margins is carried by the buccal branch of the mandibular division of the trigeminal nerve. Sensation from the mucosa lining the anterior part of the vestibule, inside the upper lip, and the adjacent mucosa lining the labial aspect of the upper alveolar margins is carried by the infraorbital branch of the mandibular division of the trigeminal nerve. Sensation from the mucosa lining the anterior part of the vestibule, inside the lower lip, and the adjacent mucosa lining the labial aspect of the lower alveolar margins is carried by the mental branch of the inferior alveolar branch of the mandibular division of the trigeminal nerve.

B. MOTOR INNERVATION

All the muscles of the palate are innervated by branches of the vagus nerve (CN X) except the tensor veli palatini, which is innervated by the mandibular division of the trigeminal nerve. All the muscles of the tongue, extrinsic and intrinsic, are innervated by the hypoglossal nerve except the palatoglossus muscle, which is considered a muscle of the palate and is therefore innervated by the vagus nerve. The mylohyoid muscle and anterior belly of the digastric muscle are innervated by the nerve to the mylohyoid muscle, a branch of the mandibular division of the trigeminal nerve. The geniohyoid muscle is innervated by fibers from the cervical spinal cord (C1), which are carried to it by the hypoglossal nerve.

■ PHARYNX

The pharynx is a muscular tube that both lies behind and communicates with the nasal, oral, and laryngeal

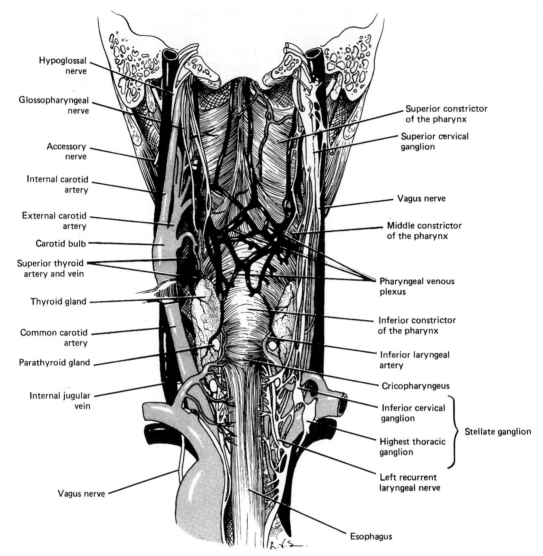

Figure 1–8. Exterior of the pharynx. (Reproduced, with permission, from Lindner HH. *Clinical Anatomy*, McGraw-Hill, 1989.)

cavities (Figure 1–8). It lies in front of the prevertebral fascia of the neck and is continuous with the esophagus at the level of the cricoid cartilage. From within, it is made of mucosa, pharyngobasilar fascia, pharyngeal muscles, and buccopharyngeal fascia.

The mucosa is lined by ciliated columnar epithelium in the area behind the nasal cavity and by stratified squamous epithelium in the remaining areas. The pharyngobasilar fascia, a fibrous layer, is attached above to the pharyngeal tubercle on the base of the skull. The muscles of the pharynx consist of the circular fibers of the constrictor muscles that surround the longitudinally running fibers of the stylopharyngeus, salpingopharyngeus, and palatopharyngeus muscles.

The buccopharyngeal fascia is a layer of loose connective tissue that separates the pharynx from the prevertebral fascia and allows for the free movement of the pharynx against vertebral structures. This layer is continuous around the lower border of the mandible, with the loose connective tissue layer that separates the buccinator muscle from the skin overlying it.

Muscles

The muscular layer of the pharynx is made of inner longitudinal and outer circular layers. The longitudinally running muscles help to shorten the height of the pharynx. As the pharyngobasilar fascia is attached to the skull, this shortening results in an elevation of the pharynx and larynx during swallowing. The salpingopharyngeus, stylopharyngeus, and palatopharyngeus muscles contribute to this layer.

The circularly running muscles help to constrict the pharynx, and their sequential contractions propel food downward into the esophagus. The superior pharyngeal constrictor muscle arises from the pterygomandibular raphe, the middle pharyngeal constrictor muscle from the hyoid bone, and the inferior pharyngeal constrictor muscle from the thyroid and cricoid cartilages. From these narrow anterior origins, the fibers of the constrictor muscles fan out as they travel back around the pharynx and attach to the corresponding muscles of the opposite side at the midline pharyngeal raphe. The pharyngeal raphe is attached along its length to the pharyngobasilar fascia and is thus anchored to the pharyngeal tubercle on the base of the skull. The orientation of the constrictor muscle fibers is such that the inferior fibers of one muscle are overlapped on the outside by the superior fibers of the next muscle down, producing a "funnel-inside-a-funnel" arrangement that directs food down in an appropriate fashion.

The narrow anterior attachments of the constrictor muscles, compared with their broad posterior insertion, create gaps in the circular muscle coat that surrounds the pharynx. Structures from without can pass into the pharynx through these gaps.

The gap between the base of the skull and the upper fibers of the superior inferior constrictor muscle allows the eustachian tube and the levator veli palatini muscle into the nasopharynx.

The gap between the lower fibers of the superior pharyngeal constrictor muscle and the upper fibers of the middle pharyngeal constrictor muscle allows the stylopharyngeus muscle and the glossopharyngeal nerve into the oropharynx.

The gap between the lower fibers of the middle pharyngeal constrictor muscle and the upper fibers of the inferior pharyngeal constrictor muscle allows both the internal laryngeal branch of the vagus nerve and the superior laryngeal branch of the superior thyroid artery into the laryngopharynx and the larynx.

The gap between the lower fibers of the inferior pharyngeal constrictor muscle and the upper fibers of the circular muscle of the esophagus allows both the recurrent laryngeal branch of the vagus nerve and the inferior laryngeal branch of the inferior thyroid artery into the larynx.

Innervation

The innervation of the pharynx is by a group of nerves whose branches form a meshwork of neurons, the pharyngeal plexus, which lies in the wall of the pharynx. The glossopharyngeal nerve, the vagus nerve, the maxillary division of the trigeminal nerve, and postganglionic fibers from the sympathetic trunk all contribute to the formation of the pharyngeal plexus.

A. SENSORY INNERVATION

The sensory innervation of the upper part of the nasopharynx is carried by branches of the maxillary division of the trigeminal nerve. The sensory innervation of the lower part of the nasopharynx, the oropharynx, and the laryngopharynx is carried by the glossopharyngeal nerve. The internal laryngeal branch of the vagus nerve carries sensation from the piriform recesses of the laryngopharynx.

B. MOTOR INNERVATION

Motor innervation of all the muscles of the pharynx, circular and longitudinal, except the stylopharyngeus, is by the pharyngeal branch of the vagus nerve, which carries motor fibers that originated in the cranial component of the accessory nerve (CN XI). The stylopharyngeus muscle is innervated by the glossopharyngeal nerve.

NASOPHARYNX

The nasopharynx extends from the base of the skull to the level of the soft palate. It is continuous with the nasal cavity through the choanae. In its lateral wall, the cartilage of the eustachian tube creates a bulge, the torus tubarius, below which is the opening of the tube. Above and behind this bulge lies a depression called the pharyngeal recess. A collection of lymphoid tissue, the pharyngeal tonsil, lies in the posterior wall and the roof of the nasopharynx. Additional lymphoid tissue, the tubal tonsil, is found around the opening of the eustachian tube. A fold of mucous membrane created by the salpingopharyngeus muscle extends down from the torus tubarius. The nasopharynx is continuous with the oropharynx below.

OROPHARYNX

The oropharynx extends from the soft palate to the epiglottis. It is continuous with the mouth through the oropharyngeal isthmus formed by the palatoglossal muscles on each side. The anterior wall of the oropharynx is formed by the posterior third of the tongue. The mucous membrane of the tongue is continuous onto the epiglottis and creates three glossoepiglottic folds—one in the midline and two placed laterally. The space on either side of the median glossoepiglottic fold is the vallecula.

The lateral wall of the oropharynx has two folds of mucous membrane, the palatoglossal and palatopharyngeal, created by the muscles of the same name, which are described with the muscles of the palate. An encapsulated collection of lymphoid tissue, the palatine tonsil, lies in the triangular recess between these two folds. The blood supply of the palatine tonsil is by a branch of the facial artery. Additional lymphoid tissue, the lingual tonsil, is located under the mucous membrane of the posterior third of the tongue. Together, the tonsillar tissues of the nasopharynx and oropharynx form a ring of lymphoid tissue that surrounds the entrances into the pharynx from the nose and the mouth. The oropharynx is continuous with the laryngopharynx below.

LARYNGOPHARYNX

The laryngopharynx extends from the epiglottis to the cricoid cartilage. It is continuous with the larynx through the laryngeal aditus, which is formed by the epiglottis and the aryepiglottic folds. On either side of these folds and medial to the thyroid cartilage are two pyramidal spaces, the piriform recesses of the laryngopharynx, through which swallowed food passes into the esophagus. The piriform recesses are related to the cricothyroid muscle laterally and the lateral cricoarytenoid muscle medially. The laryngopharynx is continuous with the esophagus below.

■ NECK

Triangles of the Neck

Bounded by the mandible above and the clavicle below, the neck is subdivided by the sternocleidomastoid muscle into an anterior and a posterior triangular region, each of which is further divided into smaller triangles by the omohyoid and digastric muscles. The surface markings of these muscles help to visibly define the borders of the triangles of the neck.

A. POSTERIOR TRIANGLE

The posterior triangle is bounded by the sternocleidomastoid muscle in front, the trapezius muscle behind, and the clavicle below. It is divided by the omohyoid muscle into an occipital triangle and a supraclavicular triangle.

1. Occipital triangle—The occipital triangle has a muscular floor formed from above, downward by the semispinalis capitis, splenius capitis, levator scapulae, and scalenus medius muscles. After emerging from behind the sternocleidomastoid muscle, the spinal accessory nerve courses across the muscular floor of the posterior triangle to pass deep to the trapezius muscle. In addition, the cutaneous nerves of the neck, discussed below, course through the deep fascia of the neck that covers the posterior triangle.

2. Supraclavicular triangle—The supraclavicular triangle lies above the middle of the clavicle. It contains the terminal portion of the subclavian artery, the roots, trunks, and divisions of the brachial plexus, branches of the thyrocervical trunk, and cutaneous tributaries of the external jugular vein. The cupola of the pleural cavity extends above the level of the clavicle and is found deep to the contents of the supraclavicular triangle.

B. ANTERIOR TRIANGLE

The anterior triangle is bounded by the sternocleidomastoid muscle behind, the midline of the neck in front, and the mandible above. It is subdivided into submental, digastric, carotid, and muscular triangles.

1. Submental triangle—The submental triangle is bounded by the anterior belly of the digastric muscle, the midline of the neck, and the hyoid bone. The mylohyoid muscle forms its floor.

2. Digastric triangle—The digastric triangle is bounded by the mandible above and the two bellies of the digastric muscle. In addition, the stylohyoid muscle lies with the posterior belly of the digastric muscle. The mylohyoid and hyoglossus muscles form the floor of this triangle. The submandibular salivary gland is a prominent feature of this area, which is also referred to as the submandibular triangle. The hypoglossal nerve runs along with the stylohyoid muscle and posterior belly of the digastric muscle, between the hyoglossus muscle and the submandibular gland, on its course into the tongue. The facial vessels course across the triangle, with the facial artery passing deep to the submandibular gland while the facial vein passes superficial to it.

3. Carotid triangle—The carotid triangle is bounded by the sternocleidomastoid muscle behind, the posterior belly of the digastric muscle above, and the omohyoid muscle below. Its floor is formed by the constrictor muscles of the pharynx. It contains the structures of the carotid sheath—namely, the common carotid artery as it divides into its external and internal carotid branches, the internal jugular vein and its tributaries, and the vagus nerve with its branches.

4. Muscular triangle—The muscular triangle is bounded by the omohyoid muscle above, the sternocleidomastoid muscle below, and the midline of the neck in front. It contains the infrahyoid muscles in its floor. Deep to these muscles are the thyroid and parathyroid glands, the larynx, which leads to the trachea, and the esophagus. The hyoid bone forms the superior attachment for the infrahyoid muscles, and the prominent thyroid cartilage and cricoid cartilage are also contained in this region.

Muscles

A. STERNOCLEIDOMASTOID MUSCLES

The sternocleidomastoid muscles act together to flex the cervical spine while extending the head at the atlantooccipital joint. Acting independently, each muscle turns the head to face upward and to the contralateral side. By virtue of their attachment to the sternum, the sternocleidomastoids also serve as accessory muscles of respiration.

B. TRAPEZIUS MUSCLES

The trapezius muscles have fibers running in several directions. The uppermost fibers pass downward from the skull to the lateral end of the clavicle, thereby playing a role in elevating the shoulder. The middle fibers pass laterally from the cervical spine to the acromion process of the scapula and help to retract the shoulder. The lowest fibers pass upward from the thoracic spine to the spine of the scapula and help to laterally rotate the scapula, making the glenoid fossa turn upward. This action assists the serratus anterior muscle in rotating the scapula when the arm is abducted overhead.

C. SCALENE MUSCLES

The scalene muscles attach to the cervical spine and pass downward to insert on the first rib. They are contained within the prevertebral layer of deep fascia and help to laterally bend the cervical spine. The roots of the brachial plexus and the subclavian artery pass between the anterior and middle scalene muscles on their course to the axilla. In contrast, the subclavian vein passes anterior to the anterior scalene muscle as it leaves the neck to pass behind the clavicle and reach the axilla. Also, the phrenic nerve lies immediately anterior to the anterior scalene muscle as it runs down the neck into the thorax.

D. INFRAHYOID MUSCLES

The infrahyoid muscles, the omohyoid, sternohyoid, sternothyroid, and thyrohyoid, are named for their attachments. Together, they act to depress the hyoid bone and the thyroid cartilage during movements of swallowing and speech.

E. SUPRAHYOID MUSCLES

The suprahyoid muscles, the mylohyoid, stylohyoid, geniohyoid, and digastric, act together to elevate the hyoid bone during movements of swallowing or speech. In addition, with the infrahyoid muscles holding the hyoid bone in place, the suprahyoid muscles help to depress the mandible and open the mouth.

Arteries

The arch of the aorta has three branches: (1) the brachiocephalic artery, (2) the left common carotid artery, and (3) the left subclavian artery. The brachiocephalic artery branches into the right subclavian and right common carotid arteries.

A. SUBCLAVIAN ARTERY

The subclavian artery gives off the vertebral artery, the internal thoracic artery, the thyrocervical trunk, and the costocervical trunk (see Figure 1–1).

1. Vertebral artery—The vertebral artery courses up through the transverse foramina of the upper six cervical vertebrae. It enters the vertebral canal, passes through the foramen magnum, and goes on to supply blood to the hindbrain, the midbrain, and the occipital lobe of the forebrain.

2. Internal thoracic artery—The internal thoracic artery leaves the root of the neck and passes into the thorax, where it supplies blood to the anterior chest wall and eventually to the upper part of the anterior abdominal wall through its superior epigastric branch.

3. Thyrocervical trunk—The thyrocervical trunk gives off the following branches: (1) the inferior thyroid artery, which supplies blood to the thyroid gland; (2) the transverse cervical artery, which passes backward across the neck to supply blood to the trapezius and rhomboid muscles; and (3) the suprascapular artery, which courses laterally across the neck toward the suprascapular notch and participates in the elaborate anastomosis of vessels that surround the scapula. The inferior thyroid artery has a branch, the inferior laryngeal artery, which enters the larynx by passing between the lowest fibers of the inferior pharyngeal constrictor muscle and the upper fibers of the circular muscle of the esophagus. The inferior thyroid artery anastomoses with the superior thyroid artery, a branch of the external carotid artery.

4. Costocervical trunk—The costocervical trunk gives off branches that supply blood to the first two intercostal spaces and the postvertebral muscles of the neck.

B. COMMON CAROTID ARTERY

The common carotid artery courses up into the neck and terminates at the level of the thyroid cartilage by dividing into the internal and external carotid arteries. It has no branches.

1. Internal carotid artery—The internal carotid artery also has no branches in the neck. It travels up to the base of the skull, where it enters the carotid canal and passes through the petrous part of the temporal bone and the cavernous sinus before turning sharply upward and backward at the carotid siphon to pierce the dura mater. It supplies blood to the frontal, parietal, and temporal lobes of the forebrain. Its main branch to the head is the ophthalmic artery, which supplies blood to the orbit and the upper part of the nasal cavity.

2. External carotid artery—The external carotid artery is the main source of blood supply to the head and neck (see Figure 1–1). In the neck, it has a number of branches.

a. Superior thyroid artery—The superior thyroid artery passes down to supply blood to the upper part of the thyroid gland. It has a branch, the superior laryngeal artery, which pierces the thyrohyoid membrane to pass into the larynx. The superior thyroid artery anastomoses with the inferior thyroid artery, a branch of the thyrocervical trunk of the subclavian artery.

b. Ascending pharyngeal artery—The ascending pharyngeal artery supplies blood to the pharynx.

c. Posterior auricular artery—The posterior auricular artery passes upward, behind the auricle, and supplies blood to the scalp.

d. Occipital artery—The occipital artery passes upward and backward to supply blood to the scalp on the back of the head.

e. Facial artery—The facial artery passes upward and forward, deep to the submandibular salivary gland. It then crosses the mandible, where its pulsations can be palpated just in front of the masseter muscle, to supply blood to the face.

f. Lingual artery—The lingual artery passes upward and forward, behind the posterior edge of the hyoglossus muscle, and into the substance of the tongue, to which it supplies blood.

g. Terminal branches—The external carotid artery then ascends into the substance of the parotid gland, where it gives off two terminal branches.

(1) Superficial temporal artery—The superficial temporal artery crosses the zygomatic arch just in front of the auricle, where its pulsations can be palpated. It then goes on to supply blood to the scalp.

(2) Maxillary artery—The maxillary artery passes medially into the infratemporal fossa and is responsible for the blood supply to both the deep structures of the face and the nose.

Veins

The venous drainage of the head and neck is best understood by comparing it with the arterial distribution described above. Many variations exist in the pattern of venous drainage, but each of the arteries has a vein that corresponds to it.

A. Retromandibular Vein

The veins that correspond to the two terminal branches of the external carotid artery, the superficial temporal

and maxillary veins, come together within the substance of the parotid gland to form the retromandibular vein. At the angle of the mandible, the retromandibular vein divides into an anterior and a posterior division.

B. External Jugular Vein

The two veins that correspond to the arteries that pass backward from the external carotid artery, the posterior auricular and occipital veins, join the posterior division of the retromandibular vein and become the external jugular vein. In addition, the suprascapular and transverse cervical veins drain into the external jugular vein.

C. Internal Jugular Vein

The two veins that correspond to the arteries that pass forward from the external carotid artery, the facial and lingual veins, join the anterior division of the retromandibular vein and drain into the internal jugular vein. The internal jugular vein drains blood from the areas to which the internal carotid artery supplies blood. The superior and middle thyroid veins drain into the internal jugular vein.

D. Inferior Thyroid Veins

The inferior thyroid veins lie in front of the trachea and drain blood from the isthmus of the thyroid gland into the left brachiocephalic vein as it lies behind the manubrium of the sternum.

E. Brachiocephalic Vein

The external jugular vein drains into the subclavian vein, which joins the internal jugular vein at the root of the neck to become the brachiocephalic vein. The two brachiocephalic veins come together to form the superior vena cava.

Lymphatics

The superficial lymph nodes of the head and neck are named for their regional location. The occipital, retroauricular, and parotid nodes drain lymph from the scalp, auricle, and middle ear. The submandibular nodes receive lymph from the face, sinuses, mouth, and tongue. The retropharyngeal nodes, although not truly superficially located, receive lymph from deeper structures of the head, including the upper parts of the pharynx. All of these regional nodes drain their lymphatic efferents into the deep cervical nodes, which lie along the internal jugular vein. Two of these deep nodes are commonly referred to as the jugulodigastric and the juguloomohyoid nodes. They lie at locations at which the internal jugular vein is crossed by the digastric and omohyoid muscles, respectively. The jugulodigastric node is concerned with the lymphatic drainage of the palatine tonsil; the juguloomohyoid node is concerned primarily with the lymphatic drainage of the tongue. The deep cervical nodes drain their lymph into either the thoracic duct or the right lymphatic duct. The thoracic duct empties into the junction of the left internal jugular vein and the left subclavian vein. The right lymphatic duct drains into a similar location on the right side of the root of the neck.

Innervation

A. SENSORY INNERVATION

The cutaneous innervation of the anterior skin of the neck is by the ventral rami of cervical spinal nerves that form the cervical plexus (C2–4), whereas the posterior skin of the neck is innervated by the dorsal rami of cervical spinal nerves (C2–5) (see Figure 1–2). The cutaneous branches of the cervical plexus emerge from just behind the sternocleidomastoid muscle, about halfway between its attachments to the sternum and the mastoid process. They are named for the areas of skin from which they carry sensation.

1. Transverse cervical nerve—The transverse cervical nerve turns forward and courses across the neck, with its branches carrying sensation from the anterior neck.

2. Supraclavicular nerves—The supraclavicular nerves course down toward the clavicle and carry sensation from the skin of the lower neck, extending from the clavicle in front to the spine of the scapula behind.

3. Greater auricular nerve—The greater auricular nerve courses up toward the auricle, with its branches carrying sensation from the skin of the upper neck, the skin overlying the parotid gland, and the auricle itself.

4. Lesser occipital nerve—The lesser occipital nerve courses upward to carry sensation from the skin of the scalp that lies just behind the auricle.

B. MOTOR INNERVATION

The infrahyoid muscles are innervated by branches of the ansa cervicalis, which is formed by the descending cervical nerve and the descending hypoglossal nerve. The descending cervical nerve (C2 and 3) arises from the cervical plexus. The descending hypoglossal nerve contains fibers from the first cervical spinal nerve, some of which first joined the hypoglossal nerve before dropping off that nerve to form the ansa cervicalis (Figure 1–9). Other fibers from the first cervical spinal nerve continue on the hypoglossal nerve and later branch off to supply the thyrohyoid muscle.

Of the suprahyoid muscles, the mylohyoid muscle and the anterior belly of the digastric muscle are innervated by the nerve to the mylohyoid muscle, which is a branch of the inferior alveolar nerve from the mandibular division of the trigeminal nerve. The stylohyoid muscle and the posterior belly of the digastric muscle are innervated by the facial nerve. The geniohyoid muscle is innervated by C1 fibers carried by the hypoglossal nerve.

The prevertebral musculature and the scalene muscles receive motor innervation from direct branches of the cervical plexus. The sternocleidomastoid muscles and the trapezius muscles are innervated by the spinal accessory nerve.

Vagus Nerve

The vagus nerve travels in the carotid sheath with the internal jugular vein and the carotid artery (Figure 1–10). In the neck, it has branches to the larynx, the pharynx, and the heart. The laryngeal and pharyngeal branches of the vagus nerve carry motor fibers that originate in the cranial component of the accessory nerve.

A. SUPERIOR LARYNGEAL NERVE

The superior laryngeal nerve gives off two branches, the external and the internal laryngeal nerves. The external laryngeal nerve provides motor innervation to the cricothyroid muscle. The internal laryngeal nerve pierces the thyrohyoid membrane to enter the larynx. It carries sensation from the part of the larynx that lies above the vocal folds and also carries sensation from the piriform recess of the laryngopharynx.

B. RECURRENT (INFERIOR) LARYNGEAL NERVE

The recurrent (inferior) laryngeal nerve provides motor innervation to all the muscles of the larynx, with the exception of the cricothyroid muscle, as previously described. In addition, it carries sensation from the part of the larynx that lies below the vocal folds and from the upper part of the trachea. It courses up the neck in the groove between the trachea and the esophagus. As a result of the differing development of the aortic arches on the right and left sides of the body, the right recurrent laryngeal nerve passes in front of the right subclavian artery and turns up and back around this vessel to course toward the larynx. In contrast, the left recurrent laryngeal nerve passes into the thorax and lies in front of the arch of the aorta before turning up and back around the aorta behind the ligamentum arteriosum to reach the larynx.

C. PHARYNGEAL BRANCHES

The pharyngeal branches provide motor innervation to all the muscles of the pharynx, with the exception of the stylopharyngeus muscle, and to all the muscles of the palate, with the exception of the tensor veli palatini muscle.

D. CARDIAC BRANCHES

The cardiac branches descend into the mediastinum and provide parasympathetic innervation to the heart.

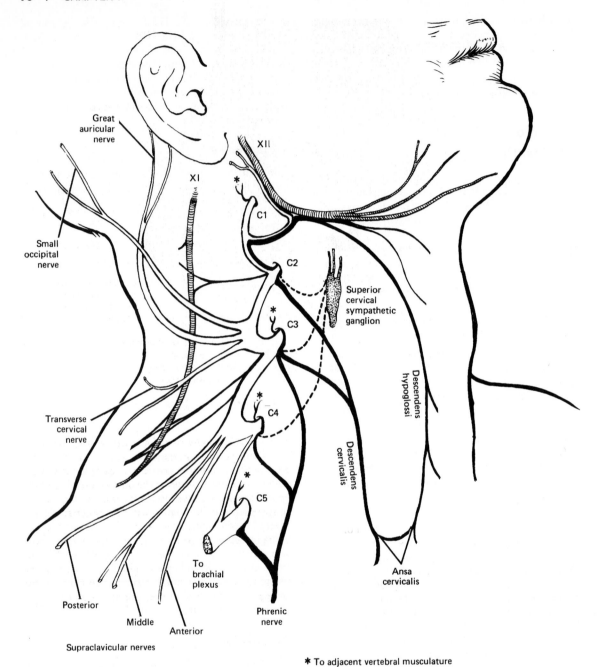

Figure 1–9. Cervical plexus. Motor and sensory innervation of the neck. (Reproduced, with permission, from Lindner HH. *Clinical Anatomy*, McGraw-Hill, 1989.)

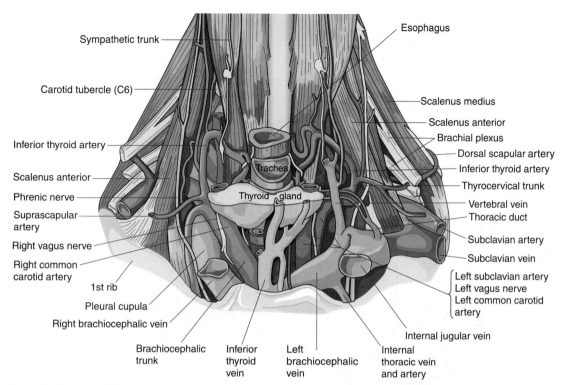

Figure 1–10. Root of the neck.

E. SENSORY BRANCHES

The vagus has sensory branches that serve the meninges and the external ear.

Phrenic Nerve

The phrenic nerve arises from the ventral rami of cervical spinal nerves C3–5 and courses down in the prevertebral fascia in front of the anterior scalene muscle, into the thorax between the subclavian artery and vein. It provides motor innervation to the diaphragm. In addition, it carries sensation from the mediastinal and diaphragmatic parietal pleura, the pericardium, and the parietal peritoneum under the diaphragm.

Sympathetic Trunk

The sympathetic trunk in the neck is an upward continuation of the thoracic part of the trunk and reaches the base of the skull, lying medial to the carotid sheath in the prevertebral fascia. Unlike the thoracic part of the trunk, which has a sympathetic ganglion associated with each spinal nerve, the cervical part of the trunk has only three ganglia. The inferior cervical ganglion lies near the first rib and is frequently fused with the

first thoracic ganglion to form the stellate ganglion. The middle cervical ganglion lies at the level of the cricoid cartilage. The superior cervical ganglion lies at the base of the skull, just below the inferior opening of the carotid canal. The cervical sympathetic ganglia get preganglionic input from fibers that originate in the thoracic spinal cord and ascend in the sympathetic trunk to reach the neck. Postganglionic outflow from these ganglia passes to the cervical spinal nerves, the cardiac plexus, the thyroid gland, the pharyngeal plexus, and as neurons that form plexuses around the internal and external carotid arteries as those vessels course up to the head.

Fascial Planes

The deep fascia of the neck is thickened into several well-defined layers that are of clinical significance.

A. INVESTING FASCIA

The investing fascia surrounds the neck, attached below to the sternum and the clavicle, and above to the lower border of the mandible, the zygomatic arch, the mastoid process, and the superior nuchal line of the occipital bone. The fascia splits to enclose the sternocleidomastoid and trapezius muscles and the submandibular and parotid salivary glands.

B. PREVERTEBRAL FASCIA

The prevertebral fascia surrounds the prevertebral and postvertebral muscles, and is attached to the ligamentum nuchae in the back. It is attached to the base of the skull above and extends down into the mediastinum below. There is a potential space, called the retropharyngeal space, between this fascial layer and the pharynx and esophagus, allowing for the free movement of these structures against the vertebral column. However, this arrangement also provides a communicating space that extends from the base of the skull down into the mediastinum, allowing for infections to easily track in either direction.

C. CAROTID SHEATH

The carotid sheath surrounds the carotid arteries, the internal jugular vein, the vagus nerve, and the deep cervical lymph nodes.

D. VISCERAL FASCIA

The visceral fascia surrounds the thyroid and parathyroid glands and the infrahyoid muscles. It extends from its attachment to the thyroid cartilage above to the pericardium below and is fused with the carotid sheath and the investing fascia.

■ LARYNX

The larynx extends from the epiglottis and the aryepiglottic folds to the cricoid cartilage (Figure 1–11). It communicates with the laryngopharynx above through the laryngeal aditus and with the trachea below. Its lateral walls have two infoldings of mucous membrane, the vestibular folds above and the vocal folds below. The space between the two vestibular folds is called the rima vestibuli, and the space between the two vocal folds is called the rima glottidis. The part of the larynx that extends from the aditus to the rima vestibuli is called the vestibule of the larynx, and the part that lies between the rima vestibuli and the rima glottidis is called the ventricle of the larynx. The ventricle has a lateral extension, the saccule, between the vestibular fold and the thyroid cartilage. The mucous membrane of the larynx is primarily ciliated columnar epithelium. The larynx is made of cartilages and ligaments that are essential to its role in phonation.

Cartilages

A. THYROID CARTILAGE

The thyroid cartilage (Adam's apple) makes up the bulk of the larynx, but is deficient posteriorly. It articulates with the cricoid cartilage below, which is narrow in front but taller in the back.

B. ARYTENOID CARTILAGES

Articulating with the posterior lamina of the cricoid cartilage and lying directly behind the thyroid cartilage are the paired arytenoid cartilages. These cartilages have

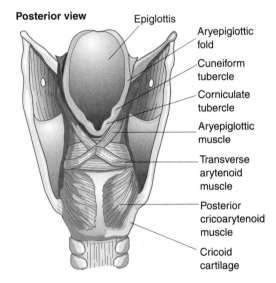

Posterior view

Epiglottis — Aryepiglottic fold — Cuneiform tubercle — Corniculate tubercle — Aryepiglottic muscle — Transverse arytenoid muscle — Posterior cricoarytenoid muscle — Cricoid cartilage

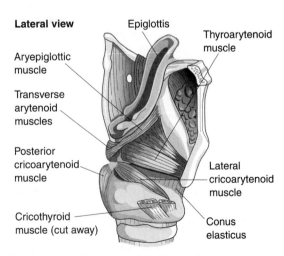

Lateral view

Epiglottis — Thyroarytenoid muscle — Aryepiglottic muscle — Transverse arytenoid muscles — Posterior cricoarytenoid muscle — Cricothyroid muscle (cut away) — Lateral cricoarytenoid muscle — Conus elasticus

Figure 1–11. Muscles and cartilages of the larynx.

laterally extending muscular processes that allow for the attachment of several muscles of vocalization and anteriorly extending vocal processes that allow for the attachment of the vocal ligaments.

C. CORNICULATE AND CUNEIFORM CARTILAGES

The epiglottis forms the roof of the larynx. The aryepiglottic folds contain two additional pairs of cartilages, the corniculate and cuneiform, which add support to the folds.

Ligaments

A. THYROHYOID LIGAMENT

The thyrohyoid ligament extends from the upper border of the thyroid cartilage to the hyoid bone above, anchoring the larynx to the hyoid bone and its associated muscles.

B. QUADRANGULAR LIGAMENT

The quadrangular ligament lies within the aryepiglottic folds, and its lower edge extends into the vestibular folds of the larynx.

C. CRICOTHYROID LIGAMENT

The cricothyroid ligament (triangular ligament) extends upward from the upper border of the cricoid cartilage. However, it is not attached to the lower border of the thyroid cartilage. Instead, it ascends medial to the thyroid cartilage and is compressed sagittally, with its top edges forming the vocal ligaments that are attached to the inside of the thyroid cartilage in front and the vocal processes of the arytenoid cartilage behind.

Muscles

The muscles of the larynx change the spatial relationships of the laryngeal cartilages during speech and swallowing.

A. POSTERIOR CRICOARYTENOID MUSCLE

The posterior cricoarytenoid muscle arises from the posterior aspect of the cricoid cartilage and courses upward and laterally to attach to the muscular process of the arytenoid cartilage. Its contraction pulls the muscular process backward and rotates the arytenoid cartilage along a vertical axis so that the vocal processes are abducted and the size of the rima glottidis is increased. In addition, the two arytenoid cartilages are approximated, an action that is similar to that of the transverse arytenoid muscle.

B. LATERAL CRICOARYTENOID MUSCLE

The lateral cricoarytenoid muscle arises from the front of the arch of the cricoid cartilage and courses upward

and laterally to attach to the muscular process of the arytenoid cartilage. Its contraction pulls the muscular processes forward and rotates the arytenoid cartilage along a vertical axis, in a direction opposite to the movement created by the contraction of the posterior cricoarytenoid muscle so that the vocal processes are adducted and the rima glottidis is closed. Additional contraction of the lateral cricoarytenoid muscle from this adducted position of the vocal ligaments, coupled with a relaxation of the transverse arytenoid muscle, pulls the two arytenoid cartilages away from each other, positioning the vocal folds for whispering, with adducted vocal ligaments but an open posterior rima glottidis.

C. TRANSVERSE ARYTENOID MUSCLE

The transverse arytenoid muscle extends between the bodies of the two arytenoid cartilages, bringing them together by its contraction.

D. THYROARYTENOID MUSCLE

The thyroarytenoid muscle has fibers that run parallel with the vocal ligaments, attaching to the deep surface of the thyroid cartilage in front and the muscular process of the arytenoid cartilage behind. Its contraction brings the arytenoid and thyroid cartilages closer, decreases the length and tension of the vocal ligaments, and lowers the pitch of the voice. A part of the thyroarytenoid muscle that lies adjacent to the vocal ligament is called the vocalis muscle. Because its fibers attach to the vocal ligaments, this muscle can provide fine control of the tension in the vocal ligaments, allowing for rapid alterations in the pitch of the voice. When the vocalis muscle contracts by itself, without an accompanying contraction of the thyroarytenoid muscle, it can pull on the vocal ligaments, increase the tension in them, and raise the pitch of the voice.

E. CRICOTHYROID MUSCLE

The cricothyroid muscle arises from the front and side of the cricoid cartilage and courses upward and backward to attach to the inferior border of the posterior part of the thyroid cartilage. Its contraction produces a rocking movement at the joints between the thyroid and cricoid cartilages, so that the front of the cricoid is pulled upward and the cricoid cartilage is tilted backward. This moves the arytenoid cartilages farther from the thyroid cartilage and increases the tension in the vocal ligaments, raising the pitch of the voice.

F. ARYEPIGLOTTIC MUSCLE

The aryepiglottic muscle arises from the muscular process of the arytenoid cartilage and extends into the epiglottis within the opposite aryepiglottic fold. Its contraction decreases the size of the laryngeal aditus and, combined with an elevation of the larynx by the suprahyoid muscles and longitudinal muscles of the pharynx as well as the push of the tongue on the epiglottis from above, prevents food from entering the larynx.

Sensory & Motor Innervation

The vagus nerve provides sensory and motor innervation to the larynx. These details are discussed with the vagus nerve in the neck. Briefly, sensation from the vestibule and ventricle of the larynx, above the vocal folds, is carried by the internal laryngeal branch of the vagus nerve, and sensation from below the vocal folds is carried by the recurrent laryngeal branch of the vagus nerve. Motor innervation of all the muscles of the larynx is by the recurrent laryngeal branch of the vagus nerve, except the cricothyroid muscle, which is innervated by the external laryngeal branch of the vagus nerve. The superior laryngeal branch of the superior thyroid artery, a branch of the external carotid artery, supplies blood to the upper half of the larynx. The inferior laryngeal branch of the inferior thyroid artery, a branch of the thyrocervical trunk from the subclavian artery, supplies blood to the lower half the larynx.

■ ORBIT

The orbit lies between the frontal bone and the anterior cranial fossa above and the maxilla and maxillary sinus below. The sphenoid bone lies behind and separates the orbit from the middle cranial fossa. The zygomatic and sphenoid bones lie lateral to the orbit, and the ethmoid and sphenoid bones lie medial to it. The orbit communicates with the infratemporal fossa through the lateral end of the inferior orbital fissure and with the pterygopalatine fossa through the medial end of this fissure. In addition, the orbit communicates with the middle cranial fossa through the superior orbital fissure and the optic canal, and with the nose through the nasolacrimal canal. The structures in the orbit receive their blood supply from the ophthalmic branch of the internal carotid artery. The corresponding veins form the ophthalmic venous plexus, which communicates in front with the facial vein, behind with the cavernous sinus through the superior orbital fissure, and below with the pterygoid venous plexus through the inferior orbital fissure. The orbit contains the eye surrounded by orbital fat, the lacrimal gland, which lies above and lateral to the eye, the muscles that help move the eye, and the nerves and vessels related to these structures.

Muscles

All of the muscles of the orbit, with the exception of the inferior oblique, arise from the sphenoid bone at or near the opening of the optic canal behind the eye (Figure 1–12). They pass forward to attach to the sclera of the eye, except for the levator palpebrae superioris muscle, which inserts on the eyelid. The inferior oblique arises from the anterior and medial part of the floor of the orbit.

A. Levator Palpebrae Superioris Muscle

The levator palpebrae superioris passes over the eye and attaches to the tarsal plate of the upper eyelid. It helps to elevate the eyelid and keep the eye open. A part of this muscle is made of smooth muscle fibers that get sympathetic innervation.

B. Superior Rectus Muscle

The superior rectus muscle passes over the eye and helps to turn the eye upward. It is assisted in this action by the inferior oblique muscle.

C. Inferior Rectus Muscle

The inferior rectus muscle passes below the eye and helps to turn the eye downward. It is assisted in this action by the superior oblique muscle.

D. Medial Rectus Muscle

The medial rectus muscle passes medial to the eye and helps to turn the eye medially.

E. Lateral Rectus Muscle

The lateral rectus muscle passes lateral to the eye and helps to turn the eye laterally.

F. Superior Oblique Muscle

The superior oblique muscle first passes around a fibrous pulley, the trochlea, which lies above and medial to the front of the eye. It then turns backward, downward, and laterally to attach to the sclera. Its contraction places the eye in a position of a downward and lateral gaze. In addition, the superior oblique muscle produces torsion of the eye around an anteroposterior axis such that the upper part of the eye is turned medially.

G. Inferior Oblique Muscle

The inferior oblique muscle passes upward, backward, and laterally from its origin to insert on the sclera. Its contraction places the eye in a position of an upward and lateral gaze. In addition, it produces torsion of the eye around an anteroposterior axis such that the upper part of the eye is turned laterally.

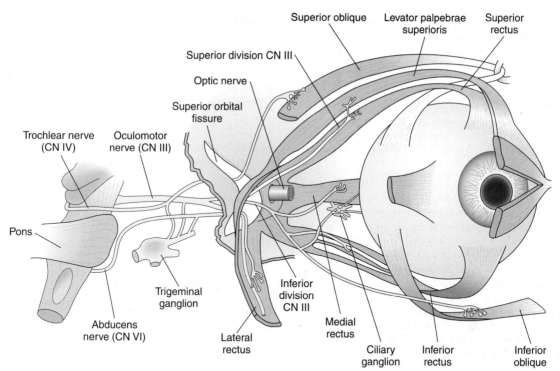

Figure 1–12. Muscles and nerves of the orbit.

Muscle Testing

During clinical examination, the rectus muscles are tested by asking a patient to follow a target with her or his eyes in the directions of the expected actions of each muscle. The superior oblique muscle is tested for its ability to turn the eye downward, but the eye is first turned medially so that the inferior rectus muscle is unable to participate in this downward movement—as it would if the eye were turned downward from its neutral position. Similarly, the inferior oblique muscle is tested by asking a patient to first turn the eye medially and then upward. With the eye placed in a direction of medial gaze, the superior and inferior rectus muscles are unable to assist as they normally would. In this situation, the superior and inferior oblique muscles are the only muscles that are optimally situated to turn the eye downward or upward, respectively, and are thus isolated and individually tested.

Innervation

The orbit is the location in which the ophthalmic division of the trigeminal nerve divides into its terminal branches after leaving the middle cranial fossa through the superior orbital fissure. The orbit also contains branches of the maxillary division of the trigeminal nerve and nerves that provide parasympathetic innervation to the lacrimal gland.

A. Sensory Innervation

1. Lacrimal nerve—The lacrimal nerve passes above and lateral to the eye and carries sensation from the lateral part of the upper eyelid.

2. Frontal nerve—The frontal nerve passes over the eye and divides into the supratrochlear and supraorbital nerves. The supratrochlear nerve exits the orbit above the trochlea and carries sensation from the skin of the forehead. The supraorbital nerve exits the orbit through the supraorbital notch (foramen) and carries sensation from the skin of the forehead that lies lateral to the area served by the supratrochlear nerve. The supraorbital nerve also carries sensation from the frontal sinuses.

3. Nasociliary nerve—The nasociliary nerve passes above and medial to the eye before giving off branches to the nose and the eye. The nasal component is made of the ethmoidal and nasal nerves that carry sensation from the roof of the nasal cavity, the skin of the nose, and the sphenoid and ethmoid sinuses. The ciliary component is made of the long and short ciliary nerves that carry sensation from the eye and cornea.

B. MOTOR INNERVATION

The orbit also contains nerves that enter the orbit through the superior orbital fissure and innervate the muscles of the eye.

1. Oculomotor nerve—The oculomotor nerve (CN III) innervates the levator palpebrae superioris; the superior, inferior, and medial recti; and the inferior oblique muscles.

2. Trochlear nerve—The trochlear nerve (CN IV) innervates the superior oblique muscle.

3. Abducens nerve—The abducens nerve (CN VI) innervates the lateral rectus muscle.

C. OPTIC NERVE

The optic nerve (CN II) enters the orbit through the optic canal and is surrounded by the meninges, which fuse with the sclera. As a result of this arrangement, the cerebrospinal fluid in the subarachnoid space can extend up to the back of the sclera along the optic nerve. The nasal retina, which has a temporal field of view, transmits its visual information through optic nerve fibers that decussate at the optic chiasm to the optic tract of the opposite side. The temporal retina, which has a nasal field of view, transmits its visual information through optic nerve fibers that remain in the ipsilateral optic tract. Thus, the left optic tract contains fibers from the temporal retina of the left eye and the nasal retina of the right eye and is responsible for carrying the visual information of objects that lie to the right of the body. Similarly, the right optic tract contains fibers from the temporal retina of the right eye and the nasal retina of the left eye and is responsible for carrying the visual information of objects that lie to the left of the body.

D. AUTONOMIC NERVES

1. Parasympathetic nerves—The ciliary muscle and the sphincter pupillae muscle of the eye receive parasympathetic innervation from the oculomotor nerve. The preganglionic fibers arise in the Edinger-Westphal nucleus of the oculomotor nerve in the midbrain, travel on that nerve, and reach the ciliary ganglion in the orbit at which they synapse. From the ciliary ganglion, the postganglionic fibers travel on the short ciliary branches of the ophthalmic division of the trigeminal nerve and reach the eye and its intrinsic musculature, namely, the ciliary and sphincter pupillae muscles. Contraction of the sphincter pupillae muscle decreases the size of the pupillary opening, diminishing the amount of light entering the eye, while at the same time increasing the depth of field through which the eye remains focused. Contraction of the ciliary muscle relieves the tension in the suspensory ligaments of the lens, allows the lens to become more convex, and increases its power. Together, the actions of the intrinsic musculature, under parasympathetic influence, are necessary for the accommodation of the eye.

2. Sympathetic nerves—The dilator pupillae muscle of the eye and a part of the levator palpebrae superioris muscle receive sympathetic innervation. The preganglionic neurons originate in the thoracic spinal cord and ascend in the sympathetic trunk to synapse in the superior cervical ganglion in the neck. Postganglionic neurons leave the superior cervical ganglion to ascend as a plexus around the internal carotid artery and then around its ophthalmic branch to reach the orbit. In the orbit, the sympathetic neurons travel on the long ciliary branches of the ophthalmic division of the trigeminal nerve to reach the eye and its dilator pupillae muscle, while the sympathetic neurons to the levator palpebrae superioris muscle reach it on further branches of the ophthalmic artery. Contraction of the dilator pupillae muscle increases the size of the pupillary opening, increasing the amount of light entering the eye. Contraction of the levator palpebrae superioris elevates the upper eyelid; therefore, the loss of either its sympathetic innervation or its innervation by the oculomotor nerve produces ptosis.

■ PTERYGOPALATINE FOSSA

The pterygopalatine fossa is a small space that lies directly in front of the pterygoid plates of the sphenoid bone and behind the maxilla. Its floor is formed by the upper end of the palatine canal, its roof by the medial half of the inferior orbital fissure, its lateral wall by the pterygomaxillary fissure, and its medial wall by the sphenopalatine foramen and perpendicular plate of the palatine bone. Through the palatine canal, which opens in the hard palate, the pterygopalatine fossa communicates with the oral cavity below; through the inferior orbital fissure, which opens behind the floor of the orbit, the pterygopalatine fossa communicates with the orbital cavity above; through the pterygomaxillary fissure, the pterygopalatine fossa communicates with the infratemporal fossa that lies lateral to it; and through the sphenopalatine foramen, which opens near the roof of the back of the nose, the pterygopalatine fossa communicates with the nasal cavity that lies medial to it. The maxillary sinus lies in front of the pterygopalatine fossa, whereas the foramen rotundum and the pterygoid canal lead into it from behind.

The maxillary artery enters the pterygopalatine fossa after branching from the external carotid artery in the substance of the parotid gland and passing through the infratemporal fossa and the pterygomaxillary fissure. The pterygopalatine fossa is the location at which the maxillary division of the trigeminal nerve divides into its terminal branches after it leaves the middle cranial fossa through the foramen rotundum. The branches of the maxillary artery essentially match the branches of the maxillary division of the trigeminal nerve that originate in and travel out of the pterygopalatine fossa.

Maxillary Nerve Branches

A. GREATER PALATINE NERVE

The greater palatine nerve courses down through the palatine canal and, on reaching the palate, turns forward to carry sensation from most of the hard palate with the exception of a small area behind the upper incisor teeth. While in the palatine canal, it sends branches that pierce through the bony medial wall of the canal, which is formed by the perpendicular plate of the palatine bone and carries sensation from the lateral wall of the nose. These are the lateral nasal nerves.

B. LESSER PALATINE NERVE

The lesser palatine nerve also courses down through the palatine canal, but on reaching the palate, it turns backward to carry sensation from the soft palate.

C. INFRAORBITAL NERVE

The infraorbital nerve courses up through the inferior orbital fissure and on reaching the orbital floor, it turns forward and runs in a bony canal in the floor of the orbit to emerge on the face through the infraorbital foramen. While running forward in the floor of the orbit, the infraorbital nerve lies in the roof of the maxillary sinus and gives branches that carry sensation from the roots of the upper premolar teeth, the middle superior alveolar nerve, and the roots of the upper canines and incisors, the anterior superior alveolar nerve. Once it reaches the face, the infraorbital nerve carries sensation from an area of skin that extends from the lower eyelid to the upper lip.

D. ZYGOMATIC NERVE

The zygomatic nerve courses up through the inferior orbital fissure and up the lateral wall of the orbit. It then branches into the zygomaticofacial and zygomaticotemporal nerves, which pierce through the zygomatic bone, turning forward onto the skin of the face and backward onto the temple, respectively, from where they carry sensation.

E. POSTERIOR SUPERIOR ALVEOLAR NERVE

The posterior superior alveolar nerve courses laterally through the pterygomaxillary fissure and, on reaching the infratemporal fossa, pierces the back of the maxilla and carries sensation from the roots of the upper molars.

F. NASOPALATINE NERVE

The nasopalatine nerve courses medially through the sphenopalatine foramen and then over the roof of the nose to reach the nasal septum. Here, it turns forward and downward and travels along the septum to reach the incisive canal, emerging behind the upper incisors. It carries sensation from the nasal septum and the anterior part of the hard palate in an area just behind the upper incisors.

Autonomic Nerves

The pterygoid canal allows the carotid canal behind to communicate with the pterygopalatine fossa in front. It passes forward in the floor of the sphenoid sinus and transmits the nerve of the pterygoid canal, which has both sympathetic and parasympathetic components.

A. DEEP PETROSAL NERVE

The sympathetic component of the nerve of the pterygoid canal is the deep petrosal nerve, which is composed of postganglionic sympathetic neurons. The preganglionic neurons originate in the thoracic spinal cord and ascend in the sympathetic trunk to synapse in the superior cervical ganglion in the neck. Postganglionic neurons leave the superior cervical ganglion to ascend as a plexus around the internal carotid artery. Some of these postganglionic sympathetic neurons branch off the carotid plexus, in the carotid canal, and form the deep petrosal nerve, which enters the pterygoid canal to reach the pterygopalatine fossa. The sympathetic neurons then join branches of the maxillary artery and travel on their walls. Because these are postganglionic neurons that reach the pterygopalatine fossa, they do not synapse in the pterygopalatine ganglion.

B. GREATER SUPERFICIAL PETROSAL NERVE

The parasympathetic component of the nerve of the pterygoid canal is the greater superficial petrosal nerve, which is composed of preganglionic parasympathetic neurons. These originate in the lacrimal nucleus of the facial nerve and course within the petrous part of the temporal bone before emerging on its superior surface as the greater superficial petrosal nerve, which then turns down into the carotid canal and forward into the pterygoid canal to reach the pterygopalatine fossa (Figure 1–13). There, the preganglionic parasympathetic neurons synapse in the pterygopalatine ganglion. The postganglionic parasympathetic neurons then join branches of the maxillary division of the trigeminal nerve and reach mucous secreting glands in the paranasal sinuses, the palate, and the nose, to which they are secretomotor. Some postganglionic parasympathetic neurons travel on the zygomatic branch of the maxillary division of the trigeminal nerve as it courses up the lateral wall of the orbit. When the zygomatic nerve leaves the orbit by piercing through the zygomatic bone, the postganglionic parasympathetic neurons leave the zygomatic nerve, con-

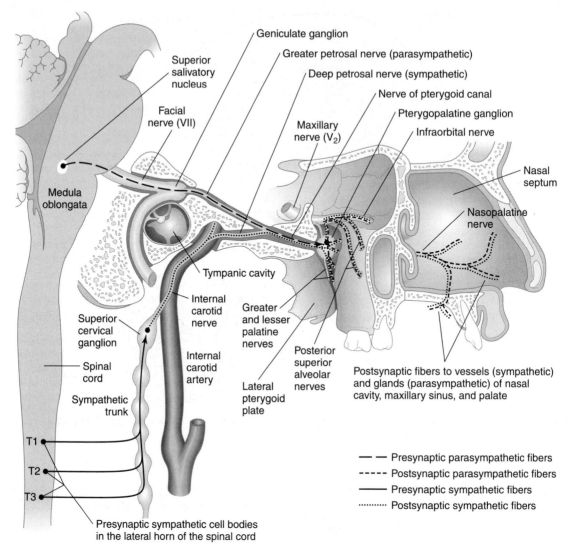

Figure 1–13. Schematic of the innervation of the glands in the nose, mouth, and orbit by the facial nerve (CN VII).

tinue up the lateral wall of the orbit, and join the lacrimal branch of the ophthalmic division of the trigeminal nerve to reach the lacrimal gland, to which they are secretomotor.

■ INFRATEMPORAL FOSSA

The infratemporal fossa lies between the mandible laterally and the lateral pterygoid plate of the sphenoid bone medially. The maxilla lies in front and the petrous part of the temporal bone behind. It is bounded above by the base of the skull and extends down to the level of the angle of the mandible. It communicates with the temporal fossa above and with the pterygopalatine fossa medial to it. The maxillary sinus lies in front of it and the temporomandibular joint behind. The maxillary artery gives off several branches here, before passing into the pterygopalatine fossa. The infratemporal fossa is the location at which the mandibular division of the trigeminal nerve divides into its terminal branches after leaving the middle cranial fossa through the foramen ovale.

Muscles

The muscles of mastication associated with this region are the temporalis, masseter, lateral pterygoid, and medial pterygoid muscles (Figure 1–14).

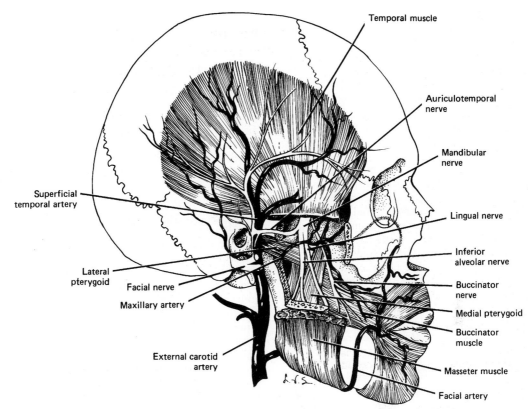

Figure 1–14. Muscles of mastication and the infratemporal fossa. (Reproduced, with permission, from Lindner HH. *Clinical Anatomy*, McGraw-Hill, 1989.)

A. TEMPORALIS MUSCLE

The temporalis muscle arises from the temporal bone and passes medial to the zygomatic arch to attach to the coronoid process of the mandible. Its anterior fibers elevate the mandible, and its posterior fibers retract the mandible.

B. MASSETER MUSCLE

The masseter muscle arises from the lower border of the zygomatic arch and attaches to the lateral aspect of the angle of the mandible. Its contraction elevates the mandible.

C. LATERAL PTERYGOID MUSCLE

The lateral pterygoid muscle arises from both the lateral aspect of the lateral pterygoid plate and the sphenoid bone above, attaching to the neck of the mandible and the articular disc of the temporomandibular joint. Its contraction protracts the mandible along with the articular disc.

D. MEDIAL PTERYGOID MUSCLE

The medial pterygoid muscle arises from the medial aspect of the lateral pterygoid plate and attaches to the medial aspect of the angle of the mandible. Its contraction, like the masseter muscle, elevates the mandible.

Temporomandibular Joint

The temporomandibular joint lies between the head of the mandible and a fossa in the temporal bone. The capsule of the joint is attached to the neck of the mandible below and the margins of the mandibular fossa above. The joint is strengthened on its medial side by the sphenomandibular ligament, on its lateral side by the temporomandibular ligament, and behind by the stylomandibular ligament.

The joint contains a fibrocartilaginous, intracapsular articular disc that divides the joint into upper and lower synovial cavities. Translational movements of the joint, produced by the protraction and retraction of the mandible, occur in the upper joint cavity such that the articular disc moves with the head of the mandible. Rotational movements of the joint, produced by elevation and depression of the mandible, occur in the lower joint cavity such that the mandibular head rotates while the articular disc remains stationary. Protraction of the mandible is produced primarily by the lateral pterygoid muscle, assisted by the medial pterygoid and masseter muscles, whereas retraction is produced by the posterior fibers of the temporalis muscle.

Elevation of the mandible (clenching the teeth) is produced by the anterior fibers of the temporalis, the masseter, and the medial pterygoid muscles. Depression of the mandible (opening the mouth) is produced by the suprahyoid muscles—namely, the geniohyoid, mylohyoid, and digastric muscles, with the infrahyoid muscles serving to hold the hyoid bone in place. As the mouth opens wide, the head of the mandible must be protracted out of the mandibular fossa; this movement is brought about by the lateral pterygoid muscle. Closing the mouth from this position requires an initial retraction of the mandible so that the head of the mandible and the articular disc are replaced into the mandibular fossa by the posterior fibers of the temporalis muscle. Side-to-side movements of the mandible are produced by contractions of the medial and lateral pterygoid muscles from one side, joined by the posterior fibers of the temporalis muscle of the other side, alternating with the opposite set of muscles.

Mandibular Nerve Branches

Unlike the ophthalmic and maxillary divisions of the trigeminal nerve, which are purely sensory in their roles, the mandibular division of the trigeminal nerve has both sensory and motor functions. Its motor branches supply all the muscles of mastication, and also the tensor veli palatini muscle, the tensor tympani muscle, the mylohyoid muscle, and the anterior belly of the digastric muscle. The mandibular division of the trigeminal nerve reaches the infratemporal fossa through the foramen ovale and gives off branches that carry sensation from the area for which they are named.

A. Buccal Nerve

The buccal nerve, which courses into the cheek, pierces the buccinator muscle but does not innervate it. This nerve carries sensation from the skin over the cheek and the mucous membrane within.

B. Lingual Nerve

The lingual nerve courses into the tongue and carries general sensation from the anterior two thirds of the tongue. The chorda tympani branch of the facial nerve reaches the infratemporal fossa by passing through the petrotympanic fissure and joins the lingual nerve. It contains preganglionic parasympathetic fibers from the superior salivary nucleus that are secretomotor to the submandibular and sublingual salivary glands. It also contains fibers that carry the sensation of taste from the anterior two thirds of the tongue. Additional details of the chorda tympani and the lingual nerve are described in the sections on the salivary glands and the mouth.

C. Inferior Alveolar Nerve

The inferior alveolar nerve courses into the mandibular canal and carries sensation from the roots of the lower teeth. It emerges onto the face through the mental foramen as the mental nerve and carries sensation from the lower lip and the skin of the chin. Before it enters the mandible, the inferior alveolar nerve gives off a motor branch, the nerve to the mylohyoid muscle, which innervates the mylohyoid and anterior belly of the digastric muscles.

D. Auriculotemporal Nerve

The auriculotemporal nerve courses backward, deep to the temporomandibular joint, and ascends onto the scalp, in front of and above the auricle, to carry sensation from that area. In the infratemporal fossa, the auriculotemporal nerve is split by the middle meningeal branch of the maxillary artery. The preganglionic parasympathetic fibers for the secretomotor pathway to the parotid gland originate in the inferior salivary nucleus, travel on the lesser superficial petrosal branch of the glossopharyngeal nerve, and synapse at the otic ganglion. Postganglionic fibers from the otic ganglion, which lies just below the foramen ovale, join the auriculotemporal nerve to reach the parotid gland. Additional details are described in the section on salivary glands.

Maxillary Artery

The maxillary artery, a branch of the external carotid artery, courses into the infratemporal fossa and passes through the pterygomaxillary fissure to reach the pterygopalatine fossa. It can pass either superficially or deep to the lateral pterygoid muscle and supplies blood, through several branches, to the structures that lie in the infratemporal fossa.

One branch, the inferior alveolar artery, enters the mandibular canal with the corresponding nerve. Another branch, the middle meningeal artery, splits the auriculotemporal nerve and passes through the foramen spinosum to enter the middle cranial fossa.

Pterygoid Venous Plexus

The veins that correspond to the branches of the maxillary artery form a plexus in the infratemporal fossa, which is continuous with the plexus of veins in the pterygopalatine fossa, and is collectively called the pterygoid venous plexus. The pterygoid venous plexus communicates with the ophthalmic venous plexus through the inferior orbital fissure and with the cavernous sinus through the foramen ovale and rotundum.

The interconnections of these venous plexuses among themselves and with the facial vein are described in the section on the face.

CRANIAL NERVES

The cranial nerves are depicted in Figure 1–15.

OLFACTORY NERVE

The olfactory nerve carries the sensation of smell. It is solely a sensory nerve. Its fibers pass through the cribriform plate of the ethmoid bone into the olfactory bulb lying in the anterior cranial fossa, carrying the sensations of smell from the olfactory mucosa in the roof of the nose. From the olfactory bulb, the olfactory tracts pass back to the cerebrum.

OPTIC NERVE

The optic nerve, which is also only a sensory nerve, carries visual information from the eye. Its fibers originate from the ganglion cells of the retina and leave the orbital cavity through the optic canal. Fibers from the nasal retina decussate at the optic chiasm, which lies just above the pituitary gland. The optic tract passes backward from the chiasm and around the midbrain to reach the lateral geniculate body, from where most fibers pass to the visual cortex.

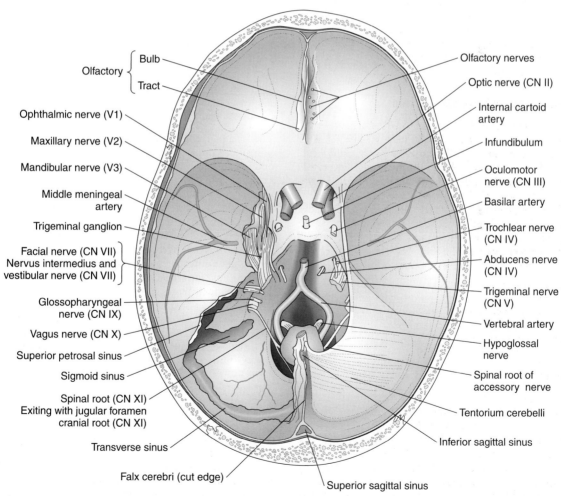

Figure 1–15. Cranial nerves in the interior of the base of the skull.

OCULOMOTOR NERVE

The oculomotor nerve innervates muscles that move the eye. It is solely a motor nerve. It also has a parasympathetic role. Its fibers originate in the midbrain and pass medial to the cerebral peduncles, through the interpeduncular cistern and between the posterior cerebral and superior cerebellar branches of the basilar artery. It then passes through the lateral wall of the cavernous sinus and enters the orbit through the superior orbital fissure, where it innervates the levator palpebrae superioris, the inferior oblique, and the superior, medial, and inferior rectus muscles.

TROCHLEAR NERVE

The trochlear nerve innervates one muscle, the superior oblique, which moves the eye. It is solely a motor nerve. It is the only cranial nerve that arises from the posterior aspect of the brain and it has a long intracranial course. It runs forward around the cerebral peduncles, lying medial to the tentorium cerebelli. It then passes through the lateral wall of the cavernous sinus and enters the orbit through the superior orbital fissure, where it innervates the superior oblique muscle.

TRIGEMINAL NERVE

The trigeminal nerve is the main sensory nerve for the face and deeper structures. It is both a sensory and a motor nerve. It innervates all the muscles of mastication and other muscles that are derived from the first branchial arch. In addition, it allows postganglionic parasympathetic fibers to travel on its branches to reach their target organs in the head. Its fibers arise from the anterolateral surface of the pons and course forward through the posterior cranial fossa to the trigeminal ganglion, which lies at the apex of the petrous part of the temporal bone in a dural cave. It is here that the cell bodies of the first-order sensory neurons from all sensory branches of the trigeminal nerve are located. The three divisions of the trigeminal nerve separate at the trigeminal ganglion.

Divisions of the Trigeminal Nerve

A. OPHTHALMIC NERVE

The ophthalmic division of the trigeminal nerve continues forward in the lateral wall of the cavernous sinus and passes through the superior orbital fissure to enter the orbit.

B. MAXILLARY NERVE

The maxillary division of the trigeminal nerve also continues forward from the ganglion and leaves the middle cranial fossa through the foramen rotundum to enter the pterygopalatine fossa.

C. MANDIBULAR NERVE

The mandibular division of the trigeminal nerve continues downward and leaves the middle cranial fossa through the foramen ovale to enter the infratemporal fossa. In addition to the sensory fibers, the motor fibers of the trigeminal nerve leave the pons and, at the trigeminal ganglion, join the mandibular division to course out of the foramen ovale and reach the infratemporal fossa. At that location, they give branches that innervate the muscles of the first branchial arch.

ABDUCENS NERVE

The abducens nerve innervates one muscle that moves the eye. It is solely a motor nerve. Its fibers originate just above the medullary pyramids, have a long intracranial course, and pass into the cavernous sinus. It courses through the middle of the sinus with the internal carotid artery, to which it is approximated. The abducens nerve enters the orbit through the superior orbital fissure, where it innervates the lateral rectus muscle.

FACIAL NERVE

The facial nerve innervates the muscles of facial expression and all other muscles that are derived from the second branchial arch. It carries the sensation of taste from the front of the tongue. It is both a sensory and a motor nerve. In addition, it has a parasympathetic role as described below. Its fibers originate at the pontomedullary junction, leave the posterior cranial fossa through the internal acoustic meatus, and enter the facial canal in the petrous part of the temporal bone. It has a motor root, and another root, the nervus intermedius, which is responsible for carrying the sensation of taste and for parasympathetic innervation.

Motor Root

The motor root travels through the facial canal and innervates the stapedius muscle. Then, the motor root turns down to emerge from the stylomastoid foramen. Here, it gives off branches to the posterior belly of the digastric and the stylohyoid muscles, whose posterior attachments are adjacent to the stylomastoid foramen. From here, the motor root lies in the substance of the parotid gland.

Nervus Intermedius

The nervus intermedius part of the facial nerve gives off two branches.

A. Chorda Tympani

The chorda tympani courses laterally through the petrous part of the temporal bone, enters the middle ear, and courses forward on the inner surface of the eardrum. It leaves the middle ear by turning down through the petrotympanic fissure and reaches the infratemporal fossa. It plays a role in carrying the sensation of taste from the anterior two thirds of the tongue. In addition, it is secretomotor to the submandibular and sublingual salivary glands. The sensory ganglion for the facial nerve is the geniculate ganglion, which lies in the petrous part of the temporal bone.

B. Greater Superficial Petrosal Nerve

The greater superficial petrosal nerve, after coursing laterally in the facial canal, turns medially in the petrous part of the temporal bone and emerges on its superior surface. Then it turns down into the carotid canal and forward into the pterygoid canal to reach the pterygopalatine fossa. It is secretomotor to the mucous glands of the sinuses and also to the lacrimal gland.

VESTIBULOCOCHLEAR NERVE

The vestibulocochlear nerve (CN VIII) carries sensory information from the vestibule and the cochlea. It is solely a sensory nerve. The vestibular fibers arise from the vestibular ganglion while the cochlear fibers arise from the spiral ganglion, in the petrous part of the temporal bone. The vestibular fibers carry sensory information about the position and angular rotation of the head, both necessary to maintain equilibrium. The cochlear fibers carry the stimuli of hearing. The sensory fibers emerge from the internal acoustic meatus and reach the brain at the pontomedullary junction.

GLOSSOPHARYNGEAL NERVE

The glossopharyngeal nerve carries sensation from the pharynx and tongue. It also innervates one muscle of the pharynx that develops from the third branchial arch. It is both a sensory and a motor nerve. In addition, it has a parasympathetic role. Its fibers arise from the medulla and leave the posterior cranial fossa through the jugular foramen. Behind the pharynx, it lies with the stylopharyngeus muscle, which it innervates. Together, the muscle and nerve enter the pharynx between the lower fibers of the superior pharyngeal constrictor muscle and the upper fibers of the middle pharyngeal constrictor muscle. In the pharynx, the glossopharyngeal nerve contributes to the pharyngeal plexus, carrying sensation from most of the pharynx and the posterior third of the tongue. In addition, as it emerges from the jugular foramen, the glossopharyngeal nerve gives off a branch that enters the petrous part

of the temporal bone and reaches the tympanic cavity to form the tympanic plexus, which carries sensation from the middle ear. These fibers then emerge on the surface of the petrous part of the temporal bone in the middle cranial fossa as the lesser superficial petrosal nerve, which exits the skull through the foramen ovale and is secretomotor to the parotid gland. The sensory ganglia for the glossopharyngeal nerve lie just below the jugular foramen.

VAGUS NERVE

The vagus nerve innervates the muscles of the palate, the pharynx, and the larynx, with some exceptions. It carries sensation from the larynx. It is both a sensory and a motor nerve and has a parasympathetic role. Its fibers arise from the medulla, are joined by the cranial root of the accessory nerve, and leave the posterior cranial fossa through the jugular foramen. Thus, the laryngeal and pharyngeal branches of the vagus nerve carry motor fibers that originated in the cranial component of the accessory nerve (XI). In addition, the laryngeal branches of the vagus nerve carry sensation from the larynx.

Innervation

A. Motor Innervation

1. Palate—All the muscles of the palate, except for the tensor veli palatini, are innervated by the vagus nerve. The tensor veli palatini is innervated by the maxillary division of the trigeminal nerve.

2. Pharynx—All the muscles of the pharynx, except for the stylopharyngeus, are innervated by the vagus nerve. The stylopharyngeus muscle is innervated by the glossopharyngeal nerve.

3. Larynx—All the muscles of the larynx, except for the cricothyroid muscle, are innervated by the recurrent laryngeal branch of the vagus nerve. The cricothyroid muscle is innervated by the external laryngeal branch of the vagus nerve.

B. Sensory Innervation

The sensory ganglia for the vagus lie just below the jugular foramen. The superior laryngeal branch of the vagus nerve carries sensation from the upper part of the larynx, above the vocal folds, whereas the recurrent laryngeal branch of the vagus nerve carries sensation from the lower part of the larynx.

ACCESSORY NERVE

The accessory nerve innervates two muscles in the neck and is solely a motor nerve. It has a cranial root and a spinal root. The fibers of the cranial root arise from the medulla. The fibers of the spinal root originate from the upper spinal cord segments (C1–5) and ascend into the skull to join the cranial root. The two roots separate almost immediately. The fibers of the cranial root join the vagus nerve in the posterior cranial fossa, exit through the jugular foramen, and are distributed in the motor branches of the vagus nerve to the pharynx, the larynx, and the palate. The fibers of the spinal root reach the neck by passing through the jugular foramen and innervate the sternocleidomastoid and trapezius muscles.

HYPOGLOSSAL NERVE

The hypoglossal nerve innervates the muscles of the tongue and is solely a motor nerve. Its fibers arise from the medulla, leave the posterior cranial fossa through the hypoglossal canal, and go on to innervate the extrinsic and intrinsic muscles of the tongue.

AUTONOMIC INNERVATION

A. SYMPATHETIC INNERVATION

The sympathetic innervation of the head and neck is from the thoracic sympathetic outflow. The preganglionic neurons originate in the thoracic spinal cord and ascend in the sympathetic trunk to synapse in the middle and superior cervical ganglia in the neck. From here, postganglionic sympathetic fibers travel as plexuses on the branches of the internal and external carotid arteries to reach target structures in the head and neck.

B. PARASYMPATHETIC INNERVATION

The oculomotor, facial, glossopharyngeal, and vagus nerves are the four cranial nerves that carry the parasympathetic outflow from the brain to most of the body. Parasympathetic innervation of the pelvic organs and lower gastrointestinal tract is from the sacral parasympathetic outflow.

1. Ciliary ganglion—Preganglionic parasympathetic fibers from the Edinger-Westphal nucleus travel on the oculomotor nerve and synapse at the ciliary ganglion (see Figure 1–12). Postganglionic fibers from the ciliary ganglion join the short ciliary branches of the ophthalmic division of the trigeminal nerve to reach the ciliary muscle and the sphincter pupillae muscle of the eye.

2. Pterygopalatine ganglion—Preganglionic parasympathetic fibers from the lacrimal nucleus travel on the greater superficial petrosal branch of the facial nerve and synapse at the pterygopalatine ganglion (see Figure 1–13). Postganglionic fibers from the pterygopalatine ganglion join branches of the maxillary division of the trigeminal nerve to reach the lacrimal gland and the mucous secreting glands of the nose and mouth.

3. Submandibular ganglion—Preganglionic parasympathetic fibers from the superior salivary nucleus travel on the chorda tympani branch of the facial nerve and synapse at the submandibular ganglion (see Figure 1–5). Postganglionic fibers from the submandibular ganglion join the lingual branch of the mandibular division of the trigeminal nerve to reach the submandibular and sublingual salivary glands.

4. Otic ganglion—Preganglionic parasympathetic fibers from the inferior salivary nucleus travel on the lesser superficial petrosal branch of the glossopharyngeal nerve and synapse at the otic ganglion (see Figure 1–4). Postganglionic fibers from the otic ganglion join the auriculotemporal branch of the maxillary division of the trigeminal nerve to reach the parotid salivary gland.

5. Visceral ganglia—The vagus nerve is the only cranial nerve that leaves the head and neck. It carries preganglionic parasympathetic fibers to the rest of the body, with the exception of the pelvic organs and organs associated with the hindgut. These fibers synapse at ganglia in the walls of the organ being innervated, from where short postganglionic fibers serve their secretomotor role.

Antimicrobial Therapy for Head & Neck Infection

Peter V. Chin-Hong, MD, & Richard A. Jacobs, MD, PhD

■ ANTIBACTERIAL AGENTS

A list of antibiotics by class and their use in otolaryngology can be found in Table 2–1.

PENICILLINS

Penicillins are a large group of β-lactam antibiotics. All share a common nucleus (6-aminopenicillanic acid) that contains a β-lactam ring, which is the biologically active moiety. The drugs work by binding to penicillin-binding proteins on the bacterial cell wall, which inhibits peptidoglycan synthesis. They also activate autolytic enzymes in the cell wall, resulting in cell lysis and death.

1. Natural Penicillins

This class includes parenteral penicillin G (eg, aqueous crystalline, procaine, and benzathine penicillin G) and oral formulations (eg, penicillin V).

Adverse Effects

The most common side effect of agents in the penicillin family is hypersensitivity, with anaphylaxis presenting in 0.05% of cases.

Clinical Uses

These drugs are most active against gram-positive organisms, but resistance is increasing. Natural penicillins are still widely used for streptococci, such as in streptococcal pharyngitis; however, 30–35% of pneumococci have intermediate- or high-level resistance to penicillin. They are also used for meningococci, *Treponema pallidum* and other spirochetes, and actinomyces.

2. Aminopenicillins

This extended-spectrum group includes ampicillin, which is administered intravenously, and amoxicillin

(only oral formulation in the United States). These agents are susceptible to destruction by β-lactamases produced by staphylococci and other bacteria.

Adverse Effects

A maculopapular rash may occur in 65–100% of patients with infectious mononucleosis who are prescribed amoxicillin. This symptom is not a true penicillin allergy.

Clinical Uses

In addition to having the same spectrum of activity against gram-positive organisms as the natural penicillins, aminopenicillins also have some activity against gram-negative rods. Because of its pharmacokinetics, amoxicillin is active against strains of pneumococcus with intermediate resistance to penicillin, but not strains with high-level resistance; it is therefore a first-line drug for the treatment of sinusitis and otitis.

3. Penicillinase-Resistant Penicillins

This class includes methicillin, dicloxacillin, and nafcillin. They are relatively resistant to β-lactamases produced by staphylococci.

Adverse Effects

Nafcillin in high doses can be associated with a modest leukopenia, particularly if given for several weeks.

Clinical Uses

These agents are used as antistaphylococcal drugs because they are less active than the natural penicillins against other gram-positives. They are still adequate in streptococcal infections.

4. Antipseudomonal Penicillins

This class includes the carboxypenicillins, such as ticarcillin (Ticar), and the ureidopenicillins, such as piperacillin (Pipracil).

Table 2–1. Examples of initial antimicrobial therapy for selected conditions in head and neck infection.

Suspected Clinical Diagnosis	Likely Etiologic Diagnosis	Treatment of Choice	Comments
Infections of the Ear			
External otitis	Gram-negative rods (Pseudomonas, Enterobacteriaceae, Proteus) or fungi (Aspergillus)	Otic drops containing a mixture of an aminoglycoside and corticosteroids, such as neomycin sulfate and hydrocortisone	In refractory cases, particularly if there is cellulitis of the adjacent periauricular tissue, oral fluoroquinolones such as ciprofloxacin 500 mg twice a day can be used for their antipseudomonal activity. However, there is increasing resistance being reported. Acute infection may be due to S aureus; dicloxacillin 500 mg four times a day may be used.
Malignant external otitis	Pseudomonas aeruginosa	Antibiotics with antipseudomonal activity (such as ciprofloxacin) for a prolonged period until there is radiographic evidence of improvement	Surgical debridement may be necessary if medical therapy is unsuccessful. It may also be necessary to rule out osteomyelitis by CT scan or MRI, as osteomyelitis requires prolonged therapy for 4–6 weeks.
Acute otitis media	S pneumoniae, H influenzae, M catarrhalis, and viruses (RSV, rhinoviruses)	Amoxicillin is the first drug of choice at 45 mg/kg/d in two or three divided doses. If drug resistance is suspected, a higher dose of amoxicillin or amoxicillin-clavulanate (90 mg/kg/d) may be used. Prevention of recurrent acute otitis media may be treated with oral doses of sulfisoxazole 50 mg/kg or amoxicillin 20 mg/kg at bedtime. If this strategy fails, the insertion of ventilating tubes may be necessary.	Treatment is a combination of antibiotics and nasal decongestants. Without treatment, there may be a spontaneous resolution of illness (less likely with S pneumoniae).
Mastoiditis	S pneumoniae, S pyogenes, H influenzae, and P aeruginosa	Myringotomy for culture and drainage and ceftriaxone, 1 g IV every 24 hours	Antibiotics may be modified based on culture results.
Infections of the Nose & Paranasal Sinuses			
Rhinitis (common cold)	Can be caused by a variety of viruses, including several serologic types of rhinoviruses and adenoviruses	Mainly reassurance of the patient and supportive therapy, such as decongestants (pseudoephedrine 30–60 mg every 4–6 hours). Nasal sprays such as oxymetazoline or phenylephrine can be immediately effective but must not be used for more than a few days at a time since rebound congestion may occur.	Secondary (bacterial) infection may occur and present as acute sinusitis.
Acute sinusitis	S pneumoniae, H influenzae, M catarrhalis, Group A streptococcus, anaerobes, viruses, and S aureus	Amoxicillin or amoxicillin/clavulanate 500 mg by mouth 3 times a day are reasonable first choices. If drug-resistant S pneumoniae is suspected, an oral fluoroquinolone such as levofloxacin may be used.	Because two-thirds of untreated patients will improve symptomatically within 2 weeks, antibiotic treatment is usually reserved for those who have maxillary or facial pain (or both), and purulent nasal discharge after 7 days of decongestants and analgesics. In cases of clinical failure, endoscopic sampling or maxillary sinus puncture can yield a specimen for microbiologic evaluation and the targeted selection of antibiotics.

Sinusitis in an immunocompromised host	Various molds, including *Aspergillus* and *Mucormycosis*	Wide surgical debridement and amphotericin B. Liposomal amphotericin, the echinocandins, and the new broad-spectrum azoles may be alternatives in appropriate patients.	These molds are highly angioinvasive and rapid dissemination and death can occur if they are not recognized in a timely fashion.

Infections of the Oral Cavity & Pharynx

Candidiasis (thrush)	*Candida albicans* (usually)	Fluconazole (100 mg by mouth daily for 7–14 days) or an oral solution of itraconazole (200 mg by mouth once daily)	AIDS patients may have fluconazole-resistant disease and may be treated with higher doses of fluconazole or itraconazole solution, or with amphotericin B administered intravenously.
Necrotizing ulcerative gingivitis (trench mouth, Vincent infection)	Usually coinfection with spirochetes and fusiform bacilli	Penicillin, 250 mg three times a day orally, with peroxide rinses	Clindamycin for patients with penicillin allergies.
Aphthous stomatitis (canker sore, aphthous ulcers)	Unknown, though human herpesvirus 6 is suspected	Mainly untreated. Options include topical steroids (eg, Kenalog in Orabase), other compounds such as mouthwashes containing amyloglucosidase and glucose oxidase, or a short course of systemic steroids.	Immunocompromised hosts, such as HIV-positive patients, may have more severe disease.
Herpetic stomatitis	Reactivation of herpes simplex virus 1 or 2	Oral acyclovir 400 mg three times daily, famciclovir 125 mg 3 times daily for 5 days, or valacyclovir 500 mg twice a day for 5 days may decrease healing time if initiated within 48 hours from the onset of symptoms. For recurrent disease, suppression with acyclovir 400 mg twice a day, famciclovir 250 mg twice daily, or valacyclovir 1 g daily is effective.	Most adults require no intervention. Immunocompromised hosts, such as HIV-positive patients, may have more severe and acyclovir-resistant disease and should be treated.
Pharyngitis	Group A, C, and G (β-hemolytic) streptococci, viruses (EBV-related infectious mononucleosis), *Neisseria gonorrhoeae*, *M pneumoniae*, human herpesvirus 6, *Corynebacterium diphtheriae*, *Arcanobacterium haemolyticum*, and *Chlamydia trachomatis*	Penicillin V (500 mg orally twice a day for 10 days), a single dose of benzathine penicillin intramuscularly (1–2 million units), or clarithromycin 500 mg by mouth twice a day for 10 days. If gonococcus is diagnosed, this may be treated with ceftriaxone 125 mg intramuscularly once, cefixime 400 mg orally in one dose, or cefpodoxime 400 mg orally in one dose. All patients with gonorrhea must also be treated for the possibility of concomitant genital *Chlamydia trachomatis* with azithromycin 1 g orally once, or doxycycline 100 mg orally twice daily for 7 days.	One of the main goals in management is to diagnose and treat Group A streptococcal infection and decrease the risk of rheumatic fever.
Epiglottitis	*H influenzae*, Group A streptococcus, *S pneumoniae*, and *S aureus*	Ceftriaxone (50 mg/kg daily for children) or cefuroxime. Adjunctive steroids are sometimes given but are not of proven benefit. Urgent tracheostomy in children or intubation in adults may be necessary.	

(continued)

Table 2–1. Examples of initial antimicrobial therapy for selected conditions in head and neck infection. *(Continued)*

Suspected Clinical Diagnosis	Likely Etiologic Diagnosis	Treatment of Choice	Comments
Parapharyngeal space infection (including Ludwig angina)	Often polymicrobial and include streptococcal species, anaerobes, and *Eikenella corrodens*	Clindamycin 600–900 mg intravenously every 8 hours, or a combination of penicillin and metronidazole	External drainage is sometimes necessary.
Jugular vein septic phlebitis (Lemierre disease)	*F necrophorum*	Clindamycin, or a combination of penicillin and metronidazole	Surgical drainage of the lateral pharyngeal space and ligation of the internal jugular vein may be performed as well.
Laryngitis	Viral (> 90% of cases)	Antibiotics are not usually indicated	
Sialadenitis	*S aureus*	Antistaphylococcal intravenous antibiotics such as nafcillin 2 g every 4 hours	
Acute cervical lymphadenitis	*Bartonella henselae* (cat-scratch disease), Group A streptococcus, *S aureus*, anaerobes, *M tuberculosis* (scrofula), *M avium*, toxoplasmosis, and tularemia	Depends on the specific diagnosis after fine-needle aspiration is performed	

Clinical Uses

These agents are used primarily for their activity against many strains of *Pseudomonas*. They also have better enterococcal coverage compared with penicillin, with piperacillin having better activity than ticarcillin.

5. Penicillins Combined with β-Lactamase Inhibitors

The addition of β-lactamase inhibitors to aminopenicillins and antipseudomonal penicillins can prevent inactivation by bacterial β-lactamases. These agents inactivate β-lactamases produced by *S aureus, H influenzae, Moraxella catarrhalis,* and *Bacteroides fragilis,* extending the activity of the parent drug to include these organisms. Augmentin (amoxicillin and clavulanic acid) is given orally. Unasyn (ampicillin and sulbactam), Zosyn (piperacillin and tazobactam), and Timentin (ticarcillin and clavulanic acid) are administered intravenously.

Adverse Effects

Augmentin is associated with some gastrointestinal intolerance, particularly diarrhea, which is decreased if administered twice a day.

Clinical Uses

Augmentin is used clinically for the treatment of refractory cases of sinusitis and otitis media that have not responded to less costly agents and may be due to anaerobes or *S aureus*. Unasyn, Zosyn, and Timentin are used as general broad-spectrum agents, with Zosyn having the most broad-spectrum activity. They are not active against methicillin-resistant *S aureus* and atypical organisms such as chlamydia and mycoplasma. Unasyn has no activity against *Pseudomonas*.

6. Other β-Lactam Drugs

Other β-lactam drugs include monobactams (aztreonam [Azactam]), and carbapenems (imipenem [Primaxin], meropenem [Merrem], and ertapenem [Invanz]). Monobactams have activity limited to gram-negative organisms, including *Pseudomonas*. Carbapenems have a wider spectrum. Imipenem is a broad-spectrum antibiotic and covers most gram-negative organisms, gram-positive organisms, and anaerobes, with the exception of *Stenotrophomonas maltophilia, Enterococcus faecium,* and most methicillin-resistant *S aureus* and *S epidermidis*. Meropenem has a similar spectrum of activity. Ertapenem, the most recent of the class, has a more narrow spectrum of activity, with no coverage against *Pseudomonas, Acinetobacter,* or *E faecalis*.

Adverse Effects

Despite the structural similarity of aztreonam to penicillin, cross-reactivity is limited and the drug can be given to those with a history of penicillin allergy, including IgE-mediated reactions. Patients allergic to penicillins may be allergic to imipenem and meropenem. Imipenem is associated with seizures, particularly if used in higher doses in elderly patients with decreased renal function, cerebrovascular disease, or seizure disorders. Meropenem is less likely to cause seizures and is associated with less nausea and vomiting than imipenem.

Clinical Uses

Aztreonam is useful for the treatment of confirmed pseudomonal infections in patients with allergies to penicillin and cephalosporins. Imipenem and meropenem should not be routinely used as a first-line therapy unless treating known multidrug-resistant organisms that are sensitive to these agents. However, in an appropriate patient who has been hospitalized for a prolonged period and who may experience infection with organisms resistant to multiple drugs, imipenem or meropenem may be used while awaiting culture results.

CEPHALOSPORINS

1. First-Generation Cephalosporins

These agents generally have good activity against aerobic gram-positive organisms (group A streptococcus, methicillin-sensitive *S aureus,* and viridans streptococci) and some community-acquired gram-negative organisms (*P mirabilis, E coli,* and the *Klebsiella* species). Agents in this class include the orally administered cephalexin (eg, Keflex) and the parenteral cefazolin (eg, Ancef).

Adverse Effects

In general, cephalosporins are safe. However, patients with a history of IgE-mediated allergy to a penicillin (eg, anaphylaxis) should not be administered a cephalosporin. Patients with a history of developing a maculopapular rash in response to penicillins have a 5–10% risk of a similar rash with cephalosporins.

Clinical Uses

Oral first-generation cephalosporins are commonly used for the treatment of minor staphylococcal infections such as in cellulitis. Intravenous first-generation cephalosporins are the drugs of choice for surgical prophylaxis in head and neck surgery if oral or pharyngeal mucosa is involved, such as in laryngeal tumor resection.

2. Second-Generation Cephalosporins

This is a heterogeneous group that includes cefuroxime (Zinacef). In general, they provide slightly more gram-negative coverage than the first-generation cephalosporins, including activity against indole-positive *Proteus*, *Klebsiella*, *M catarrhalis*, and the *Neisseria* species. They have slightly less gram-positive activity than the first-generation cephalosporins.

Clinical Uses

In patients with a mild allergy to ampicillin or amoxicillin, cefuroxime is an alternative agent for the treatment of sinusitis and otitis because it has activity against β-lactamase-producing strains such as *H influenzae* and *M catarrhalis*.

3. Third-Generation Cephalosporins

Examples of these agents include orally administered cefixime (Suprax), cefpodoxime (Vantin), and intravenously or intramuscularly administered ceftazidime (Fortaz), ceftriaxone (Rocephin), and cefotaxime. In general, these agents are less active against gram-positive organisms including *S aureus*, but most streptococci are inhibited. Of these, ceftriaxone has the most reliable pneumococcal coverage. They all have expanded gram-negative coverage. Ceftazidime has good activity against *Pseudomonas aeruginosa*. Ceftriaxone is the first-line agent for gonorrhea. Cefixime and cefpodoxime are oral alternatives.

Adverse Effects

Ceftriaxone is associated with a dose-dependent gallbladder sludging (which can be seen by ultrasound imaging) and pseudo-cholelithiasis; both of these disorders can be found particularly in patients who are not eating and who are receiving total parenteral nutrition.

Clinical Uses

Because of their penetration into cerebrospinal fluid, third-generation cephalosporins are widely used to treat meningitis. Ceftriaxone can be used to treat meningitis caused by susceptible pneumococci, meningococci, *H influenzae*, and enteric gram-negative rods. Ceftazidime is used for meningitis caused by the *Pseudomonas* species. Ceftriaxone, cefpodoxime, and cefixime are used for the treatment of gonorrhea, including pharyngeal disease.

4. Fourth-Generation Cephalosporins

Cefepime (Maxipime) is currently the only available fourth-generation cephalosporin. It has activity against *Enterobacter*, *Citrobacter*, and *Pseudomonas* species and similar activity to ceftriaxone against gram-positive organisms.

Clinical Uses

Cefepime is typically used for gram-negative organisms resistant to other cephalosporins, such as *Enterobacter* and *Citrobacter*. It is also used empirically in patients with febrile neutropenia.

QUINOLONES

This class has a broad spectrum of activity and generally low toxicity. Quinolones include the newer fluorinated agents such as ciprofloxacin (Cipro), levofloxacin (Levaquin), gatifloxacin (Tequin), gemifloxacin (Factive), and moxifloxacin (Avelox). The drugs inhibit bacterial DNA synthesis by blocking the action of the enzyme DNA gyrase. In general, quinolones have moderate gram-positive activity, especially levofloxacin, gatifloxacin, gemifloxacin, and moxifloxacin, and good gram-negative activity, with ciprofloxacin and levofloxacin providing the best activity against *P aeruginosa*, although resistance has been increasing. Only moxifloxacin has significant anaerobic activity (eg, *Bacteroides fragilis* and oral anaerobes).

Adverse Effects

The most commonly reported side effects are nausea, vomiting, and diarrhea. The prolongation of the QT interval has been observed in fluoroquinolones as a class. Tendonitis and tendon rupture have been reported, particularly in patients taking glucocorticoids or who have concomitant liver or renal failure. There is also a possible adverse effect on joint cartilage, which has been noted only in animal studies. Gatifloxacin has been linked to the development of both hypoglycemia and hyperglycemia requiring treatment.

Clinical Uses

Because of their broad spectrum, quinolones should not be typically used as first-line agents in relatively minor infections such as sinusitis, otitis, and pharyngitis when there are less expensive alternatives with narrower spectrums available. Although the increasing prevalence of fluoroquinolone-resistant *Neisseria gonorrhoeae* has limited their use in some areas of the United States and the rest of the world, a single dose of ciprofloxacin (500 mg) can be used to treat gonorrhea, including gonococcal pharyngitis. Ciprofloxacin has been used for the treatment of complicated soft tissue infections and osteomyelitis caused by gram-negative organisms. Ciprofloxacin, administered as 500–750 mg twice daily for at least 6 weeks, is used for the treatment of malignant external otitis. Ciprofloxacin has also been used to eradicate meningococci from the nasopharynx of carriers. Because of their superior activity against *Pneumococcus*, some of the newer quinolones such as levofloxacin can be used when drug-resistant *S pneumoniae* is suspected in cases of sinusitis. However, quinolones are not reliable in the treatment of methicillin-resistant *S aureus* infections.

SULFONAMIDES & ANTIFOLATE DRUGS

Sulfonamides are structural analogs of *p*-aminobenzoic acid (PABA) and compete with PABA to block its conversion to dihydrofolic acid. Almost all bacteria, with the exception of enterococci, that use PABA to synthesize folates and pyrimidines are inhibited by these agents. Mammalian cells use exogenous folate and are unaffected. Antifolate drugs such as trimethoprim block the conversion of dihydrofolic acid to tetrahydrofolic acid by inhibiting the enzyme dihydrofolate reductase. Typically, these agents are used in combination, such as trimethoprim-sulfamethoxazole (eg, Bactrim, Septra) to treat a variety of bacterial and parasitic infections.

Adverse Effects

At high doses, some of the antifolate drugs also inhibit mammalian dihydrofolate reductase (pyrimethamine and trimetrexate) so that these drugs are typically coadministered with folinic acid (leucovorin) to prevent bone marrow suppression. Adverse effects to sulfonamides, usually mild rashes or gastrointestinal disturbances, occur in 10–15% of patients without AIDS; in patients with AIDS, these adverse effects are experienced in up to 50% of patients and include rash, fever, neutropenia, and thrombocytopenia, all of which may be severe enough to discontinue therapy.

Clinical Uses

Sulfonamides are the drugs of choice for infections caused by *Nocardia*. Trimethoprim-sulfamethoxazole (Bactrim, Septra) is often used for the treatment of acute sinusitis and otitis, although resistant *Pneumococcus* is limiting its use.

ERYTHROMYCINS (MACROLIDES)

This class includes erythromycin, azithromycin (Zithromax), and clarithromycin (Biaxin). They inhibit protein synthesis of bacteria by binding to the 50S ribosomal subunits. In vitro data demonstrating an effect on cytokine production suggests an anti-inflammatory effect as well.

Adverse Effects

Nausea, vomiting, and diarrhea may occur, particularly with erythromycin, which can cause uncoordinated peristalsis. Azithromycin and clarithromycin cause milder symptoms. Reversible ototoxicity can occur after high doses of these agents, especially with concomitant hepatic and renal insufficiency. Macrolides (especially erythromycin and clarithromycin) inhibit cytochrome P450 and can significantly increase levels of oral anticoagulants, digoxin, cyclosporin, and theophylline with concomitant use. Levels should be monitored and doses appropriately adjusted.

Clinical Uses

Macrolides are the drugs of choice for infections caused by *Legionella*, *Mycoplasma*, and *Chlamydia*. Azithromycin and clarithromycin are approved for the treatment of streptococcal pharyngitis, but some areas are reporting high rates (20%) of resistance, and less expensive alternatives are available. Azithromycin and clarithromycin are frequently used to treat sinusitis, although amoxicillin and doxycycline are equally efficacious and less expensive.

KETOLIDES

Ketolides such as telithromycin (Ketek) are derivatives of the macrolides, but they have activity against macrolide-resistant and penicillin-resistant *S pneumoniae*. They inhibit bacterial protein synthesis by binding to two sites on the 50S bacterial ribosome. They do not have significant gram-negative activity.

Adverse Effects

Upper gastrointestinal symptoms are the most common drug-associated effect. Other potential effects include blurred vision, resulting from reversible alteration in accommodation (seen in young women in particular). There have been three reports of severe liver toxicity (one death and one requiring transplantation). Telithromycin is a potent inhibitor of cytochrome P450 and can significantly increase levels of several drugs such as warfarin and benzodiazepines. Statins should be temporarily stopped while patients are taking telithromycin.

Clinical Uses

Telithromycin is an alternative to quinolones for community-acquired pneumonia in which resistant *S pneumoniae* is suspected. However, patients should be carefully monitored for liver toxicity. Telithromycin is no longer recommended for the treatment of acute bacterial sinusitis given the risk of severe hepatotoxicity.

TETRACYCLINES

Doxycycline and other drugs in this class inhibit protein synthesis. Their spectrum of activity is similar to that of macrolides.

Adverse Effects

Gastrointestinal side effects are common. Drugs in this class can be bound to calcium in growing bones and teeth, causing discoloration and growth inhibition.

Clinical Uses

Similar to the macrolides, tetracyclines can be used to treat infections caused by *Legionella*, *Mycoplasma*, and *Chlamydia*.

GLYCYLCYCLINES

Tigecycline (Tygacil), a derivative of minocycline, is the first of this new class of antibiotics. The spectrum of activity includes resistant gram-positive organisms (eg, methicillin-resistant *S aureus*, penicillin-resistant *S pneumoniae*, and vancomycin-resistant enterococci) as well as several gram-negative organisms and anaerobes, but not *P aeruginosa*.

Adverse Effects

Nausea and vomiting are the most commonly reported effects reported with glycylcyclines. Like tetracyclines, tigecycline may also cause photosensitivity and pseudotumor cerebri. Its use is contraindicated in children and pregnant women.

Clinical Uses

These agents constitute another intravenously administered option against complicated skin and soft tissue infections with resistant gram-positive organisms.

AMINOGLYCOSIDES

This group includes gentamicin and tobramycin. They inhibit protein synthesis in bacteria by attaching to the 30S ribosomal subunit.

Adverse Effects

All aminoglycosides can cause ototoxicity and nephrotoxicity. Ototoxicity can be irreversible and is cumulative. It can be manifested both as cochlear injury (eg, hearing loss) and vestibular injury (eg, vertigo and ataxia). Nephrotoxicity is more common and is frequently reversible.

Clinical Uses

These agents are generally used in serious infections caused by gram-negative bacteria. Their use is limited by toxicity.

CLINDAMYCIN

Clindamycin (Cleocin) acts by inhibiting the initiation of peptide chain synthesis in bacteria. It resembles the macrolides in its spectrum and structure.

Adverse Effects

These drugs are the most frequently implicated in causing *Clostridium difficile* colitis.

Clinical Uses

Clindamycin is one of the first-line drugs for the treatment of parapharyngeal space infections (including Ludwig angina), as well as jugular vein septic phlebitis (eg, Lemierre disease). It is recommended as an alternative to amoxicillin as prophylaxis against endocarditis following oral procedures. Clindamycin has good anaerobic activity, but resistance has been reported in up to 25% of *B fragilis* isolates, thus limiting its use in serious anaerobic infections due to these organisms. Because of existing evidence suggesting that clindamycin reduces toxin production in several organisms, it is often used concomitantly with penicillin in the treatment of group A streptococcal toxic shock syndrome. Clindamycin can also be used in the treatment of brain abscesses, although it is not effective in treating meningitis.

METRONIDAZOLE

Metronidazole (Flagyl) is an antiprotozoal drug that has excellent anaerobic activity, particularly against anaerobic gram-negative organisms.

Adverse Effects

Alcohol must be avoided for the duration of the antibiotic and for 48 hours afterward to prevent a disulfiram-like reaction. Metronidazole can also decrease the metabolism of warfarin and increase the prothrombin time, necessitating careful monitoring during concomitant use.

Clinical Uses

This agent can be used in the treatment of brain abscesses, parapharyngeal space infections (including Ludwig angina), as well as septic phlebitis of the jugular vein (Lemierre disease), in combination with either penicillin or a third-generation cephalosporin. It is more predictable than clindamycin and second-generation cephalosporins in the treatment of *B fragilis* infections.

VANCOMYCIN

Vancomycin activity is limited to gram-positive organisms, and it is used as a bactericidal for most of these organisms, including staphylococci and streptococci.

Vancomycin-resistant enterococcal strains have become a major problem.

Adverse Effects

This agent is rarely ototoxic when given with aminoglycosides. There is also potential nephrotoxicity when coadministered with aminoglycosides. The rapid infusion of vancomycin can result in diffuse hyperemia ("red man syndrome").

Clinical Uses

Vancomycin is the drug of choice for methicillin-resistant *S aureus* and *S epidermidis*. Serious staphylococcal, enterococcal, and other gram-positive infections in patients allergic to penicillin can also be treated with vancomycin.

STREPTOGRAMINS

These agents are structurally similar to macrolides. They work by binding to bacterial ribosomes and include Synercid (a combination of quinupristin and dalfopristin). Synercid has a spectrum of activity primarily against gram-positive organisms, including *E faecium* (but not *E faecalis*) and methicillin-resistant *S aureus*.

Adverse Effects

Phlebitis occurs with peripheral administration, so a central line is recommended. The most common adverse effects are myalgias and arthralgias.

Clinical Uses

Streptogramins are rarely used and only in cases of serious infections secondary to vancomycin-resistant *E faecium*.

OXAZOLIDINONES

Linezolid (Zyvox) is the first agent of this class of antibiotics. It is active against aerobic gram-positive infections, including *E faecium, E faecalis,* and methicillin-resistant *S aureus* and *S epidermidis*.

Adverse Effects

Nausea, vomiting, and diarrhea are the most common adverse effects. Reversible thrombocytopenia, neutropenia, and anemia can occur if treatment is prolonged. If more than 2 weeks of treatment are planned, blood counts should be monitored.

Clinical Uses

These agents are used in cases of serious infections secondary to vancomycin-resistant *E faecium* and *E faecalis,* and in patients with methicillin-resistant *S aureus* infections who are intolerant to vancomycin.

DAPTOMYCIN

This bactericidal lipopeptide works by inserting itself into the bacterial cell membrane, causing depolarization, efflux of potassium, and cell death. Its spectrum of activity is similar to that of linezolid, targeting resistant gram-positive organisms (eg, methicillin-resistant *S aureus* and vancomycin-resistant enterococci). It is available only as a parenteral agent.

Adverse Effects

The main potential drug-related effect is reversible, dose-dependent myopathy, which is seen more than 7 days after initiating therapy.

Clinical Uses

Daptomycin is used in complicated skin and soft tissue infections with known or suspected resistant gram-positive organisms.

■ ANTIFUNGAL AGENTS

AMPHOTERICIN B

Amphotericin B has a broad spectrum of activity against many fungi that can cause systemic disease, such as *Aspergillus, Histoplasmosis, Coccidioides,* and *Candida*. Notable exceptions are *Pseudallescheria boydii* and *Fusarium*. Lipid-based amphotericin B products, such as amphotericin B lipid complex, amphotericin B colloidal dispersion, and liposomal amphotericin B, have less nephrotoxicity than amphotericin.

Adverse Effects

Amphotericin B often produces fever, chills, vomiting, and headaches. Premedication with acetaminophen and diphenhydramine may help, and the addition of 25 mg of hydrocortisone to the infusion may decrease the incidence of rigors. Nephrotoxicity and electrolyte disturbances are common side effects, and close monitoring is essential.

Clinical Uses

In immunocompromised patients, this agent is used as an initial therapy for sinus disease or other invasive disease caused by *Aspergillus*, Zygomycetes, and other molds. Amphotericin is sometimes used in the treatment of resistant thrush.

TRIAZOLES

These drugs inhibit ergosterol synthesis, resulting in inhibition of membrane-associated enzyme activity and cell wall growth and replication. Fluconazole (Diflucan) can be effective in treating infections due to *Candida* (albicans in particular), *Cryptococcus*, and *Blastomyces*. Itraconazole (Sporanox) has a similar spectrum to fluconazole, but may also be used to treat invasive disease caused by *Aspergillus*. There is no activity against *Fusarium* and zygomycetes. Newer-generation azoles such as voriconazole (Vfend) have a broader spectrum of activity, including *Aspergillus* and *Fusarium*, but not Zygomycetes. Posaconazole has a similar spectrum of activity as voriconazole, but can also be used to treat Zygomycetes.

Adverse Effects

Triazoles are generally well tolerated. Itraconazole and voriconazole have several drug interactions. Itraconazole can increase levels of cyclosporin, digoxin, and warfarin with concomitant use, necessitating the dose adjustment of these medications. Voriconazole is a potent inhibitor of cytochrome P450 isoenzymes, also mandating the dose adjustment and monitoring of cyclosporin and warfarin, as well as tacrolimus. Sirolimus is contraindicated. The most common adverse effects associated with voriconazole were reversible visual disturbances and liver toxicity.

Clinical Uses

Itraconazole, voriconazole, and posaconazole can be used in the treatment of sinus disease caused by *Aspergillus*. Voriconazole can also be used in disease caused by *Fusarium*. Fluconazole is typically a first-line treatment of thrush. Itraconazole and voriconazole also have activity against *Candida*, including some of the non-albicans species. Posaconazole is an alternative amphotericin for the treatment of Zygomycetes.

CANDINS

These drugs act by inhibiting fungal wall synthesis. Caspofungin (Cancidas), micafungin (Mycamine), and anidulafungin (Eraxis) are FDA-cleared agents in this class. They are active against *Candida*, including non-albicans species, and *Aspergillus*. They are not active against the other molds.

Adverse Effects

Candins are remarkably well-tolerated drugs and are associated with few significant drug interactions.

Clinical Uses

These drugs are recommended for patients intolerant of or refractory to treatment of *Aspergillus* disease with amphotericin or itraconazole.

■ ANTIVIRAL AGENTS

ACYCLOVIR, FAMCICLOVIR, & VALACYCLOVIR

In cells infected with herpes virus, these drugs are selectively active against viral DNA polymerase, inhibiting viral proliferation. They are useful for infections caused by herpes simplex and in herpes zoster-varicella infections. Famciclovir (Famvir) is selectively active against herpes DNA polymerase and inhibits viral proliferation. It is a prodrug of penciclovir. Herpes simplex and varicella zoster strains resistant to acyclovir are also resistant to famciclovir. Valacyclovir (Valtrex) is the prodrug of acyclovir and has increased oral bioavailability, allowing less frequent dosing.

Adverse Effects

These drugs are relatively nontoxic.

Clinical Uses

Antiviral agents are used for the treatment and prophylaxis of mucocutaneous oral lesions caused by herpes simplex. Oral acyclovir is significantly more effective than the currently available topical ointment, 5% acyclovir. Penciclovir 1% cream is effective but must be applied every 2 hours to work.

Radiology

Nancy J. Fischbein, MD, & Kenneth C. Ong, MD

◼ DIAGNOSTIC IMAGING TECHNIQUES

Diagnostic imaging is an essential element in the evaluation of many otolaryngologic problems. Computed tomography (CT) and magnetic resonance imaging (MRI) are the most commonly used imaging modalities, with positron emission tomography (PET) playing an ever-increasing role.

COMPUTED TOMOGRAPHY

CT scanning uses ionizing radiation to generate cross-sectional images based on differences in the x-ray attenuation of various tissues. Modern scanners are typically helical, meaning that x-ray source rotation and patient translation occur simultaneously; this results in the acquisition of a "volume" of data that is then partitioned and reconstructed into individual slices. Helical scanning is significantly faster than traditional slice-by-slice acquisition, thereby diminishing artifacts related to motion (eg, breathing, swallowing, and gross patient motion). The rapid data acquisition also allows for more and thinner slices to be obtained, which facilitates diagnosis by decreasing partial-volume averaging effects and allows for improved quality of multiplanar reconstructions. The most recent advance in CT imaging has been the introduction of "multislice" scanners. Multislice scanners have a variable number of parallel arcs of detectors that are capable of simultaneously acquiring volumes of data. The increased speed that results from multislice sampling can be traded for improved longitudinal resolution, an increased volume of coverage, or an improved signal-to-noise ratio.

CT scanning of the head and neck is ideally performed with thin sections, usually ≤ 3 mm, in the axial plane. Direct coronal imaging or coronal reformations are useful in some situations, notably in imaging of the paranasal sinuses and the skull base. CT scanning of the neck is usually performed following injection of iodinated contrast material because opacification of vessels helps to separate them from other structures such as lymph nodes and also helps to delineate and character-

ize pathology. If bony anatomy is the focus of the imaging study, as in imaging of the paranasal sinuses or temporal bones, then intravenous contrast material is not required.

MAGNETIC RESONANCE IMAGING

MRI exploits differences in tissue relaxation characteristics and spin density to produce an image that is exquisitely sensitive to soft tissue contrast. Depending on the parameters that are selected, variable tissue characteristics and contrast are produced. At least two different types of sequences in two planes are generally necessary to characterize lesions of the head and neck. The slice thickness should be no more than 5 mm. A gadolinium-based contrast agent is generally used to enhance the detection of pathology and improve tissue characterization, and also to aid in the generation of a differential diagnosis. In some circumstances, thinner sections covering a smaller anatomic area may be necessary for more precise diagnosis.

In the head and neck, the following imaging sequences are typically obtained: (1) sagittal, axial, and coronal T1-weighted images; (2) axial fast spin-echo T2-weighted images with fat saturation; and (3) axial and coronal postgadolinium T1-weighted images with fat saturation.

Additional planes may be useful in some circumstances, such as coronal fast spin-echo T2-weighted images with fat saturation for the assessment of paranasal sinus and anterior skull base pathology. Additional sequences such as magnetic resonance angiography (MRA) may be useful in certain circumstances (eg, paragangliomas and dural fistulas), but are not necessary for evaluating most processes of the head and neck. MR venography may be useful in the assessment of patients with pulsatile tinnitus and in the assessment of the patency of the sigmoid sinus in patients with adjacent neoplastic or inflammatory disorders. Advanced modalities in widespread use in the brain (eg, MR spectroscopy, diffusion-weighted imaging, functional MR imaging) have for the most part not found a place in routine head and neck imaging, with the exception of diffusion-weighted imaging in the evaluation of epidermoid cysts and cholesteatomas.

On a T1-weighted image, fat is bright and fluid (eg, cerebrospinal fluid [CSF]) is relatively dark. Muscle and

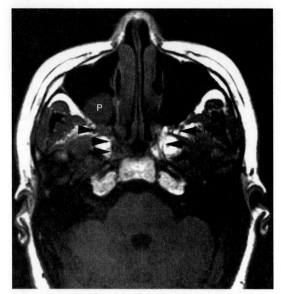

Figure 3–1. Axial T1-weighted image. Note the high signal intensity of subcutaneous fat and the marrow of the central skull base. Infiltrative neoplasm replaces normal fat in the right pterygopalatine fossa, the vidian canal, and portions of the sphenoid body (black arrowheads). The normal left pterygopalatine fossa (PPF) and vidian canal (VC) are indicated. A maxillary sinus polyp (P) is incidentally noted.

most pathologies are of intermediate signal intensity. The large amount of fat in the head and neck provides intrinsic tissue contrast, which makes the T1-weighted image very sensitive to infiltrative processes that obliterate tissue planes or that replace marrow fat (Figure 3–1). Some hemorrhagic or proteinaceous lesions cause shortening of T1 relaxation time and appear bright on a T1-weighted image. On a T2-weighted image, fluid is very bright and most pathologies are relatively bright, whereas normal muscle is quite dark. The fast spin-echo technique is very useful in limiting artifacts related to motion and magnetic susceptibility compared with conventional spin-echo T2-weighted imaging. Because fat remains bright on a fast spin-echo image, however, fat saturation should ideally be applied. In the nasal cavity and paranasal sinuses, T2-weighted images are particularly useful in distinguishing neoplastic masses from polyps, thickened mucosa, and retained secretions (Figure 3–2). Gadolinium is very useful for demonstrating pathology and tailoring a differential diagnosis based on enhancement characteristics. In a patient with head and neck cancer, postgadolinium imaging is also very useful in assessing cavernous sinus invasion, meningeal infiltration, and perineural spread of tumor (Figure 3–3). Fat saturation should ideally be applied on a postgadolinium T1-weighted image; other-

wise, the contrast between an enhancing lesion and the high signal intensity of surrounding fat may actually be reduced compared with the pregadolinium image. Because low-field scanners often do not have fat saturation capability, high-field imaging (1.5 T) is generally preferred for assessing the head and neck and skull base. If a patient is severely claustrophobic, sedation may be necessary to accomplish the scan on a high-field system.

It should be kept in mind that MRI requires more time and more patient cooperation than does CT, and therefore it is not necessarily suitable for acutely ill or uncooperative patients. In addition, there are certain absolute contraindications to MRI, including ferromagnetic intracranial aneurysm clips, cardiac pacemakers, and many cochlear implants. Therefore, patients must be carefully screened for these and other contraindications before undergoing MRI.

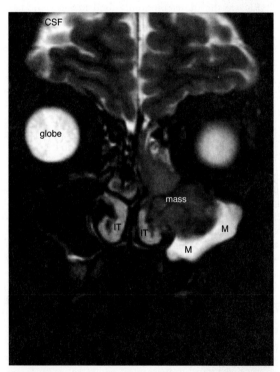

Figure 3–2. Coronal fast spin-echo T2-weighted image with fat saturation (FS). Note the high signal intensity of the vitreous humor of the ocular globe, the high signal intensity of the CSF, and the lack of signal from subcutaneous fat. In this patient with squamous cell carcinoma, the intermediate signal intensity tumor (mass) stands in contrast to the very high signal intensity of edematous mucosa and retained secretions (M) in the left maxillary sinus and the mildly high signal intensity of the inferior turbinates (IT).

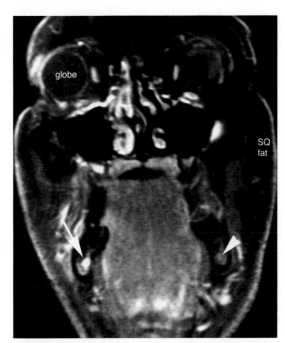

Figure 3–3. Coronal T1-weighted image, postgadolinium, with fat saturation. Note the vitreous humor is dark as in a T1-weighted image, but subcutaneous and orbital fat are also dark due to fat suppression. The high signal intensity of the nasal mucosa, as well as the enhancement of vessels and extraocular muscles, indicates that gadolinium has been given. In this patient with a history of squamous cell carcinoma of the gingivobuccal sulcus and new chin numbness, the abnormal enlargement and enhancement of V3 in the inferior alveolar canal is seen (white arrow), consistent with perineural spread of tumor. The contralateral normal canal is also indicated (white arrowhead).

POSITRON EMISSION TOMOGRAPHY

PET provides a functional view of tissues rather than simply depicting anatomy. In the head and neck, it is used primarily for oncologic diagnosis and evaluation and is performed with the radiopharmaceutical ^{18}F-fluorodeoxyglucose (FDG). FDG is taken up into tissues in proportion to the glycolytic rate, which is generally increased in neoplastic processes. Focal asymmetric uptake is suggestive of a tumor but is nonspecific, since FDG is also concentrated in areas of inflammation. FDG PET scanning is particularly helpful in the following situations: (1) the search for an unknown primary lesion in a patient presenting with metastatic neck disease (Figure 3–4), (2) the assessment of residual or recurrent disease after primary therapy, and (3) the search for synchronous or metachro-

nous primary lesions or distant metastases. FDG PET scanning can also be useful for staging the neck, but there may be a significant number of false-negative studies in patients with clinically N0 necks because small tumor deposits (approximately 1–3 mm) are generally not detectable on an FDG PET scan. These small tumor deposits are found if a neck dissection is performed. At present, most FDG PET scanning is done on dedicated PET-CT scanners, such that precise anatomic localization of FDG uptake can be achieved.

AAssar OS, Fischbein NJ, Caputo GR et al. Metastatic head and neck cancer: role and usefulness of FDG PET in locating occult primary tumors. *Radiology.* 1999;210:177. [PMID: 9885604] (FDG PET allows for the effective localization of the unknown primary site of origin in many cases of metastatic head and neck cancer and can contribute substantially to patient care.)

Anzai Y, Carroll WR, Quint DJ et al. Recurrence of head and neck cancer after surgery or irradiation: prospective comparison of 2-deoxy-2-[F-18]fluoro-D-glucose PET and MR imaging diagnoses. *Radiology.* 1996;200:135. [PMID: 8657901] (An early study demonstrating that PET metabolic imaging, compared with anatomic methods, has improved diagnostic accuracy for recurrent head and neck cancer.)

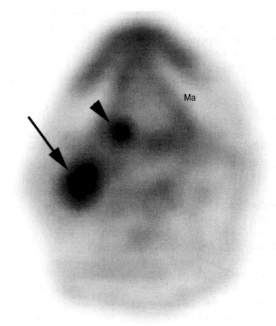

Figure 3–4. Axial FDG PET image in a patient presenting with metastatic cervical adenopathy and no primary site visible on clinical examination or MRI. A large focus of activity (black arrow) is related to known level II lymphadenopathy, and a smaller focus of activity (black arrowhead) is suspicious for a primary site at the right base of the tongue. This was confirmed by panendoscopy and biopsy. The photopenic mandible (Ma) is indicated for orientation.

Blodgett TM, Fukui MB, Snyderman CH et al. Combined PET-CT in the head and neck: Part 1. Physiologic, altered physiologic, and artifactual FDG uptake. *Radiographics.* 2005;25(4):897. [PMID: 16009814] (Combined PET-computed tomography (CT) is a unique imaging modality that permits anatomic and functional imaging on a single scanner with nearly perfect coregistration. Physiologic and artifactual uptake is reviewed.)

Fukui MB, Blodgett TM, Snyderman CH et al. Combined PET-CT in the head and neck: Part 2. Diagnostic uses and pitfalls of oncologic imaging. *Radiographics.* 2005;25:913. [PMID: 16009815] (Combined PET-CT helps prevent the misinterpretation of FDG PET findings in patients with head and neck cancer. Superior localization of FDG uptake with this technique can improve diagnostic accuracy and help avoid interpretative pitfalls.)

Hendrick RE. The AAPM/RSNA physics tutorial for residents. Basic physics of MR imaging: an introduction. *Radiographics.* 1994;14(4):829. [PMID: 7938771] (An introduction to the basic physics of MRI.)

Kanal E, Borgstede JP, Barkovich AJ et al. American College of Radiology White Paper on MR Safety. *AJR Am J Roentgenol.* 2002;178:1335. [PMID: 12034593] (A current update on MRI safety considerations.)

Mahesh M. The AAPM/RSNA Physics Tutorial for Residents: Search for Isotropic Resolution in CT from Conventional through Multiple-Row Detector. *Radiographics.* 2002;22:949. [PMID: 12110725] (An overview of the physics of CT scanning, with an emphasis on current technology.)

Plewes DB. The AAPM/RSNA physics tutorial for residents. Contrast mechanisms in spin-echo MR imaging. *Radiographics.* 1994;14(6):1389. [PMID: 7855348] (An introduction to the basic MR imaging sequences.)

Saloner D. The AAPM/RSNA physics tutorial for residents. An introduction to MR angiography. *Radiographics.* 1995;15(2):453. [PMID: 7761648] (A discussion of the basic principles and applications of MRA.)

▎IMAGING THE HEAD & NECK

SPATIAL ANATOMY OF THE HEAD & NECK

The spaces of the suprahyoid head and neck are defined by the three layers of the deep cervical fascia: the superficial, middle, and deep layers. The spaces so defined include the pharyngeal mucosal space, the parapharyngeal space, the masticator space, the parotid space, the carotid space, the retropharyngeal space, and the perivertebral space. The infrahyoid neck has traditionally been clinically defined by a series of surgical triangles, but can also be described as a series of fascia-defined spaces, which facilitates the understanding and interpretation of cross-sectional imaging modalities such as CT and MRI.

The spaces of the infrahyoid neck are also defined by the three layers of the deep cervical fascia and include the superficial space (external to the superficial layer of the deep cervical fascia), the visceral space (including the thyroid gland,

the larynx, and the esophagus), the carotid space, the retropharyngeal space, and the perivertebral space. The nasal cavity, paranasal sinuses, skull base, and temporal bone are considered unique subregions of the head.

MUCOSAL DISEASE OF THE HEAD & NECK

For mucosal disease of the head and neck, of which squamous cell carcinoma (SCC) is by far the dominant lesion, the traditional subdivisions are the nasopharynx, oropharynx, oral cavity, larynx, and hypopharynx. The pharyngeal mucosal space includes the nasopharynx, oropharynx, and hypopharynx.

NASOPHARYNX

Anatomy

The nasopharynx is bounded anteriorly by the posterior nasal cavity at the posterior choana; posterosuperiorly by the lower clivus, upper cervical spine, and prevertebral muscles; and inferiorly by a horizontal line drawn along the hard and soft palates (Figure 3–5). The lateral wall of the nasopharynx is composed of the torus tubarius, the eustachian tube orifice, and the lateral pharyngeal recess, also known as the fossa of Rosenmüller (Figure 3–6). In addition to squamous mucosa, the contents of the nasopharynx include lymphoid tissue (adenoids), minor salivary glands, the pharyngobasilar fascia, and the pharyngeal constrictor muscles. The pharyngobasilar fascia represents the aponeurosis of the superior constrictor muscle and attaches it to the skull base. A gap in the upper margin of the pharyngobasilar fascia is known as the sinus of Morgagni. The distal eustachian tube and levator palatini muscle normally pass through this gap, which also serves as a potential route of spread for nasopharyngeal carcinoma to access the skull base.

Pathology

Lesions that may be encountered on imaging studies of the nasopharynx are listed in Table 3–1. Adenoidal hypertrophy (Figure 3–7) is commonly seen in children, young adults, and patients who test positive for the human immunodeficiency virus (HIV), although in the latter group, lymphoma must be considered in the differential diagnosis. Nasopharyngeal carcinoma is the most common malignant lesion of the nasopharynx, and the spectrum of imaging findings that may be encountered with nasopharyngeal carcinoma is illustrated in Figure 3–8. Important issues to consider in the imaging assessment of a patient with nasopharyngeal carcinoma include the presence of extension to the parapharyngeal space and pterygopalatine fossa, the presence of skull base invasion,

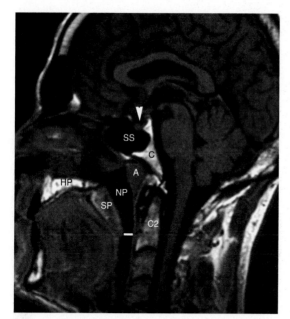

Figure 3–5. Midline sagittal T1-weighted image indicates the bony and soft tissue anatomy related to the nasopharynx (NP), with the approximate inferior margin of the nasopharynx indicated by the horizontal white line. Indicated are the adenoids (A), clivus (C), C2 vertebral body (C2), sphenoid sinus (SS), soft palate (SP), hard palate (HP), and pituitary gland in the sella turcica (white arrowhead).

and the presence of extension to the cranial nerves or the cavernous sinus.

Key Imaging Points

- The lateral pharyngeal recesses may be asymmetric owing to mucosal coaptation rather than a true mass lesion. This "pseudomass" can be diagnosed when the clinician or radiologist identifies the "kissing" mucosal surfaces rather than a true mass lesion (Figure 3–9).

Table 3–1. Common mass lesions of the nasopharynx.

Benign	Malignant
Adenoidal hypertrophy	Nasopharyngeal carcinoma
Postinflammatory retention cyst	Non-Hodgkin lymphoma
Thornwaldt cyst	Malignant tumor of minor salivary gland
Benign tumor of minor salivary gland	Rhabdomyosarcoma (in a child)

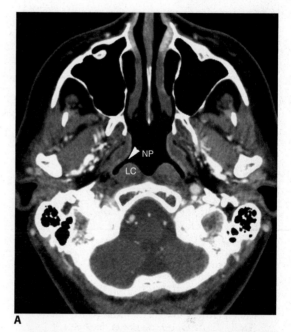

A

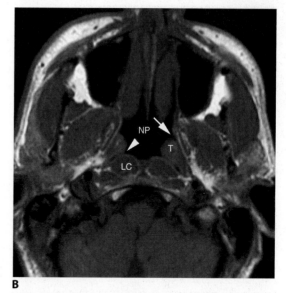

B

Figure 3–6. **(A)** Axial CT image demonstrates the nasopharyngeal airway and the lateral pharyngeal recess (white arrowhead), as well as the longus colli muscle (LC). **(B)** Axial T1-weighted image of the nasopharynx (NP) demonstrates the lateral pharyngeal recess (white arrowhead), torus tubarius (T), and eustachian tube opening (white arrow).

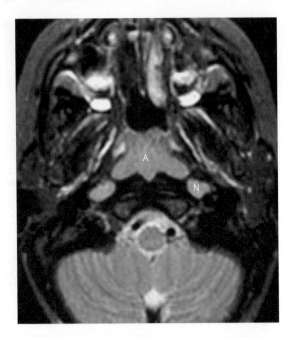

Figure 3–7. Axial T2-weighted image in a young child demonstrates prominent symmetrical hypertrophy of the adenoids (A) and prominent retropharyngeal lymph nodes (N). This degree of adenoidal enlargement is common in young children and adolescents.

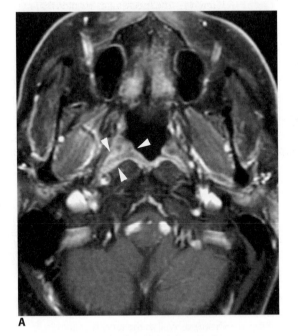

A

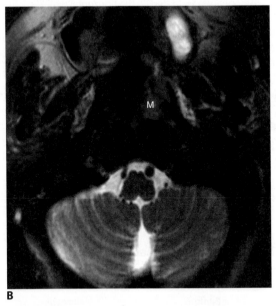

B

Figure 3–8. The spectrum of imaging findings in nasopharyngeal carcinoma (NPC). **(A)** Axial postgadolinium T1-weighted image with fat saturation demonstrates a small mass lesion (white arrowheads) filling the right fossa of Rosenmüller and outlined against adjacent soft tissues by the "white line" of the adjacent enhancing mucosa and mucosal venous plexus. This patient presented with a neck mass (not shown) that revealed poorly differentiated carcinoma on fine needle aspiration. **(B)** Axial fast spin-echo T2-weighted image with fat saturation in a 45-year-old Chinese woman with a complaint of left ear fullness demonstrates a mass (M) centered on the left fossa of Rosenmüller with extension both anteriorly and medially. *(Continued)*

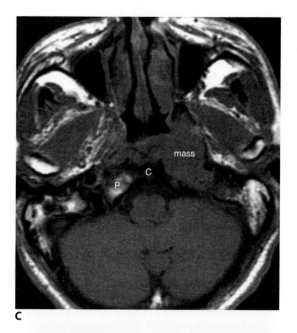

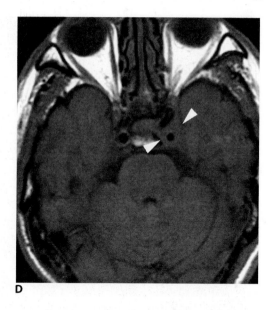

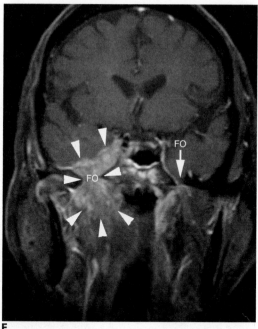

Figure 3–8 (Cont'd). The spectrum of imaging findings in nasopharyngeal carcinoma (NPC). **(C)** Axial T1-weighted image in an older Chinese man with headache, ear pain, and diplopia demonstrates a large mass centered on the left fossa of Rosenmüller, with effacement of adjacent fat planes, erosion of the left petrous bone (compare the normal petrous bone and fatty marrow shown on the right, P), and replacement of the normal high signal intensity marrow within the clivus, C. **(D)** A more superior image in the same patient shown in part C demonstrates asymmetry of the cavernous sinuses with increased soft tissue on the left (arrowheads), as well as a mild narrowing of the encased cavernous segment of the internal carotid artery, consistent with tumor extension into the cavernous sinus. **(E)** Coronal T1-weighted image postgadolinium with fat saturation in another Chinese patient with nasopharyngeal carcinoma and right facial numbness in a V3 distribution demonstrates both direct and perineural extension of tumor through a markedly widened right foramen ovale (FO) into the middle cranial fossa (arrowheads). The normal appearance of foramen ovale is demonstrated on the left (white arrow).

- The nasopharynx should be carefully scrutinized for a mass lesion obstructing the eustachian tube orifice in any adult patient with unilateral middle ear or mastoid fluid (Figure 3–10).

- Asymmetrically or unusually prominent nasopharyngeal soft tissue that is seen on an imaging study should prompt a clinical evaluation for neoplasm, especially lymphoma (particularly in the setting of HIV) or nasopharyngeal carcinoma (particularly if the patient is of southern Chinese descent) (Figure 3–11).

- Patients with nasopharyngeal carcinoma should undergo MRI rather than CT scanning for the most complete staging. In patients with nasopharyngeal carcinoma, the skull base should be carefully assessed

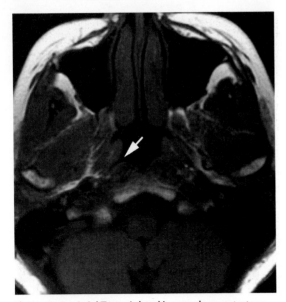

Figure 3–9. Axial T1-weighted image demonstrates a normal right fossa of Rosenmüller (white arrow). The left fossa is poorly seen, but no mass lesion is present, and the poor visualization is due to coaptation of mucosal surfaces and a lack of air in the fossa to provide contrast.

on a T1-weighted image for evidence of invasion, with particular attention to the clivus on a sagittal T1-weighted image. Postgadolinium, the cavernous sinuses and cranial nerves (notably V2 and V3) should be assessed for tumor involvement.

- Radiation necrosis of the temporal lobes may occur following high-dose radiation therapy for nasopharyngeal carcinoma, as may osteoradionecrosis of the skull base and cranial neuritis. These may mimic tumor recurrence on imaging studies (Figure 3–12).

- A patient with nasopharyngeal carcinoma may present with massive cervical lymphadenopathy yet a relatively small primary lesion. The nasopharynx should be carefully scrutinized in a patient presenting with noninfectious cervical lymphadenopathy, particularly when she or he is of southern Chinese descent.

OROPHARYNX

Anatomy

The oropharynx (Figure 3–13) is bounded anteriorly by the circumvallate papilla of the tongue, the soft palate, and the anterior tonsillar pillars, posteriorly by the superior and middle constrictor muscles, and superiorly by the soft palate. Inferiorly, it is separated from the lar-

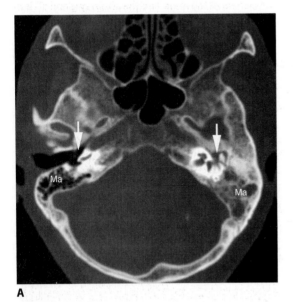

A

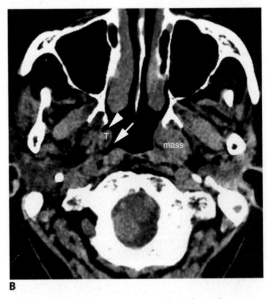

B

Figure 3–10. **(A)** Axial CT image viewed in bone window in an elderly woman presenting with unilateral serous otitis demonstrates fluid or soft tissue density in the left middle ear and mastoid. The right mastoid air cells are well pneumatized. Mastoid air cells are indicated by "Ma" and the middle ear cavities by the white arrows. **(B)** A more inferior axial noncontrast CT image viewed in a soft tissue window demonstrates a left submucosal nasopharyngeal mass that is obliterating normal anatomic landmarks. The right fossa of Rosenmüller (arrow), torus tubarius (T), and eustachian tube orifice (arrowhead) are shown for comparison. A biopsy of the lesion was suggestive of amyloidosis.

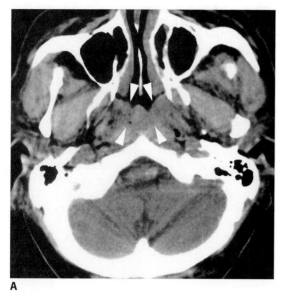
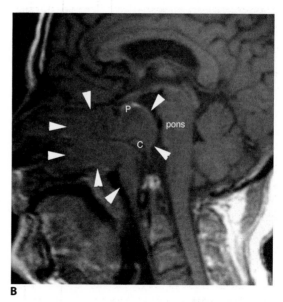

A   **B**

Figure 3–11. **(A)** Axial noncontrast CT image viewed in soft tissue window of elderly man of southern Chinese descent demonstrates abnormal fullness of the nasopharyngeal soft tissues for the patient's age (arrowheads). This was noted, but the patient was lost to clinical follow-up. **(B)** Sagittal T1-weighted image obtained 4 years later when the patient complained of nasal congestion, epistaxis, and deep pain demonstrates replacement of the clivus (C) and sphenoid sinus by a large soft tissue mass (arrowheads) that is extending anteriorly into the ethmoid sinus and nasal cavity. The pons is displaced posteriorly by a large extradural component of the mass, and the pituitary gland (P) is elevated. A biopsy was consistent with nasopharyngeal carcinoma.

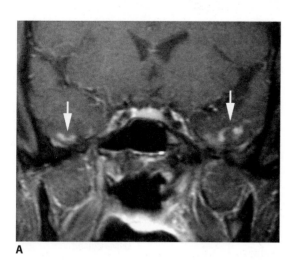
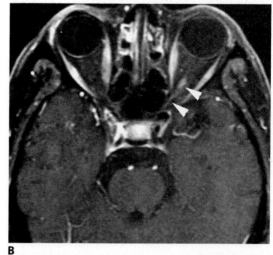

A   **B**

Figure 3–12. **(A)** Coronal postgadolinium T1-weighted image with fat saturation demonstrates irregular enhancement (white arrows) in the inferior temporal lobes bilaterally in a patient with a history of high-dose radiation therapy for nasopharyngeal carcinoma. This is a typical location and appearance of radionecrosis. **(B)** An axial postgadolinium T1-weighted image with fat saturation in the same patient demonstrates enhancement of the left optic nerve (arrowheads). The patient complained of decreased vision in the left eye, which is consistent with radiation-induced optic neuritis. The patient has been followed and has had no evidence of recurrent carcinoma.

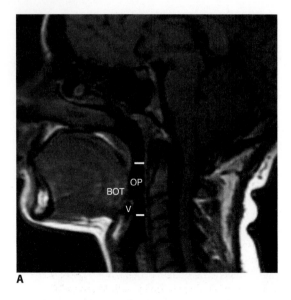

A

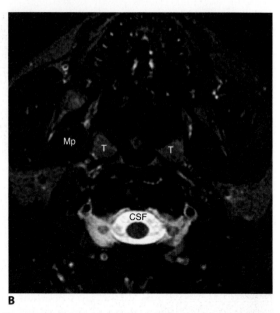

B

Figure 3–13. **(A)** Sagittal T1-weighted image demonstrates the superior and inferior limits of the oropharynx (OP), the region of the upper aerodigestive tract that can be seen posteriorly through an open mouth. Indicated are the vallecula (V) and the base of tongue (BOT). **(B)** Axial fast spin-echo T2-weighted image with fat saturation demonstrates the normal palatine tonsils (T), which, like other lymphoid tissue, are intermediate in signal intensity (note the much darker muscle [Mp, medial pterygoid muscle] and much brighter CSF) on a T2-weighted image.

ynx by the epiglottis and the glossoepiglottic fold and from the hypopharynx by the pharyngoepiglottic folds. In addition to squamous mucosa, contents of the oropharynx include the faucial and lingual tonsils, minor salivary glands, and pharyngeal constrictor muscles.

Pathology

Lesions that may be encountered on imaging studies of the oropharynx are listed in Table 3–2. Commonly encountered entities include tonsillar hypertrophy and tonsillar inflammatory processes, especially peritonsillar abscess. In a patient with inflammatory disease, it is important to look for underlying predisposing factors, such as an unsuspected foreign body, and also to look for potentially clinically occult complications, such as septic thrombophlebitis of the jugular vein (Figure 3–14). SCC of the faucial tonsil or base of tongue may present as a bulky exophytic mass lesion, an infiltrative mass lesion, or may have both infiltrative and exophytic components (Figure 3–15). It may also present as a more subtle process (Figure 3–16). The margins of the lesion are often poorly defined, and there may be infiltration of adjacent normal fat planes. SCC is typically intermediate in signal intensity on both T1- and T2-weighted images and shows moderately intense enhancement postgadolinium. In a patient with known oropharyngeal SCC, the Level

II lymph nodes should be carefully scrutinized for evidence of metastatic involvement. Imaging of lymph nodes is discussed in more detail in a later section.

Key Imaging Points

- Lymphoid hyperplasia of the palatine or lingual tonsils, especially if asymmetric, may mimic an aggres-

Table 3–2. Lesions of the oropharynx that may be encountered on imaging.

Benign	Malignant
Lingual or faucial tonsillar hypertrophy	Squamous cell carcinoma
Tonsillar or peritonsillar abscess	Non-Hodgkin lymphoma
Lingual thyroid	Malignant tumor of minor salivary gland
Postinflammatory retention cyst	Rhabdomyosarcoma (child)
Dystrophic calcification ("tonsillolith")	
Benign tumor of minor salivary gland	

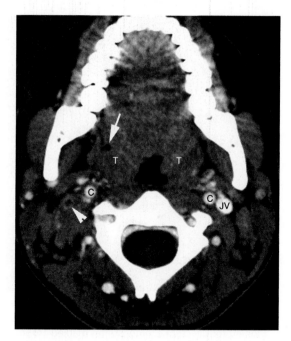

Figure 3–14. Axial contrast-enhanced CT image in a 16-year-old girl who had pharyngitis for a week as well as the recent incision and drainage of a right peritonsillar abscess demonstrates prominence of both palatine tonsils (T), right more than left. A dot of air (white arrow) is related to the recent incision and drainage. In addition, abnormal soft tissue is seen around the right internal jugular vein, and the vein itself (arrowhead) is thrombosed. The normal carotid arteries (C) and left internal jugular vein (JV) are indicated. The patient's chest CT scan (not shown) demonstrated multiple pulmonary nodules, some of which were cavitary, consistent with septic pulmonary emboli in a patient with Lemierre syndrome.

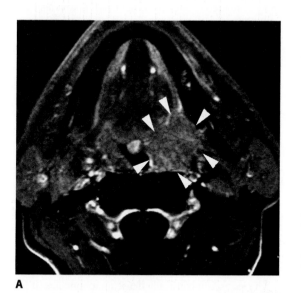

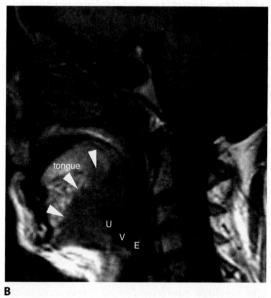

A

B

Figure 3–15. **(A)** Axial postgadolinium T1-weighted image with fat saturation demonstrates a bulky mass in the left tonsillar fossa (white arrowheads), consistent with squamous cell carcinoma. There is mass effect on the left base of tongue, but no gross invasion. **(B)** Sagittal T1-weighted image in a different patient with squamous cell carcinoma of the base of tongue demonstrates a large mass lesion (arrowheads) that is deeply infiltrative into the tongue as well as being exophytic into the vallecula (V) and displacing the epiglottis (E) posteriorly. A deep ulceration (U) is present. Note that the oral tongue shows a high signal intensity consistent with extensive fatty infiltration. This is related to denervation change secondary to neoplastic invasion of CN XII.

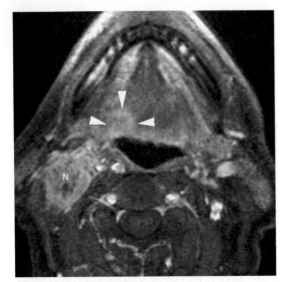

Figure 3–16. Axial postgadolinium T1-weighted image with fat saturation in an older man presenting with metastatic cervical adenopathy from squamous cell carcinoma and no clear primary site on clinical examination demonstrates a large metastatic node (N) as well as a subtle, infiltrative lesion at the right base of tongue (arrowheads) consistent with squamous cell carcinoma of the base of tongue.

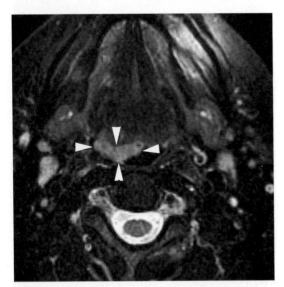

Figure 3–17. Axial fast spin-echo T2-weighted image with fat saturation in an older woman complaining of a sore throat demonstrates asymmetric soft tissue at the right base of tongue (arrowheads), which may be suggestive of lymphoma or squamous cell carcinoma, although no invasive component is identified. Operative resection for a definitive biopsy yielded only normal lingual tonsillar tissue.

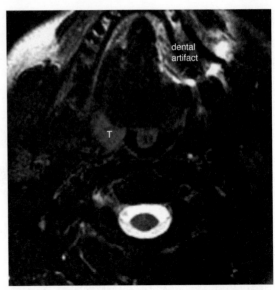

Figure 3–18. Axial fast spin-echo T2-weighted image with fat saturation in a patient who has undergone a prior left tonsillectomy demonstrates marked oropharyngeal asymmetry due to the presence of normal tonsillar tissue on the right (T) and no tissue on the left. Inhomogeneity along the left anterior aspect of the image is related to a ferromagnetic nonremovable dental appliance.

sive process such as SCC, but no invasive or infiltrative component will be identified (Figure 3–17).

- In a patient with a prior unilateral tonsillectomy, the remaining contralateral tonsil may appear to represent a mass lesion but is really a pseudomass (Figure 3–18).

- CT imaging is the modality of choice for the assessment of infectious and inflammatory processes because of its sensitivity to calcification, foreign bodies, and gas within soft tissues; it is also rapid and widely available. In the setting of peritonsillar abscess, CT scanning may show extension of the process beyond the confines of the pharyngeal constrictor muscles into adjacent deep spaces.

- Lingual thyroid tissue is seen as a rounded, midline soft tissue mass at the level of the foramen cecum. The lesion is intrinsically dense on a noncontrast CT scan because of its iodine content and enhances intensely postcontrast (Figure 3–19). The lower neck should be carefully scrutinized to assess whether any thyroid gland is present in the normal location.

- A well-circumscribed mass of the soft palate most commonly represents a pleomorphic adenoma, although a low-grade minor salivary gland malignant neoplasm may have an identical imaging appearance (Figure 3–20).

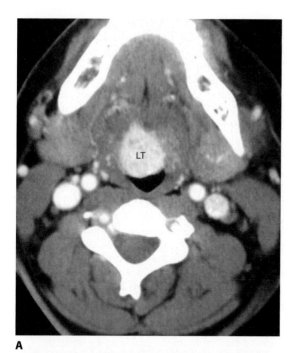

A

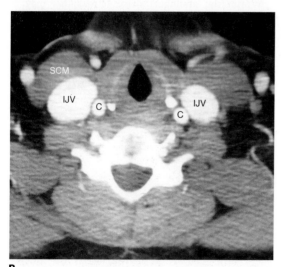

B

Figure 3–19. **(A)** Axial contrast-enhanced CT scan demonstrates a densely enhancing soft tissue mass in the midline of the base of tongue, consistent with lingual thyroid (LT). **(B)** A more inferior image through the low neck shows no normal thyroid tissue. Indicated are the common carotid artery (C), the internal jugular vein (IJV), and the sternocleidomastoid muscle (SCM).

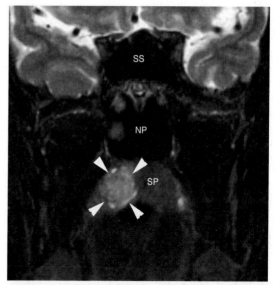

Figure 3–20. Coronal fast spin-echo T2-weighted image with fat saturation in a 50-year-old man with HIV demonstrates a fairly well-circumscribed mass (arrowheads) arising from the soft palate (SP). A pleomorphic adenoma was expected, but at resection, this mass was found to be a low-grade adenocarcinoma. The sphenoid sinus (SS) and nasopharynx (NP) are indicated.

- The palatine tonsil and base of tongue are common sites for "unknown" primary lesions in patients who present with metastatic cervical lymphadenopathy but with no obvious primary site lesions on careful head and neck examination. In some of these cases, CT scanning or MRI may demonstrate a primary site. FDG PET scanning has also been shown to play a role in the search for the unknown primary.

- The possibility of perineural spread of tumor should be evaluated. Tonsillar SCC may invade the masticator space and access V3, whereas SCC of the base of tongue may access cranial nerves IX and XII (the glossopharyngeal and hypoglossal nerves, respectively), as well as the lingual nerve. Tumors of the palate may access the palatine nerves and the pterygopalatine fossa, from which they may spread intracranially via the vidian canal and foramen rotundum.

ORAL CAVITY

Anatomy

The oral cavity (Figure 3–21) is bounded superiorly by the hard palate, the superior alveolar ridge, and the maxillary teeth, laterally by the cheek, posteriorly by the circumvallate papilla and anterior tonsillar pillars

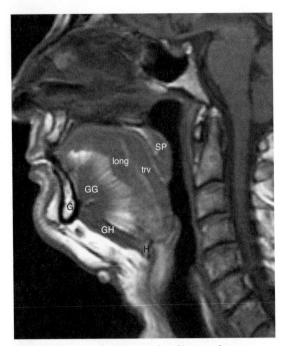

Figure 3–21. Sagittal T1-weighted image demonstrates the normal anatomy of the oral cavity. The genu (G) of the mandible and the hyoid bone (H) are indicated, along with extrinsic tongue musculature (genioglossus [GG] and geniohyoid [GH]) and intrinsic tongue musculature (longitudinal and transverse muscle fibers). The soft palate (SP) is also shown.

(which separate it from the oropharynx), and inferiorly by the mylohyoid muscle, the inferior alveolar ridge, and the mandibular teeth. The mucosal area of the oral cavity includes the oral tongue and mucosa-covered surfaces, which are readily accessible to clinical examination. The oral mucosa has buccal, gingival, lingual, sublingual, and palatal surfaces. In addition to the ubiquitous squamous epithelium, minor salivary glands are located throughout the oral cavity.

Two other major spaces are also considered in any discussion of the oral cavity: the sublingual and submandibular spaces (Figure 3–22). These spaces are separated from each other by the mylohyoid muscle, which defines the muscular floor of mouth. The sublingual space is not a true fascia-defined space; rather, it is located in the oral tongue between the mylohyoid muscle inferolaterally and the genioglossus-geniohyoid complex medially. It freely communicates with the submandibular space around its posterior edge, and its important contents include the sublingual glands and ducts, the submandibular (Wharton) duct, the lingual artery and vein, the lingual nerve, and CN IX and XII. The submandibular space is located inferolateral to the

mylohyoid muscle and superior to the hyoid bone. It is partly defined by the superficial layer of deep cervical fascia, but communicates freely with both the sublingual space around the back edge of the mylohyoid muscle and also the inferior parapharyngeal space. Important contents of the submandibular space include the submandibular gland, the Level I lymph nodes, the facial artery and vein, and CN·XII.

Pathology

The oral cavity is readily accessible to direct visualization and palpation, but imaging studies can be very helpful in assessing the deep extent of processes and guiding surgical management. In the mucosal area and oral tongue itself, the most common pathologies encountered are SCC (Figure 3–23) and extension of odontogenic infections. Benign or malignant minor salivary gland lesions may also be seen, as may congenital lesions such as venolymphatic malformations (Figure 3–24) and dermoids and epidermoids. In the setting of injury to or a lesion of CN XII, denervation change may be seen in the ipsilateral hemitongue, which may mimic a mass lesion to the unsuspecting observer.

Within the sublingual space, lesions that may be encountered on imaging studies are most frequently

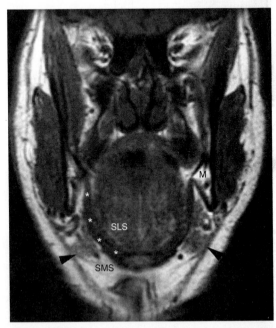

Figure 3–22. Coronal T1-weighted image demonstrates the mandible (M) and the mylohyoid muscle (*). The mylohyoid defines two spaces, the sublingual space (SLS) above and the submandibular space (SMS) below. The submandibular glands are indicated (black arrowheads).

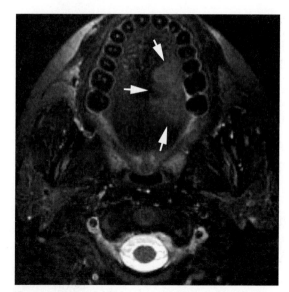

Figure 3–23. Axial fast spin-echo T2-weighted image with fat saturation in a 34-year-old woman with tongue cancer demonstrates an irregularly marginated left-sided lesion (arrows) that is deeply infiltrative into the tongue musculature.

masses of congenital, inflammatory, or malignant neoplastic etiology. As in the mucosal space, venolymphatic malformations and dermoids and epidermoids may occur. A dilated submandibular duct due to stenosis, calculus, or neoplastic obstruction may be seen (Figure 3–25), as may a ranula (Figure 3–26). Changes due to cellulitis (Ludwig angina) and frank abscess formation may also be present. Finally, SCC extending from the mucosal surface of the oral cavity (Figure 3–27) or due to deep anterior extension from the tongue base may be encountered. A similar list of diagnostic considerations can be applied in the submandibular space, with a few important additions: notably, a second branchial cleft cyst (see Cystic Neck Masses later in chapter) and lymphadenopathy, which may be reactive, inflammatory, or neoplastic, with nodal lymphoma and metastatic SCC accounting for most cases of neoplastic submandibular lymphadenopathy. Neoplastic lesions of the submandibular gland itself most commonly represent pleomorphic adenoma, but on imaging studies alone these are often indistinguishable from carcinomas. The more common pathologies of the oral cavity and associated spaces are summarized in Table 3–3.

Key Imaging Points

- Because so much of the oral cavity is readily accessible to inspection and palpation, imaging studies must

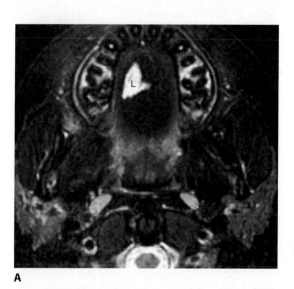

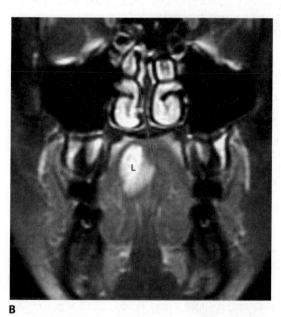

A   **B**

Figure 3–24. **(A)** Axial fast spin-echo T2-weighted image with fat saturation in a young woman with fullness in her right hemitongue and a slight bluish discoloration on clinical examination demonstrates a multilobulated, well-circumscribed, hyperintense mass lesion (L). **(B)** Postgadolinium, a coronal T1-weighted image with fat saturation demonstrates intense and homogeneous enhancement. The appearance is consistent with a venous malformation.

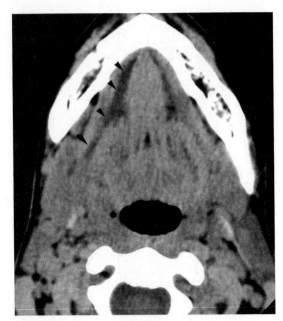

Figure 3–25. Axial noncontrast CT scan through the floor of mouth demonstrates asymmetric dilatation of the submandibular duct (black arrowheads) in a patient who has had prior removal of calculi and has a postinflammatory stenosis of the distal duct.

focus on addressing specific issues: submucosal and deep extension of neoplastic or inflammatory processes, bone involvement, and perineural spread of disease (Figure 3–28).

- Level I and II lymph nodes should be carefully assessed bilaterally in patients with oral cavity carcinoma, as bilateral nodal spread is common.

- The mucosal area of the oral cavity, particularly the buccal mucosa, can be better assessed on imaging examinations if the patient is asked to "puff out" his or her cheeks during a CT or MRI study to separate the buccal mucosa from the underlying teeth and gums (Figure 3–29).

- MRI is generally the study of choice to assess neoplasms of the oral cavity because it is less sensitive to dental artifact than CT scanning and provides superior soft tissue contrast for most processes (Figure 3–30).

- MRI is less sensitive to calcification than CT scanning; therefore, CT imaging is the study of choice for assessment of calculus disease, as well as for most infectious and inflammatory processes (Figure 3–31).

- In some cases, cellulitis and phlegmonous changes can be difficult to distinguish from an abscess. An abscess has a well-defined enhancing rim and a nonenhancing pus-filled center, and it exerts mass effect on local tissues rather than infiltrating along and obscuring fascial planes.

- A denervated hemitongue due to palsy of CN XII can mimic a mass lesion in the acute and subacute phases of denervation, when the tongue may be bright on a T2-weighted image and show enhancement postgadolinium (Figure 3–32). Denervation changes respect the midline perfectly, unlike most mass lesions. In addition, the lingual septum deviates toward rather than away from the "lesion," and the tongue flops back into the oropharynx owing to atrophy and loss of muscle tone.

- A pedunculated mass of the parotid tail (Figure 3–33) may present clinically as a mass in the posterior submandibular space.

HYPOPHARYNX

Anatomy

The hypopharynx represents the inferior continuation of the pharyngeal mucosal space, distinct from the oro-

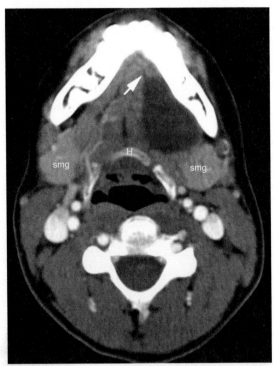

Figure 3–26. Axial contrast-enhanced CT scan through the floor of mouth in a patient with a painless swelling of the left sublingual space demonstrates a well-circumscribed fluid-density mass with a narrow extension (white arrow) to the anterior aspect of the sublingual space. A simple ranula was confirmed surgically. The submandibular glands (smg) and hyoid bone (H) are indicated.

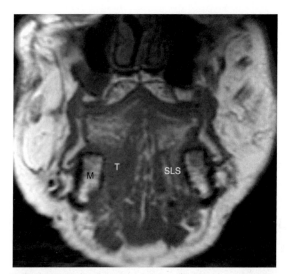

Figure 3–27. Coronal T1-weighted image in an elderly man with squamous cell carcinoma of the anterior floor of mouth demonstrates infiltration of tumor (T) into the right sublingual space; the normal fatty left sublingual space (SLS) is shown for comparison. The mandible (M) is also indicated. Note how useful a pregadolinium T1-weighted image is for demonstrating the replacement of normal fat by infiltrative soft tissue.

pharynx above and the larynx anteroinferiorly. Three major subsites of the hypopharynx are recognized: the pyriform sinus, the postcricoid area, and the posterior pharyngeal wall (Figure 3–34). The pyriform sinuses are bilaterally symmetric spaces marginated by the aryepiglottic folds anteromedially, the posterior thyroid cartilage ala laterally, and the most lateral aspect of the posterior hypopharyngeal wall posteriorly. The pyriform sinuses are shaped like inverted pyramids such that the tip of the sinus, also known as the pyriform apex, lies at the true vocal cord level. The postcricoid area forms the anterior wall of the lower pharynx at the level of the pharyngoesophageal junction, extending from the level of the arytenoid cartilages above to the inferior border of the cricoid cartilage below. This area is difficult to delineate on imaging studies because mucosal surfaces are usually coapted. The hypopharyngeal segment of the posterior pharyngeal wall extends from the bottom of the vallecula above to the esophageal inlet below. The hypopharynx contains only squamous mucosa, minor salivary glands, and the inferior constrictor muscles.

Pathology

The dominant pathology of the hypopharynx is SCC. Other lesions include retention cysts, benign and malignant tumors of minor salivary origin, and extranodal lymphoma. The pyriform sinus is the subsite most commonly involved with SCC, and these lesions are usually advanced at presentation and have a high incidence of nodal metastases (Figure 3–35).

Key Imaging Points

- The walls of the pyriform sinus are frequently coapted during imaging studies. Certain maneuvers, such as the Valsalva or "trumpet" maneuver, may help dilate the pyriform sinus and improve the imaging assessment.
- The pyriform sinus is a site where a small primary lesion may not be readily apparent in a patient who presents with metastatic cervical lymphadenopathy and no evidence of a primary lesion ("unknown primary").

Table 3–3. Lesions of the oral cavity, including the mucosal area, the sublingual space, and the submandibular space.

Congenital/Developmental	Infectious/Inflammatory	Neoplastic	
		Benign	*Malignant*
Hemangioma	Cellulitis or Ludwig angina	Pleomorphic adenoma	Squamous cell carcinoma
Venolymphatic malformation	Abscess	Other benign lesions of minor salivary origin	Malignant neoplasm of minor salivary origin
Dermoid or epidermoid	Dilated submandibular (Wharton) duct	Lipoma	Nodal metastases from SCC (SM space)
Second branchial cleft cyst (SM space)	Ranula, simple or plunging		Nodal involvement by lymphoma (SM space)

SCC, squamous cell carcinoma; SM, submandibular.

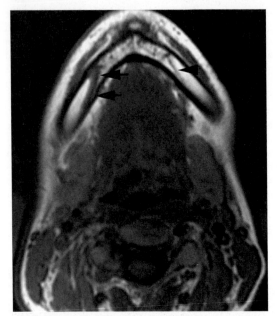

Figure 3–28. Axial T1-weighted image in a 45-year-old woman with a history of squamous cell carcinoma of the right gingivobuccal sulcus and new chin numbness demonstrates abnormal soft tissue in the right inferior alveolar canal (arrows) compared with the left (arrowhead), consistent with the perineural spread of disease. This was confirmed at the mandibulectomy.

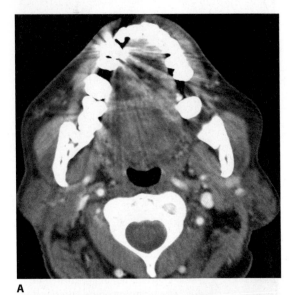

A

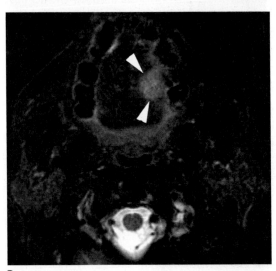

B

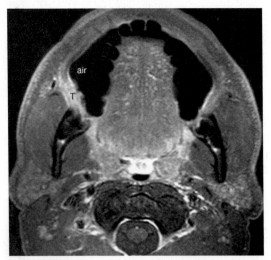

Figure 3–29. Axial postgadolinium T1-weighted image with fat saturation in a patient with squamous cell carcinoma of the right buccal mucosa obtained during a "puffed cheek" maneuver. This maneuver places air between the teeth and the tumor, making the extent of tumor (T) easier to define.

Figure 3–30. (A) Axial contrast-enhanced CT image in an older man with a left lateral squamous cell carcinoma of the tongue. The lesion is difficult to demonstrate given extensive streak artifact related to the patient's dental work as well as the relatively poor contrast between the lesion and the tongue musculature. **(B)** The tumor (arrowheads) is very well seen on an axial fast spin-echo T2-weighted image with fat saturation.

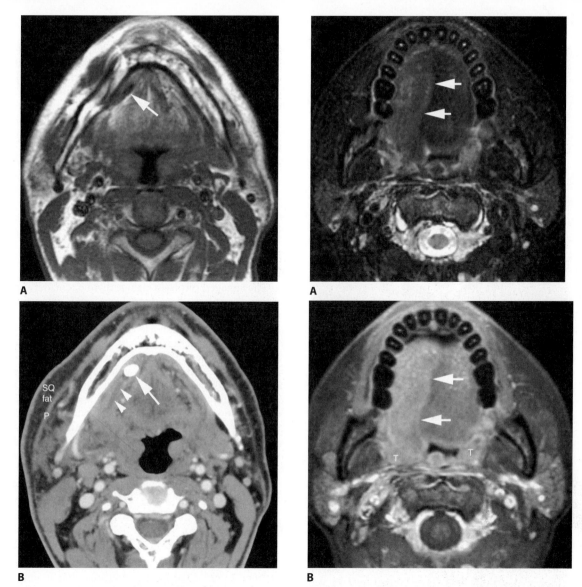

Figure 3–31. **(A)** Axial T1-weighted image in a young man complaining of fullness and slight tenderness in the right submandibular region. An ovoid low signal intensity structure in the right anterior floor of mouth (white arrow) was overlooked. This patient should probably have been referred for a CT scan rather than an MRI, given that inflammatory disease was more likely than neoplasm. **(B)** Axial contrast-enhanced CT scan obtained 4 weeks later, when the patient presented with fever and dramatic pain and swelling of the submandibular region. A calculus (arrow) obstructing the right submandibular duct (arrowheads) is seen, as well as inflammatory changes in the sublingual space with the effacement of fat planes. The platysma (P) is thickened, and the infiltration of subcutaneous fat is consistent with cellulitis. More inferiorly, a large abscess involving the submandibular gland was seen (not shown).

Figure 3–32. **(A)** Axial fast spin-echo T2-weighted image with fat saturation in a woman with a right CN XII palsy due to neoplastic infiltration of the skull base at the level of the hypoglossal canal (not shown) demonstrates sharply marginated hyperintensity of the right hemitongue (arrows) consistent with acute or subacute denervation change. Note that the lingual septum deviates toward the side of the "lesion," whereas a mass would be expected to push the lingual septum away. **(B)** Postgadolinium, an axial T1-weighted image with fat saturation demonstrates the enhancement of the right hemitongue as well as ptosis of the right tongue into the oropharynx, with compression of the ipsilateral right tonsil (T) compared with the left. These findings are typical of denervation change due to injury of CN XII.

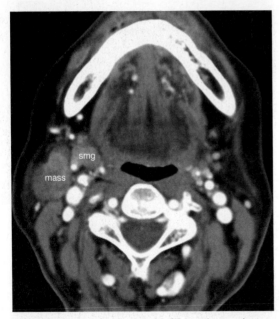

Figure 3–33. Axial postcontrast CT scan in a patient thought to have a mass arising from the submandibular gland (smg) demonstrates a well-circumscribed mass arising from the parotid tail, immediately adjacent to the submandibular gland. Fine-needle aspiration was consistent with pleomorphic adenoma.

- A lesion of the pyriform apex approaches the upper margin of the cricoid cartilage and may erode cartilage even when relatively small. Cricoid erosion may also be secondary to a primary tumor of the postcricoid region (Figure 3–36).
- Symmetric lesions of the posterior pharyngeal wall may be subtle and difficult to detect on imaging studies. A sagittal T1-weighted image can be very helpful in these cases.
- Lesions of the hypopharynx have a propensity to spread to retropharyngeal nodes, so these nodes should be carefully scrutinized in patients with hypopharyngeal cancers (Figure 3–37).

LARYNX

Anatomy

The soft tissues of the larynx (ie, the mucosa, the submucosa, and muscle) are draped over and attached to a supporting framework of cartilage, which gives the larynx its form. The endolarynx is divided into three subsites: the supraglottis, the glottis, and the subglottis (Figure 3–38). The supraglottis extends from the tip of the epiglottis above to the level of the laryngeal ventricles below and includes the epiglottis, the preepiglottic space, the aryepiglottic folds, the false vocal cords, the paraglottic space, and the arytenoid cartilages. The preepiglottic space is a fat-filled space bounded by the hyoid bone anteriorly and the epiglottis posteriorly, and halved by the hyoepiglottic ligament. The preepiglottic space communicates laterally with the paraglottic space, which is a bilateral, fat-filled space deep to the true and false vocal cords. The glottis includes the true vocal cords as well as the anterior and posterior commissures, whereas the subglottis extends from the undersurface of the true vocal cords above to the inferior surface of the cricoid cartilage below. The fibroelastic membrane known as the conus elasticus defines the lateral margin of the subglottis and extends from the cricoid cartilage below to the medial margin of the true vocal cord above.

The laryngeal cartilages include thyroid, cricoid, and arytenoid cartilages. The thyroid cartilage is composed of two anterior laminae that meet in the anterior midline. Posteriorly, the laminae elongate and form superior and inferior cornua; the superior cornua provide attachment to the thyrohyoid ligament, while the inferior cornua articulate medially with the cricoid cartilage and the cricothyroid joint. The cricoid cartilage is a complete ring that has a narrow arch anteriorly and a wide posterior lamina. The paired, pyramidal arytenoid cartilages sit atop the posterior cricoid lamina and provide attachment for the posterior margins of the vocal cords at the level of the vocal processes. The laryngeal cartilages progressively calcify and eventually ossify with age; in children and young adults they are of soft tissue density on CT scanning.

Pathology

Lesions that may be encountered on imaging studies of the larynx are listed in Table 3–4. SCC is the most common pathology of the larynx that requires an imaging assessment. Small lesions may not require imaging assessment and may, in fact, not even be visible on imaging studies, but CT scanning or MRI is useful in staging larger lesions. Involvement of preepiglottic and paraglottic spaces is well assessed on CT and MR scans, as is subglottic extension (Figure 3–39). Involvement of the laryngeal cartilages, notably the thyroid cartilage, may not be appreciated clinically but can be identified on imaging studies and has significant implications for therapy. MRI is more sensitive than CT scanning to neoplastic infiltration of the laryngeal cartilages, although neither technique is entirely reliable for detecting subtle invasion and both techniques may lead to overinterpretation of reactive changes as neoplastic infiltration. CT scanning or MRI is also useful in staging the neck and both can detect pathologic lymphadenopathy that may be missed by clinical palpation.

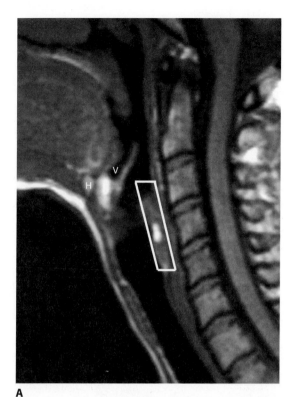

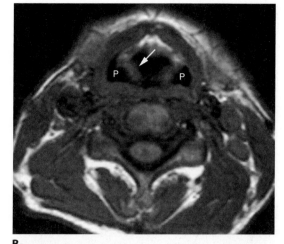

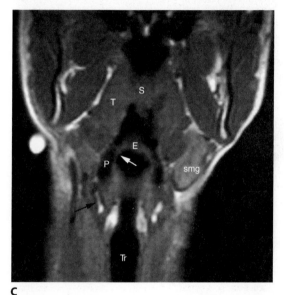

Figure 3–34. **(A)** Sagittal T1-weighted image demonstrates the hypopharynx (white lines) extending from the level of they hyoid bone (H) and vallecula (V) superiorly to the cricopharyngeus inferiorly, with the inferior extent approximated by the inferior margin of the cricoid cartilage. **(B)** Axial T1-weighted image demonstrates the pyriform sinuses (P) and the right aryepiglottic fold (arrow). **(C)** Coronal T1-weighted image demonstrates the pyriform sinus (P), epiglottis (E), aryepiglottic fold (white arrow), thyroid cartilage (black arrow), tonsil (T), trachea (Tr), soft palate (S), and submandibular gland (smg).

Lesions primary to the laryngeal cartilages are classically chondroid in nature—for example, chondroma and chondrosarcoma. These lesions are centered on the cartilage, usually the cricoid cartilage, and appear as submucosal masses on direct inspection. A calcified matrix is typically present on CT scans, and these lesions are usually extremely bright on T2-weighted MRI. Ossified laryngeal cartilages may also be involved with systemic malignant processes such as lymphoma, leukemia, multiple myeloma, and hematogenously disseminated metastases from any primary site.

Trauma to the larynx is usually assessed clinically and endoscopically, but imaging may be useful when fracture of the laryngeal cartilages or deep tissue injury is suspected. Blunt trauma to the anterior neck compresses the larynx against the cervical spine. The thyroid cartilage most commonly fractures along its anterior margin (Figure 3–40), whereas the cricoid ring, like any complete ring, tends to fracture in two or more places.

The laryngocele results from functional obstruction (eg, increased intraglottic pressures) or true anatomic obstruction (eg, post-traumatic or postinflammatory stenosis, or neoplasm) of the laryngeal ventricle or its more distal saccule. The laryngocele may be filled with air, fluid, or pus and may be internal or external. The internal laryngocele is identified in the paraglottic space and can be followed to the level of the laryngeal ventricle.

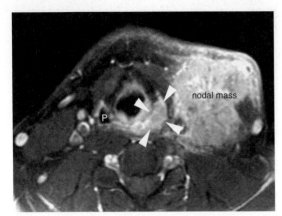

Figure 3–35. Axial postgadolinium T1-weighted image with fat saturation in a patient presenting with a left neck mass (nodal mass) shows a relatively small primary lesion in the left pyriform sinus (arrowheads). The normal right pyriform sinus (P) is indicated. Fine-needle aspiration of the nodal mass confirmed squamous cell carcinoma.

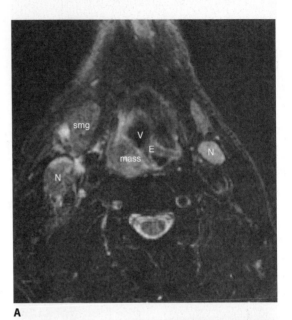

A

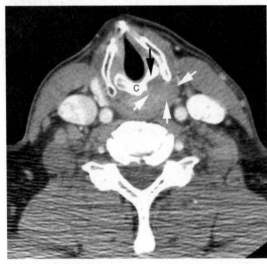

Figure 3–36. Axial postcontrast CT scan in a patient with new hoarseness and throat pain demonstrates focal erosion (black arrow) of the posterolateral cricoid cartilage (C) by a mass arising from the postcricoid hypopharynx (white arrows). This lesion could probably be better delineated from adjacent soft tissues on an MRI. Biopsy demonstrated squamous cell carcinoma.

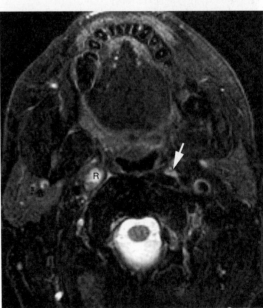

B

Figure 3–37. **(A)** Axial fast spin-echo T2-weighted image with fat saturation demonstrates a hypopharyngeal mass with associated bilateral lymphadenopathy (N). Biopsy of the mass demonstrated squamous cell carcinoma of the posterolateral pharyngeal wall. E, epiglottis; smg, submandibular gland; V, vallecula. **(B)** A more superior image demonstrates ipsilateral pathologic retropharyngeal lymph node (R) enlargement and heterogeneity. A normal contralateral retropharyngeal node (white arrow) is shown for comparison.

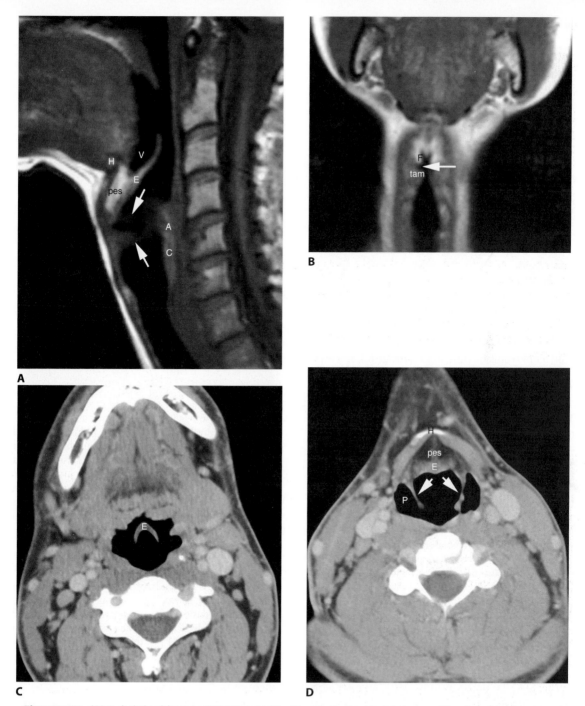

Figure 3–38. **(A)** A slightly oblique sagittal T1-weighted image demonstrates the vocal ligaments (white arrows) stretching from the vocal process of the arytenoid (A) to the anterior thyroid cartilage. Also indicated are the cricoid cartilage (C), epiglottis (E), preepiglottic space (pes), vallecula (V), and hyoid bone (H). **(B)** Coronal T1-weighted image demonstrates the thyroarytenoid muscle (tam) at the level of the true vocal cord, the laryngeal ventricle (arrow), and the fatty paraglottic space at the level of the false vocal cord (F). **(C)** Axial CT scan through the supraglottis shows the free margin of the epiglottis (E). **(D)** A slightly lower scan through the supraglottis demonstrates the fixed portion of the epiglottis (E), preepiglottic space (pes), aryepiglottic folds (white arrows), hyoid bone (H), and pyriform sinuses (P). *(Continued)*

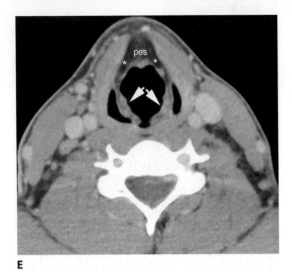

E

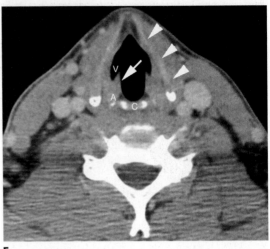

F

Figure 3–38 (Cont'd). **(E)** A slightly lower scan shows the anterior preepiglottic space (pes) merging imperceptibly with the lateral paraglottic spaces (*). The aryepiglottic folds are indicated (white arrows). **(F)** Axial CT scan at the glottic level shows the true vocal cord (white arrow) and the laryngeal ventricle (V). In this young patient, the arytenoid cartilage (A), cricoid cartilage (C), and thyroid cartilage (white arrowheads) are largely nonossified and therefore poorly seen.

The external laryngocele has both an internal component, which may be completely collapsed, and an external component that has penetrated the thyrohyoid membrane and often presents as an anterolateral neck mass (Figure 3–41).

Hoarseness is a relatively common indication for laryngeal imaging. In the absence of a mass lesion, attention should be focused on the course of the vagus nerve. When hoarseness is present along with other symptoms of lower cranial nerve dysfunction, then MRI is the study of choice to assess for a lesion of the skull base or carotid sheath (Figure 3–42). When hoarseness is the only symptom, then CT imaging is preferred, from the skull base to the aorticopulmonary window, to assess for any anatomic abnormality or mass lesion that could affect the recurrent laryngeal nerve along its course (Figure 3–43). The normal true vocal

cords are symmetrically abducted during quiet respiration, whereas the Valsalva maneuver adducts the vocal cords to an opposed, midline position. In the setting of vocal cord paralysis, the paralyzed cord is usually fixed in a paramedian position, the ipsilateral aryepiglottic fold deviates medially, the ipsilateral pyriform sinus is dilated, and the laryngeal ventricle is often patulous (Figure 3–44). Denervation atrophy of the laryngeal musculature may also be identified.

Key Imaging Points

- CT imaging is the study of choice for nonmalignant disease of the larynx (eg, trauma or laryngocele); MRI more sensitively assesses cartilage invasion and more accurately delineates the transglottic spread of tumor. However, MRI of the larynx is often compro-

Table 3–4. Common lesions of the larynx that may be encountered on imaging.

Congenital/Development	Trauma	Functional	Neoplastic	
			Mucosal	*Cartilaginous*
Hemangioma	Hematoma	Laryngocele	Squamous cell carcinoma	Chondroma
Venolymphatic malformation	Fracture of laryngeal cartilage			Chondrosarcoma
				Metastatic disease

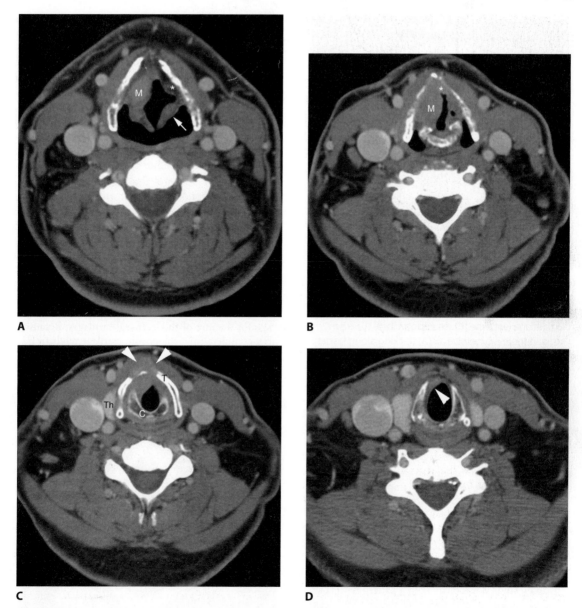

Figure 3–39. Serial axial contrast-enhanced CT images in an older man with transglottic squamous cell carcinoma with cartilage erosion. **(A)** Image through the supraglottis demonstrates a mass (M) involving the right paraglottic space and aryepiglottic fold. Normal fatty left paraglottic space (*) and aryepiglottic fold (white arrow) are indicated. **(B)** At the glottic level, the right true vocal cord is grossly enlarged by the mass (M) and the soft tissue of the anterior commissure (*) is grossly thickened. The left true vocal cord is irregular, also a consequence of tumor infiltration. **(C)** At the level of the undersurface of the vocal cords, the lesion has eroded the ventral aspect of the thyroid cartilage (T; arrowheads indicate mass) and has extended anteriorly to invade the strap muscles. **(D)** At the subglottic level, asymmetric soft tissue is seen anteriorly (arrowhead), consistent with subglottic tumor extension. Note that at the subglottic level, the air column should appear to be immediately adjacent to the cricoid cartilage with no significant intervening soft tissue.

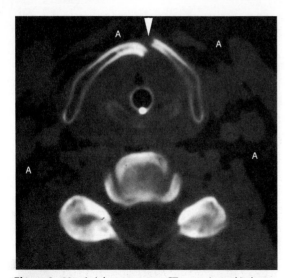

Figure 3–40. Axial noncontrast CT scan viewed in bone window obtained in a young man who was kicked in the neck demonstrates a vertical fracture of the anterior thyroid cartilage (arrowhead). An endotracheal tube is in place and there is extensive air (A) tracking along fascial planes. A more inferior image (not shown) demonstrated bilateral fractures through the posterior cricoid ring.

mised by patient motion; therefore, thin-section contrast-enhanced CT scanning may actually provide better depiction of the extent of disease in the majority of patients.

- The subsites of the hypopharynx are often confused with those of the larynx. It is important to distinguish among them as SCCs in these areas behave differently.
- The paraglottic and preepiglottic spaces are fat-filled compartments that are not separated from each other by fascia, so tumor can easily spread from one space to another.
- Imaging studies of the larynx in a patient with laryngeal carcinoma should always be assessed for preepiglottic and paraglottic space involvement, as well as for the status of the laryngeal cartilages, because these areas cannot be staged clinically except in far-advanced disease.
- New hoarseness in a patient with a history of head and neck cancer should prompt careful evaluation of the course of CN X (the vagus nerve) to look for tumor recurrence and spread along the carotid sheath and to the skull base.
- It is generally best to perform imaging of the larynx in quiet respiration, during which the true vocal cords are in their relaxed, abducted state. If indi-

cated, the scan can be repeated during a maneuver such as the Valsalva maneuver to assess for paralysis or mechanical fixation.

- The thickness of soft tissue in the anterior commissure may be as much as 2 mm in patients without disease.
- The mucosal surface of the subglottis is so closely applied to the cricoid cartilage that it is generally not appreciable on the airway side of the subglottic larynx. Visible soft tissue at this level should suggest the possible presence of tumor extension.
- A submucosal tumor of the larynx most commonly represents a chondrosarcoma or a metastatic lesion.
- In the presence of a laryngocele, the larynx should be carefully assessed clinically and radiographically for the presence of a neoplasm. Even large tumors may initially present with a neck mass secondary to a laryngocele, rather than with complaints referable to the larynx (Figure 3–45).
- In the setting of trauma to the anterior neck, particularly severe blunt trauma, CT imaging is useful to assess for fracture of the laryngeal cartilages. Because it is a complete ring, the cricoid cartilage tends to fracture in two or more places.

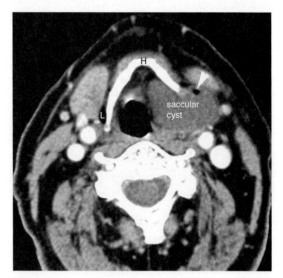

Figure 3–41. Axial contrast-enhanced CT scan through the supraglottic larynx demonstrates a fluid-filled saccular cyst protruding through the thyrohyoid membrane and demonstrating both internal and external components. A small focus of air in the cyst (arrowhead) is related to a recent aspiration. The hyoid bone (H) has been remodeled. A small air-filled external laryngocele (L) is seen on the contralateral side.

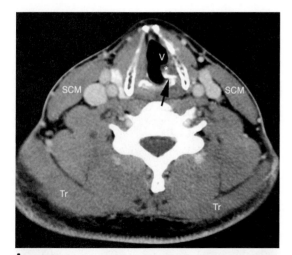

A

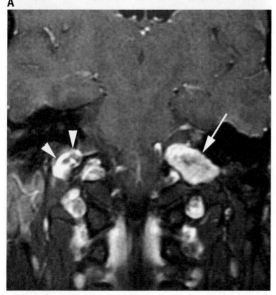

C

B

Figure 3–42. **(A)** Axial contrast-enhanced CT scan of the neck in a young man with hoarseness and left vocal cord paralysis on examination. The arytenoid (black arrow) is rotated medially, the left true vocal cord and thyroarytenoid muscle (*) show fatty atrophy compared with the contralateral side, and the left laryngeal ventricle (V) is dilated, all of which are imaging features of vocal cord paralysis. In addition, the left sternocleidomastoid (SCM) and trapezius (Tr) muscles are decreased in bulk compared with the right, suggesting also dysfunction of CN XI, although this had not been noted on clinical examination. The patient was then referred for MRI to assess for a skull base lesion. **(B)** An axial fast spin-echo T2-weighted image with fat saturation demonstrates a well-circumscribed soft tissue mass (white arrows) at the level of the left jugular foramen. The right jugular bulb (JB) and the medulla (Me) are indicated. **(C)** On a postgadolinium T1-weighted image with fat saturation, the lesion (white arrow) demonstrates slightly heterogeneous but mostly intense enhancement. The diagnosis is a lower cranial nerve schwannoma. The contralateral enhancing jugular bulb (white arrowheads) is also indicated. Note that the normal jugular bulb is a "pseudomass" that can be mistaken for significant pathology.

Becker M. Larynx and hypopharynx. *Radiol Clin North Am.* 1998;36:891. [PMID: 9747193] (Reviews the imaging anatomy and pathology of the larynx and hypopharynx.)

Chong VF, Fan YF, Mukherji SK. Carcinoma of the nasopharynx. *Semin Ultrasound CT MR.* 1998;19:449. [PMID: 9861663] (A review of the imaging of nasopharyngeal carcinoma.)

Dillon WP, Mills CM, Kjos B, DeGroot J, Brant-Zawadzki M. Magnetic resonance imaging of the nasopharynx. *Radiology.* 1984;152:731. [PMID: 6463254] (An introduction to the imaging anatomy of the nasopharynx.)

Kallmes DF, Phillips CD. The normal anterior commissure of the glottis. *AJR Am J Roentgenol.* 1997;168:1317. [PMID: 9129433] (The mean width of the anterior commissure was found to be 1.0 mm. However, 42% of patients had anterior commissures wider than 1.0 mm. Using an upper limit of 1.6 mm as a normal measurement for the anterior commissure would have included 92%

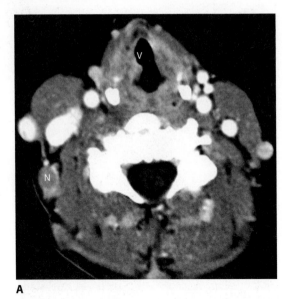

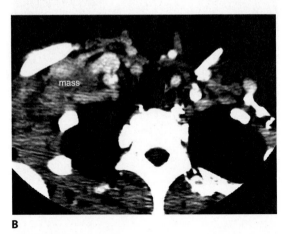

A

B

Figure 3–43. **(A)** Axial contrast-enhanced CT scan of the neck in a middle-aged woman with breast cancer and new hoarseness demonstrates a patulous right laryngeal ventricle (V) and vocal cord asymmetry consistent with a right cord paralysis. No laryngeal mass is seen. However, a metastatic node (N) is incidentally noted. **(B)** An image through the supraclavicular fossa demonstrates a metastatic nodal mass that is impinging on the course of the right recurrent laryngeal nerve.

of patients, and an upper limit of 2.1 mm would have encompassed the mean plus two standards.)

Laine FJ, Smoker WR. Oral cavity: anatomy and pathology. *Semin Ultrasound CT MR.* 1995;16:527. [PMID: 8747416] (The normal anatomy of the oral cavity, vestibule, and oral cavity proper is discussed, as is the anatomy and pathology of the sublingual and submandibular spaces.)

Pameijer FA, Mukherji SK, Balm AJ, van der Laan BF. Imaging of squamous cell carcinoma of the hypopharynx. *Semin Ultrasound CT MR.* 1998;19:476. [PMID: 9861665] (Review of imaging anatomy and pitfalls related to squamous cell carcinoma of the hypopharynx.)

Romo LV, Curtin HD. Atrophy of the posterior cricoarytenoid muscle as an indicator of recurrent laryngeal nerve palsy. *Am J Neuroradiol.* 1999;20:467. [PMID: 10219413] (Atrophy of the posterior cricoarytenoid muscle may be seen on imaging studies in patients with recurrent laryngeal nerve palsy and vocal cord paralysis. This finding is particularly useful when other imaging findings of vocal cord paralysis are absent or equivocal.)

Weissman JL, Carrau RL. "Puffed-cheek" CT improves evaluation of the oral cavity. *Am J Neuroradiol.* 2001;22:741. [PMID: 11290490] (Coaptation of mucosal surfaces can limit the assessment of oral cavity lesions, especially those of buccal origin. "Puffed-cheek" CT scans provide a clearer and more detailed evaluation of mucosal surfaces of the oral cavity than do conventional scans.)

Yates CB, Phillips CD. Oral cavity and oropharynx. *Curr Probl Diagn Radiol.* 2001;30:38. [PMID: 11300548] (An overview of the imaging anatomy and typical pathology of these areas.)

LYMPH NODES

The cervical lymph nodes must always be carefully assessed in the setting of head and neck cancer, but may also become involved by infectious, inflammatory, and granulomatous processes, as well as by systemic malignant neoplasms (eg, lymphoma or metastasis from primary sites other than the head and neck). Before discussing the normal appearance of the cervical lymph nodes on imaging studies and the differential diagnosis of nodal abnormalities, the appropriate terminology for the cervical lymph nodes is reviewed here. Over the last decade or so, clinical terminology has evolved from being anatomically based to a simpler classification based on levels. This classification has been translated into an imaging-based classification, which is summarized in Table 3–5 and Figure 3–46.

Some nodal groups are not included in this classification scheme, notably the retropharyngeal nodes, parotid nodes, the pre- and postauricular nodes, the facial nodes, and the suboccipital nodes. These nodes are still referred to by their anatomic names. Although these nodes may certainly be involved by neoplastic and nonneoplastic processes, they do not represent the most common sites of lymphatic drainage for SCC of the upper aerodigestive tract and are not included in the level classification scheme.

On noncontrast CT scans, normal lymph nodes are ovoid, homogeneous soft tissue masses with a short-axis

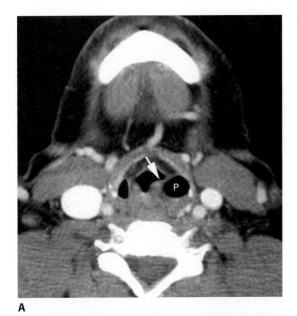

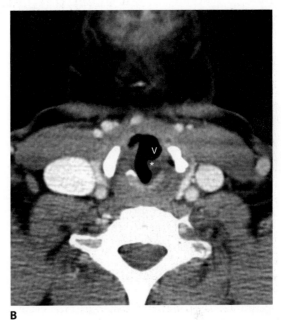

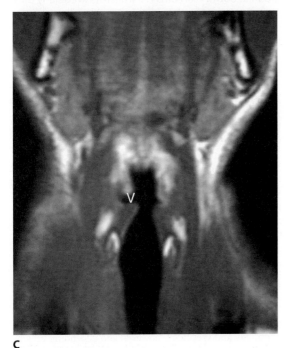

Figure 3–44. **(A)** Axial contrast-enhanced CT scan in a patient with a left true vocal cord paralysis demonstrates dilatation of the ipsilateral pyriform sinus (P) and medial deviation of the aryepiglottic fold (arrow). **(B)** A more inferior image demonstrates asymmetric enlargement of the ipsilateral laryngeal ventricle (V) and denervation change with fatty atrophy of the thyroarytenoid muscle (*). **(C)** Coronal T1-weighted image in a different patient with right vocal cord paralysis demonstrates dilatation of the right laryngeal ventricle (V) compared with the left.

diameter of 5–10 mm (Figure 3–47). A fatty hilum may be recognizable as an eccentric area of low density. Pathologic lymph nodes may be enlarged and focally or diffusely hypodense if there is cyst formation or necrosis. Necrotic lymphadenopathy may be seen with SCC, treated lymphoma, and other neoplastic processes, but it may also be seen with mycobacterial infection, cat-scratch disease, and other infectious processes (Figure 3–48).

Suppurative lymphadenopathy also leads to central hypodensity. In some circumstances, a lymph node may appear hyperdense before contrast administration, usually owing to partial or complete calcification (eg,

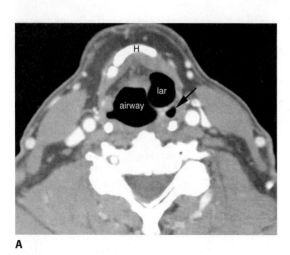

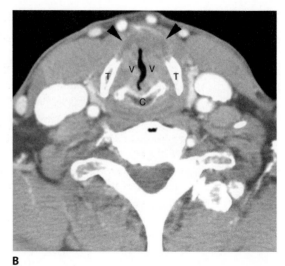

Figure 3–45. **(A)** Axial contrast-enhanced CT scan through the supraglottic larynx demonstrates an air-filled structure on the left consistent with an internal laryngocele (lar). The left pyriform sinus (black arrow) is displaced posteriorly. **(B)** A more inferior image demonstrates neoplastic infiltration of both vocal cords (V), which are irregularly thickened, as well as neoplastic erosion (black arrowheads) of the anterior thyroid cartilage (T). C, cricoid cartilage.

old granulomatous disease, metastatic tumoral calcification, or irradiated metastatic nodes). After contrast administration, normal lymph nodes show moderate homogeneous enhancement. Areas of cyst formation or necrosis appear hypodense and are more easily appreciated than on the noncontrast scan. In some cases, a focus of tumor may appear hyperdense to normal nodal tissue after contrast administration. This is most commonly seen with vascular metastases from thyroid or renal cell carcinoma but may also be seen with inflammatory processes. If extracapsular spread of tumor has occurred, then the node will have a poorly defined border and an irregular margin with surrounding soft tissue structures.

On MRI, normal lymph nodes are intermediate in signal intensity on T1-weighted images and hyperintense to muscle on T2-weighted images, and they show mild or moderate homogeneous enhancement postgadolinium (Figure 3–49). Fat may be identified at the nodal hilum. If a lymph node shows high signal intensity on a T1-weighted image before the administration of gadolinium, then metastatic thyroid cancer and metastatic melanoma should be considered. A cystic-appearing node may be due to infection or to tumor and will be of low signal intensity on T1-weighted images and of high signal intensity on T2-weighted images, and will show smooth peripheral enhancement postgadolinium. The neoplasms that typically result in cystic

nodal metastases are SCC and thyroid carcinoma, but many primary cancers may lead to cystic-appearing nodal disease. A potential pitfall is that a single cystic metastasis may be mistaken for a benign process such as a branchial cleft cyst. Nodal necrosis due to metastatic cancer usually leads to a thick, irregular, enhancing wall and central nonenhancement. In a patient with known head and neck cancer, the presence of necrotic lymphadenopathy is considered to represent metastatic disease. In some cases of metastatic SCC, areas of abnormally low signal intensity representing keratin pools are seen on T2-weighted images.

The assessment of the cervical lymph nodes for metastatic involvement in patients with head and neck cancer is an important role for CT and MRI. Because a non-necrotic node may still contain foci of tumor, size criteria have been developed for predicting the likelihood of metastatic nodal involvement. These criteria represent a trade-off between sensitivity and specificity, however, and depending on what cut-off is chosen for minimal axial diameter, there may be significant numbers of false-positive or false-negative nodes. The most widely accepted cut-off for reporting metastatic lymphadenopathy is a short-axis diameter ≥ 10 mm, but this yields a positive predictive value of only approximately 50% and a negative predictive value of approximately 80%. The development of functional and metabolic methods such as FDG PET and iron oxide-enhanced MR lymphography shows

Table 3–5. Summary of image-based nodal classification.

Level & Subclassification	Boundaries	Previous Terminology
I	Above hyoid bone, below mylohyoid muscle, anterior to a transverse line drawn through the posterior edge of the SMG	Submental and submandibular nodes
IA	Between medial margins of anterior bellies of digastric muscles	Submental nodes
IB	Posterior and lateral to medial edge of anterior belly of digastric muscle, anterior to posterior edge of SMG	Submandibular nodes
II	From skull base to the lower body of the hyoid bone, anterior to the posterior edge of the SCM and posterior to the posterior edge of the SMG*	Upper internal jugular and spinal accessory nodes
IIA	Lie anterior, lateral, or medial to the IJV, or lie posterior to the IJV and are inseparable from it	Upper internal jugular nodes
IIB	Lie posterior to the IJV and have a fat plane separating the nodes and the vein	Upper spinal accessory nodes
III	Between the lower body of the hyoid bone and the lower margin of the cricoid arch; anterior to the posterior edge of the SCM and lateral to the medial margin of the CCA or ICA	Mid-jugular nodes
IV	Between the lower margin of the cricoid cartilage arch and the level of the clavicle; anterior and medial to an oblique line drawn between the posterior edge of the SCM and the posterolateral edge of the anterior scalene muscle; lateral to the medial margin of the CCA	Low jugular nodes
V	From the skull base at the posterior border of the attachment of the SCM to the clavicle; anterior to the anterior edge of the trapezius muscle and posterior to the posterior edge of the SCM (skull base to bottom of cricoid), or posterior and lateral to an oblique line through the posterior edge of the SCM and the posterolateral edge of the anterior scalene muscle (bottom of cricoid to clavicle)	Posterior cervical
VA	From skull base superiorly to lower margin of cricoid cartilage inferiorly	Upper posterior cervical
VB	From lower margin of cricoid cartilage to level of clavicle	Lower posterior cervical
VI	Inferior to body of hyoid, superior to top of manubrium, and between the medial margins of the ICAs or CCAs	Visceral nodes
VII	Caudal to the top of the manubrium in the superior mediastinum, between the medial margins of the left and right common carotid arteries and superior to the innominate vein	Superior mediastinal

SMG, submandibular gland; SCM, sternocleidomastoid muscle; IJV, internal jugular vein; CCA, common carotid artery; ICA, internal carotid artery.
*A node located within 2 cm of the skull base and medial to the internal carotid arteries is classified as a retropharyngeal node. A node located within 2 cm of the skull base but anterior, lateral, or posterior to the ICA is classified as a level II node. More than 2 cm below the skull base, level II nodes can lie in any position relative to the internal jugular vein.
Modified, with permission, from Som PM, Curtin HD, Mancuso AA. Imaging-based nodal classification for evaluation of neck metastatic adenopathy. *AJR Am J Roentgenol* 2000;174:837.

promise in improving lymph node staging, but these techniques are not widely applied at present and also have significant limitations.

Adams S, Baum RP, Stuckensen T, Bitter K, Hor G. Prospective comparison of 18F-FDG PET with conventional imaging modalities (CT, MRI, US) in lymph node staging of head and neck cancer. *Eur J Nucl Med.* 1998;25:1255.

[PMID: 9724374] (1284 lymph nodes in 60 patients were assessed. FDG PET correctly identified lymph node metastases with a sensitivity of 90% and a specificity of 94%, whereas CT and MRI visualized histologically proven lymph node metastases with a sensitivity of 82% [specificity of 85%] and 80% [specificity of 79%], respectively. This prospective, histopathologically controlled study confirms FDG PET as the procedure with the highest sensitiv-

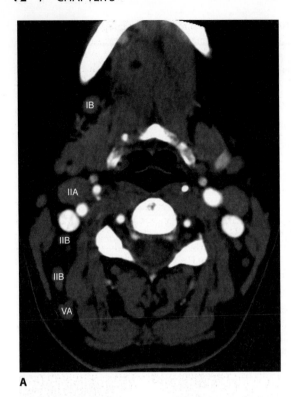

A

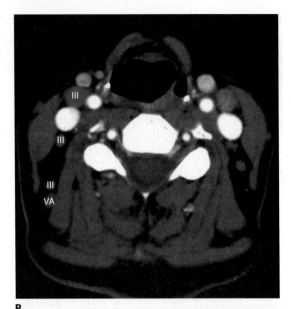

B

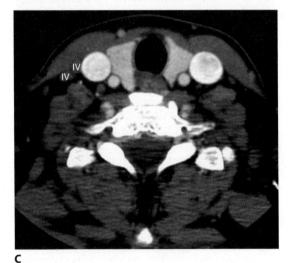

Figure 3–46. **(A, B,** and **C)** Serial contrast-enhanced axial CT scans through the neck demonstrate the image-based nodal classification system summarized in Table 3–5. Nodes in each of the five levels commonly involved by head and neck cancer are labeled.

C

ity and specificity for detecting lymph node metastases of head and neck cancer.)

Bellin MF, Beigelman C, Precetti-Morel S. Iron oxide-enhanced MRI lymphography: initial experience. *Eur J Radiol.* 2000;34:257. [PMID: 10927166] (Ultrasmall superparamagnetic iron oxide particles (USPIO) are novel contrast agents specifically developed for MRI lymphography. Early clinical experience suggests that USPIO-enhanced MRI lymphography improves the sensitivity and specificity for the detection of nodal metastases and suggests that micrometastases could be detected in normal-sized nodes.)

Curtin HD, Ishwaran H, Mancuso AA, Dalley RW, Caudry DJ, McNeil BJ. Comparison of CT and MR imaging in staging of neck metastases. *Radiology.* 1998;207:123. [PMID: 9530307] (With use of a 1-cm size or an internal abnormality to indicate a positive node, CT scanning had a negative predictive value of 84% and a positive predictive value of 50%, and MRI had a negative predictive value of 79% and a positive predictive value of 52%. Overall, CT scanning performed slightly better than MRI for all interpretative criteria, but a high negative predictive value was achieved only when a low-size criterion was used and was therefore associated with a relatively low positive predictive value.)

Sakai O, Curtin HD, Romo LV, Som PM. Lymph node pathology. Benign proliferative, lymphoma, and metastatic disease.

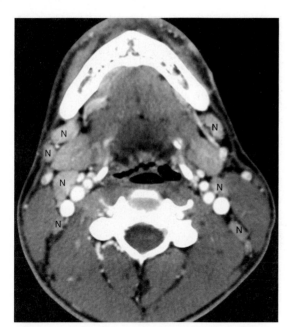

Figure 3–47. Axial contrast-enhanced CT scan of the neck in a normal young man demonstrates multiple normal-sized, homogeneously enhancing lymph nodes (N) in Levels I and II.

Radiol Clin North Am. 2000;38:979. [PMID: 11054964] (CT and MR imaging characteristics of both malignant and nonmalignant nodal diseases are reviewed and the differential diagnosis of nodal pathologies based on specific imaging findings is discussed.)

Som PM, Curtin HD, Mancuso AA. Imaging-based nodal classification for evaluation of neck metastatic adenopathy. *AJR Am J Roentgenol.* 2000;174:837. [PMID: 10701636] (Discusses the application of cross-sectional imaging to accurate and reproducible terminology for lymph node localization.)

Som PM, Curtin HD, Mancuso AA. An imaging-based classification for the cervical nodes designed as an adjunct to recent clinically based nodal classifications. *Arch Otolaryngol Head Neck Surg.* 1999;125:388. [PMID: 10208676] (A discussion of the imaging correlate to nodal levels.)

◼ NONMUCOSAL DISEASE OF THE HEAD & NECK

SPATIAL APPROACH TO THE SUPRAHYOID & INFRAHYOID HEAD & NECK

The terminology used to describe the traditional pharyngeal subdivisions of the head and neck is best suited to the assessment and staging of SCC. Because nonsquamous masses tend to spread within fascia-defined spaces, the head and neck can also be viewed as a series of deep spaces, an approach that facilitates an analysis of cross-sectional imaging of the head and neck. To simplify the discussion, the extracranial head and neck are divided into supra- and infrahyoid compartments because fascial attachments to the hyoid bone functionally cleave this region into two segments.

1. Suprahyoid Head & Neck

The spaces of the suprahyoid head and neck are defined by the three layers of the deep cervical fascia: superficial (investing), middle (buccopharyngeal), and deep (prevertebral). The spaces defined by these three fascial layers are shown diagrammatically in Figure 3–50.

Pharyngeal Mucosal Space

The pharyngeal mucosal space has complex fascial margins and is not completely circumscribed by the three

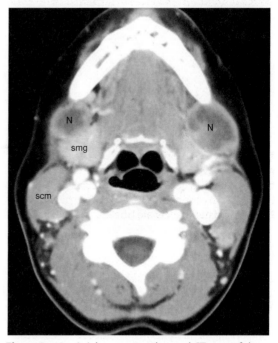

Figure 3–48. Axial contrast-enhanced CT scan of the neck in a young immunosuppressed woman demonstrates large, centrally necrotic lymph nodes (N) anterior to the submandibular glands (smg) anteriorly. Needle aspiration and culture were consistent with cat-scratch disease; scm, sternocleidomastoid muscle.

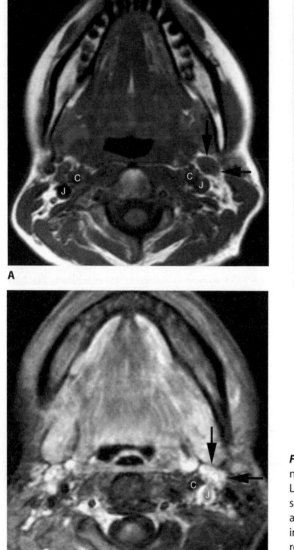

A

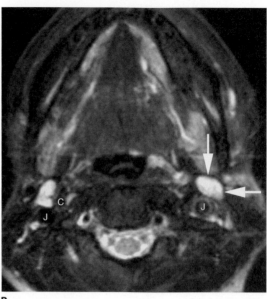

B

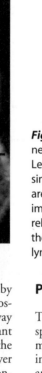

C

Figure 3–49. **(A)** Axial T1-weighted image through the neck of a young woman demonstrates a normal, left, Level IIA node (black arrows), which has a signal intensity similar to muscle. The carotid artery (C) and jugular vein (J) are indicated. **(B)** On an axial fast spin-echo T2-weighted image with fat saturation, the node is homogeneous and relatively high in signal intensity. **(C)** Postgadolinium, there is a mild and homogeneous enhancement of the lymph node on this slightly motion-degraded image.

layers of deep cervical fascia. This space is bounded by the middle layer of deep cervical fascia along its posterolateral margin, whereas on its luminal or airway side, it has no fascial boundary. The most important components of the pharyngeal mucosal space are the squamous mucosa, the lymphoid tissue of the Waldeyer ring, the minor salivary glands, and the pharyngeal constrictor muscles. The dominant pathology in this space is SCC and the pharyngeal mucosal space, divided into its traditional subdivisions of nasopharynx, oropharynx, larynx, and hypopharynx, was reviewed previously.

Parapharyngeal Space

The parapharyngeal space (PPS) is a central, fat-filled space of the deep face that is frequently displaced by masses of the surrounding spaces (Figure 3–51). Assessing the center of a deep facial mass relative to the PPS and observing the direction in which this mass displaces the fat of this space indicates the site of origin of a mass of the head and neck and helps to tailor a differential diagnosis. The PPS is defined medially by the middle layer of the deep cervical fascia and borders the pharyn-

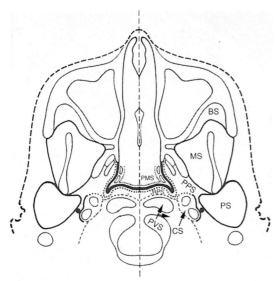

Figure 3–50. Diagrammatic representation of the fascia-defined spaces of the suprahyoid neck at the level of the nasopharynx. The dashed line represents the deep layer of deep cervical fascia, also known as the prevertebral fascia. The dotted line represents the middle layer of deep cervical fascia, and the thick solid line represents the superficial layer of deep cervical fascia, also known as the investing fascia. The heavy solid line outlining the pharyngeal mucosal space represents the pharyngobasilar fascia, which connects the superior constrictor muscle to the skull base. PMS, pharyngeal mucosal space; PPS, parapharyngeal space; MS, masticator space; PS, parotid space; CS, carotid space; RPS, retropharyngeal space; PVS, perivertebral space; BS, buccal space. (Note that the buccal space does not represent a true fascia-defined space, but is often considered as a distinct space for the purposes of anatomic localization and differential diagnosis.) (Modified and reproduced, with permission, from Harnsberger HR. CT and MRI of masses of the deep face. *Curr Probl Diagn Radiol* 1987;16:141.)

geal mucosal space. Laterally, it is defined by the superficial layer of deep cervical fascia and borders the masticator space and the parotid space. Posteriorly, the PPS is defined by the anterior part of the carotid sheath and is bordered by the carotid space. Superoinferiorly, it runs from the skull base to the hyoid bone. At its inferior extent, this space is not separated by fascia from the submandibular space, and so a process in one space may extend to the other.

The PPS contains fat, arteries, veins, and nerves; therefore, few lesions are primary to this space. Primary lesions of the parapharyngeal space include lipomas,

tumors of minor salivary rests, and atypical second branchial cleft cysts (Figure 3–52). Most lesions that appear to be primary to the PPS in fact originate from adjacent spaces and compress the PPS. Therefore, fat should be identified around the circumference of a lesion before it is said to be primary to the PPS, although peripheral fat may be difficult to identify if a lesion primary to the PPS is large. Aggressive processes that are not constrained by fascial boundaries may also involve the PPS by direct spread, notably SCC, other aggressive neoplasms (eg, sarcomas, malignant neoplasms of the salivary glands, and lymphoma; Figure 3–53), and phlegmon or abscess.

Parotid Space

The parotid space is defined by a splitting of the superficial layer of the deep cervical fascia. It abuts the masticator space anteriorly, the PPS anteromedially, the carotid space posteromedially, the temporal bone posteriorly and superiorly, and the subcutaneous fat laterally (see Figure 3–51). Its contents include the parotid gland, the facial nerve, blood vessels, and the intraparotid lymph nodes. Although the intraparotid facial nerve cannot be directly identified on cross-sectional imaging studies, it is known to lie adjacent to the retromandibular vein, and this structure serves as a rough dividing point between the

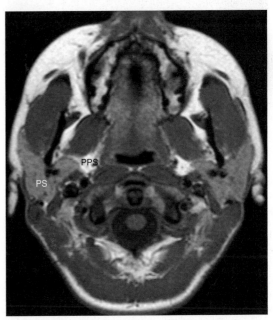

Figure 3–51. Axial T1-weighted image demonstrates high signal intensity fat in the centrally located parapharyngeal space (PPS). Also indicated is the parotid space (PS).

superficial and deep lobes of the gland. When a mass involves both the superficial and deep lobes, the distance between the mandible and the styloid process is typically widened, especially if the mass is slow growing. The parotid duct exits the anterior aspect of the parotid space, traverses the masticator space over the masseter muscle, and then pierces the buccinator muscle to enter the oral cavity at the level of the second maxillary molar.

A differential diagnosis of parotid space masses is presented in Table 3–6, and the imaging appearance of some of the more common pathologies is discussed in more detail below. It should also be noted that the presence of multiple parotid space lesions, either unilateral or bilateral, suggests a more limited differential diagnosis that includes reactive or metastatic lymphadenopathy, lymphoepithelial lesions, Warthin tumors, and recurrent pleomorphic adenoma.

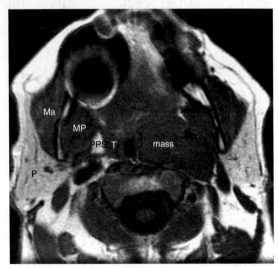

Figure 3–53. Axial T1-weighted image in a patient with lymphoma demonstrates a left oropharyngeal mass with lateral extension to obliterate the parapharyngeal fat. The normal right tonsil (T) and right parapharyngeal space (PPS) are shown for comparison. Masseter (Ma), medial pterygoid muscle (MP), and parotid gland (P) are indicated.

A. PAROTID HEMANGIOMAS

The parotid hemangioma is a vascular proliferative mass of infancy and childhood that may grow to a large size and replace the entire parotid gland before slowly involuting. The classic imaging appearance is of a multilobulated holoparotid mass that enlarges the parotid gland, is isointense to muscle on a T1-weighted image, is bright on a T2-weighted image, and enhances intensely and homogeneously postgadolinium (Figure 3–54). It usually contains prominent flow voids, and the external carotid artery and its branches are often enlarged.

B. FIRST BRANCHIAL CLEFT CYSTS

Abnormalities of the first branchial apparatus account for more than 10% of branchial complex anomalies and include cysts, sinuses, and fistulas. Typically, a cystic mass is seen within or adjacent to the parotid gland (Figure 3–55), with a tract leading to the external auditory canal visible in some cases. The cyst wall may be thickened if there has been prior infection, and adjacent soft tissues may show inflammatory change if there is active infection.

C. LYMPHOEPITHELIAL CYSTS AND LESIONS

Benign lymphoepithelial lesions are seen most commonly in association with HIV, but they also occur in

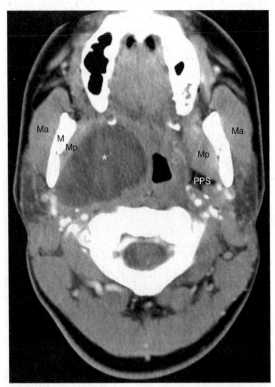

Figure 3–52. Axial contrast-enhanced CT scan demonstrates a well-circumscribed cystic lesion (*) centered on the right parapharyngeal space, deviating the airway and the pharyngeal mucosal space medially and displacing the muscles of mastication laterally. The normal left parapharyngeal space is indicated. The pathology was most consistent with a branchial cleft cyst. Ma, masseter; M, mandible; Mp, medial pterygoid; PPS, parapharyngeal space.

Table 3–6. Lesions of the parotid space.

Congenital/Developmental	Inflammatory/Infectious	Neoplastic	
		Benign	*Malignant*
Hemangioma	Parotitis or parotid abscess	Pleomorphic adenoma	Mucoepidermoid carcinoma
Venolymphatic malformation	Reactive lymphadenopathy	Warthin tumor	Adenoid cystic carcinoma
First branchial cleft cyst	Lymphoepithelial cysts or lesions	Lipoma	Acinic cell carcinoma
		Facial nerve schwannoma	Carcinoma ex pleomorphic adenoma
		Oncocytoma	Salivary ductal carcinoma
			Squamous cell carcinoma
			Extranodal or nodal non-Hodgkin lymphoma
			Nodal metastases

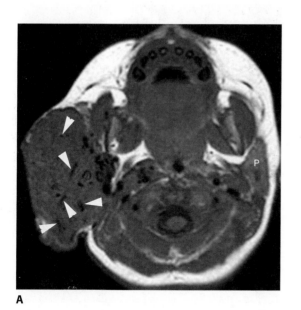

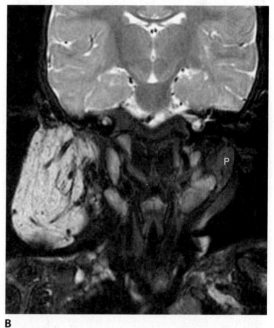

Figure 3–54. **(A)** Axial T1-weighted image in a 13-month-old female with a parotid region mass and overlying skin discoloration demonstrates a large, multilobulated, well-circumscribed mass centered on the parotid gland. Internal serpiginous hypointensities (arrowheads) are consistent with vessels. The contralateral parotid gland (P) is shown for comparison; note that the parotid gland in an infant and young child is not as fatty as in an adult and therefore not as bright on a T1-weighted image. **(B)** The mass is high in signal intensity on a T2-weighted image. Again, note the prominent vessels within the lesion. Postgadolinium (not shown), the lesion demonstrated intense and homogeneous enhancement. These imaging features are diagnostic of a parotid hemangioma.

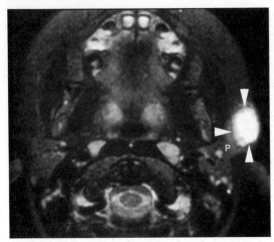

Figure 3–55. A 3-year-old girl with a left parotid-region mass and slight drainage from her external ear canal. Axial fast spin-echo T2-weighted image with fat saturation demonstrates a well-circumscribed, very high signal intensity mass (arrowheads) in the left parotid gland (P). Other images (not shown) confirmed the cystic nature of the lesion and a first branchial cleft cyst was found at surgery.

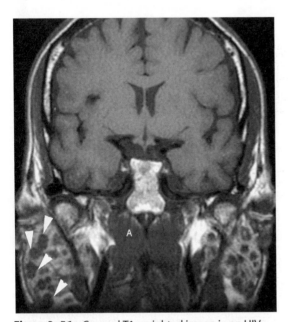

Figure 3–56. Coronal T1-weighted image in an HIV-positive patient with bilateral parotid gland enlargement demonstrates multiple small cysts (arrowheads) in both parotid glands as well as adenoidal hypertrophy (A). Findings are consistent with multiple lymphoepithelial cysts.

connective tissue disorders, notably Sjögren syndrome. In the setting of HIV, there is typically associated hypertrophy of the lymphoid tissue of Waldeyer ring (Figure 3–56) and also reactive cervical lymphadenopathy. Lesions may be purely cystic or have both cystic and solid elements, and they are typically bilateral.

D. Parotitis and Calculus Disease

Glandular enlargement, edema, and increased enhancement are seen in the setting of acute parotitis, often with inflammatory changes in adjacent fat (Figure 3–57). If the process progresses to abscess formation, a ring-enhancing mass will be present. A calculus may be identified along the parotid duct or within the gland, best detected on thin-section (1–3 mm) noncontrast CT images. The intra- or extraparotid glandular system may be dilated.

E. Pleomorphic Adenomas

The pleomorphic adenoma typically presents as a round or ovoid, well-circumscribed soft tissue mass. It may have

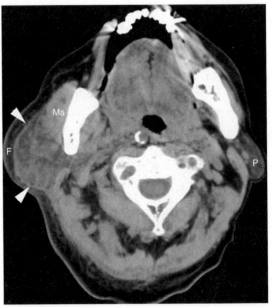

Figure 3–57. Noncontrast CT scan of the neck in an elderly patient with clinical acute parotitis demonstrates marked enlargement of the right parotid gland (arrowheads) compared with the left (P), as well as enlargement of the ipsilateral masseter muscle (Ma) and infiltration of overlying subcutaneous fat (F) due to associated myositis and cellulitis. No calculi were identified. Contrast was not administered due to the patient's underlying renal insufficiency.

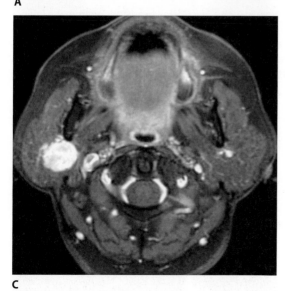

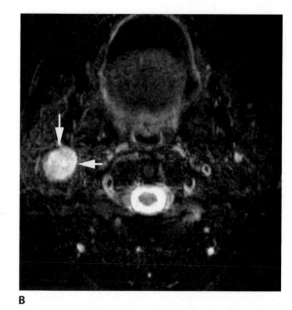

Figure 3–58. **(A)** Axial T1-weighted image in a young patient with a slowly enlarging right parotid mass shows a round, well-circumscribed lesion of intermediate signal intensity. Also indicated are the parotid glands (P), parapharyngeal space (PPS), internal jugular vein (IJV), internal carotid artery (C), lateral mass of C1 (C1), and the spinal cord (SC). **(B)** The mass is very bright on a fast spin-echo T2-weighted image with fat saturation.
(C) Following gadolinium, the lesion enhances intensely and homogeneously. These are the typical imaging features of a pleomorphic adenoma and this diagnosis was confirmed pathologically.

areas of low density on CT and is typically high signal intensity on T2-weighted MRI caused by areas of mucoid matrix or cystic degeneration (Figure 3–58). Contrast enhancement is usually intense and homogeneous, and the homogeneity typically increases over time when early and delayed postcontrast CT images are compared.

F. Warthin Tumor

A Warthin tumor is typically multilobulated, well circumscribed, and heterogeneous owing to its mixed cystic and solid nature (Figure 3–59). Areas of hemorrhage may be seen as well, and bilateral lesions are not uncommon.

G. Malignant Parotid Tumor

A low-grade malignant parotid tumor may appear well circumscribed and homogeneous, and based on imaging criteria can be difficult to distinguish from a benign lesion such as a pleomorphic adenoma. Malignant tumors do, however, tend to be somewhat lower in signal intensity on T2-weighted images than benign lesions. Higher-grade lesions are often ill marginated (Figure 3–60) and invade adjacent structures such as the temporal bone, adjacent fat, and the muscles of mastication. They may also demonstrate perineural spread proximally along the facial nerve (Figure 3–61). Note that a pregadolinium T1-weighted

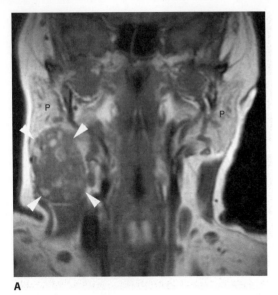
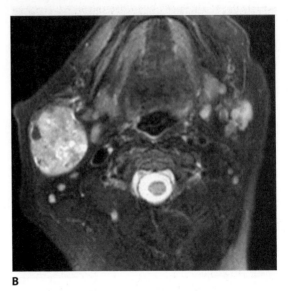

A
B

Figure 3–59. **(A)** Coronal T1-weighted image in a 55-year-old woman with a mass (arrowheads) arising from the inferior aspect of the right parotid gland (P). The lesion is well circumscribed but quite heterogeneous, with internal areas of high signal intensity representing areas of hemorrhage or proteinaceous cysts. **(B)** The lesion is hyperintense on an axial fast spin-echo T2-weighted image with fat saturation, but also somewhat heterogeneous. The heterogeneity of the lesion and the areas of intrinsic T1 shortening are suggestive of a Warthin tumor, which was confirmed pathologically.

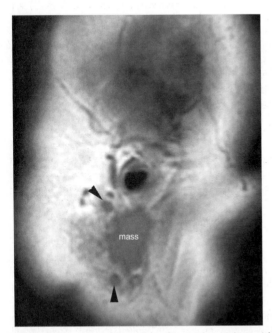

Figure 3–60. Sagittal T1-weighted image in a patient with a mucoepidermoid carcinoma of the parotid. The mass has an irregular, spiculated margin. In addition, two parotid lymph nodes (black arrowheads) are seen, which are suggestive of local metastases.

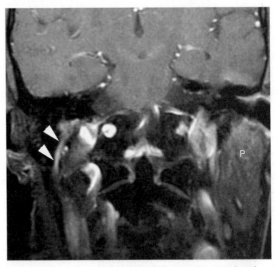

Figure 3–61. Coronal postgadolinium T1-weighted image with fat saturation in an older man who had undergone a prior right parotidectomy for carcinoma ex pleomorphic adenoma demonstrates abnormal thickening and intense enhancement of the descending mastoid segment of the right facial nerve (arrowheads), consistent with the perineural spread of disease. The normal left parotid gland (P) is indicated. The patient had a progressive right facial palsy.

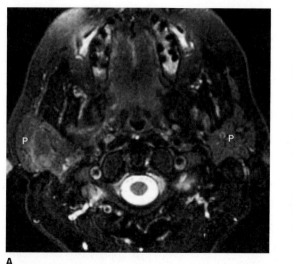 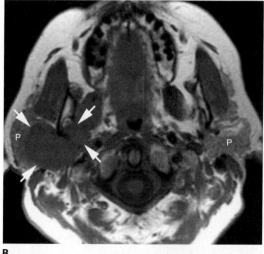

A   **B**

Figure 3–62. **(A)** Axial fast spin-echo T2-weighted image with fat saturation in a 60-year-old woman who has noted fullness in her right parotid region. Both parotid glands (P) are indicated, but the large right parotid mass is difficult to detect on this sequence. **(B)** Axial T1-weighted image demonstrates a large right parotid mass (arrows), which is easy to identify in contrast to the fatty glandular parenchyma. The low signal intensity on the T2-weighted image is suggestive of a malignant histology, and squamous cell carcinoma of the parotid gland was pathologically confirmed.

image may be the best sequence on which to identify a parotid mass as the fatty glandular parenchyma contrasts well with the intermediate signal intensity of most parotid neoplasms (Figure 3–62).

Masticator Space

The masticator space is defined by a splitting of the superficial layer of deep cervical fascia. Its coronal extent is from the inferior surface of the mandible to the skull base medially and the calvarial convexity laterally. Superomedially, the fascia attaches to the skull base just medial to the foramen ovale; superolaterally, it attaches to the zygomatic arch and then continues superiorly over the surface of the temporalis muscle, defining the suprazygomatic masticator space (Figure 3–63). The masticator space is bordered by the parapharyngeal space medially, the parotid space posteriorly, and the subcutaneous tissues laterally. Anteriorly, it abuts the buccal space. The buccal space has no true fascial boundary and is in close proximity to the masticator space, so these two spaces are often involved together by infectious or neoplastic processes. Key contents of the masticator space include the ramus and the posterior body of the mandible, the muscles of mastication (eg, the masseter, temporalis, medial pterygoid, and lateral pterygoid muscles), the motor and sensory branches of the third division of the trigeminal nerve, and the inferior alveolar vein and artery.

Lesions of the masticator space (Table 3–7) are most commonly infectious (usually of odontogenic origin) or neoplastic. In all cases of neoplastic involvement of the masticator space, V3 should be carefully assessed for evidence of perineural spread of tumor. Perineural spread, when radiologically visible, may lead to the enlargement of V3 and the foramen ovale (Figure 3–64), the asymmetric enhancement of V3 (which may extend back along the main trunk of V3 to the pons), the obliteration of fat at the extracranial aperture of the foramen ovale, and possibly the replacement of CSF in Meckel cave by abnormal soft tissue. In addition, denervation change in the muscles of mastication may be seen. In the acute and subacute phases of denervation, the muscles typically demonstrate a high signal intensity on T2-weighted images and enhancement on postgadolinium images, whereas in the more chronic phases, fatty atrophy sets in (Figure 3–65). Several "pseudomasses" of the masticator space should also be considered. Benign masseteric hypertrophy may be unilateral or bilateral and is generally seen in patients with bruxism. Accessory parotid tissue may also be unilateral or bilateral, is seen overlying the masseter muscle, and is isodense or isointense to a normal parotid gland on all imaging sequences. Denervation atrophy due to V3 injury or pathology may make the contralateral nonatrophic muscles appear masslike.

The buccal space is not a true fascia-defined compartment. It is located immediately anterior to the mas-

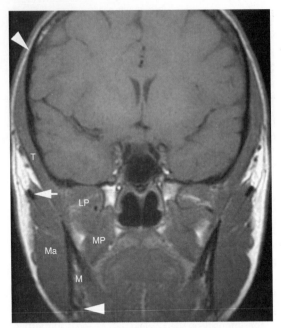

Figure 3–63. The masticator space demonstrated on a coronal T1-weighted image. The space extends from the inferior edge of the mandible below (lower white arrowhead) to the superior attachment of the temporalis muscle above (upper white arrowhead); the zygoma (white arrow) represents the inferior margin of the suprazygomatic masticator space. The mandible (M) is indicated, as are the muscles of mastication: temporalis (T), masseter (Ma), medial pterygoid (MP), and lateral pterygoid (LP).

ticator space and is often involved by extension of neoplastic or inflammatory processes from the masticator space. Important contents include the buccal fat pad, the buccinator muscle, the distal portion of the parotid duct, and the facial artery and vein. Venous malformations of the head and neck not uncommonly involve the buccal space (Figure 3–66).

A. Odontogenic Infection

Patients with an odontogenic infection usually have a history of poor dentition or recent dental manipulation. CT scanning is the study of choice and may show changes related to periodontal disease, frank mandibular osteomyelitis, and adjacent soft tissue changes with cellulitis, phlegmon, or abscess formation (Figure 3–67). CT scanning is more sensitive than MRI to calculi, foreign bodies, and gas formation.

B. Rhabdomyosarcoma

A solid mass lesion arising in the masticator space of a child is considered a rhabdomyosarcoma until proven otherwise. These lesions may appear fairly well circumscribed, although they are aggressive. They are typically isointense to muscle on T1-weighted images and intermediate in signal intensity on T2-weighted images, as is typical of small, round, blue-cell tumors owing to their high nuclear-to-cytoplasmic ratio. Postgadolinium, they enhance homogeneously or heterogeneously if areas of necrosis are present (Figure 3–68). There may be accompanying destruction of the mandible, and spread to the skull base and intracranial compartment may occur.

Carotid Space

All three layers of the deep cervical fascia contribute to the fascial boundary of the carotid space, known as the carotid sheath. The carotid space extends from the skull base to the aortic arch, and therefore spans both the supra- and the infrahyoid neck. At the level of the skull base, the carotid space communicates directly with the carotid canal and jugular foramen. The suprahyoid

Table 3–7. Lesions of the masticator space.

| Congenital/Developmental | Inflammatory/Infectious | Neoplastic | |
		Benign	*Malignant*
Hemangioma	Odontogenic infection: —Abscess —Cellulitis	Benign tumor of muscle or bone	Osteosarcoma
Venolymphatic malformation	Myositis	Nerve sheath tumor	Rhabdomyosarcoma
Masseteric hypertrophy			Non-Hodgkin lymphoma
			Deep extension of mucosal squamous cell carcinoma
			Metastatic disease

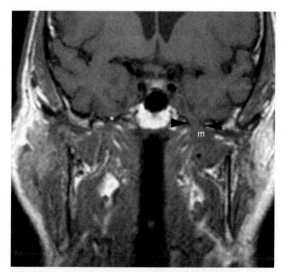

Figure 3–64. Coronal T1-weighted image in a patient with a history of carcinoma involving the left masticator space and new lower facial numbness demonstrates marked enlargement of the foramen ovale on the left (arrowheads) and a masslike enlargement of V3 (m) due to the perineural spread of tumor. The normal right foramen ovale (*) is shown for comparison.

carotid space relates laterally to the parotid space, anteriorly to the parapharyngeal space, and medially to the retropharyngeal space. Posteriorly, it borders the vertebral bodies of the cervical spine.

The contents of the carotid space include the carotid artery (common or internal, depending on the level), the internal jugular vein, the sympathetic plexus, and cranial nerves (Figure 3–69). The upper (nasopharyngeal) carotid space contains CN IX (the glossopharyngeal nerve), X (the vagus nerve), XI (the accessory nerve), and XII (the hypoglossal nerve). Only CN X traverses the oropharyngeal and infrahyoid carotid space, since the other lower cranial nerves have already exited the carotid space. CN X is typically located posteriorly between the carotid artery and the internal jugular vein, whereas the sympathetic plexus runs along the medial aspect of the carotid space. Lymph nodes are also present in the carotid space, with the highest carotid space nodes constituting the jugulodigastric nodes—or, more correctly, the upper Level IIA nodes. The most common lesions of the carotid space are vascular or neoplastic. "Pseudomasses" are typically vascular in origin and relate to the asymmetry or tortuosity of the carotid artery or the asymmetry of the jugular veins. Common lesions of the carotid space are indicated in Table 3–8.

A. PARAGANGLIOMAS

Paragangliomas arise from neuroendocrine cells of the autonomic nervous system. In the head and neck, subtypes include the carotid body tumor, the glomus vagale (arising from the nodose ganglion of the vagus nerve), the glomus jugulare (arising from the jugular ganglion), and the glomus tympanicum (arising in association with the Jacobsen nerve along the cochlear promontory). These lesions may present as a palpable neck mass or with lower cranial neuropathy, pulsatile tinnitus, or both. On CT scans, these lesions enhance intensely postcontrast. The glomus jugulare typically shows an irregular erosion of adjacent bone. On MRI, paragangliomas typically show macroscopic flow voids when they are > 2 cm and also show intense enhancement. The carotid body tumor classically splays the internal and external carotid arteries (Figure 3–70), whereas the glomus vagale displaces the internal carotid artery anteriorly (Figure 3–71). MRA and catheter angiography demonstrate a hypervascular mass, with the usual vascular supply being the ascending pharyngeal artery.

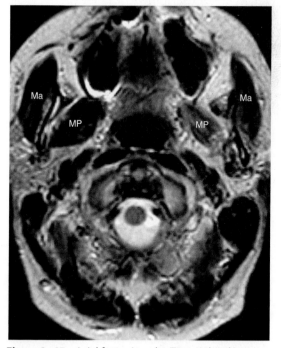

Figure 3–65. Axial fast spin-echo T2-weighted image (no fat saturation) in a patient with a left-sided perineural spread of squamous cell carcinoma along V3 demonstrates marked asymmetry of the masseter (Ma) and medial pterygoid (MP) muscles, consistent with long-standing denervation atrophy on the left.

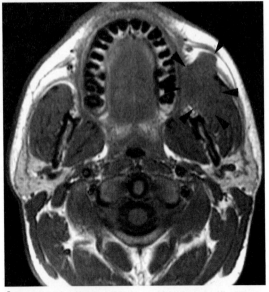

A

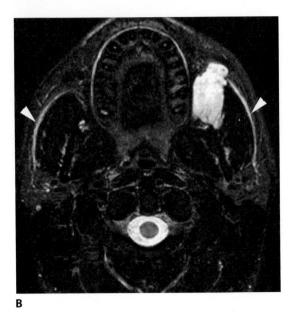

B

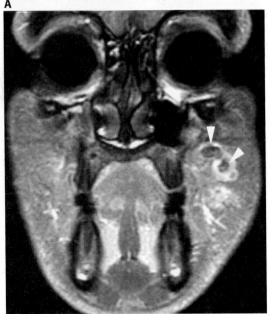

C

Figure 3–66. **(A)** Axial T1-weighted image in a young man with a soft, slowly enlarging mass of the left buccal region demonstrates a well-circumscribed, slightly lobulated soft tissue intensity mass (black arrowheads). **(B)** Axial fast spin-echo T2-weighted image with fat saturation demonstrates the lesion to be very bright. Also demonstrated are the parotid ducts bilaterally (arrowheads), running over the surface of the masseter muscles toward the buccal space. **(C)** Coronal postgadolinium T1-weighted image with fat saturation through the most anterior aspect of the lesion demonstrates two low signal intensity, rounded masses (arrowheads) within what was otherwise a homogeneously and intensely enhancing lesion. These are consistent with phleboliths, confirming the diagnosis of a venous malformation.

B. Schwannomas

Schwannomas of the lower cranial nerves may be asymptomatic and present as a neck mass or may present with lower cranial neuropathy. On imaging, these lesions are typically round or ovoid and well circumscribed (Figure 3–72). Adjacent bony structures may be smoothly remodeled but do not show infiltrative or permeative changes. Schwannomas may be homogeneous or heterogeneous owing to cyst formation and hemorrhage. They are typically moderately and homogeneously enhancing. Rarely, macroscopic flow voids may be seen in "hypervascular" schwannomas, making them difficult to distinguish from paragangliomas.

C. Squamous Cell Carcinoma

SCC may access the carotid space via direct invasion from the primary site or via nodal metastases. A pri-

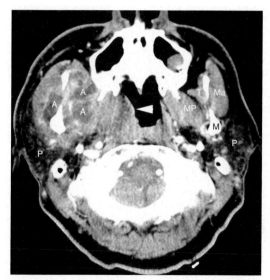

Figure 3–67. Axial contrast-enhanced CT scan of the neck in a patient with poor dentition, fever, pain, and facial swelling. Extensive abscess formation (A) is seen in the right masticator space. The normal left masticator space (M, mandible; MP, medial pterygoid; Ma, masseter; T, temporalis) is shown for comparison. The right pharyngeal wall is bowed medially, the parapharyngeal fat is obliterated, and the right parotid gland (P) is displaced posteriorly.

mary squamous carcinoma of the upper aerodigestive tract may be deeply infiltrative at the time of the first diagnosis, extending to involve the carotid artery and thereby rendering the tumor unresectable without carotid sacrifice; more commonly, recurrent disease at the primary site may infiltrate adjacent deep tissues and extend back to the carotid space. Metastases to the lymph nodes along the jugular vein (Levels II, III, and IV) are common with mucosal SCCs, and if there is extracapsular extension, the metastatic tumor may extend all the way to the skull base along the carotid sheath (Figure 3–73). New hoarseness or difficulty with articulation may be seen if CN X or XII is affected by metastatic tumor in the carotid space, and these symptoms should raise concern for recurrent disease in a patient previously treated for SCC.

D. LESIONS OF THE SYMPATHETIC CHAIN

The cervical segment of the sympathetic trunk extends from the base of the skull down to the first rib, where it becomes continuous with the thoracic segment. The cervical sympathetic chain lays posteromedial to the internal and common carotid arteries and is embedded in the deep fascia between the carotid sheath and the prevertebral fascia. Neuroblastic tumors are the third most common cause of early childhood neoplasia, and lesions originating from the

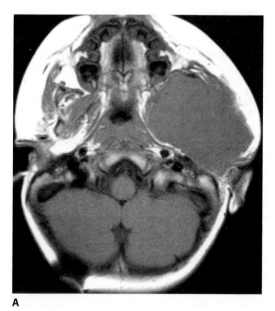

A

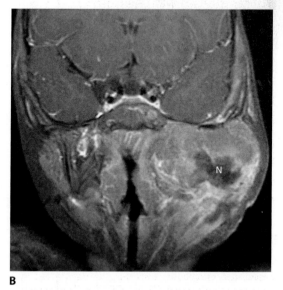

B

Figure 3–68. **(A)** Axial T1-weighted image demonstrates a large, homogeneous mass, which is isointense to muscle and centered on the left masticator space. The mandible has been largely destroyed. **(B)** Postgadolinium, a coronal T1-weighted image with fat saturation demonstrates an area of irregular central nonenhancement, consistent with necrosis (N). The lesion abuts and erodes the floor of the left middle cranial fossa, but no gross intracranial extension is seen. A rhabdomyosarcoma was confirmed pathologically.

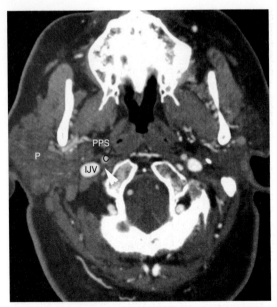

Figure 3–69. Axial contrast-enhanced CT scan of the neck demonstrates the contents of the carotid space: the internal jugular vein (IJV), carotid artery (C), and cranial nerves (arrowhead). Note that the cranial nerves cannot be individually resolved and appear as a focal soft tissue density posterior and slightly lateral to the carotid artery. Also indicated are the bordering parotid (P) and parapharyngeal (PPS) spaces.

cervical sympathetic chain account for 2–5% of neuroblastic lesions. There are three histologic subgroups, neuroblastoma, ganglioneuroblastoma, and ganglioneuroma, with neuroblastoma the least differentiated and most malignant form. A helpful diagnostic clinical feature may be the presence of Horner syndrome (Figure 3–74).

Retropharyngeal Space

The retropharyngeal space is a potential space between the middle and deep layers of the deep cervical fascia that extends from the skull base to the T4 level (Figure 3–75). Anatomically, a slip of deep cervical fascia separates the retropharyngeal space from a more posterior potential space known as the "danger space," which extends more caudally into the mediastinum and provides a conduit to this space for disease processes, notably infection. For practical purposes, however, the retropharyngeal and danger spaces are indistinguishable on imaging studies of the neck, and both are included when the retropharyngeal space is discussed. The retropharyngeal space is bordered by the pharyngeal mucosal space anteriorly, the carotid space laterally, and the danger space and prevertebral space posteriorly. The only notable contents of the retropharyngeal space are fat and lymph nodes; therefore, the retropharyngeal space is usually affected by the direct spread of tumor or infection or by the spread of tumor or infection to retropharyngeal lymph nodes. The extension of tumor beyond the confines of a retropharyngeal node may lead to skull base invasion and lower cranial nerve dysfunction, whereas the extension of infection beyond the nodal capsule may lead to retropharyngeal abscess formation.

The lateral retropharyngeal nodes are present at the level of the nasopharynx and upper oropharynx and are seen well on MRI even when nondiseased (Figure 3–76). The medial retropharyngeal nodes are present from the nasopharynx to the hypopharynx, but no retropharyngeal nodes are found below the level of the hyoid bone. Retropharyngeal lymph nodes are normally quite prominent in children and gradually decrease in size. In adults, normal retropharyngeal nodes are typically < 6 mm in short-axis dimension.

A. PYOGENIC INFECTION

Retropharyngeal nodes are commonly involved with infection in the context of pharyngitis in children and spine infections in adults. With infection, the nodes

Table 3–8. Lesions of the carotid space.

| Vascular | Inflammatory/Infectious | Neoplastic | |
		Benign	Malignant
Internal jugular vein thrombosis	Abscess	Paraganglioma	Neuroblastoma
Carotid artery thrombosis		Schwannoma	Non-Hodgkin lymphoma
Carotid artery aneurysm or pseudoaneurysm		Meningioma (from posterior fossa via the jugular foramen)	Direct extension of mucosal squamous cell carcinoma
			Nodal metastases

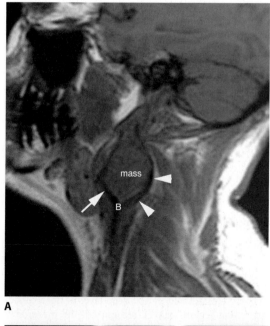

A

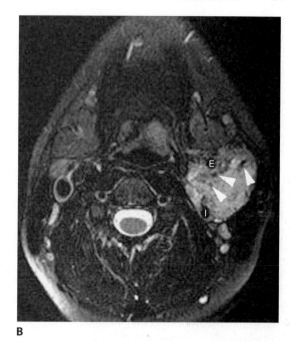

B

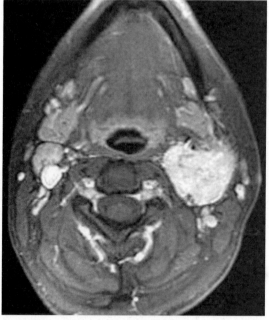

C

Figure 3–70. **(A)** Sagittal T1-weighted image demonstrates a soft tissue mass arising at the level of the carotid bifurcation (B) and displacing the internal carotid artery posteriorly (arrowheads) and the external carotid artery anteriorly (arrow). **(B)** The mass is mildly bright on an axial fast spin-echo T2-weighted image with fat saturation and also demonstrates prominent vessels (arrowheads). The internal carotid artery (I) is displaced posteriorly and the external carotid artery (E) is displaced anteriorly. **(C)** Postgadolinium, the mass enhances intensely and homogeneously. These findings are classic for a carotid body tumor.

initially enlarge and may eventually suppurate. As the infection progresses, the retropharyngeal fat becomes edematous because of retropharyngeal cellulitis, and if the nodal capsule ruptures, a retropharyngeal abscess develops (Figure 3–77). A CT scan should be performed if there is concern for a retropharyngeal abscess, since these patients generally require surgical drainage and intravenous antibiotics. In some cases, the retropharyngeal space may simply be filled with noninfected fluid (retropharyngeal edema) owing to jugular venous or lymphatic obstruction, prior radiation therapy, or noninfectious inflammatory processes; it is therefore

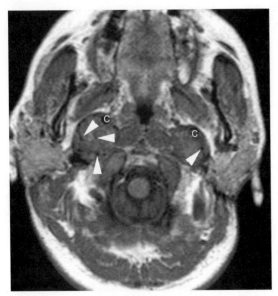

Figure 3–71. Axial T1-weighted image in a patient with bilateral glomus vagale tumors demonstrates round, well-circumscribed soft tissue masses displacing the internal carotid arteries (C) anteriorly. Prominent flow voids (arrowheads) are seen within both lesions.

important to distinguish retropharyngeal edema from retropharyngeal infection (Figure 3–78), as this will influence patient management.

B. Neoplasms

Retropharyngeal nodal metastases are most commonly seen with nasopharyngeal carcinoma and with SCC of the posterior oropharyngeal wall and hypopharynx. Non-Hodgkin lymphoma of the Waldeyer ring also commonly leads to neoplastic enlargement of the retropharyngeal nodes. The retropharyngeal space may also be involved with direct extension of a primary tumor from the pharyngeal mucosal space, the carotid space, or the vertebral column and perivertebral space.

Perivertebral Space

The space around the spinal column has generally been referred to as the prevertebral space, but an argument has been made to adopt the more encompassing term perivertebral space. Within the perivertebral space, enclosed and defined by the deep layer of deep cervical fascia, two regions can be recognized: the prevertebral and the paraspinal portions of the perivertebral space. The prevertebral portion is defined by the deep layer of the deep cervical fascia as it arches from one transverse process to the other transverse process in front of the

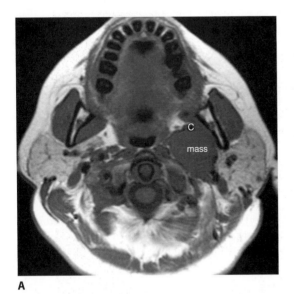

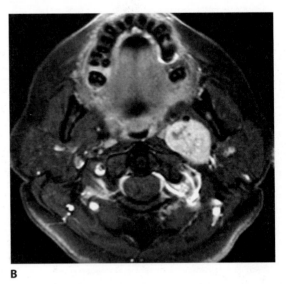

A   **B**

Figure 3–72. **(A)** Axial T1-weighted image demonstrates a well-circumscribed, homogeneous mass arising from the left carotid space, displacing the left internal carotid artery (C) anteriorly. No vessels are seen within the lesion. **(B)** Postgadolinium, the lesion enhances intensely. A few small areas of nonenhancement most likely represent small areas of cystic degeneration, as flow voids should have been seen on the T1-weighted image. The diagnosis of schwannoma was favored and was confirmed pathologically.

vertebral body, enclosing the prevertebral muscles as well as the vertebral artery, the vertebral vein, and the vertebral body. The paraspinal portion is defined by the deep layer of deep cervical fascia, extending back on each side from the transverse process to the nuchal ligament in the midline; it therefore includes only the paraspinal muscles, the posterior elements of the vertebra, and fat. The prevertebral portion of the perivertebral space is bordered by the retropharyngeal and danger spaces anteriorly and the carotid space anterolaterally. A mass in the prevertebral portion of the perivertebral space displaces the retropharyngeal space anteriorly; if the lesion is primary to the vertebral body, it also displaces the prevertebral muscles anteriorly, confirming its localization to the prevertebral portion of the perivertebral space.

The perivertebral space is most commonly involved by infectious processes originating from the vertebral bodies and the intervertebral discs (Figure 3–79), and neoplasia of the spinal column—most commonly metastatic disease, but also primary bone tumors and hematologic processes such as leukemia and myeloma (Figure 3–80). Because the deep layer of the deep cervical fascia is very tough and resists violation by tumor and infection, it is unusual for retropharyngeal space processes to extend into the perivertebral space, and vice versa.

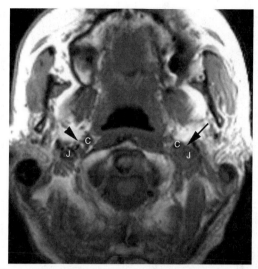

Figure 3–73. Axial T1-weighted image in a patient with recurrent squamous cell carcinoma and new cranial neuropathy demonstrates abnormal soft tissue (black arrow) infiltrating the left carotid space between the internal carotid artery (C) and a thrombosed jugular vein (J). Normal fat between the vessels (arrowhead) is demonstrated on the contralateral side. Fine-needle aspiration confirmed squamous cell carcinoma in the carotid sheath.

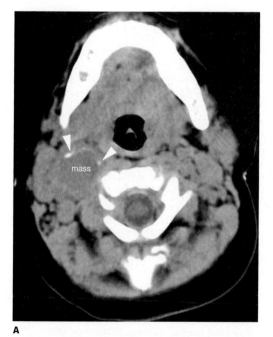

A

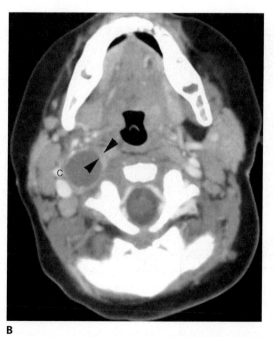

B

Figure 3–74. **(A)** A noncontrast CT scan of the neck in a 9-month-old girl with a neck mass and Horner syndrome demonstrates a relatively low-density lesion with some peripheral calcification (arrowheads). **(B)** Postcontrast, the mass is seen to be located medial to the internal carotid artery (C) in the right carotid space. The mass appears of low density and possibly cystic, but with some irregular thickness to its wall (black arrowheads). Fine-needle aspiration confirmed neuroblastoma.

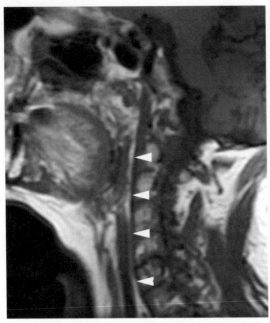

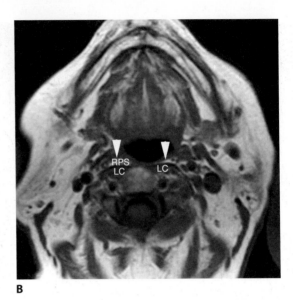

Figure 3–75. **(A)** Sagittal T1-weighted image demonstrates a hyperintense stripe of retropharyngeal fat in this slightly off-midline image. **(B)** Axial T1-weighted image demonstrates fat in the retropharyngeal space (RPS, arrowheads), which lies just anterior to the prevertebral muscles (longus colli [LC]).

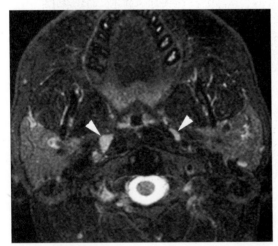

Figure 3–76. Normal, nonenlarged lateral retropharyngeal lymph nodes (arrowheads) are well seen on this axial fast spin-echo T2-weighted image with fat saturation.

Posterior Cervical Space

The posterior cervical space has complex fascial margins and is defined by both superficial and deep layers of the deep cervical fascia. It extends from the skull base to the clavicle, spanning the supra- and infrahyoid neck, but having a relatively small suprahyoid segment. It abuts the carotid space anteriorly, the perivertebral space medially, and the sternocleidomastoid muscle and subcutaneous fat laterally. Its suprahyoid contents include fat, cranial nerve XI, and lymph nodes in Levels II and V. Pathology in the posterior cervical space is most commonly nodal (Figure 3–81).

Babbel RW, Harnsberger HR. The parapharyngeal space: the key to unlocking the suprahyoid neck. *Semin Ultrasound CT MR.* 1990;11:444. [PMID: 2275807] (Reviews important anatomic relationships of this centrally located space.)

Chong VF, Fan YF. Pictorial review: radiology of the carotid space. *Clin Radiol.* 1996;51:762. [PMID: 8937318] (Illustrates the imaging features of carotid space lesions.)

Davis WL, Harnsberger HR, Smoker WR, Watanabe AS. Retropharyngeal space: evaluation of normal anatomy and diseases with CT and MR imaging. *Radiology.* 1990;174:59. [PMID: 2294573] (The review addresses the spectrum of lesions of the retropharyngeal space, the imaging features that mark a lesion as originating in this space, and whether there is a dif-

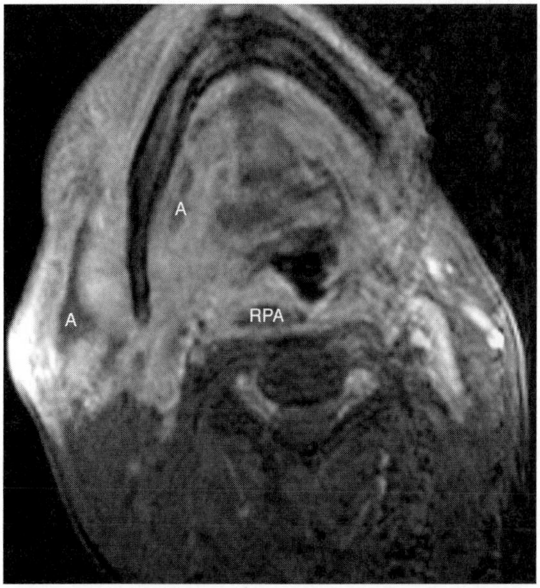

A

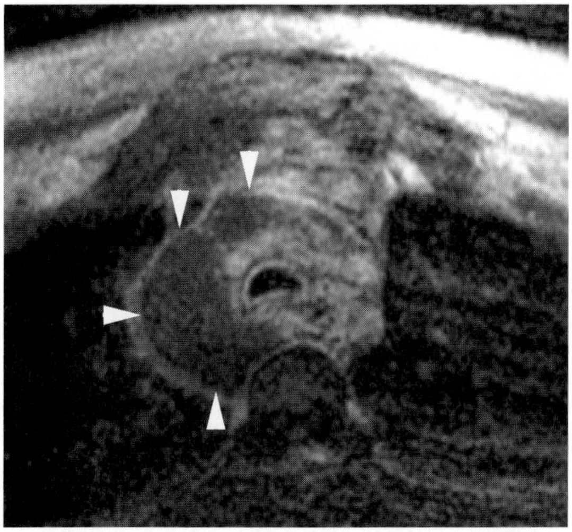

B

Figure 3–77. **(A)** Axial postgadolinium T1-weighted image with fat saturation in a young male with diabetes and extensive neck infection shows abnormal enhancement throughout the right masticator space, oral cavity, and parapharyngeal space. Focal areas of abscess formation are present (A), including in the retropharyngeal space (RPA). **(B)** Postgadolinium image through the upper mediastinum demonstrates the inferior extension of the process and a large mediastinal abscess (arrowheads).

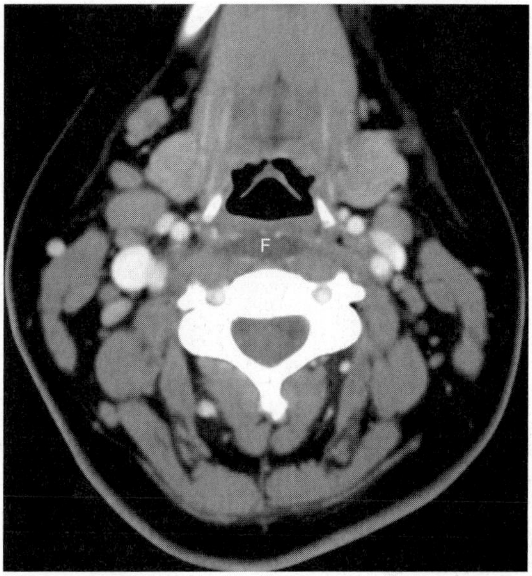

A

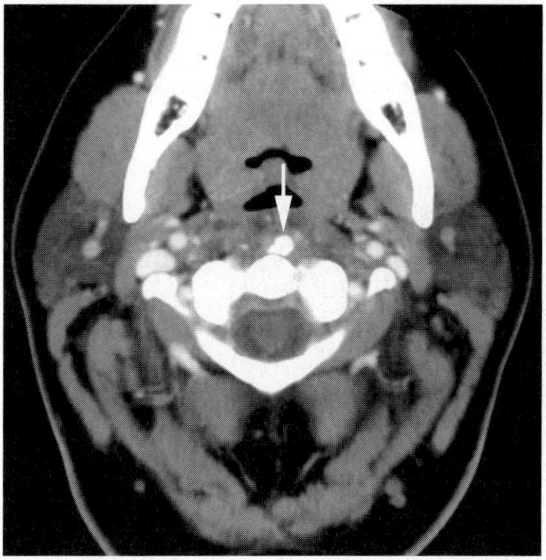

B

Figure 3–78. **(A)** Axial contrast-enhanced CT scan of the neck in a young woman with 5 days of torticollis, odynophagia, a low-grade fever, and a slightly elevated white blood cell count demonstrates a fluid collection (F) in the retropharyngeal space. A few displaced contrast-enhancing vessels are seen around the collection, but the peripheral enhancement that might be expected with a retropharyngeal abscess is not present. **(B)** Axial image at a more cephalad level demonstrates an irregular calcification anterior to the C2 vertebral body, consistent with calcific tendinitis of the longus colli muscle. The fluid collection seen in part A represents an associated retropharyngeal effusion.

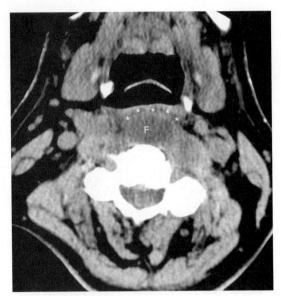

Figure 3–79. Axial noncontrast CT scan of the neck in a patient with known cervical vertebral diskitis and osteomyelitis demonstrates a prevertebral fluid collection (F) displacing the retropharyngeal fat stripe (*) anteriorly. A prevertebral abscess was drained transcervically.

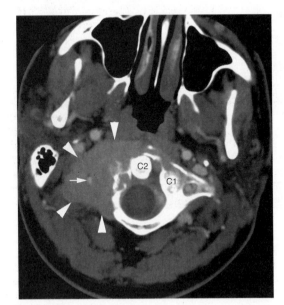

Figure 3–80. Axial contrast-enhanced CT scan of the neck demonstrates a large soft tissue mass (arrowheads) arising from and destroying the right lateral mass of the C1 vertebral body. The mass encases the right vertebral artery (small white arrow) and displaces the right prevertebral muscle and retropharyngeal fat anteriorly. The pathology demonstrated a plasmacytoma.

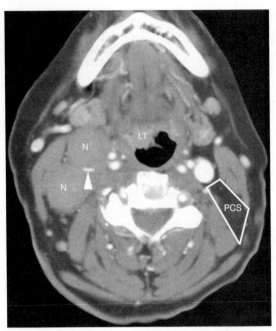

Figure 3–81. Axial contrast-enhanced CT scan of the neck in a patient with lymphoma and multiple enlarged cervical lymph nodes (N) in the right neck. The right lingual tonsil (LT) is also somewhat prominent. The right jugular vein (arrowhead) is severely compressed. The normal fat-filled posterior cervical space (PCS) is outlined on the left.

ference between the radiologic pattern of the suprahyoid and infrahyoid portions of the neck.)

Davis WL, Harnsberger HR. CT and MRI of the normal and diseased perivertebral space. *Neuroradiology.* 1995;37:388. [PMID: 7477840] (A retrospective analysis of patients with lesions in the perivertebral space to identify the imaging features that mark a lesion as originating in the perivertebral space and to define the spectrum of pathology that occurs in this space.)

Moukheiber AK, Nicollas R, Roman S, Coze C, Triglia JM. Primary pediatric neuroblastic tumors of the neck. *Int J Pediatr Otorhinolaryngol.* 2001;60:155. [PMID: 11518594] (Reviews clinical, imaging, and management issues related to pediatric cervical neuroblastic tumors.)

Mukherji SK, Castillo M. A simplified approach to the spaces of the suprahyoid neck. *Radiol Clin North Am.* 1998;36:761. [PMID: 9747188] (This article presents a simplified approach to the various spaces of the suprahyoid neck and their anatomic components. Each space is discussed separately and is accompanied by a table that lists a differential diagnosis based primarily on the normal anatomic contents of the space.)

Pollei SR, Harnsberger HR. The radiologic evaluation of the parotid space. *Semin Ultrasound CT MR.* 1990;11:486. [PMID: 2275810] (Reviews the radiologic anatomy and appearance of pathology of the parotid space.)

Tart RP, Kotzur IM, Mancuso AA, Glantz MS, Mukherji SK. CT and MR imaging of the buccal space and buccal space masses.

Radiographics. 1995;15:531. [PMID: 7624561] (Reviews the imaging anatomy and pathology of the buccal space.)

Tryhus MR, Smoker WR, Harnsberger HR. The normal and diseased masticator space. *Semin Ultrasound CT MR.* 1990;11:476. [PMID: 2275809] (Reviews the radiologic anatomy and pathology of the masticator space.)

2. Infrahyoid Neck

As in the suprahyoid neck, the infrahyoid neck is cleaved into a series of spaces by the three layers of the deep cervical fascia. These spaces are illustrated in Figure 3–82. There are five major spaces of the infrahyoid neck, four of which also traverse the suprahyoid neck, and their suprahyoid segments have already been discussed: the carotid space, the retropharyngeal space, the perivertebral space, and the posterior cervical space. Only the visceral space is unique to the infrahyoid neck.

Visceral Space

The visceral space extends from the hyoid bone to the mediastinum, and its circumference is defined by the middle layer of deep cervical fascia. This complex space contains the thyroid and parathyroid glands, the larynx and trachea, the hypopharynx and esophagus, the recurrent laryngeal nerves, and visceral (Level VI) lymph nodes.

Infrahyoid Carotid Space

The infrahyoid carotid space includes the common carotid artery, the internal jugular vein, the vagus nerve, and the sympathetic chain. Level III and IV lymph nodes are intimately associated with the infrahyoid carotid space, although they do not lie within the fascial boundaries of this space. The infrahyoid carotid space apposes the visceral space anteromedially, the perivertebral space posteromedially, and the posterior cervical space posterolaterally.

Infrahyoid Posterior Cervical Space

As in the suprahyoid neck, the infrahyoid posterior cervical space has complex fascial boundaries derived from the superficial and deep layers of the deep cervical fascia, as well as the posterior aspect of the carotid sheath. It contains primarily fat and lymph nodes, but the trunks of the brachial plexus also traverse the posterior cervical space. This space is most commonly involved with nodal pathology.

Infrahyoid Retropharyngeal Space

The only significant difference between the supra- and infrahyoid retropharyngeal space is that the infrahyoid

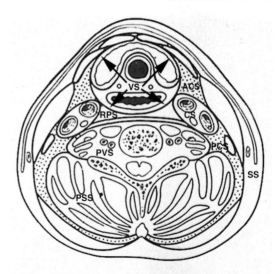

Figure 3–82. Major spaces of the infrahyoid neck. Visceral space (VS; black arrows), retropharyngeal space (RPS), perivertebral space with prevertebral (PVS) and paraspinal (PSS) compartments, and posterior cervical space (PCS). Also indicated are two minor spaces, the fat-filled anterior cervical space (ACS) and the fat-filled superficial space (SS). (Modified and borrowed, with permission, from Smoker WR, Harnsberger HR. Differential diagnosis of head and neck lesions based on their space of origin. 2. The infrahyoid portion of the neck. *AJR Am J Roentgenol* 1991;157:155.)

retropharyngeal space contains only fat, whereas the suprahyoid retropharyngeal space also contains lymph nodes. There are, therefore, almost no processes that are primary to the infrahyoid retropharyngeal space, except, occasionally, lipoma. Pathology in the retropharyngeal space, whether inflammatory, infectious, or neoplastic, accesses this space either by direct extension from adjacent spaces across fascial boundaries or by inferior extension of a process centered in the suprahyoid retropharyngeal space.

Infrahyoid Perivertebral Space

The infrahyoid perivertebral space also occurs as two distinct areas, the prevertebral and the paraspinal portions of the perivertebral space, which are enclosed by the deep layer of deep cervical fascia. In the infrahyoid neck, in addition to the prevertebral muscles and vertebral vessels, the prevertebral portion of the perivertebral space contains the phrenic nerve, the scalene muscles, and the roots of the brachial plexus. The roots of the brachial plexus actually pierce the deep layer of deep cervical fascia on their way to the posterior cervical space.

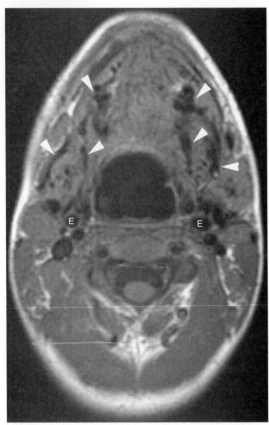

Figure 3–83. Axial T1-weighted image in a 6-year-old girl with a submental vascular malformation demonstrates marked enlargement of the external carotid arteries (E) bilaterally, as well as multiple large flow voids (arrowheads) throughout the submandibular and sublingual spaces bilaterally. No associated soft tissue mass was seen and angiography (not shown) confirmed extensive arteriovenous malformation.

Babbel RW, Smoker WR, Harnsberger HR. The visceral space: the unique infrahyoid space. *Semin Ultrasound CT MR.* 1991;12:204. [PMID: 1892686] (Reviews the anatomy and pathology of the visceral space.)

Fruin ME, Smoker WR, Harnsberger HR. The carotid space of the infrahyoid neck. *Semin Ultrasound CT MR.* 1991;12:224. [PMID: 1892687] (Reviews the anatomy and pathology of the infrahyoid carotid space.)

Shah RR, Lewin JS. Imaging of the infrahyoid neck. *Neuroimaging Clin N Am.* 1998;8:219. [PMID: 9449762] (Reviews the complex anatomy and pathology of the infrahyoid neck with updated imaging techniques.)

Smoker WR. Normal anatomy of the infrahyoid neck: an overview. *Semin Ultrasound CT MR.* 1991;12:192. [PMID: 1892685] (Reviews the complex anatomy and pathology of the infrahyoid neck.)

3. Trans-Spatial Masses

Some pathologies classically involve multiple spaces and can be considered within a unique group of multispatial or "trans-spatial" processes. These are typically lesions of structures that normally pass from one space to another, such as blood vessels, lymphatics, and nerves. Although aggressive infectious or neoplastic processes may also traverse spatial boundaries, they do so by virtue of their destructive nature rather than as a consequence of the tissue of origin. The entities that commonly present as trans-spatial processes include capillary hemangiomas, vascular malformations (venous or arteriovenous), lymphatic malformations, and plexiform neurofibromas. The latter are typically seen in patients with neurofibromatosis type I.

The soft tissue vascular lesions of the head and neck fall into two categories: hemangiomas and vascular malformations. The term *hemangioma* should be limited to vascular lesions of infancy, which grow rapidly in early infancy and then undergo fatty replacement and involution by adolescence. Vascular malformations result from abnormal blood or lymphatic vessel morphogenesis and are classified by the predominant type of vessel involved (ie, capillary, venous, lymphatic, or arteriovenous malformations). Hemangiomas are typically an intermediate signal intensity on T1-weighted images, bright on T2-weighted images, and enhance intensely postgadolinium (see Figure 3–54, parotid hemangioma). Flow voids may be seen within larger lesions and feeding arteries may be enlarged. As hemangiomas involute, they may show an increasingly high signal on T1-weighted images due to fatty replacement. In patients with a large, segmental, plaque-type facial hemangiomas, PHACE syndrome should be considered. PHACE is an acronym coined to describe a neurocutaneous syndrome that encompasses the following features: **p**osterior fossa malformations, large facial **h**emangiomas, **a**rterial anomalies, **c**ardiac anomalies and aortic coarctation, and **e**ye abnormalities. Children at risk should receive careful ophthalmologic, cardiac, and neurologic assessments. Venous malformations have similar signal characteristics, but are typically multilobulated and contain venous lakes and also rounded calcifications (phleboliths). (See Figure 3–66, venous malformation of the buccal space.) Venous malformations are not high-flow lesions and do not demonstrate enlargement of feeding vessels or internal flow voids. Lymphatic malformations are discussed later in this chapter in Cystic Neck Masses. Arteriovenous malformations have serpiginous signal voids and lack a dominant mass (Figure 3–83).

Baker LL, Dillon WP, Hieshima GB, Dowd CF, Frieden IJ. Hemangiomas and vascular malformations of the head and neck: MRI characterization. *Am J. Neuroradiol.* 1993;14:307.

[PMID: 8456703] (Characterizes the MRI appearance of a common hemangioma of infancy as well as the low- and high-flow vascular malformations of the head and neck.)

Metry DW, Dowd CF, Barkovich AJ, Frieden IJ. The many faces of PHACE syndrome. *J Pediatr.* 2001;139:117. [PMID: 11445804] (Reviews the spectrum of anomalies encountered with the PHACE syndrome.)

Mulliken JB, Glowacki J. Hemangiomas and vascular malformations in infants and children: a classification based on endothelial characteristics. *Plast Reconstr Surg.* 1982;69:412. [PMID: 7063565] (A classic paper that clarifies the categorization of hemangiomas versus vascular malformations. A cell-oriented analysis provides a useful classification of vascular lesions of infancy and childhood and serves as a guide for the diagnosis, management, and further research.)

Vogelzang P, Harnsberger HR, Smoker WR. Multispatial and trans-spatial diseases of the extracranial head and neck. *Semin Ultrasound CT MR.* 1991;12:274. [PMID: 1892690] (Reviews the imaging and differential diagnosis of multispatial processes of the head and neck.)

4. Thyroid & Parathyroid

Thyroid

The thyroid gland consists of right and left lobes connected across the midline by a narrow isthmus. A pyramidal lobe is frequently present, projecting upward from the isthmus and in some cases connecting to the hyoid bone via a fibrous or muscular band. The thyroid is a highly vascular organ that is supplied mainly by the superior and inferior thyroid arteries, the former a branch of the external carotid artery and the latter a branch of the thyrocervical trunk. Because of its high iodine concentration, the thyroid gland is intrinsically dense on a noncontrast CT scan (Figure 3–84). Following the administration of iodinated contrast material or

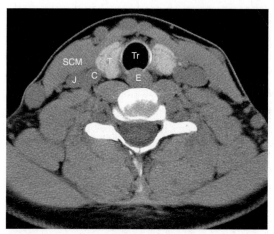

Figure 3–84. Axial noncontrast CT scan of the neck demonstrates the intrinsic high density of the thyroid gland (T). Also shown are the esophagus (E), trachea (Tr), common carotid artery (C), internal jugular vein (J), and sternocleidomastoid muscle (SCM).

gadolinium, the normal thyroid gland enhances homogeneously (Figure 3–85).

Nonspecific, incidental thyroid lesions such as cysts and adenomas are very commonly seen on cross-sectional imaging studies. The primary evaluation of a thyroid mass is typically done with ultrasound and nuclear medicine scanning, with CT scanning or MRI reserved to assess the extent of a process and evaluate the rest of the neck. If there is a concern about possible thyroid carcinoma, then the cross-sectional imaging evaluation should be done with a noncontrast CT scan or, ideally,

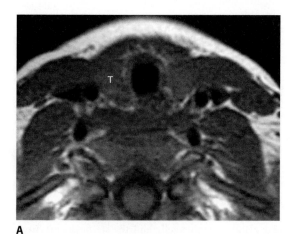

A

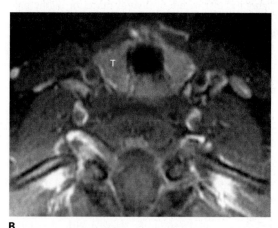

B

Figure 3–85. Axial T1-weighted image of the neck before **(A)** and after **(B)** the administration of gadolinium demonstrates homogeneous enhancement of the thyroid gland (T) following contrast administration.

gadolinium-enhanced MRI. Because the thyroid gland concentrates iodine, the bolus of iodinated contrast material that is given during a CT scan of the neck can take many months to clear from a patient's system and can delay radioiodine therapy for as long as 6 months.

A. Benign Thyroid Lesions

Benign thyroid lesions include goiter, colloid cyst, and adenoma. The goiter appears on the CT scan or MRI as a diffuse or multinodular enlargement of the gland, often with areas of heterogeneous density on CT scan and intensity on MRI. Dramatic enlargement of the gland may result in the displacement and compression of vital structures such as the trachea (Figure 3–86). A colloid cyst is a well-circumscribed cystic lesion that may appear bright on a pregadolinium T1-weighted image owing to an elevated protein content or hemorrhagic contents. A thyroid adenoma is a generally well-circumscribed mass that may have areas of calcification, hemorrhage, or cystic degeneration within it; adenomas are indistinguishable from low-grade thyroid carcinomas on the basis of imaging alone.

B. Thyroid Carcinoma

Thyroid carcinoma has a number of pathologic subtypes that are generally not distinguishable from one another on imaging studies (Figure 3–87). Less aggressive carcinomas generally present as well-circumscribed masses, whereas more aggressive lesions such as anaplastic carcinomas are highly invasive and destructive of adjacent tissues. Of note, the nodal metastases of thyroid carcinoma may appear cystic and metastatic thyroid cancer should be included in the differential diagnosis of a cystic neck mass. Because these nodal metastases may be either hemorrhagic because of the highly vascular nature of thyroid cancer or highly proteinaceous because of their thyroglobulin content, they may show a high signal intensity on a pregadolinium T1-weighted image (Figure 3–88). This appearance is highly suggestive of metastatic thyroid cancer.

Parathyroid

The parathyroid glands are ovoid bodies measuring approximately 6 mm long that are intimately related to the posterior border of the thyroid gland and lie within its fascial capsule. There are typically two superior and two inferior parathyroid glands, but in some cases, a parathyroid gland may be found some distance caudal to the gland, in association with the inferior thyroid veins or even in the superior mediastinum. Parathyroid pathology is most commonly assessed with ultrasound and with nuclear medicine scanning (sestamibi). The normal glands are usually not identified on a CT scan or MRI and are identified only when pathologically

enlarged, typically by parathyroid adenoma. A pathologically enlarged parathyroid gland may look very similar to a lymph node on a CT scan, but on MRI, the parathyroid adenoma is typically high in signal on T2-weighted images, which is a helpful feature.

Loevner LA. Imaging of the thyroid gland. *Semin Ultrasound CT MR.* 1996;17:539. [PMID: 9023867] (The embryology, anatomy, and physiology of the thyroid are discussed; congenital, autoimmune, inflammatory, metabolic, and neoplastic diseases are reviewed; and the diagnostic utility of various radiologic imaging modalities is addressed.)

Loevner LA. Imaging of the parathyroid glands. *Semin Ultrasound CT MR.* 1996;17:563. [PMID: 9023868] (The embryology, anatomy, and physiology of the parathyroid glands are reviewed. The diagnostic utility of radiologic imaging is discussed, particularly as it pertains to the evaluation of primary hyperparathyroidism.)

Yousem DM, Huang T, Loevner LA, Langlotz CP. Clinical and economic impact of incidental thyroid lesions found with CT and MR. *Am J Neuroradiol.* 1997;18:1423. [PMID: 9296181] (Incidental thyroid lesions are frequently present and often overlooked on cross-sectional images of the neck in patients being examined for other reasons. The cost of pursuing a workup of these lesions and their high prevalence in the population raise questions regarding appropriate management strategies.)

5. Cystic Neck Masses

The identification of a neck mass as cystic presents a limited differential diagnosis and often permits the differential considerations to be narrowed to a list of one or several entities when the specific clinical, CT scan, or MRI features are taken into consideration. A list of the more common cystic neck masses is presented in Table 3–9. To be considered in this differential, a mass should be of fluid density or intensity and lack enhancement. The mass should have a thin, regular rim, although prior infection may lead to thickening of the wall. It is important to note that hemorrhage into a cyst or increased protein content within a cyst may affect its density or intensity. Some lesions that are not truly cystic may mimic a cystic neck mass because of central nonenhancement—notably, a thrombosed jugular vein, a thrombosed aneurysm or pseudoaneurysm, or a necrotic mass with a nonenhancing center.

Pathology

A. Branchial Cleft Cysts

The second branchial apparatus accounts for 95% of all branchial cleft anomalies. On a CT scan or MRI, a unilocular cystic mass is seen displacing the submandibular gland anteromedially and the sternocleidomastoid muscle posterolaterally (Figure 3–89). In some cases, a "beak" pointing between the internal and external carotid arteries will be identified and, very rarely, a tract leading to the tonsillar fossa will also be identified. A sinus tract or fistula extending inferiorly in the neck to drain just above the clavicle may also be identified (Figure 3–90). If infection has occurred in the past, the cyst wall may show thickening and enhancement. If the infection is active, there may also be inflammatory changes in adjacent soft tissues.

B. Thyroglossal Duct Cysts

During embryogenesis, the thyroid anlage descends from the level of the foramen cecum at the tongue base to its normal position in the infrahyoid neck. Thyroid elements may remain at any level along this pathway (the thyroglossal duct) and may give rise to cysts, fistulas, or solid nodules of thyroid tissue. Thyroglossal duct cysts are usually located at or just below the hyoid bone, in which case a midline or paramedian cystic mass that is embedded in the strap muscles is seen (Figure 3–91). There is typically no associated enhancement unless prior or active infection has occurred. In some cases, carcinoma may arise within a thyroglossal duct cyst;

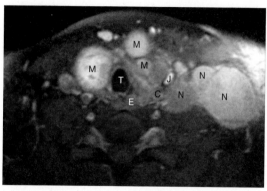

Figure 3–87. Axial postgadolinium T1-weighted image with fat saturation demonstrates multiple lobulated enhancing masses (M) in the thyroid gland and multiple nodal masses (N) lateral to the carotid artery (C) and jugular vein (J). No invasion of the trachea (T) or esophagus (E) is seen. Fine-needle aspiration confirmed papillary carcinoma of the thyroid with multiple nodal metastases.

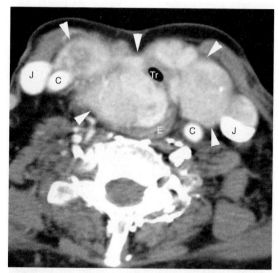

Figure 3–86. Axial contrast-enhanced CT scan of the neck in an elderly woman with a gradually enlarging neck mass demonstrates massive enlargement of a heterogeneously enhancing thyroid gland (arrowheads). There is maintenance of a smooth margin, however, and no evidence of any invasion of adjacent structures. No abnormal lymph nodes are identified. Adjacent structures are displaced and compressed by this large mass, notably, the trachea (Tr), esophagus (E), and carotid (C) and jugular (J) vessels. The surgical pathology confirmed diffuse goiter.

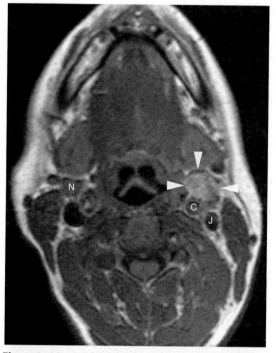

Figure 3–88. Axial T1-weighted image in a young woman who presented with an enlarged left Level IIA lymph node (arrowheads) demonstrates that the node is intrinsically bright. Compare a normal intermediate signal intensity node on the right (N). Fine-needle aspiration confirmed metastatic papillary carcinoma of the thyroid. Also shown are the carotid artery (C) and jugular vein (J).

Table 3–9. Cystic lesions of the neck.

| Congenital/Developmental | Infectious/Inflammatory | Neoplastic | | Miscellaneous |
		Benign	*Malignant*	
Branchial cleft cyst	Ranula	Cystic schwannoma	Cystic nodal metastases	Saccular cyst
Thyroglossal duct cyst	Necrotic lymphadenopathy		Cystic thyroid carcinoma	
Lymphatic malformation	Abscess			
Epidermoid or dermoid				
Foregut cyst				

clues to this include the presence of calcification and solid tissue components.

C. LYMPHATIC MALFORMATIONS

Lymphatic malformations, also known as cystic hygromas or lymphangiomas, result from the maldevelopment of lymphatic vessels and the failure of these abnormal vessels to communicate with normal lymphatic drainage channels. This leads to a fluid-filled mass that is characteristically multilobulated and multiloculated. The lymphatic malformation may involve multiple spaces, but most commonly involves the posterior cervical space. These lesions are typically of low density on CT scans, but are often heterogeneous in signal intensity on T1- and T2-weighted MRI sequences because of their variable protein content and

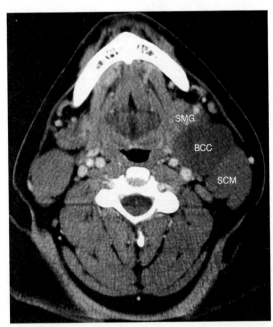

Figure 3–89. Axial contrast-enhanced CT scan of the neck demonstrates a unilocular, well-circumscribed cystic mass (BCC) between the submandibular gland (SMG) and the sternocleidomastoid (SCM) muscle, anterolateral to the carotid space. This appearance is characteristic of a second branchial cleft cyst.

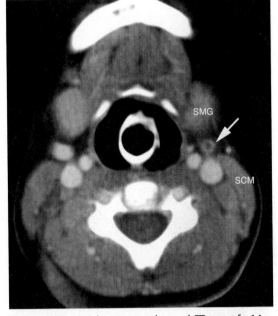

Figure 3–90. Axial contrast-enhanced CT scan of a 14-month-old girl with recurrent redness and swelling of her left neck, as well as a draining pit just above her left clavicle. A peripherally enhancing tubular structure (arrow) could be followed from the upper neck down to the level of the clavicle, representing a second branchial apparatus sinus tract. Note its location between the submandibular gland (SMG) and the sternocleidomastoid (SCM) muscle.

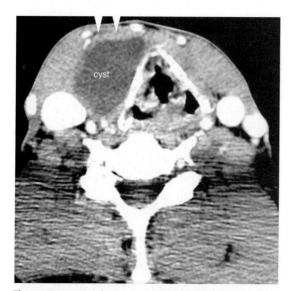

Figure 3–91. Axial contrast-enhanced CT scan of a young man with right anterior neck swelling demonstrates a well-circumscribed cystic mass adjacent to the right thyroid lamina, embedded in the strap muscles, which are displaced around the periphery of the lesion (arrowheads). Surgical excision confirmed a thyroglossal duct cyst.

their propensity to hemorrhage. In fact, fluid-fluid levels due to hemorrhage are characteristic of lymphatic malformations (Figure 3–92). Lymphatic malformations do not enhance postcontrast, although fibrous septa separating fluid spaces may normally enhance and the lesion may demonstrate peripheral enhancement if infection has occurred.

D. Epidermoid and Dermoid Lesions

Dermoid and epidermoid lesions result from the sequestration of ectodermal tissue. In the head and neck, they most commonly occur in the floor of mouth (Figure 3–93). Both are lined by squamous epithelium, but the dermoid also contains skin appendages (eg, sebaceous glands and hair follicles) within its wall. These lesions are typically midline, unilocular, and slowly growing. Both contain cheesy material due to desquamated keratin, but the dermoid may contain fatty material as well. Epidermoids are typically low density on CT scans, low signal intensity on T1-weighted images, and high signal intensity on T2-weighted images—hence, their "fluidlike" appearance. The rim of the lesion may enhance postcontrast. Dermoids are similar in appearance except that their fatty contents may result in a very low density on CT scans and a high signal on T1-weighted MRI.

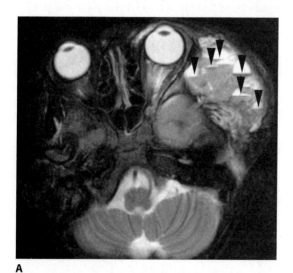

A

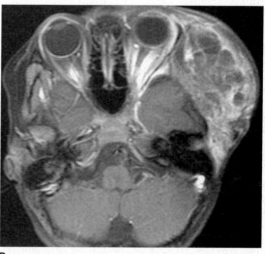

B

Figure 3–92. **(A)** Axial fast spin-echo T2-weighted image with fat saturation demonstrates a lobulated lesion of the left face with evidence of prior internal hemorrhage and multiple fluid-fluid levels (arrowheads) in its multiple cystic spaces. This is a typical appearance for a lymphangioma. **(B)** Postgadolinium, there is linear enhancement of the fibrous septa bordering some of these cystic spaces, which is often present in lymphangiomas. Some ill-defined enhancement more posteriorly and laterally is likely related to inflammation as this patient had a prior infection of the lesion as well as prior hemorrhage into it.

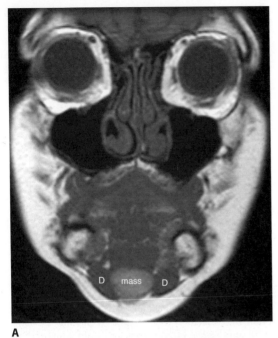

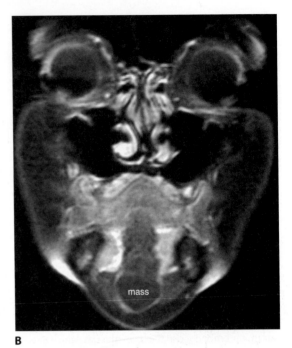

A **B**

Figure 3–93. **(A)** Coronal T1-weighted image in a 55-year-old woman with a submental mass demonstrates a rounded, well-circumscribed mass located in the midline between the anterior bellies of the digastric muscles (D). The lesion is somewhat bright on the T1-weighted image, suggesting fatty, proteinaceous, or hemorrhagic content. **(B)** On a postgadolinium coronal T1-weighted image with fat saturation, the lesion is seen to decrease in signal intensity. Hemorrhagic or proteinaceous material would not be expected to lose signal on a fat saturation image, but fatty material does. This suggests the diagnosis of dermoid cyst, which was confirmed surgically.

E. FOREGUT CYSTS

Foregut cysts are uncommon congenital defects of the developing airway and gut that may occur from the mouth to the anus. They are relatively rare in the neck, but may present with a neck mass or, if large, with airway obstruction or the compression of other vital structures. The imaging is nonspecific (Figure 3–94), although there is often high signal within the cyst fluid on a T1-weighted image owing to an elevated protein content. These lesions tend to be located in the low neck and may extend into the superior mediastinum.

F. RANULAS

The simple ranula is a mucous retention cyst that is confined to the floor of mouth and is presumed to be caused by the obstruction of a sublingual gland. In some cases, there is a rupture of the capsule or pseudocapsule and extension into the neck, and the lesion is then referred to as a plunging or diving ranula. This extension to the neck may occur along the deep lobe of the submandibular gland, between the mylohyoid and hyoglossus muscles, or via a congenital dehiscence in the mylohyoid muscle itself. A simple ranula

appears as a unilocular cyst in the floor of mouth on both CT scans (see Figure 3–26) and MRI and may be difficult to distinguish on imaging from an epidermoid or a lymphangioma. A plunging ranula usually shows a "tail" leading back to the sublingual space, which is very suggestive of the diagnosis.

G. LARYNGOCELES

A laryngocele develops when the laryngeal ventricle or its appendix is functionally or anatomically obstructed. The mass that develops may be filled with air, fluid, or pus. The internal laryngocele is confined to the paralaryngeal space, whereas the external laryngocele penetrates the thyrohyoid membrane and may present as a neck mass. The imaging characteristics depend on the laryngocele contents (see Figures 3–41 and 3–45). In all cases, the larynx should be closely inspected clinically and on imaging studies to assess for a causative obstructing lesion.

Cohen SR, Thompson JW, Brennan LP. Foregut cysts presenting as neck masses. A report on three children. *Ann Otol Rhinol Laryngol.* 1985;94:433. [PMID: 4051397] (Three patients are presented in detail, and the histopathology and differential diagnosis are discussed. Surgical extirpation of the cyst should be curative.)

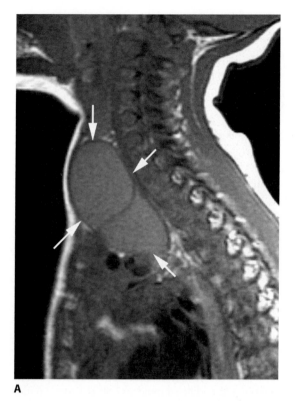

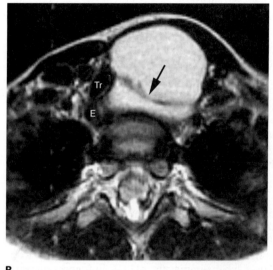

A **B**

Figure 3–94. **(A)** Sagittal T1-weighted image of the neck in a 22-month-old boy with a gradually increasing neck mass demonstrates a well-circumscribed, bilobed mass that is slightly bright on the T1-weighted image and extends inferiorly into the superior mediastinum. **(B)** Axial fast spin-echo T2-weighted image with fat saturation shows that the mass is extremely bright and has a slightly irregular internal septation (black arrow). It displaces the trachea (Tr) and esophagus (E) to the right. The mild hyperintensity on T1-weighted image is likely due to elevated protein content of the cyst fluid. On a postgadolinium image (not shown) there was mild enhancement of the internal septation, but no other enhancement. A foregut cyst was diagnosed at surgery.

Davison MJ, Morton RP, McIvor NP. Plunging ranula: clinical observations. *Head Neck.* 1998;20:63. [PMID: 9464954] (Reviews the etiology, clinical presentation, imaging, and surgical management of plunging ranulas.)

Glastonbury CM, Davidson HC, Haller JR, Harnsberger HR. The CT and MR imaging features of carcinoma arising in thyroglossal duct remnants. *Am J Neuroradiol.* 2000;21(4):770. [PMID: 10782794] (The presence of a solid nodule or invasive features in association with a thyroglossal duct lesion visible on CT scans or MRI raises the question of thyroglossal duct carcinoma. Calcification is also associated with carcinoma.)

Koeller KK, Alamo L, Adair CF, Smirniotopoulos JG. Congenital cystic masses of the neck: radiologic-pathologic correlation. *Radiographics.* 1999;19:121. [PMID: 9925396] (Reviews the clinical and radiologic features of cervical congenital cystic masses.)

6. The Pediatric Neck

The imaging evaluation of the pediatric neck raises a limited differential diagnosis, which is heavily weighted toward congenital-developmental and infectious-inflammatory processes, but also includes a limited list of neoplastic or neoplasm-like considerations. A differential diagnosis of the more common pediatric neck masses is presented in Table 3–10. The appropriate imaging workup of neck masses depends on the category of disease. Infectious-inflammatory processes are typically evaluated with CT scanning, with MRI reserved to assess complications such as spinal epidural or intracranial extension. Congenital and neoplastic processes are most completely assessed with MRI, which may also provide more specificity regarding a particular diagnosis; however, a good-quality, thin-section, contrast-enhanced CT scan may also be adequate for many of these lesions. In general, a child under the age of 5 requires monitored anesthesia care or general anesthesia for CT scanning or MRI to obtain a high-quality study. Over the age of 5, many CT studies can

Table 3–10. Limited differential diagnosis for more common pediatric neck masses.

Congenital/Developmental	Infectious/Inflammatory	Neoplastic	
		Benign or Neoplasm-like	*Malignant*
Lymphatic malformation	Suppurative lymphadenopathy	Fibromatosis colli	Neuroblastoma
Venous malformation	Abscess	Neurofibroma	Rhabdomyosarcoma
Branchial cleft cyst		Hemangioma	Lymphoma
Thyroglossal duct cyst			
Epidermoid or dermoid			

be done without sedation, but most children are not able to cooperate with a more lengthy MRI study without sedation until at least age 8 or 10.

Fibromatosis Colli

This benign disorder presents as torticollis or as a palpable neck mass in neonates and young infants. Because of its association with traumatic delivery, it is thought to be related to perinatal muscle trauma with a fibroinflammatory response within the sternocleidomastoid muscle. Imaging features are nonspecific but characteristic. On ultrasound, the mass is fusiform, expanding the belly of the sternocleidomastoid muscle and tapering at the ends; it is noncalcified and varied in its echogenicity. On MRI, the mass is similarly fusiform and oriented along the course of the sternocleidomastoid muscle. It is intermediate in signal intensity on T1-weighted images and heterogeneous on T2-weighted images, and it demonstrates enhancement postgadolinium (Figure 3–95). The adjacent soft tissues are normal and there is no associated lymphadenopathy. Its appearance is characteristic, but the clinical and imaging differential diagnosis of fibromatosis colli includes rhabdomyosarcoma.

Jaber MR, Goldsmith AJ. Sternocleidomastoid tumor of infancy: two cases of an interesting entity. *Int J Pediatr Otorhinolaryngol.* 1999;47:269. [PMID: 10321783] (Reviews the diagnostic modalities and treatment options for this entity.)

Koch BL. Imaging extracranial masses of the pediatric head and neck. *Neuroimaging Clin N Am.* 2000;10:193. [PMID: 10658162] (A thorough review that emphasizes the imaging characteristics of lesions by location: the orbit, the sinonasal cavity, the nasopharynx, the face and jaw, and the neck.)

PARANASAL SINUSES & NASAL CAVITY

Paranasal Sinuses

The paranasal sinuses and nasal cavity are well suited to assessment by thin-section (≤ 3 mm) coronal CT imaging, which clearly delineates the delicate bony anatomy

of this region (Figure 3–96). The paired maxillary sinuses lie on either side of the nasal cavity, with the orbit above, the maxillary alveolus below, and the pterygopalatine fossa behind. Drainage is via the maxillary ostium into the infundibulum. The ethmoid sinus is a series of air cells, usually divided into anterior, middle, and posterior air cells, which are intimately related to the orbit laterally and the anterior cranial fossa superiorly. The roof of the ethmoid, also known as the fovea ethmoidalis, forms part of the floor of the anterior cranial fossa and lies just lateral and superior to the cribriform plate (the roof of the nasal cavity). Drainage of the anterior and middle ethmoid air cells is into the middle meatus, whereas the posterior ethmoid air cells drain via the sphenoethmoidal recess. The frontal sinuses abut the orbit inferiorly and the anterior cranial fossa posteriorly. They drain via the nasofrontal "duct" into the frontal recess of the middle meatus. The sphenoid sinuses arise from the body of the sphenoid bone and are intimately associated with the structures of the central skull base: the sella turcica above, the cavernous sinuses laterally, and the nasopharynx inferiorly. Drainage is via the sphenoethmoidal recess into the superior meatus (Figure 3–97).

Ostiomeatal Unit of the Nasal Cavity

The lateral nasal wall is anatomically complex. The superior, middle, and inferior turbinates project from the lateral nasal wall and each overlies its respective meatus (Figure 3–98). The inferior turbinate arises from the junction of the uncinate process and the medial wall of the maxillary sinus, and the inferior meatus lies medial to it. The ostium of the nasolacrimal duct opens into the inferior meatus. The middle turbinate has more complex attachments, with a superior attachment to the cribriform plate, a lateral attachment to the lamina papyracea, and a posterior attachment to the ethmoid crest of the palatine bone. The maxillary sinuses, anterior and middle ethmoid air cells, and frontal sinuses drain into the middle meatus. The superior

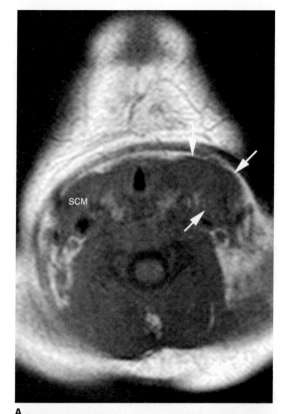

A

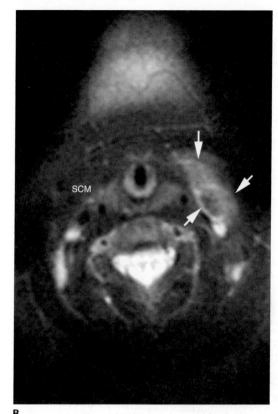

B

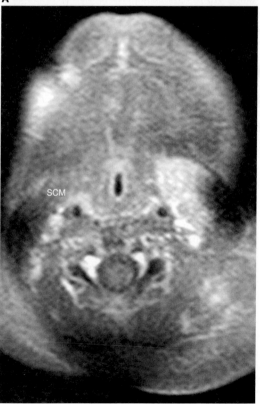

C

Figure 3–95. **(A)** Axial T1-weighted image in a 2-week-old boy with torticollis and a left neck mass (arrows) demonstrates prominent soft tissue in the expected location of the sternocleidomastoid muscle. The right sternocleidomastoid muscle (SCM) is shown for comparison. **(B)** On an axial fast spin-echo T2-weighted image with fat saturation, the normal muscle is dark, whereas the left-sided mass (arrows) has areas of mixed high and low signal. **(C)** Postgadolinium, an axial T1-weighted image with fat saturation demonstrates the diffuse enhancement of the mass, whose location and morphology paralleled that of the sternocleidomastoid muscle on every image. These imaging features are consistent with fibromatosis colli, though rhabdomyosarcoma must be considered in the differential diagnosis.

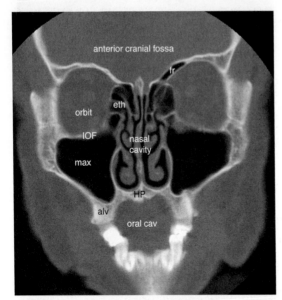

Figure 3–96. Coronal CT scan through the paranasal sinuses viewed in bone window demonstrates the anatomic relationships of the anterior paranasal sinuses. Indicated are the maxillary (max), ethmoid (eth), and frontal (fr) sinuses, as well as the maxillary alveolus (alv), hard palate (HP), and infraorbital foramen (IOF), which transmits the infraorbital nerve, a branch of V2.

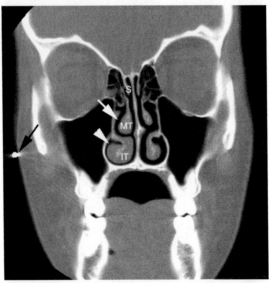

Figure 3–98. Coronal CT scan through the paranasal sinuses viewed in bone window demonstrates the inferior (IT), middle (MT), and superior (S) turbinates projecting from the lateral nasal wall. Also indicated are the middle meatus (white arrow) and inferior meatus (white arrowhead). The black arrow points to a metallic ball bearing, which has been affixed to the skin of the patient's right cheek so that there is no confusion of right and left, a not uncommon problem with sinus CT scans.

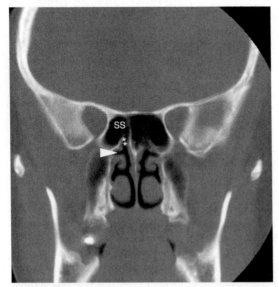

Figure 3–97. Coronal CT scan through the sphenoid sinuses (SS) viewed in bone window demonstrates the sphenoethmoidal recess (*) and the superior meatus (arrowhead).

turbinate attaches to the skull base superiorly (often merging with the attachment of the middle turbinate), the lamina papyracea laterally, and the inferior portion of the anterior wall of the sphenoid sinus posteriorly. The superior meatus receives drainage from the posterior ethmoid air cells.

The ostiomeatal unit includes the maxillary ostium and the structures of the middle meatus, and defines the region into which the frontal, anterior, and middle ethmoid and maxillary sinuses drain. When the ostiomeatal unit is diseased, a characteristic pattern of obstructive sinus disease is present, with involvement of the aforementioned areas. Important components of the ostiomeatal unit that are well visualized on coronal CT scans include the infundibulum, the uncinate process, and the ethmoid bulla (Figure 3–99). The infundibulum is a channel defined by the orbital wall laterally, the uncinate process medially, and the ethmoid bulla superiorly; it connects superomedially to the hiatus semilunaris and functions as the conduit for secretions from the maxillary and ethmoid sinuses. The uncinate process is the thin, hook-shaped bony process that forms the medial wall of the infundibulum. The ethmoid bulla receives drainage from the middle ethmoid air cells.

Anatomic Variations

The concha bullosa or pneumatized middle turbinate is seen commonly on screening CT scans of the sinus (Figure 3–100). Usually an incidental finding, a large concha bullosa may encroach on the infundibulum or become primarily diseased with mucosal inflammation, polyps, or mucocele formation (Figure 3–101). The middle turbinate may be paradoxically curved and the uncinate process may deviate medially or laterally or may be pneumatized. Variations in ethmoid air cells are also common, notably the presence of infraorbital ethmoid air cells (so-called Haller cells, Figure 3–102) and agger nasi cells, which are extensions of anterior ethmoid air cells into the lacrimal bone.

Anatomic Relationships

The nasal cavity is closely related to the pterygopalatine fossa, and these anatomic relationships are well delineated on cross-sectional imaging studies. Because the pterygopalatine fossa has connections to multiple deep facial and intracranial spaces (Figure 3–103), infection and neoplasm originating in the sinonasal cavity not uncommonly extend via this pathway. The nasal cavity connects with the pterygopalatine fossa via the sphenopalatine foramen, which is found on the high posterolateral nasal wall. Medially, therefore, the pterygopalatine fossa connects to the nasal cavity via the sphenopalatine foramen. The pterygopalatine fossa is bounded anteriorly by the posterior wall of the maxillary sinus, but anterosuperiorly, the pterygopalatine fossa connects to the orbit via the inferior orbital fissure. The pterygopalatine fossa communicates laterally with the masticator space via the pterygomaxillary fissure. Posteriorly, there are two important connections to the skull base and the cranial vault: the pterygopalatine fossa connects posteroinferiorly to the region of the foramen lacerum and the carotid canal via the vidian canal, while posterosuperiorly, it connects to the cavernous sinus and the middle cranial fossa via the foramen rotundum. The pterygopalatine fossa connects inferiorly to the palate and oral cavity via the palatine foramina.

Pathology

The paranasal sinuses and nasal cavity may be affected by a wide variety of pathologic processes, including congenital-developmental processes, inflammatory mucosal disease, and neoplasms.

A. Congenital and Developmental Disorders

The embryology of the sinonasal region is complex, and maldevelopment may lead to nasal gliomas, dermoids,

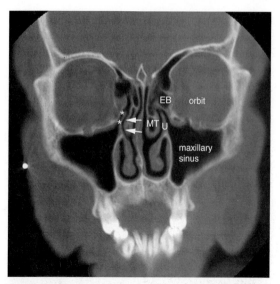

Figure 3–99. Coronal CT scan through the paranasal sinuses viewed in bone window demonstrates the anatomy of the ostiomeatal unit. Indicated on the patient's left are the uncinate process (U), ethmoid bulla (EB), and middle turbinate (MT; note that it is partially pneumatized, consistent with concha bullosa). On the patient's right, the infundibulum (*) and middle meatus (arrows) are indicated.

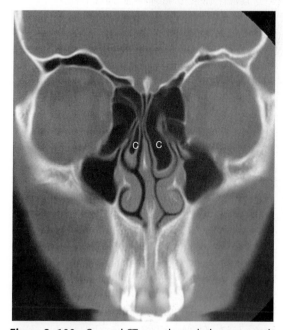

Figure 3–100. Coronal CT scan through the paranasal sinuses viewed in bone window demonstrates pneumatization of the middle turbinates bilaterally, consistent with bilateral concha bullosa (C).

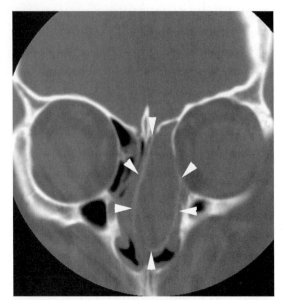

Figure 3–101. Coronal CT scan through the paranasal sinuses viewed in bone window in a patient with left nasal obstruction demonstrates an ovoid, well-circumscribed mass with a thin peripheral shell of bone (arrowheads). Note the superior attachment to the cribriform plate and the superolateral attachment to the lateral orbital wall. Surgery confirmed a mucocele arising in a pneumatized middle turbinate.

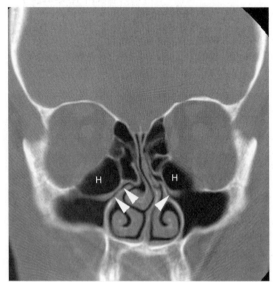

Figure 3–102. Coronal CT scan through the paranasal sinuses viewed in bone window in a patient with large bilateral Haller cells (H). The infundibula (arrowheads) are indicated.

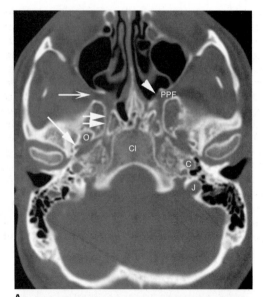

A

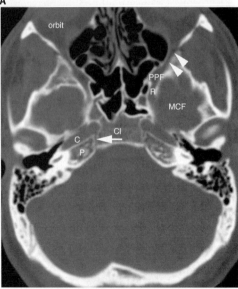

B

Figure 3–103. Axial thin-section CT scans through the skull base viewed in bone window illustrate the skull base anatomy and the interconnections of the pterygopalatine fossa. **(A)** Indicated are the pterygopalatine fossa (PPF), sphenopalatine foramen (white arrowhead), pterygomaxillary fissure (concave white arrow), vidian canal (double short white arrows), foramen ovale (O), foramen spinosum (long single white arrow), clivus (Cl), carotid canal (C), and jugular foramen (J). **(B)** At a slightly more superior level, foramen rotundum (R) is seen connecting the middle cranial fossa (MCF) to the pterygopalatine fossa at the level of the inferior orbital fissure (arrowheads). Also indicated are the petrous bone (P) and the petroclival fissure (white arrow).

sinus tracts, and cephaloceles. It is critical that a cephalocele be recognized before a surgical procedure is undertaken in order to avoid unexpected penetration of the central nervous system. In this circumstance, CT scanning and MRI often play complementary roles. CT scans show the skull base defect and may suggest the possibility of cephalocele, but MRI helps to assess exactly which tissues have herniated through the skull base defect (Figure 3–104). Congenital abnormalities of the nasal cavity such as choanal atresia (Figure 3–105) and pyriform aperture stenosis (Figure 3–106) are well assessed with CT scanning, which should be performed with very thin sections (1–2 mm). In the setting of choanal atresia, the temporal bones, which typically are included on the same scan, should be carefully assessed for anomalies that would help to support a diagnosis of the CHARGE syndrome (ocular **c**oloboma, **h**eart defects, **a**tretic choanae, **r**etarded growth or development, **g**enital hypoplasia, and **e**ar anomalies or hearing loss).

B. INFLAMMATORY DISEASE

Smooth or lobulated thickening of sinus mucosa is commonly seen on imaging studies of the brain, head, and neck. Air-fluid levels may be due to an acute bacterial sinusitis, but they are also seen commonly in the setting of sinus obstruction, such as from a nasogastric or endotracheal tube, notably in the ICU setting (Figure 3–107). With chronic sinusitis, there is often thickening of the bony walls of the sinus as well as mucosal thickening (so-called "mucoperiosteal" thickening). The pattern of inflammatory sinus disease provides insight into the level of blockage of the normal routes of mucociliary drainage, and the ostiomeatal unit and sphenoethmoidal recess should be assessed on all coronal sinus CT scans. If the ostiomeatal unit is obstructed, then inflammatory changes in the ipsilateral maxillary sinus, the anterior and middle ethmoid air cells, and the frontal sinus, as well as opacification of the middle meatus, are expected (Figure 3–108). When obstruction is at the level of the sphenoethmoidal recess, then inflammatory changes in the ipsilateral sphenoid sinus and, to a lesser degree, the posterior ethmoid air cells, are expected.

C. MUCOUS RETENTION CYSTS AND POLYPS

Mucous retention cysts and polyps are very common and often indistinguishable on imaging studies, appearing as lobulated masses of low-to-intermediate density on CT scans. On MRI, they are intermediate in signal on T1-weighted images, bright on T2-weighted images, and show a variable enhancement that is typically peripheral (Figure 3–109) if present at all.

D. MUCOCELES

A mucocele results from the obstruction of a sinus ostium, leading to the accumulation of secretions and the gradual,

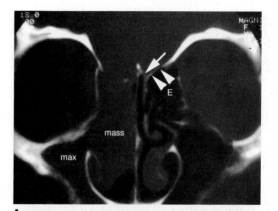

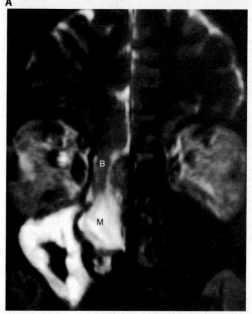

Figure 3–104. **(A)** Coronal CT scan through the paranasal sinuses viewed in bone window in a 30-year-old woman with chronic right nasal obstruction demonstrates a large soft tissue mass in the right nasal cavity. Opacification of the right maxillary sinus (max) is presumably due to outlet obstruction with the accumulation of mucoid secretions. Note that the right bony ethmoid roof is largely absent. The left cribriform plate (arrow) and ethmoid roof (arrowheads) are shown for comparison. It is unclear from the CT scan whether the mass has originated in the nasal cavity and extended up or if the mass has originated intracranially and extended down. MRI is indicated for further evaluation prior to any biopsy. **(B)** Coronal fast spin-echo T2-weighted image with fat saturation demonstrates inferior herniation of brain tissue (B) and a CSF-filled meningocele sac (M) through the skull base defect. This patient's previously unrecognized meningoencephalocele was subsequently repaired.

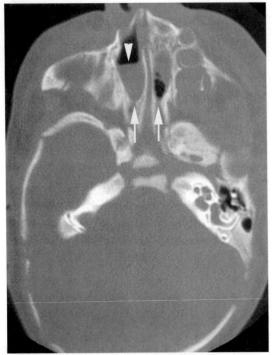

Figure 3–105. Axial CT scan through the nasal cavity viewed in bone window in a neonate with difficulty feeding and nasal obstruction demonstrates severe bony stenosis (arrows) and presumed membranous atresia of the posterior choana bilaterally. An air-fluid level (arrowhead) is seen in the right nasal cavity. The visualized temporal bone is normal.

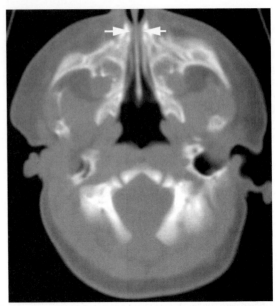

Figure 3–106. Axial CT scan through the nasal cavity photographed in bone window in a 4-year-old boy with facial dysmorphism and respiratory difficulty demonstrates tapered narrowing of the anterior nasal cavities bilaterally (white arrows), consistent with pyriform aperture stenosis. A more inferior image (not shown) demonstrated a centrally located mega-incisor, as is often seen in conjunction with pyriform aperture stenosis. This constellation of findings has been associated with holoprosencephaly, which was not present in this case.

smooth expansion of the sinus (Figure 3–110). The mucocele contents often become increasingly desiccated and have an increasing protein content over time; therefore, they may show an increased density on CT scanning and variable degrees of hyperintensity on T1-weighted MRI sequences and hypointensity on T2-weighted MRI (Figure 3–111). If sinus contents show marked hypointensity on T2-weighted images, fungal infection should be considered in the appropriate clinical setting. Thin, linear enhancement may be seen around the margin of the expanded sinus under normal circumstances, but if there is marked enhancement, then a mucopyocele should be considered.

E. Sinonasal Polyposis

Sinonasal polyposis refers to the presence of multiple polyps in the sinuses and nasal cavities, often with accompanying mucosal thickening and mucocele formation. On imaging studies, the extensive soft tissue abnormalities and bone erosion and remodeling that often accompany sinonasal polyposis may mimic an aggressive neoplastic process (Figure 3–112). The diffuse nature of the process and the lack of any focal or dominant destructive mass suggest polyposis and not a malignant tumor. Other nonneoplastic lesions that may lead to significant sinonasal bone destruction and soft tissue abnormalities include Wegener granulomatosis (Figure 3–113) and invasive fungal infections such as aspergillus and mucormycosis.

F. Complications of Sinusitis

Imaging studies may be ordered to assess the complications of sinusitis. These may be local, such as orbital cellulitis, orbital abscess, or osteomyelitis of the sinus wall, or they may involve intracranial extension. Intracranial complications include meningitis, subdural empyema, brain abscess (Figure 3–114), and cavernous sinus thrombosis. In most cases, intracranial complications are more completely assessed with MRI than with CT scanning.

G. Fungal Sinusitis

Fungal sinusitis can be classified into invasive and noninvasive forms, with the invasive forms usually affecting

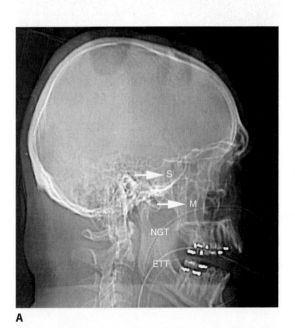

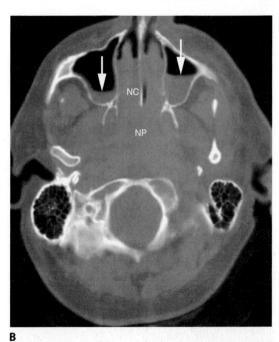

A

B

Figure 3–107. **(A)** Lateral scout digital radiograph of an ICU patient with an endotracheal tube (ETT) and nasogastric tube (NGT) suggests air-fluid levels (arrows) in the sphenoid (S) and maxillary (M) sinuses. **(B)** Axial CT scan through the paranasal sinuses photographed in bone window demonstrates bilateral maxillary sinus air-fluid levels (arrows) as well as soft tissue, fluid, or both opacifying the nasal cavity (NC) and nasopharyngeal airway (NP).

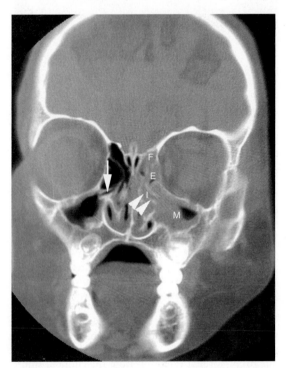

Figure 3–108. Coronal CT scan through the nasal cavity and paranasal sinuses photographed in bone window in a young boy with chronic sinusitis demonstrates thickened mucosa in the infundibulum (I, arrowheads) and middle meatus, with mucosal thickening in the maxillary (M), ethmoid (E), and frontal (F) sinuses. This is consistent with an ostiomeatal unit pattern of disease. The contralateral normal infundibulum (arrow) is indicated just below the ethmoid bulla.

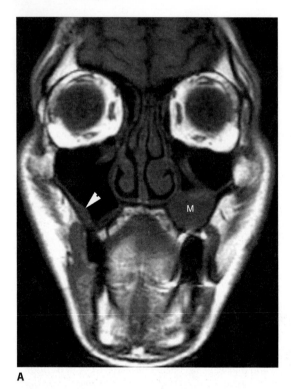

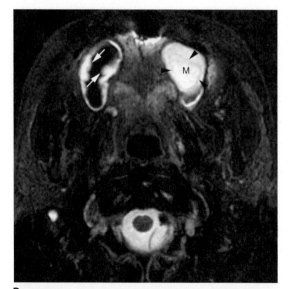

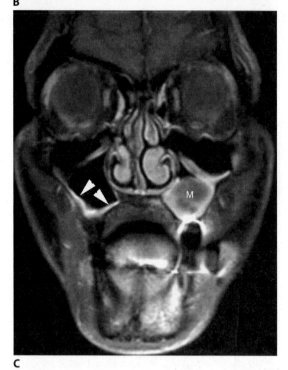

Figure 3–109. **(A)** Coronal T1-weighted image of the paranasal sinuses demonstrates a lobulated soft tissue mass (M) in the inferior aspect of the left maxillary sinus, as well as mild mucosal thickening in the right maxillary sinus (arrowhead). **(B)** Axial fast spin-echo T2-weighted image with fat saturation demonstrates a very bright mass (M) with a slightly darker rim (black arrowheads) and surrounding hyperintense material representing thickened mucosa, mucoid secretions, or both. Contralateral mild lobulated mucosal thickening is also seen (white arrows). **(C)** Postgadolinium, a coronal T1-weighted image with fat saturation shows that the mass (M) does not enhance, though there is enhancement of the adjacent mucosa, as is also seen contralaterally (white arrowheads). This mass is typical of a polyp or mucous retention cyst.

immune-compromised hosts and the noninvasive forms affecting either immune-compromised or immune-competent hosts. *Aspergillus* species are most commonly isolated, but many fungal species have been implicated. Invasive forms include acute or fulminant fungal sinusitis, granulomatous invasive fungal sinusitis, and chronic invasive fungal sinusitis. Acute fungal sinusitis is char-

acterized by extensive tissue destruction and necrosis (Figure 3–115). Tissue enhancement may be scant or absent due to the angioinvasive nature of the infection. Chronic invasive disease is also characterized by tissue destruction, but the course is far more indolent than the acute form (Figure 3–116). Orbital apex syndrome due to intraorbital extension from the ethmoid sinuses

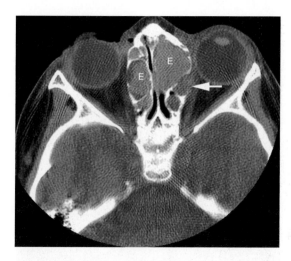

Figure 3–110. Axial noncontrast CT scan (intermediate window) of the paranasal sinuses in a 2-year-old girl with cystic fibrosis demonstrates the expansion of multiple ethmoid air cells (E) and the absence of the bony margin of one of the air cells (arrow). The material within the air cells is mildly hyperdense, consistent with inspissation and increased protein content. Findings are consistent with multiple ethmoid mucoceles.

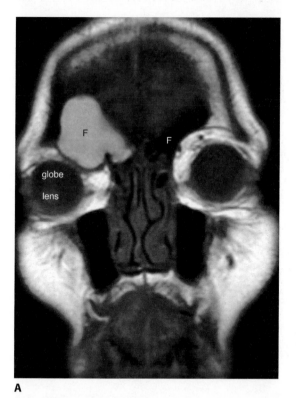

A

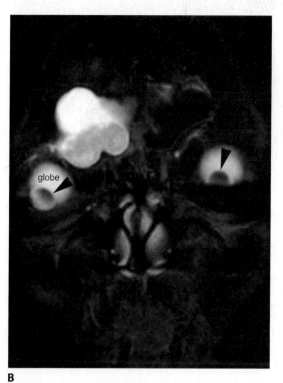

B

Figure 3–111. **(A)** Coronal T1-weighted image in an older woman with gradually progressive proptosis and double vision demonstrates smooth expansion of the right frontal sinus (black F), which encroaches on the orbit and displaces the right globe inferolaterally. The right frontal sinus is filled with hyperintense material consistent with desiccated, proteinaceous secretions. The normal aerated left frontal sinus (white F) is shown for comparison. **(B)** On a coronal fast spin-echo T2-weighted image with fat saturation, the sinus contents have variable signal intensity owing to differences in actual protein content. Findings are typical of a frontal sinus mucocele. The globes and lenses are seen to be asymmetrically positioned due to the mass effect of the expanded sinus (arrowheads).

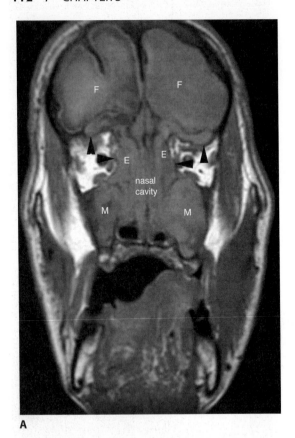

A

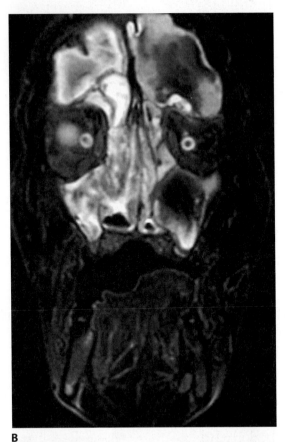

B

Figure 3–112. A 55-year-old mentally challenged man with chronic sinus congestion. **(A)** Coronal T1-weighted image demonstrates diffuse abnormal soft tissue filling the nasal cavity and paranasal sinuses (F, frontal; E, ethmoid; M, maxillary). The material within the paranasal sinuses is of a mixed signal intensity due to variable protein content. Note the remodeling of the orbital roofs and medial orbital walls (black arrowheads) due to mucocele formation and sinus expansion. **(B)** On a coronal fast spin-echo T2-weighted image with fat saturation, the heterogeneous signal intensity of the thickened mucosa and proteinaceous secretions can be well appreciated. **(C)** Postgadolinium, an axial T1-weighted image with fat saturation demonstrates enhancement around the periphery of the markedly expanded frontal sinuses (F), but no enhancement of the centrally located mucoid material. These findings are typical of severe sinonasal polyposis and mucocele formation.

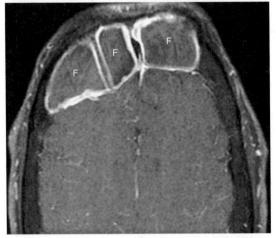

C

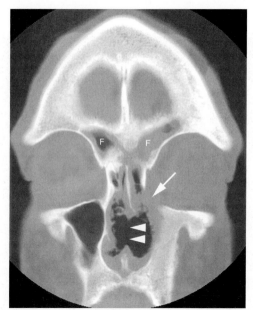

Figure 3–113. Coronal CT scan of the sinuses viewed in bone window in a patient with known Wegener granulomatosis demonstrates the loss of the membranous septum (arrowheads) as well as focal destruction of a portion of the medial orbital wall (arrow). Mucosal thickening and reactive bony thickening is seen in the frontal sinuses (F).

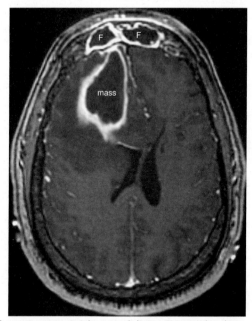

Figure 3–114. Axial postgadolinium T1-weighted image of the brain in a patient with headache and lethargy who was suspected to have a brain tumor. The imaging characteristics of the frontal lobe mass were felt to be more consistent with a brain abscess, and severe bilateral frontal sinus disease (F) was noted. In the operating room, pus was found in both the brain mass and the frontal sinuses. The patient did well after drainage and antibiotic treatment.

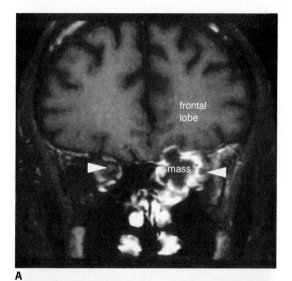

A

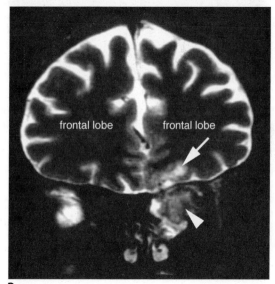

B

Figure 3–115. **(A)** Coronal postgadolinium T1-weighted image with fat saturation in a patient with AIDS, declining vision in the left eye, and a painful supraorbital mass. An ill-marginated, peripherally enhancing lesion with central necrosis is seen involving the left orbit and extending superiorly into the anterior cranial fossa. The optic nerves are indicated (arrowheads), with the left nerve significantly displaced laterally by the mass. **(B)** A coronal fast spin-echo T2-weighted image with fat saturation demonstrates a relatively low signal intensity in the necrotic center of the mass lesion (arrowhead). Although this may represent proteinaceous or hemorrhagic material, a low signal intensity is also suggestive of a fungal process, since many fungi concentrate paramagnetic ions that shorten T2 relaxation times. Focal edema (arrow) is present in the left frontal lobe. Invasive aspergillosis was confirmed at the time of surgery and the patient died 2 days later.

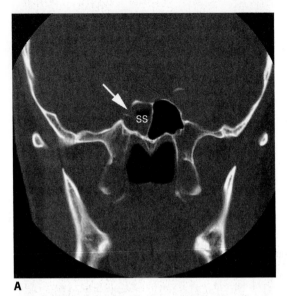

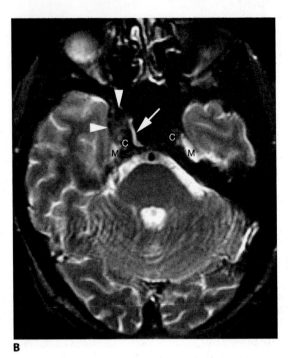

A   B

Figure 3–116. **(A)** Coronal CT scan of the paranasal sinuses viewed in bone window of an HIV-positive patient with chronic sinus symptoms demonstrates mucosal thickening in the right sphenoid sinus (SS). Also present is a focal area of bone destruction (arrow) along the lateral sphenoid sinus wall, which was not noted prospectively. **(B)** Axial T2-weighted image performed 3 months later when the patient presented with new diplopia and palsy of the right cranial nerve VI on exam demonstrates a relatively low signal intensity expansile mass (white arrowheads) involving the anterior aspect of the right cavernous sinus. Sphenoid sinus mucosal disease is minimal (white arrow) and improved from the prior examination. Indicated are the cavernous internal carotid arteries (C) and Meckel cave (M). Endoscopic sphenoidotomy and biopsy confirmed a diagnosis of invasive aspergillosis, which behaved clinically in an indolent, chronic manner.

is a common association of chronic invasive disease. Noninvasive forms of fungal sinusitis include mycetoma and allergic fungal sinusitis. Mycetoma is usually seen as a mass lesion in the maxillary sinus, often in association with chronic mucosal thickening and polyps, and the mass is typically dense or even grossly calcified on a noncontrast CT scan. Mycetomas may also occur in the nasal cavity (Figure 3–117). Allergic fungal sinusitis involves multiple sinuses, shows extensive mucosal thickening (often with complete opacification), expansion and remodeling of the sinuses, and also demonstrates increased intrasinus attenuation. Its appearance is nonspecific.

H. NEOPLASMS

Benign and malignant neoplasms may occur in the nasal cavity and paranasal sinuses. Benign lesions tend to slowly enlarge and therefore remodel bone rather than destroy it. Malignant processes are more likely to

show frank bone erosion and destruction, as well as infiltration of adjacent tissues, evidence of perineural spread, or evidence of regional metastases. On MRI, a T2-weighted sequence is particularly helpful in separating an intermediate signal intensity tumor from the high signal of edematous mucosa or mucoid secretions; this sequence often best characterizes the full extent of disease within the nasal cavity and paranasal sinuses. MRI is also very useful for the accurate assessment of orbital or intracranial extension of aggressive sinonasal lesions, as well as perineural spread of disease.

1. Inverting papillomas—Inverting papillomas are the most common benign tumors of the nose and paranasal sinuses, and usually arise in the lateral wall of the nasal cavity and the middle meatus. CT scanning typically shows a mass extending from the middle meatus into the adjacent maxillary antrum through a widened maxillary ostium (Figure 3–118). Areas of calcification may be seen within the mass, and the surface of the

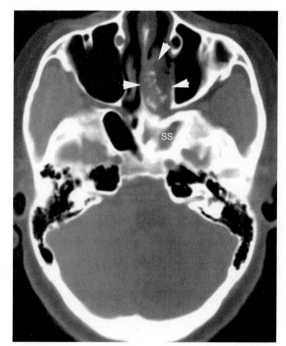

Figure 3–117. Axial noncontrast CT scan of the sinonasal region viewed in bone window demonstrates an expansile mass of the left nasal cavity (arrowheads) with dense, central calcification. The left sphenoid sinus (SS) is chronically obstructed and demonstrates mucoperiosteal thickening. Differential considerations included mycetoma and fibro-osseous lesions of the nasal cavity. A mycetoma was confirmed at the time of surgery.

lesion is typically lobulated. The appearance is nonspecific on MRI, but an inverting papilloma is typically intermediate in signal intensity on both T1- and T2-weighted images, and homogeneously enhances postgadolinium. A convoluted "cerebriform" pattern on T2- or enhanced T1-weighted images may suggest an inverting papilloma. MRI is also helpful in showing the full extent of disease, especially at the skull base, as the tumor can be more clearly delineated from adjacent mucosal thickening and inflammatory secretions on MRI than on CT scanning.

2. Juvenile nasal angiofibromas—These benign tumors arise on the posterolateral wall of the nasal cavity, at the level of the sphenopalatine foramen, and tend to extend early into the pterygopalatine fossa. Juvenile nasal angiofibromas are often large at the time of presentation and may extend into the nasopharynx, the sphenoid and ethmoid sinuses, and the middle cranial fossa. On CT scans, this tumor is multilobulated and enhances intensely postcontrast. It tends to show bone remodeling rather than aggres-

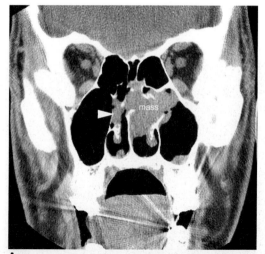

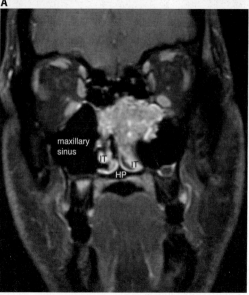

Figure 3–118. **(A)** Coronal noncontrast CT scan of the paranasal sinuses viewed in intermediate window of a 50-year-old man with left nasal obstruction. A mass visible on clinical examination appears as a lobulated, benign-appearing lesion centered on the lateral nasal wall but extending through the left maxillary ostium and also through the nasal septum into the right nasal cavity (arrowhead). **(B)** On an MRI, a postgadolinium coronal T1-weighted image with fat saturation demonstrates a moderately intense but somewhat heterogeneous enhancement of this multilobulated transseptal lesion. The mass is separate from the right inferior turbinate (IT) but does involve the left inferior turbinate. The mass has a somewhat "cerebriform" and convoluted surface appearance. An inverting papilloma was confirmed at surgery.

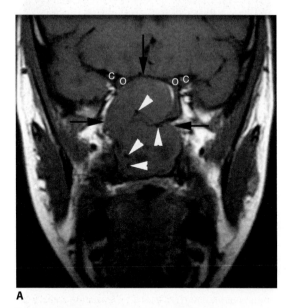

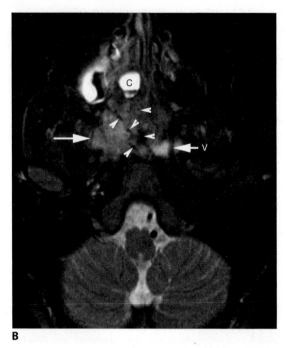

A   **B**

Figure 3–119. **(A)** Coronal T1-weighted image in a teenage male with epistaxis and nasal obstruction demonstrates a large soft tissue mass (black arrows) filling the posterior nasal cavity and nasopharynx and extending up into the sphenoid sinuses in close proximity to the optic nerves (O) in the optic canals, just medial to the anterior clinoid processes (C). Macroscopic flow voids (arrowheads) are seen within the mass. **(B)** Axial fast spin-echo T2-weighted image with fat saturation shows that the tumor is mostly intermediate in signal intensity but has a focal area of cystic degeneration (C). The tumor has invaded the right skull base (white arrow), with the contralateral skull base and vidian canal (V) shown for comparison. Flow voids are again seen within the lesion (small white arrowheads). Angiography and embolization were performed, followed by resection; pathology confirmed juvenile angiofibroma.

sive destruction, but the tumor may directly invade bone. On MRI, prominent flow voids are characteristic of these lesions, which may also be somewhat heterogeneous due to cyst formation and areas of hemorrhage (Figure 3–119). At catheter angiography, these lesions are highly vascular and preoperative embolization is an important intervention to minimize operative blood loss, increase the likelihood of total resection, and reduce surgical complications.

3. Squamous cell carcinoma—SCC of the sinonasal cavity most commonly arises in the maxillary sinus and tends to present when far advanced as early symptoms are often attributed to inflammatory sinus disease. Both CT scanning and MRI show a unilateral mass with aggressive bone destruction and irregular margins with adjacent soft tissue (Figure 3–120). If the disease has broken through the back wall of the maxillary sinus into the pterygopalatine fossa, then orbital and intracranial extension should be carefully sought. As with all neoplasms of the sinonasal cavity, T2-weighted images are particularly helpful with distinguishing tumor from inflamed mucosa.

4. Esthesioneuroblastomas—Esthesioneuroblastomas arise from the olfactory epithelium, which is located in the high nasal vault and upper nasal septum. This site of origin is intimately associated with the cribriform plate, and esthesioneuroblastomas have a high incidence of intracranial extension (Figure 3–121). Although this site of origin is highly suggestive of esthesioneuroblastoma, the imaging appearance is nonspecific and the diagnosis must be confirmed histologically. Peripheral cysts along the intracranial margin of a sinonasal mass have been noted, however, to be highly suggestive of esthesioneuroblastoma. Because there is a significant incidence of neck metastases even at the time of presentation, the neck should be scanned in these patients to assess for metastatic cervical lymphadenopathy.

5. Mucosal melanomas—Malignant melanoma arising from the mucosa of the nasal cavity and paranasal sinuses is rare, but should be considered in an older patient presenting with unilateral nasal obstruction, particularly with a history of epistaxis. The imaging findings may be nonspecific, but if the lesion contains melanin or

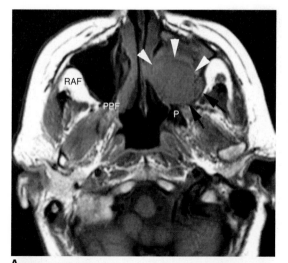

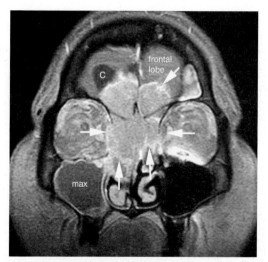

Figure 3–121. Coronal T1-weighted image postgadolinium with fat saturation in a 45-year-old woman with anosmia and nasal obstruction demonstrates an intensely enhancing soft tissue mass (white arrows) that is centered on the upper nasal vault, involves the nasal cavity bilaterally and extends into both orbits, and extends intracranially to invade brain. A peripheral intracranial cyst (C) is noted, as are obstructed secretions in the right maxillary (max) sinus. An esthesioneuroblastoma with extensive intracranial and bilateral orbital involvement was confirmed at surgery.

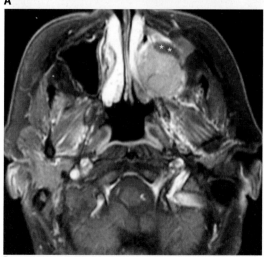

Figure 3–120. (A) Axial T1-weighted image in a 55-year-old woman with left facial pain and pressure demonstrates a soft tissue mass (white arrowheads) centered in the left maxillary sinus and extending posteriorly through the back wall of the sinus into the retroantral fat (black arrows) and pterygopalatine fossa. The normal retroantral fat (RAF) and pterygopalatine fossa (PPF) are indicated on the patient's right side. In addition, there is sclerosis of the pterygoid body and plates (P) related to tumor infiltration. Anteriorly, within the left maxillary sinus, mixed signal intensity material is consistent with inspissated proteinaceous material due to sinus obstruction. **(B)** Postgadolinium, an axial T1-weighted image with fat saturation demonstrates enhancement of the lesion and its posterior extension into the adjacent fat and bone. More anteriorly in the maxillary sinus, inspissated proteinaceous material (**) does not enhance. Invasive squamous cell carcinoma was confirmed surgically.

there has been prior hemorrhage within the lesion, it may appear focally or diffusely bright on a T1-weighted image (Figure 3–122). Mucosal melanomas are variable in signal intensity on T2-weighted images and show enhancement postgadolinium; both of these features are nonspecific. The metastatic workup of these patients is particularly important, as lymph node and distant metastases are common even at initial presentation. Perineural spread of disease is also common.

6. Non-Hodgkin lymphoma—Primary non-Hodgkin lymphoma of the sinonasal cavity has a variable and nonspecific appearance, but should be considered high among differential possibilities when the abnormal soft tissue involving the nasal cavity, the paranasal sinuses, or both is diffuse and infiltrative, often involving multiple locations, rather than presenting as a dominant mass lesion (Figure 3–123). The infiltration of adjacent fat (ie, premalar, retroantral, or within the pterygopalatine fossa) is common, as is a permeative rather than grossly destructive pattern of bony involvement. Lymphomas are typically of low-to-intermediate signal intensity on T2-weighted images owing to a high nuclear to cytoplasmic ratio. This is, however, a nonspecific finding because many paranasal sinus tumors are intermediate in signal intensity on T2-weighted images. When a lymphoma simply presents as a mass lesion, it can-

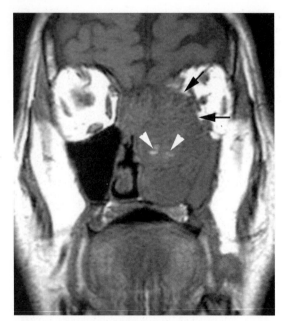

Figure 3–122. Coronal T1-weighted image in an elderly man presenting with epistaxis and left nasal obstruction demonstrates a large soft tissue mass filling the left nasal cavity, invading the left orbit (black arrows), and extending through the skull base into the anterior cranial fossa. Focal areas of a high signal intensity (arrowheads) are seen, consistent with hemorrhage or melanin. Mucosal melanoma was confirmed by biopsy.

not be confidently distinguished from many other sinonasal pathologies without tissue sampling. Lymphomas of T-cell origin predominate in the nasal cavity, whereas those of B-cell origin predominate in the paranasal sinuses. Nasal natural killer (NK)/T-cell lymphoma should be specifically considered when there is diffuse involvement of the nasal cavity, often accompanied by necrosis and midline destruction. Recall that the differential diagnosis of midfacial destruction includes Wegener granulomatosis, sarcoidosis, cocaine abuse, and infection (eg, syphilis, tuberculosis, leprosy, and fungus), as well as NK/T-cell lymphoma.

Bayram M, Sirikci A, Bayazit YA. Important anatomic variations of the sinonasal anatomy in light of endoscopic surgery: a pictorial review. *Eur Radiol.* 2001;11:1991. [PMID: 11702133] (A review of imaging anatomy and anatomic variations with emphasis on the course of the anterior ethmoidal artery, the roof of the ethmoid, the lamina papyracea, the uncinate process, the optic nerve and the internal carotid artery.)

Dillon WP, Som PM, Fullerton GD. Hypointense MR signal in chronically inspissated sinonasal secretions. *Radiology.* 1990;174:73. [PMID: 2294574] (Sinonasal secretions may have a spectrum of MRI signal intensity, ranging from hyperintense to signal void. This is related to the protein content of the material and must be kept in mind when interpreting images of patients with suspected chronic sinusitis.)

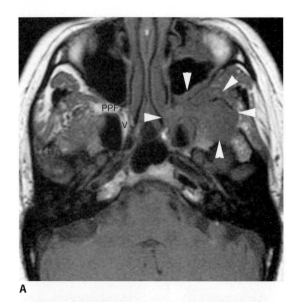

A

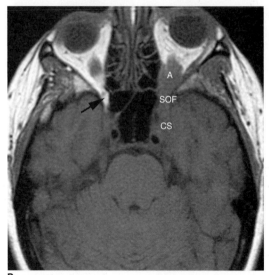

B

Figure 3–123. **(A)** Axial T1-weighted image in a 50-year-old woman with numbness in the left V2 distribution demonstrates abnormal soft tissue (arrowheads) infiltrating the posterior mucosa of the maxillary sinus, the fat of the pterygopalatine fossa, and the muscle and fat of the nasopharyngeal masticator space just below the skull base. The normal right pterygopalatine fossa (PPF) and vidian canal (V) are shown for comparison. **(B)** A more cephalad axial T1-weighted image shows abnormal soft tissue infiltrating the orbital apex (A), superior orbital fissure (SOF), and cavernous sinus (CS). The normal right superior orbital fissure is shown for comparison (black arrow). Biopsy of the posterior wall of the maxillary sinus via a Caldwell-Luc approach confirmed the diagnosis of B-cell lymphoma.

Fatterpekar G, Mukherji S, Arbealez A, Maheshwari S, Castillo M. Fungal diseases of the paranasal sinuses. *Semin Ultrasound CT MR.* 1999;20:391. [PMID: 10634589] (Reviews the various types of fungal sinusitis with emphasis on the CT and MR imaging features.)

Kim SS, Lee JG, Kim KS, Kim HU, Chung IH, Yoon JH. Computed tomographic and anatomical analysis of the basal lamellas in the ethmoid sinus. *Laryngoscope.* 2001;111:424. [PMID: 11224770] (Investigates the exact anatomic structure of the lamellas in the ethmoid sinus by CT scanning and anatomic analysis. Indicates that lamellas of the ethmoid sinus have relatively uniform patterns, although there is variability in shape.)

King AD, Lei KI, Ahuja AT, Lam WW, Metreweli C. MR imaging of nasal T-cell/natural killer cell lymphoma. *AJR Am J Roentgenol.* 2000;174:209. [PMID: 10628480] (Shows that nasal T-cell/natural killer cell lymphoma frequently exhibits diffuse invasion of the nasal cavity with necrosis, midline destruction, and extension into the nasopharynx.)

Nakamura K, Uehara S, Omagari J et al. Primary non-Hodgkin lymphoma of the sinonasal cavities: correlation of CT evaluation with clinical outcome. *Radiology.* 1997;204:431. [PMID: 9240531] (Primary B-cell lymphoma of the maxillary sinus tended to have a good prognosis in contrast to T-cell lymphomas originating from midline structures. The primary site determined at imaging appears to be correlated with the histologic phenotype and clinical outcome.)

Ojiri H, Ujita M, Tada S, Fukuda K. Potentially distinctive features of sinonasal inverted papilloma on MR imaging. *AJR Am J Roentgenol.* 2000;175:465. [PMID: 10915695] (Suggests that a sinonasal mass with a convoluted cerebriform pattern on T2- or enhanced T1-weighted images most likely represents inverted papilloma.)

Savy L, Lloyd G, Lund VJ, Howard D. Optimum imaging for inverted papilloma. *J Laryngol Otol.* 2000;114:891. [PMID: 11144847] (Reviews CT and MR imaging characteristics of inverted papilloma and how to distinguish them from other benign or aggressive sinonasal masses.)

Som PM, Lidov M, Brandwein M, Catalano P, Biller HF. Sinonasal esthesioneuroblastoma with intracranial extension: marginal tumor cysts as a diagnostic MR finding. *Am J Neuroradiol.* 1994;15(7):1259. [PMID: 7976934] (Most sinonasal masses have nonspecific imaging characteristics. The presence of cysts seen on MRI along the intracranial margin of a sinonasal mass strongly suggests esthesioneuroblastoma.)

Vanzieleghem BD, Lemmerling MM, Vermeersch HF et al. Imaging studies in the diagnostic workup of neonatal nasal obstruction. *J Comput Assist Tomogr.* 2001;25:540. [PMID: 11473183] (This review emphasizes the need for performing imaging studies in the diagnostic workup of neonates born with nasal obstruction and reviews causes of neonatal nasal obstruction.)

Yousem DM, Li C, Montone KT et al. Primary malignant melanoma of the sinonasal cavity: MR imaging evaluation. *Radiographics.* 1996;16:1101. [PMID: 8888393] (The signal intensity of sinonasal melanoma varies according to the histopathologic components of the tumor, with a high signal intensity within the lesion on T1-weighted images suggesting the presence of melanin.)

SKULL BASE

The skull base separates the extracranial head and neck from the intracranial contents. Multiple important neurovascular structures traverse the skull base, and knowledge of the complex anatomy of the skull base is essential to accurately evaluate and characterize this region. When CT scanning of the skull base is performed, both axial and coronal planes should be used, with sections no thicker than 3 mm. CT scanning of the skull base is useful for planning operative approaches, assessing many infectious, inflammatory, and congenital lesions, assessing and characterizing processes intrinsic to bone, and narrowing a differential diagnosis (ie, Is a lesion calcified or not? Does the lesion remodel or destroy bone?). MRI should also be done in multiple planes, with fat saturation on fast spin-echo T2-weighted images and postgadolinium T1-weighted images, as in the extracranial head and neck. MRI provides additional information regarding lesion extent, lesion characterization, and the involvement of brain or important neurovascular structures by disease.

The skull base can be considered in three major sections: anterior, central, and posterolateral. The major apertures of the skull base that provide communication between the intracranial compartment and the extracranial head and neck are reviewed in Table 3–11, which lists each foramen or canal and its relevant contents. These apertures and foramina can be demonstrated on CT scanning and MRI (see Figures 3–103 and 3–124).

Table 3–11. Major openings of the skull base.

Aperture	Contents
Cribriform plate	Olfactory nerves, ethmoid arteries
Optic canal	Optic nerve-sheath complex
	Ophthalmic artery
Superior orbital fissure	Cranial nerves III, IV, VI and V1 (ophthalmic nerve)
	Superior ophthalmic vein
Foramen ovale	V3 (mandibular nerve)
Foramen rotundum	V2 (maxillary nerve)
Foramen spinosum	Middle meningeal artery
Vidian canal	Vidian artery
	Vidian nerve
Carotid canal	Internal carotid artery
	Sympathetic plexus
Jugular foramen, pars nervosa	CN IX and inferior petrosal sinus
Jugular foramen, pars vascularis	Internal jugular vein
	CN X and XI
Stylomastoid foramen	CN VII
Hypoglossal canal	CN XII

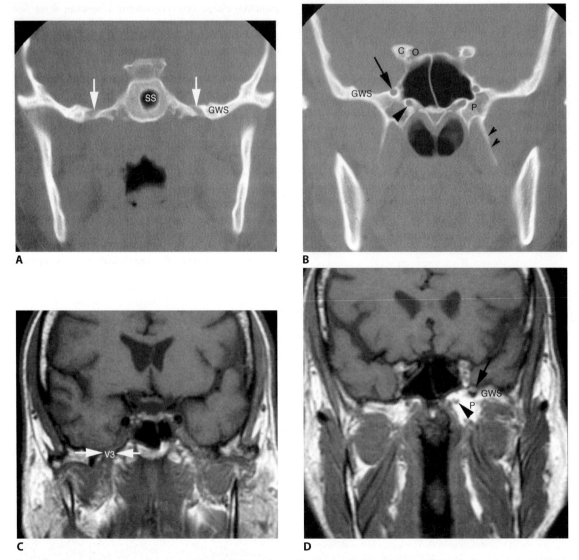

Figure 3–124. **(A)** Coronal CT scan of the skull base viewed in bone window demonstrates the foramen ovale bilaterally (white arrows) and the sphenoid sinus (SS) and greater wing of the sphenoid bone (GWS). **(B)** A more anterior image demonstrates foramen rotundum (black arrow) and the vidian canal (black arrowhead), as well as the anterior clinoid process (C) and the optic canal (O). Also seen are the greater wing of the sphenoid (GWS), the pterygoid process (P), and the lateral pterygoid plate (small double arrowheads). **(C)** A coronal T1-weighted image demonstrates the corresponding soft tissue anatomy, with V3 seen passing through the foramen ovale (arrows). **(D)** A more anterior image demonstrates foramen rotundum (black arrow) and the vidian canal (black arrowhead). Fatty marrow in the left pterygoid process of the sphenoid bone (P) and the greater wing of the sphenoid is indicated.

Anterior Skull Base

The anterior skull base makes up the floor of the anterior cranial fossa and includes the orbital plate of the frontal bone, the roof of the ethmoid bone, and the cribriform plate. From the ENT perspective, the anterior skull base is most commonly involved by superior extension of neoplasms of the nasal cavity and ethmoid sinuses (see Figure 3–121), intrinsic bony processes (such as fibrous dysplasia, Figure 3–125), and trauma.

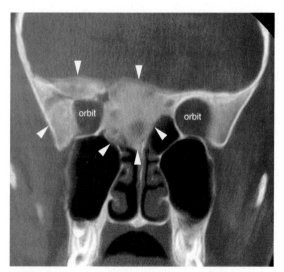

Figure 3–125. Coronal CT scan of the skull base viewed in bone window demonstrates a benign-appearing expansion of the central and right anterior skull base and right lateral orbital wall (arrowheads), which also has a somewhat "ground glass" texture. This appearance is diagnostic of fibrous dysplasia. Note that the right orbit is smaller than the left because of encroachment on the orbit by the expanded bone.

Because of the fragility of the cribriform plate, it is at high risk for traumatic disruption from accidental trauma or functional endoscopic sinus surgery, and this area should be carefully assessed in patients suspected of having CSF rhinorrhea (Figure 3–126).

Central Skull Base

The central skull base is formed by the sphenoid and occipital bones. The sphenoid bone is anatomically complex and has five distinct parts. The basisphenoid includes the sphenoid sinus, the sella turcica, the dorsum and tuberculum sella, and the posterior clinoid processes; in combination with the basilar part of the occipital bone, the basisphenoid also forms the clivus. The paired greater wings of the sphenoid form much of the floor and anterior wall of the middle cranial fossa, whereas the paired lesser wings give rise to the anterior clinoid processes and contribute to the formation of the orbital fissure. The pterygoid process of the sphenoid bone gives rise to the pterygoid plates. The planum sphenoidale is a flat plane that extends from the tuberculum sella posteriorly to the posterior edge of the cribriform plate anteriorly. The occipital bone has three major segments. The basilar part of the occipital bone is centrally located and fuses with the basisphenoid to

form the clivus; the synchondrosis between these two structures is easily visible in early childhood (Figure 3–127), but is usually completely fused by age 25. The occipital condyles are laterally located, and the squamous portion is posteriorly located and forms the majority of the floor of the posterior fossa.

The central skull base may be involved by several categories of disease processes: (1) those that extend upward and centrally from the deep spaces of the extracranial head and neck, (2) those that extend inferiorly from the intracranial compartment, and (3) those that are intrinsic to the tissues of the central skull base. The deep facial spaces that abut the central skull base include the parapharyngeal, masticator, and prevertebral portion of the periverterbal space. Disease processes primary to these spaces, notably neoplastic and infectious disorders, may access and involve the central skull base from below. Intracranial processes that may extend inferiorly to involve the central skull base are beyond the scope of this chapter.

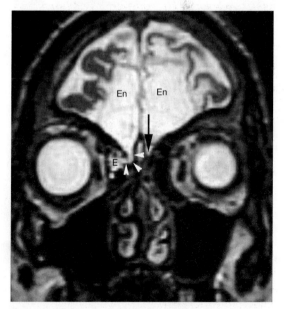

Figure 3–126. Coronal thin-section (1.5 mm) fast spin-echo T2-weighted image in a young male with post-traumatic cognitive dysfunction, anosmia, and a right-sided CSF leak. Bifrontal encephalomalacia (En) is seen. The normal left cribriform plate is demonstrated (black arrow). On the right, the cribriform plate is disrupted, and high signal intensity material consistent with CSF is seen to track from the anterior cranial fossa to the ethmoid sinus (arrowheads leading to E). At surgery, a focal defect in the right cribriform plate was confirmed and repaired.

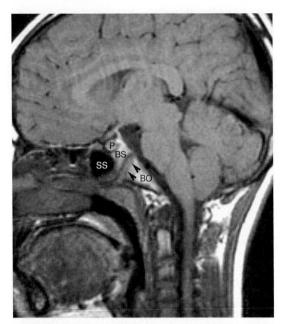

Figure 3–127. Sagittal T1-weighted image in a normal 8-year-old girl demonstrates the sphenooccipital synchondrosis (small black arrowheads) between the basisphenoid (BS) and the basilar part of the occipital bone (BO). Also shown are the sphenoid sinus (SS) and the pituitary gland (P) in the sella turcica.

A. LESIONS INVOLVING THE CENTRAL SKULL BASE FROM BELOW

1. Direct extension—Deep face infection or neoplasm may involve the central skull base by direct extension, in which case a process or mass centered in a space of the suprahyoid head and neck extends to involve the central skull base by contiguous growth. This typically leads to remodeling or frank destruction of bone, marrow infiltration, and, possibly, gross intracranial extension if the skull base is breached (Figure 3–128).

2. Perineural spread of disease—Perineural spread implies tumor extension to noncontiguous areas along nerves. In the head and neck, this most commonly involves branches of cranial nerves V and VII (the trigeminal and facial nerves, respectively). Although many malignant tumors may spread in a perineural fashion, the common head and neck lesions implicated in the perineural spread of disease include SCC of both cutaneous and mucosal origin, adenoid cystic carcinoma, lymphoma, melanoma, basal cell carcinoma, and mucoepidermoid carcinoma.

The perineural spread of tumor may result in clinical symptoms (eg, pain, dysesthesia, and hypesthesia), but may be asymptomatic even when demonstrable on imaging studies. Radiologic findings in perineural tumor spread include nerve and foraminal enlargement (Figure 3–129), foraminal destruction, obliteration of fat planes adjacent to the nerve, abnormal nerve enhancement (Figure 3–130), convexity of the lateral wall of the cavernous sinus, replacement of CSF in Meckel cave by soft tissue (Figure 3–131), and denervation changes in muscles innervated by the affected nerve (Figure 3–132). Perineural spread may occur in both antegrade and retrograde directions—for example, tumor that has spread back along V3 may reach the Gasserian ganglion and then spread in an antegrade manner along V1, V2, or both, as well as continuing to spread in a retrograde manner back along the cisternal segment of the trigeminal nerve to the pons.

B. LESIONS INTRINSIC TO THE CENTRAL SKULL BASE

The central skull base is composed primarily of cartilage and bone and is therefore subject to disease processes involving these tissues, especially neoplasm and infec-

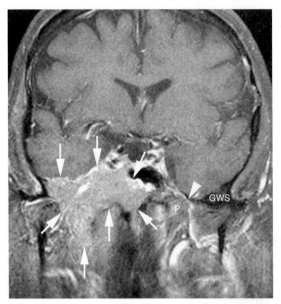

Figure 3–128. Coronal postgadolinium T1-weighted image with fat saturation in a patient with deep-seated skull base pain and right V3 dysfunction demonstrates a large soft tissue mass (arrows) destroying the right greater wing of the sphenoid. This was eventually proved to be a nasopharyngeal carcinoma that had grown primarily superolaterally to destroy the skull base and invade the middle cranial fossa (note the elevation of the right temporal lobe). Shown for comparison on the left are the greater wing of the sphenoid (GWS), the pterygoid process (P), and V3 (arrowhead).

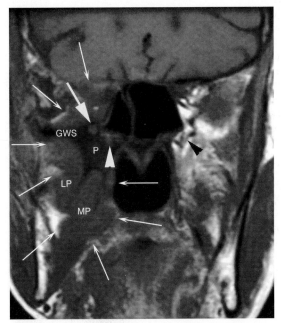

Figure 3–129. Slightly oblique coronal T1-weighted image in a patient with adenocarcinoma of the palate and extensive perineural spread of disease. Normal fat planes of the skull base and infratemporal fossa have been obliterated on the right by infiltrative tumor. The extent of tumor infiltration on the right is indicated by the thin concave white arrows. The right pterygoid process (P) and greater sphenoid wing (GWS) are low in signal intensity due to tumor infiltration instead of showing the expected high signal of fatty marrow; the medial and lateral pterygoid muscles (MP, LP) are also infiltrated. Foramen rotundum (white arrow) and the vidian canal (white arrowhead) are enlarged on the right due to the perineural spread of disease. The normal left vidian canal is indicated (black arrowhead).

tion. Certain congenital-developmental abnormalities of the central skull base may also be clinically relevant, primarily from the point of recognizing "don't touch" lesions such as fibrous dysplasia. In addition, adjacent vascular and soft tissue structures may give rise to lesions (eg, aneurysms, meningiomas, and nerve sheath tumors) that are intimately associated with the central skull base and need to be considered in the differential diagnosis of masses in this area.

1. Neoplasms—The central skull base may be involved with primary or metastatic lesions. Among the more common primary lesions are chordomas, chondrosarcomas, plasmacytomas, and lymphomas, as well as diffuse marrow infiltrative processes such as leukemia. MRI is

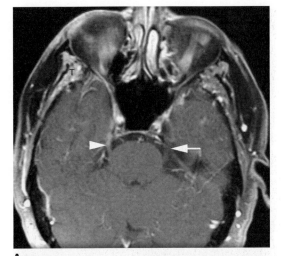

A

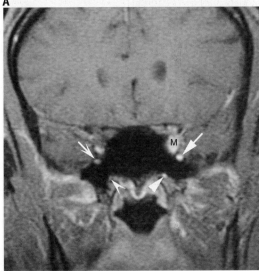

B

Figure 3–130. **(A)** Axial postgadolinium T1-weighted image with fat saturation demonstrates asymmetric enhancement of the cisternal segment of the right trigeminal nerve (arrowhead) compared with the normal left trigeminal nerve (arrow) in a patient with known perineural spread of carcinoma. The asymmetric enhancement of the right temporalis muscle (T) is a consequence of acute denervation change. **(B)** Coronal postgadolinium T1-weighted image with fat saturation in a different patient with the perineural spread of tumor demonstrates asymmetric enhancement and enlargement of left V2 (straight white arrow) compared with the right (concave white arrow) and asymmetric enhancement and enlargement of the left vidian nerve (straight white arrowhead) compared with the right (concave white arrowhead). Also shown is a soft tissue mass (M) in the left orbital fissure.

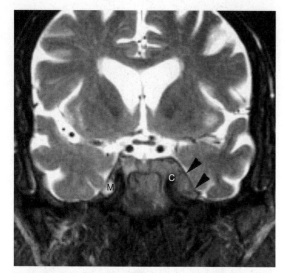

Figure 3–131. Coronal fast spin-echo T2-weighted image with fat saturation in a patient with perineural spread of squamous cell carcinoma demonstrates normal fluid intensity in the right Meckel cave (M), but the replacement of normal fluid by abnormal soft tissue (black arrowheads) on the left. The abnormal soft tissue also invaded the left cavernous sinus and surrounded the cavernous segment of the internal carotid artery (C).

generally far more sensitive than CT scanning in the detection of these lesions because T1-weighted images are very sensitive to marrow-replacing processes and become abnormal far earlier than CT scanning, which requires gross bone destruction before a lesion can be appreciated. Although the clival marrow is relatively hypointense in very young children (less than 3 years old), the marrow becomes progressively more fatty in children between 3 and 10 years and is homogeneously fatty by the teenage years. Therefore, lesions of the clivus are often best appreciated on a sagittal T1-weighted image. The normal adult clivus and, in contrast, clival marrow infiltration are demonstrated in Figure 3–133.

a. Chordomas—Chordomas arise from notochordal remnants within the clivus and are typically centered on the midline. Chordomas of the central skull base account for 35% of these lesions, which are locally aggressive and often abut or engulf vital structures by the time they are diagnosed, making surgical resection difficult or impossible. They also metastasize in approximately 40% of cases, most commonly to bone, liver, and lymph nodes. On CT scanning, a destructive mass is seen that may contain fragments of destroyed bone. On MRI, the lesions are typically intermediate in signal on T1-weighted images and markedly hyperintense on T2-weighted images (Figure 3–134), although the presence of bone fragments or hemor-

rhage may alter the signal characteristics. Postgadolinium, enhancement varies from absent or mild and heterogeneous to intense and homogeneous.

b. Chondrosarcomas—Because the skull base is derived from cartilage, chondrosarcomas not uncommonly take origin here; in fact, 75% of all cranial chondrosarcomas are located in the skull base. These slow-growing malignant cartilaginous tumors typically spread by local invasion and may cause extensive destruction of the skull base. Skull base chondrosarcomas are most commonly centered on the petrooccipital fissure and their off-midline location is a helpful feature in distinguishing them from chordomas. CT scanning shows a destructive mass that may have matrix calcification. MRI shows a mass that is intermediate on T1-weighted images and hyperintense on T2-weighted images, with intense enhancement postgadolinium (Figure 3–135). If there is significant matrix calcification, then there may be areas of heterogeneously low signal on T2-weighted images and enhancement will be heterogeneous as well.

c. Metastatic disease—Hematogenous metastases to the skull base are more common than primary neoplasms, and most frequently originate from lung, breast, prostate, and kidney. CT scanning shows lytic bone destruction if the process is advanced enough, but may

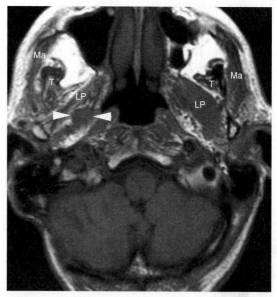

Figure 3–132. Axial T1-weighted image in a patient with perineural spread of squamous cell carcinoma along the right V3, which is massively enlarged (arrowheads). Denervation atrophy (decreased bulk, fatty infiltration) is seen in the right muscles of mastication compared with the left. Indicated are the lateral pterygoid (LP), masseter (Ma) and temporalis (T) muscles.

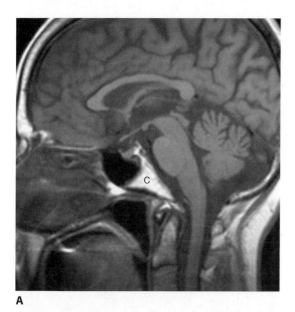 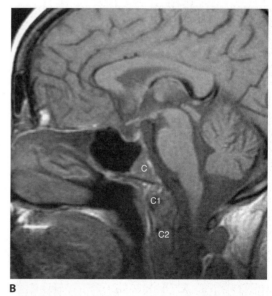

A   B

Figure 3–133. **(A)** Sagittal T1-weighted image demonstrates the normal, homogeneously fatty adult clivus (C). **(B)** Sagittal T1-weighted image in a different patient demonstrates abnormal hypointensity of the marrow spaces of the clivus (C) and C1 and C2 vertebral bodies in this patient with chronic myelogenous leukemia.

appear normal early on. MRI is far more sensitive to the replacement of normal fatty marrow by tumor. Most metastases are intermediate in signal on T1- and T2-weighted images and show enhancement postcontrast.

2. Infection—Osteomyelitis of the skull base most commonly involves the temporal bone, but may also involve the central skull base. It may result from the direct extension of sphenoid or ethmoid sinus inflammatory disease, iatrogenic or accidental trauma, or hematogenous dissemination. Infection may also spread centrally from a more lateral temporal bone focus. Diabetic and otherwise immunocompromised patients are at higher risk for skull base osteomyelitis, which may be a difficult and subtle diagnosis to render on imaging studies. The careful assessment of pregadolinium T1-weighted images for the loss of a normal, bright, fatty marrow signal and the subtle infiltration of fat planes adjacent to the skull base is particularly useful (Figure 3–136). MRI is the study of choice if this diagnosis is being considered.

3. Vascular lesions—A large or giant aneurysm, usually of the cavernous segment of the internal carotid artery, may present with headache, cranial neuropathy, or both, and may cause considerable remodeling of the sphenoid bone, thereby mimicking a neoplastic process. It is important that such a lesion be properly diagnosed rather than embarking on a biopsy, which could be fatal. On CT scanning, the lesion appears to smoothly remodel bone and may have a peripherally calcified rim. On MRI, layers of lamellated thrombus are seen if the aneurysm is partly

thrombosed, and phase artifact related to pulsatile flow may be noted (Figure 3–137). In addition, MR angiography may directly demonstrate flow within the aneurysm.

4. Congenital and developmental disorders—A cephalocele refers to a protrusion of intracranial contents through a congenital defect in the skull; it may contain meninges and CSF only (meningocele) or may contain brain tissue as well (encephalocele). Basal cephaloceles account for approximately 10% of all cephaloceles and may present as a mass visible on examination (see Figure 3–104) or may be detected incidentally on a CT scan or MRI. Patients may also present with meningitis or other complaints. It is important to avoid unintentional violation of these lesions since this may lead to meningitis, CSF leak, and other complications (Figure 3–138).

5. Other disorders—A number of conditions that affect the skull base may present a potentially confusing picture on imaging studies.

    a. Fibrous dysplasia—Fibrous dysplasia commonly involves the skull base and may be focal, multifocal, or diffuse. Fibrous dysplasia causes bone expansion and, on CT scans, a classic "ground glass" appearance of hazy sclerosis; focal lytic or cystic areas may also occur. On MRI, the hallmark is also bone expansion. The signal is typically intermediate on T1-weighted images and intermediate to dark on T2-weighted images, with prominent enhancement postgadolinium. Signal characteristics vary with the extent of the fibrous component and the presence of cystic areas. This diagnosis is

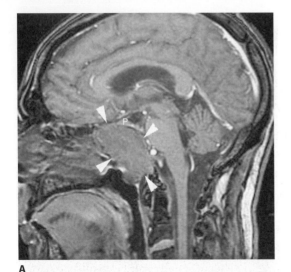

A

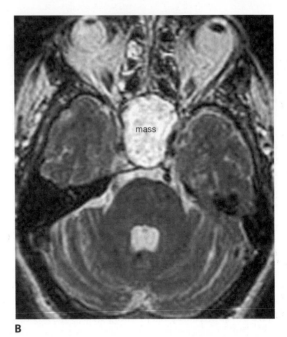

B

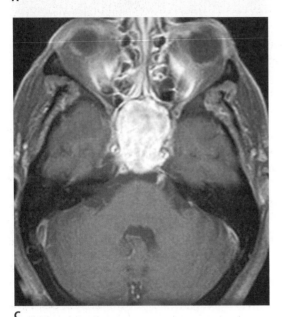

C

Figure 3–134. **(A)** A sagittal T1-weighted gradient echo image acquired as part of a surgical navigation study demonstrates an intermediate signal intensity soft tissue mass (arrowheads) obliterating the sphenoid sinus and clivus, and elevating the pituitary gland (P). **(B)** On an axial fast spin-echo T2-weighted image, the mass is high in signal intensity. **(C)** Postgadolinium, a T1-weighted image with fat saturation demonstrates intense and homogeneous enhancement. The pathology confirmed the diagnosis of chordoma.

often much more difficult to make on MRI than on a CT scan and is a potential pitfall of skull base imaging because this benign "don't touch" condition may be misdiagnosed as a skull base neoplasm. If MRI presents a confusing picture, then CT scanning may be very helpful for confirming the diagnosis of fibrous dysplasia (Figure 3–139).

b. Paget disease—Paget disease is typically seen in older patients and appears as bone thickening and sclerosis on CT scans; on MRI, bone is expanded and often quite heterogeneous in signal intensity. Although this potentially mimics fibrous dysplasia, it is typically diffuse rather than focal.

c. Osteoradionecrosis—Osteoradionecrosis of the skull base may be seen in patients who have received prior high-dose radiation therapy for head and neck cancer (notably of the nasopharynx) or for sellar or parasellar pathology. This typically appears as a mixed lytic and sclerotic process on CT scans and as heterogeneous marrow signal intensity on MRI. The differentiation from chronic osteomyelitis can be difficult, and, in fact, infection may complicate osteoradionecrosis.

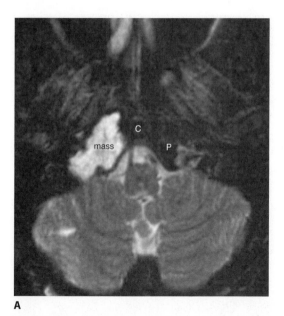

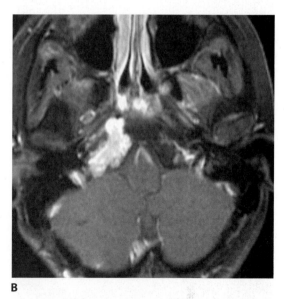

A   **B**

Figure 3–135. **(A)** Axial fast spin-echo T2-weighted image with fat saturation in a young woman with a sixth nerve palsy demonstrates a multilobulated, high signal intensity lesion involving the right lateral clivus (C) and petrous bone. The left petrous bone is identified (P). **(B)** Postgadolinium, a T1-weighted image with fat saturation demonstrates intense and homogeneous enhancement of the lesion. Imaging and pathology were consistent with chondrosarcoma.

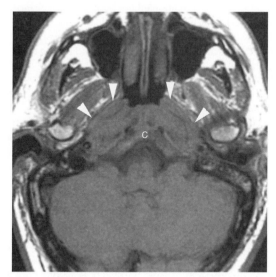

Figure 3–136. Axial T1-weighted image in a 56-year-old diabetic man with headache, low-grade fever, and lower cranial neuropathy demonstrates abnormal hypointensity of clival marrow (C). In addition, the soft tissues anterior to the central skull base (arrowheads) are abnormally full and normal fat planes are obliterated, further supporting an infiltrative neoplastic or inflammatory process. Skull base osteomyelitis was eventually confirmed by tissue sampling.

Caldemeyer KS, Mathews VP, Righi PD, Smith RR. Imaging features and clinical significance of perineural spread or extension of head and neck tumors. *Radiographics.* 1998;18:97. [PMID: 9460111] (Reviews the normal cranial nerve anatomy and the radiologic appearance and assessment of perineural tumor extension.)

Ginsberg LE. Neoplastic diseases affecting the central skull base: CT and MR imaging. *AJR Am J Roentgenol.* 1992;159:581. [PMID: 1503031] (Reviews some of the more commonly encountered tumors that can affect the skull base and describes their CT and MR imaging appearance.)

Laine FJ, Nadel L, Braun IF. CT and MR imaging of the central skull base. Part 1: Techniques, embryologic development, and anatomy. *Radiographics.* 1990;10:591. [PMID: 2198631] (The embryologic development of the central skull base, normal gross anatomy, and cross-sectional radiologic anatomy are presented.)

Laine FJ, Nadel L, Braun IF. CT and MR imaging of the central skull base. Part 2. Pathologic spectrum. *Radiographics.* 1990;10:797. [PMID: 2217972] (The authors present examples of congenital, benign, and malignant lesions that affect the central skull base.)

Laine FJ, Smoker WR. Anatomy of the cranial nerves. *Neuroimaging Clin N Am.* 1998;8:69. [PMID: 9449754] (The anatomy of CN I and III through XII is presented diagrammatically and with CT scanning and MRI correlations.)

Posterolateral Skull Base

The posterolateral skull base can be equated with the temporal bone. Certain imaging techniques and disease processes are unique to the temporal bone.

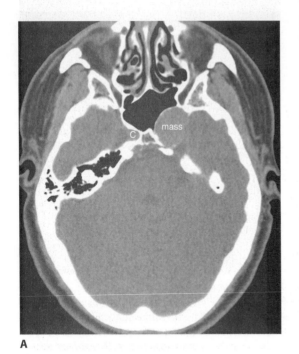 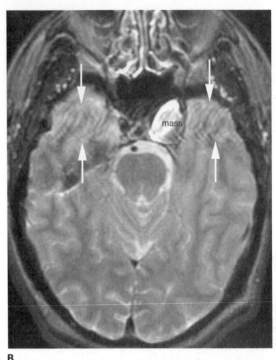

A

B

Figure 3–137. (A) Axial noncontrast CT scan of the skull base viewed in bone window in a young man with headache demonstrates a rounded mass with faint peripheral calcification that has remodeled the bone of the skull base. The mass is centered on the left carotid canal. The contralateral carotid canal (C) is demonstrated. (B) Axial T2-weighted image in the same patient demonstrates heterogeneous signal intensity within the left mass, consistent with lamellated thrombus. Phase artifact (white arrows) confirms the vascular nature of the lesion, and a large aneurysm of the cavernous carotid artery was confirmed with angiography.

A. CT SCANNING

Computed tomography is the dominant imaging modality for depicting the bony anatomy of the temporal bone. CT imaging of the temporal bone is usually performed in the axial and coronal planes with a slice thickness of ≤ 1 mm. Ideally, the source images are retargeted to a small display field of view of 10 cm for both the right and left sides individually. For the depiction of bony anatomy, intravenous contrast is not needed. The normal anatomy of the temporal bone depicted on CT scans is demonstrated in Figure 3–140.

B. MRI

Magnetic resonance imaging is useful for imaging the soft tissues and fluid compartments of the temporal bone. For suspected neoplastic and inflammatory pathologies, the intravenous administration of gadolinium is important to identify areas of abnormal enhancement. The following sequences are routinely used in examining the temporal bone:

Axial T1-weighted imaging

Axial 3D fast spin-echo T2-weighted imaging with fat saturation or axial FIESTA (Fast Imaging Employing Steady-State Acquisition) imaging

Pregadolinium axial T1-weighted imaging

Postgadolinium axial T1-weighted imaging with fat saturation

Postgadolinium coronal T1-weighted imaging with fat saturation

To best depict the detailed anatomy of the temporal bone, a field of view of 17 cm by 17 cm with a slice thickness of 2 mm with a 0 mm skip and a matrix size of 256 by 192 for T1-weighted images, both pre- and postgadolinium, is used. For T2-weighted imaging, submillimeter slices are acquired with either a three-dimensional fast spin-echo sequence or a FIESTA sequence. A pregadolinium T1-weighted imaging sequence is useful in order to identify areas of fat (such as a lipoma), hemorrhage, or elevated protein content within the inner ear, as

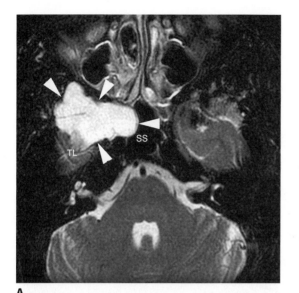

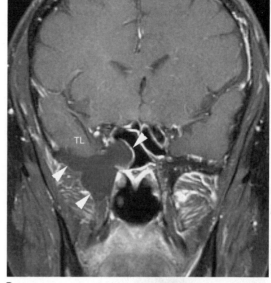

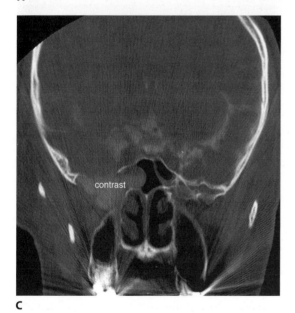

Figure 3–138. A 22-year-old man underwent MRI for evaluation of headache and was referred for treatment of a skull base "mass" that was discovered. **(A)** Axial fast spin-echo T2-weighted image with fat saturation demonstrates a well-circumscribed, strikingly hyperintense mass (arrowheads) involving the right skull base and encroaching on the sphenoid sinus (SS). It is located immediately adjacent to the temporal lobe (TL). **(B)** On a coronal postgadolinium T1-weighted image with fat saturation, the lesion is centered just below the temporal lobe at the level of the greater wing of the sphenoid and is isointense to cerebrospinal fluid. The diagnosis of lateral sphenoid meningocele was questioned and the planned biopsy was cancelled. **(C)** The patient underwent CT cisternography. Complete filling of the skull base "lesion" with contrast confirmed the diagnosis of lateral sphenoid meningocele. Note the absence of much of the greater wing of the sphenoid on the right, presumably secondary to congenital deficiency and thinning and remodeling over time due to CSF pulsations.

might be seen with a process such as labyrinthitis. Fat saturation is extremely important for postgadolinium sequences in order to identify enhancement that might otherwise be obscured by fatty marrow in the petrous bone. In many centers, diffusion-weighted imaging is now added to the temporal bone MR imaging protocol to evaluate temporal bone cholesteatomas and CPA epidermoid cysts. These lesions typically demonstrate reduced diffusion of water molecules, which is seen as localized high signal intensity on a diffusion-weighted image.

Fitzek C, Mewes T, Fitzek S et al. Diffusion-weighted MRI of cholesteatomas of the petrous bone. *J Magn Reson Imaging.* 2002;15:636. [PMID: 12112513] (Discusses the utility of DWI for evaluating cholesteatomas of the temporal bone.)

Gunlock MG, Gentry LR. Anatomy of the temporal bone. *Neuroimaging Clin N Am.* 1998;8(1):195. [PMID: 9449760] (Description of normal temporal bone anatomy.)

Nayak S. Segmental anatomy of the temporal bone. *Semin Ultrasound CT MR.* 2001;22(3):184. [PMID: 11451096] (Description of normal temporal bone anatomy.)

Stone JA, Chakeres DW, Schmalbrock P. High-resolution MR imaging of the auditory pathway. *Magn Reson Imaging Clin N*

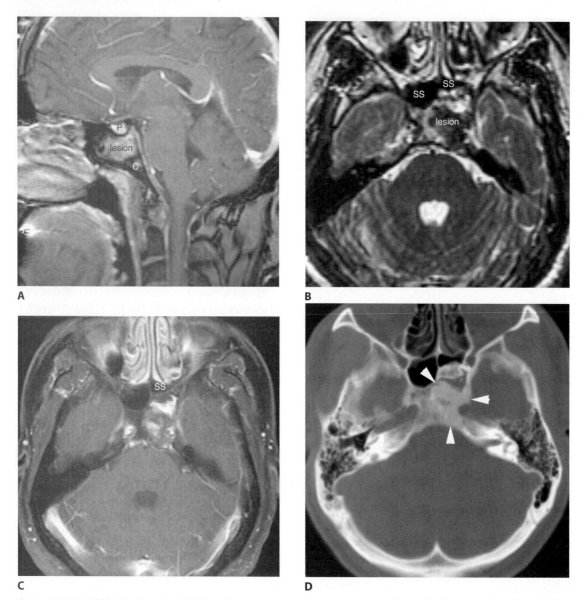

Figure 3–139. **(A)** Sagittal postgadolinium T1-weighted gradient echo image of the skull base acquired as part of a preoperative surgical navigation protocol on a patient referred for a biopsy of a skull base mass. Indicated are the normal clivus (C, which appears dark on a gradient echo image), the pituitary gland (P), and the enhancing lesion. **(B)** Axial fast spin-echo T2-weighted image shows that the lesion is quite low in signal intensity and the left sphenoid sinus (SS) appears small compared to the right. A more anterior component of the left-sided lesion is heterogeneously hyperintense. **(C)** On an axial postgadolinium T1-weighted image with fat saturation, it is clear that the left clivus is expanded, the left sphenoid sinus (SS) is small, and the bony lesion demonstrates heterogeneous but fairly intense enhancement. No destructive or aggressive features are noted. The diagnosis of fibrous dysplasia was questioned and a CT scan was recommended. **(D)** Axial CT scan of the skull base viewed in bone window demonstrates expansion of the left sphenoid bone and areas of ground glass opacity, consistent with a diagnosis of fibrous dysplasia. The unnecessary biopsy was cancelled.

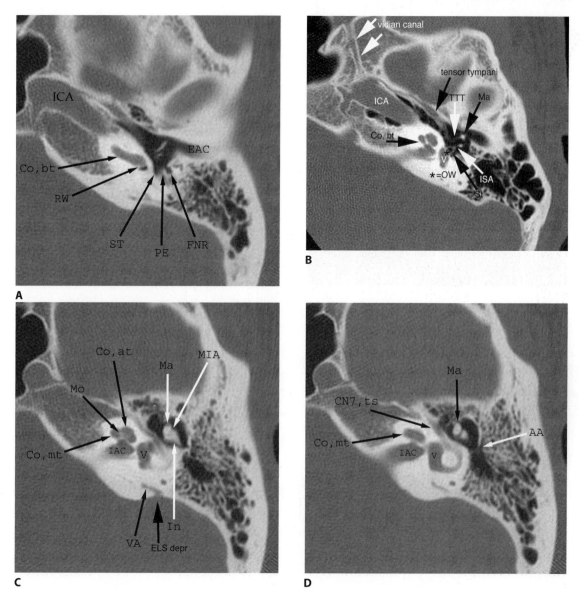

Figure 3–140. CT scan of normal temporal bone, photographed in bone window. Axial images **(A)** to **(G)** are inferior to superior. Legend for parts **(H)** to **(K)** appears on page 133. *(Continued)*

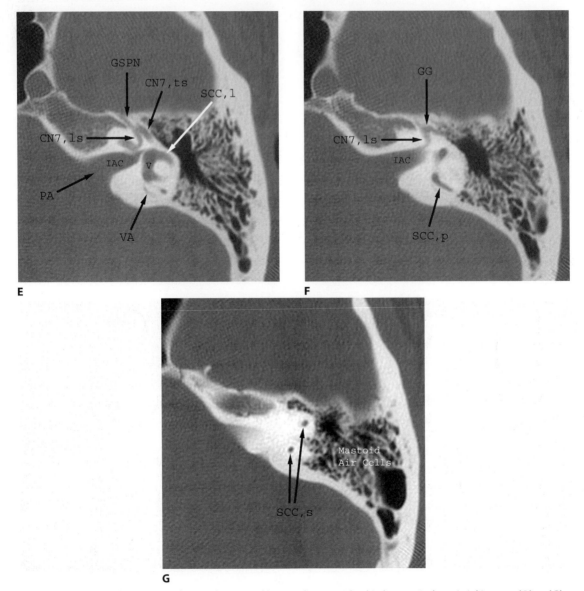

Figure 3–140 (Cont'd). CT scan of normal temporal bone, photographed in bone window. Axial images **(A)** to **(G)** are inferior to superior. *(Continued)*

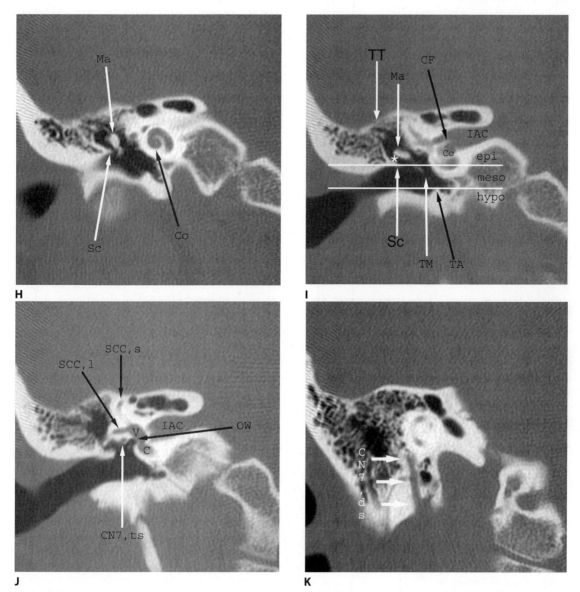

Figure 3–140 (Cont'd). CT scan of normal temporal bone, photographed in bone window. Coronal images **(H)** to **(K)** are anterior to posterior. Abbreviations: AA, aditus ad antrum; CF, crista falciformis; CN7,ds, CN VII, descending mastoid segment; CN7,ls, CN VII, labyrinthine segment; CN7,ts, CN VII, tympanic segment; Co, cochlea; Co,at, cochlea, apical turn; Co,bt, cochlea, base turn; Co,mt, cochlea, middle turn; EAC, external auditory canal; ELS dep, endolymphatic sac depression; epi, epitympanum; FNR, facial nerve recess; GG, geniculate ganglion; GSPN, greater superficial petrosal nerve; hypo, hypotympanum; IAC, internal auditory canal; ICA, internal carotid artery; In, incus; ISA, incudostapedial articulation; Ma, malleus; meso, mesotympanum; Mo, modiolus; MIA, malleoincudal articulation; OW, oval window; PE, pyramidal eminence; PA, porus acusticus; *, Prussak space; RW, round window; Sc, scutum; SCC,l, semicircular canal, lateral; SCC,p, semicircular canal, posterior; SCC,s, semicircular canal, superior; St, stapes; ST, sinus tympani; TA, tympanic annulus; TM, tympanic membrane; TT, tegmen tympani; TTT, tensor tympani tendon; V, vestibule; VA, vestibular aqueduct.

Table 3–12. Abnormalities of the external auditory canal.

| Congenital Aural Dysplasia | Inflammatory | Neoplastic | |
		Benign	*Malignant*
Atresia	Chronic external otitis (swimmer's ear)	Exostoses (surfer's ear)	Basal cell carcinoma
Stenosis	Malignant otitis externa (necrotizing external otitis)	Osteoma	Squamous cell carcinoma
	Keratosis obturans	Ceruminous gland origin tumor	Melanoma
	Cholesteatoma		Metastasis
			Ceruminous gland origin tumor

Am. 1998;6(1):195. [PMID: 9449749] (The current techniques in high-resolution MRI of the temporal bone are presented, followed by a review of normal anatomy.)

DISEASES OF THE TEMPORAL BONE

The temporal bone has five anatomic components: squamous, mastoid, petrous, tympanic, and styloid portions. It can be subdivided into three major clinically relevant compartments: the external auditory canal, the middle ear cavity, and the inner ear.

1. External Auditory Canal

Anatomy

The external auditory canal extends from the external pinna to the tympanic membrane. It includes the fibrocartilaginous ear canal and the bony ear canal.

Pathology

Abnormalities that may be encountered on imaging studies of the external auditory canal are listed in Table 3–12.

A. Atresia and Stenosis

Both atresia (Figure 3–141) and stenosis of the external auditory canal are secondary to failure of canalization of epithelial cells during the formation of the canal. Atresias of the external auditory canal can be bony, membranous, or mixed. When external auditory canal stenosis or atresia is encountered, associated deformities of the pinna and ossicles are often present. In addition, the facial nerve often has an abnormal course, being more anteriorly located than usual and exiting into the glenoid fossa rather than more medially into the stylomastoid foramen.

B. Exostoses

Exostoses (Figure 3–142) can form within the external auditory canal. This is commonly known as "surfer's

ear" because this condition appears to be induced by chronic exposure to cold water. This condition is usually bilateral and the exostosis has a broad base against the adjacent bone. Osteoma of the external auditory canal can be difficult to differentiate from an exostosis, but it is typically unilateral and pedunculated.

Davis TC, Thedinger BA, Greene GM. Osteomas of the internal auditory canal: a report of two cases. *Am J Otol.* 2000; 21(6):852. [PMID: 11078075] (Surgical intervention may be warranted to remove an osteoma of the internal auditory canal if symptoms are present.)

Swartz JD, Faerber EN. Congenital malformations of the external and middle ear: high-resolution CT findings of surgical import. *AJR Am J Roentgenol.* 1985;144(3):501. [PMID: 3871559] (Description of surgically important findings in congenital malformations of the external and middle ear.)

2. Middle Ear

Anatomy

The middle ear is separated from the external auditory canal by the tympanic membrane (see Figure 3–140). In the coronal plane, the tympanic membrane extends from the scutum to the tympanic annulus. The middle ear cavity contains three ossicles: the malleus, the incus, and the stapes. Sound is mechanically transmitted from the tympanic membrane to the malleus to the incus to the stapes and finally to the cochlea via the oval window. The oval window and the round window provide access from the middle ear cavity to the inner ear structures.

The middle ear can be further divided into three compartments: the epitympanum, the mesotympanum, and the hypotympanum. In the coronal plane, these compartments are defined by drawing imaginary extensions of the superior and inferior borders of the bony external canal across the middle ear cavity. These two lines effectively divide the middle ear cavity into three compartments. The most cephalad compartment is the epitympanum, the middle compartment is the meso-

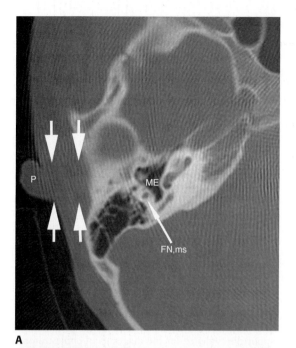

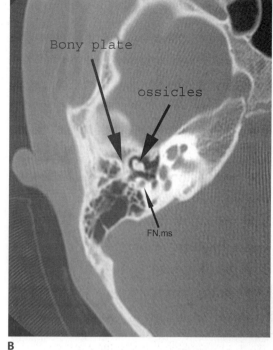

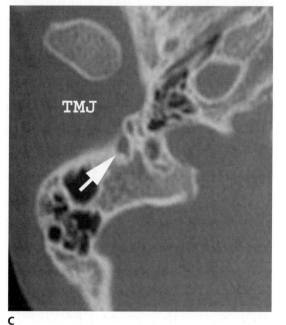

Figure 3–141. External auditory canal atresia. **(A)** Axial CT scan viewed in bone window demonstrates a malformed pinna (P) and absence of the external auditory canal (white arrows indicate expected position of the EAC). The middle ear (ME) and descending mastoid segment of facial nerve (FN, ms) are indicated. **(B)** A more superior image in the same patient demonstrates a small middle ear cleft, a bony atresia plate, and dysplastic-appearing ossicles. The inner ear is normal. **(C)** At a more inferior level, the facial nerve (arrow) exits into the posterior aspect of the temporomandibular joint (TMJ), more anterior and lateral than normal.

tympanum, and the most caudad compartment is the hypotympanum.

A. EPITYMPANUM

The epitympanum is bounded superiorly by the tegmen tympani. The relatively thin tegmen tympani separates the middle ear cavity from the middle cranial fossa. Within the epitympanum is the head of the malleus and the body and short process of the incus. Prussak space is the space between the lateral wall of the epitympanum and the neck of the malleus. Prussak space is the most common site of acquired pars flaccida cholesteatomas.

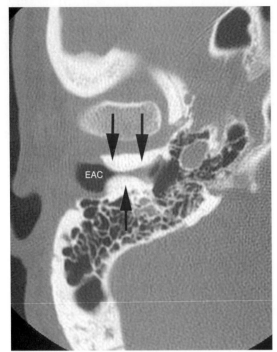

EAC

Figure 3–142. Exostosis ("surfer's ear"). Axial CT scan viewed in bone window demonstrates a marked narrowing of the external auditory canal by bony overgrowths (black arrows) representing exostoses. Abnormal soft tissue is secondary to impacted cerumen. The opposite side (not shown) was identical.

B. Mesotympanum

The mesotympanum contains the manubrium of the malleus, the long process of the incus, and the stapes. Two muscles are located in the mesotympanum. The stapedius and tensor tympani muscles serve to dampen sound transmission. The tensor tympani tendon inserts on the manubrium of the malleus. The stapedius muscle is located in the pyramidal eminence, and the stapedius tendon inserts on the head of the stapes. An important anatomic site is the sinus tympani, a clinical blind spot where cholesteatomas may hide.

C. Hypotympanum

The hypotympanum is the smallest compartment of the middle ear and contains no normal structures.

Pathology

Abnormalities that may be encountered on imaging studies of the middle ear are listed in Table 3–13.

A. Congenital Vascular Abnormalities

Congenital vascular abnormalities of the middle ear are important lesions to exclude before considering either a biopsy or surgery for a retrotympanic mass. An aberrant internal carotid artery (Figure 3–143) and a persistent stapedial artery are rare; they can be seen together or separately. The theories of development of an aberrant internal carotid artery include the presence of a persistent stapedial artery that "fixes" or "pulls" the internal carotid artery laterally into the middle ear. A second theory is that agenesis of a segment of the internal carotid artery results in the redirection of blood flow into the inferior tympanic and hyoid arteries in the middle ear. These arteries would typically have minor blood flow, but, in this situation, these arteries dilate and provide an alternate pathway through the middle ear cavity to bypass the absent segment of the internal carotid artery.

B. Cholesteatomas

Cholesteatomas arise from ectopic rests of epithelial tissue. The presence of bony erosion on imaging is strong supportive evidence for the diagnosis of cholesteatoma. A cholesteatoma can be present, however, without any evidence of bony erosion on imaging. In those cases, it is very difficult to distinguish cholesteatoma from the soft tissue changes that are seen with chronic otitis media. Cholesteatomas can be divided into congenital and acquired varieties (Figure 3–144). A congenital cholesteatoma is considered on imaging when there is a globular lesion within the middle ear with adjacent bone erosion, but without evidence or history of an inflammatory or infectious process or trauma. Acquired cholesteatomas occur when epithelial tissue gains entry to the middle ear cavity via infection or trauma that violates the tympanic membrane. The presence of a globular mass with adjacent erosions is typical. There are two types of acquired cholesteatomas. The more common type is the pars flaccida cholesteatoma, whereby the cholesteatoma arises near the pars flaccida of the tympanic membrane and extends into the Prussak space. The erosion of the scutum is one of the signs of this entity. A pars tensa cholesteatoma arises in posterosuperior retraction pockets of the tympanic membrane and often involves the sinus tympani. On MRI, the cholesteatoma has intermediate signal intensity on T1-weighted images, high signal intensity on T2-weighted images, and, on postgadolinium images, either no enhancement or a thin rim of enhancement representing adjacent granulation tissue. Diffusion weighted images also show high signal intensity. In contrast, a cholesterol granuloma of the middle ear has a high signal on T1-weighted sequences and the hyperintense signal does not diminish with fat saturation.

Table 3–13. Abnormalities of the middle ear.

Congenital Vascular Abnormalities	Congenital Masses	Inflammatory Abnormalities	Infectious Abnormalities	Neoplastic Masses		Ossicular Abnormalities
				Benign	*Malignant*	
Aberrant internal carotid artery	Congenital cholesteatoma	Acquired cholesteatoma —Pars flaccida —Pars tensa	Otomastoiditis (including complications)	Paraganglioma	Squamous cell carcinoma	Ossicular fixation
Persistent stapedial artery		Cholesterol granuloma		Hemangioma	Adeno-carcinoma	Ossicular erosion
Dehiscent jugular bulb		Langerhans cell histiocytosis (eosinophilic granuloma)		Meningioma	Adenoid cystic carcinoma	Ossicular dislocation
		Tympanosclerosis		Osseous tumors	Metastasis	Ossicular deformity
						Ossicular prosthesis

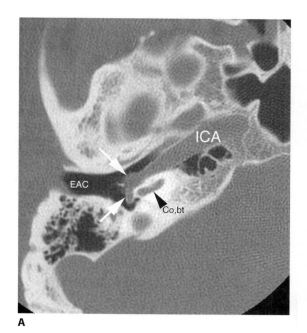
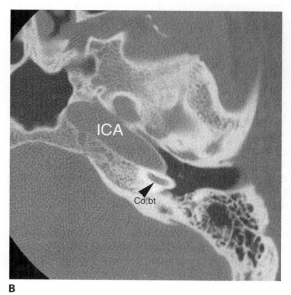

Figure 3–143. Aberrant internal carotid artery (ICA) in a patient presenting with right pulsatile tinnitus and a vascular retrotympanic mass. **(A)** Axial CT scan viewed in bone window demonstrates the aberrant ICA coursing through the middle ear cavity (white arrows) and overlying the cochlear promontory. The base turn of the cochlea is indicated (black arrow). The course of this carotid artery is more posterolateral than normal. **(B)** Contralateral ICA in the same patient shows the normal course of the horizontal segment of the ICA and a normal bony covering over the carotid canal.

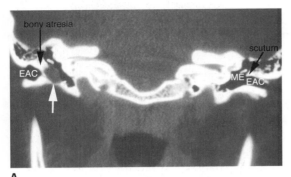

A

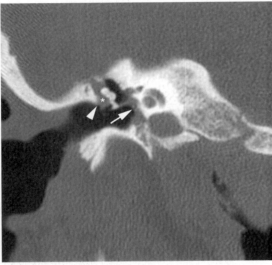

B

Figure 3–144. Cholesteatomas, congenital and acquired. **(A)** Coronal CT scan (intermediate window) demonstrates bony atresia of the right external auditory canal (EAC). Medial to the atretic plate is a rounded soft tissue mass (white arrow) that has caused some bone remodeling. At surgery, a congenital cholesteatoma was confirmed. ME, middle ear. **(B)** Coronal CT scan viewed in bone window in an adult with long-standing inflammatory disease of the right middle ear and mastoid demonstrates retraction of the right tympanic membrane (white arrow) and abnormal soft tissue in the middle ear. Soft tissue fills the right Prussak space (*), displacing the ossicles medially, and there is erosion of the scutum (arrowhead). Cholesteatoma was confirmed at surgery.

C. LANGERHANS CELL HISTIOCYTOSIS

Langerhans cell histiocytosis is a disease of children and young adults. It most commonly presents as solitary or multiple lytic lesions of bone. The temporal bone is a common location for these lesions, which appear as nonspecific unilateral or bilateral enhancing soft tissue masses on MRI.

D. INFECTION

Infection of the middle ear cavity frequently occurs in conjunction with infection of the mastoid air cells since these two compartments are connected via various channels, the largest being the aditus ad antrum. These spaces are vulnerable to infection with bacteria from the upper respiratory tract via the eustachian tubes. Coalescent mastoiditis (Figure 3–145) is diagnosed when there is erosion of the bony septa of the mastoid air cells and an abscess develops in the mastoid bone. Complications that need to be recognized include subperiosteal abscesses, thrombosis of adjacent dural venous sinuses (Figure 3–146), and intracranial extension.

E. NEOPLASMS

The most common benign tumor of the middle ear is a paraganglioma. If a paraganglioma is in the middle ear, it is called a glomus tympanicum. Often, there is a component of the lesion near the jugular bulb. The combined lesion is known as a glomus jugulotympanicum (Figure 3–147). A facial nerve schwannoma may also present as a middle ear mass.

Malignant tumors of the middle ear cavity are not common. Metastases to bone or dura may erode into the middle ear and present as a middle ear mass.

F. OSSICULAR CHAIN ABNORMALITIES

The ossicular chain consists of the malleus, the incus, and the stapes. Abnormalities of this chain lead to a conductive hearing loss. Acquired abnormalities are typically from inflammation or trauma. These processes can lead to ossicular fusion, fracture, dislocation (Figure 3–148), and erosion. Ossicular prostheses can be used to reconstruct some or all of the ossicular chain (Figure 3–149).

G. ABNORMAL COMMUNICATIONS

Abnormal communication between the middle ear cavity and the middle cranial fossa can occur from inflammation, infection, trauma, or postoperative complications. Infections can spread from the middle ear cavity into the intracranial compartment. Brain, meninges, or both may herniate through the defect into the middle ear cavity or external auditory canal (or both) (Figure 3–150).

Jackson CG, Pappas DG Jr, Manolidis S et al. Brain herniation into the middle ear and mastoid: concepts in diagnosis and surgical management. *Am J Otol.* 1997;18(2):198. [PMID: 9093677] (Prompt and effective surgical repair is successful

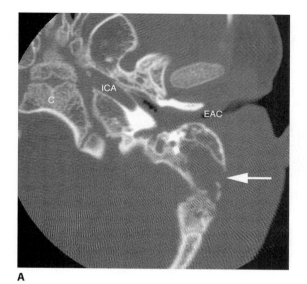

A

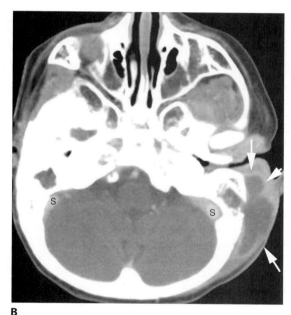

B

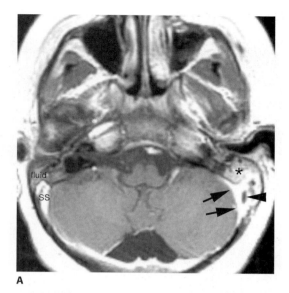

A

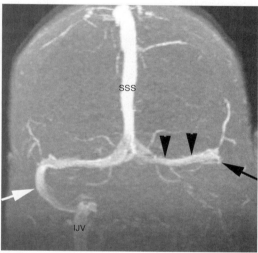

B

Figure 3–145. Coalescent mastoiditis. **(A)** Axial CT scan viewed in bone window demonstrates soft tissue narrowing of the external auditory canal, abnormal soft tissue in the middle ear cavity, and opacification of mastoid air cells. Erosion of multiple mastoid septa is consistent with coalescent mastoiditis. A focal defect is present (white arrow) in the lateral mastoid cortex, and marked overlying soft tissue swelling is seen. C, clivus; ICA, internal carotid artery; EAC, external auditory canal. **(B)** Postcontrast CT scan in the same patient demonstrates a large abscess (white arrows) involving the mastoid and extending laterally into adjacent soft tissues. The sigmoid sinuses (S) are patent bilaterally.

Figure 3–146. Mastoiditis and sigmoid sinus thrombosis. **(A)** Postgadolinium axial T1-weighted sequence shows enhancement in the left mastoid air cells (*) with adjacent intracranial extension and intense enhancement of dura at the level of the sigmoid sinus (arrows). Nonspecific mastoid fluid and a normal sigmoid sinus (SS) are indicated on the right. A focal area of nonenhancement (arrowhead) is suggestive of a partial or complete sigmoid sinus thrombosis. **(B)** MR venogram of the same patient shows a lack of flow-related enhancement of the left sigmoid sinus and internal jugular vein, confirming sigmoid sinus thrombosis. The black arrow indicates the junction of the patent transverse sinus (black arrowheads) with the thrombosed sigmoid sinus. Note the normal and patent right sigmoid sinus (white arrow). The patent superior sagittal sinus (SSS) and right internal jugular vein (IJV) are also indicated.

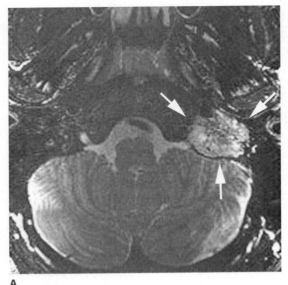

A

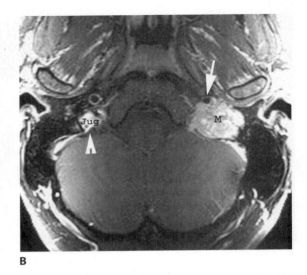

B

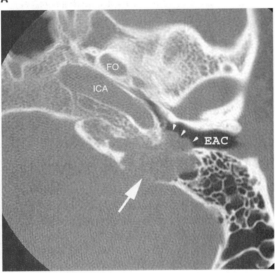

C

Figure 3–147. Paraganglioma. **(A)** Axial T2-weighted image shows a soft tissue mass centered at the jugular foramen (white arrows) with a "salt-and-pepper" appearance. The "pepper" represents small flow voids in this vascular tumor. **(B)** Axial postgadolinium T1-weighted image in the same patient shows the avid enhancement of this highly vascular mass lesion (M). The close relationship to the anteriorly displaced left ICA (white arrow) is demonstrated. The normal right jugular bulb (white arrowhead) is shown for comparison. **(C)** Axial CT scan viewed in bone window in the same patient demonstrates a lobulated lesion (white arrow) that has eroded the bone of the adjacent petrous apex, mastoid, and external auditory canal, and has extended into the hypotympanum (white arrowheads). This is consistent with a glomus jugulotympanicum type of paraganglioma. FO, foramen ovale; ICA, internal carotid artery; EAC, external auditory canal.

and integral to preventing complications in cases of temporal bone encephaloceles.)

Lo WW, Solti-Bohman LG, McElveen JT Jr. Aberrant carotid artery: radiologic diagnosis with emphasis on high-resolution computed tomography. *Radiographics.* 1985;5(6):985. [PMID: 3880011] (Classic text describing the imaging of aberrant internal carotid arteries.)

Maroldi R, Farina D, Palvarini L et al. Computed tomography and magnetic resonance imaging of pathologic conditions of the middle ear. *Eur J Radiol.* 2001;40(2):78. [PMID: 11704355] (Description of middle ear pathologies as seen on CT scanning and MRI.)

Soderberg KC, Dornhoffer JL. Congenital cholesteatoma of the middle ear: occurrence of an "open" lesion. *Am J Otol.* 1998;19(1):37. [PMID: 9455945] (Investigation of the occurrence of an "open" form of congenital cholesteatoma.)

Swartz JD. Imaging diagnosis of middle ear lesions. *Curr Probl Diagn Radiol.* 2002;31(1):4. [PMID: 11859313] (A review and description of middle ear lesions.)

Veillon F, Riehm S, Emaschescu B et al. Imaging of the windows of the temporal bone. *Semin Ultrasound CT MR.* 2001;22(3):271. [PMID: 11451100] (Detailed description of anatomy and pathology involving the round window.)

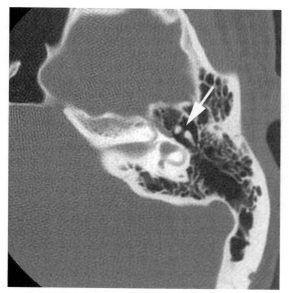

Figure 3–148. Ossicular dislocation. The head of the malleus is dislocated from the short process of the incus. The normal "ice cream cone" appearance is disrupted, and the "ice cream" has fallen off the "cone." The white arrow indicates the widened, disrupted malleoincudal articulation.

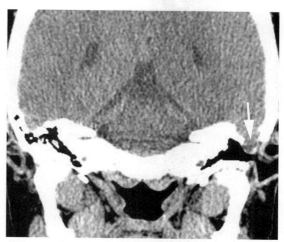

Figure 3–150. Coronal CT scan viewed in bone window in a patient who has undergone a prior mastoidectomy demonstrates the inferior herniation of brain tissue and meninges (white arrow) through a surgical defect into the external auditory canal.

3. Inner Ear

Anatomy

The inner ear contains structures for hearing and balance (see Figure 3–140). The cisternal portions of CN VII and CN VIII exit the pons near the level of the middle cerebellar peduncles. The nerves enter the internal auditory canal through the porus acusticus. The internal auditory canal, in cross-section, can be divided into four quadrants, each of which contains a nerve. The crista falciformis divides the upper two quadrants from the lower two quadrants, and "Bill's bar" divides the anterosuperior quadrant from the posterosuperior quadrant. In the anterosuperior quadrant is the facial nerve, which cannot be visualized in the internal auditory canal on CT scans but can be well seen on a fast spin-echo T2-weighted MRI. Below it, in the anteroinferior quadrant, is the cochlear nerve. In the posterosuperior quadrant is the superior division of the vestibular nerve. In the posteroinferior quadrant is the inferior division of the vestibular nerve. The vestibular nerves are posterior to the facial and cochlear nerves. The mnemonic "seven-up, coke down" reminds us to place cranial nerve VII (the facial nerve) superior to the cochlear nerve. The nerves in the posterior quadrants are easy to arrange since one has the superior and inferior divisions of the vestibular nerve. High-resolution sagittal and axial T2-weighted images demonstrating this anatomy are shown in Figure 3–151.

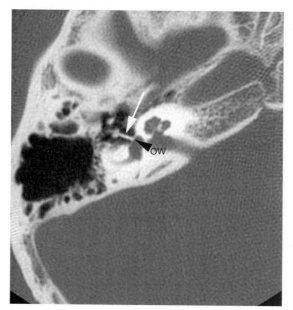

Figure 3–149. Axial CT scan viewed in bone window demonstrates a partial ossicular reconstruction prosthesis (arrow) extending from the oval window (OW) (arrowhead) toward the undersurface of the incus.

In any discussion of the anatomy of the inner ear, understanding the compartmentalization of endolymph and perilymph is useful. The structures that are visualized on CT scans represent the bony shell of the inner ear structures. An inner membrane lines the bony walls and forms a "soft shell" of ducts that essentially parallels the bony structures. Endolymph is the fluid that fills the membranous shell. Perilymph is the fluid that fills the space between the inner membranous soft shell and the outer bony shell. The oval window and the round window are openings onto the perilymphatic space.

The cochlear nerve arises from the spiral ganglion, which resides in the bony modiolus of the cochlea. On imaging studies, it is important to inspect the cochlea for $2^1/_4$ to $2^1/_2$ turns. On axial imaging, the base turn, middle turn, and apical turn of the cochlea can be identified. Within the cochlea, the scala vestibuli begins at the oval window, spirals to reach the helicotrema at the apex of the cochlea, and then spirals back down as the scala tympani. The scala tympani terminates at the round window. The scala vestibuli and scala tympani contain perilymph. The cochlear duct spirals between the scala vestibuli and scala tympani to the helicotrema.

The cochlear duct is part of the membranous labyrinth and contains endolymph. Differentiating the scala vestibuli, cochlear duct, and scala tympani is not possible on routine CT and MRI examinations, but may be possible with very high-resolution MRI.

The superior and inferior divisions of the vestibular nerve enter the bony vestibule and synapse in the vestibular ganglion. The bony vestibule contains the utricle and the saccule. The utricle and the saccule contain a motion-sensitive structure called the macula, which helps to determine head position and information about acceleration and deceleration. Nerve fibers from the utricle and saccule originate from the vestibular ganglion.

There are three horseshoe-shaped semicircular canals: the lateral, the superior, and the posterior semicircular canals, which are at right angles to one another. The posterior and superior semicircular canals share a common crus. Therefore, there are five (instead of six) connections to the utricle. Each canal contains a semicircular duct, which is part of the membranous labyrinth, surrounded by perilymph. Each semicircular duct has an ampulla that contains cristae that are sensitive to movements of the head. Nerve fibers run from the

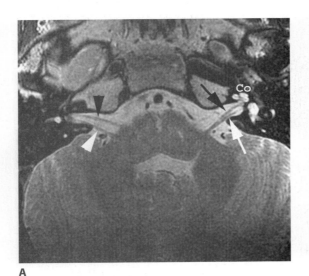

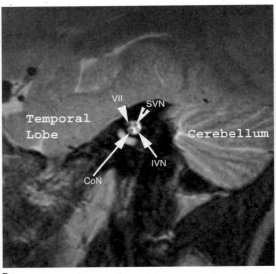

A   **B**

Figure 3–151. **(A)** Axial T2-weighted image shows the four nerves of the internal auditory canal. On this asymmetrically positioned image, the right internal auditory canal (IAC) is at a slightly higher level than the left. Therefore, the two nerves entering the right IAC are the facial nerve (black arrowhead) and the superior division of the vestibular nerve (white arrowhead). In the left IAC, the more anterior nerve that enters the cochlea (Co) is the cochlear nerve (black arrow) and the posterior nerve is the inferior division of the vestibular nerve (white arrow). **(B)** Sagittal T2-weighted image through the IAC shows the four nerves in cross-section. The anterior and superior nerve is the facial nerve (VII, arrowhead). The anterior and inferior nerve is the cochlear nerve (CoN, long arrow). The posterior and superior nerve is the superior division of the vestibular nerve (SVN, notched arrowhead). The posterior and inferior nerve is the inferior division of the vestibular nerve (IVN, short arrow). (Image courtesy of Dr. Christine Glastonbury, University of California, San Francisco.)

ampullae to the vestibular ganglion. The superior semicircular canal normally protrudes into the middle cranial fossa. This small bony protrusion is called the arcuate eminence. In some cases, a dehiscence of the bony covering of the superior semicircular canal may be present, a condition that has been associated with sound and/or pressure-induced vertigo. There is normally only a thin bony covering over the lateral aspect of the lateral semicircular canal, and this can potentially be a site of fistulous connection between the middle ear and inner ear structures.

The facial nerve has a complex course through the inner ear. After it leaves the internal auditory canal, it curves anteromedially for a short distance to the geniculate ganglion. This first segment of the facial nerve is called the labyrinthine segment. From the geniculate ganglion, the greater superficial petrosal nerve continues forward in the anteromedial direction. From the geniculate ganglion, the facial nerve reverses course and heads in an almost straight line posterolaterally, just under the lateral semicircular canal, until it reaches the posterior genu. This second segment is called the horizontal or tympanic segment. From the posterior genu, the facial nerve takes an almost 90° turn and heads directly downward, just posterolateral to the facial nerve recess. This is known as the vertical or descending mastoid segment of the facial nerve. The stapedius nerve branches from the high mastoid segment of the facial nerve to innervate the stapedius muscle. The chorda tympani branches from the inferior aspect of the vertical segment of the facial nerve and enters the middle ear cavity, where it then crosses between the manubrium of the malleus and the long process of the incus. The chorda tympani innervates the tongue (for taste) and the submandibular and sublingual glands. The vertical segment exits the stylomastoid foramen, located between the styloid process and the mastoid tip. The nerve then enters the substance of the parotid gland.

The cochlear aqueduct is a bony canal that connects the cochlea to the intracranial subarachnoid space. This aqueduct appears like a "mini" version of the internal auditory canal because it is oriented parallel with the internal auditory canal, but is located more caudally. The cochlear aqueduct, which is ultimately in communication with the scala vestibuli, the scala tympani, and the semicircular canals, contains perilymph. The function of the cochlear aqueduct is not well understood, but it is a potential route for meningitis to spread to the inner ear.

The vestibular aqueduct is another bony connection between the cerebral subarachnoid space and the inner ear. This bony canal is located at the level of the lateral semicircular canal and is oriented almost perpendicular to the internal auditory canal. It extends from the posterior petrous face at the level of the depression for the endolymphatic sac to the vestibule. The vestibular aqueduct contains the endolymphatic duct which, as the name suggests, contains endolymph. The upper limit of the normal size of the vestibular aqueduct is approximately 1.5 mm in diameter at the midpoint between the common crus and the bony aperture of the vestibular aqueduct.

Pathology

Abnormalities that may be encountered on imaging studies of the inner ear are listed in Table 3–14. Nar-

Table 3–14. Abnormalities of the inner ear.

Congenital	
Internal auditory canal	Narrow (Figure 3–152)
Bony labyrinth	Michel (labyrinthine aplasia)
	Mondini (incomplete partition of the cochlea)
	Common cavity (Figure 3–153)
	Cochlear aplasia/hypoplasia
	Semicircular canal dysplasia/aplasia
	Large vestibular aqueduct syndrome (Figure 3–154)
Membranous labyrinth	Scheibe
	Alexander
Otodystrophies	Otosclerosis/otospongiosis
	Fenestral (Figure 3–155)
	Retrofenestral (Figure 3–156)
	Paget's
	Fibrous dysplasia
	Osteopetrosis
	Osteogenesis imperfecta
Masses	Intralabyrinthine schwannoma (Figure 3–157)
	Facial nerve schwannoma (Figure 3–158)
	Hemangioma (Figure 3–159)
	Endolymphatic duct tumors (Figure 3–160)
	Metastases/with perineural spread of tumor (Figure 3–161)
Inflammation	Labyrinthitis and labyrinthitis ossificans (Figure 3–162)
	Postradiation labyrinthitis (Figure 3–163)
Trauma	Fracture/pneumolabyrinth (Figure 3–164)

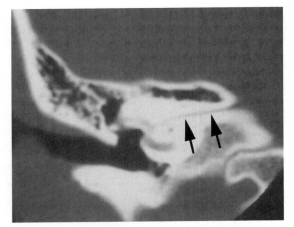

Figure 3–152. Narrowing of the internal auditory canal (IAC). Coronal CT scan viewed in bone window in a young girl with congenital sensorineural hearing loss demonstrates marked narrowing of the internal auditory canal. In these cases (if MRI is performed), very often only the facial nerve runs through the IAC and the vestibular and cochlear nerves are absent.

plasia and aplasia, one or all of the canals may be abnormal. As the lateral semicircular canal develops after the other two canals have already developed, abnormal development can affect the lateral semicircular canal in isolation after the other two semicircular canals have already developed normally, whereas an abnormality earlier in development that affects the posterior or superior semicircular canals generally also affects the subsequently developing lateral semicircular canal. Enlarged vestibular aqueduct syndrome (Figure 3–154) is the most common imaging abnormality in sensorineural hearing loss presenting in infancy or childhood. At the midpoint between the opening of the aqueduct to the subarachnoid space and the common crus, the vestibular aqueduct should measure no more than 1.5 mm. Comparing the diameter with the width of the lateral semicircular canal may also be useful, because they are normally equivalent, or the vestibular aqueduct is smaller. Sometimes the bony vestibular aqueduct appears normal on a CT scan, but an MRI may show an enlarged endolymphatic sac. The large vestibular aqueduct is often associated with cochlear abnormalities, notably a deficiency of the modiolus.

rowing of the internal auditory canal (Figure 3–152) in the setting of congenital sensorineural hearing loss has been associated with cochlear nerve deficiency or absence. An oblique sagittal high-resolution MRI can visualize and evaluate the cochlear nerve within the internal auditory canal to assess directly for its presence and its caliber.

A. Congenital Abnormalities

Congenital abnormalities of the bony labyrinth represent a spectrum of bony abnormalities that are thought to be caused by developmental arrest at specific time points. Since the development of the inner ear is separate from the development of the external and middle ears, congenital malformations of the inner ear are usually not associated with malformations of the external and middle ears. However, this separation is not absolute, and inner ear malformations can occur with external and middle ear malformations (and vice versa). Michel deformity is complete aplasia of the labyrinth. On imaging, there is total absence of the normal inner ear structures. In the Mondini malformation, or incomplete partition of the cochlea, there are only $1\frac{1}{2}$ turns of the cochlea owing to the confluence of the middle and apical turns. The basal turn is normal. The common cavity is seen when the cochlea, the vestibule, and the semicircular canals appear to merge into one large cavity (Figure 3–153). In semicircular canal dys-

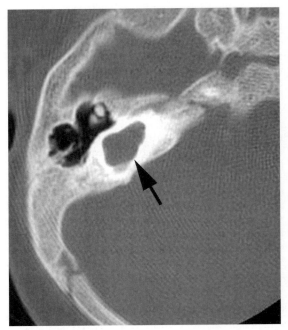

Figure 3–153. Common cavity. Axial CT scan viewed in bone window demonstrates that the cochlea, vestibule, and semicircular canals appear "merged" into a common cavity rather than having developed into distinct structures.

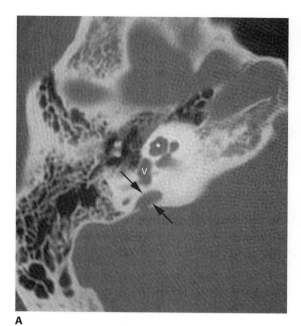

A

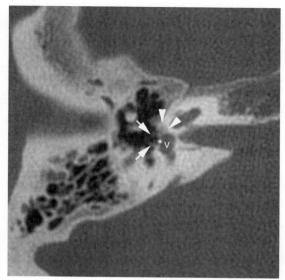

Figure 3–155. Fenestral otosclerosis. Axial CT scan viewed in bone window demonstrates the focal rarefaction of bone (white arrowheads) lateral to the cochlea and anterior to the vestibule. The oval window is indicated (*), as are the crura of the stapes (white arrows).

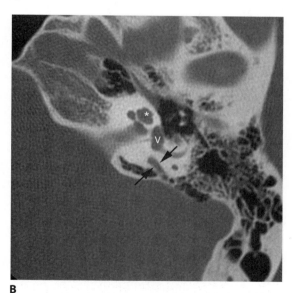

B

Figure 3–154. Enlarged vestibular aqueduct syndrome in a 40-year-old man with bilateral sensorineural hearing loss. **(A)** Axial CT scan viewed in bone window of the right temporal bone demonstrates enlargement of the vestibular aqueduct (black arrows) as well as deficiency of the cochlear modiolus (*). **(B)** The left temporal bone shows similar changes, but with less severe enlargement of the vestibular aqueduct. The vestibule (V) is also indicated.

B. OTOSCLEROSIS

Otosclerosis is divided into two types: fenestral and retrofenestral.

1. Fenestral otosclerosis—Fenestral otosclerosis (Figure 3–155) is the most common form and involves the oval window and the footplate of the stapes. The most common imaging finding is a subtle bony rarefaction at the anterior wall of the oval window. This rarefaction is due to the replacement of normal bone with hypodense spongiotic bone. The bony abnormality extends to the stapes footplate. Eventually, sclerotic changes develop and fix the stapes to the oval window. This entity presents with a conductive hearing loss.

2. Retrofenestral otosclerosis—Retrofenestral otosclerosis (Figure 3–156) is also known as cochlear otosclerosis and presents as a sensorineural or mixed hearing loss. On CT scanning, a ring of lucency around the cochlea is characteristic of this disease. On MRI, the abnormal bone shows a high signal intensity on T2-weighted images and enhancement postgadolinium.

C. SCHWANNOMAS

Schwannomas can occur in the labyrinth as well as in the more common location of the internal auditory canal. They may arise in the vestibule or cochlea (Figure 3–157) or along the course of the facial nerve (Figure 3–158). Facial nerve schwannomas tend to occur at the geniculate ganglion. Occasionally they can enlarge significantly and extend into the middle cranial fossa, presenting with seizures due to brain compression.

D. TEMPORAL BONE HEMANGIOMAS

Temporal bone hemangiomas are benign vascular tumors that tend to occur along the course of the facial nerve and also at the level of the internal auditory canal. Some produce bony spicules and are called ossifying hemangiomas. On CT scanning, the focal enlargement of the facial nerve canal and the presence of irregular calcification or ossification suggest this lesion. On MRI, these lesions are typically bright on T2-weighted images and enhance intensely postgadolinium (Figure 3–159).

E. ENDOLYMPHATIC SAC TUMORS

Endolymphatic sac tumors (Figure 3–160) arise from the endolymphatic duct, sac, or both and aggressively erode and remodel bone along the posterior petrous

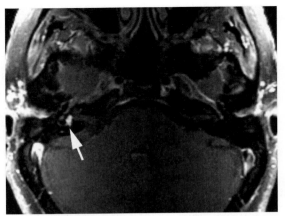

Figure 3–157. Schwannoma of the vestibule in a young man with an acute right-sided sensorineural hearing loss. Postgadolinium T1-weighted image with fat saturation shows a masslike enhancement in the vestibule (arrow) with extension into the semicircular canals. Initial considerations included intralabyrinthine schwannoma versus labyrinthitis. Over months of follow-up, the lesion gradually progressed and an intralabyrinthine schwannoma was eventually confirmed surgically.

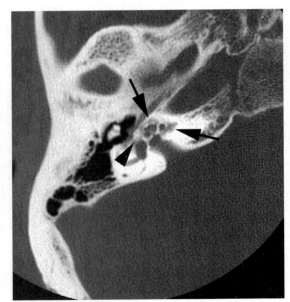

Figure 3–156. Retrofenestral otosclerosis. Axial CT scan viewed in bone window demonstrates rarefied bone (black arrows) surrounding the cochlea. Note that the abnormality also involves bone adjacent to the oval window (black arrowhead).

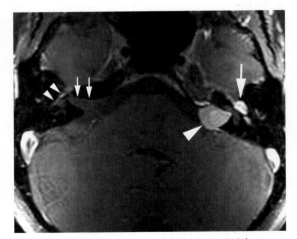

Figure 3–158. Facial nerve schwannoma. Axial postgadolinium T1-weighted image with fat saturation shows an enhancing mass in the internal auditory canal (IAC; white arrowhead) and also along the horizontal portion (tympanic segment) of CN VII (white arrow). The normal right IAC (double small arrows) and normal right tympanic segment of the facial nerve (double small arrowheads) are indicated for comparison.

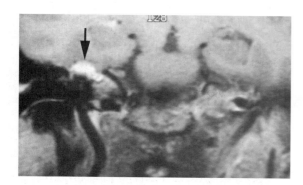

Figure 3–159. Hemangioma in a 40-year-old woman with right-sided hemifacial spasm. Postgadolinium coronal T1-weighted image demonstrates an intensely enhancing mass (arrow) at the level of the geniculate ganglion extending up into the middle cranial fossa. The overlying dura is intact and there is no brain involvement. The diagnosis of hemangioma was confirmed at surgery.

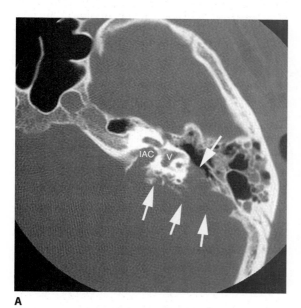

A

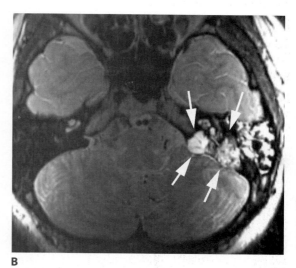

B

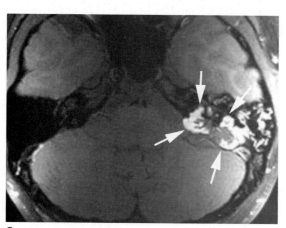

C

Figure 3–160. Endolymphatic sac tumor. **(A)** Axial CT scan viewed in bone window demonstrates a destructive lesion (arrows) centered along the posterior petrous bone, eroding the dense bone of the otic capsule and extending into the middle ear and mastoid. IAC, internal auditory canal; V, vestibule. **(B)** Axial T2-weighted image in the same patient shows a very heterogeneous but predominantly hyperintense lesion (arrows). Some of the linear and round areas of signal void represent enlarged vessels, while other areas represent bone fragments. Fluid is present more laterally in the mastoid air cells. **(C)** Axial T1-weighted fat-saturated image shows a heterogeneous, lobulated lesion in the temporal bone (arrows) with areas of intrinsic high signal due to hemorrhagic and proteinaceous material. Note that this is a pregadolinium image. The lack of signal suppression with fat saturation confirms that the high signal intensity areas do not represent fat. Postgadolinium (not shown), enhancement of the center of the lesion was seen.

face and the otic capsule. They can cause signal abnormalities within the structures of the inner ear secondary to fistulization and hemorrhage. These lesions are heterogeneous on MRI and show prominent flow voids and marked enhancement. An increased incidence of these lesions is seen in von Hippel-Lindau syndrome.

F. Perineural Spread

Perineural spread from a malignant parotid tumor extending back along the facial nerve (Figure 3–161) is important to identify. These patients usually present with a parotid mass, but, in some cases, only a new or progressive facial palsy or even a middle or inner ear mass may be noted initially.

G. Inflammation and Infection

Inflammatory and infectious processes of the inner ear can be classified by origin and etiology: tympanogenic, meningogenic, hematogenic, autoimmune, or post-traumatic. In tympanogenic labyrinthitis, inflammatory processes of the middle ear can spread by direct extension into the inner ear, usually through the oval or round windows. Infection can also spread through a fistula, most commonly involving the lateral semicircular canal. Tympanogenic labyrinthitis is usually unilateral. Meningogenic labyrinthitis is usually bilateral, with organisms and inflammatory cells entering the inner ear via the internal auditory canal or the cochlear aqueduct.

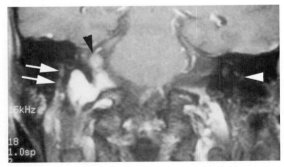

Figure 3–161. Perineural spread of parotid adenocarcinoma. Coronal postgadolinium T1-weighted image with fat saturation demonstrates asymmetric thickening and enhancement extending centrally along the descending mastoid segment of the right facial nerve (white arrows). The normal left descending facial nerve is barely seen (white arrowhead). The tumor spread all the way back to the level of the cerebellopontine angle (black arrowhead).

The classic pathogens that cause hematogenic labyrinthitis are mumps and measles, and this is also typically bilateral. Acute labyrinthitis can be identified on MRI when it causes a change in the signal intensity of inner ear fluid, enhancement of inner ear structures, or both. Labyrinthitis can lead to an increased intensity on T1-weighted images within the membranous labyrinth from elevated protein content or hemorrhage secondary to inflammation. Postgadolinium, there is typically intense contrast enhancement within the labyrinth, which may persist over weeks or even months. Pregadolinium T1-weighted images are especially helpful to determine that the hyperintensity seen on postgadolinium T1-weighted images in the membranous labyrinth is due to hemorrhage and not actually abnormal enhancement due to an intralabyrinthine mass. If no abnormality on a pregadolinium T1-weighted image is seen and fairly focal enhancement postgadolinium is evident, it is wise to get a follow-up study to make sure that the patient does not have an intralabyrinthine schwannoma that is presenting acutely. Post-labyrinthitis, sclerosis of the bony labyrinth may eventually result. This latter situation is termed labyrinthitis ossificans (Figure 3–162). Labyrinthitis can also be caused by radiation therapy (Figure 3–163) and other noninfectious insults.

H. Anomalous Course of the Facial Nerve

Occasionally, the facial nerve can have an anomalous course through the inner ear. This is most often seen in association with external auditory canal atresia (see Figure 3–141), but it may occur sporadically or in association with syndromic malformations. Knowledge of the course of the facial nerve is important for preoperative planning.

I. Fractures of the Petrous Bone

Fractures of the petrous bone can traverse and injure the structures of the inner ear, as well as disrupting the ossicular chain. In a trauma setting, the finding of fluid in the mastoid air cells on a CT scan of the head suggests that a temporal bone fracture may be present, as does pneumocephalus in proximity to the mastoid air cells. A dedicated CT scan of the temporal bone should be obtained to more sensitively assess a trauma patient for temporal bone fracture. In some cases, frank pneumolabyrinth may be seen (Figure 3–164).

Casselman JW, Offeciers EF, De Foer B, Govaerts P, Kuhweide R, Somers T. CT and MR imaging of congenital abnormalities of the inner ear and internal auditory canal. *Eur J Radiol.* 2001;40(2):94. [PMID: 11704356] (A description of imaging of inner ear and internal auditory canal abnormalities.)

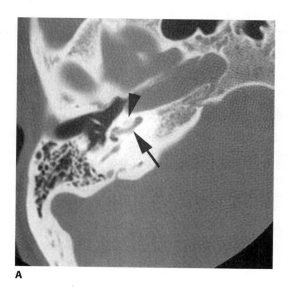

A

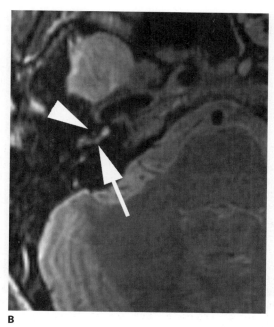

B

Figure 3–162. Labyrinthitis ossificans. **(A)** Axial CT scan viewed in bone window demonstrates ossification and therefore poor visualization of the middle and apical turns of the cochlea (arrowhead) as well as narrowing and subtle sclerosis of the base turn of the cochlea (arrow). **(B)** Axial T2-weighted image in the same patient shows absence of expected fluid signal in the middle and apical turns of the cochlea (expected position indicated by arrowhead), consistent with ossification. The base turn is narrowed, but still has some fluid signal within it (arrow). The information about patency of fluid spaces that is obtained on MRI can be useful to determine if a patient is a candidate for cochlear implantation.

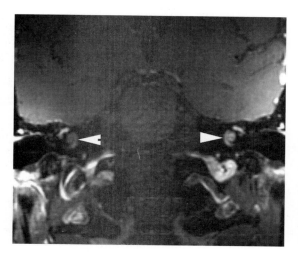

Figure 3–163. Radiation-induced labyrinthitis. A patient with bilateral hearing loss who had received radiation therapy 10 years earlier after the resection of a medulloblastoma in the posterior fossa. Postgadolinium T1-weighted image with fat saturation shows mild enhancement in the right cochlea (notched arrowhead) and intense enhancement in the left cochlea (arrowhead).

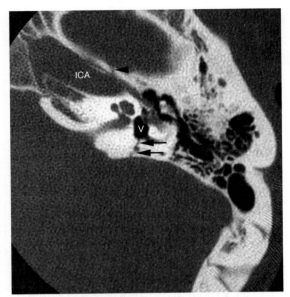

Figure 3–164. Fracture. Axial CT scan viewed in bone window demonstrates a transverse fracture (black arrows) traversing the vestibule and causing pneumolabyrinth. The fracture also traversed the carotid canal (black arrowhead), and this finding should raise a clinical suspicion of a vascular injury. ICA, internal carotid artery; V, vestibule.

Glastonbury CM, Davidson HC, Harnsberger HR, Butler J, Kertesz TR, Shelton C. Imaging findings of cochlear nerve deficiency. *AJNR Am J Neuroradiol.* 2002;23(4):635. [PMID: 11950658] (Exquisite imaging of anatomy and cochlear deficiency in the internal auditory canal.)

Inanli S, Tutkun A, Ozturk O, Ahyskaly R. Endolymphatic sac tumor: a case report. *Auris Nasus Larynx.* 2001;28(3):245. [PMID: 11489369] (Presentation of a 50-year-old man with endolymphatic sac tumor with a left-sided sensorineural hearing loss.)

Lemmerling M, Vanzieleghem B, Dhooge I, Van Cauwenberge P, Kunnen M. CT and MRI of the semicircular canals in the normal and diseased temporal bone. *Eur Radiol.* 2001;11(7): 1210. [PMID: 11471615] (A description of the normal and abnormal imaging of the semicircular canals.)

Naidich TP, Mann SS, Som PM. Imaging of the osseous, membranous, and perilymphatic labyrinths. *Neuroimaging Clin N Am.* 2000;10(1):23. [PMID: 10658153] (This article provides a detailed review of the neonatal anatomy and development of these structures, knowledge of which derives in great part from advances in CT scanning and sophisticated MR imaging.)

Swartz JD. Temporal bone trauma. *Semin Ultrasound CT MR.* 2001;22(3):219. [PMID: 11451097] (Temporal bone trauma is subdivided into fractures and pseudofractures, fistulous communication, hearing loss, and facial nerve involvement.)

CEREBELLOPONTINE ANGLE & INTERNAL AUDITORY CANAL

Anatomy

The cerebellopontine angle (CPA) is the region where the pons and the cerebellum meet and form an obtuse angle; the adjacent subarachnoid space is referred to as the cerebellopontine cistern. Lesions at the CPA are usually centered near the level of the middle cerebellar peduncle.

Pathology

Some of the more common abnormalities that may be encountered on imaging studies of the CPA are listed in Table 3–15, and a number of these entities are illustrated in Figures 3–165 through 3–169. Imaging characteristics of four of the most common CPA tumors are summarized in Table 3–16.

A. VESTIBULAR SCHWANNOMAS

Vestibular schwannomas (Figure 3–167) are also known as acoustic neuromas. These lesions typically present with asymmetric sensorineural hearing loss, but they may also present with tinnitus or may be noted incidentally on imaging studies obtained for other purposes. These lesions appear as well-circumscribed, round or ovoid masses that are relatively dark on T2-weighted images compared with the high signal intensity of surrounding CSF. They typically enhance intensely and homogeneously, except in areas of cyst formation or hemorrhage. These lesions may be small and completely confined to the internal auditory canal, but as they grow, they tend to widen the internal auditory canal and to expand medially into the cistern of the CPA. Large lesions may compress the brainstem and result in obstructive hydrocephalus, in which case the patient may present with headache or gait ataxia.

Table 3–15. Selected abnormalities of the cerebellopontine angle and internal auditory canal.

Schwannoma
Meningioma
Arachnoid cyst
Epidermoid
Vascular loop
Lipoma
Superficial siderosis

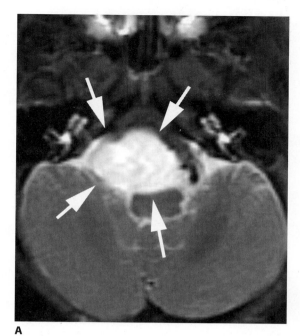

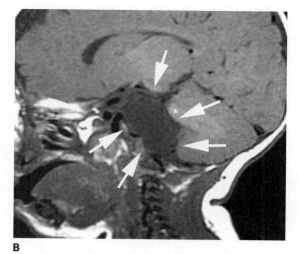

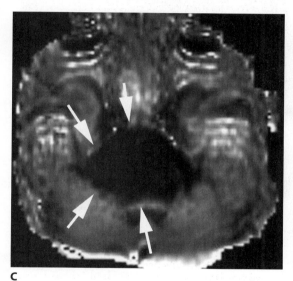

Figure 3–165. Arachnoid cyst. **(A)** Axial T2-weighted image shows a hyperintense extra-axial lesion (arrows) causing a mass effect on the medulla and cerebellum. Note the signal intensity is the same as cerebrospinal fluid. **(B)** Sagittal T1-weighted image shows the extra-axial mass (arrows) causing a mass effect on the cerebellum, notably, the middle cerebellar peduncle (*). Again, the signal intensity is the same as cerebrospinal fluid. Following gadolinium administration (not shown), there was no enhancement of the lesion. **(C)** Axial diffusion-weighted image shows a low signal intensity consistent with increased diffusion in the lesion (arrows). Diffusion-weighted imaging is very useful to separate purely cystic lesions from solid masses. In this case, the imaging characteristics on conventional MRI sequences and diffusion-weighted imaging paralleled CSF exactly, confirming the diagnosis of an arachnoid cyst.

B. FACIAL NERVE SCHWANNOMAS

Facial nerve schwannomas can also occur in the CPA but are far less common than those arising from the vestibular nerve. It can be helpful to know preoperatively if a presumed schwannoma arises from the facial nerve. Identifying abnormal enhancement extending along the labyrinthine segment of the facial nerve, or even more distally along the tympanic or descending mastoid segments, may be a helpful clue on MRI.

Bonneville F, Sarrazin JL, Marsot-Dupuch K et al. Unusual lesions of the cerebellopontine angle: a segmental approach. *Radiographics.* 2001;21(2):419. [PMID: 11259705] (Using CT and MRI to distinguish among the many cerebellopontine angle lesions.)

Curtin HD, Hirsch WL Jr. Imaging of acoustic neuromas. *Otolaryngol Clin North Am.* 1992;25(3):553. [PMID: 1625865] (A negative high-quality, high-resolution, contrast-enhanced MRI is excellent evidence that a patient does not have an acoustic neuroma.)

Heier LA, Communale JP Jr, Lavyne MH. Sensorineural hearing loss and cerebellopontine angle lesions. Not always an acous-

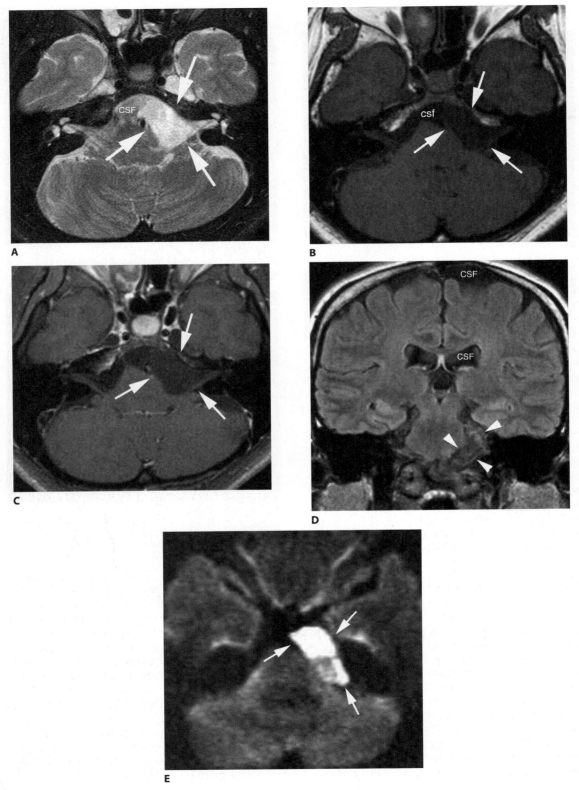

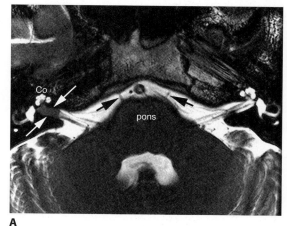

A

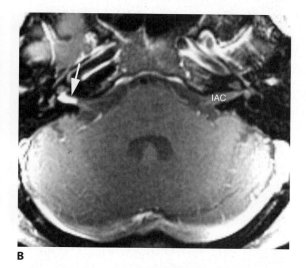

B

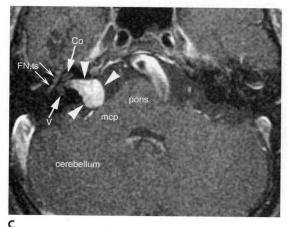

C

Figure 3–167. Vestibular schwannoma. **(A)** Axial thin-section heavily T2-weighted image shows a right intracanalicular vestibular schwannoma (white arrows) in stark contrast to the high signal of normal CSF. The lesion extends to the fundus of the internal auditory canal (IAC). Note the subtle extension of the lesion into the cochlea. Also indicated on this thin-section, high-resolution image are the bilateral sixth cranial nerves (black arrows). **(B)** An axial postgadolinium T1-weighted image with fat saturation in the same patient demonstrates intense and homogeneous enhancement of the intracanalicular lesion (white arrow) and also demonstrates the subtle extension into the cochlea. **(C)** Axial postgadolinium T1-weighted image with fat saturation in a different patient shows the classic "ice cream cone" or "mushroom" appearance of a vestibular schwannoma that has both IAC and cerebellopontine angle components. Indicated are the pons, cerebellum, and middle cerebellar peduncle (mcp), as well as the cochlea (Co), vestibule (V), and the tympanic segment of the facial nerve (FN, ts; white arrows). The pons is the pons, this is NOT an abbreviation, it is the name of a structure. FN,ts; facial nerve, tympanic segment.

Figure 3–166. *(Previous page)* Epidermoid. **(A)** Axial T2-weighted image shows an extra-axial hyperintense mass (arrows) in the left cerebellopontine angle that displaces the left seventh and eighth cranial nerve complex posteriorly and slightly compresses the brainstem. Note the slightly darker signal in the CSF to the right of the lesion. This is due to CSF pulsation artifact that causes a signal loss in the normally flowing CSF. **(B)** Axial T1-weighted image shows the lesion (arrows) to be of low signal intensity, though it is actually slightly hyperintense to CSF on this T1-weighted image. **(C)** Axial postgadolinium T1-weighted image with fat saturation shows no enhancement of this lesion (arrows). At this point, it is still not possible to distinguish between an arachnoid cyst and an epidermoid, as an arachnoid cyst that has slightly increased protein content compared with normal CSF may be slightly brighter than CSF on a T1-weighted image. **(D)** A coronal FLAIR image (fluid-attenuated inversion recovery) shows an increased signal intensity in the lesion (arrowheads) compared with CSF in the subarachnoid space and ventricles, now strongly suggesting the diagnosis of epidermoid. The FLAIR sequence is a heavily T2-weighted image with the signal from CSF suppressed. **(E)** Axial diffusion-weighted image shows a markedly increased signal intensity of the lesion, consistent with reduced diffusion. This signal is very different from CSF (which is dark on diffusion-weighted images), and the diffusion-weighted image is very useful in distinguishing an arachnoid cyst (Figure 3–165) from an epidermoid.

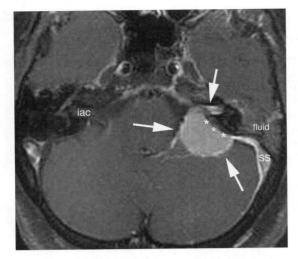

Figure 3–168. Meningioma. Axial postgadolinium T1-weighted image with fat saturation shows a homogeneously enhancing left cerebellopontine angle mass (arrows) that has a broad dural base (***) against the back of the petrous bone. Dural enhancement extends into a nonwidened internal auditory canal, and also posteriorly over the sigmoid sinus (SS) and occipital bone. Fluid is present in the left mastoid air cells, probably unrelated to the presence of the tumor.

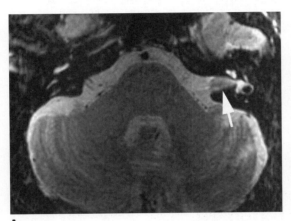

A

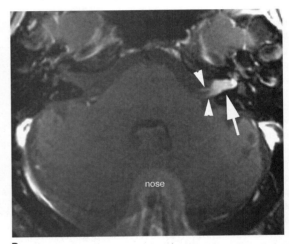

B

Figure 3–169. Inflammatory pseudotumor. **(A)** Axial T2-weighted image shows an apparent internal auditory canal (IAC) mass (arrow) that has an intermediate signal intensity. This could be a vestibular schwannoma in this patient with sensorineural hearing loss. **(B)** Axial postgadolinium T1-weighted image shows intense enhancement of the lesion (arrow). Note, however, the linear enhancement extending more proximally along the cisternal segments of the cochlear and vestibular nerves (arrowheads). This indicates that this may be an inflammatory or infiltrative lesion (such as sarcoid or lymphoma) and not a typical vestibular schwannoma. Note also the nose "wrapping around" into the posterior fossa; this is a common MRI artifact related to selection of the field of view. **(C)** After several months of steroids, a follow-up axial postgadolinium T1-weighted image shows decreased enhancement (arrow) in the IAC and the lack of more proximal enhancement. The T2-weighted image (not shown) appeared essentially normal. The diagnosis in this case was considered to be an inflammatory neuritis of uncertain etiology.

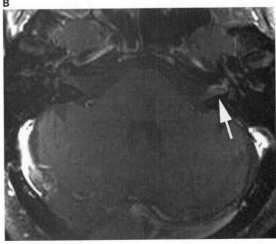

C

Table 3–16. Imaging characteristics of common cerebellopontine angle tumors ("SAME").

"SAME"	General Characteristics	CT Scan	MRI, T1-Weighted Imaging	MRI, T2-Weighted Imaging	MRI, FLAIR	MRI, DWI	MRI, Gadolinium
Schwannoma	Typically expands internal auditory canal (IAC); may be cystic; infrequently calcifies	Intermediate density on ST window; wide IAC on bone window	Intermediate (cysts may be low, hemorrhage high)	Intermediate (cysts high, hemorrhage variable)	Intermediate (cysts low)	No reduction	Avid, homogeneous enhancement (unless cysts or hemorrhage is present)
Arachnoid cyst	Follows CSF on all sequences	Fluid density	Low	High	Low	Increased diffusion, decreased signal	No enhancement
Meningioma	Look for broad dural base; may calcify	Intermediate density, ± adjacent hyperostosis	Intermediate	Intermediate (low if calcification)	Intermediate	No or mild reduction	Avid, homogeneous (unless calcification is present)
Epidermoid	Use FLAIR and DWI to differentiate from arachnoid cyst	Low density	Low	High	Intermediate	Reduced diffusion, increased signal	No enhancement

DWI, diffusion-weighted image; FLAIR, fluid-attenuated inversion recovery.

tic neuroma—a pictorial essay. *Clin Imaging.* 1997;21(3):213. [PMID: 9156313] (There are many etiologies of sensorineural hearing loss other than acoustic neuroma, with characteristic imaging features.)

Lalwani AK. Meningiomas, epidermoids, and other nonacoustic tumors of the cerebellopontine angle. *Otolaryngol Clin North Am.* 1992;25(3):707. [PMID: 1625871] (The preoperative differentiation among cerebellopontine angle lesions based on the clinical history, physical examination, and audiovestibular testing is difficult. CT scanning and gadolinium-enhanced MRI reveal the characteristic appearance of these tumors and make an accurate diagnosis possible.)

Tsuruda JS, Chew WM, Moseley ME, Norman D. Diffusion-weighted MR imaging of the brain: value of differentiating between extra-axial cysts and epidermoid tumors. *AJNR Am J Neuroradiol.* 1990;11(5):925. [PMID: 2120997] (Diffusion-weighted MRI can be useful in distinguishing between arachnoid cysts and epidermoid tumors.)

PETROUS APEX

Pathology

Some of the more common abnormalities that may be encountered on imaging studies of the petrous apex are listed in Table 3–17 and are shown in Figures 3–170 through 3–172. Imaging characteristics of

Table 3–17. Abnormalities of the petrous apex.

Fluid in aerated apex

Mucocele

Cholesterol granuloma

Arachnoid cyst or meningocele

Cholesteatoma, congenital or acquired

Chondrosarcoma

Metastasis

selected petrous apex lesions and pseudolesions are reviewed in Table 3–18. Note that it is very important to distinguish "don't touch" lesions such as simple fluid in an aerated apex or a simple meningocele from lesions that might require operative intervention such as cholesterol granulomas, cholesteatomas, or neoplasms.

Curtin HD, Som PM. The petrous apex. *Otolaryngol Clin North Am.* 1995;28(3):473-96. [PMID: 7675465] (Description and distinguishing features of petrous apex lesions.)

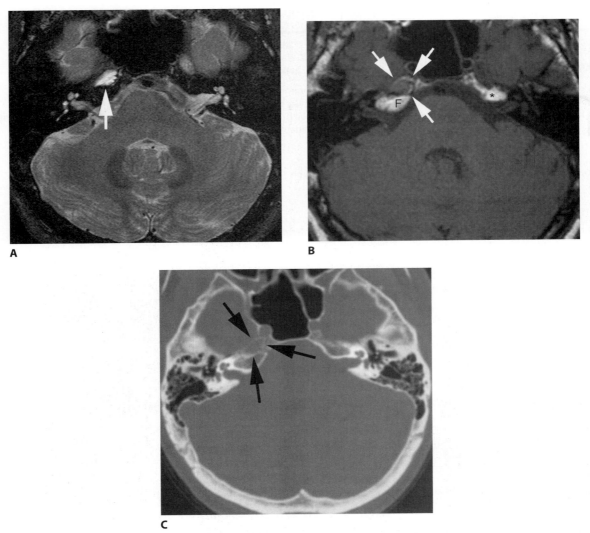

Figure 3–170. Fluid in aerated petrous apex. **(A)** Axial fast spin-echo T2-weighted image with fat saturation shows hyperintense material (arrow) at the petrous apex, with preservation of apical septa and no apical expansion. **(B)** Axial T1-weighted image shows this "lesion" (arrows) has intermediate signal intensity, consistent with slightly proteinaceous fluid. The high signal intensity posterior to the lesion represents normal apical marrow fat (F). Fat is also present in the left petrous apex (*). Postgadolinium (not shown), there was no enhancement of this lesion. At this point, the differential includes fluid in a petrous air cell, mucocele, and epidermoid, with both a mucocele and an epidermoid seeming unlikely given the apparent preservation of apical septa and a lack of expansion. In some cases, a CT scan can help differentiate among these possibilities and a follow-up scan may also be useful. **(C)** Axial CT scan viewed in bone window demonstrates a nonexpanded but opacified petrous apex air cell (arrows). CT scanning is useful to show that there is no bony destruction, which would suggest an epidermoid or a cholesteatoma, or expansion, which would suggest a mucocele or cholesterol granuloma. Follow-up imaging at 6 months showed resolution of this fluid.

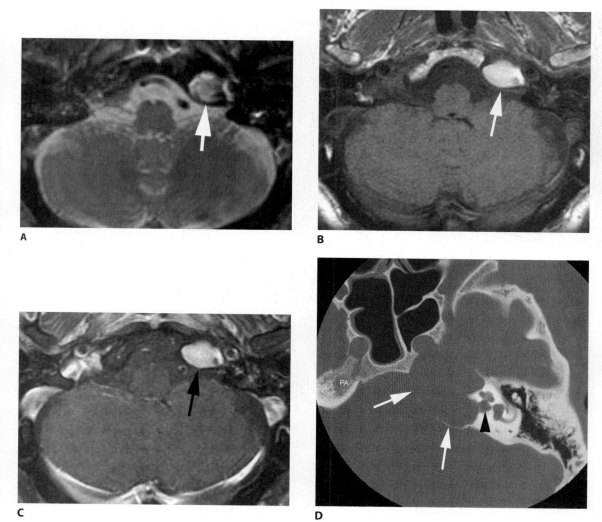

Figure 3–171. Cholesterol granuloma. **(A)** Axial T2-weighted image shows an expansile hyperintense lesion (arrow) in the inferior aspect of the petrous apex. **(B)** Axial T1-weighted image shows the lesion (arrow) to be intrinsically hyperintense. This could represent hemorrhagic debris, proteinaceous material, or fat. **(C)** Axial postgadolinium T1-weighted image with fat saturation shows the lesion (arrow) remains hyperintense and is therefore not fatty in nature. **(D)** Axial CT scan viewed in bone window in a different patient with a large left petrous apex cholesterol granuloma demonstrates an expansile lesion (arrows) that has eroded and remodeled the left petrous apex as well as parts of the adjacent clivus and otic capsule. The internal auditory canal (black arrowhead) has been partly eroded. Note the normal right petrous apex (PA) for comparison.

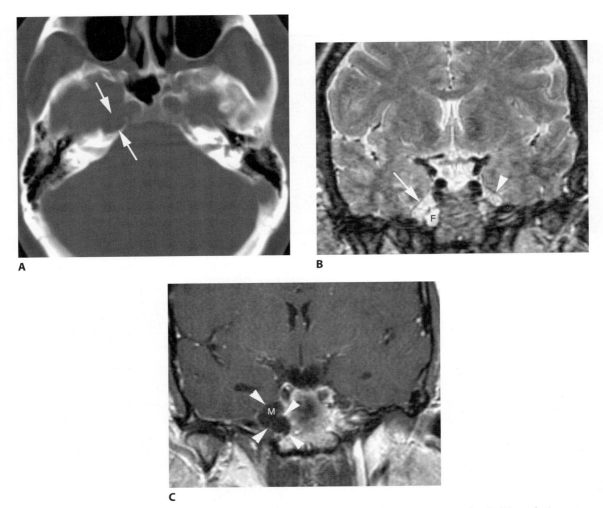

Figure 3–172. A young woman underwent CT scanning with a complaint of headache, and a skull base lesion was incidentally noted. **(A)** Axial CT scan viewed in bone window demonstrates a right petrous apex lesion (arrows) that has smoothly eroded and remodeled adjacent bone. This appearance suggests a benign lesion but is nonspecific. **(B)** A thin-section coronal fast spin-echo T2-weighted image demonstrates that the lesion is fluid-filled (F) and appears to communicate with a slightly enlarged Meckel cave (arrow). The normal left Meckel cave (arrowhead) is shown for comparison. **(C)** Coronal postgadolinium T1-weighted image demonstrates the fluid-filled lesion (arrowheads) clearly in communication with the Meckel cave (M). The imaging characteristics are consistent with a meningocele that has remodeled the petrous apex. This is a "don't touch" lesion. CT cisternography would confirm free communication between this "lesion" and the subarachnoid space, but is not necessary. In some cases these lesions can result in a CSF leak, with complicating meningitis or intracranial hypotension, and in that setting may require confirmation with CT cisternography and operative intervention.

Table 3–18. Imaging characteristics of selected petrous apex lesions and pseudolesions.

Lesions or Pseudolesion	CT Scan	MRI, T1-Weighted Image	MRI, T2-Weighted Image	MRI, Gadolinium T1-Weighted Image
Normal marrow	Normal nonaerated bone; diagnostic	High because of normal marrow fat	Low on fat saturated image	No enhancement; low if fat saturation used
Fluid-filled air cell	No destruction No expansion	Intermediate to low intensity	High	No enhancement
Mucocele (can mimic cholesterol granuloma)	Expansile No bony destruction	Variable, typically low unless proteinaceous	High	No enhancement
Acute petrous apicitis	Air-fluid levels in air cells without bony destruction	Low	High	May be mild, peripheral
Acute petrous apicitis with osteomyelitis (Gradenigo syndrome)	Opacified air cells with bony breakdown; nonexpansile	Low	High	Can show rim enhancement or enhancement of adjacent meninges
Cholesterol granuloma	Expansile	High (fat saturation does not reduce signal)	Variable, classically high	No enhancement
Cholesteatoma	Bony erosion, remodeling	Intermediate to low intensity	High	No enhancement
Chondrosarcoma	Look for bony erosions and mineralized matrix	Intermediate to low intensity	High ± some heterogeneity if calcified matrix	Avid enhancement

Moore KR, Fischbein NJ, Harnsberger HR et al. Petrous apex cephaloceles. *AJNR Am J Neuroradiol.* 2001;22(10):1867. [PMID: 11733318] (Presents the clinical and imaging features of petrous apex cephaloceles.)

Moore KR, Harnsberger HR, Shelton C, Davidson HC. "Leave me alone" lesions of the petrous apex. *AJNR Am J Neuroradiol.* 1998;19(4):733. [PMID: 9576664] (Asymmetric fatty marrow in the petrous apex and petrous air-cell effusions have characteristic MRI and CT scanning features that facilitate their correct diagnosis.)

Muckle RP, De la Cruz A, Lo WM. Petrous apex lesions. *Am J Otol.* 1998;19(2):219. [PMID: 9520060] (The clinical features, diagnostic evaluation, imaging, and treatment outcomes of patients with petrous apex lesions are reviewed.)

Anesthesia for Head & Neck Surgery

4

Errol Lobo, MD, PhD, & Francesca Pellegrini, MD

◼ ANESTHETIC DRUGS

In head and neck surgery, anesthetists use a number of drugs in monitored conditions. These drugs may be used in procedures requiring conscious sedation. Although a large majority of office-based procedures are accomplished with the use of conscious sedation, a number of procedures performed at same-day surgery centers are also done with conscious sedation.

ANALGESICS, SEDATIVES, & HYPNOTICS

OPIOIDS

General Considerations

Opioids mediate analgesia through a complex interaction of opioid receptors in the supraspinal central nervous system (CNS). They produce reliable analgesia as well as provide some sedation and euphoria. There is no impairment of myocardial contractility, but sympathetically mediated vascular tone is reduced. Ventilation is depressed because of elevation of the carbon dioxide threshold for respiration. Opioids given at recommended doses do not reliably produce unconsciousness. They may, however, cause decreased bowel motility, biliary spasm, nausea, and pruritus.

Routes of Administration

Opioids may be given by intermittent intravenous or intramuscular routes. Plasma level peaks and valleys may lead either to variations in the desired analgesia or excessive side effects. Continuous infusions or patient-controlled analgesia with smaller, more frequent doses has been shown to lead to better analgesia, with fewer side effects and less total drug use. Fentanyl and morphine may also be administered by an intrathecal or an epidural route. Either of these administration routes allows the placement of opioids in the vicinity of spinal cord receptors. A growing body of information supports the use of these routes in high-risk patients to provide superior analgesia, less sedation, and less decrement in pulmonary function.

Drug Tolerance

Tolerance developed by the induction of hepatic microsomal enzymes may occur over the course of days or weeks. The narcotic effects may be reversed with a variety of antagonists (eg, naloxone). Acute reversal may be accompanied by agitation, pulmonary and systemic hypertension, and pulmonary edema.

1. Morphine

Morphine is relatively hydrophilic and thus has a slow onset with a fairly long clinical effect. Only a small amount of administered morphine gains access to the CNS, but it accumulates rapidly in the kidneys, liver, and skeletal muscles. Profound vein vasodilatation may be induced owing to the effects of histamine release and the reduction of sympathetic nervous system tone.

2. Fentanyl

A synthetic opioid, fentanyl has effects similar to morphine but it is more lipid soluble, has a more rapid onset, and has a shorter duration of action. These factors contribute to faster entrance into the CNS and the prompt redistribution away from the CNS. Elevated doses may lead to progressive saturation in adipose tissues. When this occurs, plasma concentrations do not decline promptly. Thus, pharmacodynamic effects, including ventilatory depression, may be prolonged.

3. Remifentanil

Remifentanil was recently introduced and has a much more rapid onset and offset than fentanyl. With the initial dose, anesthesia may be achieved in approximately

160

30–60 seconds; the offset of the drug can occur within 5–10 minutes after the infusion is discontinued. Because remifentanil is metabolized in blood and skeletal muscle, it can be administered as a single dose or in an infusion. Because of the potency of this opioid and because chest wall rigidity may result, this drug should be administered by an anesthesiologist or an anesthetist.

4. Meperidine

Commonly known as Demerol, meperidine has one tenth the potency of morphine and a shorter duration of action. In low doses it has been shown to decrease the shivering associated with rewarming after surgery and after amphotericin B administration. Several metabolites are excreted by the kidney and may accumulate in the presence of renal disease. The major metabolite, normeperidine, is a proconvulsant and may cause seizures in patients with renal insufficiency.

BENZODIAZEPINES

General Considerations

Benzodiazepines produce anxiolysis and sedation by facilitation of the inhibitory actions of GABA on nerve conduction in the cerebral cortex. They may be used to produce sedation and amnesia, facilitate patient cooperation, attenuate alcohol withdrawal syndrome, treat seizures, and relieve muscle spasm.

Benzodiazepines have no analgesic properties. They may cause transient decreases in blood pressure due to decreased catecholamine levels and systemic vascular resistance, but with little effect on contractility. Respiratory depression is usually minimal and well tolerated in clinical doses, but it may be accentuated in the elderly and patients with chronic obstructive pulmonary disease. Titration to a cooperative, oriented, and tranquil state (level 2 on the Ramsey Scale) is the desired effect. Patients with a history of heavy alcohol or sedative use may require considerably more drug to achieve this response. Diazepam, midazolam, and lorazepam are three of the more commonly used benzodiazepines.

Drug Tolerance

Tolerance to benzodiazepines develops in a manner similar to prolonged alcohol and opiate use. Withdrawal may result in profound sympathetic autonomic response. The replacement of benzodiazepine plasma levels and transient autonomic control would be indicated for the control of withdrawal symptoms.

Sedation Reversal

The reversal of benzodiazepine-induced sedation has been reported with physostigmine and aminophylline.

Flumazenil, a specific benzodiazepine-receptor antagonist, provides a consistent reversal of sedation within 2 minutes of intravenous administration. The duration of reversal is short; therefore, resedation is a possibility in cases of benzodiazepine overdose. Flumazenil has also been reported to transiently reverse the somnolence of hepatic encephalopathy. Therapy with this agent should be gradual to avoid excitatory symptoms. Convulsions have been reported in patients who are seizure prone and benzodiazepine dependent.

1. Diazepam

Diazepam has a long clinical duration because of the long half-life of several active metabolites. It is not water soluble, and the parenteral suspension of propylene glycol is irritating when given intravenously or intramuscularly. Because diazepam requires microsomal nonconjugative pathways for degradation and elimination, it should not be administered to patients with acute hepatitis.

2. Midazolam

Midazolam is the most commonly used benzodiazepine in the intensive care unit. It is water soluble, with short clinical duration, and it has fewer active metabolites. Midazolam offers a more rapid onset and a greater degree of amnesia than other benzodiazepines, which makes it a good choice for brief procedures such as esophagogastroduodenoscopy (EGD) and bronchoscopy.

3. Lorazepam

Lorazepam is another frequently used long-acting benzodiazepine. There is no pain on injection and no active metabolites. This agent has become a popular choice for patients with liver disease because its metabolism is not dependent on microsomal enzymes.

ALPHA$_2$-AGONIST

The α_2-agonist dexmedetomidine is a class of sedative drug that has been approved by the FDA for use as a sedative and analgesic in the operating room and in the intensive care unit. Dexmedetomidine has pharmacologic actions similar to those of clonidine except that its affinity for the α_2-receptor is eight times greater, making dexmedetomidine five to ten times more potent than clonidine. In the past few years, the use of dexmedetomidine for the management of sedation and analgesia in the perioperative setting has increased significantly. Dexmedetomidine also possesses several properties that may additionally benefit postoperative patients who have an opioid tolerance or who are sensitive to opioid-induced respiratory depression. In spontaneously breathing volunteers, intravenous dexmedetomidine caused marked sedation with only mild reductions in resting ventilation at higher doses. Head and neck surgeons will find this drug useful for conscious sedation cases, augmented sleep studies, and fiberoptic intubations and tracheostomy placement.

Dexmedetomidine does cause some cardiovascular instability, which can be avoided when the drug is titrated carefully. Nevertheless, it should be appreciated that dexmedetomidine does cause some moderate reductions in blood pressure and heart rate.

ANESTHESIA INDUCTION DRUGS

INJECTED ANESTHETICS

1. Barbiturates

Once a mainstay in sedation management, barbiturates now seem to have fallen out of favor, mainly because of the availability of more titratable alternatives. They have numerous sites of action, but they most likely promote the inhibitory effects of GABA on neuronal function. They have no analgesic effect and cause dose-related CNS, cardiac, and respiratory depression. Short-acting agents such as methohexital and thiopental sodium are useful to produce unconsciousness for very short procedures, such as cardioversions and intubations. Both agents also can be used for short-term procedures such as examining the oropharynx of a noncooperative patient. As with most anesthetic induction drugs, patients should be adequately monitored (ie, heart rate, blood pressure, electrocardiogram, and pulse oximetry), and supplemental oxygen should be given. Emergency endotracheal intubation equipment should be readily available together with emergency medications. Dosage measures must be judicious because of the increased likelihood of respiratory and hemodynamic depression, especially in elderly patients.

Both medium-acting agents (eg, pentobarbital IV/PO) and long-acting agents (eg, phenobarbital PO) have been used for violent agitation refractory to other agents, *status epilepticus,* and the induction of barbiturate coma to treat increased intracranial pressure.

2. Propofol

Propofol is an ultra-short-acting intravenous anesthetic agent. Unconsciousness may be induced in less than 30 seconds followed by awakening in 4–8 minutes. It has potent sedative hypnotic activity, but unlike with other agents, awakening is markedly rapid from even deep sedation, with minimal residual sedative effects and good antiemetic qualities. The hepatic metabolism of propofol is rapid, but rapid redistribution also plays a role in

early awakening. It has no pharmacologic active metabolites. Propofol has been shown to decrease systemic blood pressure as a result of myocardial depression and vasodilatation. When used in low doses (eg, 10–50 mcg/kg/min) as a continuous infusion for sedation, these effects are minimal. Propofol has no analgesic effects but has been shown to decrease narcotic requirements.

One of the disadvantages in using this agent is that propofol is only slightly water soluble. It must be formulated in an oil and water emulsion of soybean oil, egg lecithin, and glycerol. This formulation is similar to a 10% intralipid solution. Thus, this agent is contraindicated in patients with the potential for allergic responses to the emulsion components. Pain is common on injection but often can be attenuated by pretreatment of the vein with a 20- to 40-mg lidocaine bolus before infusion. With prolonged used, blood lipid levels should be assessed to rule out hypertriglyceridemia.

Propofol should be treated with the same degree of caution as parenteral nutrition solutions. Multiple reports of bacterial contamination due to manipulations of the emulsion medium demonstrate that it supports rapid bacterial growth. Recent formulations of propofol have included bacteriostatic agents such as EDTA or sulfites, which have made this issue less of a clinical concern. Nonetheless, clinical guidelines still limit the handling of opened vials to less than 24 hours and, when used as an infusion, advocate line changes at regular (usually 12-hour) intervals.

A soluble cousin of propofol marketed as Aquavan (fospropofol disodium) is undergoing phase III studies and should be available for use in 2007. The drug is described to have similar properties as propofol without the pain experienced during injection. The drug has been used for conscious sedation for colonoscopies with success in several phase III studies. Like propofol, Aquavan can also cause respiratory depression and hence should be used with care and in a monitored setting with emergency airway equipment.

3. Ketamine

Ketamine is a phencyclidine derivative (similar to LSD) that produces a docile, dissociative state that may be exploited as a sedative. Agitated patients may be given an IM injection of 3–5 mg/kg or a titration of 10-mg intravenous boluses to produce a cataleptic state in which the eyes remain open with a slow nystagmic gaze. Amnesia is present and analgesia is intense. The additional advantages of using ketamine include the maintenance of airway reflexes, cardiovascular stimulation, and bronchial relaxation. The disadvantages include increased airway secretions, transient increases in intracranial pressure, and associated unpleasant visual or auditory illusions. The addition of benzodiazepines may attenuate some of these untoward sensory effects. Examples of the clinical utility of this drug include conscious sedation for burn wound dressing changes and facilitating endotracheal intubation in the hypotensive patient.

INHALED ANESTHETICS

In the operating room, general anesthesia is commonly maintained with inhaled anesthetics. These agents also provide some analgesia, amnesia, and muscle relaxation. In pediatric patients in whom there is no intravenous access, anesthesia may be induced by inhalation. All of the inhaled anesthetics, with the exception of nitrous oxide, are bronchodilators and may be useful in patients with reactive airways. Most inhaled agents reduce blood pressure owing to either direct cardiac depression (eg, halothane) or vasodilation (eg, isoflurane, sevoflurane, or desflurane). The rapidity of anesthetic induction as well as emergence from anesthesia is based on the lipid solubility characteristics of the inhaled anesthetic. The more insoluble the anesthetic agent, the faster the induction of anesthesia. The agents with high lipid solubility prolong the emergence from anesthesia.

1. Nitrous Oxide

Nitrous oxide produces general anesthesia through interaction with the cellular membranes of the CNS. Nitrous oxide is the only nonorganic inhaled anesthetic in clinical use. Although it is nonvolatile, it does support combustion and caution should be taken in the event of airway fires. The uptake and elimination of nitrous oxide are relatively rapid compared with other inhaled anesthetics and are primarily the results of its low blood-gas partition coefficient. It produces analgesia, amnesia (with a concentration greater than 60%), mild myocardial depression, and mild sympathetic nervous system stimulation. It does not significantly affect heart rate or blood pressure. Nitrous oxide is a mild respiratory depressant, although less so than the volatile anesthetics. The elimination of nitrous oxide is via exhalation.

2. Isoflurane

Until recently, isoflurane was the most commonly used inhaled anesthetic in the United States. Isoflurane causes minimal cardiac depression. Like other volatile anesthetics, isoflurane causes respiratory depression with a decrease in minute ventilation. The ventilatory response to hypoxia and hypercapnia is diminished. Another characteristic that isoflurane shares with other volatile anesthetics is its ability to cause bronchodilation; this effect occurs despite its ability to cause airway irritation.

Isoflurane increases skeletal muscle blood flow, decreases systemic vascular resistance, and lowers arterial blood pressure. High concentrations of isoflurane may increase cerebral blood flow and intracranial pressure. These effects are effectively reduced by hyperventilation. At even higher concentrations, isoflurane reduces cerebral metabolic oxygen requirements and provides cerebral protection. It also decreases renal blood flow, glomerular filtration rate, and urinary output.

3. Desflurane

The structure of desflurane is very similar to that of isoflurane except for the substitution of a fluorine atom for a chlorine atom. This composition makes desflurane highly insoluble. Its low solubility in blood and body tissues causes a very rapid "wash-in" and "wash-out" of the gas. The time required for patients to awaken is approximately half as long as that observed following isoflurane administration. Desflurane has cardiovascular and cerebral effects similar to those of isoflurane.

4. Sevoflurane

Sevoflurane has begun to replace halothane as a primary inhaled anesthetic agent used in anesthesia induction when an intravenous induction cannot be performed. It is used primarily in pediatrics where intravenous access is not available and induction has to be achieved by other means. Nonpungency and a rapid increase in alveolar anesthetic concentration make it an excellent choice for smooth and rapid inhalation induction of anesthesia. The blood solubility of sevoflurane is slightly greater than that of desflurane. Sevoflurane mildly depresses myocardial contractility and systemic vascular resistance and arterial blood pressure decline slightly less than with isoflurane or desflurane. As with isoflurane and desflurane, sevoflurane causes slight increases in cerebral blood flow and intracranial pressure at normocarbia. Sevoflurane is reported to have potential for nephrotoxicity and therefore should be used with a gas flow of > 2 L.

5. Halothane

Halothane is a halogenated alkane that is used primarily for inducing anesthesia in patients when an intravenous induction is not possible. The nonpungent and sweet-smelling odor of halothane makes it especially suitable for this purpose. Halothane causes a dose-depression reduction in arterial pressure by myocardial depression. It also causes respiratory depression. This anesthetic drug has been associated with a drug-induced hepatitis known as halothane hepatitis. This condition is extremely rare, with an incidence of 1 in 35,000 patients. The risk of halothane hepatitis is increased in (1) patients exposed to multiple doses of halothane anesthesia within short intervals, (2) middle-aged obese women, and (3) patients with a genetic predisposition to halothane hepatitis.

ANTIEMETICS

DROPERIDOL

Droperidol has greater antiemetic and sedative effects than other anesthetic agents, but it may also produce respiratory depression. If administered alone, dysphoria can result; at clinical doses, it is used in combination with a narcotic or benzodiazepine for sedation. More recently, the FDA has discouraged the use of droperidol in unmonitored settings.

ONDANSETRON & DOLASETRON

Ondansetron and dolasetron are selective antagonists of serotonin 5-HT$_3$ receptors with little or no effect on dopamine receptors. Unlike droperidol, they do not cause sedation, extrapyramidal signs, or alterations of GI motility and lower esophageal sphincter tone. 5-HT$_3$ receptors are found in the chemoreceptor trigger zone of the area postrema, in the nucleus tractus solitarius, and also along the gastrointestinal tract. The most common reported side effect is headache. Dolasetron can also prolong the QT interval.

NEUROMUSCULAR BLOCKERS

Neuromuscular blocking agents are used most commonly for facilitation of endotracheal intubation and in the operating room when patient movement is detrimental to the surgical procedure. The clinical pharmacology of the most frequently used neuromuscular blocking agents can be found in Table 4–1. The most prominent side effect of neuromuscular blockers is that they cause paralysis of the respiratory muscles. Hence, patient ventilation must be ensured by the anesthesiologist and can be achieved with a mask or a secured endotracheal tube.

Most muscle relaxants induce paralysis by blocking acetylcholine receptors at the neuromuscular junction of skeletal muscle. They have no intrinsic sedative or analgesic properties and must be used in concert with other medications. At a minimum, these agents should be used in conjunction with an anxiolysis agent. Inadequate sedation and hypnosis while using neuromuscular blockers can produce unpleasant recall by patients, with long-term side effects.

VECURONIUM

Vecuronium is a relaxant that is popular because of its short clinical duration (30–60 minutes) and lack of hemodynamic side effects. It may be given as a bolus or as a continuous infusion. It is metabolized by the liver and excreted by the kidneys.

CISATRACURIUM

Cisatracurium undergoes degradation in plasma at physiologic pH and temperature by organ-independent Hofmann elimination. Metabolism and elimination appear to be independent of renal or liver failure. It does not affect heart rate or blood pressure nor does it produce autonomic effects.

PANCURONIUM

Pancuronium has a longer duration of action (60–90 minutes) and is eliminated primarily by renal mechanisms. The major limiting factor of its use is the side effect of tachycardia, which results from a vagolytic effect, especially after bolus administration.

ROCURONIUM

Rocuronium has an onset of action similar to but slightly longer than that of succinylcholine, making it suitable for rapid-sequence inductions; however, the duration of action is much longer. This intermediate duration of action is comparable to that of vecuronium. Rocuronium undergoes no metabolism and it is eliminated primarily by the liver and slightly by the kidneys; its duration of action is modestly prolonged by severe hepatic failure and pregnancy.

Table 4–1. Pharmacokinetics of the more commonly used neuromuscular blockers. Only vecuronium is used as an infusion.

Agent	Intubation Dose	Time to Onset	Time to Recovery	Infusion Rate
Vecuronium	0.1 mg/kg	2–3 minutes	25–30 minutes	1–2 mcg/kg/min
Cisatracurium	0.2 mg/kg	1–2 minutes	50–60 minutes	---
Pancuronium	0.1 mg/kg	5 minutes	80–100 minutes	---
Rocuronium	1.2 mg/kg	1–2 minutes	40–150 minutes	---

OTHER DRUGS OF VALUE TO THE OTOLARYNGOLOGIST

KETOROLAC

Ketorolac is a recently released potent parenteral nonsteroidal analgesic without opioid-related side effects such as respiratory depression. An intramuscular dose of 60 mg is reported to be equivalent to a morphine dose of 10 mg for up to 3 hours. Clinical dosing is every 8 hours, and it appears to be the most effective in situations where swelling contributes to pain (ie, dental, gynecologic, and orthopedic surgery). It has minimal impact on ventilation, hemodynamics, and bowel motility. The disadvantages of its use include a limited analgesic effect beyond the recommended doses and an impaired platelet function. Substantial gastrointestinal mucosal breakdown may occur with use over a period as short as 1 week.

ANTICHOLINERGIC AGENTS

Anticholinergic agents are sometimes used to produce sedation and amnesia. They also have an antisialagogue effect and prevent reflex bradycardia. Atropine and scopolamine are tertiary amines that cross the lipid barrier protecting the CNS. In terms of centrally induced sedation and amnesia, scopolamine has 10 times the potency of atropine. Because scopolamine produces tachycardia as its major hemodynamic side effect, it is a popular choice as an urgent amnestic agent for the hemodynamically unstable or hypovolemic patient (eg, a trauma victim).

Undesirable side effects include (1) toxic delirium (known as central cholinergic syndrome), (2) tachycardia, (3) the relaxation of lower esophageal sphincter tone (with the associated potential for regurgitation), (4) mydriasis, and (5) the potential elevation of temperature via suppression of sweat gland function.

ANESTHETIC EQUIPMENT

The basic equipment for airway management used by the anesthesiologist should be familiar to the otolaryngologist. This equipment includes laryngoscope blades, endotracheal tubes, and breathing circuits.

LARYNGOSCOPE BLADES

In general, laryngoscope blades may be classified as either straight or curved. With proper head positioning, both types of blades provide a direct pathway to the vocal cords for endotracheal intubation. There are several designs of laryngoscope blades as shown in Figure 4–1. Some blades, like the Bainton blade, may be used in special situations in which redundant tissue or airway edema is present and the vocal cords are not easily visible.

ENDOTRACHEAL TUBES

Otolaryngologists often require specialized endotracheal tubes, depending on the procedure performed. The standard endotracheal tube is made of polyvinyl chloride and

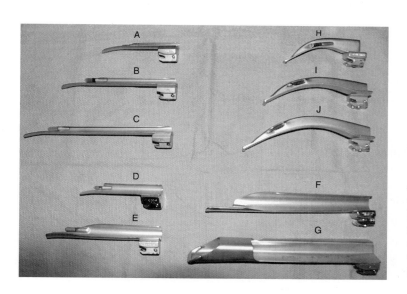

Figure 4–1. Laryngoscope blades used by anesthesiologists. Straight blades include the Miller blades **(A, B, C)**, the Wisconsin blades **(D, E, F)**, and the Bainton blade **(G)**. The Bainton blade was designed especially for situations in which ed0ematous or redundant tissue obstructs a view of the vocal cords. Curved blades include the Macintosh blades **(H, I, J)**.

Table 4–2. Recommended endotracheal tube sizes for pediatrics.

Patient Age	Patient Weight	Cuff Size	Cuff Length
< 1 month	2–4 kg	2.5–3.5 mm	10–12 cm
1–6 months	4–6 kg	4.0–4.5 mm (uncuffed)	12–14 cm
6–12 months	6–10 kg	4.5–5.0 mm (uncuffed)	14–16 cm
1–3 years	10–15 kg	5.0–5.5 mm (uncuffed)	16–18 cm
4–6 years	15–20 kg	5.5–6.5 mm (uncuffed)	18–20 cm
7–10 years	25–35 kg	6.5–7.0 mm (uncuffed)	20–22 cm
10–14 years	40–50 kg	7.0–7.5 mm (cuffed)	22–24 cm

is disposable. It can be made of clear silicon. Reusable rubber tubes are also available; these tubes have to be cleaned and autoclaved before reuse. Endotracheal tubes come in various sizes and may be **cuffed** or **uncuffed.** Uncuffed endotracheal tubes are used in neonates, infants, and children usually up to the age of 12 years. Suggestions for tube sizes in children are shown in Table 4–2. The tracheal end is usually beveled and may contain a Murphy eye. Endotracheal tube cuffs may be either high volume or low volume; both types of cuffs may cause tracheal necrosis with long-term intubation. Endotracheal tubes have gradations, usually in centimeters, to allow the

clinician to keep track of the correct position of the tube and to prevent endobronchial migration or extubation. For common procedures of the larynx, the use of a small-diameter endotracheal tube allows for better exposure. The recommended size is 5.0 mm ID for women and 5.5 mm ID for men.

For a variety of head and neck procedures, specially designed endotracheal tubes may be required. These tubes are designed to provide optimal exposure for the surgeon working in the oral and nasal cavities. The anatomic design of these tubes prevents their kinking during surgery.

Classification of Endotracheal Tubes

Three of the more commonly used endotracheal tubes are RAE endotracheal tubes, armored endotracheal tubes, and laser-resistant endotracheal tubes (Figure 4–2). These tubes are commonly used for head and neck surgery.

A. RAE ENDOTRACHEAL TUBES

RAE endotracheal tubes, named after the inventors of the tube (Ring, Adair, and Elwyn), have a preformed shape to fit the mouth or nose. The tubes are available in a variety of pediatric and adult sizes and may be cuffed or uncuffed. Nasal RAE tubes are commonly used in surgery of the oral cavity, since they do not obstruct the surgical field. Oral RAE tubes are commonly used for surgeries of the oral cavity, particularly those involving the tonsils. A drawback to RAE tubes use is that their shape may result in an inadvertent endobronchial intubation, particularly in patients with short necks.

B. ARMORED ENDOTRACHEAL TUBES

Armored endotracheal tubes are commonly used in head and neck surgery. The primary advantage of using

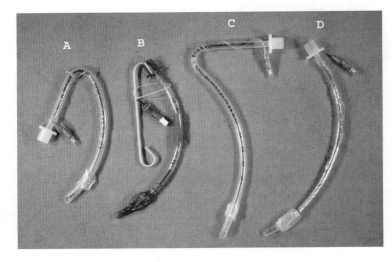

Figure 4–2. Tracheal tubes used in ENT procedures. Included are an oral RAE tube **(A)** and a nasal RAE tube **(C)**, both used for tonsillectomies and procedures in the oral cavity; an Armored tracheal tube **(B),** commonly used in laryngectomies; and a wrapped tracheal tube **(D),** used in laser procedures.

these tubes is that they can withstand the constant moving of the head without kinking.

C. LASER-RESISTANT ENDOTRACHEAL TUBES

Laser-resistant endotracheal tubes are used in laser surgery (eg, in the treatment of vocal cord papillomas). Regular endotracheal tubes can be converted to laser-resistant tubes by wrapping the ends with aluminum foil.

BREATHING CIRCUITS

After an airway is secured, oxygen is provided to the patient either (1) via a ventilator in the operating room and the intensive care unit or (2) manually, by a breathing circuit connected to an oxygen tank. The otolaryngologist should understand the components of a breathing circuit commonly used both for transporting ventilated patients and in office-based practice. The most common breathing circuit used for adults is the Mapelson F or Jackson-Rees circuit. The circuit contains a reservoir bag with a valve, a corrugated circuit, and a fresh gas flow near the attachment to the mask or the endotracheal tube (Figure 4–3). This device is used for manual ventilation either by a mask or by an endotracheal tube. This circuit can also be used to ventilate patients in emergency situations, when a ventilator is unavailable.

■ AIRWAY MANAGEMENT

A high percentage of cases involving the head and neck involve patients with "difficult airways." A patient with

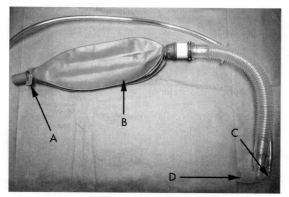

Figure 4–3. The Jackson-Rees circuit, also known as the Mapelson D circuit, is composed of **(A)** a valve, **(B)** a reservoir bag, **(C)** an ingress for fresh gases, and **(D)** a connector for attaching a mask or a tracheal tube.

Table 4–3. Conditions that may help the physician identify patients with potential airway difficulties.

Prior difficulty with endotracheal intubation
Cervical immobility (limited or no range of neck motion)
Hoarseness or stridor
Trauma
Radiation therapy
Prior surgery of the head, neck, or both
Morbid obesity
Dyspnea or dyspnea on exertion
Dysphagia
Shortness of breath

a difficult airway may pose a challenge for both manual ventilation and the placement of an endotracheal tube. Patients with difficult airways should be identified prior to surgery, especially before the induction of general anesthesia; in particular, these patients should be identified before neuromuscular blockers are used. Preoperative evaluation by the otolaryngologist, either by directly viewing the airway or by other diagnostic tools such as a CT scan or MRI, may provide invaluable information to the anesthesiologist, particularly if a difficult airway is involved.

IDENTIFICATION OF POTENTIAL AIRWAY PROBLEMS

With improvements both in record keeping and communications between patient and physician, the patient history should provide important information about the patient's airway and any potential problems for securing the airway in the operating room. Knowledge of a history of difficult intubation, prior head and neck surgery, the immobility of cervical vertebrae, and radiation therapy to the airway should alert the physician about a potentially difficult airway. Other alert items should include dysphagia, trauma to the head and neck, hoarseness, and stridor (Table 4–3).

PHYSICAL EXAMINATION

In most cases involving head and neck surgery, a detailed preoperative assessment of the airway may be performed by the otolaryngologist. This assessment is extremely helpful in determining which patients may have difficulties with endotracheal intubation. The preoperative exam should therefore include (1) a detailed frontal and profile view to assess mandibular size and mobility; (2) an examination and assessment of the mental-alveolar process and either the mental-hyoid bone or the mental-thyroid cartilage distance; (3) an assessment of neck rotation and flexion-extension mobility; and (4) an examination of the neck for evidence of masses, tracheal deviation, the size of tracheal and cricoid cartilage, and tissue plasticity. Carefully assessing patient breathing patterns and phonation may also provide the physician with important clues about airway patency and potential difficulties with endotracheal intubation (Figure 4–4).

An intraoral examination also should be performed as part of the preoperative assessment. It should include an assessment of tongue size, protrusive occlusion, and the degree of overbite (Table 4–4). Examining the oral cavity and assessing the structures that can be seen when the patient's mouth is opened wide can assist the physician in recognizing a potentially difficult airway. The classification of these views is called the Mallampati classification (Figure 4–5). In about 80% of oral (Mallampati) Class I views, a Grade 1 laryngoscopic view is observed. For Mallampati Class II, only the posterior vocal cords may be visualized in about 50% of cases. Class III and IV merit special attention as intubation of the trachea in these patients may be difficult and may indicate intubating patients while they are awake. The degree of vigilance should also be increased for patients in Classes III and IV, since manual ventilation may be a challenge.

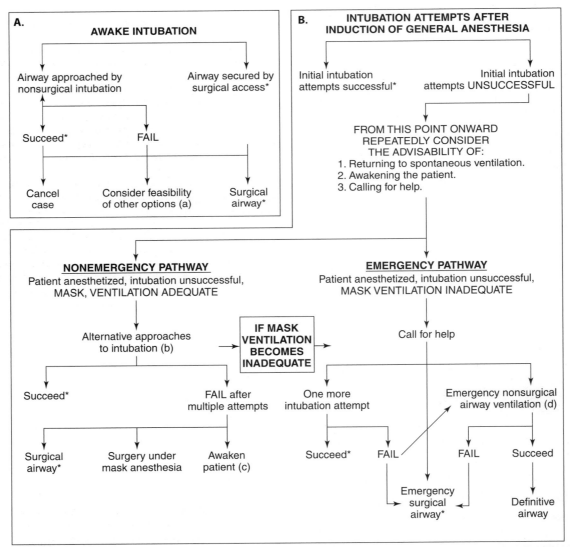

Figure 4–4. An algorithm suggested by the American Society of Anesthesiologists for dealing with airway difficulties. Asterisks denote that the airway is secured.

Table 4–4. An intraoral examination can provide important information regarding potential airway difficulties.

Loose, missing, or overly large teeth
Degree of overbite or protrusive occlusion
Size of the tongue
Visibility and size of facial structures
Patency and size of the nares; deviation of nasal septum

INTUBATION OF THE CONSCIOUS PATIENT

Patient Preparation

In patients with anticipated difficult airways or patients who are unable to either open their mouths or have cervical spine precautions, an intubation while they are awake is often necessary. The first step is to numb the oropharynx with a local anesthetic. The use of 2% lidocaine sprayed into the patient's mouth and throat may cause the loss of a gag reflex and allow the patient to be awake during the procedure. In other situations, tracheal intubation either via the oral or nasal route should be performed when the patient is awake, using a fiberoptic scope. In this situation, facilitating fiberoptic intubation may require the blockade of specific nerves.

Nerve Blocks

In the mouth, sensation to the anterior aspect of the tongue is innervated by the lingual nerve. In contrast, the posterior third of the tongue and the oropharynx are innervated by the pharyngeal branches of the glossopharyngeal nerve (the ninth cranial nerve) and by the vagus nerve (the tenth cranial nerve). Spraying the oral cavity with a local anesthetic and asking the patient to gargle and swallow the anesthetic spray can easily anesthetize these nerves. Alternately, these nerves are easily blocked by a 2-mL bilateral injection of a local anesthetic into the base of the palatoglossal arch, using a 25-gauge spinal needle. The superior laryngeal nerve, a branch of the vagus nerve, innervates the inferior aspect of the larynx to the level of the vocal cords. This nerve can be blocked by placing gauze soaked with a local anesthetic in the pyriform sinuses. In addition, this nerve may be blocked externally by locating the hyoid bone and injecting 3 mL of 2% lidocaine 1 cm below each greater cornu, where the internal branch of the superior laryngeal nerves penetrates the thyrohyoid membrane.

The recurrent laryngeal nerve innervates the mucosa below the vocal cords. This nerve may be blocked with a transtracheal injection of a local anesthetic. A transtracheal block is performed by identifying and penetrating the cricothyroid membrane while the neck is extended. The aspiration of air can confirm an intratracheal position; 4 mL of 4% lidocaine is then injected into the trachea at the end of an expiration. A deep inhalation and cough immediately following the injection distribute the anesthetic throughout the trachea.

Using a local anesthetic to block the above nerves may facilitate an endotracheal intubation in a patient who is conscious by depressing both the protective cough reflex and the swallowing reflex. Special precautions should be taken with patients at high risk for aspiration. In some patients, the use of anesthesia may be limited to the nasal passages and may be administered with either a blind nasal intubation or a fiberoptic nasal intubation. Using local anesthetics in the nares protects the airways of patients who are at high risk for aspiration.

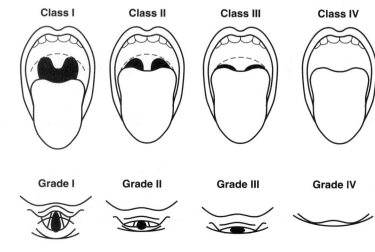

Figure 4–5. Correlation between views obtained before laryngoscopy with the naked eye (Mallampati Classification, Classes I–IV, top row) and views with laryngoscopy (Grades I–IV, bottom row).

Manual Ventilation

After a patient has been administered anesthetic induction drugs and neuromuscular blockers and cannot be awakened, maintaining a patent airway and adequate ventilation can be challenging when a difficult airway is encountered. Mask ventilation does add air to the stomach and may predispose patients to vomit. This risk is significant in patients with acid reflux disease. If manual ventilation by mask is adequate, the patient can continue to be ventilated until he or she awakens and can be intubated by an alternate technique.

In situations in which manual ventilation is difficult—even with the use of oral or nasal airways—then aggressive intervention may become necessary: a surgical airway may need to be created. The laryngeal mask airway is used when conventional methods of endotracheal intubation with a laryngoscope are unsuccessful and respiratory compromise is imminent. The laryngeal mask airway was designed as a compromise between the face mask and the endotracheal tube. It is used extensively throughout the world and has been included in the algorithm created by the American Society of Anesthesiologists to treat the difficult airway. This device requires no direct visualization of the vocal cords. However, a disadvantage of this device is that it does not prevent aspiration. Therefore, in patients who are at high risk for aspiration, a small endotracheal tube can be placed with fiberoptic guidance. Two new laryngeal mask airways have been introduced: the "fast-track" laryngeal mask airway and the ProSeal laryngeal mask airway. The fast-track laryngeal mask airway can be used much as the original laryngeal mask airway. The primary advantage of the fast-track device is that it allows endotracheal tube placement without direct laryngoscopy (Figure 4–6). The ProSeal device is very similar to the original laryngeal mask airway; however, it contains an extra lumen to suction the stomach and the intestinal contents. None of the three types of laryngeal mask airways provide protection against aspiration in a patient who vomits.

Esophageal-Tracheal Combitube

The esophageal-tracheal Combitube is another device that can be used in emergency situations. The Combitube is a hybrid of the traditional endotracheal tube and the former esophageal obturator airway. This device can prevent aspiration because of the presence of a tracheal cuff (Figure 4–7).

The GlideScope

The GlideScope (Saturn Biomedical Systems, Inc., Burnaby, British Columbia) is a new video laryngoscope that can be a useful alternative to the conventional fiberoptic scope for placement of an endotracheal tube in the trachea when confronted with a difficult airway. The GlideScope has a high-resolution digital camera incorporated in the blade, which displays a view of the vocal cords on a monitor. The blade is fashioned after the Macintosh blade with a 60° curvature to match the anatomic alignment. The blade is made of a soft plastic material and has a thickness of 18 mm. The blade also has an embedded antifogging mechanism. The GlideScope can be used with minimal treatment of the oropharynx with local anesthetic and is useful for not only endotracheal intubation, but also as a diagnostic tool.

■ PATIENT PREPARATION: ANESTHESIA & SURGERY

PREOPERATIVE ASSESSMENT

Patients scheduled for surgery should have a preoperative evaluation by the surgeon and the anesthesiologist, especially if general anesthesia will be administered. These patients should have a baseline laboratory assessment, which should include a complete blood count. In patients with coexisting disease, an evaluation of other functions is necessary. Patients over the age of 50 and patients with heart disease should also have an electrocardiogram (ECG). A preoperative pulmonary function assessment in patients with pulmonary disease is also warranted. These tests may determine postoperative care requirements and assess whether preoperative treatment may reduce the perioperative risks. Therefore, in a high percentage of cases, a cardiac or pulmonary consultation is necessary in the preoperative assessment.

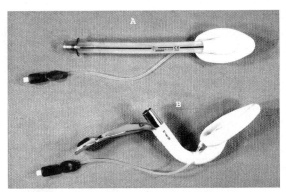

Figure 4–6. **(A)** The laryngeal mask airway. **(B)** The fast-track laryngeal mask airway.

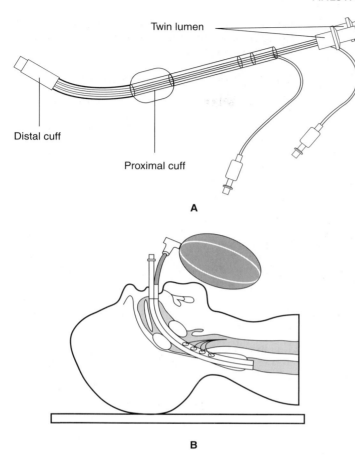

Twin lumen

Distal cuff

Proximal cuff

A

B

Figure 4–7. The Combitube is one of the more recently developed airways that can be placed without laryngoscopy and in emergency situations. The airway contains two lumens: a distal lumen that sits in the esophagus and a proximal lumen for ventilation. **(A)** There are two inflatable balloons; one is placed in the esophagus and the other in the oropharynx. **(B)** Placement of the Combitube.

Table 4–5 provides a list of tests with the sensitivity, specificity, and approximate cost of each.

Tests for Patients with Cardiac Disease

A. ELECTROCARDIOGRAM

All patients over age 50 and patients with cardiac disease should have an ECG. A preoperative ECG can provide important information on the status of the patient's cardiac circulation. Patients with abnormal Q waves seen on their ECG suggest a past myocardial infarction. These patients may be at an increased risk of a perioperative cardiac event and may need further preoperative assessment. Approximately 30% of infarctions are silent and only detected on routine ECGs, most notably in patients with diabetes or hypertension. In addition to the ECG, history taking can provide important information about the patient's cardiac status. Assessing the patient's functional status by knowing the patient's exercise tolerance may determine the need for a cardiac evaluation. The information from cardiovascular testing may allow for optimizing preoperative medications, provide information on perioperative monitoring, or determine the need for coronary revascularization.

Table 4–5. Tests performed in the preoperative patient evaluation.

Test	Sensitivity (%)	Specificity (%)	Cost (Approximate)
Ambulatory ECG (24 h)	70	85	$280
ECG (stress test)	65	80	$450
Stress echo	80	85	$600
Thallium (planar)	90	80	$1,200
Thallium (SPECT)	90	90	$1,200
Dipyridamole thallium	90	90	$1,200
Cardiac catheterization	95	95	$2,500

B. 24-Hour Ambulatory ECG

The 24-hour ambulatory ECG requires the placement of a Holter monitor, which records a continuous 12-lead ECG for 24 hours. This monitor detects arrhythmias and ischemic changes during a 24-hour period. This test often requires further testing, particularly if ischemic changes are noted.

C. Exercise Stress Test

In an exercise stress test, the patient exercises with ECG leads attached; the patient's heart rate and blood pressure are monitored. The test is considered positive if any of the following signs and symptoms are present: myocardial ischemia, patient complaints of chest pain or dyspnea, and clinical signs of left ventricular dysfunction. Even more significant is a decrease in the patient's blood pressure in response to exercise; this finding may be associated with global ventricular dysfunction. Syncope during the test also signifies decreased cardiac output. A positive exercise ECG stress test should alert the anesthesiologist that the patient is at risk for ischemia, within a wide range of heart rates, which may occur during surgery. These patients may require further workup and medical management.

D. Thallium Exercise Test

The sensitivity and specificity of a noninvasive stress test can be increased by nuclear imaging techniques. Thallium-201 (Tl-201) is a radioactive compound that mimics potassium uptake by viable myocardial cells. The sensitivity of exercise Tl-201 imaging depends on the imaging technique. For detecting coronary artery disease, qualitative visual Tl-201 imaging has an average sensitivity of 84% and a specificity of 87%, although these rates are improved with better imaging techniques. The drawback to Tl-201 imaging is that patients have to remain stationary to avoid artifacts. Thallium defects are reported as normal, fixed, or reversible. Other important measures noted by stress Tl-201 imaging are the size of the defect, lung uptake, and left ventricular cavity size. A large lung uptake of isotope has been associated with myocardial ischemia; this ischemia produces left ventricular dysfunction, which may result in pulmonary edema. The presence of a distended left ventricular cavity on the immediate post-stress image is another marker of severe coronary artery disease, presumably as a result of myocardial ischemia.

E. Coronary Testing with Pharmacologic Agents

The use of pharmacologic agents to induce cardiac stress in patients who cannot exercise can also detect coronary artery disease. These agents can be divided into two categories: (1) those that result in coronary artery vasodilatation (eg, dipyridamole and adenosine) and (2) those that increase myocardial oxygen demand (eg, dobutamine and isoproterenol). Coronary artery vasodilators are useful for defining the potential risk of myocardial disease by causing differential flows in normal coronary arteries compared with arteries that have a stenosis. The use of dobutamine is an alternative method of increasing myocardial oxygen demand without exercise. The goal is to increase heart rate and blood pressure.

F. Echocardiography

The use of echocardiography for preoperative cardiac evaluation has increased in recent years. Echocardiography can evaluate left ventricular function, pulmonary vascular pressures, and valvular competence. In most cases, a transthoracic approach is used. Transesophageal echocardiography may provide more detailed measures of valvular abnormalities and left ventricular function. Echocardiography can also be performed with exercise. In patients who are unable to exercise, dobutamine has been used to mimic the stress effects of exercise.

G. Coronary Angiography

Coronary angiography has been called the gold standard for defining coronary anatomy. Angiography can assess valvular function and hemodynamic indices, including ventricular pressure and the gradients across valves. In most cases, angiography is performed after a positive stress test to determine whether coronary revascularization will both improve cardiac function and reduce perioperative cardiac morbidity after noncardiac surgery. One major difference between the stress tests and coronary angiography is that the latter provides the clinician with anatomic, not functional, information. However, it is an expensive test with potential complications.

Tests for Patients with Pulmonary Disease

A. Preoperative Pulmonary Evaluation

Patients scheduled for head and neck surgery may present with coexisting pulmonary disease. The presence of pulmonary disease may increase perioperative morbidity and mortality. Patients with acute pulmonary disease who are scheduled for elective surgery may choose to postpone the surgery until the pulmonary disease resolves. Patients with chronic pulmonary disease may benefit from a preoperative pulmonary workup that includes a measure of arterial blood gases, a chest x-ray, and pulmonary function tests.

B. Pulmonary Function Tests

Preoperative pulmonary function tests (1) measure the severity of lung disease, (2) measure the efficacy of bronchodilator therapy (to improve pulmonary function), and (3) can predict the need for postoperative mechanical ventilation. Pulmonary disease may be classified as obstructive or restrictive.

1. Obstructive pulmonary diseases—Obstructive pulmonary disease includes asthma, emphysema, chronic bronchitis, bronchiectasis, and bronchiolitis. These disorders are characterized by an increase in expiratory airflow resistance that results in varying degrees of labored breathing. The most typical finding of pulmonary function tests is that both the forced expiratory volume per second (FEV_1) and the ratio of forced expiratory volume to forced vital capacity (FEV_1/FVC) are less than 70% of the predicted values. The expiratory airflow resistance results in air trapping. In addition, the residual volume (RV) and total lung capacity (TLC) are increased. Wheezing is a common clinical finding and represents turbulent airflow. In mild obstructive disease, wheezing may be absent but can be elicited by prolonged exhalation.

2. Restrictive pulmonary diseases—Restrictive lung diseases may be either acute or chronic intrinsic disorders and include pulmonary edema, acute respiratory distress syndrome (ARDS), infectious pneumonia, and interstitial lung diseases. Restrictive pulmonary disease may also represent extrinsic disorders involving the pleura, the chest wall, the diaphragm, and neuromuscular function.

Restrictive pulmonary disease is marked by decreased lung compliance that increases the work of breathing due to a characteristic rapid-shallow breathing pattern. Lung volumes are typically reduced, as are the FEV_1 and the FVC; however, the FEV_1/FVC ratio is normal. The expiratory flow rates are unchanged.

■ SPECIAL SURGICAL CONSIDERATIONS

SURGERY OF THE ORAL CAVITY & AIRWAY

1. Tonsillectomy & Adenoidectomy

Preoperative Considerations

A. OBSTRUCTIVE SLEEP APNEA

Most patients who undergo tonsillectomy and adenoidectomy are young and healthy. A few present with symptoms of obstructive sleep apnea. Patients with obstructive sleep apnea are often obese and may have potentially difficult airways. They may have short, thick necks, large tongues, and redundant pharyngeal tissue; the latter may require the patients to be awake during endotracheal intubation. Sedative premedication may be avoided in children with obstructive sleep apnea, intermittent obstruction, or very large tonsils.

B. UPPER RESPIRATORY TRACT INFECTIONS

Patients may present with upper respiratory tract infections. Surgery for these patients should be postponed until the infection is resolved, usually 7–14 days. These patients may develop a laryngospasm with airway manipulation. This complication carries the potential for significant morbidity and even mortality.

Intraoperative Considerations

In some patients, endotracheal intubation may be significantly difficult; therefore, the presence of an otolaryngologist may be helpful at the time of intubation. The use of an oral RAE tube for endotracheal intubation may optimize visualization of the surgical field. In younger children in whom an uncuffed tracheal tube is used, in order to avoid inhalation blood from the pharynx area, the supraglottic area may be packed with a petroleum gauze tube provided an appropriate leak around the endotracheal tube is obtained.

Patients should be awake when they are extubated, after protective airway reflexes have returned. In patients with reactive airway disease, including asthma, deep extubation may be warranted to prevent airway reactivity complications such as bronchospasm and laryngospasm.

Postoperative Complications

A. THROAT PACK RETENTION AND PULMONARY EDEMA

Retention of the throat pack is one complication of tonsillectomies and adenoidectomies. Another complication is acute airway obstruction, such as a laryngospasm, which can lead to pulmonary edema. This edema occurs when the patient breathes against a closed glottis, creating a negative intrathoracic pressure. This pressure is transmitted to the interstitial tissue, increasing the hydrostatic pressure gradient and enhancing fluid out of the pulmonary circulation into the alveoli.

B. HEMORRHAGE

Hemorrhage may result from a bleeding tonsil. Reintubations often may be difficult. Care should be taken not to oversedate the patient, who may aspirate large quantities of blood. If the bleeding is not controlled, then the patient should be returned to the operating room for exploration and surgical hemostasis.

2. Laser Surgery of the Airway

Laser surgery for lesions in the airway (1) provides precision in targeting lesions, (2) minimizes bleeding and edema, (3) preserves the surrounding structures, and (4) provides rapid healing. The carbon dioxide laser has particular application in treating laryngeal or vocal cord papillomas, treating laryngeal webs, resecting redundant subglottic tissue, and treating hemangioma coagulation.

Preoperative Considerations

The appropriate preoperative equipment should include a laser-resistant endotracheal tube; other endotracheal tubes should be available for emergency situations. Anesthesia during laser surgery may be administered with or without an endotracheal tube. All standard PVC endotracheal tubes are flammable and can ignite and vaporize when they come in contact with the laser beam. Some surgeons may prefer using a Dedo or Marshall laryngoscope and intermittent ventilation with a Sanders ventilator. The Sanders ventilator is a jet ventilator that delivers oxygen at < 50 psi directly through a port in the laryngoscope.

Intraoperative Considerations

The patient's eyes must be protected by taping them shut, followed by the application of wet gauze pads and a metal shield to prevent laser penetration of the eyes. All operating room personnel should wear special protective glasses.

Airway fires are a risk with laser surgery. A plan to handle a fire, if one occurs, is necessary. In some centers, the tracheal balloon is filled with blue methylene gas; therefore, rupture of the balloon is an early indication of a hazard. Both oxygen and nitrous oxide support combustion and a mixture of 30% oxygen and nitrogen may be used. If a fire occurs, ventilation should be discontinued, oxygen turned off, and the endotracheal tube removed. If the flame persists, the field should be flooded with normal saline. A direct examination of the pharynx and larynx provides information about the extent of the burn.

If a Dedo or Marshall laryngoscope is used, maintenance anesthesia should be administered with an intravenous anesthetic to prevent inadvertently anesthetizing the surgeon and other surgical staff. The patient should be reintubated with a regular endotracheal tube after the bronchoscope is removed. The use of the Sander's jet ventilator is contraindicated; it is associated with the risk of pneumothorax and pneumomediastinum due to the rupture of either alveolar blebs or a bronchus.

Postoperative Considerations

In the event of an airway fire during surgery, the patient should be monitored for at least 24 hours. Steroids and antibiotics should be considered for severe burns. If respiratory problems are encountered, then the patient should be observed in an intensive care setting.

SURGERY OF PATIENTS WITH ACUTE EPIGLOTTITIS

Acute epiglottitis is an infectious disease caused by *Haemophilus influenzae* B. It can progress rapidly from sore throat to airway obstruction to respiratory failure and death if the proper diagnosis and treatment are delayed. Patients are usually between the ages of 2 and 7, although acute epiglottitis has been reported in children younger than age 2; it has also been reported in adults. Characteristic signs and symptoms of acute epiglottitis include the following: the sudden onset of fever; dysphagia; drooling; thick, muffled voice; and a preference for the sitting position, leaning forward and with the head extended. Retractions, labored breathing, and cyanosis may be observed in cases where respiratory obstruction is present.

Preoperative Considerations

Direct visualization of the epiglottis should not be attempted in a patient who is not anesthetized—it could lead to airway compromise and death. The patient should be kept calm, since agitation is likely to have an adverse effect on the patient's respiratory abilities. The differential resulting from negative pressure inside and atmospheric pressure outside the extrathoracic airway results in a slight narrowing during normal inspiration. In a patient with airway obstruction, the pressure differential is exaggerated during inspiration. The likely collapse of the airway may become life threatening in the struggling and agitated patient.

Intraoperative Considerations

The intraoperative considerations for patients with acute epiglottitis include the following steps: (1) securing the airway; (2) inducing anesthesia with halothane or sevoflurane while maintaining spontaneous ventilation; (3) having an emergency airway cart and tracheostomy tray available and open; and (4) if the patient is a child, allowing his or her parent into the operating room to help keep the patient calm.

Postoperative Considerations

Postoperative care should be handled in the intensive care unit for continued observation and radiographic confirmation of tube placement. Tracheal extubation is usually attempted 48–72 hours after a significant leak around the endotracheal tube is present. At the same time, visual inspection of the larynx by flexible fiberoptic bronchoscopy can confirm a reduction in swelling of the epiglottis and surrounding tissues.

PAROTID GLAND SURGERY

Parotid gland surgery is usually performed for tumors but it can also be performed for infectious disorders. Some diseases of the parotid gland have been associated with alcohol use; these patients may exhibit the signs and symptoms of alcohol-related diseases. Parotid gland surgery is performed under general anesthesia. In most cases, the facial nerve needs to be preserved and nerve monitoring is therefore necessary. When a radical parotidectomy is performed, the facial nerve may be sacrificed and reconstructed with a graft from the contralateral greater auricular nerve.

Muscle relaxants should be avoided if nerve monitoring is used. In addition, nasal intubation may be necessary if the mandible has to be dislocated.

NASAL SURGERY

A significant percentage of nasal surgery is performed to improve cosmesis, although a large percentage is performed for functional restoration of the airway. Functional restoration is usually performed for either congenital or post-traumatic deviations of the septum. Nasal surgery is office based and performed with local anesthesia and intravenous sedation. It is important to note that patients with nasal polyps and asthma often have a hypersensitivity to aspirin, which can precipitate bronchospasm.

Intraoperative & Postoperative Considerations

The most important consideration of nasal surgery is achieving profound vasoconstriction in the nares to minimize and control bleeding. This vasoconstriction can be achieved with cocaine packs, local anesthetics, and epinephrine infiltration. Since these drugs have a profound effect on the cardiovascular system, a careful evaluation of the patient's cardiovascular functioning is essential, especially for older patients or patients with known cardiac disease. A vasoconstrictor can also precipitate dysrhythmias.

A moderate degree of controlled hypotension combined with head elevation decreases bleeding in the surgical site. Blood may passively enter the stomach. Placing an oropharyngeal pack or suctioning the stomach at the conclusion of surgery may attenuate postoperative retching and vomiting.

EAR SURGERY

The ear and its associated structures are target organs for many pathologic conditions. One of the most common ear surgeries is the placement of myringotomy tubes; tympanoplasties and the placement of cochlear implants are also common procedures. The surgeries usually require general anesthesia and in some cases rely on neuromonitoring. When nerve monitoring is undertaken, muscle relaxants should not be used. Patients are often nauseous as a result of surgery; therefore, adequate pretreatment with antiemetics and the use of anesthetics such as propofol and sevoflurane can reduce the incidence of nausea and vomiting.

For myringotomies and tube insertions, anesthetic premedication is not recommended because most sedative drugs far outlast the duration of the surgical procedure. Anesthesia may effectively be accomplished with a potent inhalation drug, oxygen, and N_2O administered by mask. As with other ear surgeries, the patient should be pretreated for nausea and vomiting.

MIDDLE EAR & MASTOID SURGERY

Tympanoplasty and mastoidectomy are two of the most common procedures performed on the middle ear and accessory structures. To avoid intrusion into the surgical field, an oral or nasal RAE endotracheal tube may be considered. Although not totally contraindicated, N_2O should be discontinued at least 30 minutes before placement of a tympanic membrane graft to avoid pressure-related displacement. In addition, extubation should be smooth to avoid straining, which may unseat the tympanic membrane graft or disrupt other repairs.

Postoperative nausea and vomiting are the most common postoperative problems. They can be reduced by (1) decompressing the stomach after inducing general anesthesia, thereby emptying the stomach of gas and fluid; (2) limiting the use of opioids; and (3) using antiemetics.

NECK SURGERY

Neck dissection may be complete, modified, or functional. The sternocleidomastoid muscle is the primary muscle involved. The primary nerve is the accessory or spinal nerve (CN XI), and the primary vascular structures are the internal and external jugular veins and the carotid artery. Often a neck dissection is performed to remove a tumor and may also involve a partial or total glossectomy.

Preoperative Considerations

Patients who present with tumors in this area may have a history of tobacco use and pulmonary disease and may need a preoperative pulmonary workup. In a large percentage of cases, the dissection may be bilateral and a tracheostomy may be performed to maintain a patent airway.

Intraoperative Considerations

Patients who undergo neck surgery may be a challenge to intubate if they have either a history of radiation treatment to the larynx and pharynx or a significant mass in the oral cavity. If nerve monitoring is undertaken, muscle relaxants should be avoided. Dissection around the carotid bulb may precipitate bradycardia, which may be treated with either an injection of a local anesthetic into the bulb or intravenous atropine or glycopyrrolate. Laryngeal edema can be a significant problem if no drains are placed.

Postoperative Considerations

Nerves injured in neck surgery can include the facial nerve, resulting in a facial droop. Injury to the recurrent laryngeal nerve can cause vocal cord dysfunction; if this injury is bilateral, airway problems may result. Since the phrenic nerve also traverses through the operative field, paralysis of the hemidiaphragm can occur if this nerve is injured. If injury to the phrenic nerve is bilateral, breathing will be impaired.

With a low neck dissection, pneumothorax can occur. In addition, excessive coughing or agitation can result in hematoma formation and airway compromise.

Al-Shaikh B, Stacey S. *Essentials of Anaesthetic Equipment*, 2nd ed. Philadelphia: Churchill Livingstone, 2002.

Barasch PG, Cullen BF, Stoelting RK. *Clinical Anesthesia*, 5th ed. Philadelphia: Lippincott, Williams & Wilkins, 2005.

Jaffe RA, Samuels, SI. *Anesthesiologist's Manual of Surgical Procedures*, 3rd ed. Philadelphia: Lippincott Williams & Wilkins, 2003.

Miller RD. *Miller's Anesthesia*, 6th ed. Philadelphia: Churchill Livingstone, 2005.

Morgan CE Jr, Mikhail MS, Murray MJ, Larson CP Jr. *Clinical Anesthesiology*, 4th ed. New York: McGraw-Hill Medical, 2005.

Lasers in Head & Neck Surgery

Bulent Satar, MD, & Anil R. Shah, MD

5

DEFINITIONS

The word "laser" is an acronym for **L**ight **A**mplification by **S**timulated **E**mission of **R**adiation. A laser is a device that produces an intense beam by amplifying light.

Radiation

The radiation produced for surgical lasers is in the electromagnetic spectrum with a wavelength that ranges from 200 to 400 nm (near-UV radiation), 400 to 700 nm (visible radiation), 700 to 1000 nm (near-infrared radiation), and more than 1000 nm (infrared radiation). The most prominent physical feature of the radiation is its wavelength, which determines its visibility. The three most commonly used types of surgical lasers are (1) the Argon laser, which is within the visible portion of the electromagnetic spectrum; (2) the neodymium:yttrium-aluminum-garnet (Nd:YAG) laser; and (3) the carbon dioxide (CO_2) laser.

Amplification

Stimulated emission is the main source of laser energy. However, the energy of stimulated emission needs to be amplified to produce an intense beam. When the laser pump activates the active medium, the active medium starts having more atoms in an excited state. As atoms in the excited state release photons, this induces the emission of the photons from other atoms through a chain reaction.

Light

One of the distinctive features of the light is its highly concentrated energy per unit area. Beams forming the light synchronously occur parallel with each other, which makes it possible for the laser to travel for certain distance without divergence. It is monochromatic. The wavelength of the light is one of the factors determining the physical characteristics of the laser and its interaction with tissue.

Stimulated Emission

The current model of stimulated emission is described by quantum physics, which defines different energy levels of electrons while revolving around the nucleus in different levels of orbit. In this model, a stable electron in a normal state makes a transition to a higher but unstable level by absorbing a photon (absorption). This unstable electron with high energy ultimately may return to the original stable level spontaneously (spontaneous emission). Alternately, this emission can be induced by a forced interaction between one photon and the unstable electron to release a new photon (stimulated emission), which is the basis of laser energy.

LASER COMPONENTS

A laser primarily consists of three main components: (1) an active medium; (2) a stimulation (excitation) mechanism, which is the power source or a laser pump; and (3) an optical chamber (feedback mechanism) (Figure 5–1). The active medium is the component where the laser radiation is generated. The function of the active medium is to supply a source of stimulated atoms, molecules, and ions. It may be in a solid, gaseous, or liquid state. Different types of lasers are named based on what is used as an active medium. Lasers with a solid state of active medium are the Nd:YAG, ruby, and diode lasers. Lasers using a gaseous active medium are the CO_2, argon, and helium-neon lasers. The helium-neon laser is used as an aiming beam in lasers with an invisible beam (as in the CO_2 laser) in order to create a visible beam. A laser with a liquid active medium uses organic dye.

The activation status of the laser medium is operated by the operation mode of the laser device. Three operational modes are available currently. In the **continuous mode,** the active medium is kept in a stimulated mode, which provides constant and stable energy. In the **pulsed mode,** the active medium is intermittently activated for a very short time, which allows tissue to cool off between pulses, thereby decreasing thermal damage. However, a much higher maximum of instantaneous energy is delivered with pulses compared with that of the continuous mode in which average power output is greater. In **Q-switched mode,** very short pulses of the laser are produced in a controlled manner. The second component of the laser is the power source that is used to activate the medium. The optical chamber is used to

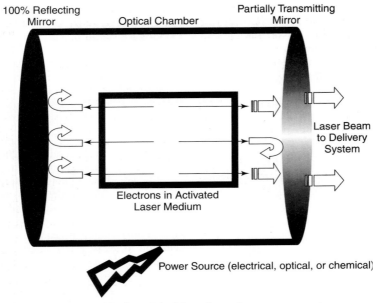

Figure 5–1. A simplified model of the primary laser components.

direct the output and also to provide feedback from amplification and collimation. The optical chamber contains the active medium.

Besides these major components of the laser, it must contain a cooling system, a delivery system, a control unit, and a remote control. Delivery systems are important in the selection of a laser. They can be an articulated arm (for the CO_2 laser), optical fibers (for near-infrared and visible lasers) or a connection between the laser and the operation microscope (for the CO_2 laser).

COMMONLY USED LASERS

CO_2 Laser

The wavelength of the CO_2 laser is 10,600 nm, which is not visible. Its power is between 0.1 and 100.0 W. A cooling system is required to couple to the main system because of the high heat energy produced by the laser. Also, the helium-neon laser beam is used as an aiming beam to make it visible. Its delivery system may be a handpiece at the end of an articulated arm consisting of reflective mirrors, a wave guide, or a micromanipulator to be coupled to an operating microscope. Practically, its energy is absorbed by the tissue within a 0.2-mm depth. Any tissue with a high water content selectively absorbs the CO_2 laser. For an incision, a small spot size with a high power density is preferred. New CO_2 laser systems have a spot size as small as 160 μm. For vaporization purpose, a low-power density is applied with a large spot size. This also creates a heat energy that coagulates blood and lymph vessels. However, its hemostasis capability is limited to vessels < 0.5 mm. In skin resurfacing, the CO_2 laser ablates 20–60 μm of tissue and up to 150 μm of residual thermal damage per pass. Generally speaking, the CO_2 laser is used for excision of laryngeal lesions and deep skin resurfacing for rhytids and acne scarring.

Argon Laser

The Argon laser is typically used for the coagulation of hemangiomas. Its beam emits a green-blue light, visible in the range of the electromagnetic spectrum (458–515 nm) and has a penetration depth of 1 mm. Because of its wavelength, it is almost completely absorbed by hemoglobin, melanin, and myoglobin.

Nd:YAG Laser

The Nd:YAG laser is a solid-state laser that delivers a 1060-nm beam (near infrared), thereby requiring an aiming beam. The penetration depth is 3–5 mm because of its low absorption by water and tissue pigments. This low absorption also causes scattering and reflection. Therefore, its use for coagulation purposes requires high power, making the thermal coagulation of vessels and hemangiomas possible. Its delivery system is a fiberoptic carrier, which provides a hemostatic effect at contact. However, it can be used for ablation in a noncontact mode. The Nd:YAG laser is used for tracheobronchial lesions, particularly for its excellent hemostatic qualities; nonablative skin resurfacing; and hair removal in ethnic patient populations.

KTP-532 Laser

The KTP-532 (potassium titanyl phosphate) laser works by passing an Nd:YAG laser through a KTP crystal, resulting in the emission of half its wavelength (532 nm), which becomes visible. The delivery system is a fiberoptic carrier (for vaporizing and coagulation effects) or a contact quartz tip (for cutting). Since this laser is primarily absorbed by oxyhemoglobin, it is mainly used in the treatment of vascular lesions (including superficial skin lesions and telangiectasias) and the surgical reduction of turbinate tissue.

Erbium:YAG Laser

The Erbium:YAG laser emits a 29–40 W, which is highly absorbed by water (12–18 times more efficiently than CO_2 laser). It has the advantage of precise tissue ablation, 5–20 μm per pass, a small zone of residual thermal damage compared with the CO_2 laser. The Erbium:YAG laser has the disadvantage of poor hemostatic qualities and limited collagen tightening compared with the CO_2 laser. It is primarily used for superficial skin resurfacing for fine wrinkles, brown spots, and acne scars.

LASER-TISSUE INTERACTION

The effects of laser on tissue rely on one of the following interactions: absorption, scattering, transmission, or reflection (Figure 5–2). The type of interaction between a laser beam and any tissue is determined by the wavelength of the laser beam, the operation mode of the laser, the amount of energy applied, and tissue characteristics. The interaction of the laser on tissue can be summarized with the general statement that "the shorter the wavelength, the greater the effect on the tissue." Table 5–1 shows lasers with their elec spectrum and penetration depth. Lasers whose lengths are within 0.1–0.8 μm (UV and visible region of the spectrum) cause minimal water absorption but considerable hemoglobin-melanin absorption. Lasers with a wavelength > 3 μm absorb water.

The visible lasers penetrate into tissue at approximately 1 mm. However, the Nd:YAG laser goes into tissue at 4 mm and absorbs minimal water. In contrast, the penetration depth of the CO_2 laser is only 30 μm, which makes it superb as a cutting tool.

Changes in tissue exposed to a laser relate to the temperature created by the laser. In temperatures higher than 50° C, enzymatic activity decreases. Protein denaturation occurs at temperatures over 60° C, the point at which physical changes are seen. However, tissue can still recover with the healing process. Over 80° C, the collagen degrades; 100° C is the temperature at which the water vaporizes, which results in expansion of the steam and finally tissue ablation. Although providing perfect hemostasis, a laser incision causes a delay in wound healing. Collateral thermal damage, though inevitable, can be minimized by using infrared lasers. Lasers can be used for incision, vaporization, or coagulation. Laser beams can be focused to spot sizes < 1 mm in diameter or defocused. A focused beam is used for cutting and a defocused beam for ablation and coagulation.

LASER SAFETY RULES

Currently, there are two main federal regulations regarding the safe use of the laser in the United States. These are the American National Standard for Safe Use of Lasers (ANSI Z 136.1), which regulates the laser industry, and Safe Use of Lasers in Health Care Facilities (ANSI Z 136.3), which regulates the installation, operation, and maintenance of lasers in health care units. There is one other standard, Safe Use of Lasers in Educational Institutions, which regulates safe use during educational activities (ANSI Z 136.5).

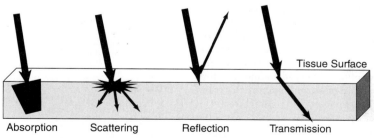

Figure 5–2. Types of laser-tissue interaction.

...urrently used lasers with their electromagnetic spectrum and ...n depth.

180 / ...CK SURGE...

Electromagnetic Spectrum	Laser Type	Wavelength	Penetration Depth
Visible lasers	Argon	514 nm	0.8 mm
	KTP-532	532 nm	0.9 mm
	Flashlamp-Excited Dye	577 nm	0.9 mm
Near infrared lasers	Nd: YAG	1060 nm	4.0 mm
Infrared lasers	Ho: YAG	2100 nm	0.4 mm
	Er: YAG	2940 nm	3.0 μm
	CO_2	10,600 nm	30.0 μm

Lasers can harm not only the patient but also the surgeon and other personnel in the operating room. Laser system hazards can be related either directly to the effect of the beam on tissue, such as the retina, the corneas, or skin, or secondary conditions such as fire, electrocution, toxic waste, and plume radiation.

Beam Hazards

A primary concern of unsafe laser use is eye injury. It can occur as a result of direct exposure to either a laser beam or a reflected beam. The best protection is for all personnel to wear approved laser safety glasses. If possible, the patient also needs to wear the same eyewear. If it interferes with the operation field or the procedure, moistened sterile cotton eye pads with moistened towels or metallic eye protectors are needed to cover the eyelids. All operating room windows must be covered with an opaque material at the wavelength of the laser used. An ANSI-approved warning sign at the entrance to all operating rooms should be placed with protective eyewear for those who enter the operating room.

Plume Hazards

Plume hazards relate to plume radiation and plume content. Plume radiation occurs when the laser beam contacts the smoke plume, which is a by-product of laser beam use. The smoke plume results from heat effect of the laser beam. Some of the energy may shift in wavelength, resulting in secondary emission and often in the visible portion of the spectrum. This secondary emission can cause temporary blindness. Continuous or frequent smoke evacuation is the only solution. Plume content biohazard relates to the direct toxic effect of the plume. In addition to laser smoke elimination, a surgical mask can minimize this risk.

Fire Hazards

Laser systems may cause airway burns from an endotracheal tube fire when the laser beam strikes an endotracheal tube, which is made of PVC. Therefore, tubes wrapped with reflective tape or made of reflective metals are preferred. Likewise, surgical drapes made of flame-retardant material are advised. The immediate surgical field should be covered with saline-soaked towels.

Precautions in Anesthetic Procedures

These precautions for anesthetic procedures are important when the operation is performed on the larynx or trachea. A closed ventilatory system that is provided with a small-cuff endotracheal tube is preferred unless the tube obstructs the surgical view. This type of system reduces the possibility of an anesthetic gas leak into the operative field, where the laser beam is present. The cuff may be filled with methylene blue. Ventilation with a high concentration of O_2 and nitrous oxide should be avoided. Jet ventilation is often necessary for glottic and subglottic lesions.

American National Standards Institute. For the safe use of lasers. ANSI Z 136.1;2000. (Provides guidance for the safe use of lasers and laser systems.)

American National Standards Institute. For the safe use of lasers in health care facilities. ANSI Z 136.3;1996. (Provides guidance for the safe use of lasers and laser systems in health care facilities.)

American National Standards Institute. For the safe use of lasers in educational institutions. ANSI Z 136.5;2000. (Describes control measures for institutions ranging from elementary schools through colleges and universities.)

Reinisch L. Laser physics and tissue interactions. *Otolaryngol Clin North Am.* 1996;29:893. [PMID: 8890123] (Describes the laser, laser beam, and delivery systems, as well as laser-tissue interactions after briefly reviewing the history of the laser.)

WEB SITES

Laser Institute of America
www.laserinstitute.org
(Aims at fostering lasers, laser applications, and laser safety worldwide, offering technical information.)

LASERS IN OTOLOGY-NEUROTOLOGY

Ear Canal

Ear canal lesions that are treatable with lasers include chronic infections, tumors, atresia, scar tissue, and webs. Chronic skin infections of the ear canal may require surgical intervention if medical treatment fails. If the full removal of canal skin is necessary, the argon or KTP-532 laser with low power is used to spot weld the edges or corners of the skin graft, which holds them in position. If whole-skin removal is not required, weeping areas of canal skin can be cauterized under local anesthesia with the argon or KTP-532 laser. Either laser is set at 1.5–2.0 W with a 1-mm spot size.

Polyps or other suspicious soft tissue in the ear canal can be biopsied with the same laser systems. Currently, there is no benefit to using lasers in canal skin carcinoma. Subcutaneous fibrous tissue in acquired ear canal atresia or stenosis can be dissected and vaporized with good hemostasis. This helps to keep the skin of the ear canal intact. In transcanal tympanoplasty, skin incision of the ear canal can be made with the laser without compromising visibility.

Tympanic Membrane

Fenestration of the tympanic membrane can be performed with a laser (laser-assisted myringotomy) under local anesthesia as an alternative to cold-knife myringotomy under general anesthesia. A CO_2 laser is set at 3–18 W with a single 100-ms pulse through a hand-held otoscope or 200-mm objective of the microscope. A spot size of 2.0–2.6 mm is preferred. Diode laser was reported to be effective in this application as well. Myringotomy opening made by either laser may be used for endoscopic examination of the middle ear. Patients with a single attack of otitis media with effusion may be candidates for laser-assisted myringotomy instead of ventilation tube placement. However, short duration (average 15 days) of myringotomy patency and recurrence should be kept in mind for chronic cases.

A minimally invasive treatment option was described for tympanic membrane atelectasis and called "laser contraction myringoplasty." In this technique, CO_2 laser set at 0.1–1 W with a spot size of 0.2 mm is applied to the perimeter of the atelectasis. It has been reported that the laser causes tightening of tympanic membrane tissues, which reduces or eliminates atelectasis.

Repairing a tympanic membrane perforation with a laser by spot welding is still far from a routine clinical practice. Nonetheless, in recurrent perforations with unresponsiveness to tympanoplasty, welding the temporalis fascia into the anterior canal skin may be effective.

Middle Ear

The KTP-532, argon, and CO_2 lasers are useful in middle ear surgery. The CO_2 laser has a small spot size (0.1–0.2 mm), which provides precision and safe handling.

Controversy exists as to which laser system is optimal; each has advantages and disadvantages. Visible lasers ensure the accurate aiming of the laser light. A handpiece eases the manipulation. The light of these lasers can pass through the overlying fluid environment. The spot size and power can vary by changing the distance between the tissue and the probe. The disadvantages of these lasers include the fact that their absorbency depends on pigment, which necessitates cautious work on white bones and tendons because of the possible inner ear damage. Therefore, in revision stapedotomy, visible lasers should not be used. In contrast, there is no inner ear damage risk in using the CO_2 laser given its depth of penetration. However, with the CO_2 laser, the aiming and treatment beams need to be accurately aligned. The lack of penetration through liquid may cause the beam to be weakened if fluid is overlying the target tissue. Visible lasers have better optical precision but less ideal tissue characteristics, and the CO_2 laser has better tissue characteristics but less ideal optical precision.

Recently, the Er:YAG laser was found safe in middle ear procedures given its high absorption rate by water, weak penetration through the otic bone, and weak transmission through the perilymph. Laser applications in middle ear surgery are not without complications. Facial nerve injury, severe vertigo, chorda tympani burn, and hearing loss can occur.

Small glomus tympanicum tumors can be vaporized with good hemostasis. Visible lasers are advantageous in this application. Although not commonly used, granulation tissue in the mastoid cavity can be removed with the argon laser at 4–6 W on continuous mode.

Laser stapedotomy was first introduced in 1979. Since then, it has gained growing acceptance. Although there are studies showing no difference in the hearing gain between classic and laser stapedotomy, laser stapedotomy appears to be advantageous over classic stapedotomy. Laser stapedectomy eliminates mechanical trauma to the inner ear as well as minimizing the prerequisite fine-hand skills. It provides precision in surgery. Postoperative vertigo is also diminished. Its benefits become more obvious in revision surgery and obliterative otosclerosis. Laser stapedotomy can be performed under local or general anesthesia. The laser is first used on the stapes tendon, and then the posterior crus of the stapes is vaporized. The latter should be done as close to the footplate as possible. Either a rosette pattern of spots with a series of laser shots or

0.6-mm fenestra with a single shot is used in the center of the footplate. After every shot, the char is wiped away. If a series of shots is to be used, the firings of the laser beam should be a few seconds apart. Recommended laser settings are as follows: (1) the spot size is 0.15 mm for the CO_2 laser and 0.20 mm for the KTP-532 and argon lasers; (2) the power is 1.5 W for the CO_2 laser and 1.6 W for the KTP-532 and argon lasers; and (3) the pulse duration is 0.1 s for each. With laser stapedotomy, closure of the air-bone gap within 10 dB is obtained in 90–95% of cases. No superiority of any laser system over another is mentioned.

For cases with otosclerosis confined to the fissula ante fenestram only, a novel technique has been described, laser stapedotomy minus prosthesis (STAMP). The technique simply includes vaporization of anterior crus first and later anterior one third of the footplate with a handheld probe of argon laser. Use of a prosthesis is not needed. If the otosclerosis is limited to the fissula ante fenestram only, this should free the remainder of the stapes. If so, the stapedotomy opening is sealed with adipose tissue. The technique may be converted to classic laser stapedotomy in appropriate cases. With this novel technique, it has been stated that high-frequency hearing (6–8 kHz) was better preserved compared with standard laser stapedotomy and also lasted as long as standard laser stapedotomy. Low incidence of refixation was also noteworthy.

In chronic ear surgery, a fixed malleus can be freed from the attic with a laser. Scar tissue, cholesteatomas, and adhesions close to the facial nerve or the stapes can be vaporized and removed. This is one of the most useful applications of the laser in otology. Diseased mucosa or granulation tissue in the mastoid bone can be removed by vaporizing with a defocused laser. A recent study showed that ancillary use of KTP laser significantly improved the rate of cholesteatoma eradication as evidenced in staged intact canal wall surgery.

Chronic intractable eustachian tube dysfunction is the new area of interest in laser use. For this condition, endoscopic transnasal laser-assisted surgery (laser eustachian tuboplasty) has been recently described with promising results. In this technique, mucosa and underlying soft tissue of the posterior wall (medial cartilaginous lamina) of the eustachian tube are vaporized through its free border using a 980-nm contact tip diode laser (7 W power, continuous-pulsed mode with 0.2 s on and 0.08 s off) or a wave guide of CO_2 laser (12 W power on superpulse mode and 0.05-s pulse).

An interesting area in which the laser is included is laser-Doppler vibrometry, which draws increasing attention in diagnostic otology. The system consists of a helium-neon laser, a joystick-controlled aiming prism both mounted on a microscope, ear speculum-sound coupler assembly with nonreflective glass covering at back, sound generator, and probe-tube microphone. Details of how the system works is beyond the scope of this chapter. The resultant parameter is the umbo velocity, which has been stated to be a useful tool in patients with intact drum to differentiate causes of conductive hearing loss.

Inner Ear

Until recently, experiences in the inner ear have been limited to the CO_2 and argon lasers, which have been used for the treatment of benign paroxysmal positional vertigo (BPPV). Despite promising results, further clinical experience is necessary to prove the superiority of laser use to the current treatment modalities. A recent animal study was aimed to investigate whether there was any difference in hearing thresholds following cochleostomy that was performed with CO_2 laser, Er:YAG laser, or a microdrill. Comparative results showed that the safest method was microdrill cochleostomy. Some degree of hearing loss, more than with microdrill and less than with Er:YAG laser, resulted from CO_2 laser application. Thus, Er:YAG laser was found to have a greater potential to cause damage.

Even classic posterior canal occlusion is reserved for patients unresponsive to repositioning or liberating maneuvers. The occlusion with a laser still does not seem an alternative to these treatment modalities in routine practice.

The argon laser is one of the laser systems used in patients with BPPV with the aim of partitioning the posterior semicircular canal. In the procedure, after a mastoidectomy and blue-lining the posterior semicircular canal, the argon laser at 4–12 W and with a 0.1–0.5 pulse duration is applied 1–3 times to create a hole on the canal. The handpiece is held 1 mm away from the canal. After the application, the hole created is covered with the temporalis fascia. It is believed that this application occludes the membranous semicircular canal, which may prevent the cupular movement that results from gravity. The CO_2 laser is also applied directly to the endolymphatic space after removing the bone of the posterior semicircular canal; the opening is then occluded with bone wax.

Partial labyrinthectomy and labyrinthine ablation, with the preservation of hearing, have been tried in a very small group of patients with promising results. The argon and CO_2 lasers were used to either weld the open ends of the semicircular canals or ablate the macula. However, this procedure is still not an alternative to labyrinthectomy.

Tinnitus is another issue of interest in terms of investigating efficacy of low-power laser treatment. Despite inconsistent results reported, a recent placebo-controlled double-blind study showed that 60-mW laser was not effective in alleviating tinnitus in patients with Ménière disease, presbycusis, and sudden hearing loss.

Neurotology

Laser systems are not commonly used for tumors in the posterior fossa. The main concern is possible thermal injury of the surrounding structures (the facial nerve and cerebellum) and the transfer of the heat via the cerebrospinal fluid (CSF). However, when taking the necessary measures to protect these structures (ie, covering them with saline-soaked cottonoid), the laser can be used safely for hemostasis on the tumor surface and debulking of the tumor. The KTP-532 (3–15 W) or CO_2 laser (5 W) with a 1-mm spot size on continuous mode can be an alternative to the ultrasonic surgical aspirator to debulk tumors. Even experienced surgeons prefer accurately applied bipolar coagulation for hemostasis near critical neural structures.

Argon and Nd:YAG lasers have some promise for the treatment of vascular tumors. In a vestibular nerve section, the KTP-532 laser at 3 W or CO_2 laser at 1 W is an option to using a scalpel.

Anthony PF. Laser applications in inner ear surgery. *Otolaryngol Clin North Am.* 1996;29:1031. [PMID: 8890133] (Reviews previous laser techniques in the inner ear and particularly addresses the use of CO_2 and argon lasers in paroxysmal vertigo and labyrinth surgery.)

Antonelli PJ, Gianoli GJ et al. Early post-laser stapedotomy hearing thresholds. *Am J Otol.* 1998;19:443. [PMID: 9661752] (Compares hearing results with CO_2 and KTP lasers in patients who have undergone laser stapedotomy.)

Brodsky L, Cook S, Deutsch E et al. Optimizing effectiveness of laser tympanic membrane fenestration in chronic otitis media with effusion: clinical and technical considerations. *Int J Pediatr Otorhinolaryngol.* 2001;58:59. [PMID: 11249981] (Addresses the issues of patient selection, disease factors, and technical factors of lasers.)

Buchman CA, Fucci MJ, Roberson JB Jr et al. Comparison of argon and CO_2 laser stapedotomy in primary otosclerosis surgery. *Am J Otolaryngol.* 2000;21:227. [PMID: 10937907] (Compares hearing results obtained with argon and CO_2 laser stapedotomy.)

Hamilton JW. Efficacy of the KTP laser in the treatment of middle ear cholesteatoma. *Otol Neurotol.* 2005;26:135. [PMID: 16232250] (Presents results of ancillary use of KTP laser in cholesteatoma surgery.)

Huber A, Linder T, Fisch U. Is the Er:YAG laser damaging to inner ear function? *Otol Neurotol.* 2001;22:311. [PMID: 11347632] (Investigates effect of Er:YAG laser on air and bone conduction thresholds.)

Kakehata S, Futai K, Sasaki A et al. Endoscopic transtympanic tympanoplasty in the treatment of conductive hearing loss: early results. *Otol Neurotol.* 2006;27:14. [PMID: 16371841] (Describes laser-assisted myringotomy and endoscopic transtympanic tympanoplasty through the myringotomy fenestration.)

Kiefer J, Tillein J, Ye Q. Application of carbon dioxide and erbium:yttrium-aluminum-garnet lasers in inner ear surgery:

an experimental study. *Otol Neurotol.* 2004;25:400. [PMID: 15129125] (Compares hearing thresholds in guinea pigs in which cochleostomy was performed either with CO_2 laser, Er:YAG laser, or microdrill.)

Kujawski OB, Poe DS. Laser eustachian tuboplasty. *Otol Neurotol.* 2004;25:1. [PMID: 14724483] (Describes a novel method to manage chronic eustachian tube dysfunction and presents its results in 56 patients with middle ear atelectasis and effusion.)

Nakashima T, Ueda H, Misawa H et al. Transmeatal low-power laser irradiation for tinnitus. *Otol Neurotol.* 2002;23:296. [PMID: 11981384] (Presents no beneficial effect obtained from low-power laser use in tinnitus.)

Nissen AJ, Sikand A, Welsh JE, Curto FS. Use of the KTP-532 laser in acoustic neuroma surgery. *Laryngoscope.* 1997;107:118. [PMID: 9001275] (This study reports favorable facial nerve outcome following acoustic neuroma surgery using the KTP-532 laser in a large-case population.)

Ostrowski VB, Bojrab DI. Minimally invasive laser contraction myringoplasty for tympanic membrane atelectasis. *Otolaryngol Head Neck Surg.* 2003;128:711. [PMID: 12748566] (Describes a novel technique of CO_2 laser to manage tympanic membrane atelectasis.)

Prokopakis EP, Lachanas VA, Christodoulou PN et al. Implications of laser assisted tympanostomy in adults. *Otol Neurotol.* 2005;26:361. [PMID: 15891634] (Presents outcome of patients with OME and AOM undergoing laser assisted tympanostomy with no ventilation tube placement.)

Rhoton AL Jr. Operative techniques and instrumentation for neurosurgery. *Neurosurg.* 2003;53:907. [PMID: 14519224] (Describes laser microsurgery in posterior fossa lesions as well as other special instrumentation.)

Rosowski J, Mehta RP, Merchant SN. Diagnostic utility of laser-Doppler vibrometry in conductive hearing loss with normal tympanic membrane. *Otol Neurotol.* 2003;24:165. [PMID: 12621328] (Evaluates efficacy of laser-Doppler vibrometry in differential diagnosis of conductive hearing loss.)

Saeed SR, Jackler RK. Lasers in surgery for chronic ear disease. *Otolaryngol Clin North Am.* 1996;29:245. [PMID: 8860923] (Summarizes laser types and reviews their usage in the middle ear for chronic otitis media.)

Sedwick JD, Loudon CL, Shelton C. Stapedectomy vs stapedotomy: do you really need a laser? *Arch Otolaryngol Head Neck Surg.* 1997;123:177. [PMID: 9046285] (Comparison of air-bone gap closure and the incidence of sensorineural hearing loss with regard to the use of the drill and KTP and argon lasers to make small fenestra.)

Silverstein H, Hoffmann KK, Thompson JH et al. Hearing outcome of laser stapedotomy minus prosthesis (STAMP) versus conventional laser stapedotomy. *Otol Neurotol.* 2004;25:106. [PMID: 15021768] (Compares hearing results in STAMP technique and laser stapedotomy, and concludes better high-frequency hearing preservation in STAMP technique.)

Vernick DM. Laser applications in ossicular surgery. *Otolaryngol Clin North Am.* 1996;29:931. [PMID: 8890125] (Reviews laser types and gives their optimal settings in middle ear surgery.)

Wiet RJ, Kubek DC, Lemberg P, Byskosh AT. A meta-analysis review of revision stapes surgery with argon laser: effectiveness and safety. *Am J Otol.* 1997;18:166. [PMID: 9093671] (Presents a meta-analysis of hearing results in revision stapes cases which have undergone either non-laser or argon laser surgeries.)

Zanetti D, Piccioni M, Nassif N et al. Diode laser myringotomy for chronic otitis media with effusion in adults. *Otol Neurotol.*

2005;26:12. [PMID: 15699714] (Analyzes the closure time of diode laser-assisted myringotomy and recurrence rate of OME.)

LASERS IN HEAD & NECK

Paranasal Sinuses & Nose

The introduction of the laser into nasal surgery has resulted from a need for good hemostasis in a narrow operative field. In using the Nd:YAG, KTP-532, and argon lasers, neighboring structures (eg, the medial rectus muscle, anterior cranial fossa, and optic nerve) are at great risk of thermal damage. Therefore, the versatility of the CO_2 and Ho:YAG lasers in this setting have received much recognition.

Reducing turbinate hypertrophy and resecting polyps, papillomas, and synechiae can be performed with the CO_2 laser. The physician should be careful not to expose the turbinate bone secondary to thermal damage, which causes scarring, prolonged pain, and persistent crusting. In turbinate resection, the anterior part of the turbinate should always be preserved. The CO_2 laser can be used in superpulse mode to provide gradual vaporization. Using an optical wave guide, the laser beam can be directed at the posterior aspect of the turbinate. During the procedure, the laser plume should be vigilantly evacuated. Although the CO_2 laser provides good hemostasis and less thermal collateral damage in resecting the previously mentioned lesions, the lack of flexibility in its delivery system constitutes a serious problem. The Ho:YAG laser has tissue interaction characteristics similar to the CO_2 laser. It is used on pulse mode. Since it can be transferred through a fiberoptic system, it is more advantageous than the CO_2 laser. Wedge resection of the inferior turbinate using consecutive interstitial and contact beams from an Nd:YAG laser is also efficient.

Holmium:YAG laser has been used to correct nasal septal cartilage without elevation of the mucoperichondrial flap. Under local anesthesia using a modified speculum, deviated septum was corrected, and then the laser via an optical fiber was applied through the mucosa. Hereditary hemorrhagic telangiectasia can be undergone with Nd:YAG laser therapy to reduce frequency of epistaxis. It should be noted that, overall, although laser systems offer some advantages, they have not replaced the classic surgical approaches.

Katz S, Schmelzer B, Vidts G. Treatment of the obstructive nose by CO_2 laser reduction of the inferior turbinates: technique and results. *Am J Rhinol*. 2000;14:51. [PMID: 10711333] (Presents techniques of the CO_2 laser for inferior turbinate reduction and comparative rhinomanometry results.)

Kuhnel TS, Wagner BH, Schurr CP, Strutz J. Clinical strategy in hereditary hemorrhagic telangiectasia. *Am J Rhinol*. 2005;19:508. [PMID: 16270607] (Investigates efficacy of Nd:YAG laser treatment in patients with hereditary hemorrhagic telangiectasia in terms of frequency of nasal bleeding.)

Ovchinnikov Y, Sobol E, Svistushkin V et al. Laser septochondrocorrection. *Arch Facial Plast Surg*. 2002;4:180. [PMID: 12167077] (Presents results of nasal septal cartilage reshaping using holmium:YAG laser in 110 patients.)

Rathfoot CJ, Duncavage J, Shapshay SM. Laser use in the paranasal sinuses. *Otolaryngol Clin North Am*. 1996;29:943. [PMID: 8890126] (Reviews laser use and its advantages and disadvantages in paranasal sinus surgery.)

Vagnetti A, Gobbi A, Algieri GM et al. Wedge turbinectomy: a new combined photocoagulative Nd:YAG laser technique. *Laryngoscope*. 2000;110:1034. [PMID: 10852526] (Describes a new method in inferior turbinate reduction using two consecutive applications of interstitial and contact Nd:YAG laser beams.)

Oral Cavity & Oropharynx

A. LASER-ASSISTED UVULOPALATOPLASTY

The treatment of snoring and sleep apnea is one of the fields in which the laser has gained great popularity. The CO_2 laser has been shown to be an effective treatment instrument for snoring and sleep apnea when the obstruction is at the level of soft palate. Although no difference is found in the postoperative snore index between laser-assisted uvulopalatoplasty (LAUP) and conventional uvulopalatopharyngoplasty, LAUP helps avoid most of the postoperative morbidity, as well as providing a good hemostatic benefit during surgery. However, it has been reported that long-term results of snoring and respiratory disturbance index were not as satisfactory as short-term results and tended to deteriorate over time, which was explained with velopharyngeal narrowing and palatal fibrosis caused by the laser.

LAUP can be performed under local-topical or general anesthesia, even in an office setting. The operation can also be staged. The CO_2 laser is the laser most commonly used by otolaryngologists for this operation. Since the diameter of the vessels encountered during the procedure is smaller than 0.5 mm, the CO_2 laser is effective for hemostasis. Basically, in a LAUP, redundant soft tissue is either excised or ablated. In a typical CO_2 laser application, the system is set to a power of 15–20 W. A backstop is used to protect the pharynx from scattering the beam. The system is used in the focused mode for excision and in the defocused mode for vaporization. Bilateral incisions at both sides of the base of the uvula are made with a handpiece. The uvula is shortened to 15 mm, excising redundant soft tissue and preserving its curved shape. The wound then heals within 3–4 weeks. Figure 5–3 shows a postoperative view of immediately after LAUP.

B. LASER TONSILLOTOMY

Laser tonsillotomy is reserved for patients who are unable to tolerate general anesthesia or unwilling to

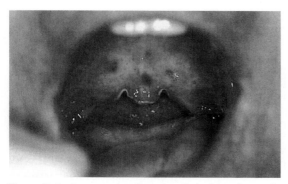

Figure 5–3. Laser-assisted uvulopalatoplasty, immediately after the application of a CO_2 laser. (Photo courtesy of Andrew N. Goldberg, MD, University of California, San Francisco, Department of Otolaryngology–Head & Neck Surgery.)

undergo classic tonsillectomy. The technique requires ablation of tonsillar crypts and gross reduction of tonsillar tissue, which can be staged many times until the level of palatoglossus muscle is achieved. The CO_2 laser is set at 15–20 W on continuous mode and applied preferably with a handpiece.

C. Laser Tonsillectomy

Laser tonsillectomy is not indicated unless a coagulation disorder is diagnosed because of the cost of the laser. The KTP-532 laser is considered the instrument of choice for tonsillectomy because it provides adequate cutting with good hemostasis and little thermal damage. Its optical fiber is held very close to the tonsillar tissue. The first incision is made in a curvilinear fashion along the anterior pillar from the superior pole to the inferior pole to define the dissection plane. Medially and inferiorly, the retracted tonsil is then dissected from the superior pole to the inferior pole.

D. Lingual Tonsillectomy

The excision of the lingual tonsil in the classic fashion is somewhat cumbersome owing to excessive bleeding, postoperative edema, and pain. The use of a laser offers resection with minimal edema, less bleeding, improved visibility during surgery, and less pain postoperatively. The need for a tracheostomy is therefore less likely. The CO_2, KTP-532, or Nd:YAG laser can be used along with a rigid laryngoscope. The operation can be staged.

E. Benign Lesions

CO_2 laser excision or ablation of gingival hyperplasias, pyogenic granulomas, and papillomas is possible with an excellent response rate, good hemostasis, and low morbidity. For especially vascular lesions, photocoagulation with an Nd:YAG laser is preferred. It is set at 32–

48 W with a pulse duration of 0.3 s. A 2-mm spot size is used with a 2-mm separation between spots.

Oral mucositis associated with chemotherapy or radiation therapy may be prevented with low-level laser use. A few mechanisms underlie the healing effect of the laser. The low-level laser has been demonstrated to increase energy production in the mitochondria. It also facilitates conversion of fibroblasts into myofibroblasts from which fibroblast growth factors are released, and these play a role in epithelial repair. The last effect is that of reducing the formation of free oxygen radicals that are stomatotoxic. The most studied form of low-level laser therapy has been helium-neon laser. The CO_2 laser is an alternative. Studies have used low-level laser either prophylactically (before radiation therapy or chemotherapy) or after the appearance of mucosal lesions during the course of radiation therapy or chemotherapy. A recent review showed that even though there is not sufficient evidence to recommend laser use, evidence of its potential usefulness is accumulating.

F. Premalignant Lesions

The CO_2 laser is often used for premalignant lesions, including leukoplakia and erythroplakia. Because these lesions are confined to the epithelium, only the superficial layer of the mucosa is removed by leaving 2–3 mm margins of normal mucosa. The wound is left to granulate and be covered by a new mucosal layer. These lesions can also be ablated. For ablation, a defocused laser at 10–20 W with a 100-ms pulse is used.

G. Malignant Lesions

The oncologic literature related to head and neck procedures is encouraging with regard to laser use. Compared with traditional methods, the advantages obtained with laser systems are improved visibility, hemostasis, decreased postoperative edema and pain, and better functional results, including speech and swallowing functions. It allows the surgeon to protect the muscular support of the tongue and the floor of mouth. However, no inherent oncologic benefits result from the laser use. Transoral CO_2 laser resection is recommended for superficial T1 and T2 tumors, considering the difficulty in defining the depth of excision with lasers. It is generally accepted that deeply infiltrative tumors, tumors > 4 cm, and tumors involving the maxilla or mandible are not suitable for laser resection. Transoral CO_2 laser excision of oral cavity carcinomas can be performed with the handpiece or a micromanipulator mounted to the operating microscope. Microscopically abnormal tissues can be detected by using 1% toluidine blue. Normal tissue margins generally measure 1–2 cm beyond the microscopically abnormal tissue.

Resection starts by outlining the margins with the CO_2 laser at 6 W and a 100-ms pulse duration. The incision is then made at 10 W on continuous mode.

The defect is left for secondary healing or is sutured. The local control rates of T1 and T2 disease addressed with transoral CO_2 laser resection is 80–100% at a 2- to 5-year follow-up. The disease-free survival rate is 83–88% at a 5-year follow-up.

Burkey BB, Garrett G. Use of the laser in the oral cavity. *Otolaryngol Clin North Am.* 1996;29:949. [PMID: 8890127] (Addresses the indications, techniques, results, and complications of laser use in the oral cavity.)

Finkelstein Y, Stein G, Ophir D et al. Laser-assisted uvulopalatoplasty for the management of obstructive sleep apnea: myths and facts. *Arch Otolaryngol Head Neck Surg.* 2002;128:429. [PMID: 11926920] (Presents medium- and long-term subjective and objective results of LAUP.)

Genot MT, Klastersky J. Low-level laser for prevention and therapy of oral mucositis induced by chemotherapy or radiotherapy. *Curr Opin Oncol.* 2005;17:236. [PMID: 15818167] (Presents literature review on low-level laser use for prevention of oral mucositis.)

Kaluskar SK, Kaul GH. Long-term results of KTP/532 laser uvulopalatopharyngoplasty. *Rev Laryngol Otol Rhinol.* 2000;121:59. [PMID: 10865488] (Presents satisfactory results of KTP-laser uvulopalatopharyngoplasty in 84% of the patients who were evaluated in the 4th year after surgery.)

Linder A, Markstrom A, Hultcrantz E. Using the carbon dioxide laser for tonsillotomy in children. *Int J Pediatr Otorhinolaryngol.* 1999;50:31. [PMID: 10596884] (Demonstrates the method using the CO_2 laser in tonsillotomy and its results.)

Osman EZ, Osborne JE, Hill PD et al. Uvulopalatopharyngoplasty versus laser assisted uvulopalatoplasty for the treatment of snoring: an objective randomised clinical trial. *Clin Otolaryngol.* 2000;25:305. [PMID: 10971538] (Investigates if there was any difference in the snore index following LAUP and UPPP.)

Rathfoot CJ, Coleman JA. Laser utilization in the oral pharynx. *Otolaryngol Clin North Am.* 1996;29:963. [PMID: 8890128] (Laser use in the oropharynx is reviewed in a detailed manner from tonsillectomy to malignant disorders.)

Saito T, Honda N, Saito H. Advantage and disadvantage of KTP-532 laser tonsillectomy compared with conventional method. *Auris Nasus Larynx.* 1999;26:447. [PMID: 10530741] (Compares pain, intraoperative blood loss, and healing time following conventional and KTP laser tonsillectomy.)

White JM, Chaudhry SI, Kudler JJ et al. Nd:YAG and CO_2 laser therapy of oral mucosal lesions. *J Clin Laser Med Surg.* 1998;16:299. [PMID: 10204434] (Describes the use of the contact Nd:YAG and CO_2 lasers in a variety of benign oral lesions.)

Larynx

Laser surgery in the respiratory tract requires additional equipment and safety precautions. Microlaryngeal instruments have a black finish to prevent the reflection or misdirection of the laser beam. A microlaryngoscope with smoke evacuation channels is used. Platforms that act as a backstop have been developed to absorb the laser energy and to prevent the spread of the laser beam down into the trachea. In addition, vocal cord protectors are used to protect the other vocal fold.

The delivery systems of various lasers are important considerations in choosing the type of laser for laryngeal surgery. The CO_2 laser can be used through a rigid laryngoscope. The spot size of the CO_2 laser has been reduced to 160 μm in new systems when it is used at a distance of 400 mm. This offers better precision and prevents collateral damage. The argon, KTP-532, and Nd:YAG lasers can be transmitted through the laryngoscope to the tissue via a fiberoptic cable. They are not preferred for nonvascular glottic lesions because of excessive energy absorption by the surrounding tissue; however, good results are reported in glottic lesions with the contact Nd:YAG laser.

A. Bilateral Vocal Cord Paralysis

The current therapy for bilateral vocal cord paralysis focuses on static airway enlargement procedures at the posterior glottis; these procedures include posterior cordotomy, medial arytenoidectomy, and total arytenoidectomy. The laser provides better hemostasis compared to classic methods.

In a posterior cordotomy, laser can be used to incise the vocal cord anterior to the vocal process. The anterior vocal process is then excised or vaporized unilaterally or bilaterally. In a medial arytenoidectomy, the vocal process and medial portion of the arytenoid body are vaporized, preserving the lateral arytenoid body and the aryepiglottic fold. A total arytenoidectomy can also be performed with the CO_2, KTP-532, and Nd:YAG lasers.

B. Benign Lesions

The use of laser for the excision of nodules, polyps, and cysts is not advantageous over microsurgical techniques in terms of preserving uninvolved mucosal layer and lamina propria. However, the surgical precision of the laser has been increased in new systems by adding a microspot manipulator. For these lesions, the laser is set at as low as 4 W of power in the focused mode. As small a spot size as possible should be used. The cautious excision of the lesion with the involved mucosa is necessary. For submucosal lesions, especially cysts and large sessile polyps, a mucosal incision can be made with the laser. The mucosa is then elevated and the lesion is removed in a standard fashion. However, the additional cost of the laser should be taken into account in these cases.

For vascular lesions, the laser is far superior to microsurgical interventions in terms of surgical precision and hemostasis. The CO_2 laser is preferred for small vascular lesions such as symptomatic dilated blood vessels and angiomatous clusters of capillaries. During laser surgery for these lesions, and after achieving endoscopic exposure, the defocused laser with a spot size of 300–400 μm and at 1–2 W is used with a single pulse of 0.1 s to coagulate the blood supply. This reduces the size of the capillary lesion. The main capillary lesion is then excised with a focused laser at the same level of power. Large vascular lesions are treated with the Nd:YAG laser for palliation. Under endoscopic exposure, a fiberoptic laser cable is introduced and secured. The lesion is then coagulated with the laser in a noncontact mode (a few millimeters away from the lesion) at 20 W and a 0.5-s pulse. The application can be staged in order to observe the response of the lesion and surrounding tissue.

Granulation tissue around the arytenoid cartilage, which arises from mucosal defects caused by gastric reflux or sustained mechanical trauma, can be excised with the CO_2 laser when surgery is warranted. The CO_2 laser can also be used to treat superior tracheal granulation tissue.

Recurrent respiratory papillomatosis can be ablated with the CO_2 laser, even though it does not provide a better recurrence rate than microlaryngeal surgery. Because the eradication of the virus is not possible, the area of active expression should be addressed. If possible, a 1-mm normal mucosal margin can be included. This intervention should be performed as infrequently as possible to avoid scarring. The laser permits a precise and bloodless excision with less scarring compared with other surgical options. The CO_2 laser can be used for either the excision of bulky disease or superficial vaporization. For excision, a focused laser is set at 4 W with 0.1-s pulse and a 0.5-s pulse interval. The same setting can be used in a defocused mode for superficial vaporization. Recurrences are addressed in the same manner. A comparative study showed that excision by microdebrider was less time-consuming compared with CO_2 laser.

Laryngeal stenosis can be addressed with a laser for cutting or coagulating purpose. However, its only advantage over standard treatment methods (ie, scalpel incision and electrocoagulation) is good hemostasis. To prevent reformation, an anterior membranous or thick glottic web can be incised with a CO_2 laser before interposing the tissue flap, keel, or stent placement. In a posterior glottic web, a CO_2 laser is used to incise the arytenoid mucosa (the micro-trapdoor flap) and vaporize the submucosal scar tissue between the arytenoids. Subglottic stenosis < 1 cm in vertical length can also be addressed with a laser to make radial incisions before bronchoscopic dilatation.

C. MALIGNANT LESIONS

The CO_2 laser offers surgical precision, minimal bleeding, less surgical trauma, and rapid healing in the endoscopic management of carcinoma in situ and early glottic carcinoma. For carcinoma in situ, the local control rate and quality of life obtained in using the CO_2 laser are close to what is achieved with radiation therapy and better than with vocal cord stripping. Also, better ultimate laryngeal preservation is obtained with the CO_2 laser compared with radiation therapy. This holds true when laser CO_2 cordectomy is compared with open surgery. In a typical application, mucosal disease is excised with the CO_2 laser in the superpulse mode at a spot size of 0.5–0.8 mm. The output power is set to 2–3 W. If invasion is found in a histopathologic examination, the underlying vocal ligament should also be excised (subligamentous cordectomy), leaving a 1- to 2-mm normal tissue margin. Studies regarding the efficacy of endoscopic laser use for more aggressive disease and tumors invading the anterior commissure are not conclusive.

The transoral excision of the supraglottic carcinoma and selected piriform sinus carcinomas can be facilitated with a laser in the context of organ preservation. The neck is addressed in a staged manner. These techniques offer less postoperative morbidity, including the avoidance of tracheotomy and improved swallowing function.

Brown DH. The versatile contact Nd:YAG laser in head and neck surgery: an in vivo and clinical analysis. *Laryngoscope*. 2000;110:854. [PMID: 10807364] (Demonstrates comparable tissue and healing effects of the CO_2 and Nd:YAG lasers in rats and presents favorable results obtained with the use of Nd:YAG laser for laryngotracheal lesions and oral-oropharyngeal carcinoma.)

Courey MS, Ossoff RH. Laser applications in adult laryngeal surgery. *Otolaryngol Clin North Am*. 1996;29:973. [PMID: 8890129] (Reviews safety measures and laser choice, and its use in vocal cord paralysis and benign and malignant lesions.)

Damm M, Sittel C, Streppel M et al. Transoral CO_2 laser for surgical management of glottic carcinoma in situ. *Laryngoscope*. 2000;10:1215. [PMID: 10892699] (Investigates the effectiveness of the CO_2 laser in glottic carcinoma in situ.)

Dedo HH, Yu KC. CO_2 laser treatment in 244 patients with respiratory papillomas. *Laryngoscope*. 2001;111:1639. [PMID: 11568620] (Presents results of frequent excision of respiratory papillomas using the CO_2 laser.)

Eckel HE, Thumfart W, Jungehulsing M et al. Transoral laser surgery for early glottic carcinoma. *Eur Arch Otorhinolaryngol*. 2000;257:221. [PMID: 10867839] (Includes analyses of rates of local control, regional control, organ preservation, and survival in patients with carcinoma in situ and T1 and T2 laryngeal lesions.)

El-Bitar MA, Zalzal GH. Powered instrumentation in the treatment of recurrent respiratory papillomatosis: an alternative to the carbon dioxide laser. *Arch Otolaryngol Head Neck Surg*. 2002;128:425. [PMID: 11926919] (Compares the advantages of microdebrider with CO_2 laser in juvenile laryngeal papillomatosis.)

Gluth MB, Shinners PA, Kasperbauer JL. Subglottic stenosis associated with Wegener's granulomatosis. *Laryngoscope*. 2003;113:1304. [PMID: 12897550] (Evaluates the outcomes of subglottic stenosis in 27 patients with Wegener's granulomatosis with emphasis on CO_2 laser and other treatment modalities.)

Maurizi M, Almadori G, Plaudetti G et al. Laser carbon dioxide cordectomy versus open surgery in the treatment of glottic carcinoma: our results. *Otolaryngol Head Neck Surg*. 2005;132:857. [PMID: 15944555] (Analyzes oncologic results in patients with glottic cancers treated by either laser CO_2 or open surgery.)

Rudert HH, Hoft S. Transoral carbon dioxide laser resection of supraglottic carcinoma. *Ann Otol Rhinol Laryngol.* 1999;108:819. [PMID: 10527270] (Describes the use of the CO_2 laser in supraglottic malignant disorders with the intents of cure and palliation, and gives outcome results comparable to the conventional surgery.)

Steiner W, Ambrosch P, Hess CF et al. Organ preservation by transoral laser microsurgery in piriform sinus carcinoma. *Otolaryngol Head Neck Surg.* 2001;124:58. [PMID: 11228455] (Presents the operative technique of transoral excision of piriform sinus carcinoma and its oncologic results with approaches to the neck.)

Tracheobronchial System

Laser use in the tracheobronchial system is limited to CO_2 and Nd:YAG lasers. In fact, use of the CO_2 laser in bronchoscopy remains restricted by the articulated arm. Another limitation of the CO_2 laser is its hemostatic capability. In contrast, an advantage of the Nd:YAG laser is the ability to use it with both rigid and flexible bronchoscopes. In addition, better hemostasis, even for deeper lesions, is obtained with the Nd:YAG laser.

Characteristics of the CO_2 laser confine its use to superficial lesions, including recurrent respiratory papillomatosis involving the tracheotomy site and the trachea, subglottic and tracheal stenosis, and capillary hemangiomas. The use of the CO_2 laser in these lesions is similar to what is described previously for laryngeal applications. For bulky lesions, the Nd:YAG laser is preferred for its vaporization and coagulation effects. In a typical application, the Nd:YAG laser is set at < 30 W and exposure should be kept to < 90 s. Laser use higher than these levels may cause necrosis and perforation in the tracheobronchial wall.

Debulking malignant disorders that obstruct the tracheobronchial system can be performed with the CO_2 or Nd:YAG laser for palliation purpose. Photodynamic therapy is useful only for patients with small lesions of squamous cell carcinoma and carcinoma in situ that can be reached with a flexible fiberoptic bronchoscope.

Esophagus

CO_2 laser has been introduced to endoscopic management of Zenker's diverticulum. The approach has been called "CO_2 laser-assisted diverticulotomy," and it is preferred in rather primary cases. With this approach, a specially designed endoscope with double lips is introduced into the esophageal lumen. At the level of diverticulum, while the anterior lip of the endoscope is directed toward the esophageal lumen, the posterior lip remains at the bottom of the diverticulum, thereby leaving the common wall and cricopharyngeus muscle between the two lips of the endoscope. Then, through an operation microscope with 400-mm lens and CO_2 laser micromanipulator, the common wall is transected with a CO_2 laser set at 5–10 W on continuous mode. The transection is recommended to continue down to the distal-most part of the common wall. This procedure also transects the hypertonic cricopharyngeus muscle, which is thought to contribute to the pathogenesis of the diverticulum. Thus, both transecting the common wall and relieving the muscle prevent food entrapment. During the procedure, one should be cautious not to violate fascia that envelops the diverticulum. Compared with open technique, this technique reduces operative time. However, one should be aware of the greater possibility of repeated surgery in this approach.

Chang CW, Burkey BB, Netterville JL et al. Carbon dioxide laser endoscopic diverticulotomy versus open diverticulectomy for Zenker's diverticulum. *Laryngoscope.* 2004;114;519. [PMID: 15091228] (Describes CO_2 laser use in the management of Zenker's diverticulum and compares the results with those of open technique.)

Cholewa D, Waldschmidt J. Laser treatment of hemangiomas of the larynx and trachea. *Laser Surg Med.* 1998;23:221. [PMID: 9829433] (Describes Nd:YAG laser technique and its results in laryngeal and tracheal hemangiomas.)

Rebeiz EE, Shapshay SM, Ingrams DR. Laser applications in the tracheobronchial tree. *Otolaryngol Clin North Am.* 1996;29:987. [PMID: 8890130] (Reviews use of the CO_2, Nd:YAG, and KTP lasers in tracheobronchial tree as well as photodynamic therapy.)

Savary JF, Monier PF, Fontolliet C et al. Photodynamic therapy for early squamous cell carcinoma of the esophagus, bronchi, and mouth with m-tetra (hydroxyphenyl) chlorin. *Arch Otolaryngol Head Neck Surg.* 1997;123:162. [PMID: 9046283] (Describes the methodology of the photodynamic therapy using m-tetra (hydroxyphenyl) chlorin in carcinoma in situ and microinvasive carcinoma of the upper aerodigestive tract.)

Sipila J, Scheinin H, Grenman R. Laser bronchoscopy in palliative treatment of malignant obstructing endobronchial tumors. *ORL J Otorhinolaryngol Relat Spec.* 1998;60:42. [PMID: 9519381] (Describes use of the CO_2 and Nd:YAG lasers with the intent of palliation in malignant endobronchial tumors as well as their fatal complications.)

LASERS IN FACIAL SKIN SURGERY

Dermatology is one of the fields in which lasers are most commonly used. Cutaneous lesions present a wide spectrum from vascular lesions to malignant disorders. The use of the laser in dermatology offers surgical precision, improved hemostasis, good preservation of the lesion for histopathologic diagnosis, the facilitation of postoperative wound care, and less scarring. The particular laser selection is based on the histologic nature of the lesion, the lesion site, and the laser characteristics. In dermatology, the cosmetic result is as important as the cure. Patients need to be well informed regarding possible drawbacks of the application, such as a temporary or permanent hypo- or hyperpigmentation, unsightly scarring, and the potential success rate.

Skin Resurfacing Ablative

Indications for laser surfacing include scars, rhinophyma, actinic cheilitis, superficial squamous cell carcinoma, and wrinkles. For a better result, the depth of thermal damage should be < 100 μm. In a typical CO_2 laser application, the pulse duration and power density are adjusted to < 10 ms and 5 J/cm², respectively. With hypertrophic scarring, the scar is ablated with nonoverlapping and intermittent pulses along the lesion. After the application, hyperpigmentation that lasts as long as a few months is expected and is usually reversible. In cases of deep thermal injury, hypopigmentation may occur and is permanent. Because of the significant risk of post-treatment skin dyschromias, CO_2 laser treatment should be limited to lighter-skinned patients. A major advantage of laser resurfacing over classic dermabrasion techniques is less crust formation. Er:YAG laser may be used for superficial resurfacing of fine rhytids and photodamage. Er:YAG laser offers less dramatic change than CO_2 laser with less risk of significant sequelae. Complications reported following laser surfacing are early and late infections by a wide spectrum of agents as well as eruption, prolonged erythema, acne, milia formation, contact dermatitis, hypertrophic scar formation, ectropion, delayed healing, pigmentary abnormalities, inflammatory reactions, and unusual granulomatous reaction.

Nonablative Skin Resurfacing

Nonablative resurfacing is the use of a laser to induce dermal remodeling without removal of the superficial layers of the epidermis and dermis. Currently, studies have shown minimal improvement in skin quality, tone, and rhytid formation with a variety of Nd:YAG lasers.

Rhinophyma

In rhinophyma, argon and CO_2 laser systems are alternate options to serial shave incisions and cryosurgery. Compared with serial shave incisions and cryosurgery, under local anesthesia, laser treatments have superior results with better hemostasis. Because the argon laser is absorbed by hemoglobin, the hypervascular form of the disease better responds to the argon laser. The argon laser is set at 1.0–2.5 W power with a 2-mm spot size and a 0.5-s pulse. A total of 150 pulses is required to treat the entire nose. Treatment sessions should be at least 2 months apart. It takes 10 days to heal after the application.

Actinic Cheilitis

In actinic cheilitis, CO_2 laser systems with a pulse duration shorter than the thermal relaxation time of the epidermis and dermis provide a better outcome. A typical new CO_2 system for this superficial lesion is set at 250 mJ and 3 W of power at 12 Hz. Conventional CO_2 laser systems with a continuous mode cause thermal damage because they require a longer healing time and may cause more scarring.

Vascular Skin Lesions

Port-wine stains are the most common vascular lesions. Laser systems are absolutely advantageous in the treatment of these lesions. The goal is to destroy the underlying blood vessels selectively without scarring. For light-colored skin, the flashlamp-excited dye laser is absorbed by red blood cells with minimal absorption in the skin, which causes only minimal thermal damage to epidermis. Its pulse duration is set at 450 μs. KTP laser is another alternative. It causes less purpura than flashlamp-excited dye laser. Figure 5–4A and B show pre- and postoperative views, respectively, of the patient with port-wine stains. The patient underwent three sessions of KTP laser treatment. For dark skin, thrombosis of the vessels is difficult to obtain without damaging the skin because of high melanin absorption. Therefore, infrared lasers are preferred. It should not be used in patients with dark skin or seizure disorders, or in patients receiving anticoagulant or photosensitizing therapy. However, purpura inevitably develops and lasts 10–14 days. Temporary or permanent hypopigmentation, transient hyperpigmentation, and scar formation may also develop.

In hemangioma and telangiectasia, flashlamp-excited dye is essential to treat the superficial component during both the proliferative phase and the phase of involution of the lesion. Nd:YAG, argon, and KTP-532 laser are other options. Superficial telangiectasias and spider capillaries can be treated effectively with either KTP-532 laser or an intense pulsed light source.

Benign Lesions

Controversy still exists about whether the CO_2 laser is superior to scalpel excision in treating keloids. However, the advantages of the CO_2 laser to the scalpel include hemostatic superiority and precision when used in the focused mode. In a typical application, a 1-mm spot handpiece is fitted. The laser is set at 10 W in the continuous mode. Excessive tissue is excised with the laser, as with a scalpel. Debris should be cleaned off when necessary; otherwise, the resultant wound would be almost twice as large as the original lesion. The physician should avoid using sutures. However, until reepithelization occurs, the wound should be watched closely.

Café au lait maculas and lentigines are the most common benign lesions. With these lesions, cosmetically better outcomes are obtained with laser systems compared with scalpel excision. Shorter wavelength lasers are preferred because of the pigment content of the lesions. Q-switched laser systems (eg, the pulsed dye laser of 504 nm, or the ruby or Nd:YAG lasers) are ideal for targeting pigmented cells. The CO_2 laser is another option in spite of its much longer wavelength. In terms of scar formation and healing time, CO_2 laser systems with a short

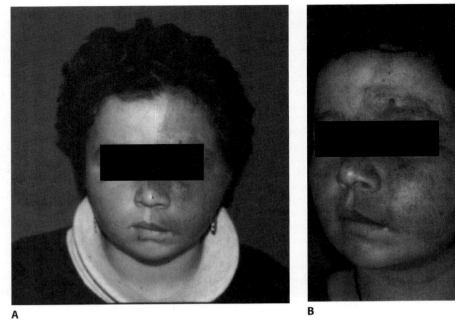

A   **B**

Figure 5–4. **(A)** Port-wine stain involving the left side of the patient's face. **(B)** Postoperative view of the regressed lesion after three KTP laser treatment sessions.   (Photo courtesy of Mustafa Sengezer, MD, Gulhane Military Medical Academy, Ankara, Department of Plastic and Reconstructive Surgery.)

pulse duration (200-ms pulses at 250 Hz and 80-W power) provide slightly better outcomes compared with conventional continuous CO_2 systems.

Facial verrucae and rosacea are also successfully treated with flashlamp-excited dye laser.

Malignant Lesions

Basal cell carcinoma, squamous cell carcinoma, and melanoma are the three most common malignant lesions encountered. Laser use is one option among scalpel excision, Mohs micrographic excision, and radiation therapy. The CO_2 laser is ideal, especially for small to moderate lesions. It is also advantageous for use in patients with coagulation defects. In addition, the CO_2 laser is good in preserving margins. The recommended margin of excision is 4–7 mm for basal cell carcinoma, 3–4 mm for squamous cell carcinoma, and 1–3 cm for melanoma.

LASER-ASSISTED HAIR REMOVAL

Lasers in hair removal induce selective damage to hair follicles, while avoiding the competing chromophobe of melanin. Temporary hair reduction is a delay in hair growth, typically lasting 1–3 months. Permanent hair reduction reduces the number of terminal hairs after a given treatment, usually lasting 6 months. Complete hair loss is the reduction of number of regrowing hairs to zero. Lasers initially produce complete but temporary hair loss. Eventually, the laser creates partial but permanent hair loss (a permanent reduction in the total number of terminal hairs). In patients with light skin, the 694-nm ruby laser and 755-nm Alexandrite laser are used. In patients with darker skin, 800-nm diode laser, 1064-nm Nd:YAG laser (long-pulse and Q-switched), and intense pulsed lights are favored because of less competition with melanin.

Alora MB, Anderson RR. Recent developments in cutaneous lasers. *Lasers Surg Med.* 2000;26:108. [PMID: 10685084] (Describes developments in skin cooling between laser applications, laser use in vascular and pigmented lesions, laser resurfacing, and hair removal.)

Alster TS, Lupton JR. Prevention and treatment of side effects and complications of cutaneous laser resurfacing. *Plast Reconstr Surg.* 2002;109:308. [PMID: 11786830] (Describes potential side effects of laser resurfacing and management.)

Dijkema SJ, van der Lei B. Long-term results of upper lips treated for rhytides with carbon dioxide laser. *Plast Reconstr Surg.*

2005;115:1731. [PMID: 15861082] (Presents an evaluation of long-term outcome of CO_2 laser use in upper lips for rhytides.)

Doctoroff A, Oberlender SA, Purcell SM. Full-face carbon dioxide laser resurfacing in the management of a patient with the nevoid basal cell carcinoma syndrome. *Dermatol Surg.* 2003;29:1236. [PMID: 14725671] (Presents CO_2 laser use in a particular case with multiple basal cell carcinoma on the face.)

Lonne-Rahm S, Nordlind K, Edstrom DW et al. Laser treatment of rosacea. *Arch Dermatol.* 2004;140:1345. [PMID: 15545543] (Presents results of flashlamp pulsed dye laser use in 32 patients with rosacea.)

Rendon-Pellerano MI, Lentini J, Eaglstein WE et al. Laser resurfacing: usual and unusual complications. *Dermatol Surg.* 1999;25:360. [PMID: 10469072] (Presents early and late complications in seven cases of patients who have undergone laser skin resurfacing.)

Ries WR, Speyer MT. Cutaneous applications of lasers. *Otolaryngol Clin North Am.* 1996;29:915. [PMID: 8890124] (Describes particular laser selection and laser use in a wide spectrum of dermatologic lesions from keloid and pigmented lesions to malignant lesions.)

Vargas H, Hove CR, Dupree ML et al. The treatment of facial verrucae with the pulsed dye laser. *Laryngoscope.* 2002;112:1573. [PMID: 12352665] (Describes pulsed dye laser use in facial verrucae.)

Waner M. Recent developments in lasers and the treatment of birthmarks. *Arch Dis Child.* 2003;88:372. [PMID: 12716698] (Presents advances in management of port wine stains, hemangiomas, and other pigmented lesions.)

SECTION II

Face

Hemangiomas of Infancy & Vascular Malformations

6

Joseph L. Edmonds, Jr., MD

Hemangiomas are true tumors with pathologic endo-thelial cell proliferation; vascular malformations are distinguished by this distinct absence.

▓ HEMANGIOMA OF INFANCY

 ESSENTIALS OF DIAGNOSIS

- *Absent at birth or history of small premonitory mark at birth.*
- *Rapid neonatal growth of the lesion.*
- *Cutaneous lesions develop either a typical "strawberry" appearance or a bluish hue ("deep bruise" appearance).*
- *Magnetic resonance imaging (MRI) is diagnostic when the diagnosis is uncertain or when serial exam is not possible.*
- *Visceral involvement is suspected if there are more than three cutaneous lesions.*
- *Progressive stridor in the appropriate age group (2–9 months) is suspicious for airway hemangioma.*

General Considerations

Hemangiomas are the most common tumors of infancy. They are more common in females than in males (3:1), in white populations, and in premature infants. Most of these neoplasms are located in the head and neck. In addition, most are single lesions; however, about 20% of patients have multiple lesions. Hemangiomas exhibit a period of rapid postnatal growth. The duration of the proliferative period is variable, but is usually confined to the first year of life. The proliferative period rarely extends to 18 months. The involutional phase is also variable, occurring over a period of 2 to 9 years. After complete involution, normal skin is restored in about 50% of patients. In other patients, the skin has evidence of telangiectasia, yellowish hypoelastic patches, sagging or fibrofatty patches, and scarring if the lesion has ulcerated.

Hemangiomas can be classified as superficial (Figure 6–1), deep (Figure 6–2) or combined. The term *superficial hemangioma* replaces the older terms *capillary hemangioma* and *"strawberry" hemangioma* and refers to hemangiomas located in the papillary dermis. The deep hemangioma, often slightly blue in color, originates from the reticular dermis or the subcutaneous space and in the past was referred to as a *cavernous hemangioma*. The combined hemangioma has elements of both the superficial and the deep hemangioma.

Pathogenesis

Proliferative hemangiomas have been shown to express high levels of indolamine 2,3-dioxygenase (IDO), basic

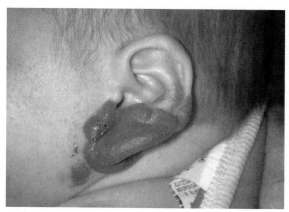

Figure 6–1. A typical superficial hemangioma of infancy.

fibroblast growth factors (β-fgf), proliferating cell nuclear antigen, type IV collagenase, urokinase, and, most recently, insulin-like growth factor 2. Involuting hemangiomas have been characterized by exhibition of tissue inhibitor of metalloproteinase 1 (TIMP1), thrombospondin, interferon-α, and decreased levels of other factors seen in the proliferative hemangioma.

In addition, it has recently been shown that endothelial cells are of clonal origin and the defect that leads to tumor growth and the altered expression of growth factors is intrinsic to the endothelial cell. These clonal endothelial cells have also been shown to have characteristics similar to placental endothelial cells, which may suggest that hemangiomas are of placental origin. A higher rate of hemangioma is found in children whose mother underwent chorionic villus sampling, which gives additional weight to placental origin theories.

Recently, the primary clonal cell of the hemangioma has been shown to have characteristics of a myeloid cell, demonstrating that it is not a typical endothelial cell.

Clinical Findings

Most commonly, the diagnosis of hemangioma is determined by the history and physical examination. The history typically reveals that more than 50% of hemangiomas are seen at birth as a prominent cutaneous mark. This mark may manifest as a whitish patch, an anemic nevus, a faint telangiectasia, or a blue spot. The rapid proliferation of this initial lesion is highly suggestive of a hemangioma. A superficial hemangioma assumes the typical "strawberry" appearance, making the diagnosis obvious. In a subcutaneous, intramuscular, or visceral tumor, the diagnosis may be uncertain. In these instances, various radiologic modalities can be very helpful. MRI is the most informative of the available modalities.

When an infant age 2–9 months presents with progressive stridor or persistent crouplike symptoms, consideration should be given to the possibility of a subglottic hemangioma. This neoplasm is said to be more common in children with a cutaneous hemangioma in a facial or "beard" distribution. The diagnosis of a subglottic hemangioma should be made with a direct laryngoscopy and a bronchoscopy.

Special consideration should be given to the child with three or more hemangiomas. In these children, abdominal ultrasounds should be obtained to evaluate for visceral hemangiomas, especially hepatic hemangiomas. If the screening ultrasound is positive, MRI of the entire body is indicated to detect other internal hemangiomas.

Another special diagnostic situation arises when a child presents with extensive facial hemangiomas, sometimes referred to as *segmental hemangiomas*. The term segmental hemangioma relates to the approximate distribution that may correspond to sensory innervation patterns. The acronym PHACE can help the clinician recall the findings seen in these children, which include the following:

Posterior fossa malformations

Hemangiomas

Arterial anomalies

Coarctation of the aorta and cardiac defects

Eye abnormalities

Differential Diagnosis

Congenital hemangiomas are rare vascular tumors that are fully developed at birth and in that way are distinguished from the more typical hemangioma of infancy. There are two types of congenital hemangiomas. One type does not involute—the noninvoluting congenital hemangioma (NICH). The other type invo-

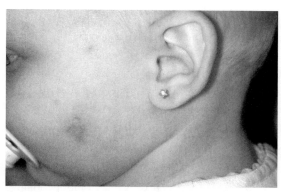

Figure 6–2. A deep hemangioma demonstrating the typical blue discoloration to the skin, similar to a bruise.

lutes quickly—rapidly involuting congenital hemangioma (RICH). These tumors are also pathologically distinguishable from the hemangioma of infancy in that they are glucose transporter-1 protein(glut-1)–negative.

A **pyogenic granuloma** is often confused with a hemangioma. A pyogenic granuloma is often the result of a minor trauma. The lesion is usually sessile and as it grows it becomes pedicled, often bleeding impressively. The treatment is surgical excision.

A **vascular malformation** is another typical diagnostic alternative to consider when attempting to diagnose a potential hemangioma. However, the natural history of the hemangioma (not present at birth with rapid growth in the first months of life) is usually adequate evidence to support a confident diagnosis.

Kaposiform hemangioendothelioma (KHE) is a rare vascular tumor closely associated with Kasabach-Merritt syndrome. Differentiation from hemangioma of infancy is typically based on recognition of aggressive behavior such as compression and invasion of surrounding tissue. These are large abnormal vascular tumors, and early recognition and treatment can be life saving.

Tufted angiomas (known in Japanese literature as angioblastoma of Nakagawa) are benign erythematous plaques that grow slowly over several years. They often stabilize after the slow growth period. A pathologic specimen is usually diagnostic.

MRI with contrast is the most useful of all radiologic evaluations of hemangiomas. MRI can differentiate a hemangioma from a vascular malformation. A discussion of clinical suspicions with the radiologist may help determine the need for concomitant magnetic resonance angiography, which is especially helpful in locating feeder vessels of high-flow arteriovenous malformations.

The ultimate method of differentiating all diagnostic possibilities is with a histologic study of the tissue. A biopsy should be done whenever there is a possibility that the lesion in question is a **malignant tumor;** however, a biopsy is rarely necessary because there is usually ample epidemiologic, clinical, and radiologic information that can facilitate a reliable diagnosis.

Complications

Although rare, the complications of hemangiomas dictate a need for treatment. These complications include:

(1) Ulceration (most common in the perineum and lip/perioral area).
(2) Airway obstruction.
(3) Visual loss. Obstruction of the visual axis for 1 week in the first year of life can cause permanent amblyopia.
(4) External auditory canal obstruction.

(5) Bleeding. Bleeding is usually low flow and therefore can be managed simply with pressure.
(6) Heart failure. This complication is managed with medical therapy (usually by a cardiologist) and with attempts to control the growth of the hemangioma. Steroids should be the initial medical therapy, with vincristine and other chemotherapies used for steroid failures. Surgical therapy combined with embolization would be a second tier of therapy if medical treatment is not effective and the problem becomes life threatening.

Treatment

The decision to intervene and attempt to treat the patient without an active or inevitable complication from hemangioma must be weighed against the fact that most hemangiomas resolve completely or with minimal long-term sequelae. For hemangiomas with active or inevitable complications, multiple treatment options exist. The most appropriate treatment depends on the location and the nature of the impending complication as well as the child's specific medical and social situation. For example, if follow-up is not possible, early definitive surgical management may be more strongly considered.

A. STEROIDS

Steroids are the usual first line of treatment. Typical initial doses are 2–5 mg/kg/d of prednisolone or prednisone. Steroids are best administered in a single morning dose. This initial therapy is usually used for 4–12 weeks, then tapered over the next several months according to what the patient can tolerate. Rebound growth may necessitate a second course of therapy. Alternate-day dosing or rest periods of several weeks may lessen troublesome side effects such as cushingoid appearance, growth retardation, decreased appetite, and susceptibility to infection. Monitoring of blood glucose and blood pressure are recommended. Adrenal suppression can be a result of therapy. Concomitant use of a proton pump inhibitor is also suggested.

Intralesional steroid injections may be used as an initial therapy, especially for orbital or periorbital lesions, tumors of the nasal tip, and globular tumors of the lips, ears, and cheeks and parotid hemangiomas. A 1:1 ratio of long-acting steroids (eg, triamcinolone 40 mg/mL) and short-acting steroids (eg, betamethasone 6 mg/mL) yields the best results. Three injections of triamcinolone, at doses of 3–5 mg/kg per procedure mixed with an equal volume of betamethsone spaced 4–6 weeks apart, are the suggested course. Injections of long-acting corticosteroids in a suspension in the periorbital tissues can result in blindness. Great caution is needed in this area, especially in the upper lid. Low-pressure injection technique is thought to decrease the risk of embolization. When effective, injection therapy usually leads to a dramatic reduction in the size of the lesion within 1 week. In general, steroid therapy (systemic or intralesional) can be extremely effective in one third of patients, partially effective in another third, and ineffective for the final third of patients.

B. INTERFERON

Interferon alfa-2a is a comparatively new agent for the treatment of hemangiomas. Although it is effective in most cases, its use is limited because of cost, route of administration, and potential side effects. The treatment is generally reserved for pulmonary hemangioma, life-threatening hemangioma, and diffuse neonatal hemangioma. Transient side effects include fever, elevated liver enzymes, and neutropenia. Spastic diplegia and other permanent neurologic complications associated with the use of interferon alfa-2a have resulted in the cautious application of this therapy. The typical dose is 3 million units/m^2 injected subcutaneously daily. The therapy is generally administered for 6–12 months.

C. VINCRISTINE

Vincristine is gaining popularity as another efficacious treatment for complicated or refractory hemangiomas. There are relatively few side effects compared with interferon. The therapy should be coordinated by a clinician experienced in using the medication. One drawback of the therapy is the need for central venous access for up to 12 weeks.

D. LASER

Laser therapy for hemangiomas is becoming widely practiced to combat mucosal lesions and cutaneous lesions with or without ulceration. In the United States, laser debulking of mucosal lesions is the typical treatment of obstructing lesions such as subglottic hemangiomas. The goal is to reduce the lesion size to allow for an adequate airway. Recurrence is anticipated and the treatment is repeated until the hemangioma stops proliferating and involutes. Various laser therapies are used, but all share the drawback of causing a mucosal ulceration in the airway.

Ulceration is a controversial indication for cutaneous laser therapy. The yellow light emitted by pulsed dye lasers is selectively absorbed by hemoglobin and melanin. In an ulcerated hemangioma, the laser light does not need to pass through the skin and the melanin within the skin to reach the hemangioma; therefore, the risks of scarring due to absorption by melanin are considered lessened. Recent advances in the flashlamp pulsed dye laser include longer wavelengths, longer pulse durations, and the very important dynamic cooling of the surface tissues. These advances have allowed for higher energy treatments, deeper penetration, fewer complications, and better overall responses. They have in turn led to increased confidence is using flashlamp pulsed-dye laser for the treatment of select nonulcerated cutaneous lesions. The KTP and Nd:YAG lasers have been used for intralesional therapy by using bare fibers to deliver high energies to the deep components of the lesions. The use of these laser technologies, although gaining in acceptance and recognition of their usefulness, is not standardized and is limited by the experience of the practitioner.

E. EXCISION

It is common to consider excision in a completely involuted lesion when the residuum causes a functional or esthetic problem.

Baggy fibrofatty tissue is recontoured for improved cosmesis.

The early surgical excision of an actively proliferating lesion is appropriate in an area (eg, the glabella, eyelid, airway, the nasal wall) that will certainly lead to complications or impaired function. This may also prevent the need for protracted systemic therapy and spare the child and family the anticipated psychosocial difficulty.

Some surgeons also advocate surgical intervention of lesions that have stopped proliferating rather than waiting for a protracted involution phase. Physicians who advocate earlier removal do so with the hope of diminishing psychosocial stress. This technique also takes advantage of the natural tissue expansion of the surrounding skin and soft tissue, which occurs in the proliferative phase.

Regardless of the timing, the procedures are typically accomplished using routine techniques. Special preoperative planning and imaging should be carried out when operating on actively proliferating or recently quiescent lesions to minimize blood loss. In addition to standard techniques, circular excision with purse-string closure and subsequent lenticular removal of scarring as needed has been advocated. This technique may lead to smaller eventual scarring.

F. TREATMENT OF ULCERATION

Local wound care consisting of topical and oral antibiotics, topical steroids, barrier creams, and wound dressings are the mainstay of treatment. Treatment to minimize the ongoing proliferation of the hemangioma remains necessary. Management of pain is also very important. Reports of the use of topical recombinant platelet-derived growth factor (Regranex) are new and promising.

Boye E, Yu Y, Paranya G, Mulliken JB, Olsen BR, Bischoff J. Clonality and altered behavior of endothelial cells from hemangiomas. *J Clin Invest.* 2001;107:165. [PMID: 11254674] (A recent development in the understanding of the pathogenesis of hemangiomas.)

Chang CJ, Kelly KM, Nelson JS. Cryogen spray cooling and pulsed dye laser treatment of cutaneous hemangiomas. *Ann Plast Surg.* 2001;46:577. [PMID: 11405354] (A description of current laser techniques and the efficacy of this treatment).

Marchuk DA. Pathogenesis of hemangioma. *J Clin Invest.* 2001;107:665. [PMID: 11254664] (A review article discussing the latest theories on pathogenesis.)

Metry DW. The many faces of PHACE syndrome. *J Pediatr.* 2001;139:117. [PMID: 11445804]

Metz BJ. Response of ulcerated perineal hemangioma of infancy to becaplermingel, a recombinant human platelet growth factor. *Acta Dermatol.* 2004;140;867. [PMID: 15262700]

Mulliken JB, Fishman SJ, Burrows PE. Vascular anomalies. *Curr Probl Surg.* 2000;57:517. [PMID: 10955029] (An extensive review of current management strategies of vascular anomalies.)

Mulliken JB, Enjolras O. Congenital hemangiomas and infantile hemangioma: missing links. *J Am Acad Dermatol.* 2004;50:875. [PMID: 15153887] (A recent paper describing the new entities, RICH and NICH.)

Mulliken JB, Glowarki J. Hemangiomas and vascular malformations in infants and children: a classification based on endothelial characteristics. *Plast Reconstr Surg.* 1982;69:412. [PMID: 706356] (A classic article describing the basis for a modern understanding of these tumors and malformations.)

North PE, Waner M, Mizerarki A, et al. A unique microvascular phenotype shared by juvenile hemangiomas and human placenta. *Arch Dermatol.* 2001;137:559. [PMID: 11346333] (New research that may shed light on the origin of these tumors.)

Ritter MR, Dorrell MI, Edmonds J, Friedlander SF, Friedlander M. Insulin-like growth factor 2 and potential regulators of hemangioma growth and involution identified by large-scale expression analysis. *Proc Natl Acad Science.* 2002;99:7455.

Ritter MR, Reinisch J, Friedlander SF, Friedlander M. Myeloid cells in infantile hemangioma. *Am J Pathol.* 2006;168:621. [PMID: 16436675]

■ VASCULAR MALFORMATIONS

CAPILLARY MALFORMATIONS

 ESSENTIALS OF DIAGNOSIS

- *Present at birth.*
- *Distribution remains constant, although the color may darken.*
- *Overlying skin is unaffected in childhood but may change in adulthood with the development of a nodular skin surface and ectatic dermal vessels.*
- *Capillary malformations must be differentiated from commonplace fading macular stains of infancy (nevus flammeus neonatorum), which are referred to as stork bites, angel kisses, or salmon patches.*
- *Lesions roughly follow cutaneous sensory nerve distributions.*

General Considerations

Capillary malformations are the most common of the vascular malformations and occur in 0.3% of newborns. These lesions are also known as *nevus flammeus* or *port-wine stains*. MRI with contrast is the most useful radiologic modality for evaluation of vascular malformations, although it is unnecessary for most lesions.

Pathogenesis

The improper sympathetic neuronal control of the capillaries may lead to chronic dilatation of dermal capillaries and their development into ectatic vessels. Clinical observation provides evidence that these lesions somewhat follow cutaneous sensory nerve distributions. Although an autosomal dominant mode of inheritance with variable penetrance has been suggested, this finding is not observed in most clinical situations.

Clinical Findings

A capillary malformation is usually not associated with other abnormalities, but it may point to other problems. When capillary malformations are associated with other vascular malformations, these combined situations are recognized as syndromes. A facial capillary vascular malformation in the ophthalmic distribution of the trigeminal nerve (CN V) may indicate that the patient has **Sturge-Weber syndrome.** This syndrome is a congenital condition consisting of the aforementioned cutaneous vascular malformation associated with a similar malformation of the underlying meninges and cortex. Children with Sturge-Weber syndrome have an increased risk for developing seizures and glaucoma as well as soft tissue and bony overgrowths in the midface. Children with a capillary malformation located in the V_1 division (the first division of the trigeminal nerve) should have both an MRI scan of the brain and screening ophthalmologic exams.

A capillary malformation that overlies a deep venous or lymphatic malformation (a mixed vascular malformation) of the extremity is referred to as **Klippel-Trenaunay syndrome.** The overlying skin is often involved with ulceration and infection. The underlying bone becomes overgrown, adding to limb hypertrophy and often necessitating surgical intervention.

A capillary malformation that overlies a deep high-flow arteriovenous malformation is referred to as **Parkes-Weber syndrome.**

Lumbosacral capillary malformations may indicate that spinal cord abnormalities exist and should also be investigated further.

Differential Diagnosis

The typical capillary malformation must be differentiated from the commonplace fading **macular stains of infancy** (eg, "stork bite"). These lesions, in contrast to a true capillary malformation, fade by the age of 1 year and are usually seen in the nuchal region, the eyelid, the glabella, or the lips. Location is the best clue to differentiation.

Complications

The primary complications of capillary malformations are skin changes and bleeding. If untreated, a significant percent of patients will manifest a change in the surface appearance of the skin. The skin can become nodular and the increasingly dilated and ectatic dermal vessels may bleed spontaneously.

Treatment

The treatment of choice for a capillary malformation is laser photocoagulation. Both cosmetic improvement and the prevention of complications in adulthood are possible with laser therapies. These therapies often require multiple treatments and are more efficacious when started early in life. The flashlamp pulsed dye laser is reported to give a 50–70% response rate. These rates range from complete to partial resolution. In a previously untreated adult patient with both progression of the lesion to a nodular appearance and troublesome bleeding, excision and skin grafting may be necessary.

Breugem CC, van der Horst CMAM, Hennekam RCM. Progress toward understanding vascular malformations. *Plast Reconstr Surg.* 2001;107:1509. [PMID: 11335828] (A detailed review of the current understanding of the pathogenesis of these birth defects.)

Enjolras O, Mulliken JB. The current management of vascular birthmarks. *Pediatr Dermatol.* 1993;10:311. [PMID: 8302734] (A review of current treatments of vascular birthmarks.)

VENOUS MALFORMATIONS

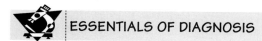 **ESSENTIALS OF DIAGNOSIS**

- *Usually present at birth, but not detected.*
- *As they become apparent, venous malformations are bluish-purple, raised, and easily compressible.*
- *Enlarge when dependent.*
- *Gradually dilate, giving the appearance of a growing lesion.*

Pathogenesis

Some venous malformations occur in families and are inherited in an autosomal dominant fashion. This occurrence has been mapped to chromosome 9q. **Blue rubber bleb nevus syndrome** (cutaneous venous malformations associated with gastrointestinal bleeding) may be genetically similar.

Clinical Findings

Craniofacial venous malformations cause symptoms dependent on location. They are almost always a cosmetic problem, and thrombosis often makes these lesions painful, impairing basic activities. MRI scanning is the single best modality to evaluate the three-dimensional complexity of a craniofacial venous malformation. Some patients also have intracranial involvement; therefore, the initial study should always include an MRI of the brain. Coagulation studies should also be done because these patients often have low-grade disseminated intravascular coagulopathy; however, this condition typically requires no therapy.

Differential Diagnosis

A venous malformation can be confused with a "deep" hemangioma, although an MRI should easily differentiate the two. Several syndromes are also included in the differential diagnoses of venous malformations: (1) Blue rubber bleb nevus syndrome. Affected patients have multiple cutaneous venous malformations and sometimes also problematic gastrointestinal bleeding from intestinal lesions. (2) Maffucci syndrome. This syndrome of multiple venous malformations associated with enchondromas begins in adolescence. The skeletal lesions often degenerate into malignant tumors.

Glomangiomas may also be misdiagnosed as venous malformations. The solitary type of glomangioma is the most common and is characterized by five classic symptoms: (1) severe pain that is seemingly out of proportion to the lesion; (2) localized tenderness; (3) sensitivity to cold; (4) the ability to localize pain to a pinpoint location (Love sign); and (5) painful symptoms eradicated by a proximal tourniquet (Hildreth sign).

Complications

Rapid growth is usually secondary to hemorrhage and hematoma formation, which can be the result of minimal trauma.

These patients may have chronic consumptive coagulopathy. An evaluation of the coagulation parameters and a platelet count are warranted.

Treatment

A. COMPRESSION

If a patient with a venous malformation of the extremities is able to wear a compressive garment, he or she may avoid the long-term morbidity of chronic engorgement. This approach is a primary therapy for extremity lesions, especially simple lesions (eg, benign varicose veins) and lesions of a combined nature (eg, Klippel-Trenaunay syndrome).

B. SCLEROTHERAPY

Sclerotherapy is the mainstay of treatment for craniofacial lesions and for extensive extremity lesions. Sclerosants are effective for these lesions because the sclerosant stays in the lesion or can be made to stay in the lesion with compression of the outflow pathway. Alcohol-based sclerosants are the most commonly used type of sclerosing agent. The sclerosant, in any formulation, is intended to do extensive endothelial damage, induce clotting, and induce eventual vascular obliteration. Complications of sclerotherapy can occur, most commonly skin necrosis with alcohol-based agents. Alcohol is typically not used in and around the eye to avoid complications leading to damaged vision.

C. LASER THERAPY

Laser treatment with the Nd:YAG can be used in selected cases. The goal of laser therapy is also to cause endothelial injury sufficient to lead to coagulation and partial resolution. Percutaneous laser use avoids damaging the skin, so it may be most beneficial at the lip vermilion. The mucosal component of lesions can also be effectively managed with the Nd:YAG laser.

D. SURGICAL MEASURES

Surgical therapy of venous malformations is generally reserved for resection of previously sclerosed areas for improved cosmesis or for lesions that respond poorly to sclerosant therapy. Surgical therapy may also be necessary for dental malocclusion or other secondary problems after primary sclerosant or laser management.

Berenguer B, Burrows PE, Zurakowski D, Mulliken JB. Sclerotherapy of craniofacial venous malformations: complications and results. *Plast Reconstr Surg.* 1999;104:111. [PMID: 10597669] (A review of a large study with detailed descriptions of techniques.)

Breugem CC, van der Horst CMAM, Hennekam RCM. Progress toward understanding vascular malformations. *Plast Reconstr Surg.* 2001;107:1509. [PMID: 11335828] (A detailed review of the current understanding of the pathogenesis of these birth defects.)

Clymer MA, Fortune DS, Reinisch L, Toriumi DM, Werkhaven JA, Ries WR. Interstitial Nd:YAG photocoagulation for vascular malformations and hemangiomas in childhood. *Arch Otolaryngol Head Neck Surg.* 1998;124:431. [PMID: 9559692] (A description of the laser technique.)

ARTERIOVENOUS MALFORMATIONS

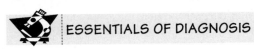 ESSENTIALS OF DIAGNOSIS

- *Commonly noted at birth and confused with a hemangioma or a capillary malformation.*
- *Eventually, local warmth and pulsation lead to diagnosis.*
- *Not easily compressible.*
- *Overlying skin changes usually precede heart failure.*

General Considerations

Arteriovenous malformations (AVMs), excluding intracranial lesions, are uncommon and are most often found in the head and neck. They are sometimes referred to as "fast-flow" lesions. Trauma or the onset of puberty may precipitate a growth of the malformation.

An AVM is a diffuse lesion with a myriad of microscopic and macroscopic components (Figure 6–3). In contrast, an arteriovenous fistula is a smaller, more localized shunt from a large artery to nearby veins. Because they are localized, an AV fistula should be considered as a separate but related entity.

Clinical Findings

Lesions are staged in four categories (Table 6–1). Clinical suspicion is easy to confirm with ultrasound or color Doppler. Either MRI or MRA (magnetic resonance angiography) is the best modality to visualize the extent of the lesion. Arteriography is often reserved for the eventual treatment phase.

Differential Diagnosis

AVMs are commonly noted at birth but are confused with hemangiomas or capillary malformations. Ultrasound can differentiate these lesions.

Complications

Congestive heart failure may necessitate urgent embolization. Echocardiography should be used to evaluate patients in stage III and at least yearly thereafter to screen for progression to stage IV.

Treatment

Ligating a large feeding vessel is always contraindicated. This procedure shifts the blood flow to collateral vessels and serves only to accelerate the growth of the malformation.

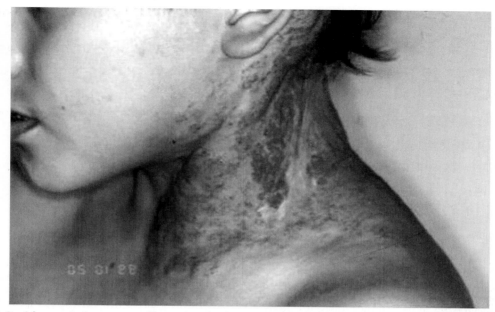

Figure 6–3. A large arteriovenous malformation that has progressed to Schobinger stage IV. Skin changes are obvious, which are present in both stages III and IV.

Complete surgical excision is the only way to ensure a permanent, successful treatment. With early diagnosis, surgical excision of a stage I malformation is possible. Early lesions have a greater chance for complete and successful surgical excision. However, because of frequent late diagnosis or the perceived risk of excising lesions, patients are typically treated in later, symptomatic stages. Super-selective arterial embolization using permanent material can be used palliatively to relieve pain or other symptoms, or as part of a combined treatment plan intended to completely eliminate the lesion. These combined treatments usually consist of either serial embolization followed by surgical resection, which is most commonly used, or embolization followed by sclerotherapy. If the overlying skin is normal, it can be saved; however, this is often not the case.

Table 6–1. Schobinger clinical staging system for arteriovenous malformations.

Stage	Description	Hallmark
I	Quiescent	Skin discoloration
II	Expansion	Pulsation
III	Destruction	Overlying skin change
IV	Decompensation	Heart failure

Long-term follow-up is essential as these lesions have a tendency for recurrence even when treated by an experienced physician.

Breugem CC, van der Horst CMAM, Hennekam RCM. Progress toward understanding vascular malformations. *Plast Reconstr Surg.* 2001;107:1509. [PMID: 11335828] (A detailed review of the current understanding of the pathogenesis of these birth defects.)

Kohout MP, Hansen M, Pribaz JJ, Mullkien JB. Arteriovenous malformations of the head and neck: natural history and management. *Plast Reconstr Surg.* 1998;102:643. [PMID: 9727427] (A description of the treatment outcome of 81 patients.)

■ LYMPHATIC MALFORMATIONS

 ESSENTIALS OF DIAGNOSIS

- *Incorrectly known as cystic hygroma or lymphangioma.*
- *Typically thought of as microcystic or macrocystic based on the size of the lymphatic spaces within the malformation.*
- *Macrocystic lesions are soft, compressible, and transilluminant.*

- *Microcystic disease is almost always present at birth and is associated with distortion of the cervicofacial soft tissue and eventually the maxillofacial bones.*

General Considerations

The commonly used term *lymphangioma* implies cellular proliferation, which is incorrect. The tissue structure of these lesions, like all vascular malformations, demonstrates no proliferative component. In the simplest terms, lymphatic malformations and all vascular malformations are birth defects.

Fifty to sixty percent of lymphatic malformations are recognized at birth; 90% are recognized by the second year. Eighty percent of all lymphatic malformations are located in the head and neck. There is no gender predilection. A lymphatic malformation tends to be slowly progressive, growing with the child. In some instances, it is apparent that the lymphatic malformation rapidly increases in size. In these cases, it is likely that the lesion has either hemorrhaged into itself or has become infected. There are reports of spontaneous regression, although they are far from typical. With adequate follow-up, a regression is usually followed by a recurrence. The incidence of lymphatic malformations is unknown.

Pathogenesis

Lymphatic malformations are thought to arise from sequestrations of the developing lymphatic system.

Clinical Findings

An MRI scan with contrast is the typical and best means for evaluating patients with a presumed lymphatic malformation. A lymphatic malformation is hyperintense on a T2-weighted image and has only a slight increase in intensity on a T1-weighted image. A

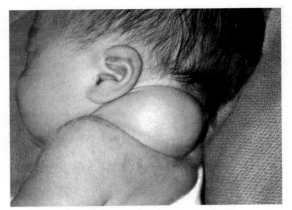

Figure 6–4. A macrocystic localized lymphatic malformation in an infant.

lymphatic malformation does not enhance on gadolinium contrast images. Based on the radiographic appearance of the size of the lymphatic spaces located within the lesion, lymphatic malformations are then broadly categorized as either macrocystic or microcystic. Further categorization may then be made based on the location of the lesion (Table 6–2). This type of staging system does offer some important prognostic information: generally, as the stage increases, the prognosis for the cure decreases. It is also generally true that facial and oropharyngeal involvement is associated with a poor prognosis.

Although the lymphatic malformations classification system is helpful prognostically, the staging system does not simplify the clinical complexities of dealing with children who have lymphatic malformations. A more practical classification designates these malformations as either **localized** and macrocystic (Figure 6–4), or **diffuse** and interdigitating (Figure 6–5). The therapeutic goals and appropriate treatments for the two groups are dramatically different.

The increased use of prenatal ultrasound has led to the diagnosis of lymphatic malformations in patients in utero, which has led to some treatment dilemmas at very early stages of life. Not all fetal ultrasound diagnoses of cystic hygroma equate with the postnatal condition of lymphatic malformation. Posterior nuchal swellings are often referred to as cystic hygromas on ultrasonography. This finding is associated with chromosomal abnormalities and increased fetal death rates. These posterior nuchal swellings are not necessarily associated with lymphatic malformation.

Anterior and lateral neck swellings identified on fetal ultrasound, which remain persistent on repeat ultrasound, likely represent congenital lymphatic malformations and are sometimes massive (see Figure 6–4). This

Table 6–2. de Serres classification of lymphatic malformations.

Stage	Location
I	Unilateral infrahyoid
II	Unilateral suprahyoid
III	Unilateral suprahyoid and infrahyoid
IV	Bilateral suprahyoid
V	Bilateral suprahyoid and infrahyoid

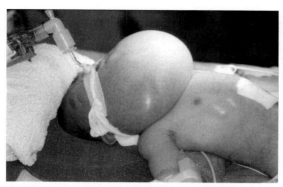

Figure 6–5. An interdigitating, macrocystic, diffuse lymphatic malformation.

distinction is well known to the experienced radiologist; however, the terminology can lead to confusion. At the time of birth, children with massive congenital lymphatic malformations usually undergo an "exit procedure" in which the airway is stabilized by intubation, bronchoscopy, or tracheostomy. These neonates should not undergo massive neonatal dissection unless symptoms dictate the need. These procedures are more likely to result in surgical complications and require, at the least, a dedicated surgical team to perform this procedure as completely as possible.

Differential Diagnosis

When lymphatic malformations become infected or hemorrhage into themselves, their rapid enlargement can be misdiagnosed as an infected branchial cyst or acute lymphadenitis. A plunging ranula or a branchial cyst can be confused with a lymphatic malformation clinically and on CT or MRI. Aspiration and examination of the cyst fluid should differentiate these lesions.

Complications

Diffuse microcystic cervicofacial disease often results in mandibulomaxillary hypertrophy, which is due to the involvement of the bone and growth of the lymphatic malformation along with the bone. After the child has matured, this hypertrophy can be managed with mandibular osteotomy and, if necessary, Le Fort osteotomies.

A secure airway is essential in patients with diffuse microcystic cervicofacial disease. It is often necessary to perform a tracheostomy to avoid obstructive airway problems.

A lymphatic malformation often swells with the onset of a general viral infection or a remote bacterial infection. This swelling typically resolves with the reso-

lution of the infection. Occasionally, the malformation itself becomes infected, which may require IV antibiotics and steroids.

Treatment

Many treatments have been used for the management of the lesions, which indicates that none has been completely effective. It is helpful here to consider treatment of the localized and diffuse groups separately.

A. LOCALIZED MALFORMATIONS

The treatment of localized malformations relies essentially on sclerosis or surgery, except in some specialized locations. Both surgery and sclerosis are very effective for localized lesions; choosing between these two modalities depends on the surgeon's experience and the specifics of the patient's situation.

1. Sclerosis—Numerous agents have been used to sclerose these lesions, including boiling water, tetracycline, cyclophosphamide, sodium tetradecyl sulfate, bleomycin, doxycycline, alcohol, and OK-432. OK-432 is a medication developed in Japan with extensive worldwide use. In the United States, the medication is under FDA investigation. The medication, a streptococcus culture treated and killed with penicillin, incites an immune response (delayed hypersensitivity reaction) in the location of the lymphatic malformation. OK-432 has been shown to be highly effective.

2. Laser resurfacing—Other localized lesions may present within the tongue. The tongue may have small blebs that bleed and become infected. An old term used to describe this type of lesion is "lymphangioma circumscriptum." These lesions can be managed with CO_2 laser resurfacing or with coblation resurfacing.

3. Tongue reduction surgery—The tongue can also become massively enlarged due to lymphatic malformation (Figure 6–6). Children with this condition cannot be treated with laser and generally require tongue reduction surgery.

4. CO_2 laser surgery—Glottic involvement is best managed with a CO_2 laser to open lesions and debulk airway obstruction. A tracheostomy tube should always be in place for this type of airway surgery.

B. DIFFUSE MALFORMATIONS

The management of diffuse cases is much more complex and may be a lifelong endeavor. For this reason, initial management decisions should not increase the morbidity of the disease by causing iatrogenic injury. The first goals of managing diffuse cervicofacial disease are to allow for an adequate airway and feeding, which often require a tracheostomy and possibly a gastrostomy. Surgical management is the mainstay of treatment for these lesions. If complete

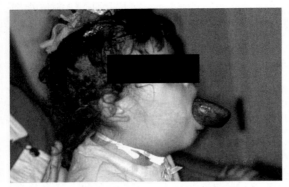

Figure 6–6. An interdigitating, microcystic, diffuse lymphatic malformation, with involvement of the neck, mandible, floor of mouth, and near-total infiltration of the tongue.

resection is not possible, it may be helpful to manage different anatomic areas as individual problems. The mylohyoid muscle is a typical boundary used to divide these massive lesions into several "zones." It is also advisable to approach the divided components of the total malformation from the "top down," if possible. For instance, the physician should attempt to deal with the tongue before dealing with the floor of mouth and then approach the neck; this approach prevents superior swelling of the untreated zone. In addition, children with diffuse cervicofacial disease also frequently require maxillomandibular reconstruction owing to overgrowth of the facial bones.

It is also advisable in the care of children with diffuse disease to involve a child psychiatrist. These children will likely have long-term morbidity, and a means for dealing with the psychosocial implications is essential.

Berenguer B, Burrows PE, Zurakowski D, Mulliken JB. Sclerotherapy of craniofacial venous malformations: complications and results. *Plast Reconstr Surg*. 1999;104:111. [PMID: 10597669] (A review of a large study with detailed descriptions of techniques.)

Breugem CC, van der Horst CMAM, Hennekam RCM. Progress toward understanding vascular malformations. *Plast Reconstr Surg*. 2001;107:1509. [PMID: 11335828] (A detailed review of the current understanding of the pathogenesis of these birth defects.)

de Serres LM, Sie KCY, Richardson MA. Lymphatic malformation of the head and neck. *Arch Otolaryngol Head Neck Surg*. 1995;121:577. [PMID: 7727093] (An outline of a novel staging system.)

Fisher R, Partington A, Dykes E. Cystic hygroma: comparison between prenatal and postnatal diagnosis. *J Pediatr Surg*. 1996;31:473. [PMID: 8801294] (A discussion of prenatal diagnosis and its implications.)

Greinwald JH, Burke DK, Sato Y. Treatment of lymphangiomas in children: an update of Picibanil (OK-432) sclerotherapy. *Otolaryngol Head Neck Surg*. 1999;121:381. [PMID: 10504592] (An update on the American drug trial.)

Marler JJ, Fishman SJ, Upton J et al. Prenatal diagnosis of vascular anomalies. *J Pediatr Surg*. 2002;37:318. [PMID: 11877641] (A discussion of prenatal diagnosis and its implications.)

Orford J, Baker A, Thonell S, King P, Murphy J. Bleomycin therapy for cystic hygroma. *J Pediatr Surg*. 1995;30:1282. [PMID: 8523225] (A description of clinical experience with a novel treatment.)

Padwa BL, Hayward PG, Ferraro NF, Mulliken JB. Cervicofacial lymphatic malformation: clinical course, surgical intervention, and pathogenesis of skeletal hypertrophy. *Plast Reconstr Surg*. 1995;95:951. [PMID: 7732142] (A convincing explanation for skeletal hypertrophy in patients with diffuse lymphatic malformation of the cervicofacial area.)

Wong GB, Mulliken JB, Benacerraf BR. Prenatal sonographic diagnosis of major craniofacial anomalies. *Plast Reconstr Surg*. 2001;108:1316. [PMID: 11604640] (A discussion of prenatal diagnosis and its implications.)

Maxillofacial Trauma

7

Andrew H. Murr, MD, FACS

Patients with maxillofacial trauma are seen everyday in emergency rooms throughout the United States. The cause of the trauma can be quite variable, ranging from industrial and motor vehicle accidents to interpersonal trauma involving either fists or weapons. It is common for trauma to be related to substance abuse or to behavior that can be linked to substance abuse. Sometimes trauma is related to sports activities or simply to accidental or work-related occurrences. The principles of management are directed at stabilizing a patient's medical condition and providing safe reconstruction to maximize both functional and aesthetic rehabilitation.

THE ABCS OF TRAUMA

It can be disconcerting when a patient is brought into the emergency room with severe craniofacial trauma. Patients may be covered with blood and have distorted anatomy that may divert attention from the initial principles of Advanced Trauma Life Support (ATLS). In these circumstances, it is critically important to follow the basic tenets of initial trauma stabilization, also known as the ABCs of trauma:

Airway management and assessment
Breathing
Circulation

Tamponade of bleeding and C-spine clearance are also critical factors when the patient initially presents to the emergency room. In the initial management period, even occurrences of severe craniofacial trauma may be examined after cases of abdominal, thoracic, and—at times—limb trauma. A neurosurgical examination and clearance are frequently desirable in severe high-velocity injuries. When ocular injury is suspected, an examination by an ophthalmologist can be indispensable. Patients on the most severe end of the injury spectrum often require airway control via orotracheal intubation or, in certain cases, via cricothyroidotomy or tracheotomy.

Most attempts to repair maxillofacial trauma will be considered after the patient is stabilized. Almost all skeletal trauma repair is guided by the information provided by fine-cut computed tomography (CT) scans. Fine-cut scans take more time and require more medical condition stability than the initial screening provided by head CT scans, which are often obtained during the initial, acute evaluation period. In contrast, soft-tissue injuries are often repaired as soon as it is practically possible. Low-velocity injuries, such as isolated nasal and mandible fractures, do not usually require the same highly consultative and collaborative team approach, especially if no other injuries are found or suspected. With isolated injuries, which tend to be more minor than multisystem injuries, treatment can be better directed; it can proceed on a pace both commensurate with and concentrated upon the direct injury.

Committee on Trauma, *Advanced Trauma Life Support for Doctors, Instruction Manual,* 6th ed. Chicago, Illinois: American College of Surgeons; 1997. (This is the best resource for individuals interested in the basics of ATLS training and initial trauma management.)

■ SOFT TISSUE TRAUMA

TREATMENT

Managing Blood Loss

Although the ABCs of trauma take precedence over most of the issues associated with maxillofacial trauma, sometimes the soft tissue injuries of the face or scalp can add substantially to blood loss. A temporal injury may lacerate the superficial temporal artery or a scalp laceration may contribute to the loss of many units of blood. Under these circumstances, it is desirable to halt bleeding immediately. The discrete clamping of an arterial vessel in a laceration may be necessary if the physician is unable to gain adequate control of blood loss by applying simple pressure. Scalp injuries usually respond to closure with a few simple mattress sutures or a pressure dressing. This blood loss management allows time for the rest of the trauma evaluation to proceed and for the patient to be stabilized.

Prophylactic Treatment Measures

A. ANTIBIOTICS

Lacerations of the scalp, face, and neck should be closed as soon as the patient is stable. In cases in which the tissue loss is minimal, which is the most common circumstance, primary closure is utilized. Primary closure is direct edge-to-edge skin approximation using fine sutures with precise suture approximation of deeper tissue layers. Protecting the patient prophylactically with tetanus immunoglobulin and tetanus toxoid should be considered. In contaminated wounds, which are extremely common, prophylactic antibiotic administration should also be strongly considered.

B. Anesthesia

It is important to administer adequate anesthesia for wound closure if the closure is to be made under local sedation. Typically, injectable 1% lidocaine with epinephrine mixed 1:100,000 is adequate to obtain anesthesia for closure. This preparation can be injected with a fine, 27-gauge needle and a control-type syringe. The toxic dose of lidocaine with epinephrine is 7 mg/kg and should be noted. During the procedure, it is often possible to keep the patient comfortable with a small amount of sedation if no contraindication exists. Sometimes topical EMLA cream (lidocaine 2.5% and prilocaine 2.5%) can be used if it is difficult to inject the patient (eg, a child) with a local anesthetic agent.

Wound Irrigation

Once anesthesia takes effect, the wound should be irrigated to help prevent future infection. However, irrigation can only be done effectively if the patient is comfortable. Saline can usually be used to irrigate the wound with a 60-mL syringe. If glass, gravel, or other foreign material is suspected to be in the wound, a finger can be used to probe the wound and remove the foreign material. Sometimes the skin is abraded so badly that the area needing to be anesthetized would be too large to safely administer lidocaine to the patient without causing lidocaine toxicity. In these cases, it is best to proceed to the operating room so that general anesthesia can be administered and the wound can be manipulated without the risk of excessive local anesthesia (Figure 7–1). In some wounds contaminated by tar, as sometimes occurs in motorcycle accidents or other road injuries, administering general anesthesia is the best recommended option for wound manipulation that is comfortable for the patient. Once the wound is thoroughly clean, povidone-iodine, commonly known as Betadine, can be used to create a sterile environment for wound closure. Any small bleeding areas can be handled with a disposable electric cautery or by using individual clamps and suture ties.

Wound Closure

Facial wound closure should heal by first intention (primary) healing whenever possible; lacerations should be closed with direct suturing to approximate skin edges. This closure can be improved with the discrete undermining of skin flaps, where necessary, to produce a tension-free closure. The key elements to obtaining good results with wound closure are (1) having a clean and sterile wound, (2) respecting anatomic boundaries, (3) avoiding tension on the suture line, and (4) having atraumatic surgical technique. The wound should be closed in layers, in the following order: (1) muscle, (2) subcutaneous tissue, (3) subcuticular tissue, and (4) superficial skin. Chromic gut sutures are useful for deep closure; fine nylon or proline stitches are useful for skin closure. Although polyglactin (eg, Vicryl) and polyglycolic acid (eg, Dexon) can also be used for deep stitches, they can sometimes become infected due to sluggish absorption, which can lead to their eventual migration out of the wound. Other dissolvable monofilament sutures may also be used for deep closure. In areas where it is difficult to remove stitches, such as around the eyelid, fast-absorbing 6–0 gut sutures or 6–0 mild chromic sutures can be used. These sutures have the advantage of leaving little trace of their placement and dissolving without requiring removal. These types of stitches may also be useful in children to prevent the need for future stitch removal or when patient follow-up is doubtful. When taking care of patients with heavy beards or dark facial hair, it is best to use a skin suture color other than black to facilitate future removal. Blue proline suture works well in these circumstances.

If wound coverage is difficult because of lost skin, transposition flaps can be used to create closure. However, these flaps are rarely necessary. If they are required, it is often best to accomplish the closure in the operating room setting as instrument sets and nursing assistance become more critical. The risk in using transposition flaps is that the wound is usually contaminated; utilizing these flaps may increase the risk of tissue loss if the wound becomes infected. In these cases, wounds may be allowed to heal by second intention (secondary) healing through the granulation and contracture process with a subsequent plan, if necessary, for wound revision.

A special circumstance of trauma involves **bite injuries,** which may be of animal, insect, or human origin. Allowing a bite injury to heal by first-intention healing should be considered carefully because the wound is likely to be contaminated. Although infection may ensue, primary closure is still recommended for these wounds after thorough irrigation and with concomitant antibiotic administration. The antibiotic coverage should be directed at a polymicrobial spectrum including α-hemolytic streptococci, *Staphylococcus aureus,* and anaerobes such as *Bacteroides.* β-lactamase stable antibiotics such as amoxicillin-clavulanic-acid combination drugs are

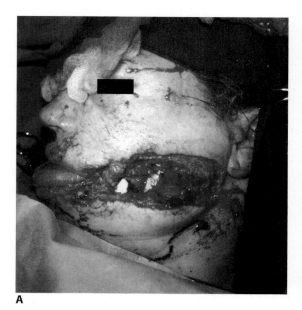

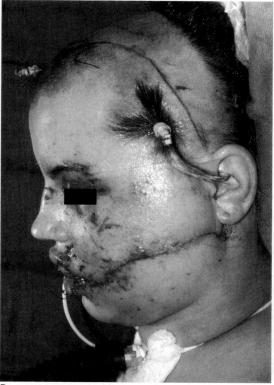

Figure 7–1. A severe laceration may sometimes require general anesthesia to properly identify cut nerves and provide a stable condition for operative closure.

B

good targeted medications for prophylaxis of these types of injuries. It is likely that the result will be no worse if an attempt at closure is made, even if the wound eventually becomes infected compared with leaving the wound open to heal by second intention.

Lackmann GM, Draf W, Isselstein G, Tollner U. Surgical treatment of facial dog-bite injuries in children. *J Craniomaxillofacial Surg.* 1992;20:81. [PMID: 1569219] (A good review of wound principles in bite injuries.)

Maas C, ed. *Wound Management and Suturing Manual.* American Academy of Facial Plastic & Reconstructive Surgery; Alexandria, VA. 2001. (An excellent overview of wound closure technique.)

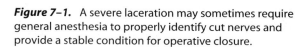

■ BURN MANAGEMENT OF THE HEAD AND NECK

During the acute management of patients with facial burns, the fundamental principles of trauma are fol-

lowed. Special attention must be directed to evaluation of the airway because airway obstruction may develop rapidly after inhalation injury. Delayed onset of obstruction within 24–48 hours may occur from progressive edema. Specific risk factors for airway compromise include a history of burn injury within a confined space, evidence of soot in the oral cavity, production of carbonaceous sputum, and concomitant facial and body burns. Laboratory evidence, including arterial blood gases and carboxyhemoglobin levels, may further suggest potential airway impairment. If time permits, serial flexible fiberoptic nasolaryngoscopy exams allow for diagnosis of oropharyngeal, true and false vocal fold edema. In management of burn patients, there should be a low threshold for early intubation.

Burns are broadly classified according to depth of penetration. First-degree burns involve the epidermis only (eg, sunburn), and clinical findings include erythema. Second-degree or partial-thickness burns involve the epidermis and a portion of the dermis. These burns are extremely painful and present with blistering and open, weeping surfaces of skin. Third-degree or full-thickness burns represent involvement of all layers of skin, including nerve endings, blood vessels, and skin appendages. As such, they are characterized as insensate, swollen, and white or gray in color. Extent of burn injury is estimated by the "rule of nines," whereby the head and neck region represents approximately 9% of total body surface area.

Inpatient management is universally required for second- or third-degree burns of the face. Early treatment goals involve the prevention of infection via sterile dressings, burn excision, and wound closure if permissible. To attenuate contracture and scar formation, temporary wound cover may be accomplished with cadaver grafts, porcine grafts, and a variety of synthetic skin substitutes. Permanent wound coverage is obtained by split-thickness skin grafts, local flaps, or microvascular free tissue transfer. Microstomia commonly results from perioral facial burns, or thermal burns that occur when small children chew electric cords. Oral splints are available for prevention of microstomia, but the efficacy of these appliances is controversial. Contracture of the eyelid, or ectropion, occurs when the eyelids are everted from the globes following burn injury. Early ophthalmologic consultation is recommended. To prevent corneal damage, early reestablishment of lid position is imperative.

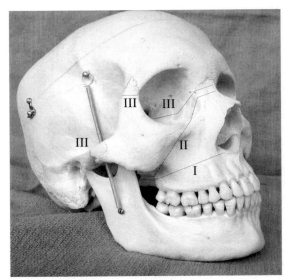

Figure 7–3. Lateral view of Le Fort midface fractures.

Bouchard CS, Morno K, Perkins J, McDonnell JF, Dicken R. Ocular complications of thermal injury: a 3-year retrospective. *J Trauma-Inj Infect Crit Care*. 2001;50:79. [PMID: 11231674]

Madnani DD, Steele NP, De Vries E. Factors that predict the need for intubation in patients with smoke inhalation injury. *Ear Nose Throat J*. 2006;85:278. [PMID: 16696366]

Yowler CJ, Fratianne RB. Current status of burn resuscitation. *Clin Plast Surg*. 2000;27:1. [PMID: 10665352]

■ SKELETAL TRAUMA

The forces of traumatic impact have a fairly predictable effect on the facial skeleton: Most force is directed through the buttress system. The buttresses consist of both vertical and horizontal systems. The horizontal buttresses are (1) the zygomatic arches, (2) the supraorbital and infraorbital rims, and (3) the glabella or nasal root (Figure 7–2). The vertical buttresses consist of (1) the frontozygomatic buttresses; (2) the maxillary buttress of the pterygoid plate; (3) the posterolateral maxillary sinus wall, which is known as the zygomaticomaxillary buttress; and (4) the frontoethmoid maxillary buttress (Figure 7–3). The successful repair of midface skeletal fractures requires an understanding of the impact of forces on the skeletal buttresses; it also requires a recognition of the weakness patterns common to this buttress system. In general, the midface creates a vertical maxillary dentition and palate height that needs to be maintained if the repair process is to maximize function.

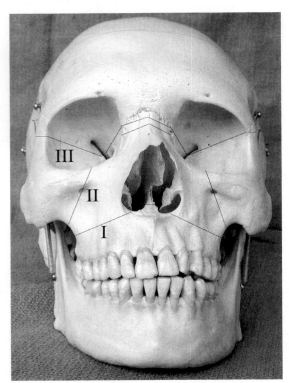

Figure 7–2. Anterior view of Le Fort midface fractures.

ORBITAL FRACTURES

Orbital fractures may occur either as a part of massive facial trauma, in conjunction with Le Fort fractures, or they may occur as isolated fractures. Orbital floor fractures known as **"blowout" fractures** are commonly encountered as isolated fractures. The mechanism of injury for these fractures is usually from direct anterior orbital trauma, such as from a fist or from a ball during a sporting activity. The orbit is made up of buttresses connected by very thin bones that include maxilla, sphenoid, lacrimal, frontal, zygomatic, ethmoid, and palatine bones. The orbital floor is also the roof of the maxillary sinus and has a natural weakness where the second division of the trigeminal nerve traverses it; the bone in this area is quite thin. Sudden anterior pressure on the orbital contents can cause a fracture of the orbital floor, which results in periorbital fat sagging into the maxillary sinus. In some cases, the inferior orbital rim may be involved at the level of the infraorbital foramen, which may also result in numbness in the V2 distribution (ie, the second division of the trigeminal nerve).

Not all orbital floor fractures require exploration and repair. Orbital fractures need surgical intervention under the following circumstances: (1) they cause entrapment of the extraocular muscles, resulting in gaze limitation or diplopia; (2) the patient has sagging of the orbital contents, causing enophthalmos and subsequent diplopia; or (3) imaging studies reveal a greatly increased relative orbital volume (greater than 5–10% relative increase when compared with the noninjured side) due to the loss of the orbital floor and sagging of the contents into the maxillary sinus. In this latter scenario, the patient is at risk for late enophthalmos, and repair would be more easily accomplished within a few weeks of the injury rather than months later, when scarring will cause the procedure to be more difficult. It is highly recommended to obtain a baseline ophthalmologic exam of vision acuity and range of motion for all patients with orbital fractures, especially before proceeding with operative repair. A fine-cut axial and coronal CT scan of the orbits is essential for operative planning. The ideal time for the repair is often 7–14 days after the injury; much of the edema from the trauma will have subsided and the repair technique will be easier to precisely gauge. The operative technique involves either a subciliary or transconjunctival incision, both of which give access to the orbital periosteum. The orbital contents are then raised out of the fracture line and supported with a titanium plate, cartilage, bone, absorbable plate, or other material. Many permanent orbital implant materials have a long history of use, including Medpore (ie, porous polyethylene), Marlex (ie, polypropylene mesh), silicone, and other materials. They all have the possibility of late extrusion. Titanium has the advantage of being able to be fixed to bone via screws, which decreases the chance of late migration. Titanium is also biocompatible. Conchal or nasal cartilage is autologous and is therefore a good material for supporting orbital repairs of this type. After the repair is completed, a forced duction test of extraocular motility should be performed to ensure that any entrapment of the extraocular muscles is relieved.

Manolidis S, Weeks BH, Kirby M, Scarlett M, Hollier L. Classification and surgical management of orbital fractures: experience with 111 orbital reconstructions. *J Craniofac Surg.* 2002;(6):726. [PMID: 12457084] (An excellent review of methods of orbital fracture repair.)

Manson PN, Clark N, Robertson B et al. Subunit principles in midface fractures: the importance of sagittal buttresses, soft-tissue reductions, and sequencing treatment of segmental fractures. *Plast Reconstr Surg.* 1999;103:1287. [PMID: 10088523] (A definitive and well-organized review article that emphasizes treatment principles.)

NASOETHMOID COMPLEX FRACTURES

The nasoethmoid complex involves both a horizontal and a vertical buttress. The horizontal buttress is the nasal root and the vertical buttress is the frontonasal maxillary pillar. Nasoethmoid complex fractures usually require high velocity and a more powerful force in order to be produced compared with isolated nasal fractures or orbital floor fractures. The key physical findings are often severe orbital swelling and ecchymosis with traumatic telecanthus (widening of the intercanthal distance), which gives the impression of widening of the eyes. Because of the close proximity of the ethmoid bone to the skull base, skull base trauma and cerebrospinal fluid (CSF) leak should be suspected in patients who sustain nasoethmoid complex fractures; neurosurgical consultation is therefore advisable.

Because the anterior ethmoid cells have an impact on frontal sinus drainage, patients with severe nasoethmoid complex fractures may require follow-up to ensure that the frontal sinus drainage is physiologically functional. If it is not, a late frontoethmoid or frontal sinus mucocele may occur, with the potential for eye or brain involvement. The key to repairing nasoethmoid complex fractures is the reestablishment of the midline vertical height of the nasal root. Reestablishing the midline vertical height prevents late deformity and restores the medial canthal tendon to an anatomically functional position. It is important to keep in mind that the normal intercanthal distance is 30–35 mm.

The surgical approach to repair a nasoethmoid complex fracture is often accomplished through a bicoronal forehead flap, which gives an excellent exposure of the nasal root to allow fracture reduction. Alternative techniques include a midfacial degloving incision or a bilateral external ethmoidectomy incision with a connection via the glabella; the latter procedure is known as the "open sky" approach. Small midface plates in various configurations can be used to painstakingly replace the shattered nasal and ethmoid bones into their anatomic positions. Occasionally, the medial canthal tendons must be retrieved and reapproximated with fine-gauge stainless-steel wire, either to titanium plates or to holes drilled in the lacrimal bone. Late diplopia can occur if the medial orbital attachments are not replaced optimally.

Cultrara A, Turk JB, Har-El G. Midfacial degloving approach for repair of naso-orbital-ethmoid and midfacial fractures. *Arch Facial Plast Surg.* 2004;6(2):133. [PMID: 15023802] (An excellent discussion of a useful surgical approach to facial trauma.)

Potter JK, Muzaffar AR, Ellis E et al. Aesthetic management of the nasal component of naso-orbital ethmoid fractures. *Plast Reconstr Surg.* 2006;117(1):10e–18e. [PMID: 16404240] (A definitive and well-organized article that emphasizes treatment principles.)

Sargent La, Rogers GF. Nasoethmoid complex fractures: diagnosis and management. *J Craniomaxillofacial Trauma.* 1999;5(1):19. [PMID: 11951221] (A good review of NEC fractures.)

ZYGOMATIC COMPLEX FRACTURES

The zygomatic complex, also known as the trimalar complex, is a facial bone commonly injured in low-velocity trauma. Lateral trauma sometimes produces an isolated zygomatic arch fracture; however, more severe force can fracture the entire zygomatic complex. Although commonly referred to as a "tripod" fracture, this name is a misnomer: a zygomatic complex fracture constitutes four discrete fractures. The components of this fracture are (1) the zygomatic arch, (2) the orbital rim, (3) the frontozygomatic buttress, and (4) the zygomatico-maxillary buttress. Patients often present with infraorbital ecchymosis and occasionally with paresthesia in the V2 distribution. There is a loss of cheek prominence, with asymmetry upon inspection. The asymmetry can be most noticeable when the patient's head is tilted back and viewed from beneath the chin. Ophthalmologic consultation should be encouraged for a patient with a zygomatic complex fracture because the repair involves manipulating the inferior and lateral orbit walls, which may affect vision. Occasionally, tooth roots can also be involved in the fracture; therefore, an inspection of the dentition is recommended as part of the presenting history and physical exam.

The repair of zygomatic fractures is often accomplished on an elective basis. Isolated arch fractures can be elevated via a classic Gillies approach. The Gillies technique involves three steps: (1) creating an incision behind the temporal hairline, (2) identifying the temporalis fascia, and (3) placing an elevator beneath the fascia to approach the arch from its deep aspect. By sliding the elevator in the plane deep to the fascia, injury to the frontal branch of the facial nerve is avoided. The arch can then be levered into a more normal anatomic position. An alternate approach, called Keen's approach, is to place an elevator via a transoral gingival buccal sulcus incision underneath the arch; the elevator then passes through the buccal space with the elevation of the arch taking place. Zygomatic complex fractures can also be approached with the same transgingival buccal sulcus incision, which can give access as high as the orbital rim. One four-hole, midface titanium plate is enough to counteract the muscular forces to reduce and fix the fracture. However, it is usually desirable to expose at least two of the four buttresses in order to allow an accurate reduction of these fractures. A small incision at the lateral brow or superior eyelid crease may be necessary to access the frontozygomatic buttress; alternately, a transconjunctival or subciliary incision may be needed to access the infraorbital rim (Figure 7–4). In rare cases, a bicoronal or a unicoronal approach may be used to obtain direct access to the zygomatic arch (1) if the fracture is very severe, (2) in cases of severe orbital-zygomatic fractures, or (3) in cases of bilateral zygomatic complex fractures. The main goals in operating on these fractures are to restore symmetry to the face and to prevent late orbital complications such as enophthalmos.

Manson PN, Clark N, Robertson B et al. Subunit principles in midface fractures: the importance of sagittal buttresses, soft-tissue reductions, and sequencing treatment of segmental fractures. *Plast Reconstr Surg.* 1999;103:1287. [PMID: 10088523] (A definitive and well-organized review article that emphasizes treatment principles.)

Rinehart GC, Marsh JL, Hemmer KM, Bresina S. Internal fixation of malar fractures: an experimental biophysical study. *Plast Reconstr Surg.* 1989;84(1):21. [PMID: 2734399] (A good study of the forces needed to stabilize ZMC fractures.)

MAXILLARY FRACTURES

Midface maxillary fractures are usually the result of high-velocity injuries (eg, motor vehicle accidents or severe and life-threatening interpersonal trauma). The primary surgical goals in repairing maxillary fractures include restoring normal contour to the facial skeleton and restoring normal dental occlusion.

Maxillary fractures were classified by René Le Fort. He subjected cadavers to various types of trauma and found that certain patterns of injury resulted. Le Fort divided these midface fractures into three discrete types: Le Fort I, Le Fort II, and Le Fort III. (Figures 7–2 and 7–3 display Le Fort fracture characteristics.)

1. Le Fort I Fractures

Le Fort I fractures are fractures that separate the palate from the midface and, by definition, involve the pterygoid plates bilaterally. This fracture type results in a mobile palate but a stable upper midface. Patients

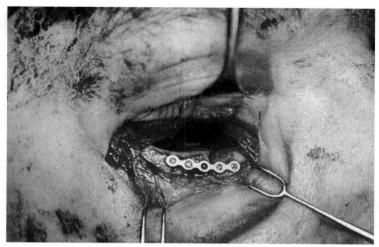

Figure 7–4. A midface reconstruction plate placed on the orbital rim via a subciliary approach.

present with malocclusion and an anterior open-bite deformity. The deformity occurs because the pull of the muscles of mastication forces the palate to slide backward, retruding the maxillary teeth. Airway compromise can occur if the palate retrusion is severe. The operative strategy in repairing Le Fort I fractures is to reduce the fracture by aligning the dentition into as normal a configuration as possible.

Normal physiologic occlusion is referred to as **Class I occlusion.** It takes place when the mesiobuccal cusp of the maxillary first molar interdigitates with the mesiobuccal groove of the mandibular first molar. **Class II occlusion** occurs when the mandible is relatively retrognathic or retruded. **Class III occlusion** occurs when the mandible is relatively prognathic or protruded. The key goal in repairing any fracture involving the dentition is to reduce the fracture to the premorbid occlusion. This goal is best accomplished with a Class I occlusion. The surgical access for the repair of a Le Fort I fracture is often obtained via bilateral maxillary gingival buccal sulcus incisions; these incisions expose the anterior maxillary wall as well as the lateral and anterior maxillary buttresses. Intermaxillary fixation using either skeletal screws or arch bars with wires is used to pull the fractures into ideal occlusion. Occasionally, reduction forceps may be necessary to bring the palate back into functional occlusion. Once the fracture is reduced and stabilized, titanium miniplates, which have low profile but great strength, are screwed directly to the maxilla both to create permanent stability and, ideally, to restore midface height and functional occlusion. The blood supply to the maxilla is quite rich and only rarely do complications such as osteomyelitis or sequestrum occur. Even small frag-

ments of bone often survive if well fixed with the miniplate systems. If the fracture is so severe that no solid bone can be used to provide stable fixation, split calvarial bone grafts or grafts from the iliac crest can be plated into position to provide a stable repair. However, if the fracture is minimally displaced, sometimes intermaxillary fixation alone for 4–6 weeks will allow an excellent recovery.

2. Le Fort II Fractures

Le Fort II fractures involve the pterygoid plates, the frontonasal maxillary buttress, and often the skull base via the ethmoid bone. This fracture, therefore, has a pyramidal appearance and results in palatal and upper-midface mobility. Because of the large amount of force required to cause Le Fort II fractures, patients who have this type of fracture often have other injuries as well, including orthopedic and neurosurgical problems (Figure 7–5). The skull base may be involved, and so nasotracheal intubation should be avoided in the acute setting because a nasal tube could potentially be forced through the fracture and into an intracranial cavity. CSF leakage is common in this type of midface fracture. The initial medical stabilization is often accomplished in the intensive care unit. Fine-cut computerized imaging, usually CT scanning (possibly with three-dimensional reconstruction), is desirable as it allows for adequate operative planning once the patient's condition has stabilized (Figure 7–6). Patient stabilization often requires several days of convalescence.

The operative approach to Le Fort II fractures requires alignment of the dentition into Class I occlusion, using wires or screws to reduce the fracture. This

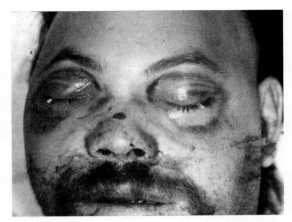

Figure 7–5. A patient with "raccoon eyes" and a mid-face fracture. Neurosurgical evaluation is important.

approach is known as intermaxillary fixation. Following intermaxillary fixation, the maxillary buttresses need to be surgically exposed to allow miniplate fixation. Many strategies can be used to accomplish the exposure, including bilateral gingival buccal sulcus incisions together with incisions designed to approach nasoethmoid complex fractures. The midface degloving incision, which uses a rhinoplasty-type intranasal exposure, combined with the gingival buccal sulcus incisions, often provides excellent access in placing the titanium miniplates in this type of fracture.

3. Le Fort III Fractures

Le Fort III fractures involve the same types of force as Le Fort II fractures; however, Le Fort III fractures result from a greater *degree* of force than type II fractures. A consultative team approach is best for these severely injured patients. In addition to injuring the pterygoid plate and the frontonasal maxillary buttress (as is found with Le Fort II fractures), Le Fort III fractures involve the frontozygomatic buttress. These fractures therefore result in complete craniofacial dislocations. In addition, associated neurosurgical injuries are often seen in patients with Le Fort III fractures.

The preoperative issues associated with Le Fort III fractures are similar to those seen in Le Fort II cases. After intermaxillary fixation, a bicoronal approach is used to facilitate the repair of the frontozygomatic buttress and zygomatic arch. This approach allows excellent access to the lateral and medial buttress systems in order both to restore the adequate vertical height of the occlusion and to provide stable fixation. A midfacial degloving approach is often combined with the bicoronal approach to allow access to the lower maxilla for plating (Figure 7–7). It is not uncommon to recom-

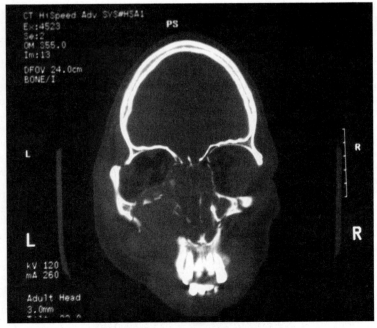

Figure 7–6. A CT scan of a midface fracture is essential for operative planning.

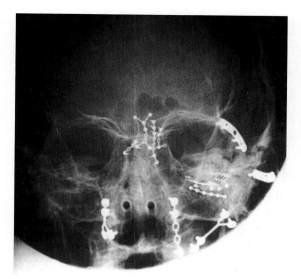

Figure 7–7. A postoperative plain film x-ray shows the locations of the plates that have stabilized the midface fracture.

mend elective tracheotomy for these patients in the postoperative period. This approach is recommended for several reasons: (1) nasotracheal intubation is usually not safe for a patient with this degree of injury because of the risk of frontal skull base injury; (2) the patient must be placed into intermaxillary fixation; (3) owing to related neurosurgical issues, the patient usually has a fairly prolonged need for the attention of an intensive care unit; and (4) the reduction of this type of severe fracture also causes temporary but significant upper airway edema. Again, a team approach to the treatment of patients with this type of severe injury often increases the prognosis for a favorable recovery.

Manson PN, Clark N, Robertson B et al. Subunit principles in midface fractures: the importance of sagittal buttresses, soft-tissue reductions, and sequencing treatment of segmental fractures. *Plast Reconstr Surg.* 1999;103(4):1287. [PMID: 10088523] (A definitive and well-organized review article that emphasizes treatment principles.)

MANDIBLE FRACTURES

Mandible fractures can be part of both high-velocity and low-velocity traumas. Mandible fractures may occur as a result of sports activities, falls, motor vehicle accidents, and interpersonal trauma. In busy inner-city emergency departments, mandible fractures are seen almost daily. Patients often present acutely and may be intoxicated by alcohol or illicit substances. Patients sometimes present the morning after the injury, when they are no longer intoxicated and realize that a problem exists due to pain and malocclusion.

Patients with mandible fractures often have pain with attempts at mastication; this symptom usually results in their seeking medical attention. Other symptoms include malocclusion and numbness of the third division of the trigeminal nerve. The initial examination should note any sensory nerve deficit and associated dental injury, such as cracked or missing teeth. The mobility of a mandibular segment is a key physical diagnostic finding in confirming a mandible fracture. However, this mobility can vary with the location of the fracture. Fractures can occur in the anterior mandible (symphysial and parasymphysial), along the body of the mandible, at the angle of the mandible, or in the ramus or condylar regions (Figure 7–8). Most fractures of the symphysis, the mandible body, and the mandible angle are open fractures that will reveal mobility upon palpation. However, condyle fractures are extremely common; they typically are not open to the oral cavity and may only present as malocclusion with some pain.

Plain x-ray films are extremely helpful in determining both the presence and type of a mandible fracture. To help delineate the extent of the fractures, a mandible series usually consists of several different views: (1) a Towne's view to examine the condyles, (2) a submental-vertex view, (3) a posteroanterior view, and (4) both left and right lateral oblique views. Often, the fracture is bilateral; therefore, the presence of a right-body fracture should alert the physician to search carefully for a fracture on the opposite side. Panorex-view plain film x-rays help to delineate the condyle and angle regions and, if available, are excellent studies (Figure 7–9).

Mandible fractures may be displaced and distracted by the pull of the muscles of mastication. When this occurs, it is termed an **unfavorable fracture.** In contrast, some fractures form in such a way that the muscles of mastication tend to help keep the fracture well aligned; this type of fracture is termed a **favorable fracture.** Fractures in adolescents are often in excellent alignment because the bone is more flexible. These fractures are referred to as **greenstick fractures** and may require less immobilization time in order to heal.

A number of approaches allow for the optimal healing of a mandible fracture; however, the first step in fracture repair is the assessment of dental occlusion. The major principle in treating a mandible fracture is to place the patient into intermaxillary fixation; this positioning approximates the premorbid occlusion. In practice, this often means that the surgeon will try to reduce the fracture to produce a Class I occlusion. Placing a patient into intermaxillary fixation requires an assessment of the existing dentition and an inspection of the way in which the teeth interdigitate. Often, wear facets on the teeth can help guide the restoration of a good functional occlusion.

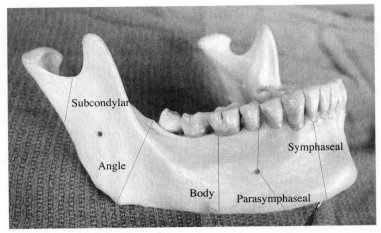

Figure 7–8. Subunit regions of the mandible.

The AO/ASIF (Arbeitsgemeinschaft Für Osteosynthesefragen, the Association for the Study of Internal Fixation), a study group that crosses a number of specialty lines, developed and continues to refine fixation techniques. They have also established guidelines for closed and open rigid fixation.

Closed splinting approaches rely either on arch bars and intermaxillary fixation or on skeletal fixation with titanium screws. Immobilization for a period of 4–6 weeks is necessary to allow secondary bone healing. Therefore, patients have their jaws wired into centric occlusion without the ability to open their mouths for an extended period of time. Patients must be on a liquid diet during the time period; many lose weight. If a patient becomes nauseated and vomits while his or her jaws are wired shut, there is a risk of aspiration with subsequent pneumonia; in the worst case, airway compromise is possible. Although this technique is the

least surgically invasive approach, the disadvantages are that it (1) requires a great deal of patient cooperation, (2) requires close and intensive patient follow-up, and (3) can lead to functional temporomandibular joint problems owing to a prolonged lack of use. In patients with substance abuse issues, the lack of postoperative cooperation can lead to malunion, nonunion, and osteomyelitis, all with devastating effects. The advantages of extended immobilization are that (1) closed intermaxillary fixation minimizes risk to the mandibular and facial nerves; (2) it allows some flexibility in achieving the exact premorbid occlusion, thus minimizing the chance of iatrogenic malocclusion; and (3) it makes wound dehiscence unlikely.

The advantage of **open rigid fixation** techniques is that fractures are stabilized with titanium plates and screws, essentially allowing functional mastication immediately after surgery. These plating systems can also allow

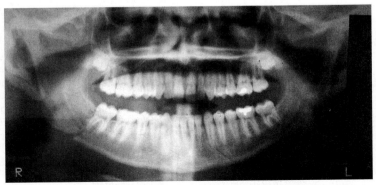

Figure 7–9. A Panorex plain film x-ray can be helpful in identifying mandible fractures.

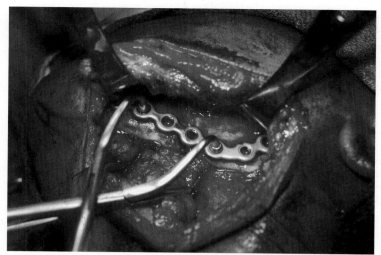

Figure 7–10. A reconstruction plate placed via an external incision on an angle fracture.

primary bone healing due to the compression of the bone fracture segments, in contrast to secondary bone healing, which occurs through callus formation that occurs with other approximation techniques. Open rigid plating techniques also allow immediate postoperative function, which can help to prevent iatrogenic temporomandibular joint fixation caused by prolonged periods of immobilization (Figure 7–10). Nevertheless, plating techniques applied to the mandible are highly technique sensitive; iatrogenic postoperative malocclusion and injury to the mandibular, mental, or facial nerve are known complications of the technique. The need for postoperative patient cooperation, however, is minimized with the adequate application of the AO principles.

Surgical approaches to mandible fractures can rely on either transoral or external incisions. Decisions must be made about whether to use compressive or noncompressive reconstruction plates, depending on the type and location of the fracture. Lag-screw and miniplate techniques can also play a role in the internal fixation of mandible fractures. The repair of these fractures is technique sensitive, however, and requires selective patient application. In addition, bilateral condylar fractures may be approached with minimally invasive endoscopic techniques.

Postoperatively, patients with mandible fractures are usually kept on oral antibiotic coverage and oral rinses with topical antimicrobial solutions such as chlorhexidine. Plate extrusion is fairly infrequent, but local infection with the loosening of screws and plates may need to be addressed with local debridement and placement of a heavier reconstruction plate system. Wound repair failures are more often due to the choice of an inadequate fixation system or a retained or cracked tooth root than to the rejection of the titanium hardware. If necessary, a transcutaneous external fixation system (known as a Joe Hall Morris appliance) may be useful, although the need to resort to this type of external fixation is rare.

Biller JA, Pletcher SD, Goldberg AN, Murr AH. Complications and the time to repair of mandible fractures. *Laryngoscope.* 2005;115(5):769. [PMID: 15867637] (Analyzes the causes of complications as it relates to the timing of repair of mandible fractures, and it relates the incidence to several types of patient factors.)

Kaplan BA, Hoard MA, Park S et al. Immediate mobilization following fixation of mandible fractures: a prospective, randomized study. *Laryngoscope.* 2001;111:1520. [PMID: 11572207] (An excellent prospective study looking at the issues surrounding alternative plating techniques for fractures.)

Murr AH. Mandibular angle fractures and noncompression plating techniques. *Arch Otolaryngol Head Neck Surg.* 2005;131(2):166. No abstract available. [PMID: 15723951] [PubMed indexed for MEDLINE] (Good summary of philosophies of managing various types of mandible fractures using several types of fixation approaches.)

Cutaneous Malignant Neoplasms

8

C. Patrick Hybarger, MD, FACS

Cutaneous malignant neoplasms encompass a large spectrum of tumors that may arise from any of the component cells in skin or its underlying structures. This chapter separates pediatric tumors from those that predominantly affect adults; it further separates nonmelanoma skin cancer from melanoma.

■ PEDIATRIC NEOPLASMS

Many lesions are present at birth or shortly thereafter. Some have the potential for malignant transformation later in life; other lesions may be mistaken for a malignant growth.

BENIGN NEOPLASMS

DERMOID CYSTS

Dermoid cysts may be seen at birth as smooth, cystic tumors that may have both solid and cystic components. The cysts are usually attached to periosteum, are lined with keratinizing epidermis, and may contain hair and fat in addition to keratinous debris. Clinical examination most often shows tumors located in the lateral periocular or nasal areas. Because of tumor fixation to the underlying periosteum, the tumor may feel immobile when palpated. Treatment is simple excision, which may be delayed until later in childhood.

PILOMATRIXOMA

Pilomatrixoma is usually a benign subcutaneous tumor that originates from the hair matrix and may show calcification. Clinical examination usually shows the tumors as stony-hard, slow-growing, deep subcutaneous masses that develop in early childhood. Rarely, invasive malignant variants with metastases have been reported. Treatment is simple excision.

SEBACEOUS NEVI

Sebaceous nevi are noted at birth as linear, raised, and tan- to yellow-colored patches on the scalp, face, or neck. The nevi may be several centimeters in size or much larger. Regression of the nevi is common until puberty, when growth of the nevi accelerates and lesions become multinodular and darker. Benign syringocystadenoma papilliferum, as well as various types of malignant neoplasms including basal cell carcinoma, squamous cell carcinoma, and adnexal tumors, may arise in adulthood. To provide optimum cosmesis and to minimize the risk of these malignant growths, patients should be treated in preadolescence with simple excision of the nevi.

NEUROFIBROMA

Neurofibroma may appear singly or may be multiple in **von Recklinghausen disease** or NF-1 (ie, neurofibromatosis with von Recklinghausen disease) and present as soft, skin-colored nodules composed of nerve cells, mast cells, and oval- to spindle-shaped nuclei in a wavy collagen matrix. The neurofibromatous nodules are usually unencapsulated and may infiltrate fat. Café au lait spots are associated with multiple neurofibromatous lesions and are usually excised for cosmetic or functional reasons. Neurofibrosarcoma may rarely develop in syndromic patients.

INFANTILE MYOFIBROMATOSIS

In infantile myofibromatosis, single or multiple fibrous, firm nodules composed of fibroblasts and smooth muscle cells are present at birth or in early childhood. The nodules are palpable, firm, and either cutaneous or subcutaneous. Lytic lesions of the cranium may occur in as many as one third of children, and visceral nodules are associated with the multicentric form. Visceral nodules may be confused with a malignant growth; indeed, the visceral form of infantile myofibromatosis is frequently fatal. Lesions occurring in the superficial, nonvisceral form usually resolve. Lesions compromising function should be treated with biopsy or excision.

CONGENITAL MELANOCYTIC NEVI

Congenital melanocytic nevi may be seen at birth or several months later as either flat or raised brown lesions, with or without hair, and usually with areas of deeper black or blue pigment. The estimated lifetime risk of developing melanocytic lesions is roughly proportional to the size of the nevus and may be as high as 8%; because of the predictable increased risk, early full-thickness surgical excision for large nevi is advocated where technically feasible.

BENIGN (TYPICAL) ACQUIRED NEVI

Benign (typical) acquired nevi begin early in childhood and are usually smaller than 5 mm. They may be flat or raised, have symmetric, smooth, and well-defined borders, and have uniform pigmentation, which may range from flesh-colored to brown. Evidence supports a higher lifetime risk of cutaneous melanoma in patients who have more than 50 benign nevi.

Wyatt AJ, Hansen RC. Pediatric skin tumors. *Pediatr Clin North Am.* 2000;47:937. [PMID: 10943267] (Comprehensive review of common childhood cutaneous malignant neoplasms and lesions that mimic malignant growths.)

MALIGNANT NEOPLASMS

In children, malignant skin tumors may develop sporadically or occur in precursor syndromes with associated abnormalities in other organ systems. The most common precursor syndromes for malignant cutaneous tumors in children are nevoid basal cell syndrome and xeroderma pigmentosum.

ATYPICAL NEVI (DYSPLASTIC NEVUS SYNDROME)

Atypical nevi (dysplastic nevus syndrome) may be familial or occur sporadically. These nevi are usually flat, but they may have a raised center; they may be dark or pigmented in a variegated distribution. The nevi increase in number over years and show histologic features, such as melanocytic atypia and hyperplasia.

Patients with atypical nevi have an increased risk for either the familial or the nonfamilial forms of cutaneous melanoma; this risk is related both to a large number of nevi and to a family history of cutaneous melanoma. Individuals without a family history of melanoma have a 184-fold increased risk for the familial form of melanoma, whereas individuals with a family history of melanoma have a 500-fold increased risk of the disease. The estimated risk for the sporadic form of melanoma is related to the number of dysplastic nevi: a 12-fold increase in risk is estimated for individuals who have more than 10 dysplastic nevi.

NEVOID BASAL CELL CARCINOMA SYNDROME

Among patients with nevoid basal cell carcinoma syndrome, inactivation of the "patched" PTC tumor suppressor gene has been found in both the sporadic and the autosomal-dominant familial forms. Multiple areas of nevoid basal cell carcinoma may develop before the patient reaches 20 years of age. Clinically, in addition to having many basal cell nevi, patients may present with frontal bossing, mandibular cysts, palmar pits, calcified falx cerebri, and one or more skeletal abnormalities. Treatment for small, well-defined areas of basal cell carcinoma is simple excision; treatment is Mohs micrographic excision for recurrent or poorly defined lesions, or lesions located in anatomic areas at high risk for malignant disease.

XERODERMA PIGMENTOSUM SYNDROME

Xeroderma pigmentosum syndrome is inherited as an autosomal-recessive trait in which defects are discovered during the repair of sun-induced DNA damage. Seven genes have been implicated in xeroderma pigmentosum, which manifests in a variety of phenotypes, depending on the specific patterns of mutation. Basal cell carcinoma, squamous cell carcinoma, and cutaneous melanoma may develop in large numbers (preceded by xeroderma pigmentosum) at an early age and in a general anatomic distribution similar to sporadic cases in adults. Clinically, children affected by xeroderma pigmentosum (1) have an onset of extensive freckling early in childhood, (2) are extremely photosensitive, and (3) have an estimated 2000-fold increase in basal cell carcinoma, squamous cell carcinoma, and cutaneous melanoma. These conditions in children occur most commonly on the face, head, and neck; squamous cell carcinoma occurs with notable frequency at the tongue tip. Treatment of xeroderma pigmentosum is total avoidance of the sun, a strategy that is necessary for reducing the number of new tumors. Recent studies with topically applied liposomal T4 endonuclease-V indicate that it may show promise in reducing the number of new skin cancers in these children.

MALIGNANT CUTANEOUS MELANOMA

Malignant cutaneous melanoma is rare in childhood but is more common among children who have a family history of melanoma, large congenital nevus, large or many dysplastic nevi, xeroderma pigmentosum syndrome, or a history of immunosuppression. In addition, convincing evidence indicates that the incidence of cutaneous melanoma is higher among children who have more than 50 benign melanocytic nevi. The essential aspects of clinical diagnosis are generally the same for children as for adults. Areas of pigment change, pain, or ulceration in large congenital nevi may indicate malignant change.

The overall treatment parallels adult guidelines and is based on the tumor thickness, the presence or absence of tumor ulceration, and the nodal status. However, the prognosis for cutaneous melanoma in children may be worse than in adults because a disproportionate number of nodular cutaneous melanoma cases in children are associated with a rapid vertical growth phase of the tumor.

In situ melanoma is excised with 7-mm margins or with Mohs micrographic frozen-section margins to minimize the surgical defect size. No further work-up is necessary.

Stage I primary tumors < 2 mm without histologic evidence of ulceration can be excised with 1-cm margins. If ulceration is present, 2-cm margins should be used and a chest x-ray should be performed.

Stage II lesions are excised with 2-cm margins where feasible; for high-risk lesions, consideration should be given to computed tomography (CT) scanning of the neck as well as sentinel lymph node biopsy or neck dissection. Recent studies have shown benefits from using high-dose interferon alfa-2b in high-risk patients.

Stage III primary neoplasms can also be excised with 2-cm margins down to the fascia, with CT scanning performed and regional lymphatics treated surgically. The postoperative treatment should include radiation as well as high-dose interferon.

Stage IV melanoma carries an extremely poor prognosis, but an attempt should be made to control local and regional disease where possible, as well as defining the extent and the location of systemic disease in order to tailor individual treatment strategies.

The overall survival in childhood melanoma is related to the stage at presentation and generally parallels that of adults: the 5-year survival rate in Stage I disease is about 95%, with the rate dropping to 65% in Stage II and 45% in Stage III disease. There are essentially no survivors in those patients who present with systemic disease.

SUBCUTANEOUS RHABDOMYOSARCOMA

Subcutaneous rhabdomyosarcoma is a poorly differentiated sarcoma; the diagnosis may require immunohistochemical staining. Clinically, the tumor usually presents singly as a firm, reddish or brown, semifixed, noncompressible subcutaneous nodule that becomes enlarged and may deform local structures. These tumors are more common in females and at a mean age of 2–3 years. Currently,

surgical excision is recommended where it is technically feasible. Alternatively, radiation and multidrug chemotherapy are recommended.

Saenz NC, Saenz-Badillos J, Busam K et al. Childhood melanoma survival. *Cancer.* 1999;85(3):750. [PMID: 100911749] (An institutional review from Sloan-Kettering of melanoma in patients younger than 18 years.)

Tsao H. Genetics of nonmelanoma skin cancer. *Arch Dermatol.* 2001;137:1486. [PMID: 11708952] (A review of the contribution of genetic processes and of mutation of DNA material to the origin of skin cancer.)

■ ADULT NEOPLASMS

Many benign lesions of childhood (eg, nevi and vascular malformations) persist into adulthood and may undergo change or be difficult to distinguish from tumors more commonly seen in adults.

BENIGN NEOPLASMS

Seborrheic keratoses and chondrodermatitis helicis are the benign tumors most commonly confused with cutaneous malignant tumors. In addition, many varieties of benign skin tumors (eg, dermatofibroma and benign adnexal tumors) may be difficult to distinguish from nonmelanoma skin cancer unless a biopsy is performed.

SEBORRHEIC KERATOSIS

Seborrheic keratosis is a tumor of unknown origin that is unique to adults. Histologically, it may exist in a variety of forms, all of which show hyperkeratosis, papillomatosis, and acanthosis. When the tumor is chronically irritated, whorls of squamous cells may be present with areas of keratin horn pearls and must be distinguished histologically from squamous cell carcinoma. Clinically, the lesions may be flat, raised, smooth, or verrucous and frequently appear to be "pasted" on the skin (Figure 8–1). Their color may vary from tan to black, and lesions containing pigment may mimic cutaneous melanoma. The lesions have no malignant potential. Treatment may be indicated for cosmetic reasons, and the lesions can be frozen with liquid nitrogen or removed by shave biopsy.

CHONDRODERMATITIS NODULARIS HELICIS

Chondrodermatitis nodularis helicis typically manifests as an ulcer filled with necrotic dermal debris as well as

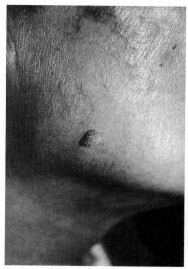

Figure 8–1. A lesion of seborrheic keratosis. (Photo courtesy of John Maddox, MD.)

adjacent granulations with degenerative changes in cartilage. Dystrophic calcification also may be present. The lesions may be seen clinically on the auricular helix as nodules that can be quite painful and may be confused with squamous cell carcinoma. Treatment is intralesional steroid therapy or simple excision.

Pariser RJ. Benign neoplasms of the skin. *Med Clin North Am.* 1998;82:1285. [PMID: 9889749] (A review of the clinical aspects of common benign cutaneous lesions.)

MALIGNANT NEOPLASMS

Cutaneous malignant lesions in adults are commonly classified as either nonmelanoma skin cancer or cutaneous melanoma. Many lesions have distinct clinical features that provide clues to the diagnosis; considerable overlap exists, however, and biopsy is almost always necessary to plan treatment. To some extent, the biopsy technique is dictated by the tentative clinical diagnosis: **shave biopsy** is an adequate treatment for exophytic nodules thought to be nonmelanoma skin cancer, whereas **punch biopsy** is necessary for flat lesions. Excisional biopsy with a 2-mm margin is preferred for pigmented lesions thought to present a high risk for cutaneous melanoma. Deep punch biopsies into subcutaneous fat in the deepest or darkest portions of the lesion also may be performed in selected lesions. Although no evidence exists showing an adverse effect of biopsy, shave biopsy in cutaneous melanoma is to be discouraged when melanoma is suspected. Moreover, wide, local excision may produce scarring that interferes with lymphatic drainage when sentinel node biopsy is later performed. An adequate amount of tissue must be obtained for processing with special stains in the event that an exact histologic diagnosis is difficult, as is frequently the case with rare or poorly differentiated nonmelanoma skin cancer. Photographs of the lesion or the biopsy defect may be valuable for identifying the exact location of the original lesion when definitive surgery is done at a later date.

NONMELANOMA SKIN CANCER

General Considerations

Nonmelanoma skin cancer may be divided into common and rare categories. Basal cell carcinoma, the most common skin cancer, constitutes about 75% of nonmelanoma skin cancer cases; squamous cell carcinoma accounts for about 20% of cases. The remaining 5% of rare nonmelanoma skin cancer cases includes fibrohistiocytic and adnexal cancers. Basal cell carcinoma, squamous cell carcinoma, and some rare types of nonmelanoma skin cancers occur more frequently in sun-exposed areas and in light-skinned individuals with light eye and hair color; they are associated with unrepaired DNA mutations induced by UV-A and UV-B radiation. The incidence of both basal cell carcinoma and squamous cell carcinoma has steadily increased during the past several decades, and nonmelanoma skin cancer is now a clinically significant health problem and a source of morbidity. Both conditions are more common in patients exposed to ionizing radiation. Basal cell carcinoma and squamous cell carcinoma also occur more frequently in patients with HIV; patients with lymphoproliferative disorders, particularly chronic lymphocytic leukemia; and patients receiving long-term immunosuppressive drug therapy after organ transplantation.

Differential Diagnosis

Rare types of nonmelanoma skin cancers include fibrohistiocytic tumors, adnexal cancers, and rare cutaneous sarcoma. Special histochemical stains are frequently necessary for distinguishing varieties of nonmelanoma skin cancer, especially adnexal tumors.

Treatment

Treatment of nonmelanoma skin cancer is determined by many factors, including the exact histologic subtype, the tumor size, the growth characteristics, and the anatomic location. Treatment is also determined by the previous treatment received, current medical problems, and patient expectations. Treatment options for nonmelanoma skin cancer can be categorized as nonsurgical and surgical.

A. NONSURGICAL MEASURES

Nonsurgical strategies include topical or injection chemotherapy (eg, with 5-fluorouracil [5-FU], a 5% preparation of imiquimod, or interferon), cryotherapy using liquid nitrogen, photodynamic therapy, and radiation therapy.

1. Topical drug therapy—Topical drug therapy is limited to lesions confined to the epidermis, such as superficial basal cell carcinoma and squamous cell carcinoma in situ (Bowen disease). A 5% preparation of 5-FU cream used in conjunction with topical retinoids may deepen the therapeutic effect and minimize the risk of the disease persisting at the adnexal level. A 5% preparation of imiquimod cream applied daily for 6 weeks has also been shown to eradicate superficial basal cell carcinoma in more than 80% of cases, but the use of imiquimod may be limited by its expense. An injection of 5-FU or methotrexate is primarily limited to lesions whose clinical characteristics and histology are consistent with keratoacanthoma. Intralesional administration of interferon has been effective for treating small basal cell carcinoma and squamous cell carcinoma, but this regimen requires multiple injections for several weeks, is expensive, and is associated with flulike side effects.

2. Cryotherapy—Cryotherapy is usually done by dermatologists or by primary care physicians. The results of this procedure are related to the skill and experience of the treating physician. The technique is especially useful for treating actinic keratoses, small nodular or superficial lesions of basal cell carcinoma, and squamous cell carcinoma in situ. Treatment is relatively inexpensive and fast but can be painful and leave dense, hypopigmented scars that may conceal deep, multifocal, persistent tumors.

3. Photodynamic therapy—Photodynamic therapy has been most extensively studied in Europe and appears to be effective for treating superficial basal cell carcinoma and Bowen disease. Currently, most regimens use a topical photosensitizer (eg, delta-aminolevulinic acid) activated by a light source. The short-term control rates for superficial basal cell carcinoma and squamous cell carcinoma in situ are comparable to cryotherapy, but the technique is currently expensive. Photodynamic therapy using intravenous dihematoporphyrin with laser photoactivation also has been reported as beneficial in a small number of patients with large, aggressive nonmelanoma skin cancer.

4. Radiation therapy—Radiation therapy is used primarily in patients older than 60 years or who are not suitable candidates for surgery. Radiation therapy is also used postoperatively for aggressive tumors or where perineural spread is noted. Because this therapy is expensive and requires frequent visits over several weeks, it is often not an option for elderly patients with a limited support system. The control rates for basal cell and squamous cell carcinoma are generally reported to be greater than 90%, and the incidence of post-therapy recurrence increases with increasing tumor size. Recent use of the electron beam and more sophisticated techniques used to model treatment fields has improved cure rates and reduced the number of complications. Long-term cosmetic results may be poor, and the complications of tissue necrosis, chondritis, and osteoradionecrosis may occur. Because of the risk of a radiation-induced malignant growth that may occur later, radiation is generally not recommended as the primary treatment modality for patients younger than 50 years of age.

B. SURGICAL MEASURES

Surgical techniques for the treatment of nonmelanoma skin cancer include curettage and desiccation, simple or wide local excision, and Mohs micrographic surgery.

1. Curettage and desiccation—Dermatologists most often perform curettage and desiccation for small, well-defined, previously untreated areas of nodular basal cell carcinoma; this procedure is also used for some squamous cell carcinomas. The advantages of this technique are its low cost and rapidity of treatment. Its 5-year recurrence rate ranges from 10% to 20%. The disadvantages of the technique are poor cosmetic results, with hypertrophic scarring as well as multifocal tumor recurrence in the scars.

2. Simple excision—Simple excision with 5-mm margins is the appropriate treatment for most well-defined, primary nodular basal cell carcinomas; it is also recommended for low-risk squamous cell carcinoma in anatomic locations where adequate excision with primary closure can be achieved with a good cosmetic result. Five-year recurrence rates of about 10% can be expected. Simple excision is not indicated for tumors that recur after radiation or surgical treatment or for high-risk tumors (eg, sclerosing basal cell carcinoma or poorly differentiated squamous cell carcinoma). It is also not indicated for rare nonmelanoma skin cancer (eg, fibrohistiocytic or adnexal cancer).

3. Wide local excision—Wide local excision generally connotes margins of 2–5 cm and is indicated primarily for (1) well-differentiated squamous cell carcinoma; (2) well-defined, large, nodular-ulcerative basal cell carcinoma; and (3) sarcomas, such as angiosarcoma and malignant fibrous histiocytoma.

4. Mohs micrographic surgery—Mohs micrographic surgery is a technique in which precise surgical margins are obtained by using inverted horizontal frozen sections in conjunction with tumor mapping. The bulk of the tumor is either excised or curetted, and the surrounding perimeter is excised around and deep to the tumor defect. The resulting disk of tissue is then separated into individual quadrants and is inked for orientation, producing a tumor map that is color-coded to represent the inked edges. Histotechnicians specially trained in the technique mount the sections, which are inverted and frozen at −30° to −50° C. Thin frozen sections are obtained, showing the base in continuity with the epidermis. The slides are stained and are examined microscopically, and tumor locations are graphically noted on the map. Additional margins are then created in the same manner, but only in areas positive for a tumor. This process is repeated until all margins are negative for a neoplasm. The process may be enhanced using rapid selective stains. Some centers perform formalin-fixed horizontal sections (1) on final margins that are shown as negative by frozen section, (2) where the tumor histology is subtle, and (3) where tumor recurrence would be catastrophic. These centers convert selected tissue blocks obtained as frozen-section margins to rush paraffin-formalin fixed slides using the same inverted tissue sectioning techniques and tumor mapping to further ensure true negative final margins on difficult cases.

An advantage of Mohs micrographic surgery is its potential to achieve the highest reported control rates for nonmelanoma skin cancer while maximally conserving normal adjacent tissue. The precise surgical margin control used in Mohs micrographic surgery has largely replaced wide local excision for most nonmelanoma skin cancer; the use of an arbitrary margin size with wide local excision does not benefit the outcome for most skin cancers. The overall cure rates using Mohs micrographic surgery are 99% for primary basal cell carcinoma, 96% for recurrent basal cell carcinoma, and 98% for primary squamous cell carcinoma. Mohs micrographic surgery is the treatment of choice for sclerosing or recurrent basal cell carcinoma, large or poorly differentiated squamous cell carcinoma, and most cases of fibrohistiocytic and adnexal cancer. The disadvantages of this technique are its high cost, lack of easy availability, and long procedure time.

Gayl Schweitzer V. Photofrin-mediated photodynamic therapy for treatment of aggressive head and neck nonmelanomatous skin tumors in elderly patients. *Laryngoscope.* 2001;111:1091. [PMID: 11404627] (Concludes that Photofrin-mediated photodynamic therapy for aggressive head and neck nonmelanomatous skin tumors provides excellent clinical and cosmetic results.)

Halpern JN. Radiation therapy in skin cancer: a historical perspective and current applications. *Dermatol Surg.* 1997;23:1089. [PMID: 9391570] (A review article that concludes that radiation therapy in skin cancer provides excellent control and cosmetic results.)

Marks R, Gebauer K, Shumack S et al. Imiquimod 5% cream in the treatment of superficial basal cell carcinoma: results of a multicenter 6-week dose-response trial. *J Am Acad Dermatol.* 2001;44:807. [PMID: 11312429] (Concludes that imiqui-

mod 5% cream has potential as a patient-administered treatment for superficial basal cell carcinoma.)

Martinez JC, Otley CC. The management of melanoma and non-melanoma skin cancer: a review for the primary care physician. *Mayo Clin Proc.* 2001;76:1253. [PMID: 11761506] (A review of management of melanoma and nonmelanoma skin cancer in primary care.)

Morton CA, Whitehurst C, McColl JH, Moore JV, Mackie RM. Photodynamic therapy for large or multiple patches of Bowen disease and basal cell carcinoma. *Arch Dermatol.* 2001;137:319. [PMID: 11255332] (Concludes that delta-aminolevulinic acid photodynamic therapy effectively treats Bowen disease and superficial basal cell carcinoma.)

Shriner DL, McCoy DK, Goldberg DJ, Wanger RF. Mohs micrographic surgery. *J Am Acad Dermatol.* 1998;39:79. [PMID: 9674401] (An updated review of history, with details of selection criteria, technique, and results with all nonmelanoma skin cancers to which technique is applicable.)

BASAL CELL CARCINOMA

Basal cell carcinoma is the most common cancer seen in adults. Historically, basal cell carcinoma has been considered most common in persons older than 60 years, but the increased incidence in younger patients has been noted and may be related to a decrease in the atmospheric ozone as well as to the use of tanning salons. Basal cell carcinoma occurs predominantly on hair-bearing skin, and most tumors arise on the face, head, and neck. No precursor lesions are known to exist. In addition to UV radiation, an increased incidence of basal cell carcinoma has been noted in patients exposed to arsenic and insecticides, and at previous vaccination sites and burn scars. Multiple sites of basal cell carcinoma may develop at an early age in patients with basal cell nevus syndrome, xeroderma pigmentosum, Rombo and Bazex syndromes, and sebaceous nevus.

If untreated or recurrent, basal cell carcinoma may produce clinically significant local destruction and cosmetic and functional morbidity. Metastatic behavior, though rare (its occurrence rate is < 0.025%), most frequently occurs in patients with cancer that is neglected for many years, who have large or recurrent tumors, who are immunosuppressed, or whose tumors have been previously irradiated. Metastases usually affect bone or lung. A careful microscopic examination of tissue to detect perineural or intravascular spread is mandatory. These histologic findings are associated with the potential for aggressive local recurrence and metastatic behavior; they require margin-controlled excision followed by radiation therapy.

Basal cell carcinoma arises from keratinocytes of the epidermis and from adnexal structures and may extend as superficial nests, cords, or filamentous strands surrounded by basement membrane and stroma. These tumors usually grow slowly, spread by direct local extension, and carry the stromal component with them.

Some tumors are highly neurotropic and are spread via superficial nerves, a phenomenon that can result in local "skip" areas with false-negative margins. Particularly dangerous anatomic areas are "embryonal fusion planes," such as those found in the nasofacial sulcus, the medial canthus, and pre- and postauricular areas: In these areas, a neoplasm can proliferate deeply before becoming clinically apparent.

Minimizing exposure to the midday sun is the most important and effective measure to reduce the lifetime risk of developing basal cell carcinoma. This practice may include the use of opaque clothing and hats (microfiber nylon fabrics in particular), as well as eyewear rated to block UV-A and UV-B radiation. Although the efficacy of sunscreens in preventing sunburn is documented, recent large studies seem to suggest that sunscreen use is associated with a reduction in new cases of squamous cell carcinoma, but not of basal cell carcinoma. No benefit has been shown with the use of oral beta-carotene or topical or systemic retinoids. Treatment for small, well-defined basal cell carcinoma is simple excision; for lesions that are recurrent, poorly defined, or located in high-risk anatomic areas, treatment is Mohs micrographic excision.

Basal cell carcinoma is most conveniently divided into four basic categories based on the clinical appearance, the tumor behavior, and the histologic differences between subtypes:

(1) Superficial basal cell carcinoma
(2) Nodular, ulcerative basal cell carcinoma
(3) Sclerosing or morpheaform basal cell carcinoma
(4) Basosquamous (keratotic or metatypical) basal cell carcinoma

These categories overlap considerably, and some tumors have features of more than one subtype.

1. Superficial Basal Cell Carcinoma

Histologically, in superficial, multicentric basal cell carcinoma, basaloid cells proliferate downward at the dermal epidermal junction. This feature also may be found in clinically normal adjacent skin. Clinically, this condition frequently presents as scaling, erythematous plaques that may be pruritic, bleed, and appear almost psoriatic or eczematoid. These plaques may be difficult to distinguish from Bowen disease clinically, and borders may be well defined or indistinct.

Previous treatment with cryotherapy, topical agents, curettage and desiccation, and other methods may render this field change multifocal and discontinuous, leading to high rates of recurrence with surgical removal. Superficial basal cell carcinoma is very slow growing and is not aggressive, but it can affect large areas of skin. Because of this characteristic, selected cases can initially be treated with a topical agent such as 5% fluorouracil or 5% imiquimod. Although most of these lesions can be cured with these regimens, many patients do not tolerate the pain and desquamation associated with topical treatment. Careful follow-up and rebiopsy are indicated if a complete clinical response is not obtained. Although effective, cryotherapy may erratically destroy lesions and produce dense scars with a buried tumor. Photodynamic therapy has been shown effective; the largest series were reported in Europe. Curettage and desiccation, radiation, or Mohs micrographic surgery is used when topical regimens fail or in areas where conservative regimens are not tolerated (eg, the eyelids or the lips).

2. Nodular, Ulcerative Basal Cell Carcinoma

Histologically, tumors of nodular, ulcerative basal cell carcinoma show solid masses of malignant basal cells with scant cytoplasm and peripheral palisading of nuclei, proliferating with an associated connective tissue stroma. A variety of histologic subtypes exist within this category, and long-neglected neoplasms may have micronodular filaments or sclerosing features at the periphery of the lesion.

Clinically, the tumors are typically discrete, painless, well-defined nodules that may be ulcerated centrally with a waxy, telangiectatic peripheral border. Small, nodular neoplasms of basal cell carcinoma must be distinguished from acneiform eruptions and common benign skin lesions such as nevi or granulomatous skin lesions. Nodular, ulcerative lesions of basal cell carcinoma carry a low risk unless they persist for long durations or are located in high-risk anatomic areas. If untreated or recurrent, these lesions may become quite large and clinically more aggressive and may pose considerable challenges both for adequate tumor removal and reconstruction.

Treatment for the lesions is dictated by patient age and expectations for cosmesis, associated medical problems, the anatomic location and size of the neoplasm, and whether the lesion is primary or has recurred after previous treatment. Curettage and desiccation may be appropriate for small nodular basal cell carcinoma, but recurrence is common and scars are typically hypopigmented and conspicuous. Simple excision with 5-mm margins is the appropriate treatment for lesions smaller than 1 cm located in low-risk anatomic areas (ie, where surgical closure is possible without using a flap or graft). Mohs micrographic surgery is ideal for optimizing the conservation of normal tissue while achieving the highest tumor control rates. It is the technique of choice for neoplasms that recur after prior treatment or where reconstruction with a flap or skin graft is anticipated. Radiation therapy for these tumors is effective, but recurrence rates with this therapy are higher than for Mohs micrographic surgery. Cosmetic results may be poor over time, and subsequent radiation-induced tumors may occur.

3. Sclerosing Basal Cell Carcinoma

In sclerosing or morpheaform basal cell carcinoma, the histologic examination may show fine, filamentous tumor strands that extend in all directions; these strands account for high tumor recurrence rates. Clinically, the lesions present as white-to-yellow, telangiectatic, indurated plaques with poorly defined margins. Dense stroma associated with the neoplasm gives it a sclerotic appearance and, over time, it may ulcerate. Although many patients have the lesions for long periods, some tumors have a more aggressive growth pattern and widely infiltrate seemingly normal adjacent tissue, resulting in large surgical defects and considerable morbidity.

In general, basal cell carcinoma with sclerosing features should be treated with Mohs micrographic surgery. Radiation may be appropriate for patients who are not suitable candidates for surgery; however, recurrence rates are higher with this mode of treatment and it may yield cosmetically poor results. To minimize the risk of tumor recurrence, which may be catastrophic in locations such as the medial canthus, Mohs micrographic surgery followed by radiation is the necessary treatment for neoplasms showing perineural spread.

4. Basosquamous Basal Cell Carcinoma

Keratotic (basosquamous or metatypical) basal cell carcinoma represents a true basal cell carcinoma and is characterized by squamous differentiation and keratinization. Clinically, these tumors can be aggressive locally and may occasionally metastasize, particularly if large or recurrent. The tumors may appear similar to nodular basal cell carcinoma and may be confused clinically with squamous cell carcinoma, fibrohistiocytic lesions, or adnexal tumors. Treatment for this form of basal cell carcinoma is Mohs micrographic surgery or wide local excision. Radiation therapy is effective but yields recurrence rates higher than for Mohs micrographic surgery.

Rubin AI, Chen EH, Ratner D. Basal cell carcinoma. *N Engl J Med.* 2005;353:2262. [PMID: 16306523] (Concise overall review of diagnosis and treatment of basal cell carcinoma.)

Thissen MR, Neumann MH, Schouten LJ et al. A systematic review of treatment modalities for primary basal cell carcinomas. *Arch Dermatol.* 1999;135:1177. [PMID: 10522664] (Literature review suggests recurrence rates for different modalities could not be compared due to differences in reporting. Mohs micrographic surgery appeared best for large morpheaform basal cell carcinoma in high-risk areas.)

SQUAMOUS CELL CARCINOMA

Lesions of squamous cell carcinoma, the second most common skin cancer, have an epidemiology and an anatomic distribution similar to basal cell carcinoma. Patients with squamous cell carcinoma may present with keratotic nodules, granular plaques, or ulcerating nodules that may or may not be painful. Common predisposing conditions for squamous cell carcinoma of the face, head, and neck are previous radiation burn scars or longstanding sinus tracts, a history of psoralen and UV-A phototherapy, and immunosuppression. The risk of local recurrence, metastasis, or both is increased by multiple factors and by each of the following:

The size and depth of the invasion: Tumors with a depth of ≥ 6 mm or a diameter of ≥ 2 cm.

The location on the lip (especially near the commissure), ear, and nasal septum.

The degree of differentiation; the risk of local recurrence and metastatic disease is generally inversely proportional to the degree of differentiation.

The rapidity of growth (except for patients with keratoacanthomatous tumors), where a history of rapid growth between the diagnoses and the time of treatment is a poor prognostic sign.

Recurrence after prior treatments; a subsequent recurrence is associated with a high risk of both local recurrence and metastatic disease.

Perineural spread, which carries a particularly poor prognosis and may be suggested by intense pruritus, pain, hypesthesia, or (rarely) paralysis.

Immunosuppression in patients with squamous cell carcinoma, either as a result of chronic disease (eg, chronic lymphocytic leukemia) or drugs (eg, cyclosporine, azathioprine); this immunosuppression is associated with an increasing number of lesions over the time of exposure, and many lesions may develop synchronously with a high cumulative risk of metastases and a very poor prognosis. Most of these patients can be shown to have human papillomavirus.

Squamous cell carcinoma may be preceded by precursor lesions such as actinic keratosis (most commonly) or Bowen disease (ie, squamous cell carcinoma in situ). A histologic examination of actinic keratoses shows superficial neoplasms consisting of defined epidermal proliferation of abnormal keratinocytes. In an estimated 1% per year of affected patients, actinic keratoses may evolve into squamous cell carcinoma. Clinically, the lesions are small, scaly, white, red, or occasionally pigmented keratotic crusts with a friable base. Treatment consists of cryotherapy with liquid nitrogen, curettage and desiccation, topical 5-FU, or simple excision.

1. Squamous Cell Carcinoma In Situ (Bowen Disease)

Bowen disease (ie, intraepidermal squamous cell carcinoma or squamous cell carcinoma in situ) appears histologically as squamous cells with acanthosis and large, hyperchromatic nuclei which proliferate radially along the epidermis. Individual cell keratinization may be present, and the basement membrane is preserved. Bowen disease generally occurs on sun-exposed areas of the face; its occurrence on areas not exposed to sunlight has been linked to arsenic exposure. If left untreated, a small percentage (perhaps 5%) of lesions will develop into invasive squamous cell carcinoma.

Lesions typically present as erythematous superficial plaques with irregular, variably defined borders and may be confused with superficial basal cell carcinoma, psoriasis, or eczema. Induration may indicate invasive squamous cell carcinoma.

If biopsy results fail to show invasion and if the lesion occurs in a suitable area, topical treatment may be administered initially. A 0.025% preparation of tretinoin gel in conjunction with 5% 5-FU is used for 4–6 weeks. Daily application of imiquimod 5% cream for 16 weeks has recently been shown to be a safe and very effective regimen in treating Bowen disease.

Excellent short-term results also have been reported with photodynamic therapy and laser. Mohs micrographic surgery is recommended for treating lesions located in anatomic areas such as the eyelids, lips, other areas where topical agents are not suitable, or when conservative treatment fails.

Patel GK, Goodwin R, Chawla M, Laidler P, Price PE, Finlay AY, Motley RJ. Imiquimod 5% cream monotherapy for cutaneous squamous cell carcinoma in situ (Bowen's disease): a randomized, double-blind, placebo-controlled trial. *J Am Acad Dermatol.* 2006;54(6):1025. [PMID: 16713457] (Controlled trial demonstrating that patients with cutaneous squamous cell carcinoma in situ receiving topical and allowed 5% cream as monotherapy experienced a high degree of clinical benefit compared with placebo.)

2. Keratoacanthoma

Squamous cell carcinoma can be usefully classified as well-differentiated or poorly differentiated tumors that vary both in terms of their histologic features and their clinical behavior. In addition to tumors in these categories, however, keratoacanthoma should be mentioned because of its clinical and histologic similarities to squamous cell carcinoma; some pathologists consider it a low-grade squamous cell carcinoma.

A biopsy of keratoacanthomatous neoplasms shows histologic features that may be indistinguishable from those of squamous cell carcinoma, except for the absence of epithelial membrane antigen. To exclude a diagnosis of invasive squamous cell carcinoma, the biopsy specimen must include the tumor junction and adjacent normal tissue. A cross section of the tumor shows a central keratinous core, an epidermal lip, and glassy keratinocytes with numerous mitoses in the proliferative phase and a few mitoses in the resolution phase.

Keratoacanthoma is generally considered a benign lesion but is characterized by explosive growth in the proliferative phase, which lasts 2–4 weeks and is associated with a central crater filled with a keratin plug (Figure 8–2). The tumors may grow to a large size and then mature over weeks to months; they usually resolve if left untreated. Special tests to distinguish keratoacanthoma from invasive squamous cell carcinoma include cytokeratin staining and epithelial membrane antigen. Tumors that are believed to be clinically obvious keratoacanthoma or that are confirmed by biopsy frequently respond to intralesional administration of either 5-FU or methotrexate. Larger lesions or those not responding to intralesional agents should be excised, and radiation therapy can be used in patients who are not suitable candidates for surgery.

3. Well-Differentiated Squamous Cell Carcinoma

In well-differentiated squamous cell carcinoma, microscopic examination shows large, malignant squamous cells that proliferate downward from the epidermis as nests or cords. Intercellular bridges are seen and keratin pearls are seen frequently; peritumoral inflammation also may be present. These tumors stain positive for cytokeratins. Inactivation of the tumor suppressor gene TP 53 appears to be involved in both actinic keratoses and squamous cell carcinoma. Primary lesions with well-defined borders are best treated by simple excision and primary

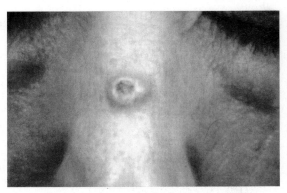

Figure 8–2. A keratoacanthoma lesion shows the central crater filled with a keratin plug. (Photo courtesy of Jeffrey Schneider, MD.)

closure. Recurrent tumors or those occurring in immunosuppressed patients should be removed using frozen-section margin control, preferably with Mohs micrographic surgery. Radiation therapy also is effective.

4. Poorly Differentiated Squamous Cell Carcinoma

In squamous cell carcinoma, the extent of cellular differentiation is directly proportional to amount of keratin and intercellular bridges: The less the differentiation, the fewer keratin and intercellular bridges are present. In anaplastic tumors, no keratin or intercellular bridges are present, and individual cells are markedly atypical with increased mitoses. Immunohistochemical stains or electron microscopy may be necessary to distinguish poorly differentiated squamous cell carcinoma from melanoma, atypical fibroxanthoma, or other poorly differentiated neoplasms. Dedifferentiated squamous cell carcinoma can appear as granular plaques, rapidly growing nodules, or areas of ulceration. Distant metastases occur but are usually preceded by nodal disease; occasionally, tumors originating in the lung present as skin metastases. Patients should be examined carefully for regional adenopathy and have an x-ray of the chest. Other tests, including imaging studies to detect occult nodes, may be indicated, especially in immunocompromised patients.

In poorly differentiated squamous cell carcinoma, the treatment of primary tumors is surgical; ideally, frozen-section margin control should be used (as in Mohs micrographic surgery) or at least 1-cm margins. Defects should be closed without a flap, if possible. Tumors that recur after surgery or after radiation should be excised with Mohs micrographic surgery. Postoperative radiation therapy to the tumor bed and regional lymph nodes is indicated for tumors larger than 2 cm, for perineural invasion, or for tumors occurring in immunocompromised patients. Neck dissection is indicated for adenopathy detected clinically or by imaging; sentinel node biopsy has been shown feasible but remains investigational.

RARE NONMELANOMA SKIN CANCER

The most frequently encountered of the many varieties of rare nonmelanoma skin cancer include three types of fibrohistiocytic tumors: (1) atypical fibroxanthoma, (2) dermatofibrosarcoma protuberans, and (3) malignant fibrous histiocytoma. Rare nonmelanoma skin cancer also includes adnexal cancers.

1. Atypical Fibroxanthoma

Atypical fibroxanthoma is a relatively common tumor thought to represent a superficial form of a low-grade malignant lesion. Histologic examination of the tumor shows densely cellular spindle cell neoplasms in the dermoepidermal junction; pleomorphic, histiocytic cells; giant cells with bizarre nuclei; and fibroblastic spindle cells. By definition, these tumors do not extend into the underlying muscle or fascia. From a histologic perspective, the differential diagnoses include spindle cell carcinoma, malignant fibrous histiocytoma, and melanoma. Special stains are frequently needed to confirm the diagnosis.

Atypical fibroxanthoma generally appears as flat plaques with pigment ranging from yellow to reddish brown in areas of sun-damaged skin; the tumor may grow rapidly. Tumors classified as atypical fibroxanthoma can recur locally if excision is inadequate and rarely metastasize. Lesions proven to invade muscle or fascia should be considered malignant fibrous histiocytoma. Treatment for atypical fibroxanthoma is excision, ideally using Mohs micrographic surgery to minimize local recurrence.

2. Dermatofibrosarcoma Protuberans

Dermatofibrosarcoma protuberans is a slow-growing, fibrous tumor that originates in the dermis, is locally invasive, and occasionally metastasizes. Histologic examination shows packed spindle cells with diffuse infiltration into the dermis and subcutaneous fat as well as (rarely) into deeper structures. Expression of CD34 antigen is positive, and expression of s100 is negative. In younger patients, dermatofibrosarcoma protuberans usually presents as a raised plaque that may appear similar to a keloid in some patients (Figure 8–3). An initial staging evaluation, including a chest x-ray and possibly a CT scan, is indicated because these tumors occasionally metastasize.

Although wide local excision has long been advocated as a treatment for dermatofibrosarcoma protuberans, local recurrence of the disease still occurs, even when 3-cm margins are used. Increasing evidence in the medical literature shows that excision using Mohs micrographic surgery in conjunction with rush paraffin sections provides the highest local control rates; in this technique, the wound is closed only after both frozen and paraffin sections show no tumor. Prophylactic nodal dissection is not indicated for the treatment of dermatofibrosarcoma protuberans because the tumors do not spread to the local nodes. Radiation therapy should be added postoperatively where local recurrence would be catastrophic, but this therapy generally is not used as the primary treatment modality. Patients should be observed at frequent intervals for early detection of local tumor recurrence.

3. Malignant Fibrous Histiocytoma

Malignant fibrous histiocytoma is predominately a tumor of adults and rarely occurs on the head and neck. The term defines a spectrum of cellular tumors that may resemble atypical fibroxanthoma or dermatofibrosarcoma

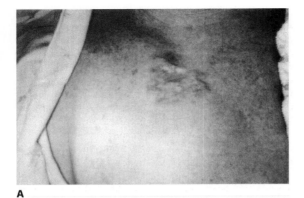

A

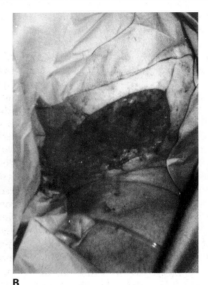

B

Figure 8–3. **(A)** A preoperative lesion of dermatofibro-sarcoma protuberans and **(B)** a postoperative defect.

protuberans (when well differentiated or superficial) or may appear as a poorly differentiated, deeply invasive fibrosarcoma. The neoplasm is considered to be of fibroblastic origin and seems to be more common in previously irradiated areas. Several general subtypes exist, including storiform pleomorphic, myxoid, giant cell, inflammatory, and angiomatoid forms; a single tumor may contain separate areas with features of each subtype.

Clinically, the tumors may appear as elevated plaques or nodules, and surgical borders may be poorly defined because of the diffuse infiltrative nature of the tumor. Rapidly growing tumors may present with hemorrhage and necrosis. The prognosis for lesions of the head and neck is generally related to the depth of the invasion, the tumor grade, and the tumor size at diag-

nosis. Tumors invading muscle or fascia have high rates of both local recurrence and metastases, whereas superficial tumors confined to the subcutis have a more favorable prognosis. The differential diagnosis includes other fibrohistiocytic tumors and sarcomas, Hodgkin disease, and pleomorphic carcinoma. Distinguishing between these conditions and malignant fibrous histiocytoma may require immunohistochemical staining.

Patients should undergo initial staging, including CT scans of the chest, head, and neck, as well as an evaluation by an oncologist. Wide excision with 3- to 5-cm margins including fascia is generally recommended. Mohs micrographic surgery with both frozen and rush paraffin sections may be of value for head and neck tumors to achieve comparable (or higher) local control rates and possibly smaller defect size; comparisons of long-term outcomes are lacking because of the rarity of the neoplasm. Nodal metastases are unusual, so neck dissection is not indicated. Postoperative radiation may further reduce the likelihood of local recurrence.

4. Adnexal Tumors

Adnexal tumors—cutaneous malignant growths arising from adnexal structures—are the rarest types of skin cancer, and several types are highly malignant. Only the more common tumors in this group, that is, proliferating trichilemmal cysts, microcystic adnexal carcinoma, Merkel cell carcinoma, and sebaceous carcinoma, are reviewed here.

Classification

A. PROLIFERATING TRICHILEMMAL CYSTS

Proliferating trichilemmal cysts or tumors are usually composed of proliferating lobules of squamous epithelium with central keratinous debris and are sharply separated from normal surrounding tissue. Malignant variants occur and are usually characterized by sudden rapid growth as well as by an invasion or an erosion of the underlying structures. Regional as well as distant metastases with transformation to invasive squamous cell carcinoma have been reported; indeed, some pathologists consider all proliferating trichilemmal cysts to be low-grade squamous cell carcinoma. The tumors usually occur singly on the scalp in older women as subcutaneous nodules or cysts and are most often confused with a wen or an inclusion cyst. Malignant transformation may be preceded by rapid growth, necrosis, and ulceration. Treatment is simple excision; malignant variants are treated like squamous cell carcinoma.

B. MICROCYSTIC ADNEXAL CARCINOMA

Microcystic adnexal carcinoma (also termed sclerosing sweat duct carcinoma) has microscopic features consisting of basaloid keratinocytes, horn cysts, and abortive

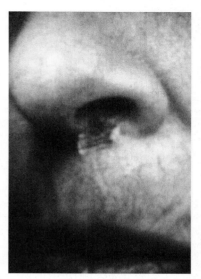

Figure 8–4. A taped lesion of microcystic adnexal carcinoma.

hair follicles in desmoplastic stroma. Perineural invasion occurs frequently; these tumors grow aggressively with extensive infiltration beyond the apparent clinical margins and rates of local recurrence are high. Nodal spread does not occur, and distant metastases have not been reported. Clinically, microcystic adnexal carcinoma usually presents as an indurated papule on the midfacial region (Figure 8–4) and may be confused with trichoepithelioma or basal cell carcinoma. A deep biopsy may be necessary to make the diagnosis.

Treatment is surgical excision, and Mohs micrographic surgery apparently provides optimal local control because of the ability to pursue the unpredictable tumor filaments at the margins (Figure 8–5). The role of radiation therapy for microcystic adnexal carcinoma remains unclear.

C. MERKEL CELL CARCINOMA

Merkel cell carcinoma is a rare, highly aggressive skin cancer that probably has a neuroendocrine origin. Histologic examination shows small- to medium-size cells with scant cytoplasm originating in the basal layer. These cells proliferate as cords and contain neuroendocrine granules. Special stains or electron microscopy may be necessary to distinguish Merkel cell carcinoma from small cell lymphoma or metastatic oat cell cancer. Large tumors consisting of small cells with numerous mitoses (10 per high-power field) have the poorest prognosis. Ultraviolet radiation has been implicated as causing Merkel cell carcinoma, which occurs most frequently in patients who received psoralen UV-A treatment.

Clinically, Merkel cell carcinoma usually presents as a bland, painless nodule on the head and neck of older patients; it is usually pink to almost purple but can appear cystic. Nodal metastases may be found in up to 15% of patients at the initial presentation and subsequently develop in over 50% of cases. Distant metastases occur frequently in patients with nodal disease and can develop rapidly; the overall mortality remains about 50% and most affected patients die within 3 years after the initial diagnosis. Therefore, the initial diagnostic examination should include not only blood tests and CT scans of the chest and neck, but also should include a positron emission tomography (PET) scan, which may cause some tumors to be reclassified into a higher stage because of the early detection of metastatic disease. When staging is reclassified, treatment strategies must be altered accordingly.

Treatment of Merkel cell carcinoma should be planned in conjunction with an oncologist and generally consists of an initial surgical excision followed by radiation to the primary site and nodes. Although excisional margins of 2 cm are generally recommended, the relation between surgical margins and successful outcome is difficult to evaluate. Available studies suggest that, like excision of melanoma, excision of Merkel cell carcinoma using larger surgical margins does not necessarily increase local disease control or the treatment outcome. Mohs micrographic surgery may therefore be a reasonable choice to minimize defect size (especially on the face); studies have shown local recurrence rates comparable with those obtained by using wide local excision. Although Merkel cell tumors are highly radiosensitive, surgery followed by radiation probably achieves locoregional control more successfully than radiation or surgery alone. However, this comparative result has not been reflected in overall survival rates.

Other treatment modalities include sentinel node technology, which has been shown to be feasible and may correctly identify the nodal basin at risk for metas-

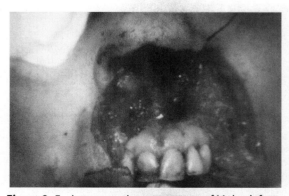

Figure 8–5. Intraoperative appearance of Mohs defect.

tases. Although sentinel node biopsy in necks without clinical signs of disease may aid in staging disease and may limit the frequency of unnecessary neck dissection, the relation between sentinel node biopsy and a successful outcome ultimately is unclear. Finally, chemotherapy is effective for palliating metastatic disease, but the role of adjuvant chemotherapy remains to be defined.

Gupta SG, Wang LC, Penas PF, Gellenthin M, Lee SJ, Nghiem P. Sentinel lymph node biopsy for evaluation and treatment of patients with Merkel cell carcinoma: the Dana-Farber experience and meta analysis of the literature. *Arch Dermatol.* 2006;142(6):685. [PMID: 16785370] (Sentinel lymph node biopsy detects Merkel cell carcinoma spread in one third of patients whose tumors would have otherwise been clinically and radiologically understaged and who may not have received treatment to the involved node bed.)

D. SEBACEOUS CARCINOMA

Sebaceous carcinoma, the fourth most common skin cancer, is more common in patients with Muir-Torre syndrome and in anatomic areas that have been previously irradiated. Histologic examination of tumor nodules shows variably sized lobules of sebaceous cells that contain lipid globules. Sebaceous carcinoma must be distinguished from basal cell carcinoma with sebaceous differentiation. Patients with sebaceous carcinoma present with tumors as nodules on the head and neck; most tumors occur on the eyelids. Symptoms of ocular irritation are common and may be confused with blepharitis or chalazion. Mortality rates increase with tumor size. About 50% of affected patients with tumors larger than 1 cm die; distant metastases occur in viscera and bone, and orbital invasion may be more common in tumors with pagetoid features. Local recurrence and nodal metastases are common. The initial diagnostic examination should include an ophthalmologic examination; magnetic resonance imaging (MRI) of the orbits and neck should be used to rule out occult metastatic disease in tumors larger than about 6 mm.

Treatment for sebaceous carcinoma is surgical excision; Mohs micrographic surgery using frozen sections followed by rush paraffin sections may optimize local control and tissue conservation. The role of radiation therapy as a primary treatment for sebaceous carcinoma is less clear, but improved technology may make this treatment an option when excision is contraindicated or refused.

Alam M, Ratner D. Cutaneous squamous cell carcinoma. *N Engl J Med.* 2001;344:975. [PMID: 11274625] (A review of the incidence, etiology, and treatment of cutaneous squamous cell carcinoma.)

Ballo MT, Zagars GK, Pollack A. The role of radiation therapy in the management of dermatofibrosarcoma protuberans. *Int J Radiat Oncol Biol Phys.* 1998;40:823. [PMID: 9531366] (Combined resection and postoperative radiation therapy should be considered for high-risk tumors.)

Chiller K, Passaro D, Schueller M, Singer M, McCalmont T, Grekin RC. Microcystic adnexal carcinoma: forty-eight cases, their treatment, and their outcome. *Arch Dermatol.* 2000;136:1355. [PMID: 11074698] (Average surgical defect size four times the clinical estimate; Mohs micrographic surgery rated superior due to the unpredictability of surgical margins.)

Clayton BD, Leshin B, Hitchcock MG, Marks M, White WL. Utility of rush paraffin-embedded tangential sections in the management of cutaneous neoplasms. *Dermatol Surg.* 2000;26:671. [PMID: 10886277] (Concludes that Mohs micrographic surgery in combination with rush formalin-fixed, paraffin-embedded tangential histologic sections provides enhanced accuracy in the surgical treatment of cutaneous neoplasms.)

Cook BE Jr, Bartley GB. Treatment options and future prospects for the management of eyelid malignancies: an evidence-based update. *Ophthalmology.* 2001;108:2088. [PMID: 11713084] (Concludes that the strongest evidence favors complete excision of the malignant neoplasm using histologic controls to determine the margins.)

Gillenwater AM, Hessel AC, Morrison WH et al. Merkel cell carcinoma of the head and neck: effect of surgical excision and radiation on recurrence and survival. *Arch Otolaryngol Head Neck Surg.* 2001;127:149. [PMID: 11177031] (No detectable effect of width of surgical margins; significant improvement in locoregional control with postoperative radiation therapy.)

Gloster HM Jr, Harris KR, Roenigk RK et al. A comparison between Mohs micrographic surgery and wide surgical excision for the treatment of dermatofibrosarcoma protuberans. *J Am Acad Dermatol.* 1996;35:82. [PMID: 8682970] (Mayo Clinic study favors Mohs micrographic surgery for dermatofibrosarcoma protuberans.)

Hill AD, Brady MS, Coit DG et al. Intraoperative lymphatic mapping and sentinel lymph node biopsy for Merkel cell carcinoma. *Br J Surg.* 1999;86:518. [PMID: 10215828] (Shows feasibility and utility in determining the prognosis; the effect on survival is not clear.)

Hochman M, Lang P. Skin cancer of the head and neck. *Med Clin North Am.* 1999;83:261. [PMID: 9927974] (A review for the clinician of skin lesions and their treatment.)

Huether MJ, Zitelli JA, Brooland DG. Mohs micrographic surgery for the treatment of spindle cell tumors of the skin. *J Am Acad Dermatol.* 2001;44:656. [PMID: 11260542] (Data support Mohs micrographic surgery for spindle cell tumors, including atypical fibroxanthoma.)

Schoelch SB, Flowers FP. Recognition and management of high-risk cutaneous tumors. *Dermatol Clin.* 1999;17:93. [PMID: 9986998] (A review concerning the recognition of cutaneous tumors requiring advanced and aggressive treatment.)

Skidmore RA Jr et al. Nonmelanoma skin cancer. *Med Clin North Am.* 1998;82:1309. [PMID: 9889750] (A review with emphasis on the diagnosis of malignant skin neoplasms that occur frequently or with significant morbidity.)

Sondak VK, Cimmino VM, Lowe LM, Dubay DA, Johnson TM. Dermatofibrosarcoma protuberans: what is the best surgical approach? *Surg Oncol.* 1999;8:183. [PMID: 11128831] (Lower recurrence rate with Mohs micrographic surgery in comparison with standard surgical excision.)

Spencer JM, Nossa R, Tse DT, Sequeira M. Sebaceous carcinoma of the eyelid treated with Mohs micrographic surgery. *J Am Acad Dermatol.* 2001;44:1004. [PMID: 11369914] (Mohs micrographic surgery results are superior to historic series of standard excision.)

Tom WD, Hybarger CP, Rasgon BM. Dermatofibrosarcoma protuberans of the head and neck: treatment with Mohs surgery using inverted horizontal paraffin sections. *Laryngoscope.* 2003;113:1289. [PMID: 12897547] (Improved outcome using addition of rush paraffin conversion of all negative frozen sections before final reconstruction.)

CUTANEOUS MELANOMA

General Considerations

Malignant melanoma of the skin is the third most common cutaneous malignant lesion; about 25% of these lesions occur on the head and neck. The incidence of cutaneous melanoma continues to increase exponentially and is currently increasing at a rate of about 5% annually. The overall mortality rate per 100,000 persons continues to increase, but survival rates among patients with lower-staged tumors have increased, and the overall cure rates for melanoma exceed 90%. Both an increased incidence and a decreased mortality may be related to an increased awareness of cutaneous melanoma and its early detection and treatment. Although most cases of the disease are sporadic, some show familial patterns and may be associated with dysplastic nevus syndrome, which carries a 100-fold increased lifetime risk for the development of cutaneous melanoma.

Other precursor lesions associated with an increased risk of cutaneous melanoma include large congenital nevi and the presence of more than 50 benign acquired nevi. A strong correlation with prior intermittent intense sun exposure exists, and active programs for prevention as well as early detection may ultimately help decrease the incidence. The role of sunscreens in preventing melanoma remains unclear. Melanoma of the head and neck can be separated into three general categories: (1) melanoma in situ (ie, lentigo maligna melanoma), (2) superficial spreading melanoma, and (3) nodular melanoma. Primary tumors are also classified using the American Joint Committee on Cancer (AJCC) nomenclature.

A. MELANOMA IN SITU

Melanoma in situ is characterized by the proliferation of atypical neoplastic melanocytes at the dermoepidermal junction along adnexal structures. A characteristically prolonged radial growth pattern is present and may last decades; approximately 0.10–0.25% of such lesions annually become invasive melanoma. These lesions are the least common form of melanoma and usually occur on the cheek, nose, or temple in elderly patients. Early lesions may be clinically indistinguishable from solar lentigo.

B. SUPERFICIAL SPREADING MELANOMA

Superficial spreading melanoma, the most common form, may evolve during a period of several years from a preexisting lesion, such as a nevus, in middle-aged individuals. The lesion is characterized histologically by a predominantly radial growth phase with eventual proliferation of malignant cells into the dermis, as well as upward growth that may present as nodularity and ulceration, which denotes the onset of the vertical growth phase.

C. NODULAR MELANOMA

Nodular melanoma occurs most commonly in children and represents approximately 15% of adulthood melanomas. It is characterized by early invasion and a vertical growth phase. The neoplasms can be black or variegated in color and are occasionally amelanotic. These tumors show no radial growth phase and are, by definition, invasive at the time of presentation.

Lesions suspected to be nodular melanomas should be either biopsied with a deep 3-mm punch or excised with a 2-mm margin. Shave biopsy should not be performed because the precise measurement of the tumor depth will not be possible and valuable staging information will not be accurate. A careful search for ulceration, induration of surrounding tissue, satellite or in-transit lesions, and regional adenopathy should be part of the initial examination. Nodular melanomas can become quite large and present significant surgical challenges, both in terms of achieving local control surgically and in reconstructing the defects after removal.

Diagnosis

The early clinical diagnosis of cutaneous melanoma requires a high index of suspicion based on family history, risk factors, and physical examination, which should include an examination for satellite lesions, the presence of ulceration, and regional nodes. To distinguish benign, pigmented lesions from high-risk lesions, the **"A-B-C-D-E"** approach to physical diagnosis is useful. This approach consists of observing five criteria:

Asymmetric lesions

Borders are irregular

Color may vary with multiple shades from brown to red-black

Diameter > 6 mm

Evolving lesions that have shown growth or change

Staging Criteria

The review of prior staging and survival data (Table 8–1 and Figure 8–6) suggests that, in addition to tumor thickness, the presence of melanoma ulceration, in-transit metastases or satellite lesions, and number of nodes (identified as positive by clinical or pathologic examination) has strong independent prognostic predictive value. The AJCC recently approved the final

Table 8–1. Survival rates for patients with melanoma, grouped by TNM and staging categories and according to year of diagnosis.

Pathologic Stage	TNM	Thickness (mm)	Ulceration	No. + Nodes	Nodal Size	Distant Metastasis	No. of Patients	Survival ± SE			
								1-Year	2-Year	5-Year	10-Year
IA	T1a	1	No	0	-	-	4,510	99.7 ± 0.1	99.0 ± 0.2	95.3 ± 0.4	87.9 ± 1.0
IB	T1b	1	Yes or level IV, V	0	-	-	1,380	99.8 ± 0.1	98.7 ± 0.3	90.9 ± 1.0	83.1 ± 1.5
	T2a	1.01–2.0	No	0	-	-	3,285	99.5 ± 0.1	97.3 ± 0.3	89.0 ± 0.7	79.2 ± 1.1
IIA	T2b	1.01–2.0	Yes	0	-	-	958	98.2 ± 0.5	92.9 ± 0.9	77.4 ± 1.7	64.4 ± 2.2
	T3a	2.01–4.0	No	0	-	-	1,717	98.7 ± 0.3	94.3 ± 0.6	78.7 ± 1.2	63.8 ± 1.7
IIB	T3b	2.01–4.0	Yes	0	-	-	1,523	95.1 ± 0.6	84.8 ± 1.0	63.0 ± 1.5	50.8 ± 1.7
	T4a	>4.0	No	0	-	-	563	94.8 ± 1.0	88.6 ± 1.5	67.4 ± 2.4	53.9 ± 3.3
IIC	T4b	>4.0	Yes	0	-	-	978	89.9 ± 1.0	70.7 ± 1.6	45.1 ± 1.9	32.3 ± 2.1
IIIA	N1a	Any	No	1	Micro	-	252	95.9 ± 1.3	88.0 ± 2.3	69.5 ± 3.7	63.0 ± 4.4
	N2a	Any	No	2–3	Micro	-	130	93.0 ± 2.4	82.7 ± 3.8	63.3 ± 5.6	56.9 ± 6.8
IIIB	N1a	Any	Yes	1	Micro	-	217	93.3 ± 1.8	75.0 ± 3.2	52.8 ± 4.1	37.8 ± 4.8
	N2a	Any	Yes	2–3	Micro	-	111	92.0 ± 2.7	81.0 ± 4.1	49.6 ± 5.7	35.9 ± 7.2
	N1b	Any	No	1	Macro	-	122	88.5 ± 2.9	78.5 ± 3.7	59.0 ± 4.8	47.7 ± 5.8
	N2b	Any	No	2–3	Macro	-	93	76.8 ± 4.4	65.6 ± 5.0	46.3 ± 5.5	39.2 ± 5.8
IIIC	N1b	Any	Yes	1	Macro	-	98	77.9 ± 4.3	54.2 ± 5.2	29.0 ± 5.1	24.4 ± 5.3
	N2b	Any	Yes	2–3	Macro	-	109	74.3 ± 4.3	44.1 ± 4.9	24.0 ± 4.4	15.0 ± 3.9
	N3	Any	Any	4	Micro/macro	-	396	71.0 ± 2.4	49.8 ± 2.7	26.7 ± 2.5	18.4 ± 2.5
IV	M1a	Any	Any	Any	Any	Skin, SQ	179	59.3 ± 3.7	36.7 ± 3.6	18.8 ± 3.0	15.7 ± 2.9
	M1b	Any	Any	Any	Any	Lung	186	57.0 ± 3.7	23.1 ± 3.2	6.7 ± 2.0	2.5 ± 1.5
	M1c	Any	Any	Any	Any	Other visceral	793	40.6 ± 1.8	23.6 ± 1.5	9.5 ± 1.1	6.0 ± 0.9
Total							17,600				

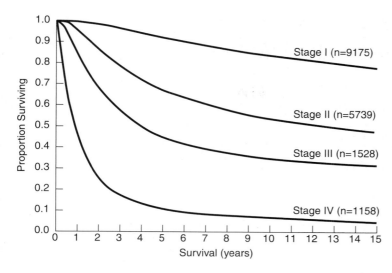

Figure 8–6. A graph of the 15-year survival curves comparing localized melanoma (Stages I and II), regional metastases (Stage III), and distant metastases (Stage IV). (Reproduced, with permission, from Balch CM, Buzaid AC, Soong SJ et al: Final version of the American Joint Committee on Cancer staging system for cutaneous melanoma. *J Clin Oncol.* 2001;19:3635.)

version of a revised staging system that incorporates several major changes relevant to head and neck surgery. These changes relate to melanoma thickness and ulceration (but not to the level of invasion) that is to be used in all but T1 categories. This strategy essentially changes the classification of tumors based on their thickness in millimeters in Stages II–IV to integers, with the substage based on the presence or the absence of ulceration. The current system for classifying primary tumors and nodes is shown in Table 8–2.

The number of metastatic lymph nodes and the delineation of clinically occult or microscopic nodes is used in the "N" category of the classification system. Macrometastases are defined as clinically, radiologically, or pathologically detectable nodes or as gross nodal extracapsular extensions. Micrometastases are detected with sentinel lymph node biopsy or elective node dissection.

As a result of these changes, the overall staging has changed (Table 8–3). As a result of the new staging criteria, some patients qualify for upgraded treatment strategies:

All patients with Stage I, II, and III disease are staged upward (or *upstaged*) when the primary melanoma is ulcerated.

Satellite metastases around a primary melanoma site and in-transit metastases are merged into a single staging entity grouped into Stage III disease.

A new convention defines clinical and pathologic staging to incorporate the staging information gained from intraoperative lymph node mapping and sentinel node biopsy.

Sites of distant metastases and the presence of an elevated serum lactic dehydrogenase (LDH) level are incorporated into the "M" category.

The role of the initial evaluation after the initial diagnosis is related to the presumed stage of disease. It has been questioned in lesions measuring < 1.0 mm because this examination may yield a high rate of false-positive results and lead to unnecessary further studies. Patients who have melanoma **in situ** or **Stage I** disease without ulceration or symptoms need no further examination. Patients who have **Stage I** or **II** melanoma with ulceration or **Stage III** lesions may benefit from the addition of CT scanning of the neck, sentinel lymph node biopsy, or both procedures. The following tests are indicated for **T4 lesions:** (1) CT imaging to include the chest, the abdomen, and the pelvis; (2) an MRI of the brain; and (3) testing of the serum LDH level before sentinel lymph node biopsy. When confirmed by repeated tests, a finding of an elevated LDH level may have an independent predictive value for a poor prognosis. The addition of PET scanning may add additional prognostic information and cause staging of intermediate-risk lesions to be revised upward, thus changing the treatment strategies in high-risk patients. (Current studies are limited to investigational centers.)

Treatment

A. SURGICAL MEASURES

Treatment of melanoma of the head and neck is based on the initial staging and generally consists of surgical excision of the primary lesion; surgical margins are determined on the basis of the T stage. The role of the surgical margin size is particularly important for the head and neck, where conservation of normal structures and function is a high priority, particularly if the effect of larger margins is not manifested in the outcome. It is

Table 8–2. Classification system for describing primary tumors and nodes.

Current Primary Tumor Classification

T0	No primary tumor located	
T1s	Melanoma in situ	
T1a	1.0 mm or less	Without ulceration and Clark's level II/III
T1b		With ulceration or Clark's level IV/V
T2a	1.01–2.0 mm	Without ulceration
T2b		With ulceration
T3a	2.01–4.0 mm	Without ulceration
T3b		With ulceration
T4a	4.0 mm or more	Without ulceration
T4b		With ulceration

Nodal Classification

N1a	1 node with micrometastasis
N1b	1 node with macrometastasis
N2a	2–3 nodes with micrometastasis
N2b	2–3 nodes with macrometastasis
N2c	In-transit/satellites without metastatic nodes
N3	4 or more nodes, matted nodes, or satellites with nodes

Adapted and reproduced with permission from the author and publisher from: Balch CM et al: Final version of the American Joint Committee on Cancer staging system for cutaneous melanoma. *J Clin Oncol* 2001;19:3635.

important to note that if wide local excision is planned, ideally, it should be done in conjunction with sentinel lymph node biopsy; however, it should not be performed before that procedure because of the potential for the altered lymphatic distribution of injected agents. (The role and technique of sentinel, elective, and therapeutic neck dissections are discussed in Chapter 27, Neck Neoplasms & Neck Dissection.)

The generally accepted surgical margins are based on the primary tumor stage. **Melanoma in situ** can be excised using a Woods light with a 5-mm margin of clinically normal skin into subcutaneous fat. Mohs micrographic surgery may be beneficial for excising melanoma in situ in certain locations where tissue conservation is of great concern (eg, the eyelid or nose).

Stage I melanomas as deep as 2 mm without ulceration can be excised with a 1-cm margin; Stage I melanoma with ulceration should have 2-cm margins and consideration should be given to the use of sentinel lymph node biopsy.

Stage II and **Stage III** lesions should have 2-cm margins and should include subcutaneous fat down to the fascia, if possible. Sentinel lymph node biopsy or elective node dissection, as well as postoperative radiation therapy, other adjuvant treatment, or a combination of these therapies, should be considered.

B. NONSURGICAL MEASURES

1. Radiation therapy—Radiation therapy can be used to treat lentigo maligna or in situ disease when surgery is not feasible. Radiation therapy also has been shown effective in decreasing locoregional recurrence postoperatively in patients with extracapsular spread or bulky nodal disease. Some centers currently recommend radiation therapy for Stage II disease if the nodes are not treated surgically; alternately, these centers recommend postoperative radiation therapy for use in node-positive or recurrent disease.

Table 8–3. Stage groupings for cutaneous melanoma.

	Clinical Staging	Pathologic Staging
0	T1s N0 M0	T1s N0 M0
IA	T-1A N0 M0	T-1A N0 M0
IB	T-1B N0 M0	T-1B N0 M0
	T-2A N0 M0	T-2A N0 M0
IIA	T-2B N0 M0	T-2B N0 M0
	T-3A N0 M0	T-3A N0 M0
IIB	T-3B N0 M0	T-3B N0 M0
	T-4A N0 M0	T-4A N0 M0
IIC	T-4B N0 M0	T-4B N0 M0
IIIA		T1-4A N1A M0
		T1-4A N2A M0
IIIB		T1-4B N1A M0
		T1-4B N2A M0
		T1-4A N1B M0
		T1-4A N2B M0
		T1-4A/B N2C M0
IIIC		T1-4B N1B M0
		T1-4B N2B M0
		Any T N3 M0
IV	Any T Any N Any M1	Any T Any N Any M1

Adapted and reproduced with permission from the author and publisher from: Balch CM et al: Final version of the American Joint Committee on Cancer staging system for cutaneous melanoma. *J Clin Oncol* 2001;19:3635.

Actic Keratosis's.

2. Adjuvant therapies—Adjuvant therapies abound, but only high-dose interferon (eg, IFN-alpha 2b) has been shown to statistically improve the rates of both disease-free survival and the overall survival in randomized trials done after surgical dissection in Stage IIB and Stage III disease. A variety of multiagent protocols for advanced disease are currently in institutional trials. Tumor vaccines have shown promise but remain experimental.

Balch CM, Soong SJ, Smith T, Ross MI et al. Long-term results of a prospective surgical trial comparing 2 cm versus 4 cm excision margins for 740 patients with 1–4 mm melanomas. *Ann Surg Oncol.* 2001;8:101. [PMID: 11258773] (Concludes that ulceration of the primary melanoma is the most significant prognostic factor for local recurrence; local recurrence has a high prognostic value for morbidity.)

Cooper JS, Chang WS, Oratz R, Shapiro RL, Roset DF. Elective radiation therapy for high-risk malignant melanomas. *Cancer J.* 2001;7:498. (PMID: 11769862] (Concludes that radiation therapy helps to control residual disease after surgery for melanoma but that better therapies for distant metastases must be sought.)

Kanzler MH, Mraz-Gerhard S. Primary cutaneous malignant melanoma and its precursor lesions: diagnostic and therapeutic overview. *J Am Acad Dermatol.* 2001;45:260. [PMID: 11464189] (A review of current, evidence-based literature on the diagnosis and treatment of primary cutaneous melanoma.)

Kirkwood JM, Ibrahim JG, Sosman JA et al. High-dose interferon alpha-2b significantly prolongs relapse-free and overall survival compared with the GM2-KLH/QS-21 vaccine in patients with resected stage IIB-III melanoma: results of intergroup trial E1694/S9512/C509801. *J Clin Oncol.* 2001;19:2370. [PMID: 11331315] (Concludes that high-dose interferon is superior to GM2-KLH/QS-21 vaccine in the treatment of patients with melanoma.)

Lentsch EJ, Myers JN. Melanoma of the head and neck: current concepts in diagnosis and management. *Laryngoscope.* 2001;111:1209. [PMID: 11568543] (Concise review of diagnosis, staging, and management from M.D. Anderson Cancer Center.)

Morton DL, Thompson JF, Mozillo N et al. MSLT Group. Sentinel node—biopsy or nodal observation in melanoma. *N Engl J Med.* 2006;355(13):1307. [PMID: 17005948] (The staging of immediate thickness 1.2 to 3.5 mm primary melanomas according to the results of sentinel node biopsy provides important prognostic information and identifies patients with nodal metastases whose survival can be prolonged by immediate lymphadenectomy.)

Reske SN, Kotzerke J. FDG-PET for clinical use. Results of the 3rd German Interdisciplinary Consensus Conference, "Onko-PET III," 21 July and 19 September 2000. *Eur J Nucl Med.* 2001;28:1707. [PMID: 11702115] (A comprehensive review of the use of fluorine-18-fluoro-2-deoxy-D-glucose position emission tomography in the diagnosis and treatment of malignant tumors.)

Sondak VK. Adjuvant therapy for melanoma. *Cancer J.* 2001;7:Suppl 1:S24. [PMID: 11504282] (A review of various adjuvant therapies and their efficacy for the treatment of melanoma.)

Tom WD, Hybarger CP, Rasgon BM. Dermatofibrosarcoma protuberans: treatment with Mohs surgery using inverted horizontal paraffin sections. *Laryngoscope.* 2003;113(8):1289–1293. (PMID: 12897547] (Improved outcome using addition of rush paraffin conversion of all negative frozen sections before final reconstruction.)

Zitelli JA, Brown CD, Hanusa BH et al. Surgical margins for excision of primary cutaneous melanoma. *J Am Acad Dermatol.* 1997;37:422. [PMID: 9308558] (Provides recommended surgical margins for excision of melanoma based on size and location of lesions.)

SECTION III
Nose

| Olfactory Dysfunction | 9 |

Anil K. Lalwani, MD

OLFACTORY LOSS

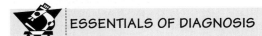

ESSENTIALS OF DIAGNOSIS

- *History of olfactory loss, often manifesting as loss of the sense of taste.*
- *Sensory evaluation with quantitative tests indicating olfactory loss.*

General Considerations

The sense of smell determines the flavor and palatability of food and drink. Along with the trigeminal system, it serves as a monitor of inhaled chemicals, including dangerous substances such as natural gas and smoke, and odors common to everyday life. The loss of smell or a decreased ability to smell affects approximately 1% of people under age 60 and more than half of the population beyond this age.

Abnormalities of olfaction include the following: (1) **anosmia** (absence of the sense of smell); (2) **hyposmia** (diminished olfactory sensitivity); (3) **dysosmia** (distorted sense of smell); (4) **phantosmia** (perception of an odorant when none is present); and (5) **agnosia** (inability to classify, contrast, or identify odor sensations verbally, even though the ability to distinguish between odorants may be normal).

Disorders of the sense of smell are caused by conditions that interfere with the access of the odorant to the olfactory neuroepithelium (transport loss), injure the

receptor region (sensory loss), or damage the central olfactory pathways (neural loss). Table 9–1 summarizes the most common causes of olfactory dysfunction.

Classification

A. TRANSPORT OLFACTORY LOSS

Transport olfactory loss can result from the following conditions: a swollen nasal mucous membrane in acute viral upper respiratory infections; bacterial rhinitis and sinusitis; allergic rhinitis; and structural changes in the nasal cavity (eg, deviations of the nasal septum, polyps, and neoplasms). It is also likely that abnormalities of mucus secretion, in which the olfactory cilia are immersed, could result in a loss of olfactory sensitivity.

B. SENSORY OLFACTORY LOSS

Sensory olfactory loss results from damage to the olfactory neuroepithelium by any of the following causes: viral infections, neoplasms, the inhalation of toxic chemicals, drugs that affect cell turnover, and radiation therapy to the head.

C. NEURAL OLFACTORY LOSS

Neural olfactory loss can occur in a number of ways: head trauma, with or without fracture of the base of the anterior cranial fossa or cribriform plate area; Parkinson disease; Alzheimer's disease; Korsakoff psychosis; vitamin B_{12} deficiency; neoplasms of the anterior cranial fossa; neurosurgical procedures; administration of neurotoxic agents (eg, ethanol, amphetamines, topical cocaine, aminoglycosides, tetracycline, cigarette smoke); and in some congenital disorders such as Kall-

Table 9–1. Causes of olfactory dysfunction.

Transport Olfactory Losses
Allergic rhinitis
Bacterial rhinitis and sinusitis
Congenital abnormality (encephalocele)
Nasal neoplasms
Nasal polyps
Nasal septal deviation
Nasal surgery
Viral infections

Sensory Olfactory Losses
Drugs
Neoplasms
Radiation therapy
Toxic chemical exposure
Viral infections

Neural Olfactory Losses
AIDS
Alcoholism
Alzheimer's disease
Chemical toxins
Cigarette smoke
Diabetes mellitus
Depression
Drugs
Huntington's chorea
Hypothyroidism
Kallmann syndrome
Korsakoff psychosis
Malnutrition
Neoplasm
Neurosurgery
Parkinson disease
Trauma
Vitamin B_{12} deficiency
Zinc deficiency

mann syndrome. Other endocrine disorders can affect smell perception, including Cushing syndrome, hypothyroidism, and diabetes mellitus.

Pathogenesis

Molecular aspects of olfaction are now becoming understood. In mammals, there are probably 300–1000 olfactory receptor genes belonging to 20 different families located on various chromosomes in clusters. The receptor genes are present at more than 25 different human chromosomal locations. Olfactory receptor proteins are G protein-coupled receptors characterized by the presence of seven alpha-helical transmembrane domains. Each olfactory neuron expresses only one, or at most, a few receptor genes, providing the molecular

basis of odor distinction. The olfactory system is thus characterized by three important features: (1) the large family of receptor genes exhibits remarkable diversity allowing response to a variety of smells, (2) the receptor proteins exhibit exquisite specificity allowing for odor discrimination, and (3) odor associations are well kept in memory long after the incident that formed the association is forgotten.

Etiology

Many patients experience olfactory dysfunction due to one or more of the following causes: obstructive nasal and sinus disease, post-upper respiratory infection, cranial trauma, and congenital causes. Aging, exposure to toxins, and idiopathic causes also account for the loss of smell.

A. NASAL OBSTRUCTION AND UPPER RESPIRATORY INFECTION

Air flows through the medial and anterior to the lower part of the middle turbinate to reach the olfactory cleft. Nasal obstruction at this area or above it caused by severe mucosal swelling, tumors, nasal polyps, or bony deformities can result in hyposmia or anosmia. In addition, patients often report a loss of sense of smell during an upper respiratory infection; generally, this loss is due to airway obstruction secondary to mucosal swelling. Olfactory ability should improve or return altogether with relief of the obstruction.

B. CRANIAL TRAUMA

Approximately 5–10% of adult patients with head trauma report olfactory loss to be in the anosmic range. The degree of olfactory loss is generally associated with two things: the severity of the trauma and the site of cranial trauma. Total anosmia is more likely to occur with occipital traumas; however, frontal blows most frequently cause olfactory loss.

C. CONGENITAL ANOSMIA

Perhaps the most well-known type of congenital anosmia is **Kallmann syndrome,** an X-linked disorder. Caused by mutation in the KAL gene, Kallmann syndrome is characterized by hypogonadotropic hypogonadism, which results when olfactory receptor neurons and neurons synthesizing gonadotropin-releasing hormone fail to migrate from the olfactory placode.

D. AGING

Aging and dementia-related diseases can result in olfactory loss. Olfactory sensitivity tends to drop sharply in the sixth and seventh decades of life. Anatomically, cellular elements associated with olfaction decrease with age, as does olfactory bulb volume (found at the base of the frontal cortex). Alzheimer disease and Parkinson disease may be associated with olfactory dysfunction. In these patients, the most likely mechanism is damage to the olfactory bulb or central olfactory cortex, which results in the loss of olfactory detection and recognition ability.

E. TOXINS AND OTHER FACTORS

Olfactory loss from toxins may occur over a period of days or years. Formalin exposure is an example of a toxicity that accumulates over a period of years. Most agents that cause olfactory loss are either gases or aerosols that enter the nose with the respiratory air stream.

Patients with depression and schizophrenia may have olfactory losses as part of their illnesses. Although depressed patients do have some altered gustatory ability, the ability to identify odorants is usually normal; when it is not, the olfactory complaints most likely stem from a problem in the central nervous system. It may be that the same chemicals that cause symptoms of depression affect the neural connections between the limbic system and the hypothalamus.

Clinical Findings

A. SIGNS AND SYMPTOMS

Knowing the onset and development of an olfactory disorder may be of paramount importance in making an etiologic diagnosis. Unilateral anosmia is rarely a complaint; it can be recognized only by separately testing smell in each nasal cavity. Bilateral anosmia, on the other hand, does bring patients to medical attention. Anosmic patients usually complain of loss of the sense of taste, even though their taste thresholds may be within normal limits. In actuality, they are complaining of a loss of flavor detection, which is mainly an olfactory function.

B. PHYSICAL FINDINGS

The physical examination should include a complete examination of the ears, upper respiratory tract, head, and neck. Pathology of each area of the head and neck can result in olfactory dysfunction. The presence of serous otitis media suggests the presence of a nasopharyngeal mass or inflammation. A careful nasal examination for nasal mass, clot, polyps, and nasal membrane inflammation is critical. When available, anterior rhinoscopy should be supplemented with endoscopic examination of the nasal cavity and nasopharynx. The presence of telecanthus on the ocular exam may suggest a sinus mass or inflammation. Nasopharyngeal masses protruding into the oral cavity or purulent drainage within the oropharynx may be seen during the oral examination. The neck should be palpated for masses or thyroid enlargement. A neurologic examination emphasizing the cranial nerves and cerebellar and sensorimotor function is essential. The patient's general mood should be assessed and signs of depression should be noted.

C. LABORATORY FINDINGS

Techniques have been developed to biopsy the olfactory neuroepithelium. However, because of the widespread degeneration of the olfactory neuroepithelium and intercalation of respiratory epithelium in the olfactory area of adults with no apparent olfactory dysfunction, biopsy material must be interpreted cautiously.

D. IMAGING

A computed tomography (CT) scan or magnetic resonance imaging (MRI) of the head is required to rule out neoplasms of the anterior cranial fossa, unsuspected fractures of the anterior cranial fossa, paranasal sinusitis, and neoplasms of the nasal cavity and paranasal sinuses. Bone abnormalities are best seen with CT, whereas MRI is useful in evaluating olfactory bulbs, ventricles, and other soft tissues of the brain. Coronal CT is optimal for assessing the cribriform plate, anterior cranial fossa, and sinus anatomy and disease.

E. SENSORY EVALUATION

The sensory evaluation of olfactory function is necessary to (1) corroborate the patient's complaint, (2) evaluate the efficacy of treatment, and (3) determine the degree of permanent impairment.

1. Step 1: Determining qualitative sensations— The first step in the sensory evaluation is to determine the degree to which qualitative sensations are present. Several methods are available for olfaction evaluation.

a. The Odor stix test—The Odor stix test uses a commercially available magic marker–like pen that produces odor. It is held approximately 3–6 inches from the patient's nose to check for gross perception of the odorant.

b. The twelve-inch alcohol test—Another test that assesses gross perception of an odorant, the twelve-inch alcohol test, uses a freshly opened isopropyl alcohol packet held approximately 12 inches from the patient's nose.

c. Scratch-and-sniff card—A scratch-and-sniff card that contains three odors to test gross olfaction is commercially available.

d. The University of Pennsylvania Smell Identification Test (UPSIT)—A far superior test to other assessments is the University of Pennsylvania Smell Identification Test (UPSIT); it is highly recommended for the evaluation of a patient with smell disorder. This test utilizes 40 forced-choice items that feature microencapsulated scratch-and-sniff odors. For example, one of the items reads, "This odor smells most like (a) chocolate, (b) banana, (c) onion, or (d) fruit punch." The patient is instructed to answer one of the alternatives. The test is highly reliable (short-term test-retest reliability r = 0.95) and is sensitive to age and gender differences. It is an accurate quantitative determination of the relative degree of olfactory deficit. Individuals with a total loss of olfactory function score in the range of 7–19 out of 40. The average score for total anosmics is slightly higher than that expected on the basis of chance alone because of the inclusion of some odorants that act by trigeminal stimulation.

2. Step 2: Determining the detection threshold— After the physician determines the degree to which qualitative sensations are present, the second step in the sensory evaluation is to establish a detection threshold for the odorant phenylethyl alcohol. This threshold is established using a graduated stimulus. Sensitivity for each side of the nose is determined with a detection threshold for phenyl-ethyl methyl ethyl carbinol. Nasal resistance can also be measured with anterior rhinomanometry for each side of the nose.

Differential Diagnosis

At the present time, there are no psychophysical methods to differentiate sensory from neural olfactory loss. Fortunately, the history of olfactory loss provides important clues to the cause. The leading causes of olfactory disorders are head trauma and viral infections. Head trauma is a more common cause of anosmia in children and young adults, and viral infections are more common causes of anosmia in older adults.

A. Viral Infection

Viral infections destroy the olfactory neuroepithelium; it is replaced by the respiratory epithelium. Parainfluenza virus type 3 appears to be especially detrimental to human olfaction. Human immunodeficiency virus (HIV) infection is associated with a subjective distortion of taste and smell that may become more severe as the disease progresses. Moreover, the loss of taste and smell may play an important role in the development and progression of HIV-associated wasting.

B. Cranial Trauma

Cranial trauma is followed by a unilateral or bilateral impairment of smell in up to 15% of cases; anosmia is more common than hyposmia. Olfactory dysfunction is more common when associated with loss of consciousness, more severe head injuries (grades II–V), and skull fracture. Frontal injuries and fractures disrupt the cribriform plate and olfactory axons that perforate it. Sometimes an associated cerebrospinal fluid rhinorrhea results from a tearing of the dura overlying the cribriform plate and paranasal sinuses. Anosmia also may follow blows to the occiput. Once traumatic anosmia

develops, it is usually permanent; only an estimated 10% of patients ever improve or recover. The perversion of the sense of smell may occur as a phase in the recovery process. Zinc sulfate therapy may enhance improvement in olfaction following trauma.

C. Congenital Anosmia

Congenital anosmias are rare but important. Kallmann syndrome is a neuronal migration defect for which the X-linked gene (KAL) has been cloned. It is characterized by congenital anosmia and hypogonadotropic hypogonadism. Anosmia also can occur in persons with albinism. The receptor cells are present but are hypoplastic, lack cilia, and do not project above the surrounding supporting cells.

D. Meningioma, Adenoma, and Aneurysm

Meningioma of the inferior frontal region is the most common neoplastic cause of anosmia; rarely, anosmia can occur with glioma of the frontal lobe. Occasionally, pituitary adenomas, craniopharyngiomas, suprasellar meningiomas, and aneurysms of the anterior part of the circle of Willis extend forward and damage olfactory structures. These tumors and hamartomas also may induce seizures with olfactory hallucinations, indicating involvement of the uncus of the temporal lobe.

Dysosmia, a subjective distortion of olfactory perception, may occur with intranasal disease that partially impairs smell or may represent a phase in the recovery from a neurogenic anosmia. Most dysosmic disorders consist of disagreeable or foul odors, and they may be accompanied by distortions of taste. Dysosmia is associated with depression.

Treatment

A. Transport Olfactory Loss

Therapy for patients with transport olfactory losses due to allergic rhinitis, bacterial rhinitis and sinusitis, polyps, neoplasms, and structural abnormalities of the nasal cavities can be undertaken rationally and with a high likelihood of improvement. The following treatments are frequently effective in restoring the sense of smell: (1) allergy management; (2) antibiotic therapy; (3) topical and systemic glucocorticoid therapy; and (4) operations for nasal polyps, deviation of the nasal septum, and chronic hyperplastic sinusitis.

B. Sensorineural Olfactory Loss

There is no treatment with demonstrated efficacy for sensorineural olfactory losses. Fortunately, spontaneous recovery often occurs. Some clinicians advocate zinc and vitamin therapy. Profound zinc deficiency undoubtedly can result in loss and distortion of the sense of smell, but it is not a clinical problem except in very limited geographic areas. Vitamin therapy has been predominantly in the form of vitamin A. The epithelial degeneration associated with vitamin A deficiency can cause anosmia, but vitamin A deficiency is not a common clinical problem in Western societies. Exposure to cigarette smoke and other airborne toxic chemicals can cause metaplasia of the olfactory epithelium. Spontaneous recovery can occur if the insult is discontinued; therefore, patient counseling is helpful in these cases.

C. AGING-RELATED OLFACTORY LOSS (PRESBYOSMIA)

As previously mentioned, more than half of people older than age 60 suffer from olfactory dysfunction. No effective treatment exists for presbyosmia, but it is important to discuss the problem with elderly patients. It can be reassuring to patients when a physician recognizes and discusses that smell disorders are common. In addition, direct benefits can be gained by identifying the problem early; the incidence of natural gas–related accidents is disproportionately high in the elderly, perhaps in part because of the gradual loss of smell. Mercaptan, the pungent odor in natural gas, is an olfactory and not a trigeminal stimulant. Many older patients with olfactory dysfunction experience a decrease in flavor sensation and find it necessary to hyperflavor food. The most common method is by increasing the amount of salt in their diet. Careful counseling can help these patients develop healthy strategies to deal with their decreased sense of smell.

Prognosis

The outcome of olfactory dysfunction is largely dependent on its cause. Olfactory dysfunction due to an obstruction caused by polyps, neoplasms, mucosal swelling, or septal deviation is reversible. When the obstruction is released, olfactory ability should return. Most patients who lose their sense of smell during an upper respiratory infection completely recover olfactory ability; however, a small number of patients never recover after the other symptoms of the upper respiratory infection resolve. For unclear reasons, these patients are mostly women in their fourth, fifth, and sixth decades of life. The prognosis for recovery is generally poor. Olfactory identification ability and thresholds progressively decline with age. Head trauma to the frontal region most frequently causes olfactory loss, although total anosmia is five times more likely with an occipital blow. Recovery of olfactory function following traumatic cranial injury is only 10%, and the quality of the olfactory ability after recovery is usually poor. Exposure to toxins such as cigarette smoke can cause metaplasia of the olfactory epithelium. Recovery can occur with removal of the offending agent.

Doty RL. Olfactory dysfunction and its measurement in the clinic and workplace. *Int Arch Occup Environ Health.* 2006;79(4):268. [PMID: 16429305] (Reviews quantitative assessment of the sense of smell in both the clinic and workplace.)

Simmen D, Briner HR. Olfaction in rhinology—methods of assessing the sense of smell. *Rhinology.* 2006;44(2):98. [PMID: 16792166] (Review of subjective and objective assessment of sense of smell.)

Zou Z, Buck LB. Combinatorial effects of odorant mixes in olfactory cortex. *Science.* 2006;311(5766):1477. [PMID: 16527983] (Cortical neurons that respond to combination of two odorants do not respond to a single odorant, thus explaining why odorant mixtures lead to novel precepts in humans.)

Congenital Anomalies of the Nose

Christina J. Laane, MD

■ CONGENITAL MIDLINE NASAL MASSES

Congenital midline nasal masses, which include nasal dermoid cysts, nasal encephaloceles, and nasal gliomas (Figures 10–1 and 10–2; see also Figure 10–5), are rare malformations; one occurs in 20,000–40,000 live births in the United States. Frontoethmoidal encephaloceles are more common in Southeast Asia, with one occurring in every 5000 births. Of the three types of anomalies, nasal dermoid cysts are the most common, accounting for 61% of all midline nasal lesions. In contrast, only about 250 nasal gliomas have been reported in the literature.

Dermoid cysts, encephaloceles, and gliomas most often occur in the nose, although these anomalies also can be found in the soft palate, the nasopharynx, and the paranasal sinuses. Dermoid cysts can occur in the tongue or neck as well. Nasal encephaloceles occur more frequently in males and have associated abnormalities in 30–40% of cases. Nasal dermoid cysts occur together with craniofacial malformations in 40% of cases; nasal dermoids are generally sporadic, although familial cases have been reported. Nasal gliomas generally occur as isolated anomalies.

NASAL DERMOID CYSTS

 ESSENTIALS OF DIAGNOSIS

- *Usually present as a slow-growing nasal mass or midline pit.*
- *Do not compress or transilluminate.*
- *Contain skin and dermal elements, including hair follicles and sebaceous glands.*
- *Magnetic resonance imaging (MRI) may reveal an intracranial connection.*

General Considerations

Nasal dermoid cysts consist of both ectodermal and mesodermal elements, including hair follicles, sweat glands, and sebaceous glands. They are probably embryologically related to nasal gliomas and nasal encephaloceles (see Figure 10–2); all three can occur as a result of an anterior skull base defect.

Clinical Findings

A. SYMPTOMS AND SIGNS

Nasal dermoid cysts are found in the midline of the nose as masses, sinus tracts, or as a combination of the two. They are usually diagnosed within the first 3 years of life and account for 1–3% of all dermoid cysts; they also account for 4–12% of head and neck dermoid cysts.

Nasal dermoid cysts are firm, slow-growing masses that do not transilluminate or compress. They demonstrate a negative Furstenberg test, meaning that these lesions don't expand with crying, Valsalva maneuver, or compression of the ipsilateral jugular veins. Nasal dermoid cysts occur anywhere along the nose from the glabella down to the nasal tip or columella, with the most common site being the lower third of the nasal bridge. They can cause broadening of the nasal dorsum and deformation of the nasal bones or cartilages. Patients may present with intermittent discharge of sebaceous material or inflammation; hair protruding from the site is pathognomonic, although this occurs in less than half of patients. Nasal dermoid cysts have an intracranial connection in up to 20–45% of cases (Figure 10–3).

B. IMAGING STUDIES

1. Computed tomography (CT) scans—As with nasal encephaloceles and nasal gliomas, CT imaging is useful for visualizing bony defects of the skull base. A bifid crista galli process and enlargement of the foramen cecum suggest intracranial involvement of the dermoid; however, up to 14% of children under the age of 1 year have incomplete ossification of these areas. With CT imaging, false-positive and false-negative results regarding intracranial involvement are not uncommon.

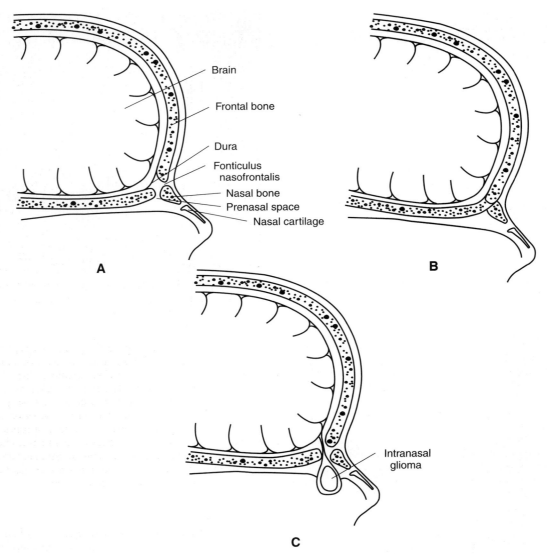

Figure 10–1. Nasal anatomy. **(A)** Early nasal anatomy. **(B)** Normal late nasal anatomy. **(C)** Intranasal glioma.

2. MRI—In general, MRI is more sensitive and specific than CT; it is superior for visualizing soft tissues and diagnosing intracranial extension and is thus the preferred imaging study. Nasal dermoid cysts appear very hyperintense on T1-weighted MRI images (Figure 10–4).

Complications

Untreated nasal dermoid cysts can lead to local inflammation or abscess formation. With the presence of an intracranial connection, they may result in cerebrospinal fluid (CSF) leakage, meningitis, cavernous sinus thrombosis, or periorbital cellulitis. Gradual expansion of nasal dermoid cysts can deform nasal bones or cartilages.

Treatment

Nasal dermoid cysts and sinuses, in general, should be surgically removed as soon as possible to avoid complications. As with nasal gliomas and nasal encephaloceles, any surgical intervention of nasal dermoid cysts should be preceded by full evaluation, including MRI imaging to determine which dermoid cysts have intracranial extension. For those that do, a neurosurgical evaluation is

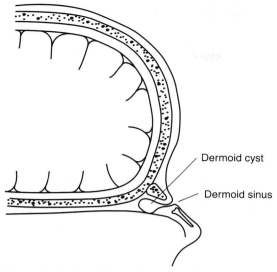

Figure 10–2. Nasal dermoid cyst and dermoid sinus.

Dermoid cyst

Dermoid sinus

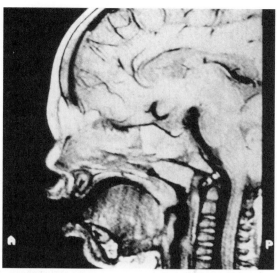

Figure 10–4. MRI of nasal dermoid cyst with intracranial involvement. (Imaging courtesy of Kristina W. Rosbe, MD, University of California, San Francisco.)

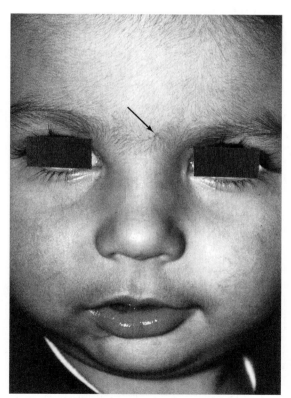

Figure 10–3. Dermoid cyst of nasal glabella, with tuft of hair visible (see *arrow*). (Photo courtesy of Kristina W. Rosbe, MD, University of California, San Francisco.)

required and craniotomy is generally performed as part of the procedure. The nasal portion of the dermoid can be removed using any one of various incisions, including midline vertical, transverse, lateral rhinotomy, or mid-brow. The external rhinoplasty approach allows good surgical exposure in combination with a superior cosmetic result. Cartilaginous grafts are needed at times for dorsal augmentation when normal nasal structures have been altered by the mass. More recently, intranasal endoscopic approaches have been used to resect nasal dermoid cysts, including their removal from the dura.

Prognosis

Recurrence rates for nasal dermoid cysts are as high as 50–100% when dermal elements are incompletely removed; however, when these elements are completely removed, the prognosis is good, although facial scarring, saddle nose deformity, or other nasal structure abnormalities can persist.

Bilkay U, Gundogan H, Ozek C et al. Nasal dermoid sinus cysts and the role of open rhinoplasty. *Ann Plast Surg.* 2001;47(1):8. [PMID: 11756796] (The etiology, diagnosis, and surgical management of nasal dermoid cysts are discussed, and advantages of the open rhinoplasty approach are described.)

Bloom D, Carvalho DS, Dory C, Brewster DF, Wickersham JK, Kearns DB. Imaging and surgical approach of nasal dermoids. *Int J Pediatr Otorhinolaryngol.* 2002;62(2):111. [PMID: 11788143] (MRI was determined to be the most accurate and cost-effective approach for imaging nasal dermoids, while the external rhinoplasty approach is recommended as the preferred surgical technique.)

Bratton C, Suskind DL, Thomas T, Kluka EA. Autosomal dominant familial frontonasal dermoid cysts: a mother and her identical twin daughters. *Int J Pediatr Otorhinolaryngol.* 2001;57(3):249. [PMID: 11223458] (This study is the first reported case of a mother and twin daughters who all had frontonasal dermoid cysts, suggesting an autosomal dominant inheritance in certain nasal dermoids.)

Lees MM, Connelly F, Kangesu L, Sommerlad B, Barnicoat A. Midline cleft lip and nasal dermoids over five generations: a distinct entity or autosomal dominant Pai syndrome? *Clin Dysmorphol.* 2006:15(3):155. [PMID: 16760735] (First described syndrome involving nasal dermoids.)

Mankarious L, Smith RJ. External rhinoplasty approach for extirpation and immediate reconstruction of congenital midline nasal dermoids. *Ann Otol Rhinol Laryngol.* 1998;107:786. [PMID: 9749549] (The external rhinoplasty approach for excision of congenital midline nasal dermoid cysts is the preferred method of treatment, although the subsequent impact on nasal growth is unknown.)

Weiss DD, Robson CD, Mulliken JB. Transnasal endoscopic excision of midline nasal dermoid from the anterior cranial base. *Plast Reconstr Surg.* 1998;102(6):2119. [PMID: 9811012] (Description of two patients, each with a nasal dermoid cyst with transcranial extension, whose masses were removed using endoscopic techniques without the need for craniotomy.)

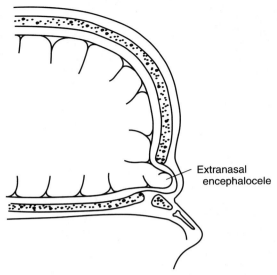

Figure 10–5. Extranasal encephalocele.

■ NASAL ENCEPHALOCELES & NASAL GLIOMAS

 ESSENTIALS OF DIAGNOSIS

- *Present, usually at birth, with midline nasal mass, nasal obstruction, or CSF leak.*
- *Nasal encephaloceles are compressible and expand with crying.*
- *Nasal gliomas are firm and noncompressible.*
- *MRI imaging may reveal intracranial extension in either anomaly.*

Nasal encephaloceles and nasal gliomas are congenital anomalies that are considered to be embryologically related. Nasal encephaloceles occur as a result of herniation of meninges, with or without brain tissue, through a congenital skull base defect (Figure 10–5). They may occur in occipital, basal, or frontoethmoidal regions. All encephaloceles involve a midline skull defect, which corresponds to the site of neural tube closure in the midline. Nasal gliomas likely have a similar origin, though they have lost their intracranial meningeal connection following closure of the anterior fontanelle (see Figure 10–1C).

Clinical Findings

A. SYMPTOMS AND SIGNS

Encephaloceles and gliomas in the nasal region generally present at birth as nasal masses. They may result in nasal obstruction, snoring, or respiratory distress. Patients may have hypertelorism or dislocation of the nasal bones or septum (Figure 10–6). Nasal encephaloceles are generally found at the root of the nose or inferior to the nasal bones. They are soft compressible masses that transilluminate and whose appearance may be confused with nasal polyps. Occasionally these lesions present with CSF rhinorrhea or meningitis.

Nasal gliomas are usually diagnosed at birth or in early childhood, although they also have been diagnosed in adulthood. With advances in ultrasound technology, gliomas can be diagnosed in utero. They most often occur without associated abnormalities. Nasal gliomas are usually firm, noncompressible masses with a negative Furstenberg test. They may be purple or gray and are sometimes covered with telangiectasias; therefore, they can be confused with nasal hemangiomas. Sixty percent of nasal gliomas are extranasal, 30% are intranasal, and 10% are both. Intranasal gliomas may be found high in the nasal vault, along the septum, or along the inferior turbinate. Approximately 15–20% of these lesions have a connection to dura by a pedicle of glial tissue. Histologically, nasal gliomas consist of mature astrocytes surrounded by fibrous connective tissue and normal nasal mucosa.

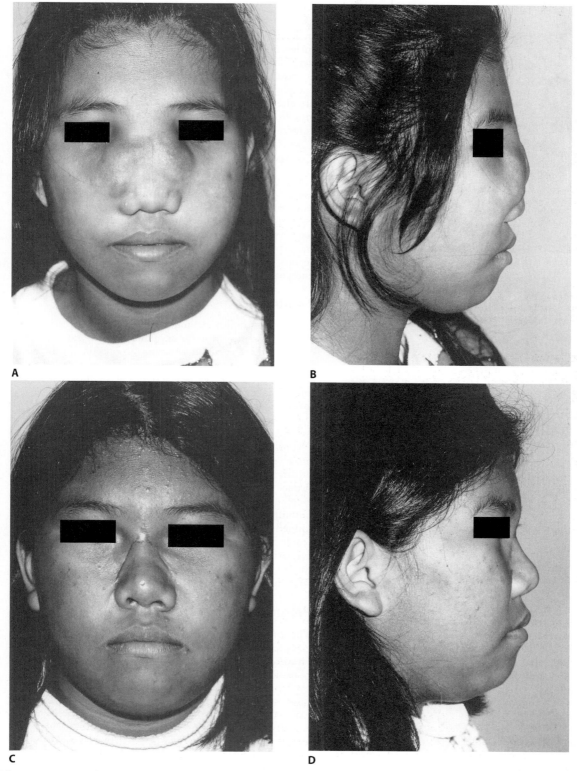

Figure 10–6. Nasal encephalocele: (**A** and **B**) Preoperative photos. (**C** and **D**) Postoperative photos. (Photos courtesy of William Y. Hoffman, MD, University of California, San Francisco.)

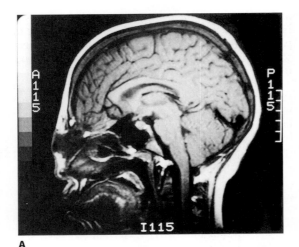

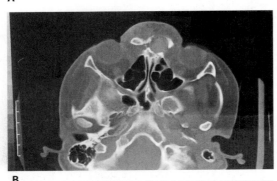

Figure 10–7. Nasal encephalocele. **(A)** MRI depicting intracranial involvement. **(B)** CT scan depicting extranasal involvement and hypertelorism. (Imaging courtesy of William Y. Hoffman, MD, University of California, San Francisco.)

B. IMAGING STUDIES

Imaging is important for detecting the presence and degree of intracranial involvement as well as for discovering associated abnormalities. Nasal gliomas appear isodense on CT scans and occasionally contain calcifications or cystic changes. On MRI scans, they usually appear hyperintense on T2-weighted images and of variable intensity on T1-weighted images. By revealing a contiguous CSF space, MRI imaging can also clearly differentiate nasal gliomas from nasal encephaloceles. CT imaging is most useful for visualizing bony defects of the skull base. MRI, however, is superior for demonstrating soft tissues and detecting intracranial extension (Figure 10–7).

Differential Diagnosis

Nasal gliomas and nasal encephaloceles may be confused with other masses found in the nasal area, including dermoid cysts, polyps, lacrimal duct cysts, hemangiomas, or malignant neoplasms. Nasal hemangiomas have a tendency for early rapid growth followed by involution, characteristics seen neither in nasal gliomas nor in nasal encephaloceles. Nasal polyps are very rare in infants and are often associated with cystic fibrosis. Polyps generally arise from the lateral nasal wall, as can nasal gliomas; in contrast, nasal encephaloceles are found in the midline.

Complications

Untreated, nasal encephaloceles carry the risk of CSF leak as well as associated infections that include meningitis and intracranial abscesses. These complications may occur in nasal gliomas as well, but with less frequency. In addition, nasal encephaloceles may increase in size over time, leading to progressive facial deformity. There are, however, no reports of malignant transformation of either nasal encephaloceles or nasal gliomas.

Treatment

Nasal masses in infants should not be biopsied or excised before a complete workup, including imaging, to determine whether there is an intracranial connection. If there is no such communication, intranasal masses may be removed endoscopically, which results in minimal trauma and minimal cosmetic deformity. External lesions may be excised using a skin incision over the mass or a coronal flap approach. More extensive lesions involving the cribriform plate may require a lateral rhinotomy.

For nasal encephaloceles and nasal gliomas with intracranial communication, a combined neurosurgical-otolaryngologic approach is most often recommended. A one- or two-stage procedure involving craniotomy in combination with an intranasal approach, lateral rhinotomy, or another external approach, may be performed. Some physicians, however, advocate endoscopic techniques for the treatment of nasal gliomas even with an intracranial connection; both resection of the lesion and repair of the CSF fistula may be achieved with endoscopic procedures.

Prognosis

The prognosis after the surgical resection of nasal encephaloceles and nasal gliomas is generally good. However, a recurrence rate of 4–10% exists as a result of the incomplete resection of nasal gliomas.

Chang KC, Leu YS. Nasal glioma: a case report. *Ear Nose Throat J.* 2001;80(6):410. [PMID: 11433845] (A case of nasal glioma removed using the lateral rhinotomy approach is described.)

De Biasio P, Scarso E, Prefumo F, Odella C, Venturini PL. Prenatal diagnosis of a nasal glioma in the mid trimester. *Ultrasound Obstet Gynecol.* 2006;27(5):571. [PMID: 16570265] (Diagnosis of glioma at 21 weeks with early resection.)

Hedlund G. Congenital frontonasal masses: developmental anatomy, malformations, and MR imaging. *Pediatr Radiol.* 2006;36(7):647. [PMID: 16532348] (MRI superior to determining extension.)

Hoeger PH, Schaefer H, Ussmueller J, Helme K. Nasal glioma presenting as a capillary haemangioma. *Eur J Pediatr.* 2001;160(2):84. [PMID: 11271395] (A case of a nasal glioma originally misdiagnosed as a capillary hemangioma is described.)

Hoving EW. Nasal encephaloceles. *Childs Nerv Syst.* 2000;16:702. [PMID: 11151720] (The pathogenesis, diagnosis, and treatment of nasal encephaloceles are reviewed.)

Mahapatra AK, Agrawal D. Anterior encephaloceles: a series of 103 cases over 32 years. *J Clin Neurosci.* 2006;13(5):536. [PMID: 16679016] (Nasal encephalocele of frontoethmoid origin all had swelling of nose, varying degrees of hypertelorism.)

Rouev P, Dimov P, Shomov G. A case of nasal glioma in a newborn infant. *Int J Pediatr Otorhinolaryngol.* 2001;58(1):91. [PMID: 11249987] (Description of glioma located along the inferior turbinate in a 1-day-old infant.)

Sciarretta V, Pasquini E, Frank G et al. Endoscopic treatment of benign tumors of the nose and paranasal sinuses: a report of 33 cases. *Am J Rhinol.* 2006;20(1):64. [PMID: 16539297] (Endonasal gliomas can be resected endoscopically in select patients with reasonable results.)

Shah J. Pedunculated nasal glioma: MRI features and review of the literature. *J Postgrad Med.* 1999;45(1):15. [PMID: 10734326] (A case of nasal glioma is presented and its MRI features described; diagnosis of nasal gliomas is discussed.)

Van Den Abbeele T, Francois M, Narcy P. Transnasal endoscopic repair of congenital defects of the skull base in children. *Arch Otolaryngol Head Neck Surg.* 1999;125:580. [PMID: 10326818] (Four cases of transnasal endoscopic resection of nasal gliomas and encephaloceles, including one that involved the repair of CSF leak, are described.)

■ NEONATAL BONY NASAL OBSTRUCTIONS

CHOANAL ATRESIA

 ESSENTIALS OF DIAGNOSIS

- *Bilateral cases present at birth with respiratory distress.*
- *Unilateral cases may present with unilateral rhinorrhea or nasal obstruction.*
- *CT scanning confirms the diagnosis.*

General Considerations

Choanal atresia occurs in one of every 5000–8000 live births. It affects females twice as often as males, and unilateral atresia is twice as common as bilateral atresia. Increased rates of choanal atresia have been suggested in patients with a history of in utero exposure to methimazole; this exposure can also lead to other malformations, including esophageal atresia and developmental delay.

Most cases of choanal atresia are sporadic, although familial cases suggest autosomal dominant or autosomal recessive modes of a single gene defect. Approximately one-half to two-thirds of patients with choanal atresia have associated malformations, which occur more frequently with bilateral atresia. The most common of these is the **CHARGE** association:

Coloboma of the eye
Heart malformations
Choanal **A**tresia
Retarded growth, development, or both
Genital hypoplasia
Ear malformations, deafness, or both

Choanal atresia is associated with as many as 20 other syndromes; other common coexisting malformations include polydactyly, tracheoesophageal fistula, craniosynostosis, high arched palate, and Treacher Collins syndrome.

Clinical Findings

A. SYMPTOMS AND SIGNS

Neonates are obligate nasal breathers during the first 3–5 months of life; therefore, choanal atresia leading to nasal obstruction may present as respiratory distress and require emergent intervention. This is particularly true of bilateral choanal atresia in which severe nasal obstruction leads to a cyclical cyanosis that improves with crying and worsens with feeding. The nose is often filled with thick mucus and the initial diagnosis is usually made by the inability to pass a small catheter through the choana. Unilateral choanal atresia occurs more frequently in the right choana and may present later in life with unilateral nasal obstruction or rhinorrhea. Frequently, nasal cavity stenosis is found in the patent side as well.

B. IMAGING STUDIES

CT imaging is the study of choice for visualizing choanal atresia (Figure 10–8). Axial images allow examination of the entire nasal cavity and help distinguish between complete and incomplete atresia. On CT imaging, choanal atresia is diagnosed if the posterior choanal orifice measures less than 0.34 cm unilaterally or if the posterior vomer measures greater than 0.55 cm. Traditionally, choanal atresia has been described as 90% bony and 10% membranous. However, more recent studies reveal that in 29% of cases, choanal atre-

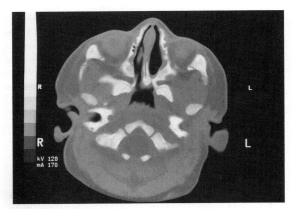

Figure 10–8. CT scan depicting left choanal atresia. (Imaging courtesy of Kristina W. Rosbe, MD, University of California, San Francisco.)

sia consists of purely bony elements; in 71% of cases, both bony and membranous materials are present. Often, widening of the vomer is noted as well.

Treatment

A. Nonsurgical Measures

The initial treatment, particularly of bilateral choanal atresia, is to secure a safe airway for the neonate. Often this can be accomplished using an oral airway or a McGovern nipple placed into the patient's mouth. The **McGovern nipple** features an enlarged hole through which the infant can breathe as well as feed. When these appliances fail, alternatives include intubation or tracheotomy.

B. Surgical Measures

When the patient is stable for general anesthesia, surgical correction of the atresia can be performed using one of several different techniques. Most commonly, transpalatal and transnasal approaches are used.

1. The transpalatal approach—The transpalatal approach is more often reserved for older patients with unilateral atresia. Although there are better visualization and higher success rates, palate growth can be disrupted, which frequently leads to palate and crossbite deformities.

2. The transnasal approach—The transnasal approach involves less blood loss and is quicker; however, there is an increased risk of CSF leakage and meningitis. A perforating instrument such as a curved trocar can be used to make an opening in the atretic plate.

3. Laser therapy—Various lasers, including carbon dioxide, KTP, and holmium:YAG, can be used to treat choanal atresia. KTP lasers have been used together with

endoscopic techniques, with good success, to create an opening. An effective method is using an operating microscope in combination with a carbon dioxide laser to create mucosal flaps on the nasal and nasopharyngeal sides of the atretic plate. These are laid into the new choanal opening to help prevent scar contracture, which could lead to closure of the circumferential epithelial defect.

C. Additional Measures

Regardless of the type of choanal atresia repair used, most physicians place either round or keel-type stents into the nasal cavity for 2–6 weeks to prevent restenosis. In addition, mitomycin applied to the posterior choanae at the completion of surgical repair, done in combination with stenting, often decreases recurrence rates as compared to stenting alone.

Prognosis

Success rates are in the range of 55–85% for surgical correction of choanal atresia. Failure results when the choanae become obliterated by granulation or scar tissue. Recurrences can occur between 2 months and 6 years and often require further surgical correction or dilations. Recently, repeated balloon dilation has been used successfully to treat recurrent choanal atresia.

Chia S, Carvalho DS, Jaffe DM, Pransky SM. Unilateral choanal atresia in identical twins: a case report and literature review. *Int J Pediatr Otorhinolaryngol.* 2002;62(3):249. [PMID: 11852129] (A case of monozygotic twins with choanal atresia is presented.)

Dedo HH. Transnasal mucosal flap rotation technique for repair of posterior choanal atresia. *Otolaryngol Head Neck Surg.* 2001;124(6):674. [PMID: 11391260] (Thirty-two cases of choanal atresia were treated using a combination of carbon dioxide laser, anterior mucosal flaps, and Teflon keels, with all patients having resultant adequate to good bilateral nasal orifice sizes.)

Goettmann D, Strohm M, Strecker EP. Treatment of a recurrent choanal atresia by balloon dilation. *Cardiovasc Intervent Radiol.* 2000;23(6):480. [PMID: 11232900] (A case report that demonstrates that recurrent choanal atresia can be treated successfully using balloon dilation.)

Holland BW, McGuirt WF Jr. Surgical management of choanal atresia: improved outcome using mitomycin. *Arch Otolaryngol Head Neck Surg.* 2001;127(11):1375. [PMID: 11701078] (Eight children with choanal atresia treated with mitomycin intraoperatively required significantly fewer postoperative dilations compared with patients not treated with mitomycin.)

Tzifa KT, Skinner DW. Endoscopic repair of unilateral choanal atresia with the KTP laser: a one-stage procedure. *J Laryngol Otol.* 2001;115(4):286. [PMID: 11276330] (Three patients with choanal atresia treated with endoscopic KTP required no dilations or further surgical repair of the atresia.)

Vanzieleghem B, Lemmerling MM, Vermeersch HR et al. Imaging studies in the diagnostic workup of neonatal nasal obstruction. *J Comput Assist Tomogr.* 2001;25(4):540. [PMID: 11473183] (Review of the imaging studies used in the diagnostic workup of 12 neonates with choanal atresia, nasal pyriform aperture stenosis, a nasolacrimal duct mucocele, or nasal hypoplasia.)

NASAL PYRIFORM APERTURE STENOSIS

ESSENTIALS OF DIAGNOSIS

- *Presents with nasal obstruction within the first few months of life.*
- *Examination reveals bony obstruction at the nasal vestibule.*
- *CT imaging confirms the diagnosis.*

General Considerations

Congenital nasal pyriform aperture stenosis was first described in 1989 as a bony overgrowth of the medial maxilla that leads to narrowing of the nasal inlet. This disorder is often considered a form of holoprosencephaly. As many as 50 cases have been described in the last decade. Pyriform aperture stenosis can be found either in isolation or together with other malformations, including submucous cleft palate, absence of the anterior pituitary gland, hypoplastic maxillary sinuses, or a central maxillary incisor.

Clinical Findings

A. SYMPTOMS AND SIGNS

Half of patients with nasal pyriform aperture stenosis present at birth with the same symptoms found in patients with bilateral choanal atresia. With severe stenosis, neonates have respiratory distress, feeding difficulties, or a cyclical cyanosis that is relieved by crying. Examination of the nose reveals a bony obstruction in the vestibule and an inability to pass a catheter into the nose. In 60% of cases, a central maxillary incisor is present, lending support for pyriform aperture stenosis being a form of holoprosencephaly. Other features of holoprosencephaly seen in these patients include hypotelorism and a flat nasal bridge.

B. IMAGING STUDIES

On CT imaging, nasal pyriform aperture stenosis is diagnosed when the transverse diameter of each aperture is less than 3 mm or when the width is less than 8 mm. In addition, brain MRI or CT imaging should be performed to rule out pituitary or midbrain abnormalities.

Treatment

The initial treatment of mild forms of nasal pyriform aperture stenosis is conservative. Attempts are made to alleviate nasal obstruction using topical nasal decongestants, corticosteroids, suctioning, or humidification. In more severe cases, stents or a McGovern nipple may be required to maintain a patent nasal airway. If the infant fails to respond to medical treatment within 10–15 days, loses weight, has cyclical cyanosis, or develops pulmonary hypertension from obstruction, surgical repair is recommended. This is generally accomplished by a superior gingivolabial incision and premaxillary degloving approach. Taking care to preserve mucosa, the aperture is widened using drills and stents are usually placed for 1–4 weeks.

Prognosis

The symptoms related to mild cases of nasal pyriform aperture stenosis may resolve as the child grows. Patients who require surgery most often achieve relief of nasal obstruction and follow-up to at least 1 year postoperatively reveals favorable outcomes.

Brown OE, Myer CM III, Manning SC. Congenital nasal pyriform aperture stenosis. *Laryngoscope.* 1989;99(1):86. [PMID: 2909825] (Congenital nasal pyriform aperture stenosis is described for the first time.)

Fornelli RA, Ramadan HH. Congenital nasal pyriform aperture stenosis: clinical review. *Otolaryngol Head Neck Surg.* 2000;122(1):113. [PMID: 10629496] (A case of nasal pyriform aperture stenosis and a review of the literature are presented.)

Lee JJ. Congenital nasal pyriform aperture stenosis: nonsurgical management and long-term analysis. *Int J Otorhinolaryngol.* 2001;60(2):167. [PMID: 11518596] (Two cases of congenital nasal pyriform aperture stenosis are reviewed, and the embryology, presentation, and treatment of this disorder are discussed.)

Van Den Abbeele T, Triglia JM, Francois M, Narcy P. Congenital nasal pyriform aperture stenosis: diagnosis and management of 20 cases. *Ann Otol Rhinol Laryngol.* 2001;110(1):70. [PMID: 11201813] (The diagnosis, treatment, outcome, and abnormalities associate with pyriform aperture stenosis are reviewed.)

Vanzieleghem B, Lemmerling MM, Vermeersch HF et al. Imaging studies in the diagnostic workup of neonatal nasal obstruction. *J Comput Assist Tomogr.* 2001;25(4):540. [PMID: 11473183] (The imaging studies used in the diagnostic workup of 12 neonates with choanal atresia, nasal pyriform aperture stenosis, a nasolacrimal duct mucocele, or nasal hypoplasia are reviewed.)

■ SELECTED ANOMALIES OF THE NOSE

HEMANGIOMAS

Hemangiomas are common tumors that occur in up to 10–12% of Caucasian children and up to 22% of premature infants. They affect females three times more

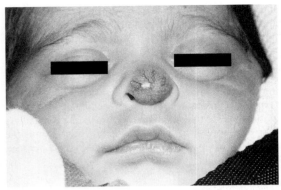

Figure 10–9. Hemangioma of the nasal tip. (Photo courtesy of Kristina W. Rosbe, MD, University of California, San Francisco.)

frequently than males. These lesions are not present at birth but appear within the first few months of life. MRI is the most appropriate imaging modality. In general, hemangiomas demonstrate an early 3–9 month proliferative phase followed by quiescence and then involution, generally by 5–7 years of age. As many as 50–98% of hemangiomas regress spontaneously, often making close observation the most appropriate treatment.

Hemangiomas may be present in any portion of the head or neck, including the nose (Figure 10–9). Here they may be found intra- or extranasally and can lead to nasal obstruction. Nasal hemangiomas, in comparison to hemangiomas found in other sites, may have lower rates of involution. Lesions that do not regress, and those that lead to airway obstruction, bleeding, or thrombocytopenia require more aggressive intervention. Severe cases may be treated with systemic or intralesional corticosteroids, surgery, or with carbon dioxide or Nd:YAG lasers. Good response rates also have been reported with interferon alpha, although neurologic complications may occur. Nasal reconstruction may be necessary when nasal cartilages or bones have been destroyed or distorted. A full discussion of hemangiomas is found in Chapter 6.

ARRHINIA

Arrhinia is defined as a congenital absence of the nose; approximately 25 cases have been reported in the literature. In this situation, the nasal bones, cribriform plate, and nasal septum are absent. The paranasal sinuses and olfactory bulbs are often absent as well, and high arched palate and hypertelorism are common findings. The embryologic abnormality is likely to be failure of the nasal placode to invaginate during the fifth week of fetal development. Most cases reported are sporadic, although familial cases with a dominant inheritance have been described. Surgical correction is often delayed until preschool age, unless problems with feeding are severe. Surgery involves both correction of the high arched palate and reconstruction of an external nose. Surgery is often performed in multiple stages, using techniques such as forehead flaps, rib grafts, and tissue expansion.

DUPLICATION ANOMALIES

Fewer than 10 cases of duplication anomalies of the nose have been reported in the literature. These include polyrrhinia and supernumerary nostrils.

1. Polyrrhinia

Polyrrhinia describes the existence of two external noses. One embryologic theory to describe this malformation involves the development of two pairs of nasal placodes, which then undergo the normal development. Frequently, bilateral choanal atresia is also present. The atresia is corrected first, followed by excision of the medial portions of each external nose for cosmetic improvement.

2. Supernumerary Nostrils

A supernumerary nostril is an extra opening lateral, medial, or superior to the normal nostril; at presentation, it may be filled with fluid. This additional orifice may be unilateral or bilateral and may or may not communicate with the nasal cavity. Embryologically, this structure may result from a localized abnormality of the lateral nasal process in which a fissure appears accidentally during mesenchymal proliferation. A supernumerary nostril may be excised as a wedge, closing the normal nasal tissue primarily.

Clymer M, Fortune DS, Reinisch L, Toriumi DM, Werkhaven JA, Ries WR. Interstitial Nd:YAG photocoagulation for vascular malformations and hemangiomas in childhood. *Arch Otolaryn Head Neck Surg.* 1998;124:431. [PMID: 9559692] (Interstitial photocoagulation of hemangiomas and vascular malformations can achieve reduction in the size of these lesions.)

Greinwald JH Jr, Burke DK, Bonthius DJ, Bauman NM, Smith RJ. An update on the treatment of hemangiomas in children with interferon alfa-2a. *Arch Otolaryn Head Neck Surg.* 1999;125:21. [PMID: 9932582] (Although interferon alfa-2a is an effective treatment in pediatric patients with massive or life-threatening hemangiomas, neurologic evaluation must be performed because this therapy leads to a high incidence of associated neurologic abnormalities.)

Hallak A, Jamjoon H, Hosseinzadeh T. Supernumerary nostrils: a case report and review. *Aesthetic Plast Surg.* 2001;25(3):241.

[PMID: 11426317] (A case of supernumerary nostril, its treatment, and the theories of the embryogenesis of this finding are discussed.)

McCarthy JG, Borud LJ, Schreiber JS. Hemangiomas of the nasal tip. *Plast Reconstr Surg*. 2002;109(1):31. [PMID: 11786788] (Early open rhinoplasty for resection of nasal tip hemangiomas can be performed safely and with minimal scarring.)

Meyer R. Total external and internal construction in arrhinia. *Plast Reconstr Surg*. 1997;99(2):534. [PMID: 9030164] (A multiple-stage surgical correction of arrhinia is described.)

Olsen OE, Gjelland K, Reigstad H, Rosendahl K. Congenital absence of the nose: a case report and literature review. *Pediatr Radiol*. 2001;31(4):225. [PMID: 11321738] (Twenty-two previously reported cases and one new case of congenital absence of the nose are reviewed.)

Williams A. Supernumerary nostril: a rare congenital deformity. *Int J Pediatr Otorhinolaryngol*. 1998;44(2):161. [PMID: 9725533] (A case of supernumerary nostril and a review of eight cases of duplication anomalies of the nose are presented.)

Nasal Trauma

Jeffrey H. Spiegel, MD, FACS, & William Numa, MD

ESSENTIALS OF DIAGNOSIS

- *History of recent trauma to midface; should assess mechanism of injury, presence of epistaxis or rhinorrhea, history of previous injury, and new onset of nasal airway obstruction or deformity.*
- *On examination, note any mucosal laceration, septal disruption, or septal hematoma.*
- *Depending on severity of insult, must rule out concurrent injury to eyes, lacrimal system, paranasal sinuses, teeth, and oral cavity.*

General Considerations

Nasal fracture as a result of trauma to the midface is considered the most common of head and neck fractures. Frequently the result of physical altercation, nasal trauma is most often not life-threatening; however, significant functional and aesthetic impairment may result if these injuries are not accurately diagnosed and addressed in a timely fashion.

The incidence of nasal fracture is high in both adults and children. Of maxillofacial injuries, fractures of the nasal bones account for up to 39–45% of cases reported in adults, and up to 45% of injuries in children. In adults, the highest rates of incidence are found among men, with a 2:1 predominance over cases reported in women. In men, nasal fracture is most often associated with intentional trauma and is clearly more common in the 15- to 25-year age group. In women, nasal trauma is usually the result of personal accidental injury, most commonly the result of falls and is often seen in patients over the age of 60.

In children, a clear gender predilection for injury is less likely, although cases are more often reported in boys. Also, more cases of nasal trauma in children are the result of accidental injury related to sports and play rather than physical confrontation. It is important to note, however, that anywhere from 30% to 50% of all pediatric victims of abuse present with maxillofacial injury, a concern not to be overlooked, particularly when evaluating the possibility of fracture concealed by the presence of facial edema.

Pathogenesis

Given the central and prominent position of the nasal bones and the significant lack of skeletal support for their position, the nose is particularly vulnerable to fracture as a result of maxillofacial injury. Reports indicate that the amount of force required to create a fracture of the nasal structure is small, possibly as little as 25 pounds of pressure. Superiorly, the structure of the nasal bones thickens with support from the underlying nasal spine of the frontal bone, an area more resistant to injury than the distal, thinning segment of the nose, which is unsupported and much more often the location of a fracture.

Trauma to the nasal cartilage, either from a directed frontal or inferior assault or from an indirect lateral injury, often results in displacement, dislocation, or avulsion rather than true fracture. The physical elasticity and flexible attachments of the nasal cartilage allow for the significant absorption and dissipation of energy, thus preventing considerable injury from a greater amount of force than the bony structure would tolerate. The nasal septum, however, is less apt to avoid injury given its rigid osteochondral junctions, which include the perpendicular plate of the ethmoid bone and the vomer anteriorly and its relatively weak association with the maxillary crest. As such, a higher incidence of true fracture can be found with the cartilaginous septum as a result of trauma to the midface, usually with a vertical orientation caudally and a horizontal orientation posteriorly.

In children, the nasal bones retain their elasticity with stability resulting from development and immature pneumatization. These factors, combined with a child's proportionally smaller nasal bones and proportionally larger cartilaginous structures, produce a greater tendency for cartilaginous injury to occur. However, in most cases of nasal trauma, the nasal cartilage fractures without significant displacement and, given the inherent flexibility of a child's nose, often returns to its anatomic position.

Classification

The classification of nasal injuries can be separated into two groups: those created by lateral or oblique impact and those created by frontal impact.

A. LATERAL INJURIES

Lateral injury, the more common variety given the absence of structural support on either side of the nasal pyramid, can be divided into three planes, with the extent of involvement dependent on the force of impact. Injury in the first plane results only in fracture of the ipsilateral nasal bone, by far the most common occurrence, which usually results in a visible depression of the bony surface two thirds of the way down its slope. With greater force, injury in the second plane would also involve the contralateral nasal bone and septum. In the third plane, enough force would be provided to fracture the frontal process of the maxilla and the lacrimal bone, possibly resulting in fragmentation, a total dislocation of the nasal architecture, or even injury to the lacrimal apparatus.

With lateral injuries, fractures of the nasal septum usually extend posteriorly into the perpendicular plate of the ethmoid bone, but without extension to the cribriform plate.

B. FRONTAL INJURIES

Frontal injuries generally require a greater amount of force and are divided into three planes as well. The first plane is limited to the nasal tip and does not extend beyond an anatomic line separating the lower part of the nasal bones from the nasal spine. With most of the impact absorbed by the nasal cartilage, injury usually involves avulsion of the upper lateral cartilages. Posterior dislocation of the septal and alar cartilages is also possible, but less likely. Injury in the second plane includes the nasal spine as well as the nasal dorsum and the nasal septum. Injuries in this plane produce a flattening and splaying of the nasal bones with deviation of the septum, overriding segmentation, mucosal tearing, and fracture of the nasal spine. Injury in plane 3 requires a substantial force of impact and may involve fractures of the orbit or extend to structures within the cranial vault. The nasal bones are often comminuted and associated with fractures of the frontal process of the maxilla, lacrimal, and ethmoid bones, and occasionally the cribriform plate. Fracture and dislocation of the nasal septum are severe, with collapse of the dorsal plane and telescoping of the septal fragments.

The nasal septum may be involved in approximately 20% of all traumatic fractures of the nose. A substantially greater impact, however, whether frontal, lateral or oblique, consistently produces a C-type fracture of the septum just posterior to the nasal spine and extending posteriorly and superiorly into the perpendicular plate. It then changes direction anteriorly, ending just before and below the cribriform plate, along the posterosuperior aspect of the nasal bones. This finding can be demonstrated on physical exam by noting displacement of the caudal septum to one side and deviation of the posterior septum to the other.

Anatomy

A. NASAL PYRAMID

The structure of the nasal pyramid projects anteriorly from the midface, attached to the facial skeleton at its base superiorly. From the apex or nasal tip, the columella projects inferoposteriorly toward the center of the superior lip, adjacent on either side to the nares. Encompassing the border of the nares are the alae of the nose superiorly and laterally, and the floor of the nose inferiorly. At the posterior aspect of the base of the nose is the piriform aperture, bordered superiorly and laterally by the frontal processes of the maxilla and the nasal bones. The inferior portion of the cartilaginous nose, otherwise considered the base of the nose, includes the lobule, which consists of the lower lateral cartilages, the tip, the alae, and the columella. In the midline, the posterior aspect of the medial crura of the lower lateral cartilages articulates with the caudal membranous septum. Anteriorly, the medial crura are enclosed within the columella. The lateral crura of the lower lateral cartilages project superiorly to overlap the inferior aspect of the upper lateral cartilages in the midline. Laterally, these crura loosely attach to the piriform aperture. The superior portion of the cartilaginous nose includes the two upper lateral cartilages and the quadrilateral cartilage of the septum, all of which are invested by a common perichondrial sheath. Laterally, the superior aspects of the upper lateral cartilages are also loosely attached to the piriform aperture.

B. NASAL VAULT

Superior to the nasal base is the bony vault of the nose, which is bound by the frontal processes of the maxilla, the nasal bones, and the alveolar process. Through the midline of this vault runs the anterior nasal spine inferiorly and the perpendicular plate of the ethmoid bone superiorly. At the superior aspect of where the nasal bones meet the frontal bone is the nasion, which is the midline portion of the nasofrontal suture. At the inferior aspect of where the nasal bones meet the nasal cartilages is the rhinion, which is also in the midline. The septum of the nose includes the quadrilateral cartilage and the anterior nasal spine anteroinferiorly, and the perpendicular plate of the ethmoid bone, the sphenoid crest, the vomer, and the maxillary crest posterosuperiorly. At the roof of the nose within the nasal cavity is the cribriform plate, and at the posterior aspect of this roof is the choana, through which the nasal cavities and the nasopharynx communicate. At the floor of the nasal cavity are the palatine process of the maxilla and the horizontal process of the palatine bone, with the medial pterygoid plates located laterally on either side.

C. NASAL TURBINATES

The nasal turbinates are found on the medial aspects of the nasal cavities. The inferior turbinate lies superior to the inferior meatus and is the largest of the three. Inferior to the turbinate within the inferior meatus is the opening of the ipsilateral nasolacrimal duct. The middle meatus lies between the inferior and middle turbinates and accepts drainage from the frontal sinus, the maxillary sinus, and the anterior ethmoid air cells. The superior turbinate lies above the superior meatus, which drains the posterior ethmoid air cells. Posterosuperior to this structure lays a sphenoethmoid recess on either side of the anterior aspect of the sphenoid sinus.

D. EXTERNAL BLOOD SUPPLY

The external blood supply of the nose includes indirect contributions from both the external and the internal carotid arteries. From the external carotid artery, branches of the facial artery supply the inferior aspects of the nose and include the superior labial and lateral nasal arteries. These branches join with the dorsal nasal artery, a terminal point for the ophthalmic artery from the internal carotid artery. The internal blood supply of the nasal pyramid and superior portion of the nasal cavity also include an indirect contribution from the internal carotid artery by way of the anterior and posterior ethmoid branches of the ophthalmic artery. The maxillary artery off of the external carotid artery provides most of the blood supply to the nasal cavity by way of the sphenopalatine artery. At the posterior aspect of the middle turbinate, the sphenopalatine artery splits into the posterolateral nasal and septal arteries, the septal branches of which communicate anteriorly with the anterior ethmoid arteries—an important anastomosis between the external and internal arterial systems.

E. VENOUS DRAINAGE

Venous drainage of the nose follows the accompanying arterial supply, with facial veins emptying into the external and internal jugular veins. In the nasal cavity, venous drainage from the ethmoid bones enters the orbit, thereby communicating via the ophthalmic veins with the cavernous sinus and dural venous system. Posteriorly, venous drainage from the nasal cavity follows the sphenopalatine veins into the pterygopalatine fossa and plexus, also communicating with the dural venous system. This posterosuperior venous drainage of the nose is thus a potential vehicle for extracranial infections to spread intracranially.

F. NERVE SUPPLY

The nerve supply of the nose includes general somatic efferent innervation from buccal branches of the facial nerve. General somatic afferent innervation is supplied by the first two branches of the trigeminal nerve. From the ophthalmic branch arise the anterior and posterior ethmoid nerves and the infratrochlear nerve. From the maxillary branch arise the posterolateral and posteroinferior nasal nerves, the nasopalatine nerve, and the infraorbital nerve, which joins with the infratrochlear nerve and external nasal branch of the anterior ethmoid nerve to innervate the skin. Sympathetic innervation to the nasal mucosa is derived from postganglionic fibers of the maxillary nerve via the nerve of the pterygoid canal, which originates via the deep petrosal nerve from the superior cervical sympathetic ganglion. Parasympathetic innervation in the nose includes zygomaticotemporal distribution to the lacrimal gland, also via the maxillary nerve and the nerve of the pterygoid canal. Special sensory innervation via the olfactory nerve pierces the cribriform plate at the roof of the nasal cavity from the inferior aspect of the olfactory bulbs to innervate the superior aspect of the nasal septum and the superior turbinate. A terminal nerve also pierces the cribriform plate to innervate the cartilaginous septum anteriorly from a terminal ganglion located medially to the olfactory bulbs.

Clinical Findings

A. HISTORY

The mechanism of injury in nasal fracture usually involves some variety of blunt traumas to the midface. However, information regarding the direction, force, and exact location of the impact is valuable in determining the probable extent of injury. Given the nature of severe edema associated with midface trauma, an evaluation of the extent of injury can be hindered if a significant delay exists between the time of injury and the time of examination. Early treatment is important because most nasal-septal fractures can be managed by closed reduction within a few hours. Thus, if the timing of the injury has allowed for a hindrance to proper inspection, repair must be delayed from 3 to 11 days, depending on the time required for the inflammation to subside. If enough time has passed for the initial insult to heal, the management required to repair the fracture could be extensive.

B. SYMPTOMS AND SIGNS

Additional history regarding the findings associated with nasal trauma can also be paramount in determining the extent of the injury. In most cases, a history of epistaxis is noted, the severity of which depends on the

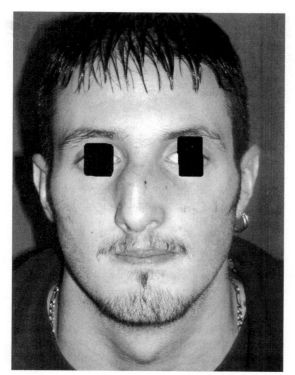

Figure 11–1. A young man 7 days after getting hit in the nose during an altercation. Note the obvious deformity and deviation.

extent of mucosal laceration sustained at the time of injury. Rhinorrhea may also be noted and, depending on the accuracy of the patient's description of his or her nasal discharge, may be indicative of trauma intracranially (eg, cerebrospinal fluid [CSF] rhinorrhea). Deformity of the nose and airway obstruction can be severe, but a history of insult, including fracture, obstruction, or reconstructive surgery, may interfere with determining the degree of the deformity sustained acutely. If the mechanism of injury is severe, a regional review of systems may be required, including a history of oculomotor or visual dysfunction, anosmia independent of mucosal injury, and dental or facial sensory deficits often associated with maxillary involvement.

C. Physical Examination

With the patient seated and comfortable, the nose should be viewed externally from all angles, with any unusual variations in contour, size, anatomic angles, lacerations of the skin, and hematomas noted. The presence and severity of epistaxis and, if applicable, CSF rhinorrhea should also be noted. A proper internal examination of the nose requires mucosal decongestion with either 0.25% phen-

ylephrine or oxymetazoline hydrochloride administered as a spray or with careful placement of cotton pledgets. If desired, 4.0% cocaine may be used, which has the advantage of providing anesthesia in addition to local vasoconstriction. Following this preparation, palpation of the nasal skeleton and cartilages may reveal abnormal variations in position and stability, as well as the presence of crepitus or point tenderness. Using a nasal speculum, each nasal cavity should be assessed either via direct visualization or, if necessary, with the aid of endoscopy. The nasal septum should be examined for the presence of deformity, dislocation, swelling, laceration, and hematoma (Figure 11–1).

During examination, an unusually wide or flat nasal base or nasal tip, along with abnormal nasal tip deflections, suggests prior injury or deformity. Injury extending to the orbit may include loss of the glabellar angle and the presence of telecanthus. CSF rhinorrhea indicates extension to the cribriform plate, frontal sinuses, or nasoethmoid complex. Medial maxillary involvement includes maxillary wall depression and a C-shaped nasal-septal deformity, with or without concurrent depression of the frontal process of the maxilla or inferior orbit. The stability of this process may be assessed further with bimanual examination using a Kelly clamp internally and a finger externally.

Unusual mobility of the nasal cartilages is consistent with avulsion, a finding often associated with mucosal laceration. Acute injury to the nasal septum is better differentiated from prior injury by the presence of motion tenderness with bimanual palpation. Pain localized to the anterior nasal spine, with or without dislocation, is also indicative of acute injury and should be assessed by sublabial palpation. A septal hematoma, if present, usually involves only the cartilaginous septum. It is associated with widening of the septum and persistent discoloration and should be pursued further with direct aspiration or mucosal incision.

D. Imaging Studies

Although still controversial, in most cases, the use of imaging studies in the diagnosis of nasal trauma is unnecessary. With radiographs, studies have demonstrated poor sensitivity and specificity in diagnosing nasal fractures; therefore, even in patients whose abnormalities were not demonstrated, management was unaffected. In addition, differentiating prior fracture from acute injury in the case of minimal displacement is unlikely. Thus, since the assessment and intervention of acute nasal injury are determined by clinical presentation, obtaining radiographs is not recommended except when legal documentation is necessary, as in the case of suspected abuse, or when the presence of additional fractures to the midface is suspected, as in more extensive injury. With severe trauma that includes involvement of the orbit, the ethmoid bones, or the cribriform plate, coronal sections with computed tomography (CT) should be obtained.

Differential Diagnosis

Although simple nasal fractures remain the most common of all facial fractures, they must be distinguished from the more serious maxillofacial and nasoethmoid fractures. As mentioned previously, nasoethmoid fractures include extension into and through the nasoethmoid complex, often resulting in dural tears and CSF rhinorrhea. Fractures of the zygoma usually involve a V-shaped deformity with three separate breaks, two occurring along each end and one in the middle of the arch. On physical exam, trismus of the temporalis muscle may be elicited, depending on the degree of bony impingement. A tripod or zygomaticomaxillary fracture may be found with force that has been directed at the cheek; it usually involves one or more of the articulations among the zygoma, the frontal bone, and the maxilla, with extension through the orbital floor. On physical exam, paresthesia may be found along the distribution of the ipsilateral infraorbital nerve. With force directed at the inferior maxilla, alveolar fractures may be found along the superior aspect of the dental margin, often associated with loosened dentition and gingival ecchymosis or hemorrhage.

In ruling out additional fractures of the midface that are seen with nasal trauma, the **Le Fort classification** denotes three classic patterns of injury associated with blunt midfacial injury. **Type I** injury involves separation of the maxillary process from the maxilla itself, with extension to the maxillary sinuses. This typically results from force directed horizontally across the midface below the level of the orbit. **Type II** injury occurs in association with fracture of the nasal bones extending through the lacrimal bone toward and through the zygomaticomaxillary junction. In addition, the fracture extends posteriorly just below the zygoma and along the superior border of the pterygoid plates. Infraorbital paresthesia and bilateral subcutaneous hematomas are often found on examination. **Type III** injury is also associated with nasal fracture, but courses posteriorly through the ethmoid bones and laterally through the orbits below the optic foramen and through the pterygomaxillary suture into the sphenopalatine fossa. This results in craniofacial dysjunction and the appearance of a long, flat, facial deformity.

In children, additional fractures of the face associated with significant nasal trauma are not uncommon. Given the lack of significant nasal projection and inherent cartilaginous flexibility of the pediatric nasal skeleton, trauma to the midface is more evenly distributed to the maxilla. This provides for a significant risk of maxillofacial and midface fracture as well as extensive facial edema, which often obscures the diagnosis. Such injuries have been associated with disturbances in the normal growth and development of the facial structure—as with premature ossification of the septovomerine suture, which is found with injuries of the nasoethmoid complex—and thus require a conservative approach to diagnosis and management.

Complications

A. Cosmetic Deformity

External physical deformities that result from nasal trauma include the creation of a dorsal hump, lateral deviation of the dorsum and tip, a widened nasal base, and depression and splaying of the nasal tip. Complex (and obstructing) septal deformities may also result, including the appearance of bony spurs, complex alterations in nasal symmetry, and angular deflections of the septum itself. Internally, synechiae may develop where mucosal lacerations are found, particularly between the septum and adjacent turbinates. Most deformities require reconstructive septorhinoplasty to restore function and cosmetic appearance. In cases of pediatric deformity, a delay of revision is often required to allow for normal facial growth and development. With obstructive scar tissue and synechiae, simple division and separation with pledgets coated with antibiotic ointment are usually effective in allowing for reepithelialization.

B. Epistaxis and CSF Leak

The initial edema and epistaxis of nasal trauma usually resolve without intervention; however, persistent epistaxis may require tamponade with nasal packing or, rarely, identification and coagulation or ligation of the bleeding vessel. With CSF leak, the injury is significantly more severe and may require consultation with a neurosurgeon. Therapy usually includes close observation and may involve bone grafting or placing a drain in the lumbar spine.

C. Septal Hematoma and Saddle Nose Deformity

Septal hematoma results from bleeding, often bilateral, within the subperichondrial plane of the septum. If left unattended, fibrosis of the septal cartilage may occur, followed by necrosis and perforation within 3–4 days. The loss of structural support leads to septal collapse, which results in a characteristic saddle nose deformity of the nasal dorsum and retraction of the columella. A hematoma is often suspected given excessive septal edema and severe localized tenderness on examination. Treatment is urgent and includes a horizontal incision made at the septal base to provide for mucoperichondrial drainage. Reaccumulation is prevented with the application of plastic splints or intranasal packing. Antibiotic prophylaxis is also required. Saddle nose deformity may require an extensive reconstruction to restore the structure and shape of the nose. We prefer split calvarial bone grafting for reconstruction of this deformity, although rib cartilage and other materials have been used with success.

D. Airway Obstruction

Fibrosis of the nasal septum, as occurs with septal hematoma, may become organized, creating cartilaginous thickening and resulting in partial airway obstruction. Obstruction may also occur at the nasal vestibule from a traumatic loss of epithelium or the malunion of a nasal fracture. The treatment of nasal septal reorganization may be accomplished with submucosal resection, although some cases require partial turbinectomy. Soft tissue injury and contracture that occur at the nasal vestibule may require excision of the resultant scar and reconstruction with composite or autologous grafts. Malunion is treated with simple osteotomy.

Treatment

A. Timing of Repair

Within 1–3 hours of the time of injury before significant edema has developed, simple closed fixation of nasal fracture is possible given a cooperative patient and uncomplicated clinical findings. However, patients rarely present this early and often require reevaluation within 3–7 days to allow for extensive facial edema to subside. In adults, closed reduction can be performed within 5–11 days after injury before the fractured nasal skeleton becomes adherent and difficult to manipulate, with fixation occurring in 2–3 weeks. In children, healing is more rapid, with adherence and fixation occurring in roughly half that time. Thus, given a significant therapeutic delay, the necessity for osteotomy and bony reconstruction becomes more likely, which is a particular concern for the pediatric population. Regardless of patient age, however, severe nasal trauma that results in more significant injury, such as septal hematoma, open fractures, or associated fractures of the midface and cranium, requires immediate surgical attention.

B. Anesthesia

In choosing a method of anesthesia to use when repairing nasal fracture, both the severity of the injury and the patient's preference should be considered. General anesthesia is necessary for significant trauma that requires operative intervention. With simple nasal trauma, local anesthesia, with or without sedation, is generally preferred. Local anesthesia is safer and considered as effective in providing for adequate fracture reduction when compared to general anesthesia. However, with nasal trauma in children, general anesthesia provides more control than is usually provided by an uncooperative minor. In either case, the physician should decide which method would provide the optimal comfort necessary to allow for the application of force necessary to reduce the nasal fracture. It has been our experience that in a properly prepared patient and with an experienced surgeon, local anesthesia using only topical cotton-soaked nasal packs is adequate for comfortable closed reduction and stabilization of most nasal fractures in all age groups. It is necessary to remember that the anesthetic-soaked cotton must be placed superiorly between the nasal bones and the septum rather than along the inferior septum or along the inferior turbinates, as is commonly done for other intranasal interventions.

C. Closed Reduction

Closed reduction is safe and easy to perform. Reasonable cosmetic and functional results are attainable with closed reduction, obviating the need, when applicable, to subject the patient to unnecessary risk, procedure, and cost. Treatment should be geared toward the best long-term results possible, given the least invasive technique available. However, the failure rate of closed-reduction procedures may require a secondary open reduction or delayed reconstruction, an inevitability that many proponents of primary open reduction strive to avoid.

Ideally, the presentation of injury suitable for closed reduction includes injury in the first plane as either a fracture of the nasal tip or depressed fracture of the nasal bone on one side. To proceed, local anesthesia should be provided along the distributions of the infraorbital and supratrochlear nerves and at the base of the anterior nasal septum. If needed, nerve blocks are achieved using 1–2% lidocaine with epinephrine. Once the nose has been anesthetized, a Boies elevator, the back of a metal knife handle, or even the closed tips of a straight Mayo scissors can be inserted under the depressed nasal fragments to within approximately 1 cm of the nasofrontal angle. Elevation is accomplished by exerting force in the direction opposite to the direction of the fracture. Pressure is then applied externally with a free hand on any segment that is displaced laterally. If manipulation of the fracture proves difficult owing to impaction or locking of the fragments, Walsham forceps may be used to directly manipulate the nasal bones and facilitate reduction. Occasionally, free-hand manipulation of more mobile fragments may be necessary to achieve adequate repositioning. It is common to need to rotate the depressed fragment first medially, then superiorly and laterally, to dislodge it. In many cases, a satisfying "click" is felt as the bone repositions into the proper location.

Adequate closed reduction of the nasal pyramid often allows for the spontaneous reduction of a displaced or fractured septum. If this is not the case, Asch forceps may be used to gently elevate the nasal dorsum and allow for replacement of the septum into its anatomic position. In the case of a difficult reduction, a perichondrial elevator may be required to expose an overriding segment of cartilage for resection.

Structural support after a successful reduction can be provided using cotton pledgets soaked in an appropriate intranasal antibiotic. It is preferable, however, not to leave in any nonabsorbable material; therefore, we recommend small pieces of surgical oxycellulose (eg, Surgicell), if necessary. Silastic splints may also be desirable to stabilize the septum. Externally, Steri-strips or other protective tape should cover the nasal dorsum before applying a malleable thermoplastic or plaster splint that has been conformed to the shape of the nasal reduction (Figure 11–2). After approximately 3–5 days, the internal packing can be removed, followed by removal of the external splint by day 7–10 if stability has been accomplished.

D. Open Reduction

The reduction of nasal fractures using open techniques is usually reserved for cases in which either a prior closed reduction has failed or malunion has occurred. Other cases where primary open reduction would be appropriate include third-plane fractures, fractures involving the orbit or maxilla, and Le Fort fractures of the midface. Depending on the indication for open reduction, most cases can be adequately reduced with a standard endonasal rhinoplasty. This approach provides for a more appealing cosmetic result while allowing for direct fragment manipulation. Operative exposure, however, is limited. For cases involving the orbit or injury to the frontal sinuses, an external approach from incisions made distal to the nose may be required. Other more complex fractures may require degloving techniques, a coronal approach, or even a lateral rhinotomy.

In most cases, nasal trauma that requires open reduction involves interlocking segments with dislocation of the quadrangular cartilage or a C-shaped septal deformity. After the appropriate administration of anesthesia, open reduction begins with hemitransfixion of the nasal septum on the affected side and septoplasty. Lateral intercartilaginous incisions are then made, allowing for both elevation of the nasal dorsum off of the upper lateral cartilages and elevation of the nasal periosteum. Lateral fracture lines may be accessed via incisions made at the piriform aperture. Affected cartilaginous segments are then exposed and reduced.

With nasoseptal injury, a Cottle elevator is used to strip cartilage from buckled or telescoping portions of the septum, allowing for the spontaneous return of the septum to the midline. Structural support may be lost with excessive resection, and aggressive periosteal eleva-

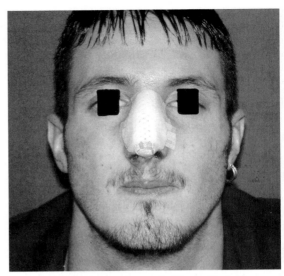

Figure 11–2. Same patient as in Figure 11–1 after closed reduction of nasal fracture in the office with local anesthesia. Note that a thermoplastic splint holds nasal bones in a "straight" reduced position.

tion may result in necrosis or subsequent malunion. For C-shaped deformities, separation of the upper lateral cartilages from the dorsal septum is necessary. Once reduction is accomplished, additional support for the septum may be provided with stay sutures placed through the periosteum at the anterior nasal spine and the inferior aspect of the septal cartilage.

If encountered, displacement of the maxilla may require the complete removal of the maxillary crest. Any unstable fragments, as seen with comminuted fractures, can be secured using fine wire or miniplate fixation and a minidrill. Using a "figure 8" configuration, wires should not be palpable below the skin. Intranasal packing is rarely necessary, although prophylactic oral antibiotics are administered for at least 5 days. With septal injury, splints may also be applied.

E. Pediatric Considerations

The treatment of nasal trauma in children must be based on the potential for developmental dysfunction as a result of therapy and the consequences of delayed intervention. In cases of minimal injury, the child's nose may spontaneously return to an anatomic position with only an external splint to protect the nasal dorsum during the healing process. The integrity of the nasal septum, however, is vital to nasal skeletal and anterior maxillary growth and therefore requires specific attention.

Operative intervention is required for nasal septal displacement that results in significant cosmetic or functional impairment. As with the adult population, closed reduction is preferred, although general rather than local anesthesia is usually necessary with children. Simple reductions can often be performed with digital manipulation; otherwise, the standard procedure for closed reduction should be used. Fracture dislocations that do not reduce with closed techniques are approached very carefully, making sure no measures are undertaken that might compromise normal growth and development. Aggressive resection is avoided altogether, and any septorhinoplasty deemed necessary to restore appearance or function is delayed until the teenage years. With reasonable conservative correction of the deformity and restoration of a patent airway, adequate surgical management will not result in a disruption of nasal growth centers or the creation of significant structural abnormalities.

Prognosis

In general, uncomplicated fractures heal within 2–3 weeks with good cosmetic and functional results. Refractory cosmetic complications, however, are possi-ble with both open and closed techniques and usually involve septal deviation. Reductions that result in malunion or deformity may require further reduction or reconstruction, depending on the severity of injury and the difficulty the reduction of the primary injury presents. Septorhinoplasty remains the standard of care for unsatisfactory results and is often necessary in cases of failed reduction attempts.

Haug RH. Maxillofacial injuries in the pediatric patient. *Oral Surg Oral Med Oral Path Oral Rad Endodontics.* 2000;90(2):126. [PMID: 10936829] (Includes discussion of relevant pediatric considerations in the diagnosis and treatment of nasal and other facial fractures.)

Rohrich RJ, Adams WP Jr. Nasal fracture management: minimizing secondary nasal deformities. *Plast Reconstr Surg.* 2000;106(2):266. [PMID: 10946923] (Methods of open and closed reduction in nasal fracture.)

Rubinstein B, Strong EB. Management of nasal fractures. *Arch Fam Med.* 2000;9(8):738. [PMID: 10927714] (Review of relevant literature on the diagnosis and management of nasal trauma.)

Staffel JG. Optimizing treatment of nasal fractures. *Laryngoscope.* 2002;112:1709. [PMID: 12368602]

Nasal Manifestations of Systemic Disease

12

Ashish R. Shah, MD, John M. Ryzenman, MD, & Thomas A. Tami, MD

■ GRANULOMATOUS & AUTOIMMUNE DISEASES

General Considerations

Granulomatous and autoimmune diseases are characterized by a systemic chronic inflammatory process and a predilection for particular organ systems. The incidence of sinonasal manifestations is variable and often nonspecific; the common clinical findings consist of nasal obstruction, rhinorrhea, and recurrent sinusitis. Therefore, the practitioner must often include these diseases in the differential diagnosis of chronic sinonasal symptoms and assess for systemic manifestations in the history and physical examination. Occasionally, patients present with florid nasal symptoms including severe crusting, inflammation, and saddle-nose deformity, which raise suspicion early in the evaluation.

Although obtaining biopsies of suspicious lesions is essential for establishing a diagnosis, specimens often demonstrate nonspecific chronic inflammation and necrosis. Helpful adjunctive testing includes the markers of inflammation (erythrocyte sedimentation rate and C-reactive protein), complete blood cell count, various autoimmune tests, chest x-ray, and urinalysis. Bacterial and fungal infectious etiologies should also be ruled out.

The goals of managing the sinonasal manifestations of these diseases are (1) to provide maximum relief of nasal obstruction and crusting and (2) to reduce the incidence and severity of secondary sinusitis from ostial obstruction by facilitating mucociliary clearance and reducing mucosal edema.

WEGENER GRANULOMATOSIS

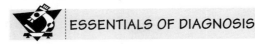

ESSENTIALS OF DIAGNOSIS

- Complete head and neck exam.
- Chest x-ray, urinalysis, and ANCA (antineutrophil cytoplasmic autoantibodies).
- Biopsy, including multiple turbinate and septal specimens; possible renal biopsy.

General Considerations

Wegener granulomatosis occurs in all age groups, with a peak incidence from ages 30–40. It predominantly affects white populations. This granulomatous disease is a vasculitis as well as an autoimmune process, with a predilection for the upper and lower respiratory tracts. The spectrum of disease presentation ranges from localized to disseminated forms. Classic Wegener granulomatosis describes a triad of necrotizing granulomas of the upper and lower airways, glomerulonephritis, and disseminated vasculitis. Upper respiratory tract symptoms may occur in up to 90% of patients, and sinonasal symptoms may be the only systemic manifestation in 30%. The previously undiagnosed patient may present with a pattern of chronic or recurrent sinusitis, managed both medically and often surgically with variable clinical improvement.

Clinical Findings

A. SYMPTOMS AND SIGNS

The more limited, localized form of Wegener granulomatosis typically presents with a several-week history of upper respiratory infection symptoms, which are unresponsive to standard medical treatment, with the presence of serosanguineous nasal drainage and pain characteristically over the dorsum. Significant bilateral nasal crusting, particularly over the nasal turbinates, with underlying friable mucosa, is noted with possible extension to the nasopharynx. Septal perforations may be found with progressive disease, which can lead to saddle-nose deformity (ie, loss of dorsal cartilaginous support, creating a concavity). Other potentially involved head and neck sites are (1) the orbit, with nasolacrimal duct obstruction from nasoethmoid disease; and (2) the ear, with otologic symptoms that can include serous otitis media, with or without mastoiditis, and possible sensorineural hearing loss. In addition, oral cavity ulcerations, subglottic stenosis, and gingival lesions have been described. Systemic symptoms may include weakness, night sweats, and migratory arthralgias. More advanced systemic disease manifests in clinically significant pulmonary and renal pathology, although most patients have renal involvement, even if it is subclinical.

The clinical diagnostic criteria for Wegener granulomatosis include the following: (1) abnormal urinalysis (which suggests renal involvement); (2) abnormal chest x-ray (which may include nodules, cavities, or fixed infiltrates); (3) oral ulcers and nasal serosanguineous discharge; (4) granulomatous inflammation evident on biopsy; and (5) laboratory studies and imaging.

B. Laboratory Findings

ANCA is very specific for Wegener granulomatosis, with a sensitivity rate of 90% in patients with active systemic disease, 60% in patients with localized disease, and 30% for patients in a remission phase. Typically, the C-ANCA (cytoplasmic) is positive on immunofluorescence followed by a confirmatory PR3-ANCA (proteinase 3) on enzyme immunoassay. After remission, a sudden rise in titers can correlate with recurrence. A positive biopsy characterized by coagulation necrosis from the vasculitis, multinucleated giant cells, and palisading histiocytes is highly suggestive of the diagnosis when fungal cultures and acid-fast bacilli stains and cultures are negative. See Table 12–1 for additional laboratory tests recommended for Wegener granulomatosis and other nasal manifestations of systemic disease.

Treatment

For active disease, high-dose steroids (eg, prednisone 1 mg/kg/d) and cyclophosphamide (2 mg/kg/d) should be maintained for a duration of 1 month. The steroids can then be tapered over several months. Cyclophosphamide should be continued for 6–12 months until symptoms disappear. Methotrexate may be considered for induction therapy in less severe disease. Treatment for the maintenance of remission is recommended, and attempts should be made to switch to methotrexate, azathioprine, or mycophenolate mofetil, which are less toxic than cyclophosphamide. Trimethoprim/sulfamethoxazole may have a role for either the limited form of Wegener granulomatosis or for prophylaxis while on immunosuppressants and thereafter to prevent recurrence.

Sinonasal manifestations may be treated medically with low-dose systemic steroids, topical nasal steroids, saline irrigations, and, when bacterial superinfection (typically *Staphylococcus* species) is suspected, with antibiotics.

Gubbels SP, Barkhuizen A, Hwang PH. Head and neck manifestations of Wegener's granulomatosis. *Otolaryngol Clin North Am.* 2003;36(4):685. [PMID: 16344616] (Review of the otolaryngology effects of the disease.)

Hellmich B, Lamprecht P, Gross WL. Advances in the therapy of Wegener's granulomatosis. *Curr Opin Rheumatol.* 2006;18:25.
[PMID: 16344616] (Contemporary discussion of pharmacotherapeutic options and future directions of treatment.)

Lynch JP, White E, Tazelaar H, Langford CA. Wegener's granulomatosis: evolving concepts in treatment. *Semin Respir Crit Care Med.* 2004;25(5):491. [PMID: 16088495] (Comprehensive overview of disease and treatment recommendations.)

Seo P, Stone JH. The antineutrophil cytoplasmic antibody-associated vasculitides. *Am J Med.* 2004;117:39. [PMID: 15210387] (The clinical and pathologic hallmarks of these diseases.)

Yucel EA, Keles N, Ozturk AS, Solmaz MA, Deger K. Wegener granulomatosis presenting in the sinus and orbit. *Otolaryngol Head Neck Surg.* 2002;127:349. [PMID: 12402017] (Review of granulomatosis in the sinus and orbit.)

SARCOIDOSIS

 ESSENTIALS OF DIAGNOSIS

- *Complete head and neck and general physical exam.*
- *Chest x-ray (bilateral hilar adenopathy).*
- *Angiotensin-converting enzyme (ACE) levels positive in 60% of patients with active disease.*
- *Serum calcium level is elevated in 15% of patients.*
- *Biopsy of suspicious mucosal lesions, transbronchial lymph nodes, or labial minor salivary gland.*

General Considerations

The incidence of systemic sarcoidosis is 6–10 persons per 100,000, whereas the incidence of symptomatic sinonasal manifestations in patients with sarcoidosis is 1–4%. A female predominance has been noted, with a peak incidence between the ages of 20 and 40 years, and a racial predilection in African American and Latin populations.

Sarcoidosis is a chronic granulomatous disease with predominantly pulmonary manifestations, although almost any organ system may become involved. Classic head and neck manifestations include xerostomia, xerophthalmia, and salivary gland enlargement. Other manifestations include lupus pernio (cutaneous sarcoid), neurosarcoidosis, and uveoparotid fever (Heerfordt's disease), which is the association of uveitis, parotitis, and facial nerve paralysis with sarcoidosis.

Pathogenesis

The cause of sarcoidosis is unknown. The histopathology reveals noncaseating granulomas without necrosis and vasculitis.

Clinical Findings

The clinical symptoms associated with sinonasal sarcoidosis are usually nonspecific and include nasal obstruc-

Table 12–1. Laboratory tests for the diagnosis of sinonasal disorders.

Diagnosis	Gold Standard Tests	Helpful or Suggested Screening Tests	Possibly Helpful or Secondary Tests
Autoimmune Disorders			
Wegener's granulomatosis	Nasal biopsy		Complete blood count
Polyarteritis nodosa	Nasal biopsy	Erythrocyte sedimentation rate	
		Perinuclear antineutrophil cytoplasmic antibody assay (p-ANCA)	
Relapsing polychondritis	Nasal biopsy		
Cystic fibrosis	Sweat test	Sweat patch test Sweat conductivity	Nasal action potential Genetic tests
Disorders of Unknown Cause			
Sarcoidosis	Nasal biopsy (diagnosis of exclusion—negative cultures for fungus and acid-fast bacilli)	Angiotensin converting enzyme level	Erythrocyte sedimentation rate
		Chest radiograph	Kveim test
Churg-Strauss syndrome	Nasal biopsy (vasculitis is not usually seen in nasal specimens); must be coupled with clinical picture and lung biopsy	Complete blood count with differential (eosinophil count)	
Immunodeficiency	Documentation of absence of function of a subset of the immune system	Total IgG, IgM, IgA, IgG subclasses	IgG1 deficiency: response to diphtheria and tetanus toxoid vaccine
		Complete blood count with differential CH50 or CH 100	IgG2 deficiency: response to pneumococcal vaccine
Neoplasms			
Lethal midline granuloma (angiocentric T-cell lymphoma)	Nasal biopsy		

Adapted with permission from Ferguson BJ and Mabry RL: Laboratory diagnosis. *Otolaryngol Head Neck Surg* 1997;117:S12.

tion, postnasal drainage, headache, and recurrent sinus infections. In patients with coexisting lung disease sarcoidosis should be in the differential diagnosis. The classic intranasal finding includes submucosal yellow nodules from granulomatous infiltration. Other intranasal features that may be highly suggestive of sarcoidosis include severe nasal obstruction and crusting with friable mucosa. A thorough history and head and neck examination may reveal other manifestations. Ultimately, directed intranasal biopsy may be needed to definitively establish the diagnosis. Chest x-ray and laboratory studies may be highly suggestive.

Treatment

Attempts have been made to stratify patients with sarcoid nasal disease into three levels in order to tailor their treat-

ment regimen: (1) mildly affected patients are treated with standard medical therapy and topical steroids, (2) patients who are significantly affected may respond to the intralesional injection of steroids, and (3) the most refractory cases may require systemic steroids. Other medication regimens may include methotrexate, chloroquine, azathioprine, thalidomide, and anticytokines. Nasal irrigation may allow for the mechanical debridement of crusting and thick mucus. Surgical intervention should be avoided when possible but may be necessary in cases of severe nasal obstruction and chronic sinusitis. Overall, therapy should be designed to minimize the use of long-term systemic steroids if the patient's systemic disease is well controlled.

Kay DJ, Har-El G. The role of endoscopic sinus surgery in chronic sinonasal sarcoidosis. *Am J Rhinol.* 2001;15:249. [PMID: 11554657] (Discussion of the risks and benefits of endoscopic sinus surgery in sarcoidosis patients.)

Krespi YP, Kuriloff DB, Aner M. Sarcoidosis of the sinonasal tract: a new staging system. *Otolaryngol Head Neck Surg.* 1995;112:221. [PMID: 7838542] (New, proposed classification staging system for nasal sarcoidosis.)

Schwartzbauer HR, Tami TA. Ear, nose, and throat manifestations of sarcoidosis. *Otolaryngol Clin North Am.* 2003;36(4):673. [PMID: 14567059] (Head and neck sarcoid manifestations.)

Tami TA. Sinonasal sarcoidosis: diagnosis and management. *Semin Respir Crit Care Med.* 2002;23(6):549. [PMID: 16088650] (Discussion of important and often subtle clinical findings and medical and surgical management.)

CHURG-STRAUSS SYNDROME

 ESSENTIALS OF DIAGNOSIS

- *The following criteria are based on definitions of the American College of Rheumatology in 1990:*
  - *(1) Asthma.*
  - *(2) Eosinophilia > 10%.*
  - *(3) Neuropathy.*
  - *(4) Migratory pulmonary infiltrates.*
  - *(5) Parasinonasal abnormalities.*
  - *(6) Tissue eosinophils.*
- *The presence of four of the above six findings results in a diagnostic sensitivity of 85%, with a specificity of 99%.*

General Considerations

Churg-Strauss syndrome is also referred to as allergic angiitis and granulomatosis. The syndrome is defined as a granulomatous vasculitis with typical eosinophil-rich granulomas and a necrotizing vasculitis of small- to medium-sized vessels, asthma, and eosinophilia. The cause of the disease is unknown, but causative factors implicated include vaccinations, desensitization, and various medications including leukotriene-receptor antagonists. ANCA may be positive in approximately 50% of patients, which is usually perinuclear (P-ANCA) on immunofluorescence and myeloperoxidase (MPO-ANCA) on enzyme immunoassay.

Clinical Findings

The symptoms and signs of Churg-Strauss syndrome generally occur within three stages, and shorter transition intervals to progressive stages are associated with a more severe occurrence of disease:

1. The **prodromal stage** may last for years with the development of adult-onset asthma and allergic

rhinitis with nasal polyposis (70%). Septal perforation is rare.

2. The second stage consists of **serum and tissue eosinophilia,** primarily in the lungs (Löffler's syndrome) and gastrointestinal system.

3. The third stage consists of the development of **systemic vasculitis,** which may affect the peripheral nervous system, integument, heart, gastrointestinal system, and kidneys, although renal dysfunction is usually not as severe as in Wegener granulomatosis.

Treatment

The administration of corticosteroids (prednisone 1 mg/kg/d) usually results in a rapid regression of symptoms. Although a steroid taper can begin at about 1 month, long-term low-dose corticosteroid treatment is often necessary owing to persistent asthma. Cyclophosphamide is indicated for first-line therapy when poor prognostic indicators are present or as second-line treatment with failure of corticosteroid therapy.

Guillevin L, Pagnoux C, Mouthon L. Churg-Strauss syndrome. *Semin Respir Crit Care Med.* 2004;25(5):535–545. [PMID: 16088497] (Comprehensive discussion of disease and its treatment.)

Ishiyama A, Canalis RF. Otologic manifestations of Churg-Strauss syndrome. *Laryngoscope.* 2001;111:1619. [PMID: 11568616] (Review of Churg-Strauss signs and symptoms.)

■ NEOPLASTIC DISEASES

T-CELL LYMPHOMA

 ESSENTIALS OF DIAGNOSIS

- *Complete head and neck and general physical exam.*
- *Nasal obstruction and epistaxis.*
- *Rapidly progressive with aggressive local destruction.*
- *Uncommon systemic symptoms include fever, chills, night sweats, and weight loss.*
- *Biopsy recommended; multiple specimens required due to large areas of secondary necrosis.*

General Considerations

Nasal T-cell lymphoma, also known as NK-cell lymphoma and lethal midline granuloma, is rare in the

United States but is common in Asia. In China, it is the second most common type of extranodal non-Hodgkin lymphoma. The ratio of male to female patients who present with T-cell lymphoma is 2.5:1.0; the average age of presentation is in the fourth and fifth decades. Overall, patients with T-cell lymphoma tend to be younger than patients with conventional lymphomas. These tumors tend to resist traditional non-Hodgkin regimens, which may result in a poor outcome.

Pathogenesis

Histologically, primary nasal natural killer cell (NK- or T-cell) lymphoma is characterized by mixed cellular infiltrates with angiocentric lymphoid invasion and occlusion of blood vessels, resulting in ischemic necrosis of normal and neoplastic tissues.

Studies from Asian and Western countries have shown a possible association between the Epstein-Barr virus (EBV) and nasal T-cell lymphomas, suggesting that EBV might play a role in the development of nasal T-cell lymphoma. The exact mechanism and potential for future treatment modalities are currently unknown. Lesions characteristically express the T-cell-lineage markers CD2(+), CD45RO(+), CD7(+), CD43(+), and the natural killer-cell–associated marker CD56 is often present. However, other T-cell antigens are often absent, such as CD3(–) and CD5(–).

Clinical Findings

A high index of suspicion is required for the diagnosis of T-cell lymphoma. The tumor is highly invasive locally. Grossly, the lesions are gray or yellow with a friable granular surface that involves the nasal septum or midline palate. Nasal septal perforation is a common finding, and eventual palatal destruction may occur. Occasionally, the tumor may infiltrate surrounding tissues and organs, such as the nasopharynx, the lateral wall of the nasal cavity, the orbits, or the oropharynx. The cranial nerves are sometimes affected. If disseminated, the tumor may be found in the skin, the gastrointestinal tract, and the testis. Cocaine abuse may present similarly as an impressive midline nasal destructive process, and its use should be ascertained in the patient's history. Table 12–2 lists the complete differential diagnosis.

Treatment

If untreated, the complications can range from local tissue destruction to death. A combination of chemotherapy and radiation therapy appears to be more effective than either modality alone. Radiation therapy alone may be sufficient in low-stage tumors.

Table 12–2. Conditions that may present clinically as midline nasal destructive lesions.

Cocaine abuse
Trauma
Infectious diseases
    Bacterial: brucellosis, syphilis, rhinoscleroma, leprosy, actinomycosis, tuberculosis
    Fungal: histoplasmosis, candida, mucormycosis, blastomycosis, rhinosporidiosis, coccidiomycosis
    Parasitic: leishmaniasis, myiasis
Inflammatory diseases
    Sarcoidosis
    Wegener's granulomatosis
    Systemic lupus
    Polyarteritis nodosa
    Hypersensitivity angiitis
    Idiopathic midline destructive disease
Neoplastic diseases
    Squamous cell carcinoma
    Basal cell carcinoma
    Esthesioneuroblastoma
    Adenoid cystic carcinoma
    Sinonasal lymphoma

Reprinted, with permission, from Rodrigo JP, Suarez C, Rinaldo A et al. Idiopathic midline destructive disease: fact or fiction. *Oral Oncol* 2005;41:340–348.

Liang R. Diagnosis and management of primary nasal lymphoma of T-cell or NK-cell origin. *Clin Lymphoma.* 2000;1:33. [PMID: 11707809] (Diagnosis and histopathologic findings of nasal T-cell lymphoma.)

Rodrigo JP, Suarez C, Rinaldo A et al. Idiopathic midline destructive disease: fact or fiction. *Oral Oncol.* 2005;41:340. [PMID: 15792605] (Evaluation of the patient with a midline destructive process.)

Rodriguez J, Romaguera JE, Manning J et al. Nasal T-cell and NK-cell lymphomas: a clinicopathologic study of 13 cases. *Leuk Lymphoma.* 2000;39:139. [PMID: 10975392] (Therapeutic outcomes of nasal T-cell lymphoma management at MD Anderson.)

■ INFECTIOUS DISEASES

RHINOSCLEROMA

 ESSENTIALS OF DIAGNOSIS

- *High index of suspicion in individuals from endemic regions.*

- *Extensive nasal polyposis adherent to nasal septum, with minimal sinus involvement.*
- *Cultures specific for Klebsiella pneumoniae rhinoscleromatis (typically is not normal nasal flora).*
- *Nonenhancing, well-defined borders on CT scans; bone and cartilage rarely involved.*
- *Biopsies of actively involved areas (septum inferior turbinates) diagnostic.*

General Considerations

Rhinoscleroma is a rare, slowly progressing granulomatous disease of the upper respiratory tract caused by *Klebsiella rhinoscleromatis*. Nasal disease presents with three typical stages: (1) **catarrhal,** with nonspecific rhinitis; (2) **proliferative,** which consists of a granulomatous reaction and the presence of Mikulicz cells; and (3) **cicatricial,** with mucosal fibrosis. The rise in the incidence of rhinoscleroma in the United States may be due to the increased number of immigrants from endemic regions such as eastern and central Europe, Central and South America, East Africa, and the Indian subcontinent. Rhinoscleroma may be found in all age groups, but typically young adults 20–30 years old are most frequently affected. Airborne transmission combined with poor hygiene, crowded living conditions, and poor nutrition contribute to its spread.

Pathogenesis

The chronicity of this disease is believed to be a result of the ability of the bacteria, in the proliferative stage, to evade the host defenses. During the catarrhal phase, the organism gains access to the subepithelial layer via ulcerations that allow deep colonization. Once this progression begins, the bacteria, which are characterized by pleomorphism and vigorous growth both intracellularly and extracellularly—coupled with incomplete phagocytosis of the neutrophil cell—prompts histiocytes to phagocytize them both. Mikulicz cells are thus formed; however, the organism continues to multiply intracellularly until the Mikulicz cells rupture and deliver viable bacteria interstitially. This cycle continues and eventually leads to clinically evident granuloma formation and pseudoepitheliomatous hyperplasia.

Clinical Findings

Rhinoscleroma manifests primarily in the nose; however, it can be found in the larynx, the trachea, and the eustachian tube. In advanced disease, nasal obstruction (94%), nasal deformity (32%), epistaxis (11%), and crusting (94%) are the main symptoms. Laryngeal symptoms may include hoarseness with interarytenoid hyperemia, exudates, and vocal cord edema. Late laryngeal fibrosis typically involves the glottis and subglottis, with subsequent stridor and potential airway obstruction.

Treatment

The organism may be difficult to eradicate, despite aggressive therapy. A combination of conservative surgical debridement and long-term antibiotic coverage is the mainstay of therapy for rhinoscleroma. Tetracycline has been shown to be effective and inexpensive for patients unless contraindicated. Fluoroquinolones may be used as an alternative, given their excellent gram-negative activity and convenient dosing regimen.

Relapse rates can be high because the organism has the ability to remain dormant in its spore form.

Ammar ME, Rosen A. Rhinoscleroma mimicking nasal polyposis. *Ann Otol Rhinol Laryngol.* 2001;110:290. [PMID: 11269777] (Clinical findings and management of rhinoscleroma.)

Canalis RF, Zamboni L. An interpretation of the structural changes responsible for the chronicity of rhinoscleroma. *Laryngoscope.* 2001;111:1020. [PMID: 11404614] (Review of the pathophysiology of rhinoscleroma.)

HIV-RELATED NASAL INFECTIONS

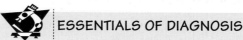 ESSENTIALS OF DIAGNOSIS

- *HIV serology is diagnostic.*
- *CD4 cell counts and viral titers are indicative; lower CD4 counts and higher viral titers predict symptomatic immunodeficiency.*
- *Opportunistic pathogens can be seen with CD4 < 50 cells/mm³. Empirically treat for P aeruginosa in HIV patients with sinusitis when CD4 < 200 cells/mm³.*
- *Endoscopic-guided cultures should be used to direct for antibiotic coverage.*
- *Nasal masses and skin lesions should be biopsied to rule out malignant neoplasms.*

General Considerations

Rhinosinusitis may affect up to 68% of patients infected with the human immunodeficiency virus (HIV), with an incidence and severity that correlate with the stage of HIV infection. As immune function deteriorates, the incidence of opportunistic infections increases, especially with CD4 counts < 50 cells/mm³.

Pathogenesis

HIV infection results in a gradual depression of humoral and cellular immunity, primarily owing to the depletion of helper T lymphocytes. The result is an increased susceptibility to infection. HIV-infected patients have also been found to have decreased mucociliary transport time, which can lead to thick, tenacious nasal secretions.

Nasopharyngeal lymphoid hypertrophy affects 56–88% of patients early in the disease course, which contributes to findings of nasal obstruction and serous otitis media. The relationship between HIV infection and increased atopy is unclear at this time.

Clinical Findings

The typical presentation of rhinosinusitis in these patients is no different from that in seronegative patients; common findings consist of fever, facial pain or pressure, headache, postnasal drip, purulent nasal discharge, periorbital swelling, and nasal congestion. As the HIV infection progresses, the inflammatory response is reduced, resulting in less mucosal edema and rhinorrhea. The microbiology is usually the same as in seronegative patients when the CD4 count is > 50 cells/mm³ with *Streptococcus pneumoniae, Haemophilus influenzae,* and *Moraxella catarrhalis* being common for acute infection and *Staphylococcus aureus, P aeruginosa,* and anaerobes being common for chronic infection. When the CD4 count falls below 50 cells/mm³, the risk of infection by opportunistic bacterial, fungal, protozoal, and viral organisms increases. Although extrasinus complications of sinusitis are not known to have a greater incidence in these patients, a high index of suspicion is required with progressive immunodeficiency. Skin lesions such as Kaposi sarcoma, herpetic ulcerations, and seborrhea-like dermatitis are common cutaneous processes that affect the nose and surrounding facial skin. These lesions may herald the progression from asymptomatic HIV infection to AIDS. Nasopharyngeal lymphoid hypertrophy, which causes nasal obstruction and serous otitis media, may warrant biopsy to rule out lymphoma.

Treatment

The level of immunodeficiency should guide initial antibiotic therapy. When the CD4 is greater than 200 cells/mm³ choices should include amoxicillin (1.5–4 g/d), amoxicillin/clavulanate (1.75–4/250 g/d), cefuroxime, trimethoprim/sulfamethoxazole, or a macrolide. With incomplete response to initial antibiotic therapy, the development of chronicity, or when the CD4 count falls below 200 cells/mm³, coverage should include *Pseudomonas, Staphylococcus,* and anaerobes. An appropriate empiric treatment regimen would include at least 3 weeks of a fluoroquinolone with clindamycin or metronidazole. Nevertheless, endoscopically obtained cultures should be performed to guide specific therapeutic decisions. In addition, patients may benefit from decongestants, mucolytics, and nasal saline irrigation. In chronic disease, topical nasal steroids may reduce inflammation and rhinorrhea. Prophylactic treatment with trimethoprim/sulfamethoxazole has been shown to decrease the risk of sinusitis and otitis media. When medical measures fail, functional endoscopic sinus surgery has been shown to be a safe and effective tool in improving and sustaining relief from sinus symptoms, whereas low CD4 counts do not serve as a contraindication for definitive surgery.

Friedman M, Landberg R, Tanyeri H, Schults RA, Kelanic S, Caldarelli DD. Endoscopic sinus surgery in patients infected with HIV. *Laryngoscope.* 2000;110:1613. [PMID: 11037812] (Indications and outcomes of functional endonasal sinus surgery in patients with HIV.)

Gurney TA, Murr AH. Otolaryngologic manifestations of human immunodeficiency virus infection. *Otolaryngol Clin North Am.* 2003;36:607. [PMID: 14567056] (Comprehensive review of the head and neck manifestations of HIV.)

Shah AR, Hairston JA, Tami TA. Sinusitis in HIV: microbiology and therapy. *Curr Infect Dis Rep.* 2005;7:165. [PMID: 15847717] (Review of findings and medical and surgical treatment recommendations.)

▓ GENETIC DISORDERS

CYSTIC FIBROSIS

 ESSENTIALS OF DIAGNOSIS

- *High index of suspicion in patients with chronic rhinitis, thick tenacious secretions, pulmonary symptoms, and pseudomonal positive cultures.*
- *Sweat chloride test is diagnostic.*
- *Genetic testing is recommended and family history is indicative.*
- *Sinus CT scan with pathognomonic findings is diagnostic.*

General Considerations

Cystic fibrosis is a common autosomal recessive genetic disorder with a prevalence of 1 in 2000 live births among Caucasians and a carrier rate of 1 in 20–25. The prevalence is significantly lower in Asians and African Americans. The incidence of nasal polyposis varies from 6% to 48%, usually occurring in patients aged 5–20. The disease causes a systemic dysfunction of exocrine glands that clinically manifests as chronic bronchial infections; these infections are due to thick, inspissated secretions with progressive pulmonary obstruction and intestinal maldigestion secondary to pancreatic insufficiency. Cardiopulmonary failure is a common cause of mortality.

Pathogenesis

Patients with cystic fibrosis have impaired mucociliary clearance, despite normal cilia. Their secretions tend to be thick and inspissated, which is thought to be due to a genetic defect in the chloride ion transport channel. This channel is coded by the cystic fibrosis transmembrane regulator (CFTR) gene. This defect alters the physiochemical properties of the mucus by decreasing its hydration. The mucus stasis leads to local inflammation, which may promote goblet cell hyperplasia and local tissue edema. The secretions become colonized, and the bacteria can secrete factors that lead to further ciliary dyskinesia. The exact mechanism for polyp formation in these patients is not known.

Prevention

The prompt treatment of sinus disease, which is often a source of opportunistic pathogens, can reduce pulmonary exacerbations and improve the outcome in lung transplant candidates and recipients.

Clinical Findings

The incidence of patient-reported symptoms in individuals with cystic fibrosis is low, especially in children who may have never had a healthy baseline and who therefore have adapted to their symptoms. Of the symptoms reported, the most common are nasal obstruction, rhinorrhea, mouth breathing, headache, facial pain, and coughing. Anterior rhinoscopy reveals congested, erythematous mucosa and thick secretions. Polyps are typically multiple and bilateral. A positive chloride sweat test for a presumptive diagnosis can be confirmed by definitive genetic testing for mutations of the CFTR gene. Characteristic radiographic findings, in addition to the universally found paranasal sinus disease, include the following: (1) frontal and sphenoid sinuses that are absent or underdeveloped, (2) lateral nasal walls and flattened middle turbinates that are displaced medially, and (3) absent or demineralized uncinate processes.

Bacterial cultures often produce *P aeruginosa* and *S aureus,* whereas more infrequently streptococci, *Haemophilus,* and other gram-negative bacteria are cultured.

Complications

The standard complications resulting from chronic sinusitis are uncommon in patients with cystic fibrosis, possibly because of the patient's concomitant pulmonary disease, which is frequently treated with antimicrobial agents. However, the sinonasal spaces of these patients tend to serve as reservoirs for bacteria such as *P aeruginosa,* which can then exacerbate or precipitate

pulmonary infections. In addition, lung transplant recipients can develop severe sepsis from sinus pathogens because they are frequently further immunocompromised by antirejection medicines.

Treatment

Conservative management is the mainstay for patients with cystic fibrosis. Maximal medical therapy includes nasal irrigations with hypertonic saline (3%, typically), which can both clear secretions and decrease mucosal edema. Mucolytic agents, intranasal steroids, and systemic steroid bursts for acute symptomatic exacerbations have been used successfully, although they do not affect the underlying pathology. Future research in gene therapy may improve or eliminate nasal disease. Until that time, prolonged courses of appropriate intravenous antibiotics are required for episodes of sinusitis. There is evidence that macrolide antibiotics may have an anti-inflammatory effect and may reduce the size of nasal polyps.

The indication for surgery in patients with cystic fibrosis must be tailored to their physical findings. In the past, surgery was conservative and limited to polypectomies, which were often required multiple times. Recent studies since the advent of FESS have shown that performing wide maxillary antrostomies with anterior ethmoidectomies—with polypectomies when needed—can provide longer periods of benefit to these patients than polypectomies alone. The use of aerosolized tobramycin for pulmonary infections of *P aeruginosa* is well established. A number of studies have shown that postoperative topical sinonasal irrigations may prolong favorable surgical results and decrease pulmonary exacerbations. Several transplant centers include such irrigations in their pretransplant protocols. However, randomized controlled studies have yet to be performed to show whether topical irrigations with tobramycin are beneficial in patients with cystic fibrosis who also have sinusitis.

Prognosis

Patients with cystic fibrosis tend to succumb to pulmonary disease, although lung transplantation can prolong life if secondary infections and complications are avoided. Sinus complications are a rare cause of direct mortality in this population.

Gysin C, Alothman GA, Papsin BC. Sinonasal disease in cystic fibrosis: clinical characteristics, diagnosis, and management. *Pediatr Pulmonol.* 2000;30:481. [PMID: 11109061] (Sinonasal disease in cystic fibrosis, including clinical characteristics, diagnosis, and management.)

Tandon R, Derkay C. Contemporary management of rhinosinusitis and cystic fibrosis. *Curr Opin Otolaryngol Head Neck Surg.* 2003;11:41. [PMID: 14515101] (Medical and surgical treatment recommendations.)

Nonallergic & Allergic Rhinitis

13

Saurabh B. Shah, MD, FAAOA, & Ivor A. Emanuel, MD

Rhinitis is defined as an inflammatory condition that affects the nasal mucosa. The symptoms of rhinitis include nasal obstruction, hyperirritability, and hypersecretion. Rhinitis can be caused by a variety of different allergic and nonallergic conditions (Table 13–1). The incidence of rhinitis seems to have increased since the industrial revolution. One in five Americans is estimated to be afflicted with rhinitis.

Allergic rhinitis is one of the most common chronic conditions in the United States. Of the approximately 50 million US individuals who have rhinitis, many do not have an allergic cause to their rhinitis. The symptoms of nonallergic rhinitis include nasal obstruction, hypersecretion, and irritability, none of which is due to allergy.

■ ANATOMY & PHYSIOLOGY

Airflow through the nose is more efficient in gas exchange and requires less energy than mouth breathing. The nose serves as the initial conduit into the airway. As such, it has important functions of warming, humidifying, and cleansing the air that we breathe. The nasal cycle consists of simultaneous sympathetic and parasympathetic modulation in opposite directions on opposite sides of the nose. The nasal cycle can alter airflow in one nostril by up to 80%, while maintaining total airflow.

From anterior to posterior, the different structural elements of the nose act together to achieve these functions. The nasal vestibule is lined by vibrissae that filter large particulates as they enter the nose. The vestibule then communicates with the nasal valve region, where the nasal mucosa becomes a ciliated, pseudostratified, columnar epithelium. This type of epithelium permeates the entire sinonasal cavity; its importance is underscored when considering conditions such as Kartagener syndrome in which immotile cilia lead to chronic crusting from mucus stasis. Under the mucosa lie stromal cells, inflammatory cells, nerves, blood vessels, and seromucous glands. Each of these elements may play a role in nasal inflammation.

The nose is divided into left and right chambers by a septum comprised of cartilage and bone. Laterally, three bony projections—superior, middle, and inferior turbinates—project into the nasal cavity. These turbinate bones are lined by mucosa, thereby increasing the nasal surface area and covering important sinus ostia. The nasolacrimal duct drains into the inferior meatus. The frontal, maxillary, and anterior ethmoid sinuses drain into the middle meatus; the posterior ethmoid sinuses drain into the superior meatus. Finally, the sphenoid sinus ostia are superior to the choana and drain medially to the superior turbinate. Inflammation in these critical drainage sites can lead to epiphora or sinus disease.

Nasal vascularity includes the internal and external carotid arteries, which feed the nose. The anterior and posterior ethmoid arteries are terminal branches of the ophthalmic artery, a branch of the internal carotid artery. The external carotid artery supplies the sphenopalatine artery. The venous drainage of the nose is primarily through the pterygoid and ophthalmic plexuses.

Finally, the character of the nasal mucus itself is significant. Nasal and sinus mucus typically exists in two layers on the epithelial surface. The deeper layer is thinner and less viscous than the outer layer and therefore allows the cilia to beat with less resistance. The outer layer traps inhaled particulates and has a greater density of inflammatory mediators and leukocytes to protect against infectious agents and foreign substances.

■ NONALLERGIC RHINITIS

Nonallergic rhinitis typically presents with clear rhinorrhea and nasal obstruction. Sneezing and itchy, watery eyes do not typically present with nonallergic rhinitis. There is an increasing incidence of nonallergic rhinitis with advancing age. Patients with nonallergic rhinitis should always be questioned about the use of over-the-counter nasal sprays, previous trauma, work or chemical exposure, and previous intranasal drug use. Epistaxis, pain, and unilateral symptoms may be harbingers of a neoplasm and should be noted.

Table 13–1. Types of rhinitis.

Allergic Rhinitis	Infectious Rhinitis	Nonallergic, Noninfectious Rhinitis	Miscellaneous
• Seasonal • Perennial	• Viral • Bacterial rhinosinusitis	Eosinophilic syndromes • NARES • Nasal polyposis Noneosinophilic syndromes • Vasomotor rhinitis • Rhinitis medicamentosa • Occupational rhinitis • Rhinitis of pregnancy • Hypothyroidism • Medication (eg, birth control pills)	• Granulomatous rhinitis • Atrophic rhinitis • Gustatory rhinitis

VIRAL RHINITIS

Viral rhinitis is very common and often associated with other manifestations of viral illness, which can include headache, malaise, body aches, and cough. Nasal drainage in viral rhinitis is most often clear or white and can be accompanied by nasal congestion and sneezing.

OCCUPATIONAL RHINITIS

A number of different indoor and outdoor pollutants may affect the nose. These agents include dust, ozone, sulfur dioxide, cigarette smoke, garden sprays, and ammonia. Irritant agents can be found in a variety of work environments. Typically, these agents cause nasal dryness, reduced airflow, rhinorrhea, and sneezing. Decreased ciliary movements within the nose have been seen in chronic cigarette smoke exposure and in exposure to wood particles. Environmental control is critical in these patients. Limiting exposure through removal of the causal agent, avoidance, improving ventilation, and the use of protective particulate respirator masks are all helpful.

VASOMOTOR RHINITIS

Patients with vasomotor rhinitis present with symptoms of nasal obstruction and clear nasal drainage. The symptoms are often associated with changes in temperature, eating, exposure to odors and chemicals, or alcohol use. Some clinicians suggest that abnormal autonomic regulation of nasal function leads to vasomotor rhinitis.

NONALLERGIC RHINITIS WITH EOSINOPHILIA

Nonallergic rhinitis with eosinophilia (NARES) is a recently described syndrome in which patients present with nasal obstruction and congestion; these patients frequently experience more severe exacerbations, including the development of sinusitis and polyposis. These patients also display marked eosinophilia on nasal smears (> 25%) but are not allergic to any inhalant allergens by skin testing or in vitro testing. The cause of NARES remains unknown.

RHINITIS MEDICAMENTOSA

Patients with rhinitis medicamentosa often present with nasal obstruction that has worsened over a number of years. They typically have been using over-the-counter topical vasoconstrictive nasal sprays. Many times these patients need increasing doses of these sprays as tachyphylaxis occurs. The use of these sprays for prolonged periods leads to rebound rhinitis in which the patient experiences severe obstruction as the effects of the topical agents subside.

RHINITIS DURING PREGNANCY

Another common presentation of nonallergic rhinitis is rhinitis associated with pregnancy. The systemic concentration of estrogen rises throughout pregnancy. This rise in estrogen leads to a rise in hyaluronic acid in the nasal tissue, which can result in increasing nasal edema and congestion. Moreover, there is an increase in mucous glands and a decrease in nasal cilia during pregnancy, both of which heighten nasal congestion decreasing mucus clearance. Rhinitis is usually most severe during the second and third trimesters of pregnancy.

VASCULITIDES, AUTOIMMUNE, & GRANULOMATOUS DISEASES

The physical examination of a patient with rhinitis should include a thorough head and neck exam. Externally, the nose is evaluated for evidence of previous trauma or saddling, which can be indicative of septal deficiency. Internally, the nasal septal position and character are examined. Signs of chronic inflammation, vasculitis, and septal perforation can be indicative of a variety of systemic problems ranging from Wegener granulomatosis to cocaine abuse. The size and character of the turbinates are also important to note, as is the character of any rhinorrhea. Moreover, the physician should examine the patient for nasal polyposis or other intranasal masses or tumors.

A more in-depth examination of the nasal cavity can be accomplished—after applying topical anesthesia—with the use of either a rigid or flexible nasal endoscope. A 4.0-mm rigid nasal endoscope may be used for adults and a 2.7-mm nasal endoscope for children. This affords visualization of the middle meatus, sphenoethmoidal recess, and nasopharynx regions otherwise not seen with anterior rhinoscopy. In addition, nasal cytology can be helpful to determine both cell types as well as the presence of ciliary motility.

Sanico A, Togias A. Noninfectious, nonallergic rhinitis (NINAR): considerations on possible mechanisms. *Am J Rhinol.* 1998;12:65. [PMID: 9513662]

Settipane RA, Lieberman P. Update on nonallergic rhinitis. *Ann Allergy Asthma Immunol.* 2001;86:494. (Detailed review of the various causes of nonallergic rhinitis.) [PMID: 11379801]

Treatment of Nonallergic Rhinitis

A. NONSURGICAL MEASURES

1. Irritant avoidance—The treatment of nonallergic rhinitis includes the avoidance of offending agents such as chemicals, perfumes, cigarette smoke, and other fumes. In addition, for patients with workplace exposure, a particulate mask can be useful in limiting irritants.

2. Saline irrigation—Saline irrigation is an important adjunctive treatment to help avert intranasal stasis and reduce crusting. The use of saline not only increases the efficacy of intranasal topical medications, but also improves ciliary function.

3. Topical steroids—A mainstay of treatment for nonallergic rhinitis is topical nasal steroid administration. Topical intranasal steroids work in the nasal mucosa to reduce eosinophil and neutrophil chemotaxis; they also reduce inflammation, suppress mast cell-related reactions, and decrease intracellular edema. With this treatment, the efficacy of nasal steroids is enhanced; in addition, the side effects of epistaxis are lessened by administering the spray away from the nasal septum in a head-down position. The newer steroid preparations, such as mometasone and fluticasone, have extensive first-pass metabolism in the liver and therefore very low systemic bioavailability. Thus, the systemic side effects seen with oral steroid administration are rarely encountered with the newer nasal steroids.

4. Adrenergic agents—Other treatments for nonallergic rhinitis include the adrenergic agents. There are two main families of adrenergic drugs: (1) phenylamines (eg, ephedrine, pseudoephedrine, phenylephrine, and phenyl-propanolamine) and (2) imidazolines (eg, xylometazoline, oxymetazoline, and naphazoline). Phenylamines are oral agents, whereas imidazolines are topical agents. The primary role of phenylamines is to decrease mucosal capacitance vessels by agonizing α-adrenergic receptors; this leads to a decongestant effect. Phenylamines can cause dose-related adverse effects such as tremulousness, irritability, tachycardia, hypertension, and urinary retention. They are contraindicated in patients with hypertension, severe coronary artery disease, and in patients on monoamine oxidase inhibitors. Topical imidazolines decrease nasal blood flow by affecting α_1- and α_2-adrenergic receptors. Potent vasoconstriction can cause rebound congestion upon withdrawal of the drug (rhinitis medicamentosa) if used for more than 5 days.

5. Additional agents—Anticholinergic agents such as ipratropium bromide can be used topically to block parasympathetic input and thereby decrease rhinorrhea. Ipratropium bromide is available in a 0.03% formulation for noninfectious rhinitis and a 0.06% concentration for viral rhinitis. Anticholinergic agents can be used in combination with intranasal steroids. They should be avoided in patients with narrow-angle glaucoma, prostatic hypertrophy, or bladder neck obstruction.

Some over-the-counter sprays, such as cromolyn sodium, are safe to be used repetitively. These intranasal sprays act to stabilize mast cell membranes. They must be given prior to mast cell degranulation to be effective and have relatively short half-lives, so their administration must be frequent. Newer therapies that have been tried for rhinitis include the use of intranasal antihistamine spray. Azelastine spray is purported to work on vasomotor rhinitis. For some patients, a bitter taste precludes frequent use of azelastine. Finally, some clinicians are using leukotriene inhibitors as adjuvant treatments in the treatment of nonallergic rhinitis. However, more studies on the efficacy of these agents in nonallergic rhinitis are warranted.

B. SURGICAL MEASURES

1. Septal procedures—The surgical treatment for nonallergic rhinitis is focused on correcting structural abnormalities that may contribute to patient symptoms. Septal deviation is a common defect that can contribute to nasal obstruction. Septoplasty or nasoseptal reconstruction is used to correct cartilaginous or bony abnormalities of the septum. Septal perforations can contribute to crusting or epistaxis. The surgical correction of septal perforations may include the placement of septal buttons, advancement flap closures of perforations, and, more recently, free-tissue transfers for large perforations.

2. Turbinate surgery—Inferior turbinate surgery is also commonly used to counteract nonallergic rhinitis. The type and extent of surgery on the inferior turbinate continues to be a source of debate. Various techniques for turbinate surgery exist and include outfracture, cauterization, radiofrequency ablation, submucous resection, submucosal reduction via a microdebrider, and partial or complete turbinate resection. In general, the current trend is to preserve as much turbinate mucosa as possible to allow normal physiologic function to continue.

Tomooka LT, Murphy C, Davidson TM. Clinical study and literature review of nasal irrigation. *Laryngoscope.* 2000;110:1189. [PMID: 10892694]

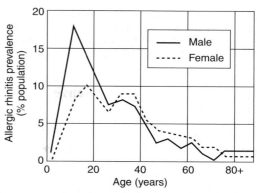

Figure 13–1. Prevalence of allergic rhinitis by age group.

■ ALLERGIC RHINITIS

 ## ESSENTIALS OF DIAGNOSIS

- *May be seasonal, perennial, or both.*
- *Characterized by sneezing, itching, rhinorrhea, and congestion.*
- *Can be associated with other chronic conditions, including asthma, otitis media with effusion (OME), rhinosinusitis, and nasal polyposis.*
- *Typical symptoms of sneezing, rhinorrhea, and nasal congestion can be associated with viral, bacterial, allergic, and nonallergic etiologies.*
- *Can have multiple triggers, both inhaled and ingested.*

General Considerations

Allergy is a clinical manifestation of an adverse immune response after repeated contact with usually harmless substances such as pollens, mold spores, animal dander, dust mites, foods, and stinging insects. Allergic rhinitis is an inflammation of the nasal mucous membranes caused by an IgE-mediated reaction to one or more allergens. The prevalence of allergic rhinitis can vary considerably among age groups and locales.

Allergic rhinitis is one of the most common allergic diseases in the United States, affecting between 20% and 25% of the population (approximately 40 million people). Allergic rhinitis may have its onset at any age, but the incidence of onset is greatest in adolescence, with a decreasing incidence with advancing age. Its peak prevalence is during the third and fourth decades (Figure 13–1).

The economic costs of allergic rhinitis, both direct and indirect, are considerable. The largest portion of the direct costs is the expenditure for both prescription and nonprescription medications (approximately 4 billion dollars annually). The largest indirect costs are from both the allergy itself and also from the negative side effects of allergy medication (primarily over-the-counter antihistamines).

Although allergic rhinitis is not life threatening, its symptomatic effects are considerable, resulting in a significantly diminished quality of life for many sufferers. A number of quality of life studies have shown that in almost every facet of daily life, including social and physical functionality, energy and fatigue levels, and a lack of sleep and mental health, patients with allergic rhinitis have a significant loss of the quality of life compared with nonallergic individuals. In fact, patients with allergic rhinitis have been shown to have a lower quality of life than many asthmatics. In addition, allergic rhinitis may contribute to sleep disorders, fatigue, and—of particular importance with children—learning problems.

Pathogenesis

The allergic response is mediated primarily by a type I hypersensitivity reaction. This response involves the excess production of IgE antibodies and is termed an atopic reaction. In addition to allergic rhinitis, most cases of asthma and atopic dermatitis are considered to have an atopic cause.

In patients with an atopic disposition (a genetic trait), an allergic reaction begins with sensitization to a specific allergen (in allergic rhinitis, these are usually airborne), which induces IgE-antibody production. This occurs through a T-cell, B-cell, and plasma cell cascade. On subsequent exposure, the specific antigen attaches to two specific IgE antibodies attached to the surface of mast cells, which are prevalent in the submucosa of the respiratory and gastrointestinal tracts, the subconjunctiva of the eye, and the subcutaneous layer of the skin. Consequently, this IgE-mediated reaction causes degranulation of the mast cell, which then provokes an inflammatory response with the release of mediators such as histamine, leukotrienes, cytokines, prostaglandins, and platelet-activating factor. This is referred to as the **early-phase** or **humeral reaction** and occurs within 10–15 minutes of allergen exposure; the release of histamine causes the symptoms of sneezing, rhinorrhea, itching, vascular permeability, vasodilatation, and glandular secretion.

The release of cytokines and leukotrienes subsequently causes an influx of inflammatory cells (mainly eosinophils) into the affected area (chemotaxis). This inflammatory response is called the **late-phase** or **cellular reaction,** which can begin 4–6 hours after the initial sensitization and may prolong and enhance the allergic cascade for as long as 48 hours. This response is the main cause of the symptoms of nasal congestion and postnasal drip in allergic rhinitis.

In addition, these mediators produce a hyperreaction to both specific allergens and nonspecific irritants such as tobacco smoke and chemical fumes, referred to as the **priming effect.**

Causes

The development of atopy may be influenced by the following: (1) genetic susceptibility (ie, family history); (2) environmental factors (eg, dust and mold exposure); (3) exposure to allergens (eg, pollens, animal dander, and foods); (4) passive exposure to tobacco smoke (especially in early childhood); and (5) diesel exhaust particles (in urban areas)—among other factors.

In infancy and childhood, food allergens such as milk, eggs, soy, wheat, dust mites, and inhalant allergies such as pet dander are the major causes of allergic rhinitis and the comorbidities of atopic dermatitis, otitis media with effusion, and asthma. In older children and adolescents, pollen allergens become more of a causative factor.

Classification

A. SEASONAL ALLERGIC RHINITIS

The symptoms of seasonal allergic rhinitis, as its name implies, occur or are increased during certain seasons, usually depending on the pollination of plants to which the patient is allergic. Trees pollinate in the spring, grasses in the late spring and summer, and weeds in the fall. In addition, molds may cause symptoms in the fall.

Characteristic symptoms of seasonal allergies include sneezing, watery rhinorrhea, itching of the nose, eyes, ears, and throat, red and watering eyes, and nasal congestion. Symptoms are usually worse in the morning and are aggravated by dry, windy conditions when higher concentrations of pollen are distributed over a wider area.

B. PERENNIAL ALLERGIC RHINITIS

The symptoms of perennial allergic rhinitis are usually constant, with little seasonal variation, although they may vary in intensity. Characteristic symptoms are predominantly nasal congestion and blockage, and postnasal drip. Rhinorrhea and sneezing are less common. Eye symptoms are less common, except with animal allergies. Seasonal pollen may cause the exacerbation of any of these symptoms.

Common allergens that cause perennial allergic rhinitis are indoor inhalants, predominantly dust mites, animal dander, mold spores, and cockroaches (in inner cities). Certain occupational allergens may also cause perennial allergic rhinitis; these are not usually constant because they depend on workplace exposure.

Food allergens may also contribute to perennial allergic rhinitis. In addition, food allergies are often associated with other symptoms, including gastrointestinal problems, urticaria, angioedema, and even anaphylaxis after food is ingested.

Infections and nonspecific irritants may influence perennial allergic rhinitis. In children with allergies, there may be a higher incidence of respiratory tract infections, which in turn tend to aggravate allergic rhinitis and may lead to the development of complications, especially rhinosinusitis and otitis media with effusion. Other irritants such as tobacco smoke, chemical fumes, and air pollutants can also aggravate symptoms.

C. OTHER CLASSIFICATIONS

Recently, other classifications of allergic rhinitis have been introduced. One of these is related to both the temporal incidence and the quality of life. Symptoms are classified (1) as being intermittent (< 4 d/wk or < 4 weeks' duration) or persistent (> 4 d/wk or > 4 weeks' duration) and (2) by the intensity of the symptoms, with either minimal or moderate to severe changes in the quality of life. In another classification system, symptoms are based according to the type of symptom (eg, patients who experience sneezing and a runny nose or those who are congested) without a temporal relationship.

Clinical Findings

A. PATIENT HISTORY

The diagnosis of allergic rhinitis should determine whether the patient is atopic and, if so, what the causative allergen is. To determine these, a basic clinical evaluation should be performed, which should consist of a patient history, a physical examination, and confirmatory tests.

A careful history provides important clues for the diagnostician. Genetic factors determine the likelihood of an individual becoming sensitized and producing IgE antibodies (ie, being atopic). A family history of allergies, eczema, or asthma increases this possibility. Children with parents who have allergies have been shown to have a > 50% chance of becoming allergic themselves. If only one parent or a sibling has allergies, this rate is lower but still significant.

A thorough allergy history should determine whether symptom patterns are seasonal or perennial. Symptoms may include clear and watery nasal discharge, nasal congestion, postnasal drip, and itching of the nose, throat, and eyes. Persistent symptoms are presumed to be due to exposure to an indoor allergen. Seasonal symptoms or symptoms that are reproducible from an inciting factor, such as cat exposure, are most likely to be allergic. If the use of medication, especially antihistamines (both prescription and nonprescription) or intranasal corticosteroids improves symptoms, allergy is probable. This is not the case with either intranasal or oral decongestants, which affect both allergic and nonallergic symptoms. A history of an anaphylactic reaction following ingestion of a particular food or being stung by an insect usually indicates an atopic patient.

Patients should be questioned about the onset, duration, type, progression, and severity of their symptoms. A relationship to the seasons is important, with seasonal symptoms usually indicating a pollen allergy or possibly a mold allergy, but temperate climates can blur these seasonal distinctions. Perennial symptoms usually mean an allergy to dust mites, mold, or animals. An increase in symptoms at night usually suggests an allergy to dust mites or pet dander.

Associated ocular, pharyngeal, and systemic symptoms, including recurrent rhinosinusitis, ear infections, asthma flare-ups, gastrointestinal symptoms, and skin rashes and hives, are important facts to ascertain in the history taking.

The patient should always be questioned about the impact of the symptoms on the quality of his or her life, because the correct diagnosis and, ultimately, symptomatic relief from the appropriate treatment will play a large part in the functional impact on the patient's life.

B. Physical Examination

A physical examination should include inspection of the ears, throat, and nasal passages (including after decongesting with a topical decongestant). Typical findings in the nose in patients with seasonal allergic rhinitis include bluish, pale, boggy turbinates; wet, swollen mucosa; and nasal congestion with nasal obstruction. With perennial allergies, nasal congestion is the predominant sign, but the nasal examination may appear normal. Anatomic abnormalities, such as a deviated nasal septum, concha bullosa, and nasal polyps, may be present. It should be determined whether these abnormalities are the main cause or merely contributing factors to the patient's symptoms. If nasal polyps are suspected, an endoscopic nasal exam is also warranted. Other possible physical findings include conjunctivitis, eczema, and, possibly, asthmatic wheezing.

In children, allergic "shiners" (dark circles under the eyes), facial grimacing, mouth breathing, and the "nasal salute" (constant rubbing of the tip of the nose with the hand) are common physical findings. In addition, in this age group, a concomitant otitis media with effusion is also a possibility.

C. Special Tests

1. Allergy testing—Allergy testing is performed to establish objective evidence of atopic disease. It also can determine the causative allergens responsible, which would then lead to specific therapeutic recommendations. Two major types of testing are available for identifying and quantifying allergen sensitivity: skin testing and in vitro serum assays.

2. Skin testing—Skin testing can be epicutaneous, intradermal, or a combination of both.

a. Skin prick test—The skin prick test is the most common epicutaneous test used. In general, it is a quick, specific, safe, and economical test. With new multitest systems available, it is an easy and simple office procedure to perform and also allows for uniformity in the testing procedure. When a test result is equivocal, it is often followed by an intradermal test.

b. Intradermal testing—Intradermal testing, using quantitative 1:5 serial dilutions, is the skin testing method of choice for most otolaryngic allergists. This type of testing, termed **intradermal dilutional testing** (IDT) and formerly known as serial endpoint titration (SET), is an excellent quantifier of allergen sensitivity, and, as such, is of significant benefit in the preparation of safe and cost-efficient immunotherapy treatment. Today, many otolaryngologists use the skin prick multitest as a screening test prior to performing IDT.

3. In vitro testing—Allergen-specific serum IgE testing is an easy and accurate method for determining the presence of atopic allergy, and with newer in vitro technology available, in vitro testing is at least equivalent to skin testing in efficacy. In vitro assays are safe, specific, cost-effective, and reproducible, and do not require the patient to be free of antihistamines and other medications that may interfere with skin testing. They are also easy and quick and are therefore preferred, especially in children and in anxious patients.

Although the original in vitro assay, the RAST test (radioallergosorbent test), is no longer performed, its name is still used today to generally describe IgE-specific blood testing. However, not all in vitro assays available today are alike. The newer assays tend to be faster, more reliable, and more efficient than previous tests. The ImmunoCap is an excellent example of this newer technology. Not using a reliable assay may affect the diagnosis of atopy and therefore the prescribing of appropriate therapy (Figure 13–2).

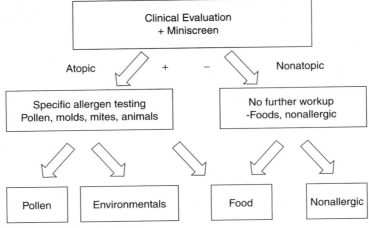

Figure 13–2. In vitro testing process.

In vitro testing can be cost-effective if an initial, appropriately chosen inhalant screening battery of 10–12 allergens consisting of the most prevalent pollens, molds, dust mites, and animals in the local environment is used. In children, common allergenic foods are substituted or added. No further testing is necessary if this battery is negative. If the screening battery is positive and if no immunotherapy is considered, additional allergy testing can be performed.

Differential Diagnosis

The differential diagnoses of allergic rhinitis include the following: (1) infectious rhinitis (acute or chronic); (2) perennial nonallergic rhinitis (eg, vasomotor rhinitis); (3) pollutants and irritants; (4) hormonal rhinitis (eg, pregnancy or hypothyroidism); (5) medication-induced topical rhinitis (rhinitis medicamentosa); (6) anatomic deformity (eg, a deviated septum, nasal polyps, or a concha bullosa); and (7) tumors or foreign bodies.

Treatment

The appropriate management of these common respiratory diseases differs substantially, particularly when allergy is a contributing component. The treatment of allergic rhinitis must consider the main symptoms, their severity, the patient's quality of life, the cost of therapy, as well as the allergens involved in order to individualize the patient's treatment options. In addition, in the treatment of nasal allergies, consideration must be given to both the patient's desire for rapid long-lasting relief of symptoms without side effects and the relief of any particular idiosyncratic symptoms, such as persistent rhinorrhea.

In general, three options are available for the management of allergic rhinitis: (1) avoidance and environmental controls, (2) pharmacotherapy, and (3) immunotherapy.

A. Environmental Controls

Even if environmental controls are not complete, reducing the allergic load may significantly decrease symptoms. Methods of minimizing exposure to pollen are to avoid outdoor activities during relevant pollen seasons (eg, mowing the lawn and gardening), to keep home and car windows closed, and to use air conditioning when possible. To control dust mites, mold, and pet dander, the following practices should be used: (1) reduce household humidity to below 50%; (2) wash bed linens in hot water; (3) remove carpets and pets from the most often used living areas, especially bedrooms; (4) encase pillows, mattresses, and box springs in hypoallergenic coverings (for dust mite protection); and (5) in poor and urban settings, eliminate cockroaches (Table 13–2). For airborne allergens (eg, animal dander), air purifiers can be used.

B. Pharmacotherapeutic Measures

When selecting a pharmacologic treatment for allergic rhinitis, consideration must be given to the patient's underlying condition, the likely pathophysiology, the dominant symptoms, the patient's age and condition, the coexistence of related airway disorders, the patient's preference, and the patient's compliance history. In addition, before initiating any pharmacotherapy, the patient's use and response to previous treatment should be considered (Table 13–3).

1. Antihistamines—Antihistamines are frequently used as a first-line therapy; many are available without a prescription. They block H_1 receptor sites and prevent histamine-induced reactions, including inhibiting increased vascular permeability, smooth muscle contraction, increased mucus production, and pruritus. Antihistamines also inhibit the "wheal and flare" response of the skin and therefore they affect skin testing unless withdrawn a few days before skin testing. They do not affect in vitro testing. Antihistamines are effective in early-phase reaction and therefore reduce sneezing, rhinorrhea, and itching. They have little effect on nasal congestion, a late-phase phenomenon.

Nonprescription, first-generation antihistamines can cause sedation and impair performance and have been associated with a higher risk of both automobile and work-related accidents, decreased work performance and productivity, and impaired learning and academic performance. These side effects can be significantly exacerbated by alcohol, sedatives, antidepressants, and hypnotics. Many have anticholinergic effects and cause dry mouth. These include diphenhydramine (eg, Benadryl), hydroxyzine (eg, Atarax), chlorpheniramine, and brompheniramine. The latter two are found in most nonprescription cold remedies.

Second-generation antihistamines have an antihistamine activity comparable to that of first-generation antihistamines but have a better safety profile with little, if any, sedation as they have little affinity for central H_1 receptors. They have no anticholinergic activity and are well absorbed, with a rapid onset of action and symptom relief usually within 1 hour. Second-generation antihistamines are typically dosed once daily and are rarely associated with drug tolerance with prolonged use. Those available orally in the United States are fexofenadine (eg, Allegra), loratadine (eg, Claritin), desloratadine (eg, Clarinex), and cetirizine (eg, Zyrtec). A second-generation intranasal antihistamine, azelastine (eg, Astelin), is also available.

2. Intranasal corticosteroids—Intranasal corticosteroids may be the most effective medications for the overall control of allergic rhinitis symptoms. They relieve sneezing, itching, and rhinorrhea, and also nasal congestion. Maximal effect may take from 1 to 2 weeks after the onset of their use. Their effectiveness depends

Table 13–3. Pharmacologic agents in the management of allergic rhinitis.

Class	Mechanism of Action
Antihistamines	Antagonize the H_1 receptor–mediated effects of histamine
Decongestants	Act predominantly on α-adrenergic receptors of the mucosa of the respiratory tract
Intranasal and oral corticosteroids	Exert a wide range of effects on multiple cell types and mediators
Mast cell stabilizers	Inhibit the release of mediators from mast cells
Anticholinergic agents	Antagonize the action of acetylcholine at muscarinic receptors
Leukotriene modifiers	Antagonize the action of leukotriene receptors or inhibit 5-lipoxygenase and the formation of leukotrienes

on regular use and an adequate nasal airway for application. They act on the late-phase reaction and therefore prevent a significant influx of inflammatory cells. The newer formulations (mentioned below) have minimal systemic absorption with no systemic side effects, and they have been approved for use in children. They have no systemic side effects with regard to HPA axis suppression and do not affect long-bone growth in children. In young adults and children, they are considered the drugs of choice in the treatment of allergic rhinitis. Local side effects, such as dryness and epistaxis, can be reduced by careful patient instruction on their use and also the regular, concomitant use of intranasal saline. Commonly available intranasal corticosteroids in the United States include triamcinolone (eg, Nasacort), budesonide (eg, Rhinocort), fluticasone (eg, Flonase), and mometasone (eg, Nasonex).

3. Systemic corticosteroids—Systemic corticosteroids may be necessary for severe, intractable symptoms. They can be administered either by intramuscular injection or orally. With the latter, a tapering dose is usually given over 3–7 days. Systemic corticosteroids act on inflammation and significantly reduce all the symptoms of allergic rhinitis. The repeated use of these agents can cause serious side effects, such as HPA axis suppression, as well as other common side effects of steroid use.

4. Decongestants—Decongestants act on α-adrenergic receptors of the nasal mucosa, producing vasoconstriction and thus reducing turbinate congestion. They improve nasal patency but do not relieve rhinorrhea,

Table 13–2. Environmental control of indoor aeroallergens.

Allergen	Environmental Control
House dust mites	• Encase mattress, box spring, and pillows in occlusive covers • Wash all bedding in water > 130° F weekly • Dehumidify (< 50% level) • Remove reservoirs (especially carpeting)
Pets	• Remove pet from home or at least from patient's bedroom • Remove reservoirs (carpeting, stuffed furniture), if feasible • Wash animal frequently

pruritus, and sneezing. These preparations are found mostly in nonprescription cold medicines and should be used with care in patients with cardiac problems and hypertension. Intranasal decongestants (eg, oxymetazoline) can cause rebound nasal congestion and cause dependency if used for more than 3–4 days (rhinitis medicamentosa).

5. Intranasal anticholinergics—These agents tend to control only rhinorrhea and have no other effects on allergy symptoms. One of the most commonly used intranasal anticholinergics is ipratropium bromide (eg, Atrovent). These agents can be combined with other allergic medications to control rhinorrhea in perennial allergic rhinitis.

6. Intranasal cromolyn—Intranasal cromolyn (eg, Nasalcrom) must be used before the onset of symptoms to be effective. This medication must be used throughout the entire exposure; it is considered to be very safe. The recommended dosage is four times daily.

7. Leukotriene inhibitors—Montelukast "Singulair" is a newer medication for the treatment of allergic rhinitis. To date, clinical studies have shown its efficacy to be greater than that of placebo, but less effective than antihistamines and intranasal steroids in the treatment of allergic rhinitis (Table 13–4).

C. Immunotherapy

Immunotherapy attempts to increase the threshold level of the appearance of symptoms after aeroallergen exposure. The exact mechanism of how immunotherapy works is still unclear; it may be the production of so-called "blocking" antibodies, as well as regulation of the immune cascade that causes allergic reactions.

Indications for immunotherapy include long-term pharmacotherapy for prolonged periods of time, the inadequacy or intolerability of drug therapy, and significant allergen sensitivities. Before beginning immunotherapy, the physician must first confirm the atopic diagnosis by testing IgE specific to the offending allergen (or allergens).

Most immunotherapy administered in the United States today is through a gradual increase in the dose of the antigen(s) given until either a mild systemic symptom or a large local reaction at the subcutaneous injection site occurs (optimal dose therapy). In some centers, sublingual immunotherapy is the method of choice. This is more common in Europe and tends to be easy and safe to administer at home by the patients themselves.

There is no adequate test available to indicate to the patient how long immunotherapy must be continued. Therefore, a clinical response with a reduction in symptoms dictates the duration of specific treatment. A minimum of 2–3 years is usually given to avoid a rapid recurrence of symptoms in uncomplicated allergic rhinitis.

D. Other Treatment Considerations

The first aspect of treating patients who have not responded well to therapeutic measures, including immunotherapy, is determining to what degree therapeutic compliance has occurred. The next steps are to adjust drug dosages, try one or two other agents, and consider combination therapy. In addition, the physician should determine whether allergy exposure has increased and should also review the environmental control measures. Finally, it may be necessary to reconsider the diagnosis and reevaluate the patient.

Baraniuk JN. Pathogenesis of allergic rhinitis. *J Allergy Clin Immunol.* 1997;99:S763. [PMID: 9042069]

Bousquet J, Vignola AM, Campbell AM, Michel FB. Pathophysiology of allergic rhinitis. *Int Arch Allergy Immun.* 1996;110:207. [PMID: 8688666]

Jarvis D, Burney P. ABC of allergies: the epidemiology of allergic disease. *BMJ.* 1998;316:607. [PMID: 9518918]

Poon AW, Goodman CS, Rubin RJ. In vitro and skin test testing for allergy: comparable clinical utility and costs. *Am J Manag Care.* 1998;4(7):969. [PMID: 10181996]

Table 13–4. Pharmacotherapies for allergic rhinitis.

Agent	Inflammation	Congestion	Rhinorrhea	Sneezing	Nasal Itch	Ocular Symptoms
Antihistamines						
1st generation	–	–	+	+	+	+
2nd generation	±	–	+	+	+	+
Topical antihistamines	±	±	+	+	+	±
Decongestants	–	+	–	–	–	–
Intranasal steroids	+	+	+	+	±	±
Oral steroids	+	+	+	+	±	+
Intranasal cromolyn	±	±	±	±	±	±

SECTION IV

Sinuses

Acute & Chronic Sinusitis

Ashish R. Shah, MD, Frank N. Salamone, MD, & Thomas A. Tami, MD

 ESSENTIALS OF DIAGNOSIS

- *Suspect acute bacterial rhinosinusitis with an upper respiratory infection that does not resolve in 10 days or worsens after 5–7 days with symptoms that may include facial pain/pressure, nasal obstruction, and discolored nasal discharge.*
- *In chronic rhinosinusitis, nasal endoscopy and/or CT scan may be necessary to make the diagnosis because symptoms do not correlate well with findings.*

General Considerations

Rhinosinusitis is by far the most common disease of the paranasal sinuses, affecting about 14%, or 31 million adults annually. The costs of chronic rhinosinusitis alone are estimated at over $4 billion per year. The appropriate and cost-effective treatment of rhinosinusitis is therefore critical.

Rhinosinusitis is broadly defined as a group of disorders characterized by inflammation of the nose and paranasal sinuses. Classification by the duration of an inflammatory episode includes acute (up to 4 weeks), subacute (4–12 weeks), and chronic (> 12 weeks). Additional categories include recurrent acute rhinosinusitis (≥ four episodes per year without evidence of chronic rhinosinusitis) and acute exacerbations of rhinosinusitis. Chronic rhinosinusitis may be subclassified as chronic rhinosinusitis with or without nasal polyps and with eosinophilic or noneosinophilic histologic features.

Paranasal Sinus Anatomy & Physiology

The paranasal sinuses are mucosa-lined structures physically contiguous with the nasal cavity. Proposed functions include (1) acting as resonating chambers for the voice, (2) providing protection to the brain from trauma, (3) moisturizing and humidifying ambient air, and (4) lightening the weight of the facial skeleton. However, there is no convincing evidence for any of these theories.

Knowledge of paranasal sinus anatomy is critical to understanding the pathophysiology, the possible complications, and the surgical treatments of sinusitis (Figure 14–1). Anteriorly, the nasal cavity opens to the outside environment through the skin-lined nasal vestibule. Moving posteriorly, the prominent inferior turbinate can be seen projecting medially from the lateral nasal wall. The nasolacrimal duct empties into the inferior meatus lateral to the inferior turbinate. Superior to the inferior turbinate, the middle turbinate hangs from its attachment to the skull base. Medial to the middle turbinate, the ethmoid bulla can be identified. Anterior and inferior to the bulla, the trough-shaped ethmoid infundibulum serves as the drainage conduit for the anterior ethmoid cells, the maxillary sinus, and the frontal sinus. The hiatus semilunaris is the crescent-shaped opening of the infundibulum into the nose.

The ostiomeatal complex, which includes those ostia that drain into the middle meatus, is an anatomically constricted region that is prone to blockage, especially in the presence of structural anomalies such as Haller cells and concha bullosa (see section on Paranasal Sinuses & Nasal Cavity in Chapter 3). In addition, the ostia themselves are small. The functional diameter of

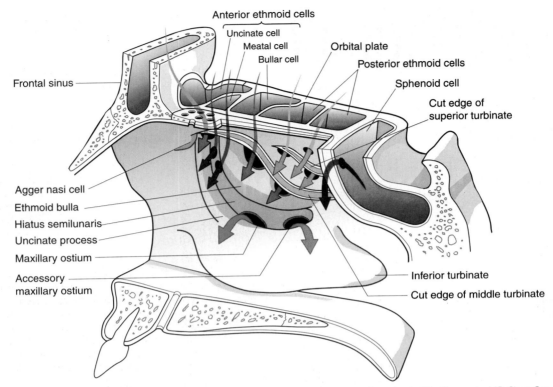

Figure 14–1. Lateral wall of the nasal cavity. (Reproduced, with permission, from Levin HL, Clemente MP. *Sinus Surgery: Endoscopic and Microscopic Approaches.* Thieme Medical Publishers, 2005.)

the maxillary sinus ostia is usually only 2–4 mm and the ostia of the ethmoid air cells are even smaller.

Posterior and superior to the middle turbinate lie the superior and, in some people, the supreme turbinates. The sphenoid sinus and the posterior ethmoid cells drain into the sphenoethmoidal recess posterior and medial to the attachment of the superior turbinate.

The relationship of the paranasal sinuses to the brain and the orbits is of critical importance. Superiorly and medially, the cribriform plate of the ethmoid bone serves as the roof of the nasal cavity and the floor of the anterior cranial fossa. More laterally, the ethmoid air cells are separated from the anterior cranial fossa by the fovea ethmoidalis, which is part of the frontal bone. The paper-thin lamina papyracea of the lateral ethmoid bone separates the ethmoid sinuses from the orbit and can serve as a route of the spread of infection from the sinuses to the periorbita.

The nose and paranasal sinuses are lined with pseudostratified columnar, ciliated epithelium with goblet and seromucous cells. Normal sinonasal mucociliary clearance is predicated on (1) ostial patency, (2) ciliary function, and (3) mucus consistency. Impairment of any of these factors at the osteomeatal complex may result in mucus stasis,

which under the proper conditions induces bacterial growth. Furthermore, cilia have a tendency to propel mucus toward the natural ostia of a sinus, which explains why surgical openings made into a sinus at places other than the natural ostia (eg, in the inferior meatus) are ineffective at draining the sinus (Figure 14–2).

Lethbridge-Çejku M, Rose D, Vickerie J. Summary health statistics for U.S. adults: National Health Interview Survey, 2004. National Center for Health Statistics. *Vital Health Stat.* 2006;10:228. (A large-scale adult health survey.)

Murphy MP, Fishman P, Short SO et al. Health care utilization and cost among adults with chronic rhinosinusitis enrolled in a health maintenance organization. *Otolaryngol Head Neck Surg.* 2002;127(5):367. [PMID: 12447229] (The impact of chronic rhinosis on the use and cost of health care.)

Pathogenesis & Clinical Features

A. ACUTE BACTERIAL RHINOSINUSITIS

Acute bacterial rhinosinusitis typically begins as a viral upper respiratory infection that persists longer than 10 days. In some cases, a secondary acute bacterial rhinosi-

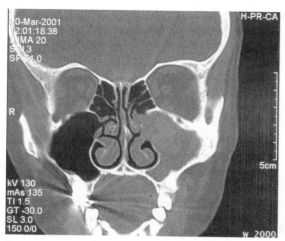

Figure 14–2. Acute maxillary sinusitis. The left maxillary sinus is completely opacified and the ostium is occluded.

nusitis may result from ostial blockage owing to mucosal edema and possible ciliary damage. The end result is mucus stasis and the creation of an environment suitable for bacterial proliferation. The most common organisms responsible for acute sinusitis include *Streptococcus pneumoniae, Haemophilus influenzae,* and *Moraxella catarrhalis.* The diagnosis of acute bacterial rhinosinusitis can be made when a viral upper respiratory infection does not resolve within 10 days or worsens after 5–7 days. Symptoms suggestive of the diagnosis are listed in Table 14–1. Severe symptoms may imply impending complication, and the patient certainly should not wait 5–7 days before receiving further evaluation and treatment.

B. Chronic Rhinosinusitis

The pathophysiology of chronic rhinosinusitis remains incompletely understood, but it is clear that a number of systemic, local, and environmental factors play important predisposing roles. The presence or absence of nasal polyps may represent different pathophysiologic mechanisms. Nasal polyps are smooth, edematous lobulated masses that usually arise from the middle meatus or sphenoethmoid recess and represent a noninfectious and most often eosinophilic inflammatory reaction. Eosinophilic chronic rhinosinusitis represents a spectrum of diseases that may have diverse causes, including both allergic and nonallergic and including allergic fungal rhinosinusitis (AFRS), eosinophilic mucin rhinosinusitis, aspirin-exacerbated respiratory disease (nasal polyps, asthma, and ASA sensitivity), and eosinophilic granuloma. Chronic rhinosinusitis with or without nasal polyps and with noneosinophilic features are thought to be the result of impaired mucociliary

clearance, abnormal sinus ventilation, or immune deficiency. Chronic rhinosinusitis with noneosinophilic nasal polyps includes antral choanal polyp, cystic fibrosis, ciliary dyskinesias, and bacterial infection. Chronic rhinosinusitis without nasal polyps may be related to many disorders including immunodeficiency, autoimmune/granulomatous diseases, allergic rhinitis, anatomic irregularities, and scarring.

Although the most common symptoms of chronic rhinosinusitis are nasal discharge, nasal obstruction, facial congestion, and facial pain/pressure, patients with chronic rhinosinusitis with nasal polyps more often have hyposmia and less pain/pressure complaints than those who do not have nasal polyps. Also, patients with chronic rhinosinusitis without nasal polyps may be more likely to have bacterial infection and may be more likely to improve with medical therapies.

The role of bacteria in the pathogenesis of chronic rhinosinusitis is controversial, although antibiotics are frequently prescribed. The most common organisms isolated in chronic rhinosinusitis subjects include *Staphylococcus aureus,* anaerobes, and gram-negative enterics such as *Pseudomonas aeruginosa.* Recent avenues of investigation about the relationship of bacteria to chronic rhinosinusitis include the roles of bacterial superantigens, biofilms, and osteitis (Figure 14–3).

C. Fungal Rhinosinusitis

1. Invasive fungal sinusitis—Invasive fungal sinusitis is usually a complication of diabetes or an immunocompromised state; it is characterized by a fulmi-

Table 14–1. Major and minor factors in the diagnosis of acute sinusitis.

Major Factors
  Facial pain or pressure
  Facial congestion or fullness
  Nasal obstruction or blockage
  Nasal discharge, purulence, or discolored postnasal drainage
  Hyposmia or anosmia
  Purulence in nasal cavity
  Fever (in acute rhinosinusitis only)
Minor Factors
  Headache
  Fever (in chronic sinusitis)
  Halitosis
  Fatigue
  Dental pain
  Cough
  Ear pain, pressure, or fullness

Adapted with permission from Lanza DC et al: Adult rhinosinusitis defined. *Otolaryngol Head and Neck Surg* 1997;117:S1.

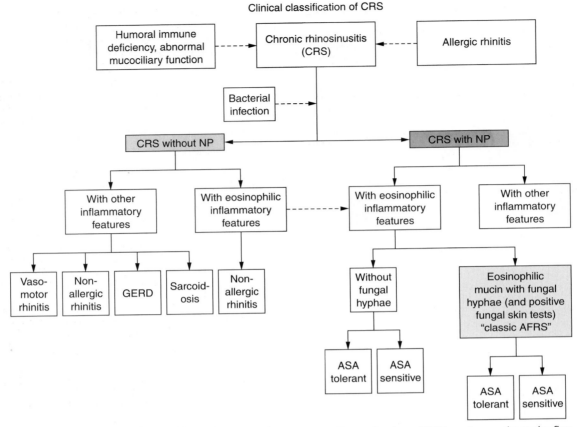

Figure 14-3. Proposed subclassification of chronic rhinosinusitis. NP, nasal polyps; GERD, gastroesophageal reflux disease; AFRS, allergic fungal rhinosinusitis; ASA, acetylsalicylic acid. (Reproduced, with permission, from Meltzer EO, Hamilos DL, Hadley JA et al. Rhinosensitivity: establishing definitions for clinical research and patient care. *Otolaryngol Head Neck Surg.* 2004;1315:51.)

nant, invasive infection. A pathologic examination of the black necrotic debris that is often seen intranasally demonstrates arterial and venous thrombosis due to direct fungal invasion. The treatment consists of (1) debriding all involved structures, including the orbital contents, if necessary; (2) aggressive intravenous antifungal therapy; (3) normalizing the underlying immunocompromised state (usually neutropenia); and (4) stabilizing the diabetes. The typical fungal pathogens are *Aspergillus, Mucor,* and *Rhizopus.*

2. Fungal ball—Fungal ball is the development of a noninvasive conglomeration of fungal hyphae into a mass. *Aspergillus* is the most common pathogen, and chronic rhinosinusitis results from paranasal sinus obstruction. Treatment is complete extirpation of the fungal mass.

3. Allergic fungal rhinosinusitis (AFRS)— Fungus can also stimulate an immune response from the sinonasal mucosa, resulting in allergic fungal sinusitis. Typically, polypoid tissue is seen anterior to a mass consisting of mucin, fungal elements, Charcot-Leyden crystals, and eosinophils. Sinus expansion and bony remodeling are hallmark features of this process. Even though this is not an invasive, infectious process, the treatment is primarily surgical with postoperative topical nasal steroids. Immunotherapy and systemic steroids may be necessary to reduce recurrence. Topical antifungals may also prove to have a role in treatment.

Anon JB, Jacobs MR, Poole MD. Antimicrobial treatment guidelines for acute bacterial rhinosinusitis. *Otolaryngol Head Neck*

Surg. 2004;130s:s1. [PMID: 147269904] (Sinus and Allergy Health Partnership Guidelines.)

Benninger MS, Ferguson BJ, Hadley JA et al. Adult chronic rhinosinusitis: definitions, diagnosis, epidemiology, and pathophysiology. *Otolaryngol Head Neck Surg.* 2003;129(3 suppl):1. [PMID: 12958561] (Task force to define chronic rhinosinusitis.)

Hunt SM, Miyamoto RC, Cornelius RS, Tami TA. Invasive fungal sinusitis in the acquired immunodeficiency syndrome. *Otolaryngol Clin North Am.* 2000;33:335. [PMID: 10736408] (Treatment of fungal sinusitis in the immunocompromised patient.)

Meltzer EO, Hamilos DL, Hadley JA et al. Rhinosinusitis: establishing definitions for clinical research and patient care. *Otolaryngol Head Neck Surg.* 2004;131S:S1. [PMID: 15577816] (Consensus statement from five organizations to define rhinosinusitis.)

Diagnostic Modalities

A. PHYSICAL EXAMINATION

A complete head and neck exam with anterior rhinoscopy is essential in all patients suspected of having rhinosinusitis. Findings of mucopurulence, edema, septal deflection, and polyps should be noted. The middle meatus is often well visualized after appropriate decongestion.

B. ENDOSCOPIC EVALUATION

Rigid or flexible nasal endoscopy may be necessary in the evaluation of rhinosinusitis. Findings to be noted include mucopurulence at the ostiomeatal complex and sphenoethmoid recess, edema, erythema, polyps/polypoid tissue, and crusting. In acute bacterial rhinosinusitis, endoscopy is useful to confirm the diagnosis and to obtain cultures at the middle meatus. Because symptoms do not correlate well with findings in chronic rhinosinusitis, endoscopy and/or imaging is essential to make the appropriate diagnosis and to obtain cultures from the middle meatus. When performed carefully to avoid contamination from the nose, middle meatus cultures correlate well with maxillary sinus aspiration, which is the gold standard. Aerobic, anaerobic, fungal, and acid-fast bacilli cultures should be obtained.

C. IMAGING STUDIES

Computed tomography (CT) scanning is currently the method of choice for sinus imaging. Because a viral upper respiratory infection may cause abnormalities on CT that are indistinguishable from rhinosinusitis, imaging in acute bacterial rhinosinusitis has limited usefulness except when complications are suspected. On the other hand, symptoms of chronic rhinosinusitis do not correlate well with findings. Therefore, CT and/or nasal endoscopy is necessary to make the diagnosis. In addition to providing excellent visualization of mucosal thickening, air fluid levels, and bony structures, coronal scans give optimal visualization of the osteomeatal complex and are conveniently oriented for the surgeon in terms of surgical planning.

Magnetic resonance imaging (MRI) of the sinuses is much less commonly performed than CT scanning largely because this modality does not image bone well. However, MRI can usually differentiate retained mucus from soft tissue masses based on signal intensity characteristics, which have an identical appearance on CT scans; therefore, MRI can be very helpful in differentiating a sinus completely filled with tumor from one partially filled with retained secretions. MRI is also a helpful modality with suspected orbital or intracranial extension.

D. LABORATORY TESTS

Laboratory tests are rarely helpful in the evaluation of sinusitis. If there is any question of an immunocompromised state, testing for HIV and IgG levels should be performed. An evaluation for sarcoidosis may be appropriate. Also, scarring in the nasal cavity can be seen in autoimmune conditions, such as Wegener granulomatosis, and therefore cytoplasmic-antineutrophil cytoplasmic antibody (C-ANCA), erythrocyte sedimentation rate (ESR), and antinuclear antibody (ANA) tests should be considered.

Hwang PH, Irwin SB, Griest SE et al. Radiologic correlates of symptom-based diagnostic criteria for chronic rhinosinusitis. *Otolaryngol Head Neck Surg.* 2003;128(4):489. [PMID: 12707650] (Correlation of CT scan and sinusitis symptom criteria from 1997 Task Force on Rhinosinusitis.)

Tantilipikorn P, Fritz M, Tanabodee J et al. A comparison of endoscopic culture techniques for chronic rhinosinusitis. *Am J Rhinology.* 2002;16(5):255. [PMID: 12422969] (Aspiration and swab of culture material are no different in this study.)

Differential Diagnosis

The differential diagnoses of acute and chronic sinusitis are many and include the following: the common cold; temporomandibular joint (TMJ) pain; headache (including migraine); tooth, nasal, and trigeminal pain; and sinus neoplasm. The symptoms of facial pressure and pain, purulent nasal discharge, nasal congestion, hyposmia, tooth pain, and a poor response to nasal decongestants can help differentiate these entities.

A. VIRAL RHINITIS (COMMON COLD)

The most difficult point in the diagnosis of sinusitis is differentiating it from the common cold. The presence of purulence on examination of the nasal cavity can assist in the diagnosis. Sinus infection is more likely if symptoms become worse after 5 days or last longer than 10 days. Acute unilateral symptoms are also more consistent with sinusitis. Allergic rhinitis may also cause rhinorrhea and postnasal drip, as seen in sinusitis.

B. TEMPOROMANDIBULAR JOINT PAIN

Because of the complex anatomy of the head and neck, many conditions may mimic sinus symptoms. Temporomandibular joint pain is common and is frequently dull and aching in quality. Palpation for joint tenderness and click is therefore important.

C. HEADACHE AND MIGRAINE

Headache, both migraine and tension type, may be confused with sinus pain. Migraine headaches are characterized by throbbing head pain, frequently unilateral, that lasts from 4 to 72 hours. Migraines can occur with or without neurologic symptoms such as visual disturbances or numbness. Noting the presence of an aura, the relatively short duration of symptoms, and the response to migraine medicines such as ergot alkaloids can help differentiate migraine headaches from sinusitis. The bandlike frontal pressure associated with tension headache typically worsens as the day goes on, whereas sinus pain remains relatively constant. Sinus pain is typically not as severe as the symptoms associated with cluster headache.

D. TOOTH, NASAL, AND TRIGEMINAL PAIN

Tooth pain may be a result of sinusitis or may be mistaken for sinus pain. Particularly in children, nasal foreign body may cause sinusitis and should be excluded. Trigeminal neuralgia is uncommon, but it can cause paroxysms of lancinating pain along the distribution of the trigeminal nerve. This sensation is in contrast to the constant dull ache of sinusitis.

E. SINUS NEOPLASM

Sinus neoplasm is relatively uncommon, but it is critical to exclude. A history of unilateral nasal obstruction and epistaxis warrants further workup, including CT scan and nasal endoscopy. Changes in vision and cranial nerve deficits, particularly in the distribution of the infraorbital nerve, should also cause suspicion. Radiographically, sinus neoplasm is identified by unilateral findings and bone erosion (see Chapter 16, Paranasal Sinus Neoplasms).

Treatment

A. ANTIBIOTICS

Antibiotic recommendations for acute bacterial rhinosinusitis have evolved based on increasing resistance patterns. Twenty-five percent of *S pneumoniae* infections are penicillin resistant, and resistance to macrolides and trimethoprim/sulfamethoxazole (TMP/SMX) is common. Thirty percent of *H influenzae* and almost all strains of *M catarrhalis* produce β-lactamase. Current guidelines for antibiotic choice in acute bacterial rhinosinusitis are dependent on the severity of the disease and whether the patient has received antibiotics in the past 4–6 weeks. Duration of treatment should be 10–14 days. With mild disease and no recent antibiotic use,

recommendations include amoxicillin/clavulanate (1.75–4 g/250 mg/d or 45–90 mg/6.4 mg/kg/d in children), amoxicillin (1.5–4 g/d or 45–90 mg/kg/d in children), or cefpodoxime, cefuroxime, or cefdinir. β-Lactam-allergic adults should receive TMP/SMX, doxycycline, or a macrolide, and β-lactam-allergic children should receive TMP/SMX or a macrolide. Failure rates, however, with these non–β-lactam antibiotics may reach 25%. With recent antibiotic use or in moderate disease, initial drug selection should include a respiratory quinolone, amoxicillin/clavulanate, ceftriaxone, or a combination to provide broad-spectrum coverage in adults and amoxicillin/clavulanate or ceftriaxone in children. β-Lactam-allergic adults should receive a respiratory quinolone or clindamycin and rifampin, whereas β-lactam-allergic children should receive TMP/SMX, a macrolide, or clindamycin.

Failure to respond to treatment within 72 hours should lead to a reevaluation and change of therapies to provide broader coverage. In this circumstance, CT scan, nasal endoscopy, or culture should be considered.

Chronic sinusitis is associated with a different set of pathogens and therefore demands an antibiotic with a spectrum that includes gram-negative organisms, *S aureus,* and anaerobes. In addition, longer courses of antibiotics, typically 3–6 weeks, are often recommended. Culture-directed therapy is highly recommended (Table 14–2).

B. NASAL SPRAYS AND IRRIGATION

Mucosal inflammation and polyposis, which lead to the obstruction of sinus ostia, are critical in the pathogenesis of most chronic rhinosinusitis. Nasal steroid sprays directly address this problem by reducing mucosal inflammation and the size of polyps, thereby limiting postoperative recurrence. Systemic side effects are uncommon (although arguably possible), and therefore nasal steroids are often prescribed for maintenance therapy in those with chronic rhinosinusitis. Nasal saline irrigation is an important component in the treatment of chronic rhinosinusitis. Frequent rinsing prevents the accumulation of nasal crusts and promotes mucociliary clearance. Hypertonic saline may increase the rate of clearance in certain cases. Antibiotic irrigations such as gentamicin (80 mg/L) may be considered in refractory cases of chronic rhinosinusitis. Although nasal saline sprays do not have the mechanical débridement effect of saline irrigation, they do help to keep the mucosa moist and to facilitate mucociliary clearance in both acute bacterial rhinosinusitis and chronic rhinosinusitis.

Oxymetazoline hydrochloride spray causes intense vasoconstriction of the nasal mucosa. Rebound swelling may incite a vicious cycle, leading to complete nasal obstruction and subsequent sinus disease. Oxymetazoline spray may be used for very short periods of time

Table 14–2. Efficacy of antibiotics in the therapy of sinusitis.

Oral Antimicrobial	Acute Sinusitis			Chronic Sinusitis		
	S pneumoniae	*Haemophilus* spp.	*Moraxella catarrhalis*	*S aureus*	Anaerobes	Enterics
Penicillin/Amoxicillin	+	0	0	0	±	0
Cephalosporins						
First-generation	±	0	0	+	0	0
Second-generation	+	+	+	+	0	±
Third-generation	±	+	+	±	0	+
Amoxicillin/Clavulanate	+	+	+	+	+	+
Macrolides	±	±	±	+	0	0
Clindamycin	+	0	0	+	+	0
Imipenem*/meropenem*	+	+	+	+	+	+
Trimethoprim/sulfamethoxazole	–	+	+	±	0	+
Quniolones (older) or aminoglycosides*	±	+	+	±	0	+
Quinolones (newer)	+	+	+	+	±	+

0, no or little (< 30%) activity; ±, some activity (30–80%); +, good activity (> 80%).
*Available in parenteral form only.

(eg, 3 days) for symptomatic relief usually in acute bacterial rhinosinusitis or acute exacerbations of chronic rhinosinusitis.

C. SYSTEMIC STEROIDS, DECONGESTANTS, AND OTHER THERAPIES

Systemic steroids are highly effective at reducing mucosal inflammation and nasal polyp bulk in chronic rhinosinusitis because of their anti-inflammatory effects. However, a thorough discussion with patients regarding the risks of systemic steroid administration is mandatory. A tapered regimen may be given during severe chronic rhinosinusitis flare-ups and in the postoperative period, but their use should be limited and carefully monitored. Systemic decongestants and mucolytic agents such as guaifenesin may provide some symptomatic relief. Given the favorable side effects of these agents, they are often added to the therapeutic regimen. Leukotriene receptor antagonists (montelukast, zafirlukast) and macrolide antibiotics, which have anti-inflammatory effects, may also prove to be useful therapeutics.

D. ALLERGY MANAGEMENT

For patients with documented allergic disease, ongoing allergy management is beneficial. Environmental controls, topical steroids, and immunotherapy may prevent exacerbations of rhinitis, therefore preventing the progression to sinusitis.

E. SINUS SURGERY

Maximal medical therapy, typically defined as 4–6 weeks of appropriate antibiotics, nasal steroids, and generally systemic steroid therapy, is prescribed prior to the consideration of surgical management. Surgical therapy may be necessary if evidence of mucosal disease or ostiomeatal unit obstruction—as determined by either CT scan or endoscopic evaluation—persists in spite of aggressive medical treatment. Patients with clear anatomic abnormalities or sinonasal polyps may be more likely to respond to surgical therapy.

1. Functional endoscopic sinus surgery—
a. Indications—Functional endoscopic sinus surgery is based on several key observations: (1) widely patent antrostomies in nonanatomic positions may fail to drain sinuses due to the directionality of mucociliary flow; (2) the ostiomeatal unit is anatomically constricted; and (3) the stripping of sinus mucosa leads to delayed healing and the loss of normal ciliary function. Thus, a conservative endoscopic technique has been developed. The keys to the technique are the use of "through-cutting" instruments that preserve sinonasal mucosa and the excellent visualization made possible with modern telescopes. Mucosal polyps can be carefully débrided, the natural ostia enlarged, and the ethmoid sinuses unroofed, which opens them to the nasal cavity. The improvement in symptoms with functional endoscopic sinus surgery may be expected in more than 90% of patients.

b. Relationship with other treatments—Functional endoscopic sinus surgery must be regarded as only one component of a total sinusitis treatment plan that must also include preoperative optimization of medical therapy, meticulous postoperative care, and, finally, long-term maintenance therapy. Any underlying medical conditions, such as diabetes mellitus, immunodeficiency, and atopic disease, must also be addressed if ultimate success in treatment is to be obtained.

c. Complications—The complications of surgical therapy are related to the close anatomic proximity of the paranasal sinuses to the brain and orbits. An intimate knowledge of this anatomy is critical to safely perform this surgery; a definite learning curve is associated with the adoption of this technique. Injury to the medial wall of the orbit may cause the prolapse of orbital fat into the nasal cavity. A violation of the orbital wall, with subsequent hemorrhage and orbital hematoma, may lead to compression of the optic nerve and blindness. Damage to the cribriform plate region may lead to cerebrospinal fluid leak, herniation of cranial contents, meningitis, or intracranial bleeding.

2. Open sinus surgery—In spite of the versatility of endoscopic procedures, open sinus surgery is sometimes needed. An example is the Caldwell-Luc antrostomy in which the maxillary sinus is entered through a sublabial incision. The Caldwell-Luc approach allows biopsy of the sinus contents; also, once the sinus is entered, a drainage window may be made into the nasal cavity.

If surgery is not an option or the disease is refractory to surgical intervention, a trial of intravenous antibiotic therapy may be appropriate.

Bonfils P, Nores JM, Halimi P, Avan P. Corticosteroid treatment in nasal polyposis with a three-year follow-up period. *Laryngoscope.* 2003;113(4):683. [PMID: 12472629] (Retrospective review demonstrating the efficacy of topical and systemic steroids for nasal polyposis.)

Graham SM, Nerad JA. Orbital complications in endoscopic sinus surgery using powered instrumentation. *Laryngoscope.* 2003;113(5):874. [PMID: 12792325] (Retrospective review of orbital injuries during sinus surgery.)

Statham MM, Seiden A. Potential new avenues of treatment for chronic rhinosinusitis: an anti-inflammatory approach. *Otolaryngol Clin North Am.* 2005;38(6):1351. [PMID: 16326930] (Discussion of potential anti-inflammatory approaches to treating sinus disease.)

Complications

A. ORBITAL INFECTION

The lamina papyracea of the ethmoid bone forms a large part of the medial wall of the orbit. The orbit, therefore, is separated from the ethmoid sinuses by the paper-thin and often dehiscent lamina. Because of the weakness of this barrier, the spread of infection

Table 14–3. Orbital complications of sinusitis.

Lid Edema
No limitation of extraocular movements and vision is normal.
Infection is anterior to the orbital septum.
Orbital Cellulitis
Infection of the soft tissue posterior to the orbital septum.
Subperiosteal Abscess
Pus collection beneath the periosteum of the lamina papyracea.
Orbital Abscess
Pus collection in the orbit.
Associated with limitation of extraocular movements, exophthalmos, and visual changes.
Cavernous Sinus Thrombosis
Bilateral eye involvement, meningeal signs, and other intracranial complications.

to the orbit is the most common complication of acute sinusitis. In addition, the ophthalmic venous system is devoid of valves and communicates with the ethmoid veins, providing a path for infection to enter the orbit. Infection of the orbital structures usually follows a stepwise sequence as described in Table 14–3.

Inflammatory edema of the lid may be treated in an outpatient setting with oral antibiotics, provided that close follow-up can be achieved. Orbital cellulitis usually responds to intravenous antibiotics, whereas subperiosteal and orbital abscesses require operative drainage and drainage of the offending sinus. Cavernous sinus thrombosis is truly life threatening and is associated with a poor prognosis even with aggressive medical and surgical management. The incidence of all orbital complications is higher in the pediatric population than in adults.

B. MENINGITIS

Meningitis usually occurs by extension of infection from the ethmoid or sphenoid sinuses. On examination, patients with this complication may have a diminished sensorium or may be obtunded. The typical signs of meningitis, such as Kernig and Brudzinski signs, may be present. If meningitis secondary to sinus infection is suspected, a high-resolution CT scan of the brain with contrast and a sinus CT scan should be obtained. A CT scan of the brain is critical both to rule out mass effect and to delineate any other intracranial complications. Lumbar puncture is diagnostic and provides material for culture. The treatment for meningitis involves intravenous antibiotics and surgical drainage of the sinuses.

C. EPIDURAL ABSCESS

An epidural abscess is a collection of purulent material between the bone of the skull and the dura, typically in

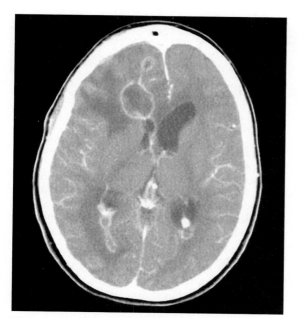

Figure 14–4. Brain abscess due to frontal sinusitis. This contrast-enhanced axial CT scan shows a left frontal brain abscess caused by frontal sinusitis.

relation to frontal sinusitis. The further spread of infection, either by direct extension or by hematogenous seeding, may lead to subdural empyema and eventually to brain abscess (Figure 14–4). Draining both the abscess and the offending sinuses is mandatory, and long-term antibiotics are often necessary. Regardless of the treatment, morbidity and mortality are high, particularly with subdural involvement.

D. CAVERNOUS SINUS THROMBOSIS

Septic emboli may flow posteriorly through the ophthalmic venous system to the cavernous sinus, causing infection, inflammation, and eventually thrombosis of the sinus. Ocular symptoms include chemosis, sluggish pupillary response, ophthalmoplegia, and blindness. These findings are often bilateral. Intravenous antibiotic treatment should be instituted immediately, and, if indicated, the involved sinuses should be surgically drained. The role of anticoagulation to prevent further thrombus formation and systemic steroid therapy is controversial.

E. POTT PUFFY TUMOR

If infection in the frontal sinus spreads to the marrow of the frontal bone, localized osteomyelitis with bone destruction can result in a doughy swelling of the forehead classically described as Pott puffy tumor. Surgical drainage and débridement must be undertaken.

Chandler JR, Langenbrunner DJ, Stevens ER. The pathogenesis of orbital complications in acute sinusitis. *Laryngoscope.* 1970;80:1414. [PMID: 5470225] (Classic article on orbital complications of sinusitis.)

Prognosis

The prognosis for acute sinusitis is excellent, with an estimated 70% of patients recovering without treatment. Oral antibiotics may decrease the time that a patient is symptomatic. Chronic sinusitis has a more variable course. If an anatomic cause is found and is rectified by surgery, the prognosis is good. More than 90% of patients have improvement with surgical intervention. However, these patients are always prone to relapse; therefore, a vigorous preventive regimen is essential.

Frontal Sinus Fractures

15

Steven D. Pletcher, MD, & Andrew N. Goldberg, MD, MSCE

 ESSENTIALS OF DIAGNOSIS

- *History of head trauma.*
- *Visible open fracture or fracture on computed tomography (CT) scans or plain x-rays.*

General Considerations

The frontal sinus begins as an outgrowth of the nasal chamber in utero but does not begin to invade the vertical portion of the frontal bone until the fourth year of life. The sinus attains adult configuration at age 15 and typically reaches adult size by age 20. A variable structure, the frontal sinuses are typically asymmetric and may be unilateral (10%) or absent altogether (5%).

The anterior wall of the fully developed frontal sinus is a thick bony arch that can withstand between 800 and 2200 pounds of force. The force required to fracture this robust structure often leads to multiple injuries; therefore, a full trauma workup of all patients with frontal sinus fractures is paramount. As with all trauma patients, the airway, circulatory system, and other organ systems must be evaluated upon arrival. All patients require ophthalmologic and neurologic examination as well as radiographic and clinical examination of the cervical spine. Intracranial injury (40–50%) and other facial fractures (75–95%) are among the most commonly associated injuries in patients with frontal sinus fractures.

Pathogenesis

Motor vehicle accidents are the most common mechanism of injury for patients with frontal sinus fractures, accounting for 60–70% of all frontal sinus fractures. Assault typically requires the use of a blunt object to fracture the frontal sinus; fists alone rarely generate sufficient force. Other mechanisms of injury include industrial accidents, recreational accidents, and gunshot wounds. Young men in their third decade of life are most at risk for frontal sinus fracture. In one study, 30% of patients with frontal sinus fractures had blood

alcohol levels over the legal limit or positive urine toxicology screens.

The anterior wall of the frontal sinus is significantly thicker than the posterior wall. Injuries that provide enough force to fracture the anterior wall of the frontal sinus often have enough force to fracture the posterior wall as well.

Prevention

The use of seatbelts and air bags for passengers and drivers can decrease the incidence of severe head trauma and frontal sinus fractures. Patients in automobile accidents in which airbags are deployed have a significant decrease in the number of facial fractures. Estimates are that only 15% of young patients with frontal sinus fractures resulting from automobile accidents were wearing a seatbelt; less than 10% of patients with frontal sinus fractures from motorcycle accidents were wearing a helmet. The use of helmets with motorcycles, bicycles, at appropriate sporting events, and in industrial situations also can protect the frontal sinuses.

Murphy RX Jr, Chernofsky MA. The influence of airbag and restraining devices on the patterns of facial trauma in motor vehicle collisions. *Plast Reconstr Surg.* 2000;105(2):516. [PMID: 10697154] (The use of restraining devices and airbags decreases the incidence of facial fractures and lacerations.)

Wright DL, Hoffman HT, Hoyt DB. Frontal sinus fractures in the pediatric population. *Laryngoscope.* 1992;102(11):1215. [PMID: 1405980] (Discussion of the similar severity and treatment of frontal sinus fractures in adult and pediatric patients.)

Clinical Findings

A. SYMPTOMS AND SIGNS

Most patients lose consciousness with the force required to sustain a frontal sinus fracture; estimates are that 25% of patients remain conscious throughout the injury, 50% regain consciousness within the first 4 hours after injury, and the final fourth develop prolonged unconsciousness.

Patients who are conscious at the time of the evaluation typically report frontal pain. Forehead lacerations occur in approximately 80% of frontal sinus fractures. Other less common signs on physical examination include the following: frontal numbness; palpable step-offs or crepitus; cerebrospinal fluid (CSF) leak; exposed bone; exposed brain; and ocular abnormalities, including diplopia, ophthalmoplegia, and decreased visual acuity. Between 5% and 10% of patients have no significant physical findings on examination.

Associated injuries are the rule with frontal sinus fractures. Other facial fractures occur in up to 95% of patients; bones of the orbit and paranasal sinuses are the most commonly involved. Intracranial injuries are seen in approximately 50% of patients; of these types of injuries, frontal contusions are the most common.

B. IMAGING STUDIES

1. CT scans—CT scanning is the imaging examination of choice for the evaluation of frontal sinus fractures. Clinicians looking for intracranial pathology after head trauma order CT scans of the head and often discover fractures.

When evaluating the extent of injury and determining the operative plan for frontal sinus fractures, thin-cut axial and coronal facial CT scans are preferable over thicker-cut 5–10 mm head CT scans. Axial and direct coronal images using 3-mm cuts and bone windows are typically used for the evaluation of frontal sinus fractures. In selected cases, thinner-cut 1.5-mm images can offer more detail. Soft tissue windows should be used to evaluate intracranial and orbital injuries, which are often seen in patients with frontal sinus trauma. Many patients with associated injuries do not tolerate direct coronal images. In these patients, 1-mm axial cuts with reformatted coronal images represent a viable alternative.

2. X-rays—The role of plain x-ray films in the evaluation of frontal sinus fractures is limited. In patients with nonoperative fractures and fluid in their frontal sinuses, serial Caldwell views may be used to monitor resolution of the fluid, insuring patency of the frontonasal recess.

Wallis A, Donald PJ. Frontal sinus fractures: a review of 72 cases. *Laryngoscope.* 1988;98:593. [PMID: 3374232] (Review of the etiology, presenting symptoms, treatments, and complications of 72 cases.)

Differential Diagnosis

Frontal sinus fractures should be distinguished from both simple forehead contusions and lacerations. Frontal bone fractures without the involvement of the frontal sinus may be mistaken for frontal sinus fractures. CT scans distinguish between these possibilities with relative ease.

Determining the extent of a fracture is more difficult than determining whether a frontal sinus fracture is present. Involvement of both the posterior table of the frontal sinus and the frontonasal recess is critical in determining the treatment of the fracture. Anterior

table fractures are often easily identified on axial CT scans; however, because of the thin nature of the posterior table, nondisplaced posterior table fractures can be less obvious. A high index of suspicion for posterior table fractures is necessary in all patients. Pneumocephalus on the CT scan may provide a clue that the posterior table has been violated, but pneumocephalus also may come from fractures of the ethmoid bones or other aerated regions of the skull.

In patients with frontal sinus fractures, the frontonasal recess is the most difficult area to evaluate. When evaluating a frontal sinus fracture, it is important to assess the future function of the frontonasal recess. In the surgeon's judgment, if disruption of frontal sinus drainage is likely, then obliteration or cranialization (ie, removal of the posterior table and mucosa of the frontal sinus) of the frontal sinus should be strongly considered. Serial imaging studies may be considered in select patients in whom reliable follow-up is likely. Certain fracture patterns can be helpful in predicting frontonasal recess damage. In isolated anterior wall fractures, involvement of the frontonasal recess is rare. Patients with anterior wall fractures and associated supraorbital rim or nasoethmoid complex fractures have associated frontonasal recess injury in 70–90% of cases. Combined anterior and posterior wall fractures are also commonly associated with injury to the frontonasal recess.

Complications

There are many complications of frontal sinus fractures. More severe complications include mucoceles, severe persistent pain, and infectious intracranial complications. Such complications are uncommon, with a reported rate of 6% for meningitis and mucocele formation and 1% for severe pain and brain abscess.

Minor complications are relatively common. Wound infections, CSF leaks, numbness over the forehead area, and mild deformity are each found in approximately 10–20% of patients. Chronic sinusitis, mild chronic pain, and diplopia (ie, double vision) are significantly less common.

Well-known complications of frontal sinus fractures include (1) mucoceles and mucopyoceles; (2) intracranial complications such as meningitis, brain abscess, and CSF leak; and (3) other complications such as chronic infection and osteomyelitis. All of these complications, particularly mucoceles, may not manifest until years after the original injury. With the evaluation of the extent of the injury and appropriate treatment, complications from frontal sinus fractures can be limited.

A. MUCOCELES AND MUCOPYOCELES

Mucoceles and mucopyoceles are well-known complications that typically appear years after the original injury. Because of their severity, these complications usually mandate surgical intervention.

Mucoceles are expansile, benign, but locally destructive lesions that occur when entrapped or segregated mucosa secretes mucus into a confined space, causing progressive expansion. Frontal sinus mucosa is distinct from normal pseudostratified ciliated respiratory epithelium both histologically and pathologically. Frontal sinus mucosa tends to have a flatter, more cuboidal epithelium with a greater propensity for mucocele formation. Conditions that tend to result in mucocele formation include frontonasal recess obstruction and mucosa entrapment, both commonly associated with frontal sinus fractures.

The **foramina of Breschet** are venous drainage channels located in the posterior wall of the frontal sinus. These foramina are significant not only in their role in the spread of infection, but also because they act as sites of mucosal invagination in the posterior wall of the sinus. Failing to completely remove mucosa in an obliterated sinus predisposes the development of mucoceles. Mucoceles tend to follow an insidious course with significant bony destruction and potential erosion into the intracranial, intraorbital, or subcutaneous space.

The entrapped, static secretions within mucoceles may become infected, resulting in a mucopyocele. Mucopyoceles tend to follow a more aggressive course than mucoceles. Expansile, infectious masses, mucopyoceles carry significant risks of intraorbital infectious complications; they also may erode directly into the intracranial space.

B. Intracranial Complications

Meningitis and brain abscesses may occur as early or late sequelae of frontal sinus fractures. Frontal sinus fractures are often compound, dirty wounds at the time of injury, with bits of glass and dirt within the wound. This early contamination combined with the frequent association of posterior table fractures and even dural tears provides a direct route for bacterial entry to the intracranial space, which results in meningitis, a brain abscess, or both. Late intracranial infections are typically associated with mucopyoceles.

Traumatic CSF leaks are another form of intracranial complications. They have been noted to seal spontaneously in 80–95% of cases; however, these data may be skewed by a high percentage of temporal bone fractures. It is estimated that in patients with a traumatic CSF leak present for more than 24 hours, approximately 53% resolved spontaneously within an average of 5 days. Those leaks that go unrecognized or are not adequately repaired may result in delayed intracranial infections.

C. Other Complications

Chronic infection and osteomyelitis may occur after frontal sinus fracture. This can result in the development of a frontocutaneous fistula and chronic drainage as well as the extrusion of hardware used during frontal sinus repair. Chronic frontal sinus pain and the sensation of frontal sinus fullness may be present after both frontal sinus fracture and obliteration. Severe or unrelenting pain may be a sign of mucocele development or infectious complication and should be evaluated thoroughly. Cosmetic forehead deformities may result after inadequate reduction of anterior table fractures or the loss of anterior table bone. Mucoceles, mucopyoceles, osteomyelitis, or hardware extrusion can also result in cosmetic deformities.

Friedman JA, Ebersold MJ, Quast LM. Post-traumatic cerebrospinal fluid leakage. *World J of Surg.* 2001;25(8):1062. [PMID: 11571972] (Forty-seven percent of patients with post-traumatic CSF leaks of 24-hour duration required surgical intervention.)

Goldberg AN, Oroszlan G, Anderson TD. Complications of frontal sinusitis and their management. *Otolaryngol Clin North Am.* 2001;34(1):211. [PMID: 11344074] (A review of frontal sinusitis complications and their management.)

Treatment

The treatment of frontal sinus fractures depends on the extent of the fracture. Fractures of the frontonasal recess and the posterior table of the frontal sinus often require operative intervention. Displaced fractures typically require open reduction. The primary goals of treatment in frontal sinus fractures include preventing complications and restoring normal forehead contour.

A. Surgical Measures

Surgical developments within the last few decades have reduced marked cosmetic deformities and a high incidence of long-term complications. The creation of an osteoplastic flap and the cranialization procedure are the two primary procedures used today to repair complex frontal sinus fractures. The choice of when to operate and which procedure to perform depends on the extent of the fracture.

More recent advances in instrumentation and technique have also allowed endoscopic methods to be used to repair and/or camouflage fractures. These techniques are performed through small incisions behind the hairline similar to the approach used for an endoscopic brow lift.

1. The osteoplastic flap—The concept of removing the frontal sinus as a functioning unit was introduced in 1958 by Goodale and Montgomery with the osteoplastic flap. This flap or hinged opening of the frontal sinus is created through either a midforehead or coronal incision and sinus obliteration; this approach may also be used through an existing forehead laceration. The procedure, which remains one of the principal means for treating frontal sinus fractures today, involves raising a subperiosteal flap from a coronal or midforehead incision down to the superior border of the frontal sinus. The anterior table of the frontal sinus is then opened at its superior and lateral margins, creating an inferiorly based bone flap. All mucosa is then stripped from the sinus and all the bony walls of the sinus are burred down with a drill to ensure complete mucosal removal. The frontonasal recess mucosa is stripped or turned down into the ostium, and the ostium is obliterated using a muscle or fascia plug. The sinus is then obliterated, most commonly using a free fat graft. Finally, the anterior wall of the frontal sinus and the coronal or midforehead flap is replaced.

2. The cranialization procedure—In the cranialization procedure, the posterior wall of the frontal sinus is removed and the frontal dura is allowed to rest against the anterior table of the frontal sinus. This procedure also involves complete stripping of the mucosa, burring any mucosal remnants from the remaining anterior sinus wall, and plugging the frontonasal recess.

3. Endoscopic repair—Using endoscopic techniques, incisions can be made smaller and morbidity from extensive dissection minimized. At this point, endoscopic techniques are used to repair and/or camouflage frontal sinus fractures involving the anterior table only, although technique development is ongoing. Small incisions behind the hairline are used to reduce and fixate fractures and camouflage contour defects through onlay grafts and other techniques for improved cosmesis.

4. Surgical grafts—There has been significant debate over which material is best for obliterating the frontal sinus. One option is to remove all mucosa, plug the frontonasal recess, and allow ingrowth of fibrous tissue without obliteration. Other options involve the use of various grafts.

a. **Autologous fat grafts**—Free-fat grafts have been both studied and used most extensively. Overall autologous fat provides a safe obliterative material with few infectious complications. Over time fat tends to be reabsorbed and replaced with fibrous material. Serial MRI scans in patients with fat-obliterated frontal sinuses show the median half-life of the obliterated adipose tissue to be 15.4 months. In addition, the incidence of seroma in fat harvests is approximately 5%.

b. **Other autologous tissue grafts**—Other autologous tissues for obliteration include cancellous bone, muscle, and pericranial flaps. Autologous grafts typically involve some donor site morbidity, such as pain, infection, or the formation of sarcomas, hematomas, or both. Pericranial flaps with an inferior or lateral base offer a living tissue option for both obliteration and recreation of the anterior table with minimal donor site morbidity.

c. **Grafts of synthetic materials**—One difficult situation in which synthetic materials may play a role is in

fractures with a loss or a severe comminution of the anterior table. In these scenarios, bone grafts (iliac, rib, or split calvarial) or **methyl methacrylate** have been used to recreate the anterior table. **Titanium mesh** offers a synthetic alternative for severely comminuted fractures, but its use is limited in cases with significant loss of anterior table bone. **Hydroxyapatite cement** is another synthetic material that has been used both to obliterate the sinus and recreate the anterior table but experience is limited.

B. LOCATION-RELATED MEASURES

1. Anterior table fractures and frontonasal recess injuries—To treat fractures of the anterior wall appropriately, a couple of key issues need to be resolved. The first is the degree of the displacement of the fracture; this question can be answered easily with a combination of physical exam and CT scan. If a displaced fracture is present, exploration of the fracture with open reduction and internal fixation is required. Figure 15–1 depicts a CT scan of a patient with a displaced anterior table frontal sinus fracture.

The second key issue in treating fractures of the anterior wall is whether there is significant injury to the frontonasal recess. The frontonasal recess is more difficult to evaluate accurately on a CT scan because the functional capability of the frontal sinus drainage path-

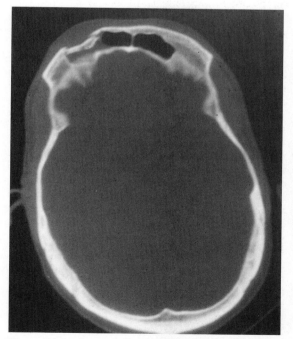

Figure 15–1. Coronal CT scan with a displaced fracture of the anterior table of the frontal sinus.

way is not clearly elucidated on CT. A 70–90% rate of frontonasal recess injury has been reported for patients who have associated fractures of the floor of the frontal sinus, the nasoethmoid complex, or the supraorbital rim. It is thus reasonable to surgically evaluate the frontonasal recess in such patients.

Traditional management of fractures involving the frontonasal recess is operative exploration and either obliteration or cranialization if injury to the frontonasal recess is noted intraoperatively. However, some studies suggest that fractures with frontonasal recess involvement do not always require obliteration or cranialization. Some physicians have managed these patients expectantly, following this approach with serial CT scans. Patients who failed to re-aerate their sinuses were treated with endoscopic frontal sinus procedures; in limited trials, favorable results were obtained.

For unilateral frontonasal recess injuries in which the contralateral duct has been demonstrated to work, some clinicians advocate the **Lothrop procedure:** removal of the intersinus septum and the use of mucosal flaps to allow drainage through the contralateral frontal sinus. This procedure can be performed endoscopically.

2. Posterior table fractures—Fractures of the posterior table often require surgical intervention. In general, posterior table fractures should be inspected for dural tears or CSF leaks. Some clinicians advocate the use of serial x-rays and close follow-up of nondisplaced posterior table fractures. Dural tears should be repaired in consultation with a neurosurgeon. The treatment of minimally displaced posterior table fractures is controversial and may require obliteration based on the surgeon's judgment. These fractures have a high incidence of frontonasal recess injury and, untreated, are at high theoretic risk for mucocele formation because of entrapped mucosa at the fracture site.

Comminuted posterior table fractures are best treated with cranialization. "Through and through" injuries involve significant injury to the skin, anterior table, posterior table, and dura. These injuries can often be diagnosed by viewing the brain through the wound and are best managed with cranialization if sufficient bone remains to recreate the anterior table. In cases of severe anterior and posterior table bone loss, ablation may be the only viable alternative.

Lakhani RS, Shibuya TY, Mathog RH, Marks SC, Burgio DL, Yoo GH. Titanium mesh repair of the severely comminuted frontal sinus fracture. *Arch Otolaryngol Head Neck Surg.* 2001;127(6):665. [PMID: 11405865] (Favorable results using titanium mesh for repair of comminuted frontal sinus fractures is discussed.)

Pariscar A, Har-El G. Frontal sinus obliteration with the pericranial flap. *Otolaryngol Head Neck Surg.* 2001;124(3):304. [PMID: 11240996] (Favorable results using pericranial flap for frontal sinus obliteration is discussed.)

Petruzzelli GJ, Stankiewicz JA. Frontal sinus obliteration with hydroxyapatite cement. *Laryngoscope.* 2002;112(1):32. [PMID: 11802035] (Favorable results using hydroxyapatite cement to obliterate the frontal sinus and recreate the anterior wall of the frontal sinus is discussed.)

Smith T. Endoscopic management of the frontal recess in frontal sinus fractures: a shift in the paradigm? *Laryngoscope.* 2002;(112):784. [PMID: 12150607] (A limited series of expectant management of frontal outflow tract injuries with endoscopic surgery for failed ventilation yields good results.)

Strong EB, Kellman RM. Endoscopic repair of anterior table frontal sinus fractures. *Facial Plast Surg Clin North Am.* 2006;14(1):25.

Weber R. Osteoplastic frontal sinus surgery with fat obliteration: technique and long-term results using MRI in 82 operations. *Laryngoscope.* 2000;(110):1037. [PMID: 10852527] (An osteoplastic flap with fat obliteration is highly effective.)

Pediatric Considerations

Frontal sinus fractures in the pediatric population are more commonly associated with orbital fractures and major intracranial injury such as intraparenchymal hemorrhage and CSF leak. Patients with intracranial injury tend to be younger than those with no intracranial injury. The cribriform plate is involved to a greater degree as a site of CSF leak than in adults, and craniotomy is commonly needed for CSF leak repair.

Whatley WS, Allison DW, Chandra RK, Thompson JW, Boop FA. Frontal sinus fractures in children. *Laryngoscope.* 2005;115(10):1741.

Prognosis

A. SHORT-TERM PROGNOSIS

The immediate prognosis for patients with frontal sinus fractures is mostly dependent on the presence and severity of the associated injuries, particularly intracranial injuries. Patients with "through and through" frontal sinus fractures have a short-term mortality rate of approximately 50% at the scene or in transport. Another 25% die in the early postoperative period.

B. LONG-TERM PROGNOSIS

The long-term prognosis for patients with frontal sinus fractures has been difficult to assess. With the significant possibility of delayed complications, long-term follow-up is required to adequately evaluate the prognosis for patients with frontal sinus fractures. These patients, however, tend to be noncompliant, making long-term follow-up problematic. Because of this dilemma, the prevalence of long-term complications is likely understated in the literature.

Paranasal Sinus Neoplasms

16

Aditi H. Mandpe, MD

ESSENTIALS OF DIAGNOSIS

- *Symptoms and signs mimic benign sinonasal disease.*
- *Malignant tumors typically present at advanced stage of disease.*
- *Immunohistochemical markers are often required for definitive diagnosis of tumors.*

General Considerations

Paranasal sinus neoplasms, both benign and malignant, are relatively rare in the head and neck. Malignant neoplasms of the paranasal sinuses account for approximately 3.0% of head and neck cancers and 0.5% of all malignant tumors. In general, these tumors are identified and treated at advanced stages as their symptoms mimic benign inflammatory conditions. The most common malignant neoplasm of the nose and paranasal sinuses is squamous cell carcinoma. This tumor most commonly arises from the maxillary antrum and secondarily from the ethmoid sinus. Treatment includes surgical resection, radiation therapy, and, rarely, chemotherapy. Benign tumors present in a similar manner and typically necessitate surgical resection and close postoperative follow-up. As nasal endoscopes are used with increasing frequency clinically, both benign and malignant tumors will ideally be identified earlier in the disease progression.

Clinical Findings

A. SYMPTOMS AND SIGNS

The most common presenting symptoms in patients with paranasal sinus neoplasms are nasal obstruction, rhinorrhea, and sinus congestion, which are similar to those of patients with benign sinonasal diseases. However, as the masses grow, paranasal sinus neoplasms lead to facial pain and epistaxis. In addition, orbital symptoms, such as diplopia, proptosis, visual loss, and epiphora, can occur with either neoplastic invasion or expansion into the orbit. Entry through the skull base

into the anterior cranial fossa can lead to headache, cranial neuropathies, and occasional frontal lobe symptoms (such as personality alterations). Tumors can also invade the maxilla and present as a hard-palate mass.

B. PHYSICAL EXAMINATION

The physical examination of a patient suspected to have a paranasal neoplasm should include a complete head and neck examination. It is unusual to find a small tumor on physical examination because paranasal neoplasms grow silently until they lead to either orbital symptoms or sinus obstruction.

1. Nose and paranasal sinus—The examination of the nose and paranasal sinus cavity can reveal a nasal mass with overlying polyps or polypoid mucosa. The septum can be markedly deviated to the contralateral side because of the expansion of the neoplasm, sometimes with tumor erosion into the contralateral nasal cavity. An endoscopic evaluation may be useful with benign neoplasms such as mucoceles or inverted papillomas in order to evaluate the mucosa and the presence of drainage.

2. Oral cavity—The teeth and hard palate need to be examined closely to determine whether invasion into the maxilla has occurred. An expanded alveolar ridge or loose maxillary dentition indicates early bony invasion of the maxilla, and a mass on the hard palate indicates frank invasion into the maxilla.

3. Face and orbit—Facial swelling and thickening of the cheek and nose skin is an indication that the neoplasm has invaded the soft tissue through the anterior bony walls. Proptosis is seen with expansion through the lamina papyracea compressing the periorbital in benign disease, such as mucocele, and in malignant disease due to intraorbital invasion. Diplopia is commonly seen with proptosis, and visual loss is a sign of progressive orbital involvement; however, visual loss also can be a sign of orbital apex involvement with compression of the optic nerve.

4. Cranial nerves—Cranial nerve (CN) involvement is common in advanced malignant neoplasms of the paranasal sinuses. The olfactory nerve, CN I, is involved in esthesioneuroblastomas. Other cranial nerves involved are the optic nerve (CN II), the oculomotor nerve (CN III), the trochlear nerve (CN IV), the abducens nerve (CN

VI), and the supraorbital and maxillary branches of the trigeminal nerve (CN V1 and CN V2).

5. Other physical findings—Other findings that can be identified by physical examination are serous otitis media due to eustachian tube involvement, and neck masses due to metastatic neoplastic spread into the regional lymph nodes. The most commonly involved lymph nodes are the upper jugulodigastric nodes.

C. IMAGING STUDIES

Imaging is vital to determine the extent of disease in patients with malignant tumors of the paranasal sinuses. A computed tomography (CT) scan can delineate the mass well and can be sufficient for both bony and benign diseases. It is excellent for determining bony invasion. Its limitations are an inability to distinguish between edematous mucosa and tumor involvement and to identify the intracranial extension of tumors. Magnetic resonance imaging (MRI) with both T1- and T2-weighted images with gadolinium enhancement is superior in determining the true involvement of the anterior cranial fossa, the skull base, and the orbit (Figure 16–1). MRI is also superior at soft tissue delineation, can distinguish a tumor from obstructed secretions in the sinus, and complements the bony architecture information obtained from the CT scan. Both scans are often needed to ensure appropriate surgical planning.

D. SPECIAL TESTS

A biopsy of the mass is critical both in diagnosing a malignant tumor and in determining its treatment. If the mass is easily visualized in the physician's office, then an in-

Table 16–1. Differential diagnosis of nasal and paranasal sinus masses.

Benign Masses	Malignant Masses
Cementoma	Adenocarcinoma
Chondroma	Adenoid cystic carcinoma
Hemangioma	Hemangiopericytoma
Inverted papilloma	Lymphoma
Juvenile angiofibroma	Malignant mucosal melanoma
Meningioma	Olfactory esthesioneuroblastoma
Neurofibroma	Sarcoma
Ossifying fibroma	Sinonasal undifferentiated carcinoma
Osteoma	Squamous cell carcinoma
Schwannoma	Teratoma or teratocarcinoma

office biopsy should be obtained of the mass itself and not just the overlying tissue. Considerations for this biopsy include the assurance that the lesion is not vascular or does not contain cerebrospinal fluid (CSF). These lesions are often soft and cystic and expand with a Valsalva maneuver. A needle biopsy of these lesions can be considered if the diagnosis is still uncertain.

Differential Diagnosis

The differential diagnosis of a paranasal sinus mass is extensive (Table 16–1). The most common benign lesion of the paranasal sinuses is the inverted papilloma. The most common malignant neoplasm of the paranasal sinuses is squamous cell carcinoma. Other tumors that are frequently seen are adenocarcinoma, adenoid cystic carcinoma, olfactory esthesioneuroblastoma, malignant mucosal melanoma, and sinonasal undifferentiated carcinoma.

Dulguerov P, Jacobsen MS, Allal AS, Lehmann W, Calcaterra T. Nasal and paranasal sinus carcinoma: are we making progress? *Cancer.* 2001;92:3012. [PMID: 11753979] (Meta-analysis suggesting an improvement in the prognosis for patients with malignant paranasal sinus disorders.)

■ BENIGN NEOPLASMS

INVERTED PAPILLOMAS
General Considerations

An inverted papilloma, also called a schneiderian papilloma from the name of the mucosa from which it arises, is

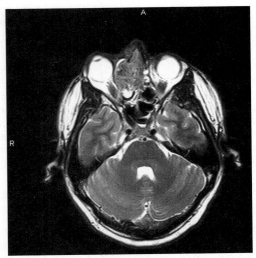

Figure 16–1. Axial T2-weighted MRI scan showing a mass in the right ethmoid sinus.

typically located on the lateral nasal wall; rarely is it found on the septum. The incidence of this tumor is between 0.5% and 7.0% of all nasal tumors. The cause of this tumor is unclear; however, there is an association with human papillomavirus (HPV) but not to allergy or nasal polyps. Inverted papillomas typically involve the middle meatus and at least one sinus cavity; the most common sinuses involved are the maxillary and ethmoid sinuses, followed by the sphenoid and frontal sinuses.

Inverted papillomas are usually unilateral, but they have been reported to be bilateral in up to 13% of cases. These tumors can extend through the septum into the contralateral nasal cavity. Multifocal tumors have been documented in approximately 4% of cases. Whether because of multicentricity or incomplete excision, these neoplasms have a high rate of recurrence with any procedure—as high as 75%. Patients also have a 5–15% risk of developing squamous cell carcinoma within the inverted papilloma.

Clinical Findings

Patients diagnosed with inverted papillomas complain about nasal obstruction, rhinorrhea, and unilateral epistaxis. Other symptoms include facial pressure, headache, and anosmia. On gross examination, there are no clear distinguishing characteristics between an inverted papilloma and an inflammatory polyp, although an inverted papilloma may be firmer and less translucent than an "average" polyp. On histopathologic examination, the distinguishing feature of inverted papillomas is the proliferation of epithelium with fingerlike inversions into the underlying epithelium.

Staging

Several staging systems have been developed that range from tumors located solely in the nasal cavity to tumors that extend to the anterior cranial fossa or orbit. Although these staging systems may be helpful in surgical planning, they do not yet have clinical significance in predicting patient outcome.

Treatment

Treatment for inverted papillomas consists of total excision of the tumor. The traditional approach has been a lateral rhinotomy or midfacial degloving approach, to a medial maxillectomy for total tumor removal. An osteoplastic frontal sinus exploration is sometimes required for disease spreading into the frontal sinus. To ensure a more complete resection, a microscope can be used to improve visualization of the mucosa. Recently, with advances in endoscopic sinus technology and techniques, endoscopic resection of the tumor has been advocated as a treatment option. The procedures range

from a transnasal resection to an endoscopic modified Lothrop and should be performed by an experienced surgeon. The advantage of an endoscopic approach is improved visualization of the diseased mucosa that requires resection. The tumors most amenable to endoscopic resection are those neoplasms with disease limited to the inferior or middle meatus or the middle turbinate.

An important feature in the management of patients with these neoplasms is that all of the excised specimens should be closely examined with multiple sections to rule out invasive squamous cell carcinoma. Endoscopic approaches tend to use microdebriders to facilitate the resection. In these cases, the débrided tissue fragments are collected into a container for histologic evaluation to ensure that no microscopic focus of squamous cell carcinoma is identified.

Prognosis

Recurrence rates for both the open and endoscopic approaches are comparable and have ranged from a low of 8–10% to a high of 49–75% in different studies.

Han JK, Smith TL, Loehrl T, Toohill RJ, Smith MM. An evolution in the management of sinonasal inverting papilloma. *Laryngoscope.* 2001;111:1395. [PMID: 11568575] (Endoscopic techniques can allow resection of most inverting papillomas, with similar recurrence rates as open techniques.)

Krouse JH. Development of a staging system for inverted papilloma. *Laryngoscope.* 2000;110:965. [PMID: 10852514] (A staging system for inverted papilloma is proposed using imaging criteria.)

Sukenik MA, Casiano R. Endoscopic medial maxillectomy for inverted papillomas of the paranasal sinuses: value of the intraoperative endoscopic examination. *Laryngoscope.* 2000;110:39. [PMID: 10646713] (An endoscopic examination in experienced hands may be better than a CT scan for preoperative mapping of the lesion.)

JUVENILE ANGIOFIBROMAS

Clinical Findings

Juvenile angiofibromas occur primarily in young boys and are highly vascular. The primary symptoms are nasal obstruction and epistaxis. They originate in the posterior nasal cavity but by the time of presentation they have grown to fill the nasopharynx, often extending into the pterygopalatine fossa and infratemporal fossa. The rate of tumor growth is slow.

Treatment

The treatment consists of surgical resection and sometimes radiation therapy for persistent disease, despite a hypothesis that regression of these tumors occurs over time. To minimize blood loss, a preoperative angiogram with embolization and hypotensive anesthesia

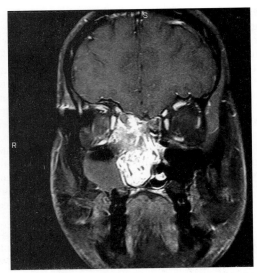

Figure 16–2. Coronal T1-weighted MRI scan showing a mass in the right ethmoid sinus.

intraoperatively are recommended. Surgical approaches consist of a lateral rhinotomy and medial maxillectomy approach; the prognosis is excellent in patients who undergo these treatment methods.

■ MALIGNANT NEOPLASMS

SQUAMOUS CELL CARCINOMAS

General Considerations

Squamous cell carcinoma is the most common malignant neoplasm of the paranasal sinuses, accounting for 60–80% of paranasal sinus tumors. The etiology and epidemiology of this tumor are poorly understood, although nickel workers are at a markedly increased risk of developing these tumors.

Clinical Findings

Squamous cell carcinomas arise from a silent location and grow insidiously with few to no symptoms. At the time of diagnosis, these tumors are very large and therefore bode a very poor prognosis. Only when these neoplasms invade adjacent structures, causing symptoms of oral, ocular, or facial involvement, are patients accurately diagnosed and treated (Figure 16–2). These symptoms include pain in the maxillary teeth, erosion of the palate, diplopia, prop-

tosis, and cheek paresthesias. Squamous cell carcinomas arise most commonly in the maxillary antrum and account for up to 80% of all paranasal sinus squamous cell carcinoma. The ethmoid sinus is the second most common site of origin. Primary squamous cell carcinomas of the frontal and sphenoid sinuses are rare.

Staging

The revised staging system for maxillary sinus carcinoma, created by the American Joint Committee on Cancer (AJCC), is clinically more relevant and better at distinguishing survival results between T2–T3 and T2–T4 diseases than its previous staging system. The N stage designates regional lymph node involvement and is identical with staging of the neck in other head and neck cancers. The staging system for ethmoid sinus cancers is shown in Table 16–2.

Treatment & Prognosis

For nearly all patients, the treatment is surgical resection followed by radiation therapy. Treatment with this combination of modalities has shown markedly improved results compared with radiation therapy alone. The 5-year survival rate for patients with maxillary sinus squamous cell carcinoma who are treated with combined surgery and radiation therapy is 46–68% versus 9–19% for patients treated with radiation therapy alone. Surgical procedures typically start with a maxillectomy and can include orbital exenteration, infratemporal fossa dissection, and craniofacial resection. Postoperative radiation therapy is administered until at least 65 Gy is delivered. Intensity-modulated radiation therapy (IMRT) allows an even greater dosage delivery while sparing crucial structures such as the optic nerve and chiasm, the pituitary gland, and the brain.

The addition of chemotherapy may improve locoregional control and 5-year disease-specific survival.

Because of the rarity of ethmoid squamous cell carcinoma, all ethmoid tumors tend to be grouped together, despite different histologic features. Patients with ethmoid tumors fare no better than patients with maxillary sinus tumors; the 5-year local control and disease-specific survival rates for both are similar.

Dulguerov P, Jacobsen MS, Allal AS, Lehmann W, Calcaterra T. Nasal and paranasal sinus carcinoma: are we making progress? *Cancer.* 2001;92:3012. [PMID: 11753979] (Meta-analysis suggesting an improvement in the prognosis for patients with paranasal sinus malignancies.)

Hayashi T, Nonaka S, Bandoh N, Kobayashi Y, Imada M, Harabuchi Y. Treatment outcome of maxillary sinus squamous cell carcinoma. *Cancer.* 2001;92:1495. [PMID: 11745227] (Multimodality therapy offers improved 5-year survival rates compared to radiotherapy alone.)

Le QT, Fu KK, Kaplan M, Terris DJ, Fee WE, Goffinet DR. Treatment of maxillary sinus carcinoma: a comparison of the 1997 and 1977 American Joint Committee on cancer staging

Table 16-2. Staging criteria of primary malignant maxillary and ethmoid sinus tumors.

Stage	Maxillary Sinus	Ethmoid Sinus
T_x	Primary tumor cannot be assessed	
T_0	No evidence of primary tumor	
T_{IS}	Carcinoma in situ	
T_1	Tumor confined to antral mucosa with no bony destruction	Tumor confined to ethmoid sinuses with no bony destruction
T_2	Tumor causing bony destruction (except for posterior wall of maxillary sinus), including extension into the hard palate or middle meatus	Tumor extends into the nasal cavity
T_3	Tumor invades any of the following: bone of the posterior wall of maxillary sinus, subcutaneous tissue, skin of cheek, floor of medial wall of orbit, infratemporal fossa, pterygoid plates, ethmoid sinuses	Tumor extends to the anterior orbit or the maxillary sinus
T_4	Tumor invades orbital contents beyond the floor or medial wall, including any of the following: the orbital apex, cribriform plate, base of skull, nasopharynx, sphenoid, frontal sinus	Tumor with intracranial extension; orbital extension including the apex or the sphenoid, the frontal external nose, or the skin of the external nose

systems. *Cancer.* 1999;86:1700. [PMID: 10547542] (The 1997 staging system is superior to the 1977 system in determining patient survival and local control. Combined modality therapy was superior to radiotherapy alone.)

Waldron JN, O'Sullivan B, Gullane P et al. Carcinoma of the maxillary antrum: a retrospective analysis of 110 cases. *Radiother Oncol.* 2000;57:167. [PMID: 11054520] (Local disease extension often determines the prognosis, despite the treatment modality. The best treatment modality is, as yet, elusive.)

ADENOCARCINOMAS & ADENOID CYSTIC CARCINOMAS

General Considerations

Adenocarcinomas arise from the epithelial surface of the sinonasal mucosa and occur more frequently than adenoid cystic carcinomas, which arise from the minor salivary glands. Together, they represent the most common mucous gland malignant neoplasms of the paranasal sinuses. Adenoid cystic carcinomas tend to arise from the maxillary antrum and can infiltrate into the surrounding tissue. They demonstrate perineural spread into the maxillary and mandibular branches of the trigeminal nerve (CN V), with extension into the foramina ovale and rotundum. Adenoid cystic carcinomas have a low incidence of regional metastases but greater distant metastases.

Clincal Findings

Adenocarcinomas arise typically from the ethmoid sinuses. There has been no correlation with smoking in the development of adenocarcinomas, but there has been a documented association with woodworkers and leather workers. Several histologic types are seen with variability in mucin production and cellular differentiation. They are similar to adenoid cystic carcinomas in their growth behavior.

Treatment

The treatment for both adenocarcinomas and adenoid cystic carcinomas consists of multimodality therapy at the advanced stages of disease. For maxillary sinus tumors, the treatment usually consists of a maxillectomy. An anterior craniofacial resection is often the recommended treatment for advanced ethmoid cancers. Postoperative radiation therapy is frequently employed in treating patients with all of these tumors.

Cantu G, Solero CL, Mariani L et al. Anterior craniofacial resection for malignant ethmoid tumors: a series of 91 patients. *Head Neck.* 1999;21:185. [PMID: 10208659] (Surgical resection for most ethmoid tumors, regardless of tumor histology encroaching the cribriform plate, necessitates an anterior craniofacial resection.)

OLFACTORY ESTHESIONEUROBLASTOMAS

General Considerations

Olfactory esthesioneuroblastomas arise from the olfactory epithelium superior to the middle turbinate. These neoplasms account for only 1–5% of all malignant tumors of the paranasal sinuses. Olfactory esthesioneuroblastomas are initially unilateral and can grow into the adjacent sinuses and the contralateral nasal cavity; they can spread to the orbit and the brain.

Classification

No TNM staging system has been created for these tumors; a clinical grouping system has been developed that has no prognostic value. This system designates the following groups: (1) Group A consists of patients with tumors limited to the nasal cavity; (2) Group B includes patients whose tumors are localized in the nasal cavity and the paranasal sinuses; and (3) patients in Group C have tumors that extend beyond both the nasal cavity and the paranasal sinuses. Metastasis to the neck is seen in approximately 10–20% of cases in all three groups.

Clinical Findings

Histologically, olfactory esthesioneuroblastomas can appear similar to both peripheral neuroblastomas and other sinonasal malignant tumors. Two features often seen on microscopy are rosettes and neurofibrillary processes. Immunocytochemical staining of the specimen, though showing tremendous variability, is an important and often necessary step in making an accurate diagnosis. Histologically, olfactory esthesioneuroblastomas do not appear to stain for keratin and epithelial membrane antigen. The most common positive immunoreactions are with neuron-specific enolase, S-100, microtubule-associated protein, Class III β-tubulin isotype, neurofilament, and synaptophysin.

Treatment & Prognosis

Patients with esthesioneuroblastomas are best treated with combined-modality therapy, even if the tumors are designated as either Kadish Group A or B neoplasms. The 5-year disease-free survival for single-modality therapy for patients in Kadish Groups A and B is 55% compared with 61% for patients in Kadish Group C. The local tumor control rate of combined therapy is 87% versus 51% for radiation alone, and 0% for surgery alone. Surgical resection may involve either local resection or craniofacial resection with radiation doses of 60–65 Gy postoperatively.

Chao KS, Kaplan C, Simpson JR et al. Esthesioneuroblastoma: the impact of treatment modality. *Head Neck.* 2001;23:749. [PMID: 11505485] (The Kadish staging system in patients with esthesioneuroblastomas did not prognosticate local control or disease-free survival.)

MALIGNANT MUCOSAL MELANOMAS

General Considerations

Respiratory tract mucosal melanomas occur in the nasal cavity and paranasal sinuses. They are exceedingly rare, with only 0.5–1.5% of all melanomas occurring in the sinonasal cavity. These neoplasms originate from melanocytes within the submucosa and from the mucosa of the paranasal sinuses. They are located most frequently in the anterior septum, followed by the middle and inferior turbinates. The maxillary sinus is the most common sinus cavity involved.

Clinical Findings

Epistaxis appears to be the most common symptom, and nasal obstruction is also common. On examination, the mass appears to be fleshy and polypoid. Tumors in the nasal cavity tend to be smaller at the time of diagnosis than tumors that arise within the sinuses. Nodal metastasis occurs in 10–20% of cases.

Staging

No TNM staging system exists for mucosal melanomas. However, a practical staging system has been developed: (1) Stage I designates localized disease, (2) Stage II indicates regional metastasis, and (3) Stage III signifies distant metastasis. The factors that influence clinical outcomes include the clinical stage, a lesion thickness > 5 mm, the presence of vascular invasion, and the development of distant metastasis.

Treatment & Prognosis

The treatment for malignant mucosal melanomas consists of surgical excision followed by postoperative

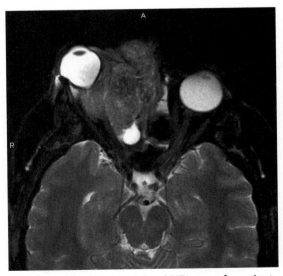

Figure 16–3. Axial T2-weighted MRI scan of a patient with a sinonasal undifferentiated carcinoma of the right ethmoid sinus. This tumor extends into the orbit with marked proptosis.

radiation therapy. As a result of this combined treatment approach, the 5-year disease-specific survival rate for sinonasal mucosal melanomas is approximately 47%.

Patel SG, Prasad ML, Escrig M et al. Primary mucosal malignant melanoma of the head and neck. *Head Neck.* 2002;24:247. [PMID: 11891956] (Fifty-nine patients at Memorial Sloan-Kettering Cancer Center, in a span of more than 20 years, were reviewed. The only prognostic factors are the stage at presentation, the tumor thickness, vascular invasion, and distant metastasis.)

SINONASAL UNDIFFERENTIATED CARCINOMAS

Sinonasal undifferentiated carcinomas are highly aggressive tumors of the paranasal sinuses and often appear to be histologically similar to olfactory esthesioneuroblastomas. Like inverted papillomas, sinonasal undifferentiated carcinomas appear to arise from schneiderian mucosa. They grow rapidly, with extensive local invasion into the sinuses, the orbit, and the brain (Figure 16–3). Histologically, they appear to stain for keratin and epithelial membrane antigen and do not appear to have an association to Epstein-Barr virus (EBV), which would distinguish these tumors from undifferentiated nasopharyngeal carcinomas. Surgical resection with postoperative radiation therapy is the mainstay of therapy, although this combined approach results in a very poor prognosis.

Cerilli LA, Holst VA, Brandwein MS, Stoler MH, Mills SE. Sinonasal undifferentiated carcinoma: immunohistochemical profile and lack of EBV association. *Am J Surg Pathol.* 2001;25:156. [PMID: 11176064] (Sinonasal undifferentiated carcinoma does not demonstrate EBV staining as do other tumors in the region [eg, nasopharyngeal carcinoma]. EBV staining can be used as a marker to distinguish these tumors from other small blue-cell tumors in the sinonasal cavity.)

Sharara N, Muller S, Olson J, Grist WJ, Grossniklaus HE. Sinonasal undifferentiated carcinoma with orbital invasion: report of three cases. *Ophthal Plast Reconstr Surg.* 2001;17:288. [PMID: 11476180] (Aggressive tumors that appear as small blue cells on histologic examination require differentiation from other tumors such as esthesioneuroblastoma.)

SECTION V
Salivary Glands

Benign Diseases of the Salivary Glands

Fidelia Yuan-Shin Butt, MD

General Considerations

The salivary glands consist of two parotid glands, two submandibular glands, two principal sublingual glands, and a large number of minor salivary glands. Combined, the salivary glands produce serous secretions, mucous secretions, or both. The serous saliva of the parotid gland and the predominantly mucous secretions of the submandibular, sublingual, and minor salivary glands provide digestive enzymes, bacteriostatic functions, lubrication, and hygienic activities. The secretions of the parotid and submandibular glands are primarily stimulated by the autonomic nervous system.

Classification

Benign diseases of the major and minor salivary glands can often be classified as nonneoplastic and neoplastic. Most clinically significant benign diseases involve primarily the parotid and submandibular glands and less frequently the paired principal sublingual and widely distributed minor salivary glands.

A. Parotid Gland

The parotid gland is the largest of the paired major salivary glands, with an average weight of 25 grams. Each gland is located lateral to the masseter muscle anteriorly and extends posteriorly over the sternocleidomastoid muscle behind the angle of the mandible. The dermis lies laterally to the gland, and the lateral parapharyngeal space lies medially. Each encapsulated gland is artificially divided into a superficial lobe and a deep lobe by the branches of the seventh cranial nerve. The parotid duct, or **Stensen duct,** courses anteriorly from the parotid gland over the masseter muscle and pierces the buccinator muscle to enter through the buccal mucosa, usually opposite the second maxillary molar. The Stensen duct can be found approximately 1.5 cm below the zygoma.

The parotid gland has two layers of draining lymph nodes. The superficial layer lies beneath the capsule, and the deeper layer lies within the parotid parenchyma.

B. Submandibular Gland

The paired submandibular glands are the second largest salivary glands in the body, each weighing approximately 10–15 grams. Each submandibular gland is divided into superficial and deep lobes by the posterior edge of the mylohyoid muscle and occupies the submandibular triangle. The submandibular duct, also known as the **Wharton duct,** courses anteriorly above the mylohyoid muscle and ends in the anterior floor of the mouth. The submandibular duct is inelastic and therefore, when obstructed, causes pain.

C. Sublingual Glands

The principal sublingual glands are paired and located in the submucosa, superficial to the mylohyoid muscle. Each gland is bounded laterally by the inner cortex of the mandible and medially by the styloglossus muscle; the paired glands meet in the midline. The sublingual glands have multiple small or "minor" sublingual ducts, referred to as the **ducts of Rivinus,** which open directly into the oral cavity. Some of these ducts unite to form the major **ducts of Bartholin.** These major ducts can also join the submandibular ducts.

The lingual nerve descends laterally to the anterior end of the sublingual gland and runs along its inferior border. Anteriorly, the lingual nerve and submandibular duct run parallel until the lingual nerve ascends into the tongue.

D. Minor Salivary Glands

The hard and soft palates contain the greatest concentration of minor salivary glands; however, these glands are also located in the oral cavity, lips, tongue, and oropharynx. Minor salivary glands may be identified in groups, such as the anterior lingual **glands of Blandin-Nuhn.**

The salivary glands consist of multiple secretory units that include an acinus at the proximal end and a distal ductal unit. The ductal unit combines a sequential array of ductal elements extending away from the acinus: the intercalated duct, the striated duct, and the excretory duct. Myoepithelial cells surround the acinus and extend to the intercalated duct. These myoepithelial cells contract, enabling the glandular cells to expel their secretions. Benign disorders of the salivary glands involve abnormalities of saliva production and secretion.

Saliva is produced by the clustered acinar cells and contains electrolytes, enzymes (eg, ptyalin and maltase), carbohydrates, proteins, inorganic salts, and even some antimicrobial factors. Approximately 500–1500 mL of saliva is produced by the acinar cells daily and transported through the ductal elements at an average rate of 1 mL per minute. Human saliva is generally alkaline.

■ NONNEOPLASTIC DISEASES

A list of nonneoplastic diseases can be found in Table 17–1.

INFECTIOUS INFLAMMATORY DISEASES

Infections can occur in an otherwise normal salivary gland or result from prolonged abnormalities of salivary function. Infections can be acute, subacute, or chronic. The primary etiologic agents include viruses and bacteria. However, infections may result secondarily from trauma, radiation, or duct obstruction, as is the case with acute sialadenitis.

Table 17–1. Nonneoplastic benign diseases of the salivary glands.

Noninfectious, Inflammatory Disease
Sialolithiasis
Chronic sialadenitis
Sjögren syndrome
Benign lymphoepithelial lesion
Kimura disease
Necrotizing sialometaplasia
Adenomatoid hyperplasia
Sarcoidosis
Infectious Disease
Mumps virus
Coxsackie virus
Influenza virus
Echovirus
Human immunodeficiency virus
Bacteria
Granulomatous infections
Noninflammatory Disease
Sialadenosis
Branchial cleft cysts
Dermoid cysts
Congenital cysts
Mucoceles

ACUTE VIRAL INFLAMMATORY DISEASE

 ESSENTIALS OF DIAGNOSIS

- *Acute, bilateral swelling of the parotid glands accompanied by pain, erythema, tenderness, malaise, fever, and occasionally trismus.*
- *Peak incidence in young children aged 4–6 years.*
- *Incubation period is 14–21 days.*
- *Disease is contagious.*
- *Diagnosis can be confirmed with serologic testing.*

General Considerations

Mumps (paramyxovirus) is the most common viral disorder causing parotitis (ie, inflammation of the parotid gland). The peak incidence occurs in children aged 4–6 years. The incubation period is 14–21 days, and the disease is contagious during this time.

Clinical Findings

In an acute viral inflammation of the parotid gland, bilateral swelling may be accompanied by pain, erythema, tenderness, malaise, fever, and occasionally trismus if an extensive inflammation of the adjacent pterygoid musculature exists. After a thorough history and physical exam, checking the antibodies for the mumps S, mumps V, and hemagglutination antigens can confirm the diagnosis.

Differential Diagnosis

The differential diagnoses of viral parotitis include the coxsackie A virus, cytomegalovirus, influenza A virus, and echoviruses. A serologic screen to test for these viruses may verify the diagnosis.

Complications

Complications of acute viral parotitis may involve other organs. Rare sequelae include meningitis, encephalitis, hearing loss, orchitis, pancreatitis, and nephritis.

Treatment & Prognosis

The disease course of viral parotitis is self-limiting and treatment is primarily symptomatic. The administration of the mumps vaccine has likely decreased the incidence of mumps. Viral infections in immunocompetent individuals often resolve with excellent prognosis.

ACUTE SUPPURATIVE SIALADENITIS

ESSENTIALS OF DIAGNOSIS

- *Acute painful swelling of the salivary glands with fever.*
- *Can occur in postoperative patients and in elderly patients with chronic medical conditions.*
- *Risk factors include dehydration, trauma, immunosuppression, and debilitation.*
- *Skin overlying the parotid may be warm, tender, and edematous.*
- *Untreated acute suppurative sialadenitis may lead to an abscess.*
- *Saliva from the affected gland should be cultured.*

General Considerations

In addition to viruses, bacteria can cause symptoms of acute painful swelling of the salivary glands, especially the parotid gland. Acute suppurative sialadenitis accounts for 0.03% of hospital admissions and can occur in up to 30–40% of postoperative patients.

Pathogenesis

An underlying pathogenesis begins with the stasis of salivary flow in patients; stricture or obstruction of the ducts then follows. The stasis decreases the ability of saliva to contribute to oral hygiene and promote antimicrobial activity.

Prevention

Predisposing factors for acute suppurative sialadenitis include dehydration, immunosuppression, trauma, and debilitation. Therefore, a higher incidence of this infection is found in postoperative and elderly patients, as well as in patients who have undergone chemotherapy or radiation.

Clinical Findings

In addition to acute parotid swelling in parotitis, there may be overlying skin erythema, pain, tenderness, trismus, purulent ductal discharge, induration, accompanying fevers, or any combination of these symptoms and signs. The common bacteria cultured from purulent saliva include *Staphylococcus aureus, Streptococcus pneumoniae, Escherichia coli,* and *Haemophilus influenzae.* Other organisms obtained from chronically ill, hospitalized patients are *Klebsiella, Enterobacter, Pseudomonas,* and *Candida.*

Complications

If left untreated, acute suppurative sialadenitis can progress to an abscess, a potentially fatal complication in severely debilitated patients. Clinical palpation of the parotid gland may reveal significant induration and a doughlike consistency of the gland. An ultrasound or a computed tomography (CT) scan of the parotid gland may aid in locating an area of loculation.

Treatment

The principal treatment of acute suppurative sialadenitis includes rehydration, intravenous antibiotics with penicillinase-resistant gram-positive coverage, warm compresses, massage, sialogogues, improved oral hygiene, or a combination of these therapies. If there is no clinical improvement within 48 hours of nonsurgical therapy, then an abscess may be presumed. Incision and drainage using a parotidectomy incision may be performed. Care must always be used to avoid injury to the facial nerve. An alternative method may use CT- or ultrasound-guided imaging to perform a fine-needle aspiration of an abscess.

Prognosis

Most patients with acute suppurative sialadenitis respond to medical therapy. However, mortality rates may be higher in patients with severely debilitating or complicated medical conditions. In the case of submandibular sialadenitis, failure of improvement warrants consideration of other pathology: duct obstruction, abscess, salivary stones, or tumors. Submandibular abscesses can mimic Ludwig angina, a severe infection involving the floor of mouth and the submental and submandibular spaces. If not treated, Ludwig angina can lead to airway obstruction.

Fattahi TT, Lyu PE, Van Sickels JE. Management of acute suppurative parotitis. *J Oral Maxillofac Surg.* 2002;60(4):446. [PMID:111928106] (A review of the medical and surgical management of acute suppurative parotitis.)

Honrado CP, Lam SM. Bilateral submandibular gland infection presenting as Ludwig angina: first report of a case. *Ear Nose Throat J.* 2001;80(4):217. [PMID: 11338645] (One potential complication of untreated acute submandibular sialadenitis and its management is discussed.)

CHRONIC GRANULOMATOUS SIALADENITIS

 ESSENTIALS OF DIAGNOSIS

- Chronic unilateral or bilateral salivary gland swelling.
- Minimal pain.
- Fine-needle aspiration biopsy of the gland can aid in diagnosis.
- Risk factors such as exposure to tuberculosis, animal exposure, trauma, and multiorgan system involvement should be considered.
- Uveitis, facial palsy, and parotid enlargement are suggestive of sarcoidosis.

Clinical Findings

Granulomatous disorders may present with acute salivary gland swelling or chronic unilateral glandular swelling. The glandular mass is not usually accompanied by significant pain. Primary tuberculosis should be considered if there are risk factors for exposure.

Differential Diagnosis

The diagnosis of tuberculous sialadenitis may be made with acid-fast staining for organisms, a culture of the saliva, and placement of a purified protein derivative skin test. A fine-needle aspirate of the gland helps to obtain material for diagnosis. Treatment of primary tuberculous sialadenitis includes multidrug antituberculous medications.

The differential diagnoses of granulomatous sialadenitis include animal cat-scratch disease, sarcoidosis, actinomycosis, Wegener granulomatosis, and syphilis.

A. CAT-SCRATCH DISEASE

Cat-scratch disease does not directly involve the parotid gland; instead, it affects the periparotid and intraparotid lymph nodes. In the submandibular gland, it can present as an acute submandibular mass without causing ductal obstruction, which suggests the involvement of the adjacent lymph nodes. The offending organism is a gram-negative rod, *Bartonella henselae,* and diagnosis may be made with the Warthin-Starry silver stain. Cat-scratch disease is usually self-limiting and treatment is supportive while the mass lesions slowly resolve.

B. SARCOIDOSIS

Sarcoidosis is noninfectious and involves the parotid gland in less than 10% of cases. It is a diagnosis of exclusion and is confirmed by histologic findings of noncaseating granulomas. Sarcoidosis may occur as part of a syndrome known as uveoparotid fever or **Heerfordt syndrome.** This syndrome is characterized by parotid enlargement, facial palsy, and uveitis. The involvement of the parotid and lacrimal glands leads to xerostomia and xerophthalmia. The disease often affects adults in their twenties and thirties with spontaneous resolution occurring in the ensuing months to years.

C. ACTINOMYCOSIS

Actinomycosis is easily diagnosed with special histologic stains that demonstrate sulfur granules. Actinomycosis should be suspected if a patient has painless parotid swelling with a history of recent dental infection or trauma. Trismus may develop with progression of the infection. Penicillin is the drug of choice for treatment of actinomycosis.

D. WEGENER GRANULOMATOSIS

Wegener granulomatosis can present as an acute unilateral mass in the gland, often with pain. This diagnosis, characterized histologically by necrotizing inflammation and vasculitis, is confirmed with serologic testing for the cytoplasmic antineutrophil cytoplasmic antibody (C-ANCA) and histopathologic examination.

The treatment of Wegener disease depends on the involvement of other organs; Wegener granulomatosis can be a rapidly fatal disease if it is untreated and involves other major organs. The initial treatment consists of several weeks of steroids with the addition of cyclophosphamide or other immunosuppressive agents. A more indolent subtype of Wegener, as often seen in the head and neck region, can be controlled with immunosuppressive therapy. The prognosis is excellent for many of the granulomatous diseases.

Crean SJ, Adams R, Bennett J. Sublingual gland involvement in systemic Wegener granulomatosis: a case report. *Int J Oral Maxillofac Surg.* 2002;51(1):104. [PMID: 11936391] (A case report of sublingual gland involvement in systemic Wegener granulomatosis is discussed.)

Garcia-Porrua C, Amor-Dorado JC, Gonzalez-Gay MA. Unilateral submandibular swelling as unique presentation of Wegener granulomatosis. *Rheumatology*. 2001;40:953. [PMID: 11511775] (A case report and description of the evaluation, diagnosis, and treatment of Wegener granulomatosis presenting in the salivary gland is presented.)

Mandel L, Surattanont F, Miremadi R. Cat-scratch disease: considerations for dentistry. *J Am Dent Assoc*. 2001;132(7):911. [PMID: 11480644] (Cat-scratch disease can mimic a salivary gland mass and should be considered in the differential diagnosis of salivary gland masses. A case report is also presented.)

Surattanont F, Mandel L, Wolinsky B. Bilateral parotid swelling caused by sarcoidosis. *J Am Dent Assoc*. 2002;133(6):738. [PMID: 12083650] (A case report and discussion of sarcoidosis involving the salivary glands are presented.)

HIV INFECTION

 ESSENTIALS OF DIAGNOSIS

- *Painless, bilateral enlarged parotid glands.*
- *Xerostomia.*
- *Known risk factors for HIV.*
- *Associated cervical lymphadenopathy may be associated.*
- *Presence of amylase in the cyst fluid helps confirm the diagnosis.*

General Considerations

Lymphoepithelial cysts associated with human immunodeficiency virus (HIV) occur almost exclusively in the parotid gland; however, anecdotal reports cite some occurrences of these cysts in the submandibular glands as an unusual finding. One possible explanation for the predominant presence of these cysts within the parotid gland is that this gland, unlike the submandibular gland, has intraglandular lymph nodes.

Clinical Findings

A. SYMPTOMS AND SIGNS

HIV infection should be considered in a young individual with bilateral symmetric parotid swelling, especially if the parotid swelling appears multicystic; this finding may be the initial presenting symptom of HIV infection for some patients.

B. DIAGNOSTIC EVALUATION

A CT scan or ultrasound may reveal bilateral multiple cystic masses in the parotid gland. Serologic testing for HIV antibodies confirms the diagnosis. Fine-needle aspiration of these cysts can reveal amylase in the fluid, which also leads to the diagnosis (see Figure 17–1).

Treatment

Observation or serial drainage of symptomatic cysts is the recommended treatment. A recent treatment modality includes sclerotherapy of the cysts. Rarely is parotidectomy indicated; however, when it is performed, the histopathology often shows multiple lymphoepithelial lesions and florid follicular hyperplasia with follicle lysis. Similarly, cysts involving the submandibular gland may require gland excision.

Prognosis

The parotid cysts found in HIV-infected patients are often associated with the histologic finding of benign lymphoepithelial lesions. There is little malignant transformation.

Langford RJ, Whear NM. Serology should be a routine investigation when presented with a major salivary gland lump. *Br J Oral Maxillofac Surg (Scotland)*. 2000;38(2):158. [PMID: 10864714] (Two cases where a serologic diagnosis may have precluded the need for the surgical biopsy of a salivary gland are discussed.)

Marcus A, Moore CE. Sodium morrhuate sclerotherapy for the treatment of benign lymphoepithelial cysts of the parotid gland in the HIV patient. *Laryngoscope*. 2005;115(4):746. [PMID: 15805892]. (A case report.)

Uccini S, D'Offizi G. Cystic lymphoepithelial lesions of the parotid gland in HIV-1 infection. *AIDS Patient Care STDS*. 2000;14(3):143. [PMID: 10763543] (A review of rare benign cystic lymphoepithelial lesions of the parotid gland in HIV-infected patients is presented.)

NONINFECTIOUS INFLAMMATORY DISEASES
SIALOLITHIASIS

 ESSENTIALS OF DIAGNOSIS

- *Acute, painful swelling of the major salivary gland, especially the submandibular gland, which may be recurrent.*
- *Aggravation of symptoms with eating; swelling may subside after approximately 1 hour.*
- *History of gout or xerostomia.*
- *A stone in the floor of the mouth may be palpated; treatment depends on the location of the calculus.*

- Calculus may be extracted intraorally, or if distal, then the submandibular gland may be indicated.
- Complications include acute suppurative sialadenitis, ductal ectasia, and stricture.

General Considerations

Approximately 80–90% of salivary calculi occur in the submandibular gland, whereas only 10–20% are reported in the parotid gland; a very small percentage of salivary calculi are found in the sublingual and minor salivary glands. Sialolithiasis is a common cause of salivary gland disease and can occur at any age with a predilection in men. Risk factors for salivary stone obstruction include long illnesses with dehydration. There are also associations with gout, diabetes, and hypertension.

Pathogenesis

Normal saliva contains abundant hydroxyapatite, the primary compound in salivary stones. Aggregates of mineralized debris in the duct can form a nidus, promoting calculi formation, salivary stasis, and eventually obstruction. The submandibular gland is more susceptible to calculi formation than the parotid gland because of the longer course of its duct, higher salivary mucin and alkaline content, and higher concentrations of calcium and phosphate.

Submandibular calculi consist primarily of calcium phosphate and hydroxyapatite; because of the high calcium content of these calculi, the majority are radiopaque and visualized on x-rays. Parotid calculi are less likely to be radiopaque. Approximately 75% of the time, a single stone is found in the gland. If the obstruction is not relieved, local inflammation, fibrosis, and acinar atrophy ensue.

Clinical Findings

A. SYMPTOMS AND SIGNS

Recurrent swelling and pain in the submandibular gland exacerbated with eating is the common presentation of salivary calculi. Prolonged obstruction can lead to acute infection with increasing pain and erythema of the gland. Patients may also report a history of xerostomia and occasionally gritty, sandlike foreign bodies in their oral cavity. A physical exam is essential as stones often are palpated in the anterior two thirds of the submandibular duct. In addition, an induration of the mouth floor is sometimes observed. Stones located within the body of the gland are not easily palpated.

B. IMAGING

X-rays with lateral and occlusal views can reveal a radiopaque stone, but these views are not always reliable. Intraoral views may be more helpful. Sialography is the most accurate imaging method to detect calculi. Sialography can be combined with CT scanning or magnetic resonance imaging (MRI), especially as CT scans are sensitive to calcium salts. Ultrasound has not proven to be useful.

C. ENDOSCOPY

Recent advances in endoscopy have allowed endoscopic examination of the submandibular duct to detect calculi.

Complications

Persistent obstruction from sialolithiasis leads to salivary stasis. It also predisposes the gland to recurrent acute infections and even abscess formation.

Treatment

A. INTRAORAL EXTRACTION

Treatment is based on the location of the salivary stone. If the stone is palpated or visualized in the anterior portion of the submandibular duct and does not pass spontaneously, it can be extracted intraorally. The ductal papilla can be dilated serially with ease using graded lacrimal probes; the stone is then expressed. If the stone is too large, a more extensive intraoral procedure under local or general anesthesia may be attempted. The duct is cannulated, and an incision over the stone is created to allow extraction. No closure of the incision is made and careful attention must be paid to the adjacent lingual nerve.

B. SURGICAL EXCISION

Larger stones embedded in the hilum or the body of the submandibular gland causing symptoms may require surgical excision of the gland. Similarly, a symptomatic stone embedded in the body of the parotid gland will necessitate a parotidectomy.

C. ENDOSCOPIC TECHNIQUES

Recent endoscopic techniques allow an intraoral endoscopic extraction of salivary calculi and excision of the submandibular gland. The procedure has been performed with minimal morbidity and carries the advantage of avoiding a transverse cervical incision.

D. OTHER MEASURES

Other methods for calculi removal include wire basket extraction under radiologic guidance, pulsed dye laser lithotripsy, and extracorporeal shock wave lithotripsy.

Prognosis

The recurrence of stones is approximately 18%. If the risk factors are corrected, this may decrease the rate of recurrence.

Guerrissi JO, Taborda G. Endoscopic excision of the submandibular gland by an intraoral approach. *J Craniofac Surg.* 2001;39(3):299. [PMID: 11358106] (A new, safe technique allowing intraoral excision of the submandibular gland in the treatment of sialadenitis is discussed.)

Marchal F, Kurt AM. Histopathology of submandibular glands removed for sialolithiasis. *Ann Otol Rhinol Laryngol.* 2001;110:464. [PMID: 11372932] (A review of the pathophysiology of sialolithiasis is discussed.)

CHRONIC SIALADENITIS

General Considerations

Chronic sialadenitis results from either a decreased production of saliva or alterations in the salivary flow leading to salivary stasis. There may or may not be associated obstruction. This slow, progressive inflammatory process is usually found in adults, but it can affect children as well.

Pathogenesis

A decreased flow or stasis compromises the salivary functions, creating an environment at risk for infection. Chronic sialadenitis may be caused by retrograde infection from normal oral flora and chronic inflammation from repeated acute infections. In the latter, chronic inflammation causes changes in the ductal epithelium, which commonly leads to increased mucin in secretions, decreased flow, and mucous plugs.

Histologically, the ductal epithelium in chronic sialadenitis may demonstrate mucous cell, squamous, or oncocytic metaplasia. There may be ductal dilatation and atrophy of the acinar cells. Prolonged inflammation can lead to fibrosis and infiltration with lymphocytes. If a stone obstruction is the cause, calculi may be seen within the ducts.

Prevention

A variety of conditions can cause chronic nonobstructive sialadenitis; these include repeated acute infections, trauma, radiation, and immunocompromised conditions. Histologic changes from radiation are likely permanent. Some patients may develop salivary gland swelling, xerostomia, and taste alterations after receiving intravenous iodine contrast. Smoking has also been found to predispose an individual to chronic sialadenitis because it reduces the antimicrobial activity of salivary secretions. Another condition known descriptively as chronic sclerosing sialadenitis or Kuttner tumor may be indistinguishable from neoplasia until a pathologic examination is done.

Clinical Findings

Presenting symptoms consist of chronic, intermittent painful swelling of the salivary gland, especially with eating. Swelling is often bilateral and may or may not be associated with an acute infection.

A thorough history and physical examination can elicit risk factors and direct the search for treatable causes, such as a salivary stone. A CT scan or MRI may help to exclude a malignant tumor, especially if there is an associated fibrous mass in the parotid gland. Sialography and fine-needle aspiration have not been consistently diagnostic; however, sialographs can be helpful in finding obstructions, acinar atrophy, and irregular dilatations of the ducts.

Differential Diagnosis

The differential diagnoses include granulomatous diseases, sialolithiasis, sarcoidosis, benign lymphoepithelial lesion, inflammatory pseudotumors, Sjögren syndrome, and Mikulicz syndrome.

Complications

As a reactive process to trauma or disease, chronic nonobstructive sialadenitis may progress to a fibrous mass formation or an inflammatory pseudotumor. Other complications of the disease include pain and permanent damage to the acinar unit and ductal epithelium. Progressive changes further compromise the function of the acinar units, which clinically manifest as bulging, irregular, nodular glands.

Treatment

Conservative therapy and surgical gland excision are the most successful treatment methods of chronic nonobstructive sialadenitis. If no treatable cause is identified, patients are encouraged to improve oral hygiene with increased hydration, massage of the affected gland, adequate nutrition, and use of sialagogues. Antibiotics are administered with acute exacerbations.

Superficial parotidectomy is the common surgical treatment of persistent symptoms in the parotid gland. Alternative treatments include iatrogenic fibrosis of the gland with 1% methyl violet and low-dose radiation therapy. Procedures such as parotid duct ligation and tympanic neurectomy, used to cease secretion, also may prove therapeutic.

Prognosis

The prognosis depends on treating an identifiable underlying cause; few recurrences have been reported following these treatments.

Huang C, Damrose E, Bhuta S, Abemayor E. Kuttner tumor (chronic sclerosing sialadenitis. *Am J Otolaryngol.* 2003;24(4): 278. [PMID: 12430136]. (A case report and discussion.)

Mandel SJ, Mandel L. Radioactive iodine and the salivary glands. *Thyroid.* 2003;13(3):265. [PMID: 12729475]. (Description of a side effect to the salivary glands from radioactive iodine therapy.)

Qi S, Liu X, Wang S. Sialoendoscopic and irrigation findings in chronic obstructive parotitis. *Laryngoscope.* 2005;115(3):541. [PMID: 15744174] (Sialoendoscopy can provide more detailed observation of the salivary ductal system.)

SJÖGREN SYNDROME

 ESSENTIALS OF DIAGNOSIS

- Salivary gland swelling with dryness of the mouth and eyes leading to oral and ocular pain and sensitivity.
- Often associated with another connective tissue disease.
- More commonly seen in postmenopausal women.
- Detection of autoantibodies SS-A and SS-B and others, along with minor salivary gland biopsy, may confirm the diagnosis.
- Slowly progressive disease.
- High risk for development of malignant lymphoma in primary Sjögren syndrome.

General Considerations

Sjögren syndrome is an autoimmune disorder classically characterized by parotid enlargement, xerostomia, and keratoconjunctivitis sicca. It also may be associated with a connective tissue disease such as rheumatoid arthritis or systemic lupus erythematosus. Sjögren syndrome occurs 90% of the time in females, usually in their sixth decade. It is the second most common connective tissue disorder; only rheumatoid arthritis occurs more frequently.

Clinical Findings

A. SYMPTOMS AND SIGNS

Patients often present with bilateral, nontender salivary gland enlargement. The parotid swelling may occur intermittently or stay constant. Other symptoms include dry eye, dry mouth, altered taste, dry skin, myalgia, vaginal dryness, vasculitis, and arthritis.

B. LABORATORY FINDINGS

Useful laboratory tests showing the presence of SS-A or SS-B autoantibodies, rheumatoid factor, or antinuclear antibodies can aid the diagnosis. The microscopic examination of a minor salivary gland biopsy such as from the lip, can confirm Sjögren disease. According to histologic criteria, a focus score of greater than 1 focus/ 4 mm^2 is diagnostic. Characteristic histopathologic findings include a lymphocytic infiltrate in acinar units and epimyoepithelial islands surrounded by lymphoid stroma.

Differential Diagnosis

The differential diagnoses include benign lymphoepithelial lesion, also known as Mikulicz syndrome, and chronic nonobstructive sialadenitis.

Complications

Complications of primary Sjögren syndrome result from chronic progression of the disease. The deterioration of salivary function can cause patients to have difficulties with speaking, swallowing, and masticating; in addition, increased dental decay with loss of teeth and oral mucosal discomfort can result. More importantly, there is an approximate 10% incidence of lymphoma in patients with primary Sjögren syndrome.

Treatment

Treatment is symptomatic and supportive. Steroids and topical steroid eyedrops may be indicated for severe symptoms. Superficial parotidectomy may be required for severe recurrent parotid infections.

Prognosis

The prognosis for those affected with Sjögren syndrome is generally favorable. However, there is an increased incidence in malignant lymphoma or lymphoepithelial carcinoma in patients with this syndrome. Therefore, careful observation with appropriate diagnostic studies is recommended.

Gannot G, Lancaster HE. Clinical course of primary Sjögren syndrome: salivary, oral, and serologic aspects. *J Rheumatol.* 2000;27(8):1905. [PMID: 10955331] (Primary Sjögren syndrome is a slow, progressive disease that affects salivary gland function. There is a high incidence of lymphoma in these patients.)

BENIGN LYMPHOEPITHELIAL LESIONS

ESSENTIALS OF DIAGNOSIS

- Unilateral firm or cystic swelling of the parotid gland, with bilateral involvement in approximately 20% of cases.
- Parotid gland most often involved, but the submandibular gland may also be involved.
- Most often seen in HIV-infected populations.
- Fine-needle aspiration aids in diagnosis, showing acinar atrophy with diffuse lymphocytic infiltration, and foci of epimyoepithelial islands.
- Disease may progress to near total or total replacement of acinar tissue in the gland.

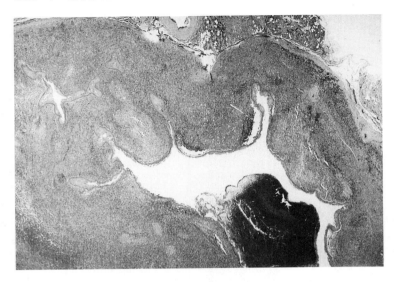

Figure 17–1. Benign lymphoepithelial cyst. (Courtesy of Christina Kong, MD, Stanford University School of Medicine, Stanford, CA.)

- *Higher probability of progression to low-grade B-cell lymphoma of mucosa-associated lymphoid tissue (MALT).*

General Considerations

Benign lymphoepithelial lesions are also known as **Godwin tumor, Mikulicz syndrome,** or punctate parotitis. Benign lymphoepithelial lesion has a predilection for females, especially in the fifth and sixth decades of life. It is also associated with multicystic disease in HIV-infected patients.

Pathogenesis

A benign lymphoepithelial lesion is an inflammatory process characterized by lymphocytic infiltration around salivary gland ducts and parenchyma (Figure 17–1). With increasing lymphocytic infiltration, progressive acinar atrophy and even replacement of the acini result. Upon further progression, the ductal epithelia proliferate and eventually cause ductal obstruction.

Clinical Findings

Patients often present with recurrent unilateral firm or cystic swelling of the parotid gland with or without pain. Bilateral involvement occurs in 20% of cases. Fine-needle aspiration of the parotid mass is helpful. Sialography is rarely indicated unless a stone is suspected.

This condition often affects the parotid gland and rarely affects the submandibular gland; when it does affect the submandibular gland, it presents as a painless mass. There may be an associated reactive lymphadenop-

athy. The diagnosis is best made on histopathologic findings of acinar atrophy with diffuse lymphocytic infiltration, with or without the presence of epimyoepithelial islands. There is an association with Sjögren syndrome.

Complications

Cases of progression to neoplastic disease can result, including lymphoepithelial carcinoma, low-grade B-cell lymphoma of MALT pseudolymphoma, and non-Hodgkin lymphoma. There is also an association with Kaposi sarcoma in HIV-infected patients.

Treatment & Prognosis

The treatment of benign lymphoepithelial lesion is symptomatic unless the parotid enlargement is severe enough to warrant a superficial parotidectomy. Complete submandibular excision is an adequate treatment of the rare benign lymphoepithelial cyst. Infrequently, there is malignant transformation; however, careful observation is warranted even after complete excision of the gland.

Carbone A. Pathologic features of lymphoid proliferations of the salivary glands: lymphoepithelial sialadenitis versus low-grade B-cell lymphoma of the malt type. *Ann Otol Rhinol Laryngol.* 2000;109:1170. [PMID: 11130833] (A histopathologic study concluding that the distinction between benign lymphoepithelial lesions of the salivary glands and low-grade B-cell lymphoma of mucosa-associated lymphoid tissues relies on evaluation of morphologic features of the gland.)

Ussmuller J, Reinecke T, Donath K, Jaehne M. Chronic myoepithelial sialadenitis: symptomatology, clinical signs, differential diagnostics. *Laryngorhinootologie.* 2002;81(2):111. [PMID: 11914948] (A retrospective chart review of patients with myoepithelial sialadenitis—ie, benign lymphoepithelial lesion—

showing that the clinical relevance of this diagnosis lies in the higher risk of developing malignant lymphoma.)

KIMURA DISEASE

 ESSENTIALS OF DIAGNOSIS

- *Slowly growing, painless mass in the major salivary gland, primarily in Asians.*
- *Commonly seen in the second and third decades; 80% of patients are male.*
- *Enlargement of gland accompanied by regional lymphadenopathy.*
- *Serologic tests often demonstrate peripheral eosinophilia and elevated IgE levels.*
- *Recurrence may occur after surgical excision of the gland.*

General Considerations

Kimura disease is a rare, benign chronic inflammatory disease mimicking a tumor in regions of the head and neck. It occurs predominantly in young Asian males in their twenties and thirties.

Clinical Findings

When Kimura disease occurs in the head and neck regions, the major salivary glands are usually involved. In the parotid and submandibular glands, this disease presents as painless superficial swellings often accompanied by regional lymphadenopathy. The formation of lymphoid follicles and the aggregation of eosinophils in the affected tissues are found on histologic examination.

Differential Diagnosis

The differential diagnoses of Kimura disease include the following: (1) angiolymphoid hyperplasia with eosinophilia, (2) reactive lymphadenopathy, (3) parotid tumor, (4) extranodal manifestations of Rosai-Dorfman disease, and (5) benign lymphoepithelial lesion. Angiolymphoid hyperplasia with eosinophilia differs from Kimura disease in the lack of lymphadenopathy and decreased eosinophilia. **Rosai-Dorfman disease** is an idiopathic benign condition characterized by histiocytic proliferation and massive lymphadenopathy, including involvement of the intraparotid lymph nodes.

Treatment

The treatment of choice when Kimura disease is found in the parotid gland is parotidectomy with continued observation for potential recurrence. Kimura disease of the submandibular gland is usually treated with excision of the gland and the adjacent lymph nodes. Because Kimura disease often affects other sites, systemic therapy with steroids and radiation also may prove beneficial.

NECROTIZING SIALOMETAPLASIA

Necrotizing sialometaplasia is a benign, self-healing inflammatory process mainly involving the minor salivary glands. It has a predilection in males and occurs over a wide age range. It presents as a spontaneously appearing, painless ulceration or swelling usually over the hard palate, but can occur wherever there are salivary gland tissues. The lesions are usually unilateral and can present with burning sensations and numbness. The cause is unknown, but there are associations with trauma and radiation therapy. The pathogenesis is thought to be ischemic.

The diagnosis of necrotizing sialometaplasia is confirmed on biopsy. Histology shows the characteristic pseudoepitheliomatous hyperplasia and squamous metaplasia. Care must be taken to avoid confusing the diagnosis with squamous cell carcinoma or mucoepidermoid carcinoma; the main complication is misdiagnosis. Lesions in necrotizing sialometaplasia are self-healing, usually by secondary intention, and recurrences are rare.

ADENOMATOID HYPERPLASIA

Adenomatoid hyperplasia is a rare swelling of the minor salivary glands that occurs most commonly in the palate. Local trauma, environmental irritation, and chronic inflammation are the proposed causes of this condition. Patients present with painless swellings that have been present for an indeterminate length of time. The overlying mucosa usually appears normal. Adenomatoid hyperplasia must be distinguished from minor salivary gland tumors. The differential diagnoses include benign and malignant tumors.

Histologic examination reveals glandular hypertrophy and inflammatory infiltrates, but no change in the general architecture of the gland and no evidence of neoplasia or atypia. Complete excision is the treatment of choice. Because of the higher incidence of malignant tumors within the hard palate, the key is to distinguish malignant tumors from benign adenomatoid hyperplasia.

Shimoyama T, Wakabayashi M. Adenomatoid hyperplasia of the palate mimicking clinically as a salivary gland tumor. *J Oral Sci*. 2001;43(2):135. [PMID: 11515598] (A case report distinguishing adenomatoid hyperplasia from salivary gland tumors based on immunohistologic findings is presented.)

NONINFLAMMATORY DISEASES
SIALADENOSIS

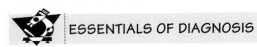

ESSENTIALS OF DIAGNOSIS

- *Bilateral, occasionally unilateral, diffuse enlargement of the salivary glands, particularly the parotid glands.*
- *Pain may or may not be associated.*
- *The condition usually begins between the ages of 20 and 60 years and may persist for more than 20 years.*
- *In half of the cases, there are associated underlying systemic factors, including endocrine disorders, malnutrition, and drugs.*
- *Biopsy of the affected gland shows acinar enlargement.*
- *The cause is peripheral autonomic neuropathy of the salivary glands; present treatments are not entirely satisfactory as they do not address this underlying cause.*
- *Surgery should be reserved if cosmetic deformity of the gland is unacceptable.*

General Considerations

Sialadenosis, or sialosis, is a rare, noninflammatory condition that causes bilateral, diffuse, and painless enlargement of the salivary glands. This condition may also cause degenerative changes to the autonomic innervation of the glands. The parotid gland is the most affected, followed by the submandibular gland.

Prevention

Although the etiology is not clear, several metabolic and medical conditions are associated with sialadenosis. These include obesity, alcoholic cirrhosis, diabetes, hyperlipidemia, hypothyroidism, anemia, pregnancy, malnutrition, menopause, and even certain medications (eg, clozapine).

Clinical Findings

A thorough physical exam and screening are necessary. Fine-needle aspiration complemented with CT scanning can establish the diagnosis. Histopathologic findings show acinar enlargement.

Treatment & Prognosis

The treatment of sialadenosis is directed at the underlying conditions. Parotidectomy is considered if the parotid enlargement is cosmetically unacceptable. Surgical resection of the affected submandibular gland is the treatment of choice; but unless correction of the underlying disorder is addressed, there may be persistent enlargement of any residual glands. The prognosis is therefore dependent on treatment of the underlying conditions.

Kastin B, Mandel L. Alcoholic sialosis. *NY State Dent J.* 2000;66(6):22. [PMID: 11132299] (Sialosis or sialadenosis is a benign salivary disorder often associated with alcoholism, endocrine disorders, and malnutrition. The presence of sialosis warrants further investigation into these unsuspected systemic disorders.)

PAROTID CYSTS

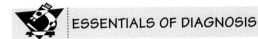

ESSENTIALS OF DIAGNOSIS

- *Fluctuant swellings of the salivary glands.*
- *Cysts of the parotid gland may be acquired or congenital.*
- *Congenital cysts may be either Type I or Type II branchial arch cysts.*
- *Acquired cysts may occur secondary to trauma, sialolithiasis, ductal stricture, or benign lymphoepithelial lesions.*
- *HIV should be considered in the differential diagnosis.*

True cysts of the parotid gland account for 2–5% of parotid lesions.

Classification

A. CONGENITAL PAROTID CYSTS

1. Branchial cleft anomalies—Congenital cysts may result from branchial cleft anomalies; these anomalies are subdivided into Type I and Type II cysts.

a. Type I cysts—Type I cysts are a duplication anomaly of the ectodermal external auditory canal. The cyst may be located anteroinferior to the ear lobule.

b. Type II cysts—Type II cysts consist of ectodermal and mesodermal elements and may open anteriorly to either the sternocleidomastoid muscle or the external auditory canal.

Both Type I and Type II branchial cleft anomalies may have sinus tracts, which are intimately related to the facial nerve. Therefore, excision of these congenital parotid cysts requires a parotidectomy approach and preservation of the facial nerve.

2. Dermoid cysts—A second type of congenital cyst occurring in the parotid gland is a dermoid cyst. This cyst results from trapped embryonic epidermis and presents as a rounded mass. It contains keratinizing squamous epithelium, sweat glands, and other associated skin appendages. Excision to prevent recurrent infections, with attention to the facial nerve, is the most successful treatment.

B. ACQUIRED PAROTID CYSTS

Acquired cysts of the parotid gland may result from other parotid disorders such as tumors, trauma, chronic sialadenitis, sialolithiasis, and radiation injury. Cysts related to HIV infection have been discussed earlier in this chapter.

Nasuti JF, Yu GH, Gupta PK. Fine-needle aspiration of cystic parotid gland lesions: an institutional review of 46 cases with histologic correlation. *Cancer.* 2000;90(2):111. [PMID: 10794160] (A retrospective study of 46 cases of patients with cystic parotid lesions was performed to determine the diagnostic accuracy of fine-needle cytology.)

Orvidas LJ, Kasperbauer JL, Lewis JE, Olsen KD, Lesnick TG. Pediatric parotid masses. *Arch Otolaryngol Head Neck Surg.* 2000;126(2):177. [PMID: 10680869] (A retrospective review of pediatric parotid masses demonstrates a variety of pathologic diagnoses, including benign tumors, branchial cleft cysts, vascular malformations, and malignant entities.)

CONGENITAL SALIVARY FISTULAS OF THE SUBMANDIBULAR GLAND

Congenital salivary fistulas and sinus tracts are exceedingly rare. They are thought to arise from aberrant salivary gland tissue or aberrant gland formation during the end of the sixth week of gestation. These fistula and sinus tracts may form cutaneous openings in the submandibular skin with discharge. A fistulogram or MRI may help with the diagnosis. Complete surgical excision is the recommended treatment.

Kapadia LA, McClay JE. Congenital midline submandibular sinus tract. *Int J Pediatr Otorhinolaryngol.* 2000;53(3):221. [PMID: 10930638] (A case report and discussion of a rare case of a salivary gland sinus tract.)

MUCOCELES

 ESSENTIALS OF DIAGNOSIS

- *Painless, cystic lesions commonly seen on the lip, oral cavity, and often with mucous extravasation.*
- *Cystic lesion in the floor of mouth may be localized or extend into the neck, presenting as a neck mass.*
- *Presentation may be preceded by minor trauma to soft tissue or oral mucosa.*

General Considerations

Mucoceles represent dilatations of the minor salivary gland ducts due to both accumulated mucous secretions and, often, mucous extravasations into the connective tissue. Mucoceles are fairly common and are seen frequently in the lip (60–70%), buccal mucosa, floor of the mouth, and palate. When a mucocele appears in the mouth floor, it is defined as a **ranula** (related to the Latin term for frog). It is also known as a **mucous retention cyst.**

Pathogenesis

Mucoceles are thought to arise from either a trauma to or a rupture of the minor salivary gland ducts with extravasation of mucus into the surrounding tissue. Sublingual glands and minor salivary glands are more susceptible to developing mucoceles owing to continuous mucous secretions in these glands, whereas the parotid and submandibular glands secrete on stimulation. The cause of ranulas is not as clear.

Clinical Findings

Mucous retention cysts generally present as pale, smooth, bluish-hued submucosal cysts. They are painless and may slowly enlarge.

Ranulas, involving the sublingual or submandibular ducts, present as round, fluctuant masses in the mouth floor. They are usually unilateral and may affect any age group with no gender preference. A **simple ranula** is a true cyst with an epithelial lining that occurs intraorally with elevation of the mouth floor. A **plunging ranula** extends below the mylohyoid muscle, beyond the sublingual space, and involves the submandibular space. It may extend further inferiorly to present as a painless submandibular or cervical neck mass. Unlike a simple ranula, a plunging ranula does not have an epithelial lining and therefore is classified as a pseudocyst.

A physical exam is usually adequate for the diagnosis, but a CT scan can provide excellent views of the extent of the cyst.

Complications

Mucoceles and ranulas cause few complications. However, infections can occur.

Differential Diagnosis

The differential diagnoses include cystic hygroma, lymphangioma, thyroglossal duct cyst, and dermoid cyst. An important differential diagnosis for a mucous retention cyst is malignant mucoepidermoid carcinoma.

Treatment & Prognosis

A complete surgical intraoral excision of a mucous retention cyst is curative with few recurrences at the site. The treatment of a simple ranula consists of either simple excision of the cyst and possible removal of the associated gland, or marsupialization of the cyst wall. Recurrences are possible with the latter procedure. In the case of plunging ranulas, treatment requires excision either intraorally or combined with a cervical incision and extirpation of the associated gland. Recurrence can occur with inadequate excision.

Anastassov GE, Haiavy J. Submandibular gland mucocele: diagnosis and management. *Oral Surg Oral Med Oral Pathol Oral Radiol Endod.* 2000;89(2):159. [PMID: 10673650] (A review of the pathophysiology of mucoceles and rare occurrences in the submandibular gland is presented.)

Kapadia LA, McClay JE. Congenital midline submandibular sinus tract. *Int J Pediatr Otorhinolarygol.* 2000;53(3):221. [PMID: 10930638] (A case report and discussion of rare congenital fistula, cysts, and sinus tracts of the salivary glands that present as head and neck masses is presented.)

XEROSTOMIA

Xerostomia is defined as dry mouth. In addition to the discomfort from dry mouth, patients with xerostomia may also experience an altered sense of taste, dysphagia, and complications related to dental decay. Disorders of salivary flow in the parotid gland can cause this condition. In addition, many systemic conditions can result in dry mouth: Sjögren syndrome, stress, diabetes, chronic infection, and irradiation. Xerostomia also results as a side effect of a variety of medications.

The treatment of xerostomia is aimed at the underlying conditions; symptomatic treatment includes an increased intake of fluids, sialagogues, mouthwashes, and artificial saliva. In addition, there are currently medications prescribed to minimize xerostomia for patients undergoing radiation.

Daniels T. Evaluation, differential diagnosis, and treatment of xerostomia. *J Rheumatol Suppl.* 2000;61:6. [PMID: 11128701] (A review of the clinical course of xerostomia, including its differential diagnosis and treatment, is presented. The treatment combines dental decay prevention, salivary flow stimulation, the treatment of chronic oral candidiasis, and the use of salivary substitutes. Also presented is a review of pharmacotherapeutics.)

PTYALISM

Ptyalism refers to the hyperproduction of saliva. It is associated with a number of medical conditions, including inflammation, cerebral palsy, and pregnancy. Medications may also produce ptyalism as a side effect.

If medications with drying agents are not effective, surgical treatment is indicated. Other treatment options include selective neurectomy of the chorda tympani nerve, excision of the salivary gland, and either ligation or transposition of the affected duct.

■ BENIGN NEOPLASTIC DISEASES

 ESSENTIALS OF DIAGNOSIS

- *64–80% percent of primary salivary tumors occur in the salivary gland, 7–15% occur in the submandibular gland, and < 1% occur in the sublingual glands.*
- *54–80% of all tumors are benign.*
- *Peak incidence of salivary tumors occurs in the sixth to seventh decades.*
- *Painless, slowly enlarging solitary mass in the salivary gland.*
- *Deep parotid lobe tumors may present as a painless, asymmetric swelling of the soft palate.*
- *Fine-needle aspiration cytology and imaging aid in the diagnosis.*
- *Complete surgical excision is most often curative.*

General Considerations

Approximately 80% of salivary gland tumors occur in the parotid gland. Of these tumors, approximately 75–80% are benign. There is no consistent correlation between the rate of tumor growth and whether a tumor is benign or malignant. Most benign tumors of the parotid gland are epithelial tumors.

In general, only 15% of diseases of the submandibular gland are neoplastic. Compared with parotid tumors, approximately 50–60% of submandibular tumors are benign.

Minor salivary gland tumors account for approximately 15% of all salivary gland tumors. It is estimated that only 35% of minor salivary gland tumors are benign, with pleomorphic adenoma being the most common neoplasm followed by basal cell adenoma.

Clinical Findings

Most benign parotid tumors present as slow-growing, painless masses often in the tail of the parotid gland. Tumors of the other salivary glands similarly present as painless masses. Fine-needle aspiration of salivary tumors, although not as sensitive or specific as in other tumors (eg, the thyroid), is extremely useful in differentiating between malignant and benign processes. The accuracy rate is approximately 85% in determining if a parotid tumor is benign or malignant; this rate is higher when determining whether or not a lesion originates from parotid tissue. CT scanning and MRI may help identify deep lobe tumors if clinically warranted.

Differential Diagnosis

The differential diagnoses of benign salivary gland tumors not only include each other, but must also alert a clinician to their malignant counterparts. Various other benign neoplastic entities involving the salivary glands must be considered: papillary ductal adenomas, sebaceous adenomas, ancient schwannomas, congenital epithelial tumors, cavernous hemangiomas, and ectopic extraglandular tissues. Fine-needle aspiration is most useful in determining whether an asymptomatic mass in the region of the parotid gland or submandibular space is of glandular origin or not. Treatment options can be tailored based on these initial findings.

Complications

Complications of pleomorphic adenomas are rare and include malignant transformation into a carcinoma ex-pleomorphic adenoma. There is rare malignant transformation of Warthin tumor, monomorphic adenomas, and the benign salivary tumors to be described. Little is known about the incidence of the malignant transformation of tumors found in the submandibular gland.

Complete excision ensures an excellent prognosis; however, recurrence occurs if there are positive margins. With the repeat excision of recurrences, the risk to the facial nerve expectedly rises. Recurrent tumors are frequently multinodular. Recurrence can be attributed to either inadequate margins, or in the case of Warthin tumor, to its multicentricity.

Treatment

Complete surgical excision with uninvolved margins is the recommended treatment of benign tumors of the salivary glands. Usually, a superficial parotidectomy with preservation of the facial nerve is adequate unless there is deep lobe involvement. Parapharyngeal space tumors require resection through a form of transcervical approach. Enucleation alone is inadequate for tumors of the parotid gland; a complete submandibular excision, with preservation of the marginal mandibular, lingual, and hypoglossal nerves, is the treatment of choice. Radiation is not indicated in the treatment of benign salivary tumors.

Prognosis

With the complete removal of the tumor and excision of the affected gland, the prognosis is excellent. Malignant transformation and recurrences are rare.

PLEOMORPHIC ADENOMAS

Pleomorphic adenomas, or **benign mixed tumors,** are the most common neoplasms of the salivary glands (Figure 17–2). They represent approximately 60–70% of all parotid tumors and 90% of submandibular benign tumors. These neoplasms affect females more than males and are commonly seen in the third to sixth decades of life. When the deep parotid lobe is involved, a pleomorphic adenoma can present as a parapharyngeal space tumor with soft palate swelling. It presents as an isolated swelling or mass in the submandibular gland

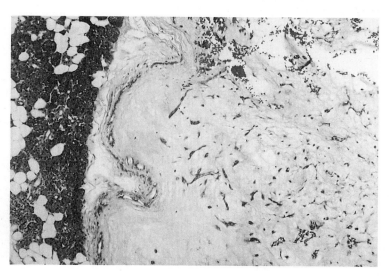

Figure 17–2. Pleomorphic adenoma. (Courtesy of Christina Kong, MD, Stanford University School of Medicine, Standford, CA.)

with little associated pain. There are no known etiologic factors.

Histologically, pleomorphic adenomas arise from the distal portions of the salivary ducts, including the intercalated ducts and acini. The mixture of epithelial, myoepithelial, and stromal elements is represented by the name, benign mixed tumor. Any of these individual components may predominate in the histology, but all three must be present to confirm the diagnosis. Both immunohistochemical stains specific for myoepithelial cells and epithelial cells can help to distinguish pleomorphic adenoma.

The differential diagnoses for pleomorphic adenomas should include malignant neoplasms: adenoid cystic carcinoma, polymorphous low-grade adenocarcinoma, deep-seated adnexal neoplasms, and mesenchymal neoplasms. Rare complications of pleomorphic adenoma include malignant transformation into a tumor known as carcinoma ex-pleomorphic adenoma, or alternately, "benign" metastasizing mixed tumors. The word "benign" describes solely the histology, but not the pathologic behavior of this rare entity.

Although radiation is not indicated in the treatment of benign salivary tumors, it has been used occasionally to control recurrent pleomorphic adenomas. Complete surgical excision of the tumor with uninvolved margins is the recommended treatment. For example, a superficial parotidectomy with clear margins is the treatment for a pleomorphic adenoma located in the superficial lobe of the parotid gland. The prognosis for pleomorphic adenomas is excellent, with a 96% rate of nonrecurrence.

Webb AJ, Eveson JW. Pleomorphic adenomas of the major salivary glands: a study of the capsular form in relation to surgical management. *Clin Otolaryngol.* 2001;26(2):134. [PMID: 11309055]

(This article provides a retrospective study that correlates capsular characteristics to histopathology. It also confirms that a parotidectomy is the treatment of choice over enucleation.)

WARTHIN TUMOR

Warthin tumor is also known as **papillary cystadenoma lymphomatosum** and is found almost exclusively in the parotid gland (Figure 17–3). It is characterized histologically by papillary structures composed of double layers of granular eosinophilic cells or oncocytes, cystic changes, and mature lymphocytic infiltration. It arises from the ectopic ductal epithelium. It represents approximately 5% of all salivary gland tumors and approximately 12% of benign tumors of the parotid gland. This tumor is more commonly seen in males in the fifth to seventh decades of life and there is an associated risk with smokers.

There is approximately 5.0–7.5% bilaterality and 14% multicentricity in Warthin tumor. CT scanning may demonstrate a well-defined mass in the posteroinferior segment of the superficial lobe of the parotid. If radiosialography is performed, increased activity is seen related to the presence of oncocytes and their increased mitochondrial content.

The diagnosis of Warthin tumor is easily arrived at based on histologic findings, with rare confusion with other tumors. The treatment requires complete excision of the affected portion of the gland with uninvolved margins.

MONOMORPHIC ADENOMAS

These slow-growing tumors represent less than 5% of all salivary gland tumors (Figure 17–4). Monomorphic adenomas differ from pleomorphic adenomas, in that they consist of only one morphologic cell type. Monomorphic

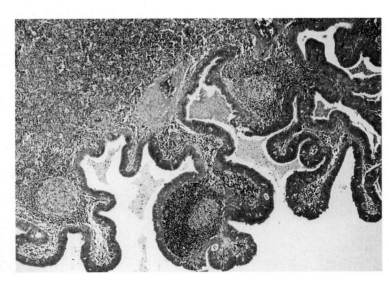

Figure 17–3. Warthin tumor. (Courtesy of Christina Kong, MD, Stanford University School of Medicine, Stanford, CA.)

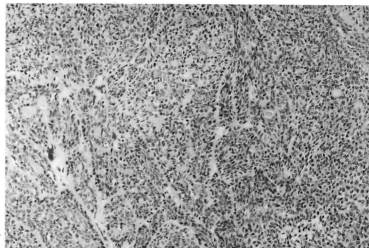

Figure 17–4. Monomorphic adenoma. (Courtesy of Christina Kong, Stanford University School of Medicine, Stanford, CA.)

adenomas are subclassified into a group of mostly epithelial and myoepithelial neoplasms that include basal cell adenomas, canalicular adenomas, oncocytomas or oxyphilic adenomas, and myoepitheliomas.

1. Basal Cell Adenomas

Basal cell adenomas account for 2% of all epithelial salivary gland neoplasms. Histologic types include tubular, trabecular, cylindroma, and solid; the latter is the most common variant. Basal cell adenomas occur equally between males and females and usually between the fourth and ninth decades of life. The parotid gland is the most common site involved.

A basal cell adenoma must be differentiated from adenoid cystic carcinoma, basal cell adenocarcinoma, and ameloblastoma.

2. Canalicular Adenomas

The canalicular adenoma is a benign neoplasm that affects the minor salivary glands. This tumor used to be a subtype of the basal cell adenoma; however, it is now recognized as a separate entity based on histologic features. It must also be differentiated from adenocarcinoma. The canalicular adenoma tends to be multifocal and often occurs in the upper lip mucosa, especially in the elderly. Complete intraoral excision is curative, although the multifocality of the disease can predispose to recurrence if all foci are not addressed.

3. Oncocytomas

These benign tumors are composed of large polyhedron-shaped epithelial cells, known as oncocytes, packed with granular eosinophilic cytoplasm and mitochondria. The cytoarchitecture of these tumors is best visualized with electron microscopy.

Oncocytomas account for < 1% of all salivary gland neoplasms. There is no gender predilection and they occur in the sixth to eighth decades of life. There remains debate on the pathogenesis of these tumors and whether they are true neoplasms; oncocytomas may result from a hyperplastic process, a metaplastic process, or both.

The parotid gland is the most common site of an oncocytoma, followed by the submandibular gland. In these sites, this tumor presents as a painless, slow-growing mass that is often solid and occasionally cystic. The swelling of the parotid gland may be diffuse with approximately 7% bilaterality. Multiple tumors have also been reported. Owing to the high mitochondrial content of the cells, radiosialography can demonstrate high uptake of technetium-99m.

The oncocytoma is easily distinguished from Warthin tumor and pleomorphic adenoma. However, it must also be considered separately from the mucoepidermoid carcinoma, acinic cell adenocarcinoma, adenoid cystic carcinoma, clear cell carcinoma, and metastatic renal cell or thyroid carcinoma. Surgical excision with uninvolved margins is the recommended treatment; oncocytomas are radioresistant.

4. Myoepitheliomas

This subtype of monomorphic adenomas accounts for less than 1% of all salivary gland neoplasms. It consists almost exclusively of myoepithelial cells. There is no gender predilection and myoepitheliomas are commonly seen in the third to sixth decades of life. The tumor occurs in the parotid gland 40% of the time.

Histologically, myoepitheliomas are well encapsulated. There are spindle cell and plasmacytoid cell types. The differential diagnoses include mixed tumor, schwannoma, leiomyoma, plasmacytoma, spindle cell carcinoma, and fibrous histiocytoma.

Mirza S, Dutt SN, Irving RM, Jones EL. Intraductal papilloma of the submandibular gland. *J Laryngol Otol.* 2000:114(6):481. [PMID: 0010962690] (Case report of intraductal papillomas in the submandibular gland; this entity is more commonly seen in the minor salivary glands.)

Toida M et al. Intraoral minor salivary gland tumors: a clinicopathological study of 82 cases. *Int J Oral Maxillofac Surg.* 2005;34(5):528. [PMID: 16053873]. (Retrospective study of 82 patients with intraoral minor salivary gland tumors at a university hospital.)

GRANULAR CELL TUMORS

The granular cell tumor is benign with malignant potential and is most commonly associated with the minor salivary glands. This tumor tends to occur in the oral cavity and is well circumscribed, mobile, and painless. Fine-needle aspiration can demonstrate a neoplastic process. A histopathologic examination shows polygonal cells with abundant eosinophilic granular cytoplasm and mildly pleomorphic nuclei that are round to oval-shaped. Because of its malignant potential, a combination of wide local excision and close observation is the most effective treatment.

Hughes JH, Volk EE, Seethala RR, LiVolsi VA, Baloch ZW. Relative accuracy of fine-needle aspiration and frozen section in the diagnosis of lesions of the parotid gland. *Head Neck.* 2005;27(3):217. [PMID: 15672359] (Clinical review of 220 cases of parotid gland fine-needle aspiration with histologic follow-up.)

Wilbur DC. Pitfalls in salivary gland fine-needle aspiration cytology. *Arch Pathol Lab Med.* 2005;129(1):26. [PMID: 15628905] (Data confirming the difficulty in interpreting cytology from salivary gland specimens to minimize diagnostic errors.)

HEMANGIOMAS

General Considerations

Although not of glandular origin, hemangiomas are significant in the differential diagnosis of a parotid mass, especially in children. These benign tumors are of endothelial cell origin and represent less than 5% of all salivary gland tumors. In children, the capillary hemangioma is the most common salivary gland tumor, accounting for more than 90% of parotid gland tumors in children less than 1 year of age. It affects females more than males and almost exclusively occurs in the parotid gland.

Clinical Findings

A hemangioma usually presents at birth as a unilateral, painless mass. It has a rapid, proliferative growth that often causes cosmetic deformity. Fine-needle aspiration is usually not necessary. CT scanning, MRI, or both may demonstrate the vascularity of the lesion. The differential diagnosis includes other vascular proliferative disorders such as lymphangioma and cavernous hemangioma.

Treatment

The possibility of spontaneous regression exists and therefore surgical excision may be delayed. However, if there is significant cosmetic or functional compromise, complete excision via parotidectomy with facial nerve preservation may be indicated. A caveat in children is the more superficial location of the facial nerve than that seen in adults, which is important to consider during intraoperative identification of the nerve. Malignant transformation has not been described.

Bentz BG, Hughes CA, Ludemman JP, Maddolozzo J. Masses of the salivary gland region in children. *Arch Otolaryngol Head Neck Surg.* 2000;126(12):1435. [PMID: 11115277] (A retrospective review of salivary masses in children demonstrating predominance of vascular lesion over solid tumors is presented.)

Zbaren P, Schar C, Hotz MA, Loosli H. Value of fine-needle aspiration cytology of parotid gland masses. *Laryngoscope.* 2001;111:1989. [PMID: 0011801984] (Fine-needle aspiration cytology is a valuable adjunct to preoperative assessment of parotid masses; it provides an 86% accuracy rate, a 64% sensitivity rate, and a specificity rate of 95%.)

Malignant Diseases of the Salivary Glands

18

Adriane P. Concus, MD, Tuyet-Phuong N. Tran, MD, & Mark D. DeLacure, MD

General Considerations

Malignant salivary gland neoplasms represent 3–4% of head and neck malignancies and < 0.5% of all cancers diagnosed yearly in the United States, with an incidence of only 1–2 per 100,000 individuals. Unlike the more common mucosal head and neck cancers, which, in general, are attributed to excessive tobacco and alcohol use, specific carcinogenic factors for malignant salivary gland growths have not been as clearly identified. Viral infections, radiation, environmental exposure, and genetic factors have been hypothesized as causes. Malignant salivary gland tumors are classified by the World Health Organization as carcinomas, nonepithelial tumors, lymphomas, metastatic or secondary tumors, and unclassified tumors (Table 18–1).

Only 20–25% of parotid gland neoplasms are malignant; approximately 45–50% of submandibular gland neoplasms, and > 70% of sublingual and minor salivary gland neoplasms are malignant. However, because 75–80% of salivary gland neoplasms are located in the parotid gland, this gland is still the most common salivary gland to be affected with a malignant neoplasm; a ratio of 40:10:1 is cited for malignant tumors of the parotid, submandibular, and sublingual glands, respectively.

Table 18–2 shows the histologic types of malignant salivary gland disease in order of frequency. The disease site also is important for predicting the histology. Mucoepidermoid carcinoma is most common in the parotid gland. Approximately half of malignant submandibular gland neoplasms are adenoid cystic carcinomas. Minor salivary gland malignant neoplasms are most often adenoid cystic carcinomas and adenocarcinomas. Prognosis varies according to histologic type, stage, and primary site.

Anatomy

The salivary gland unit is depicted in Figure 18–1. The acinus is located at the distal end of a salivary unit. It consists of pyramidal saliva-forming cells arranged around a central lumen, with myoepithelial cells interposed between the basal side of these cells and the basement membrane. Acinar cells may be serous, mucinous, or seromucinous, which explains the different chemical compositions of the saliva of each gland.

Serous cells predominate in the parotid glands. The submandibular glands have mixed populations of serous and mucinous acinar cells. The sublingual glands have mixed populations of mucinous and seromucinous cells. The minor salivary glands have mostly seromucinous cells. The acinus empties into an intercalated duct, composed of cuboidal cells similarly lined by myoepithelial cells between the basal side and the basal lamina. Intercalated ducts empty into striated ducts composed of columnar cells with fine striations. Lastly, the striated ducts empty into excretory ducts, which are composed of two layers of epithelial cells ranging in shape from cuboidal to squamous. Undifferentiated reserve cells associated with the intercalated ducts differentiate into acinar cells, intercalated duct cells, striated duct cells, and myoepithelial cells. Reserve cells associated with the excretory ducts give rise to excretory duct columnar and squamous cells.

Histologically, the salivary glands are arranged into lobules separated by connective tissue septa and encased in a connective tissue capsule; the salivary unit ducts converge in a treelike fashion into a central draining duct. Salivary gland lobules are made up of the acini, intercalated ducts, and small striated ducts. Larger striated ducts and excretory ducts are located within the connective tissue septa.

The major salivary glands are the paired parotid, submandibular, and sublingual glands. In addition, 600–1000 minor salivary glands are distributed throughout the rest of the upper aerodigestive tract.

The parotid gland is located anteroinferior to the ear, overlying the mandibular ramus and masseter muscle, extending medially between the mandibular ramus and the temporal bone to occupy the parapharyngeal space. The facial nerve travels through the substance of the parotid gland, dividing the gland into superficial and deep lobes, though this distinction is a convenience of surgical dissection and does not reflect an embryologic fusion plane or separate fascial layer. Malignant involvement of the facial nerve can result in facial weakness or paralysis and can provide an avenue for the

Table 18–1. World Health Organization classification of salivary gland malignant neoplasms.

Carcinomas
Mucoepidermoid carcinoma
Adenoid cystic carcinoma
Acinic cell carcinoma
Malignant mixed tumor
Carcinoma in pleomorphic adenoma
Carcinosarcoma
Polymorphous low-grade adenocarcinoma (terminal duct adenocarcinoma)
Epithelial-myoepithelial carcinoma
Salivary duct carcinoma
Basal cell carcinoma
Mucinous adenocarcinoma
Papillary cystadenocarcinoma
Adenocarcinoma, not otherwise specified (NOS)
Clear cell carcinoma
Sebaceous carcinoma and lymphadenocarcinoma
Oncocytic carcinoma
Malignant myoepithelioma (myoepithelial carcinoma)
Squamous cell carcinoma
Adenosquamous carcinoma
Lymphoepithelial carcinoma
Small cell carcinoma
Undifferentiated carcinoma
Other carcinomas
Tumors
Sarcoma
Malignant Lymphomas
Secondary Tumors
Melanoma
Squamous cell carcinoma
Renal cell carcinoma
Thyroid carcinoma
Unclassified Tumors

Modified, with permission, from Seifert G, Sobin LH: Histological typing of salivary gland tumours. In: *World Health Organization International Histological Classification of Tumours,* 2nd ed. New York, Berlin, Heidelberg: Springer-Verlag, 1991.

intracranial extension of tumor. In addition, the facial nerve is at risk for injury during parotid surgery. The lymphatic drainage of the parotid gland is to both intraparotid and periparotid lymph nodes, and locally

Table 18–2. Frequency of salivary gland malignant neoplasm by histologic type.

Histologic Type	Frequency of Occurrence
Mucoepidermoid carcinoma	34%
Adenoid cystic carcinoma	22%
Adenocarcinoma	18%
Malignant mixed tumor	13%
Acinic cell carcinoma	7%
Squamous cell carcinoma	4%
Other	< 3%

Modified, with permission, from Spiro RH. Salivary neoplasms: overview of a 35-year experience with 2,807 patients. *Head Neck Surg* 1986;8:177.

and regionally to the submandibular and deep jugular chain of nodes (levels I and II).

The submandibular glands are located in the submandibular triangle along with lymph nodes and branches of the facial artery and facial vein. The lingual, hypoglossal, and marginal mandibular nerves are all intimately associated with the submandibular gland. As with malignant disorders of the facial nerve and parotid gland, these nerves can be invaded by the cancer, resulting in paresis, paralysis, or numbness, as well as the intracranial extension of tumor. These nerves also are at risk for injury at the time of surgery. Submandibular gland lymphatics drain to the submandibular and deep jugular chain of nodes.

The sublingual glands are located deep in the anterior floor of mouth mucosa, adjacent to the submandibular glands. The sublingual gland lymphatics also drain to the submandibular and to the jugular chain of nodes.

Most of the minor salivary glands are located in the oral cavity and oropharynx, but minor salivary glands are distributed throughout the upper aerodigestive tract. The lymphatic drainage of the minor salivary glands is according to the lymphatic drainage of the anatomic location.

Pathogenesis

The **Reserve Cell Theory** (currently favored) of salivary gland neoplasia states that salivary neoplasms arise from reserve (or stem) cells of the salivary duct system. The type of neoplasm depends on the stage of differentiation of the reserve cell at the time at which the neoplastic transformation occurs; it also depends on the type of reserve cell. The intercalated duct reserve cells give rise to adenoid cystic and acinic cell carcinoma. The excretory duct reserve cells give rise to mucoepidermoid, squamous cell, and salivary duct carcinoma.

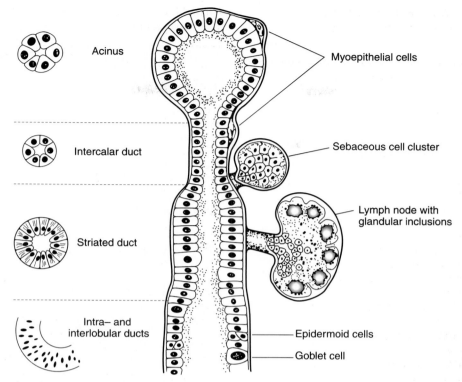

Figure 18–1. The salivary gland unit. (Adapted, with permission, from Thawley SE, Panje WR, Batsakis JG, Lindberg RD. *Comprehensive Management of Head and Neck Tumors.* Philadelphia: WB Saunders, 1999.)

The **Multicellular Theory** of salivary gland neoplasia states that salivary neoplasms arise from differentiated cells along the salivary gland unit. For example, squamous cell carcinoma arises from the excretory duct epithelium and acinic cell carcinoma arises from the acinar cells.

Batsakis JG, Regezi JA, Luna MA et al. Histogenesis of salivary gland neoplasms: a postulate with prognostic implications. *J Laryngol Otol.* 1989;103:939. [PMID: 2685148] (Classic article proposing the Reserve (Stem) Cell Theory of salivary gland histogenesis.)

Saku T, Hayashi Y, Takahara O et al. Salivary gland tumors among atomic bomb survivors, 1950–1987. *Cancer.* 1997;79(8):1465. [PMID: 9118025] (A look at Hiroshima and Nagasaki atomic bomb survivors and salivary gland neoplasms, supporting a role for ionizing radiation in salivary gland tumorigenesis.)

Staging

Table 18–3 lists the American Joint Committee on Cancer (AJCC) 2002 TNM (tumor, node, metastasis) Staging System used for malignant disorders of the major salivary glands. Malignant diseases of the minor salivary glands are staged according to the staging system for the primary site (oral cavity, pharynx, larynx, nasal cavity, and paranasal sinuses). For the first time, T4 tumors are divided into resectable (T4a) and unresectable (T4b) tumors, and, accordingly, Stage IV is now divided into IVA, IVB, and IVC (distant metastases present).

American Joint Committee on Cancer. Greene FL, Page DL, Fleming ID, Fritz AG, Balch CM, Haller DG, eds. *AJCC Cancer Staging Manual,* 6th ed. New York, Berlin, Heidelberg: Springer-Verlag, 2002. (The definitive reference for the currently used American Joint Committee on Cancer staging system.)

Clinical Findings

A. Symptoms and Signs

Patients with malignant disease of the salivary glands most often present with an incidentally noted mass. Pain, facial nerve palsy (although lingual and hypoglossal nerves can be affected by submandibular and sublingual tumors), and cervical adenopathy portend locally advanced disease and a poor prognosis. In the parotid gland, the superficial lobe refers to the parotid tissue lateral to the facial nerve and encompasses about two

Table 18–3. T (tumor), N (nodes), M (metastases) staging for major salivary gland (parotid, submandibular, sublingual) malignant neoplasms, 2002 revision.

Stage	T	N	M
I	T_1	N_0	M_0
II	T_2	N_0	M_0
III	T_3	N_0	M_0
	T_{1-3}	N_1	M_0
IVA	T_{1-3}	N_2	M_0
	T_{4a}	N_{0-2}	M_0
IVB	T_{4b}	Any N	M_0
	Any T	N_3	M_0
IVC	Any T	Any N	M_1

T_X	Primary tumor cannot be assessed
T_0	No evidence of primary tumor
T_1	Tumor ≤ 2 cm, no extraparenchymal extension
T_2	Tumor > 2 cm, ≤ 4 cm, no extraparenchymal extension
T_3	Tumor > 4 cm or extraparenchymal extension (or both)
T_{4a}	Tumor invades skin, mandible, ear canal, facial nerve, or any of these structures
T_{4b}	Tumor invades skull base or pterygoid plates, or encases carotid artery
N_X	Regional lymph node cannot be assessed
N_0	No cervical lymph node metastasis
N_1	Single ipsilateral lymph node < 3 cm
N_{2a}	Single ipsilateral lymph node metastases > 3 cm ≤ 6 cm
N_{2b}	Multiple ipsilateral lymph node metastases, each ≤ 6 cm
N_{2c}	Bilateral or contralateral lymph node metastases, each ≤ 6 cm
N_3	Single or multiple lymph node metastases > 6 cm
M_X	Distant metastasis cannot be assessed
M_0	No distant metastasis
M_1	Distant metastasis present

thirds of the gland parenchyma; the deep lobe refers to that which is medial, although there is no embryologic fascial plane between these two locations. Parotid gland tumors involving the deep lobe can have parapharyngeal space extension and present as a symptomatic or asymptomatic (usual) oropharyngeal mass with no palpable external abnormality. In the submandibular triangle, it can be difficult to distinguish between a mass in the submandibular gland itself and an enlarged submandibular lymph node. Malignant disease of the minor salivary glands is often submucosal and can be located anywhere throughout the upper aerodigestive tract.

B. LABORATORY FINDINGS

Fine-needle aspiration (FNA) biopsy of major salivary gland and neck masses is easily performed in the office. For malignant salivary gland neoplasms, FNA is 80–90% sensitive. Because the usual recommendation is for surgical removal of a salivary gland with any neoplasm, the cost-effectiveness of routinely performing FNA for salivary neoplasms is a matter of current debate.

C. IMAGING STUDIES

Computed tomography (CT) scanning and magnetic resonance imaging (MRI) are both effective modalities for imaging the size and the local and regional extension of malignant salivary gland growths, as well as highlighting potentially malignant cervical nodes. CT and MRI give more detailed information and are therefore preferred to ultrasound, which is also useful in identifying salivary gland masses as well as in distinguishing between solid and cystic masses. Positron emission tomography (PET) scanning is of use in evaluating metastatic or unknown primary site disease. Other nuclear medicine imaging that has been used for the salivary glands includes technetium radioisotope scanning, although this is more useful for benign Warthin tumors.

Batsakis JG, Sneige N, El-Naggar AK. Fine-needle aspiration of salivary glands: its utility and tissue effects. *Ann Otol Rhinol Laryngol.* 1992;101:185. [PMID: 1739267] (A look at the use of FNA biopsy in salivary gland neoplasms.)

Histologic Types

The classification of malignant salivary gland neoplasms and the relative incidence by histologic type has been listed in Tables 18–1 and 18–2. Malignant salivary gland disorders are further divided into low-grade, intermediate-grade, and high-grade histology based on clinical behavior and prognosis (Table 18–4). Below are descriptions of the more common histologic types.

A. MUCOEPIDERMOID CARCINOMA

Mucoepidermoid carcinoma is the most common type of malignant salivary gland disorder. Eighty to ninety percent of mucoepidermoid carcinoma occurs in the parotid gland. Its prevalence is highest in the fifth decade of life, with a female preponderance as high as 4:1. Histologically, mucoepidermoid carcinomas are characterized by a mixed population of cells: mucin-producing cells, epithelial cells, and intermediate cells

Table 18–4. Grade classification of salivary gland malignant neoplasms.

Low Grade
Low-grade mucoepidermoid carcinoma
Low-grade adenocarcinoma
Low-grade squamous cell carcinoma
Acinic cell carcinoma
Polymorphous low-grade adenocarcinoma
Basal cell carcinoma
Intermediate Grade
Intermediate-grade mucoepidermoid carcinoma
Intermediate-grade adenocarcinoma
Intermediate-grade squamous cell carcinoma
Adenoid cystic carcinoma
Epithelial-myoepithelial carcinoma
Oncocytic carcinoma
Myoepithelial carcinoma
Carcinoma in pleomorphic adenoma
Salivary duct carcinoma
High Grade
High-grade mucoepidermoid carcinoma
High-grade adenocarcinoma
High-grade squamous cell carcinoma
Carcinosarcoma
Undifferentiated carcinoma

Reprinted, with permission, from Therkildsen MH, Christensen M, Andersen LJ et al. Salivary gland carcinomas prognostic factors. *Acta Oncol* 1998;37:701.

(Figure 18–2). The intermediate cells are believed to be the progenitor of the other two types of cells. No myoepithelial cells are present.

Mucoepidermoid carcinomas are classified as low, intermediate, and high grade based on clinical behavior and tumor differentiation. Clinical aggressiveness, local invasion, and lymph node metastases are all greater, and the prognosis is worst for high-grade tumors. Histologically, low-grade mucoepidermoid carcinomas are well circumscribed, with pushing margins and dilated cystic areas containing mucinous material. The cystic structures are lined by mucin-producing, intermediate, or epidermoid cells. As the grade escalates, the tumors become more infiltrative and poorly circumscribed. Cystic formations seen in low-grade tumors are lost. Nests of tumor become more solid and irregular with intermediate or epidermoid cells dominating. High-grade mucoepidermoid carcinomas are characterized by the invasion of adjacent normal structures, atypical mitoses, perineural invasion, and lymph node metastases. High-grade

mucoepidermoid carcinoma is distinguished from squamous cell carcinoma by the presence of intracellular mucin.

The 5-year survival rate for low-grade mucoepidermoid carcinomas is 70%, whereas for high grade it is only 47%. The 15-year disease-free survival rate is approximately 50% for low-grade mucoepidermoid carcinoma and 25% for intermediate- and high-grade tumors.

B. ADENOID CYSTIC CARCINOMA

Ten percent of salivary gland neoplasms are adenoid cystic carcinoma. More than two thirds of them arise from the minor salivary glands. Adenoid cystic carcinoma is the most common type of malignant disorder to arise in the submandibular, the sublingual, and the minor salivary glands. It occurs with equal frequency in men and women and most often presents as an otherwise asymptomatic mass.

Adenoid cystic carcinoma is usually partially or nonencapsulated and infiltrates the surrounding normal tissue. There is basaloid epithelium clustered in nests in a hyaline stroma. The most common histologic subtype (44%) is the cribriform type, characterized by a "Swiss cheese" pattern of vacuolated areas (Figure 18–3A). The prognosis for the cribriform subtype is intermediate. The tubular subtype (35%) carries the best prognosis and is characterized by cords and nests of malignant cells (Figure 18–3B). The solid subtype (21%) has the worst prognosis and is characterized by solid sheets of adenoid malignant cells (Figure 18–3C).

Adenoid cystic carcinomas are unique among salivary gland tumors because of their indolent and protracted clinical course. Perineural spread, including "skip lesions" or discontinuous areas of spread along a nerve, occurs commonly (up to 80% of cases). For this reason, adjuvant radiation that includes the anatomic course of the regional named nerves is often recommended. Lymphatic spread is uncommon, and consequently neck dissection or wide-field radiation to regional lymphatics is rarely recommended. Distant metastases can occur up to 20 years after the initial diagnosis; disease-specific survival continues to decline for more than 20 years after the initial treatment. Prognostic factors for adenoid cystic carcinoma include site of origin, TNM staging, local spread, nodal status, distant metastasis, and recurrence. The survival rate among patients with adenoid cystic carcinomas arising from the parotid gland is higher than that for patients with similar tumors arising from the minor salivary glands.

C. ACINIC CELL CARCINOMA

Acinic cell carcinoma represents 15% of malignant parotid gland neoplasms. Eighty to ninety percent occur in the

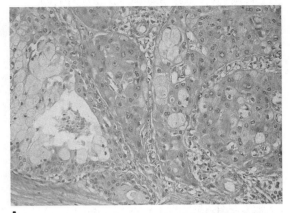

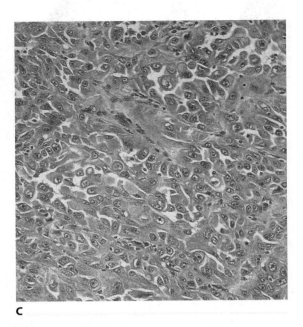

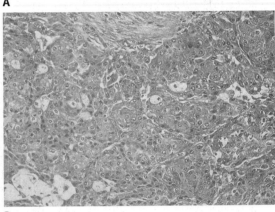

Figure 18–2. Mucoepidermoid carcinoma. **(A)** Low grade, **(B)** intermediate grade, and **(C)** high grade. (Reprinted, with permission, from Wenig BM. *Atlas of Head and Neck Pathology*. Philadelphia: WB Saunders, 1993.)

parotid gland, and most of the remaining occur in the sub-mandibular gland. Acinic cell carcinoma occurs most often in the fifth decade of life and in women more often than in men.

Acinic cell carcinomas are typically encased in a fibrous capsule. Histologically, there are two cell types: (1) serous acinar cells (explaining the predilection for the parotid gland) and (2) cells with clear cytoplasm (Figure 18–4). There are four histologic patterns: solid, micro-cystic, papillary, and follicular.

Acinic cell carcinomas are low-grade malignancies. The overall survival rate at 5, 10, and 15 years is 78%, 63%, and 44%, respectively.

D. MALIGNANT MIXED TUMORS

Malignant mixed tumors represent 3–12% of malignant salivary gland disorders. They arise in benign mixed tumors (pleomorphic adenomas). Microscopically, there may be one small malignant growth within a benign mixed tumor, or the benign tumor may be essentially replaced by the malignant lesion with destructive infiltra-tive growth.

Carcinoma ex-pleomorphic adenoma is the most common malignant mixed tumor variant (Figure 18–5A); 75% occur in the parotid gland. Histologically, there is a mixture of epithelial and mesenchymal cells, but the dis-tinguishing feature is that the malignant component is purely epithelial. The malignant part may have features of an adenocarcinoma, a squamous cell carcinoma, an undifferentiated carcinoma, or some other form of a malignant epithelial disorder. Carcinoma ex-pleomor-phic adenomas are nodular or cystic with minimal encap-sulation. Unlike pleomorphic adenomas, they typically have areas of necrosis and hemorrhage.

A true malignant mixed tumor, also called carcinosar-coma, is very rare (Figure 18–5B). It has epithelial and mesenchymal malignant elements in both the primary site and in nodal metastases.

Malignant mixed tumors are classified as high grade. If treated before they become invasive, the prognosis is

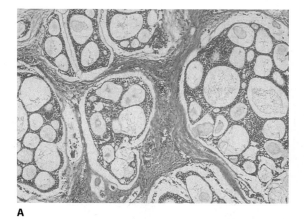

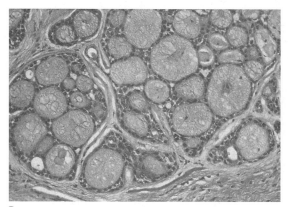

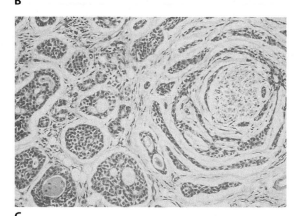

Figure 18–3. Adenoid cystic carcinoma. **(A)** Cribriform pattern and **(B)** cribriform and tubular growth pattern, **(C)** solid subtype. (Reprinted, with permission, from Wenig BM. *Atlas of Head and Neck Pathology.* Philadelphia: WB Saunders, 1993.)

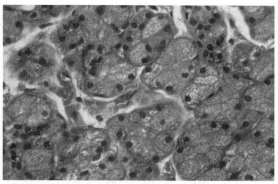

Figure 18–4. Acinic cell carcinoma. (Reprinted, with permission, from Wenig BM. *Atlas of Head and Neck Pathology.* Philadelphia: WB Saunders, 1993.)

good. However, invasion and locoregional and distant metastases are common. Surgery with adjuvant radiation is the preferred treatment. Nonetheless, the 5-year survival rate is < 10%.

E. ADENOCARCINOMA

Adenocarcinomas of the major salivary glands originate from excretory or striated ducts. In its most differentiated form, the glandular cytoarchitecture is maintained. The growth pattern can be solid or cystic, papillary or nonpapillary, with or without mucin production, and can range from low grade to high grade in histology and clinical course. With newer refinements in special staining and classification systems, many malignant disorders formerly categorized as adenocarcinomas have defined their own categories, including polymorphous low-grade adenocarcinoma, epithelial-myoepithelial carcinoma, and salivary duct carcinoma. Adenocarcinomas of the salivary glands not fitting into one of the more specific classifications are called *adenocarcinoma NOS* (not otherwise specified). Clinically, poor prognostic indicators for adenocarcinomas include advanced stage, infiltrative growth pattern, and abnormal DNA content.

F. POLYMORPHOUS LOW-GRADE ADENOCARCINOMA

Polymorphous low-grade adenocarcinoma is also termed terminal duct carcinoma or lobular carcinoma and is the second most common malignant disorder of the minor salivary glands. Fifty percent of polymorphous low-grade adenocarcinomas occur in the palate. Women are affected more often than men, typically in the sixth decade.

Polymorphous low-grade adenocarcinoma most often presents as a painless, submucosal mass. There is cytologic uniformity of myoepithelial or luminal ductal cells within one tumor, but histologic diversity of the

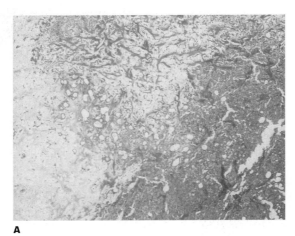 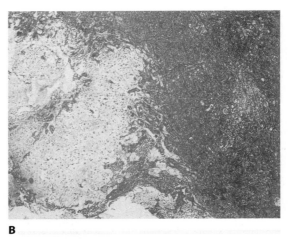

A **B**

Figure 18–5. Malignant mixed tumors. **(A)** Carcinoma ex-pleomorphic adenoma and **(B)** carcinosarcoma. (Reprinted, with permission, from Wenig BM. *Atlas of Head and Neck Pathology.* Philadelphia: WB Saunders, 1993.)

cells between tumors (Figure 18–6). Patterns of growth include tubular, papillary, glandular, and solid. Despite infiltrative growth and perineural invasion, the clinical course is typically indolent, with < 10% having lymph node metastases.

G. EPITHELIAL-MYOEPITHELIAL CELL CARCINOMA

Epithelial-myoepithelial cell carcinoma represents only 1% of salivary gland neoplasms. Most occur in the parotid gland. Histologically, there are malignant epithelial (ductal) cells and also malignant myoepithelial cells (Figure 18–7). Cribriform, tubular, or solid patterns can be formed.

Forty percent of patients experience local recurrence, 20% experience cervical metastases, and 40% die of disease.

H. SALIVARY DUCT ADENOCARCINOMA

Salivary duct adenocarcinoma is named for its histologic resemblance to intraductal carcinoma of the breast (Figure 18–8). Unlike intraductal carcinoma of the breast, this disease occurs in men three times more frequently than in women. This malignant disorder arises from the excretory duct reserve cells and is a high-grade malignant disease process with a dismal prognosis. Thirty-five percent of patients have local recurrence;

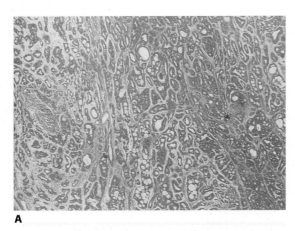 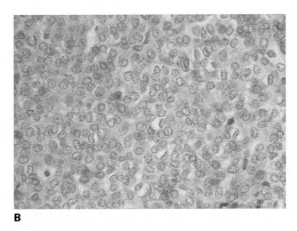

A **B**

Figure 18–6. Polymorphous low-grade adenocarcinoma. **(A)** Low power and **(B)** high power. (Reprinted, with permission, from Wenig BM. *Atlas of Head and Neck Pathology.* Philadelphia: WB Saunders, 1993.)

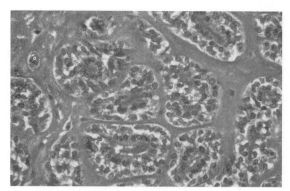

Figure 18–7. Epithelial-myoepithelial carcinoma. (Reprinted, with permission, from Wenig BM. *Atlas of Head and Neck Pathology*. Philadelphia: WB Saunders, 1993.)

62% develop distant metastases; 77% die of disease, with a mean survival of 3 years.

I. CLEAR CELL CARCINOMA

Clear cell carcinomas arise in the minor salivary glands, usually in the oral cavity. Histopathologically, trabeculae, cords, and nests of monomorphic clear cells are seen. They are glycogen-rich, but mucin-negative. This is a low-grade tumor.

J. SQUAMOUS CELL CARCINOMA

Squamous cell carcinoma (SCC) of the salivary gland is rare (Figure 18–9). Debate exists as to whether or not true primary SCC of the salivary glands exists. High-grade mucoepidermoid carcinoma must be excluded. The distinction is made with special immunohistochemical staining for mucin, which is positive in mucoepidermoid carci-

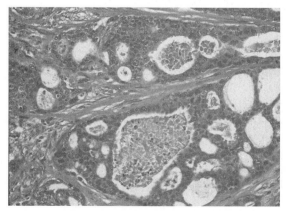

Figure 18–8. Salivary duct carcinoma. (Reprinted, with permission, from Wenig BM. *Atlas of Head and Neck Pathology*. Philadelphia: WB Saunders, 1993.)

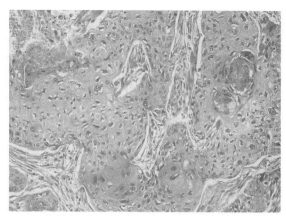

Figure 18–9. Squamous cell carcinoma. (Reprinted, with permission, from Wenig BM. *Atlas of Head and Neck Pathology*. Philadelphia: WB Saunders, 1993.)

noma but not in SCC. Metastases to the parotid gland or the direct extension of SCC from the overlying skin must also be considered. Most SCCs of the salivary glands present in advanced stage and > 50% of the time have nodal metastases at diagnosis.

K. LYMPHOMA

Salivary gland lymphoma arises from intraglandular lymph nodes or from extranodal lymphoid tissue within the salivary glands. Patients are typically in their sixth or seventh decade. Ninety percent occur in the parotid gland. Five percent of extranodal lymphomas affect the salivary glands. The majority of salivary gland lymphomas are of B-cell lineage. Upon the diagnosis of a salivary gland lymphoma, a full-body evaluation for other involved sites is performed, as with a new diagnosis of lymphoma anywhere else in the body.

There is an association between Sjögren's disease and salivary gland lymphoma, with the risk of developing a salivary gland lymphoma being 44 times higher in patients with Sjögren's disease than in the general population. The prognosis for a lymphoma associated with Sjögren's disease is worse than for salivary gland lymphoma not associated with this disease.

Some salivary gland lymphomas are immunohistochemically indistinguishable from low-grade lymphomas of the mucosa-associated lymphoid tissue (MALT) and are therefore termed salivary gland MALT lymphomas. Like the gastrointestinal tract MALT lymphomas, salivary gland MALT lymphoma is an indolent disease and affected patients have a long survival.

L. METASTASES TO THE SALIVARY GLANDS

Less than 10% of malignant salivary gland disorders are metastases from other sites. Most are lymphatic metastases to the parotid gland from skin cancers of the face, ear, or scalp. These are evenly divided between SCC and melanoma; the likelihood of metastasis depends on the stage/depth of the primary lesion. Hematogenous metastases to the salivary glands are rare, but have been reported from lung, kidney, breast, and thyroid cancers. The contiguous extension of cutaneous malignant disorders, as well as those of sarcomas arising from the facial soft tissues, is another mechanism for secondary malignant involvement of the salivary glands.

M. MALIGNANT SALIVARY GLAND NEOPLASMS IN CHILDREN

Mucoepidermoid carcinoma is the most common malignant salivary gland neoplasm in children, followed by acinic cell carcinoma. Eighty-five percent of malignant salivary gland disorders in children occur in the parotid gland.

Khafif A et al. Adenoid cystic carcinoma of the salivary glands: a 20-year review with long-term follow-up. *Ear Nose Throat J.* 2005;84(10):662,664. [PMID: 16382750] (Review of an institution's experience and analysis of prognostic indicators in patients with adenoid cystic carcinoma.)

Seifert G, Sobin LH. Histological typing of salivary gland tumours. In: *The World Health Organization Histological Classification of Tumours.* 2nd ed. New York, Berlin, Heidelberg: Springer-Verlag, 1991. (The WHO classification of salivary gland neoplasms.)

Westra WH. The surgical pathology of salivary gland neoplasms. *Otolaryngol Clin North Am.* 1999;32(5):919. [PMID: 10477796] (Review of the cellular and morphologic features of the most common salivary gland neoplasms.)

Treatment

A. SURGICAL MEASURES

Surgery with the complete removal of the tumor, including a cuff of histologically normal tissue for adequate margins, is the mainstay of treatment for both major and minor salivary gland malignancies.

1. Surgery for major salivary gland malignant neoplasms—For malignant parotid gland tumors, a total parotidectomy (or an extended parotidectomy if the tumor extends into surrounding structures) is recommended. The facial nerve is sacrificed if it is directly involved with the tumor (ie, encased in the tumor, unable to be dissected from tumor, paretic, or paralyzed preoperatively). In patients whose facial nerve is intact but the margins of resection are close to the nerve, postoperative adjuvant radiation should be considered because it has been shown to significantly improve local control. The typical surgical approach is through a Blair or modified Blair-type incision. For malignant disorders of the parotid gland with parapharyngeal space extension, surgery must include parapharyngeal space (or infratemporal fossa) dissection, sometimes requiring a submandibular or even a mandibulotomy-mandibulectomy approach. A lateral temporal bone resection may be required as well if the ear canal is involved.

For malignant disease of the submandibular and sublingual glands, formal supraomohyoid neck dissection is preferred over a simple gland excision. As with the facial nerve in parotidectomy, the lingual, hypoglossal, and marginal mandibular nerves are preserved unless there is evidence either preoperatively or intraoperatively of their direct involvement by the tumor.

2. Surgery for minor salivary gland malignant neoplasms—For malignant growths of the minor salivary glands, wide local excision is recommended. This approach may be extensive, even including a skull base resection, depending on the location, size, and extension of the tumor. Tumors involving the maxillary sinus and nasal cavity may require partial or total maxillectomy. If the ethmoid is involved with extra-sinus extension, craniofacial resection, orbital exenteration, or both may be required for more extensive tumors. A transoral or combined transoral-transcervical approach is used for malignant neoplasms of the minor salivary glands that affect the oral cavity and oropharynx. A partial or total laryngectomy or even tracheal resection is required for minor salivary gland tumors involving the larynx or trachea.

3. Neck dissection—Neck dissection is the recommended treatment of the neck for malignant salivary gland tumors (1) with clinically apparent cervical adenopathy (14% of cases); (2) for tumors > 4 cm (in which the risk of occult metastases is > 20%); or (3) for a high-grade histology (in which the risk of occult metastases is > 40%) (Table 18–5). Elective neck dissection for adenoid cystic carcinoma generally is not recommended, because the risk of occult nodal metastasis is low.

B. NONSURGICAL MEASURES

1. Radiation therapy—Both conventional and neutron-beam radiation therapy have been advocated as

Table 18–5. Incidence of occult lymph node involvement for salivary gland malignant neoplasms.

Salivary Gland Neoplasm	Incidence
Squamous cell carcinoma	40%
Adenocarcinoma	18%
Mucoepidermoid carcinoma	14%
Acinic cell carcinoma	4%
Adenoid cystic carcinoma	4%
Tumor < 4 cm	4%
Tumor > 4 cm	> 20%

single-modality treatments for T1 and T2 malignant salivary gland neoplasms. This approach is controversial, but may be considered if there are real contraindications to surgery.

Adjuvant radiation to the tumor resection bed improves local control for (1) T3 and T4 tumors; (2) tumors of high-grade histology (see Table 18–4); (3) positive nodes or perilymphatic invasion; (4) facial or other perineural involvement; (5) a close or positive surgical margin; (6) bone, cartilage, or muscle invasion; or (7) recurrent disease. The standard radiation therapy used is a unilateral mixed electron and photon technique. Postoperative radiation to the neck is recommended, as above, for major and certain minor salivary gland primary sites when there are positive neck nodes. Radiation is an acceptable alternative for a node-negative (ie, N0) neck with aggressive features (see indications for neck dissection). For minor salivary gland tumors, elective radiation of the N0 neck is advocated only for primary tumors of the tongue, floor of mouth, pharynx, and larynx. Conventional radiation has been shown to have prohibitively poor local control rates for inoperable disease.

Neutron-beam radiation has been shown to be more effective than conventional radiation against malignant salivary gland disorders; it results in a higher degree of tumor destruction with fewer toxic effects to surrounding normal tissues. In particular, neutron-beam radiation protocols have been more successful than conventional radiation in treating adenoid cystic carcinoma. Neutron-beam therapy can achieve excellent locoregional control, higher than mixed beam and photons in advanced, recurrent, as well as incompletely resected salivary neoplasms. It is also the preferred treatment for inoperable disease. Fast neutron therapy is not widely available.

2. Chemotherapy—The role for chemotherapy in the treatment of malignant salivary gland disorders is limited to the palliative setting, such as in advanced-stage or metastatic disease not amenable to local therapies including surgery and/or radiation. Partial or complete responses have been achieved in up to 50% of patients, which typically last 5–8 months and may include significant pain control. Most of these patients have adenoid cystic carcinoma, mucoepidermoid carcinoma, or high-grade adenocarcinoma. Currently, paclitaxel is the agent used most frequently. Although chemotherapy alone does not improve survival rates, the integration of radiation and chemotherapy has been shown to increase local control and represents an improvement in the management of salivary gland malignancies.

C. TREATMENT OF RECURRENCE

Recurrent, malignant salivary gland tumors are treated with the same guidelines as for primary disease. Neu-

tron-beam radiation can, in selected cases, be used when previous external beam radiation has already been administered.

D. COMPLICATIONS OF TREATMENT

The complications of the treatment of salivary gland tumors include complications of surgery and those of radiation therapy.

1. Complications related to surgery—Facial nerve (or other nerve) paralysis, hematoma, salivary fistula or sialocele, Frey syndrome, and cosmetic deformity are among the surgical complications.

2. Complications related to radiation therapy—Complications of radiation include acute mucositis, trismus and fibrosis, osteoradionecrosis, and impairment of vision. Since most radiation protocols for malignant salivary gland neoplasms involve unilateral treatment, xerostomia occurs less often than in the treatment of other upper aerodigestive tract tumors.

Cortesina G, Airoldi M, Palonta F. Current role of chemotherapy in exclusive and integrated treatment of malignant tumours of salivary glands. *Acta Otorhinolaryngol Ital.* 2005;25(3):179. [PMID: 16450774] (A look at the role of chemotherapy in the treatment of salivary gland malignancies.)

Douglas JG et al. Treatment of salivary gland neoplasms with fast neutron radiotherapy. *Arch Otolaryngol Head Neck Surg.* 2003;129 (9):944. [PMID: 12975266] (The University of Washington experience with and their evaluation of the efficacy of neutron-beam radiotherapy for adenoid cystic carcinoma.)

Huber PE et al. Radiotherapy for advanced adenoid cystic carcinoma: neutrons, photons or mixed beam? *Radiother Oncol.* 2001;59(2):161. [PMID: 11325445] (Comparison of the different radiotherapeutic treatments of advanced adenoid cystic carcinomas.)

Laurie SA, Licitra L. Systemic therapy in the palliative management of advanced salivary gland cancers. *J Clin Oncol.* 2006;24 (17):2673. [PMID: 16763282] (Review of the role of chemotherapy in advanced salivary gland malignancy of different histologies.)

Prott FJ, Micke O, Haverkamp U et al. Results of fast neutron therapy of adenoid cystic carcinoma of the salivary glands. *Anticancer Res.* 2000;20(5C):3743. [PMID: 11268448] (The University of Munster experience with neutron-beam radiotherapy and adenoid cystic carcinoma.)

Spiro JD, Spiro RH. Cancer of the parotid gland: role of 7th nerve preservation. *World J Surg.* 2003; 27(7):863. [PMID: 14509520] (A look at the management of the facial nerve in surgeries for parotid malignancies.)

Spiro RH. Management of malignant tumors of the salivary glands. *Oncol.* 1998;12(5):671. [PMID: 9597678] (Review of treatment guidelines for malignant neoplasms of the salivary glands.)

Prognosis

The indicators of a poor prognosis for malignant salivary gland tumors include pain, facial or other nerve involvement, high-grade histology, the invasion of skin

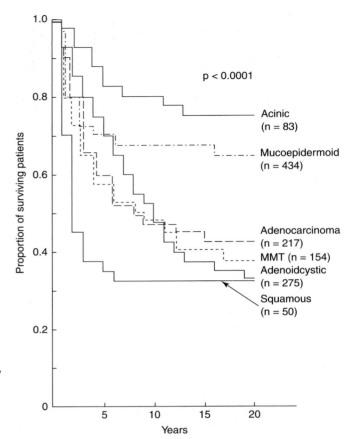

p < 0.0001

Acinic
(n = 83)

Mucoepidermoid
(n = 434)

Adenocarcinoma
(n = 217)
MMT (n = 154)
Adenoidcystic
(n = 275)
Squamous
(n = 50)

Figure 18–10. Kaplan-Meier survival curve for malignant salivary gland disorders, subdivided by histologic type. (Adapted, with permission, from Spiro RH. Salivary neoplasms: overview of a 35-year experience with 2,807 patients. *Head Neck Surg.* 1986;8:177.)

and other surrounding tissues, the presence of cervical or distant metastases, and recurrent disease. For major salivary gland tumors, distant metastases occur most often in adenoid cystic carcinoma and undifferentiated carcinoma. The lungs, liver, bone, and brain are the most common sites. Survival varies greatly with both histologic type and the initial stage. For example, malignant mixed tumors with distant metastases portend a very poor patient survival; whereas survival of more than 10 years has been reported for adenoid cystic carcinoma with distant metastases. For this reason, treatment of the primary adenoid cystic tumor and its metastatic sites is warranted. Figure 18–10 shows sur-

vival curves, subdivided by histologic type, for major and minor salivary gland tumors.

Carinci F, Farina A, Pelucchi S et al. Parotid gland carcinoma: 1987 and 1997 UICC T classifications compared for prognostic accuracy at 5 years. *Eur Arch Otorhinolaryngol.* 2001;258(3):150. [PMID: 11374257] (The 1997 T-staging found to be of greater prognostic value than the earlier 1987 T-staging system for malignant parotid lesions.)

Regis de Brito Santos I, Kowalski LP, Cavalcante de Araujo V et al. Multivariate analysis of risk factors for neck metastases in surgically treated parotid carcinomas. *Arch Otolaryngol Head Neck Surg.* 2001;127(1):56. [PMID: 11177015] (Identified risk factors for neck metastasis in parotid carcinoma include histologic type and T stage.)

SECTION VI
Oral Cavity, Oropharynx, & Nasopharynx

Cleft Lip & Palate

William Y. Hoffman, MD

In large series, the distribution of clefts is about 50% cleft lip and palate, 30% cleft palate only, and 20% cleft lip only. Cleft lip occurs most often on the left side; the distribution of left to right to bilateral cleft lip is approximately 6:3:1. Right-sided clefts are more commonly associated with syndromes. There is a slightly higher incidence in males.

Modern ultrasound can identify cleft lip by the absence of muscle fibers crossing the lip. Specific efforts must be made to obtain a frontal view to make a prenatal diagnosis. Newer ultrasounds have increasing accuracy. Although fetal surgery for clefts is not yet feasible in humans, prenatal diagnosis makes it possible to counsel parents earlier and prepare them for the care that their new child will require (Figure 19–1).

EMBRYOLOGY

It is important to remember the embryology of clefting; the primary palate includes the lip and premaxilla, whereas the secondary palate extends from the incisive foramen back. The lip and alveolus are formed by the fusion of the frontonasal process and the lateral maxillary processes; this fusion is reinforced by the migration of mesenchymal tissue derived from neuroectoderm (Figure 19–2). The stabilization of neuroectoderm by folate during the first trimester of pregnancy has been shown to reduce the incidence of clefting as well as that of other neural crest defects such as myelomeningocele.

ANATOMY

An understanding of the anatomic derangements is critical to proper repair. In the cleft lip, the orbicularis oris muscle is interrupted, and the remnants of the muscle adjacent to the cleft flow toward the upper portion of the cleft, at the base of the columella medially and at the alar base laterally. Incomplete clefts have variable amounts of muscle intact across the upper portion of the lip. In bilateral complete clefts, there is no muscle in the central portion (the prolabium).

Normally, the levator palatini muscle forms a sling that elevates the soft palate and excludes the nasopharynx from the oropharynx during speech and swallowing. In the cleft palate, the levator muscle is oriented longitudinally, parallel with the cleft margin. This abnormal orientation of the muscle is even seen in submucous cleft palate, when the mucosa is intact (Figure 19–3). The most recent techniques of cleft palate repair incorporate reorientation of the levator muscle as part of the repair, which contributes to the improved speech results seen today.

The tensor palatini muscle is also abnormally oriented, more longitudinally than normal; this results in inadequate opening of the eustachian tube in children with cleft palate. It also explains the high incidence of serous otitis media seen in these children; almost all children with clefts require myringotomy and tube placement in early development. As they grow, the eustachian tube develops stronger cartilaginous support and the need for ventilating tubes is generally outgrown.

CLASSIFICATION

Clefts are generally classified as complete or incomplete. **Complete cleft lip** implies a separation of the lip that extends through the nasal sill and the alveolus into the

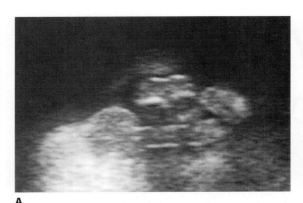
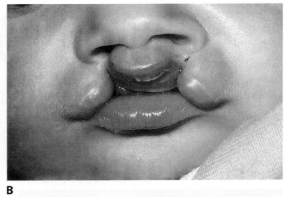

A **B**

Figure 19–1. **(A)** Ultrasound of a child with bilateral cleft, incomplete on the left. **(B)** Photo of the same child post-natally before lip repair.

palate. **Incomplete cleft lip** may present as a cleft of variable width with an intact bridge of skin below the nasal sill, known as a Simonart's band. At the other end of the spectrum is the **forme fruste** or **microform cleft lip,** which may be as little as a small notch in the ver-milion (Figure 19–4).

Clefts may also be **unilateral** or **bilateral.** As with unilateral clefts, bilateral clefts may be complete or incomplete, and these variants may be different on the two sides. In a complete bilateral cleft, the central portion of the alveolus, the premaxilla, is attached only to the nasal septum and the central lip or prolabium is attached only to the premaxilla and the columella. These cases pose a particular problem because the premaxilla

migrates anteriorly and can be virtually horizontal in orientation. The premaxilla must be brought down into a closer relationship with the lateral segments in order to achieve a bilateral cleft lip repair (Figure 19–5).

Complete cleft palate occurs in association with complete cleft lip, whereas **incomplete cleft palate** refers to a cleft of the secondary palate only. As with the lip, the presentation of incomplete clefts has a great deal of variability, from a wide cleft of the palate extending all the way forward to the incisive foramen, to a narrow cleft of the posterior portion of the soft palate. The **submucous cleft palate** represents a specific entity with separation of the levator palatini muscles but intact mucosa.

A **B**

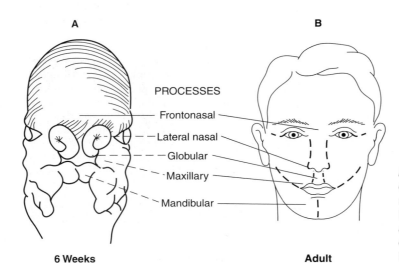

PROCESSES

— Frontonasal —
— Lateral nasal —
— Globular —
— Maxillary —
— Mandibular —

6 Weeks **Adult**

Figure 19–2. Diagram of a 6-week-old embryo. The frontonasal process will give rise to the central lip and premaxilla, the lateral nasal process will develop into the alae of the nose, and the maxillary processes will produce the lateral lip and maxillary segments.

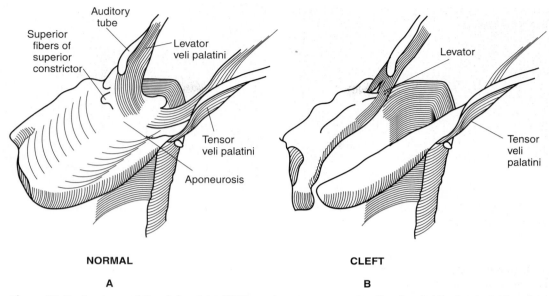

Figure 19–3. Anatomy of the cleft palate. **(A)** Normal anatomy; note the sling formed by the two sides of the levator palatini muscle. **(B)** Cleft palate; the levator muscle is oriented longitudinally, somewhat parallel with the cleft margin.

SYNDROMES

Literally hundreds of congenital syndromes include clefting as one manifestation of a genetic abnormality. Together, these make up < 20% of all clefts; those not associated with a syndrome are generally referred to as "isolated" clefts.

1. Velocardiofacial Syndrome

Velocardiofacial syndrome, or **Shprintzen syndrome,** is associated with a deletion at the 21p locus. This is the

same locus involved in the DiGeorge syndrome, and there may be overlap with this syndrome of B-cell dysfunction. As the name implies, affected children have clefts (usually of the palate only), cardiac anomalies, and characteristic facial appearance. There may be velopharyngeal insufficiency in the absence of any cleft. Children with velocardiofacial syndrome have a developmental delay that may contribute to problems with speech. It is possible to test for the genetic deletion with **fluorescent in situ hybridization** (ie, FISH testing).

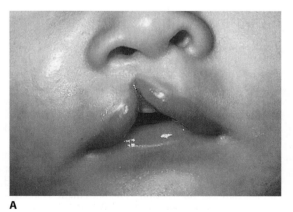
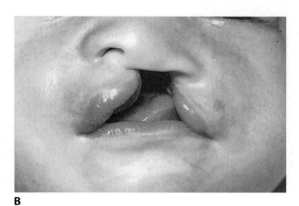

Figure 19–4. Examples of unilateral cleft lip. **(A)** Incomplete cleft. **(B)** Complete unilateral cleft lip.

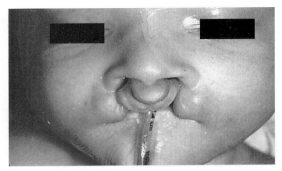

A

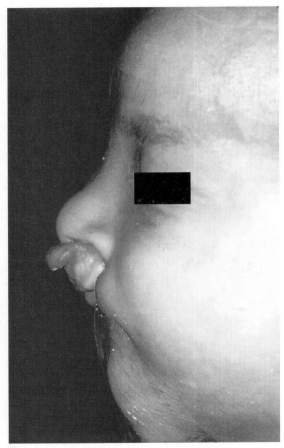

B

Figure 19–5. Bilateral complete cleft lip. **(A)** Antero-posterior view. The central portion, the prolabium, is of fairly good size in this example. **(B)** Lateral view. Note the short columella and the anterior displacement of the prolabium and premaxilla due to the interruption of the orbicularis oris muscle.

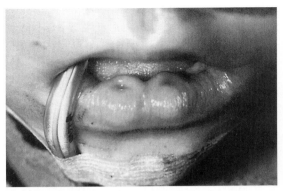

Figure 19–6. Van der Woude syndrome. This child has only a cleft palate, but the expression is variable and can include complete cleft lip and palate as well. The lip pits (sinus tracts of minor salivary glands) in this patient are particularly prominent.

2. Van der Woude Syndrome

Van der Woude syndrome is an association of clefting with lower lip sinus tracts, known as **lip pits.** This syndrome is notable for autosomal dominant inheritance and for variable penetrance; even within a single family, affected children may have different presentations (Figure 19–6).

3. Stickler Syndrome

Stickler syndrome is an association between clefts and ocular abnormalities, including fairly severe myopia presenting at an early age, as well as retinal abnormalities. Generally, an examination by a pediatric ophthalmologist is recommended for children with clefts to make or rule out the diagnosis in the first year of life.

PIERRE ROBIN SEQUENCE

Pierre Robin syndrome is characterized by a triad of retrogenia, retrodisplacement of the tongue, and respiratory insufficiency. Most children with this syndrome also have clefts of the secondary palate, which are characteristically U-shaped clefts that are quite wide. The breathing difficulties seen in Pierre Robin sequence arise from posterior positioning of the tongue and upper posterior pharyngeal obstruction (Figure 19–7).

In most cases, the respiratory obstruction is seen immediately in the neonatal period. Turning the infant to the prone position may move the tongue forward and alleviate the obstruction. The placement of a nasogastric feeding tube permits better nutrition and also breaks the seal of the tongue against the posterior pharyngeal wall. Various types of oral airways have been

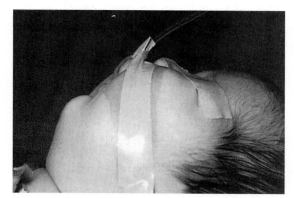

Figure 19–7. Pierre Robin sequence. Note the extremely retruded chin in this child, who is being prepared for surgical tongue-lip adhesion.

used as temporizing measures to keep the tongue down and forward. Over time, the mandible grows forward in most cases and the problem improves.

If conservative measures fail in the neonatal period, surgical intervention is warranted. The goal of surgery is to avoid infant tracheostomy, which remains the final resort in these cases. **Tongue-lip plication,** or **glossopexy,** is a simple procedure that requires an incision in the tongue just below the tip and in the wet vermilion of the lower lip; the two mucosal incisions are closed along with a retention suture that is tied over two buttons on the tongue and in the lower chin. Recently, bone distraction has been used in the infant mandible to elongate the ramus and bring the tongue forward with the mandible; there are no long-term outcomes from these cases and the effects of such early intervention remain unknown. The tongue-lip adhesion has been successful in about 80% of cases in large series; thus, the use of mandibular distraction would be very rare.

SUBMUCOUS CLEFT PALATE

Submucous cleft palate represents a special subset of clefts that remains confusing both in diagnosis and treatment. The diagnosis is made by the findings of the classic triad of a bifid uvula, central thinning of the soft palate, and a palpable notch in the posterior border of the hard palate (normally the location of the posterior nasal spine). Anatomically, there is the same separation of the levator palatini muscle that is seen in overt clefts.

In large prospective studies, most patients with submucous cleft palate do not have speech problems (ie, nasal air loss). However, it is not uncommon to see patients with nasal speech who have an unrecognized submucous cleft. Patients with submucous clefts should

be observed as speech develops; if nasal air loss occurs, surgical intervention should be considered. The **Furlow double-opposing Z-plasty** is an excellent method for repair in these cases (see Treatment section, below).

Treatment

The care of children with a cleft lip and palate requires a comprehensive treatment plan from the initial diagnosis through the completion of reconstruction in adolescence. A child with a complete cleft lip and palate requires several operations as he or she develops. In general, the goal of treatment is to have as few operations as possible with the best possible outcome. Naturally, there are a variety of approaches, any of which may produce the same final result. A comparison of outcomes has been difficult because of treatment differences, as well as the fact that the experience and ability of the individual surgeon may also influence the outcome.

It is important to emphasize the team approach to cleft care, which has developed gradually over the past 50 years. Although surgeons, speech therapists, and orthodontists, among others, may offer specific treatment, a dedicated cleft team offers the best possibility of coordinating the care among various specialists. This approach can both minimize the number and length of the various interventions as well as ensure that they are done at optimal times. The American Cleft Palate-Craniofacial Association has developed an outline of the standards for team care of cleft patients.

A. PREOPERATIVE CONSIDERATIONS

Before any surgery, it is important for the patient to have a thorough team evaluation, including genetic and pediatric examinations, which can lead to other studies to diagnose or rule out specific syndromes.

Oral intake can be compromised in children with cleft palate because of their inability to suck effectively. It is important to instruct parents in the use of a cleft nurser. There are a variety of types, all of which require less effort than a normal bottle; even a cross-cut nipple on a regular bottle may work in these cases. Most of the bottles require some squeezing to supplement flow. Adequate oral intake is assessed by weight gain.

Preoperative manipulation of the alveolar segments in complete cleft lip and palate is often used to reduce the width of a cleft, facilitating a tension-free surgical closure. Orthodontic appliances such as molding plates can be used but require frequent (weekly) modification of the plates to continue moving the segments. This is labor-intensive for the orthodontist, but can give the most accurate positioning of the segments. The use of taping across the cleft is much simpler and is still quite effective, but less predictable. This process is most important in complete bilateral clefts, in which control of the premaxilla is essential to achieving any type of repair. Once the lip is repaired, the intact orbicularis oris muscle maintains and continues to mold the position of the alveolar shelves.

Lip adhesion is a procedure in which the cleft segments are surgically united via small flaps, essentially creating an incomplete cleft lip. A successful lip adhesion molds the alveolar segment. A secondary operation is performed after an interval to convert the adhesion to a formal lip repair. Though appealing, this procedure creates scar tissue in the lip, which may impede the final lip repair.

B. Cleft Lip Surgery

1. Timing of lip repair—The classic "rule of tens" is still a reasonable guideline for lip repair: 10 weeks of age, a weight of 10 pounds, and a hemoglobin of 10 have been considered prerequisites for lip repair. This is partly based on anesthetic safety, which is probably a little better with increased age. The timing of the lip repair must be individualized for the patient. A premature infant may benefit from a later repair because of the increased incidence of apnea after general anesthesia in the first 3 months or so after gestational age. Similarly, if presurgical manipulation of the alveolus or premaxilla is required, this should be completed before the lip repair is undertaken. An incomplete cleft lip has less urgency because the alveolar segments are held in place by the intact Simonart's band.

2. Goals of lip repair—The essence of lip repair is to create a symmetrical Cupid's bow and lip fullness, without losing normal contour of the lip and the philtrum. To create length on the cleft side, some tissue from the lateral lip element must be inserted into the medial segment. Breaking up the scar also reduces scar contraction, which can create secondary shortness of the repair. This was commonly seen with the original straight-line cleft repair.

The initial efforts to break up the scar and recruit lateral tissue were so-called quadrilateral repairs, with a stair-step closure that had the disadvantage of discarding a significant amount of tissue. The triangular lip repair essentially placed a modified Z-plasty above the vermilion border. Other repairs have a Z-plasty in the central portion of the lip. The rotation advancement repair moved the Z-plasty to the area below the nasal sill.

Many fine adjustments contribute to the ideal cleft lip repair. The symmetry of the nose, including the tip, as well as the alar base and the nasal sill are critical to the final appearance. The fullness of the mucosa should be equal on the two sides. The alignment of the junction of the wet and dry vermilion (the so-called "red line") can be a subtle but important difference between a good repair and an adequate one.

3. Rotation advancement cleft lip repair—The rotation advancement cleft lip repair, also referred to as a Millard repair, is probably the most commonly performed repair today. Almost no tissue is discarded; the medial lip element is rotated downward, even with a back cut, if necessary, and the lateral lip element is advanced into the defect under the nasal sill. Mucosal flaps are used to line the nose and the vestibule of the lip (Figure 19–8).

It is important to understand that the rotation advancement repair recruits length for the lateral advancement flap by following the vermilion border. Increasing the amount of rotation (and leaving a larger secondary defect) creates length on the medial side of the repair; this length cannot be duplicated on the lateral segment unless the incision is carried along the vermilion border. This is known as a "cut-as-you-go" technique, because modifications can be made during the operation to obtain better symmetry.

The Millard repair has the advantage of creating good lip projection ("pout") by creating tension under the nasal sill rather than along the vermilion border. The most common problem is that the lip may be somewhat short after healing is complete. Placement of a tiny Z-plasty (1.0–1.5 mm) may improve this problem. Revision, if necessary, is much easier than revision after a triangular repair because of the linear nature of the lower portion of the repair.

4. Triangular cleft lip repair—The rotation advancement repair is by far the most frequently used in the United States; the triangular lip repair makes up the majority of the remainder. The triangular lip repair may also be referred to as the **Tennison-Randall cleft lip repair.**

The triangular cleft lip repair evolved from earlier quadrilateral repairs; they have in common a zigzag clo-

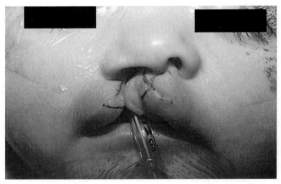

Figure 19–8. Rotation advancement (Millard) repair for unilateral cleft lip. The high point of the Cupid's bow on the central segment is brought down by the rotation; the secondary defect under the nose is filled by the lateral advancement flap.

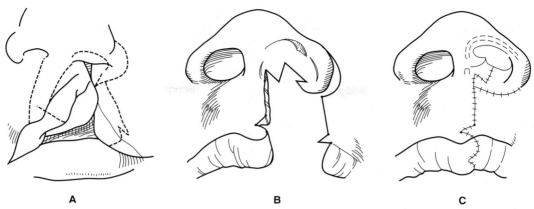

A   **B**   **C**

Figure 19–9. Triangular cleft lip repair. **(A)** Markings for triangular repair; shaded areas will be discarded. **(B)** Appearance during triangular repair. **(C)** Completed repair.

sure, which breaks up the forces of scar contracture. In the triangular repair, a nearly horizontal incision is made in the lower half of the medial cleft segment, and a triangular piece is fashioned in the lateral flap to fit in the resulting defect. This closure is essentially a modified Z-plasty placed relatively low on the lip. In some ways, the small Z-plasty discussed with the Millard repair is a modified triangular repair appended to the rotation advancement technique (Figure 19–9).

In all Z-plasties, length is borrowed at the expense of width. The placement of the triangle low on the lip results in an excellent lip length, but it has the disadvantage of creating a flat repair when viewed from the side. In contrast, the rotation advancement repair places the tightest part of the closure beneath the nasal sill, where the lip is normally the flattest, and creates a more natural pout, but at the expense of greater difficulty in obtaining adequate length.

5. Bilateral cleft lip repair—Several factors contribute to the greater complexity of bilateral cleft lip repair.

a. Premaxilla—In complete bilateral cleft lip and palate, the premaxilla is usually quite protrusive and must be controlled preoperatively to achieve an adequate repair. Resection of the premaxilla was practiced previously, but this procedure results in severe maxillary retrusion, and an extremely complex reconstruction that can be accomplished only with prosthetics. The simplest method, **taping,** can be effective but requires a great deal of parental participation. As noted previously, **alveolar molding** with orthodontic plates is also used in a number of centers. This technique generally gives better alignment of the three segments of the maxilla before surgical intervention. Severe protrusion can be approached at the time of surgery with an **osteotomy of the vomer** to allow the premaxilla to be set back surgically, but this should be done only as a last resort because it is associated with maxillary hypoplasia.

b. Nasal deformity—The second major challenge in the bilateral cleft repair is the nasal deformity. The columella is extremely short and the nasal tip is flat, with bilateral alar base widening. Alveolar molding may be combined with **nasal molding** by adding small prongs anteriorly that are gradually elongated over several weeks; this can lengthen the columella nicely. Postoperative **nasal stents** can also be useful after lip repair.

Debate still exists over the management of the short columella. Traditionally, tissue has been obtained from the lip as forked flaps or nasal alae as **V-to-Y advancement flaps.** More recently, attention has been focused on obtaining length from the nose itself, since some of the loss of length is due to the separation of the nasal tip cartilages. Thus, V-to-Y incisions at the alar rim or vertical incisions over the tip have been proposed. As noted previously, preoperative orthodontic manipulation of the segments may be combined with nasal molding to lengthen the columella, which obviates any additional scars.

c. Blood supply maintenance—The third problem in the complete bilateral cleft is the maintenance of blood supply to the central cutaneous segment, the prolabium, as well as the bony premaxilla. The more extensive lengthening procedure done in a unilateral cleft cannot be applied to both sides of a bilateral cleft simultaneously without jeopardizing this blood supply, which can come only from the nasal septum. Thus, the bilateral cleft repair is often planned in stages to prevent any possible loss of tissue.

d. Symmetrical deformities—Symmetrical deformities are best approached with a symmetrical repair. It is essential to obtain complete closure of the orbicularis oris muscle at the time of the lip repair, bringing the two segments from each side together across the middle. The intact muscle contributes greatly to later

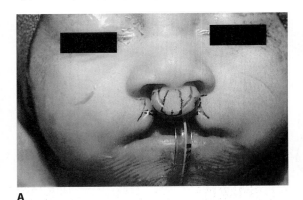

A

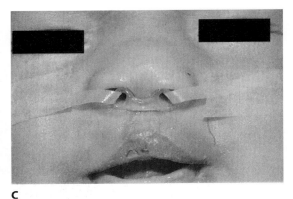

C

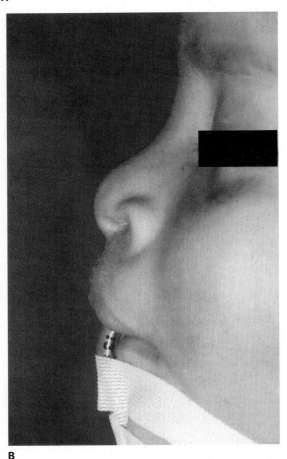

B

Figure 19–10. **(A)** Markings for bilateral cleft lip repair. The forked flaps on each side of the prolabium will be placed under the nasal sills for later lengthening of the short columella. The mucosa is step-cut on the lateral segments to close in the midline under the prolabium, avoiding a whistle deformity. **(B)** Postoperative lateral view. The short columella is demonstrated. **(C)** Postoperative anteroposterior view. This child is wearing a Silastic stent in the nose to elongate the columella and round out the nostril.

growth of the lip, so the length of the lip is less critical (Figure 19–10).

C. Primary Cleft Nasal Repair

The cleft nasal deformity in the unilateral cleft is multifactorial. There is the cleft itself, which in a complete unilateral situation extends up through the nasal sill and floor of the nose. This creates a widening of the alar base, which is further exaggerated by the decrease in bony support in the piriform aperture on the side of the cleft. The nasal septum is generally deviated toward the side of the cleft, further tipping the nasal pyramid toward the cleft

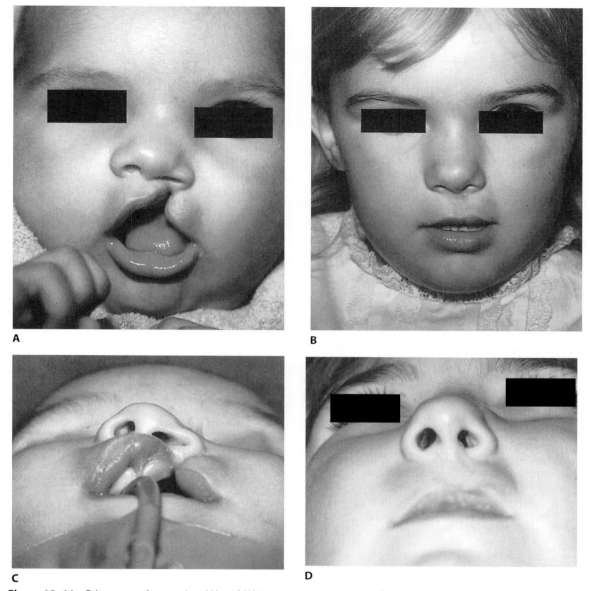

A **B**

C **D**

Figure 19–11. Primary nasal correction. **(A)** and **(B)** Anteroposterior views before and after surgery, respectively. **(C)** and **(D)** Views before and after lip repair, respectively, with primary nasal correction (one operation at 3 months of age).

side. There is decreased projection of the dome of the alar cartilage on the side of the cleft, either as a primary deformity or secondary to the above. The final result is a nasal appearance that can be the primary stigma of the cleft deformity after a well-performed cleft lip repair.

Previously, the prevailing wisdom was that any procedure performed on a cleft nasal deformity early in life would result in irreparable scarring and the loss of growth potential of the nose. Today, abundant evidence

exists that early correction of a cleft nasal deformity at the time of cleft lip repair can produce lasting improvement that grows proportionately with the child.

The common denominator in early cleft nasal correction is undermining of the nasal tip skin over the entire alar cartilage on the cleft side and over the dome of the non-cleft side, extending the dissection up onto the inferior dorsum of the nose. This is done entirely through the existing incisions for the lip repair, at the base of the columella and at the alar base. No intranasal incisions are required. Suspensory sutures are then placed to elevate the nasal dome and to anchor the lateral crus of the alar cartilage on the cleft side in an advanced position; these are tied over percutaneous bolsters. **Internal suturing techniques** have also been described. The sutures are generally removed after only a few days. This procedure can result in excellent symmetry of the nose in simpler cases and acceptable improvement in more severe cases (Figure 19–11).

More recently, **nasal molding extensions** have been added to alveolar molding plates to improve nasal contour before the lip repair. Other surgeons prefer to use postoperative nasal stents, available commercially in Silastic (ie, polymeric silicone), which can be gradually increased in size and used to help mold the nose over several weeks after the surgery for lip repair.

D. Cleft Palate Surgery

Cleft palate repair is primarily related to speech. Although there are obvious hygiene issues involved with the nasal regurgitation of food and fluids, most infants with cleft palates are able to gain weight appropriately and even to advance to solid food at about the same time as children without cleft palates. Intelligible speech, however, requires not only an intact palate but one with normal function.

1. Timing of palate repair—Again, the overriding concern is speech. The trend in timing of palate repair has been toward earlier repair, and there are data supporting palate repair earlier than a year of age. Both a decrease in compensatory articulations (habits that are developed to mimic a sound that cannot be produced because of the cleft), as well as a decreased need for secondary surgery for speech have been demonstrated with earlier repairs, even when compared to "later" repairs at 12–18 months of age.

It is critical to think of palate repair in relation to the child's development of speech and language. The cleft does not affect speech development but, rather, the ability to produce specific sounds. In particular, sounds requiring positive intraoral pressure will be most affected. Early palate repair, then, is carried out in children who are displaying normal development in motor skills as well as in speech (babbling is the norm at about 7–9 months of age). In contrast, in children with syndromes that are associated with developmental delay, speech development may well be delayed as well and palate repair will be a little safer at a later stage, even at 18–24 months of age.

2. Techniques of palate repair—It is useful to conceptualize the different types of palate repair by separating techniques used for hard palate closure from those used for the soft palate. In both the hard and soft palates, the goal is a repair of both the nasal and oral mucosa, whereas in the soft palate, the functional repair of the levator muscle is an equally important component of the repair. Historically, the first palate repairs were of the soft palate only in patients with clefts of the secondary palate. Later, the introduction of mucoperiosteal flaps became the basis of most hard palate techniques.

a. Von Langenbeck repair—Two-stage palate repairs were originally described as a means of treating wide clefts; soft palate repair was done at the same time as lip repair, with the hard palate repaired later after the cleft width had diminished. In a way, this is analogous to lip adhesion; the surgeon is committed to a second operation and has additional scar to confront at the time of the second procedure. The use of two-stage palate repair has consistently been shown to produce poorer speech results when compared with most single-stage techniques, but is still used by some surgeons.

In this technique, relaxing incisions are made on each side, just behind the alveolar ridge. The hard palate is closed with bipedicle mucoperiosteal flaps (the primary blood supply is from the greater palatine vessels). It is necessary in all of these repairs to develop corresponding flaps on the nasal side. On the non-cleft side, a superiorly based mucoperiosteal flap on the vomer is elevated to allow closure of the nasal mucosa. The open areas from the relaxing incisions are left to heal by secondary intention, which generally takes about 2 weeks.

b. V-Y pushback—In the V-Y pushback, also referred to as the **Veau-Wardill-Kilner repair**, open areas are left anteriorly to attempt to improve the length of the soft palate. Since the entire anterior border of the flap is elevated, it is imperative to preserve the greater palatine vessels for blood supply. The nasal incision is made behind the posterior border of the hard palate (Figure 19–12).

Although the pushback repair is excellent for improving length and can be used to great effect in combination with a pharyngeal flap, in complete clefts there is a substantial anterior area, which depends on nasal closure only. It is not surprising that this repair has a higher incidence of anterior fistulas, which can contribute to speech problems and are difficult to repair secondarily.

c. Two-flap palatoplasty—This technique uses more extensive bilateral flaps, which are based on the palatine vessels, and provides both greater security in the anterior closure and a decreased incidence of fistulas. Basically, this procedure extends the von Langenbeck technique by bringing the relaxing incisions behind the alveolar ridge forward to the cleft margin (Figure 19–13).

d. Double-opposing Z-plasty—The use of opposing Z-plasty procedures on the oral and nasal side of the soft palate produces increased length but also realigns the levator palatini muscle in an overlapping fashion. The tensor tendon can be divided to release some of the tension on the repair. This may be a difficult technique to use in wider clefts, but it is an excel-

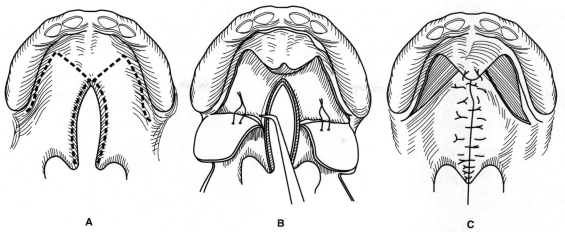

Figure 19–12. V-Y pushback palate repair. **(A)** Markings for incisions. **(B)** Mucoperiosteal flaps are developed from the oral surface based on the greater palatine vessels (shown) and on the nasal surface. **(C)** Completed repair. Note the bare areas on the anterior surface of the palate.

lent choice in narrower clefts and submucous clefts (Figure 19–14).

e. Levator muscle repair—The routine repair of the levator palatini muscle has only recently become a widely accepted technique in palate repair. The dissection of the muscle from both oral and nasal mucosa can be difficult, especially on the nasal side, and some physicians have even proposed using a microscope for the procedure.

A more aggressive approach to the levator muscle is achieved by dividing the tensor palatini tendon as it curves behind the hamulus so that the conjoined portion of the levator muscle is released. The muscle can

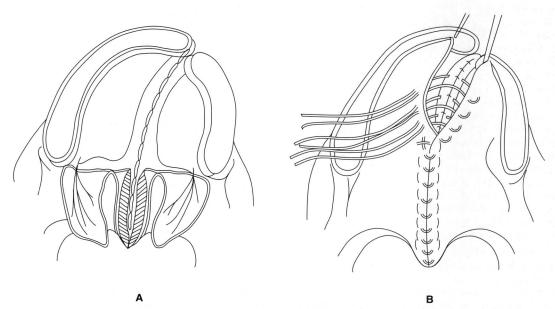

Figure 19–13. Two-flap palatoplasty. **(A)** Mucoperiosteal flaps raised with intact greater palatine vessels. **(B)** Closure completed anteriorly up to the posterior alveolar margin.

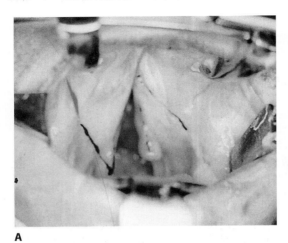 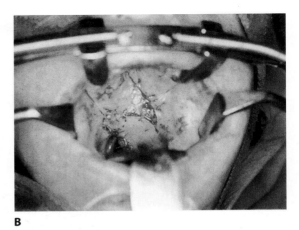

A   **B**

Figure 19–14. Furlow double-reversing Z-plasty. **(A)** Marking for Z-plasty. **(B)** Flaps transposed. Note that the nasal pattern (not seen) is the reverse pattern.

then be placed well posteriorly and even overlapped to give additional tension to the closure. Excellent speech outcomes have been reported with this technique.

E. VELOPHARYNGEAL INSUFFICIENCY

Even with the best surgical technique, some patients have nasal air escape with speech after cleft palate repair. This can be due to scarring or shortening of the soft palate, inadequate movement of the levator muscle (which can be due to preexisting neurologic factors or surgical injury), or fistula formation with air loss through the hole rather than through the posterior pharynx. This is termed velopharyngeal insufficiency, or VPI.

1. Preoperative evaluation—Careful speech evaluation by a speech pathologist, usually a member of the cleft palate team, is the cornerstone of evaluation of VPI. Diagnostic methods include lateral cephalograms, nasal manometry, video fluoroscopy, or direct evaluation by nasoendoscopy. The temporary occlusion of a fistula by a piece of foil or a stoma adhesive in a cooperative patient can help to differentiate problems with the soft palate from those caused by a fistula. It is important to differentiate global VPI from "phoneme-specific" VPI, which occurs only with certain sounds, usually sibilants; the latter can be treated with speech therapy only, whereas the former generally requires surgical intervention.

2. Surgical measures—Surgery for VPI can be broadly divided into procedures that lengthen a functioning palate and those that partially obstruct the area of closure in the posterior pharynx. Lengthening procedures include the V-Y pushback or the Furlow Z-plasty, both described

previously. Posterior procedures include the pharyngeal flap and the pharyngoplasty.

a. Pharyngeal flap—The pharyngeal flap consists of mucosa and muscular tissue taken from the posterior pharyngeal wall, generally with a superior base near the adenoid tissue (Figure 19–15). The flap can be placed into a defect in the nasal mucosa when combined with a pushback procedure, or sutured into the soft palate with a variety of techniques. All of these methods leave

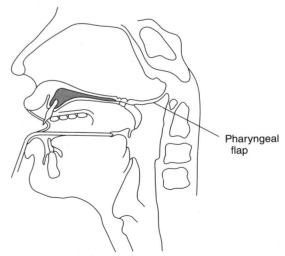

Figure 19–15. Pharyngeal flap. The flap is raised off the posterior pharyngeal wall and inset into the soft palate. Ports are left on each side of the flap for airflow.

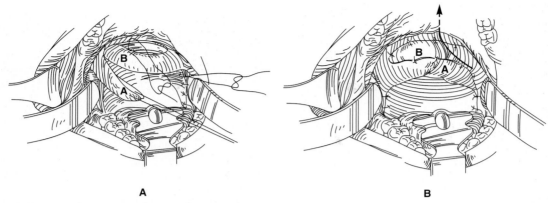

Figure 19–16. Sphincter pharyngoplasty. **(A)** Myomucosal flaps are elevated from each posterior tonsillar pillar and a transverse incision made joining the two. **(B)** The overlapping flaps are sutured to each other and to the posterior pharyngeal wall, creating a central narrow port for airflow.

the flap partially obstructing the nasopharynx with air going through "ports" on either side. If the ports are too large, VPI will persist; if they are too small, nasal obstruction and hyponasal speech may result. In most large series, the success rate in treating VPI is 80–90%. A significant rate of sleep apnea, as high as 30–40%, has been reported with pharyngeal flaps.

b. Sphincter pharyngoplasty—The sphincter pharyngoplasty uses flaps made from the posterior tonsillar pillars, including the palatopharyngeus muscle, to create a theoretically innervated flap. These two flaps are sutured into a bare area created on the posterior pharyngeal wall just below the adenoids, creating a central port of decreased size and a larger area of prominence for contact with the velum. Success rates have been reported at approximately 90%, but with a smaller rate of sleep apnea (Figure 19–16).

3. Nonsurgical measures—Nonsurgical approaches to velopharyngeal insufficiency (VPI) can be considered when patients are poor candidates for surgery either because of general health or because of specific conditions in the palate, such as scarring. Nonsurgical treatment modalities include orthodontic appliances to cover any open fistulas anteriorly or a **speech bulb prosthesis** (also known as a **palatal lift appliance**), which is a prosthetic device with a large posterior extension to lift the soft palate superiorly and posteriorly. In a palate that is not repaired, a speech bulb may itself provide a point for contact of the posterior and lateral pharyngeal walls to provide closure during speech (Figure 19–17).

F. SECONDARY SURGICAL PROCEDURES

As the child with a cleft grows, additional procedures are required. At a minimum, after lip and palate repair, bone grafting of the alveolar cleft and, later, septorhinoplasty,

usually combined with any residual lip repair, are performed. It is important to reiterate the role that team care can play in this process; by having at least annual visits, the team can monitor the child's progress and recommend appropriate interventions at the optimum time.

1. Lip revision—The ultimate goal of cleft lip repair is to avoid secondary surgery, since each revision of a cleft lip scar creates new scar tissue and, of necessity, removes at least a small amount of adjacent normal tissue. Revision of the cleft repair is a common necessity, however; the most common problems are misalignment of the white roll or the junction of the wet and dry mucosa, inadequate length of the lip on the repaired side, and disparate fullness of the lip between the two sides. The last is easiest to correct, because the new scar can be placed out of sight completely within the wet vermilion. Many techniques exist to correct the length of the lip repair, the most common being re-rotation of an advancement-rotation repair (Figure 19–18).

The timing of revision is often coordinated with school ages, since entering a new school can be traumatic for the young child. Obvious problems are best corrected before kindergarten. A minor problem that is not causing any psychological concerns can often be addressed in conjunction with other procedures, such as bone grafting or rhinoplasty.

Bilateral cleft lip repairs are often staged, and columellar lengthening is best performed at age 4 or 5 before school starts. In some bilateral clefts with severe scarring, a **cross-lip flap** (also known as an **Abbe flap**) may be necessary; this simultaneously reduces the lower lip while adding bulk and length to the central portion of the upper lip (Figure 19–19).

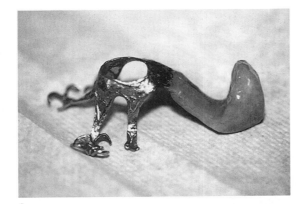

A

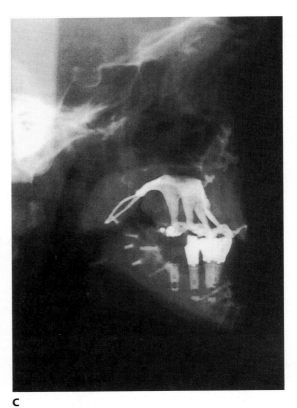

C

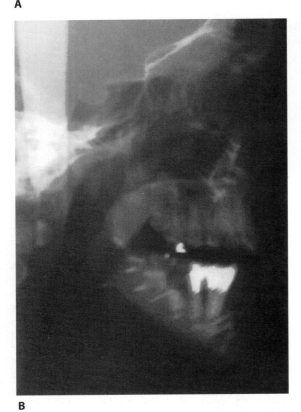

B

Figure 19–17. **(A)** Speech bulb prosthesis. The large projection on the right side of the photo is gradually built up to elevate the soft palate. **(B)** Lateral cephalogram without the prosthesis. **(C)** Lateral cephalogram with prosthesis. The reduction in the posterior pharyngeal airspace can be seen clearly.

2. Bone grafting—Bone grafting of the alveolar cleft is generally performed during mixed dentition, before eruption of the permanent cuspid. The procedure generally follows orthodontic maxillary expansion, if it is required; it is important to coordinate this procedure with the efforts of the treating orthodontist. The bone graft serves several functions: (1) stabilization of the maxilla, (2) support for the roots of the adjacent teeth, (3) closure of any residual anterior fistula, and (4) sup-port for the alar base on the cleft side. As noted above, the lateral incisor is usually absent; the bone graft will support a dental implant for replacement of the missing incisor and aid in support for other prosthetic devices, such as a fixed bridge.

The bone graft is placed between the bony margins of the two (or three) alveolar segments after elevating the mucoperiosteal flaps to close the nasal floor and the anterior palate; the anterior opening is then closed by

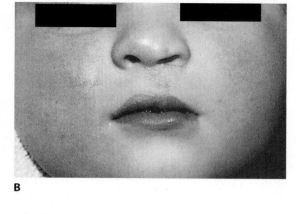

B

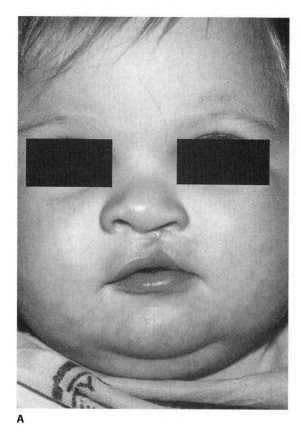

A

Figure 19–18. Revision of unilateral cleft lip repair. **(A)** A 1-year-old child several months after lip repair complicated by partial separation. **(B)** One year after revision, with complete redo of rotation advancement repair.

advancing a gingivoperiosteal flap from the lateral segment. Although cranial bone and rib have been advocated as donor sites, iliac crest cancellous bone remains the "gold standard" for this application.

Early bone grafting has also been proposed, with placement of a small rib graft in the alveolar space at the time of lip repair. This has generally been associated with increased rates of maxillary hypoplasia, although there may be significant technical variations that have an effect on long-term results.

As discussed previously, some centers are performing **gingivoperiosteoplasty,** which is the closure of the alveolar gap at the time of the primary lip repair. This can be accomplished only after careful alveolar positioning with a molding plate. Early results are promising at this stage, but it is too soon to evaluate the orthodontic and maxillary growth aspects of dentofacial development in these children.

3. Rhinoplasty—Both unilateral and bilateral clefts require rhinoplasty—usually in the early teens. If orthognathic surgery is required (see the following section), rhinoplasty is done subsequently. Every effort should be made at the time of lip repair to minimize the nasal deformity, but

this has no effect on the severe septal deviation to the side of the cleft that is seen in most patients with a unilateral cleft.

The septum is corrected with **septoplasty** or submucous resection of the septum; the latter is useful in that the removed cartilage can be used to reconstruct the nasal tip and provide graft material for a columellar strut and for the nasal tip.

Open rhinoplasty techniques are favored for cleft nasal reconstruction since they provide greater exposure for accurate correction. In unilateral clefts, the deficient cartilage on the side of the cleft can be rotated into a symmetrical position, sometimes augmented with tip grafting. In bilateral clefts, the two alar cartilages must be sutured together to achieve better tip narrowing and projection (Figure 19–20).

4. Orthognathic surgery—Approximately 10–15% of patients with clefts require **orthognathic surgery,** usually maxillary advancement. The decision regarding jaw surgery affects the orthodontic approach as well as the timing of bone grafting (this can be done at the time of maxillary surgery in some cases, rather than as a separate procedure). A large discrepancy between the two jaws may require the simultaneous setback of the mandible. Generally,

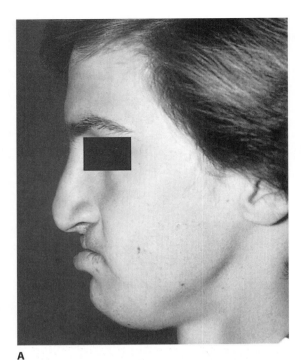
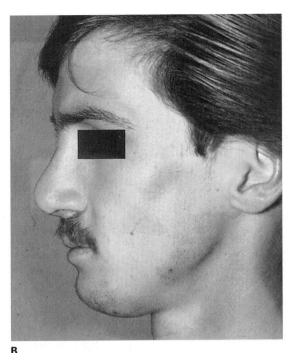

A   B

Figure 19–19.   A cleft lip reconstruction. The upper lip was reconstructed with an Abbe (cross-lip) flap, and a complete septorhinoplasty was completed. **(A)** Lateral view before surgery. **(B)** Lateral view after two operations. Note that the transfer of tissue from lower to upper lip has restored normal balance between the two.

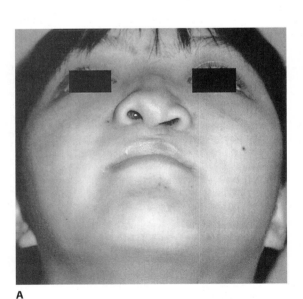
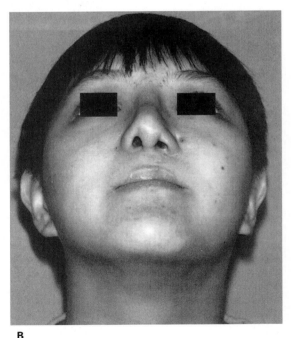

A   B

Figure 19–20.   Late nasal reconstruction. **(A)** Preoperative view. Note severe slumping of alar cartilage on the cleft (left) side, inadequate nasal dorsum. **(B)** Postoperative view after rib cartilage grafting to the dorsum and columellar strut to support the nasal tip.

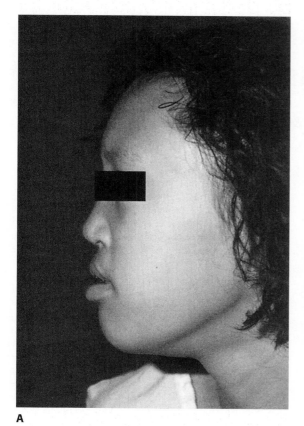
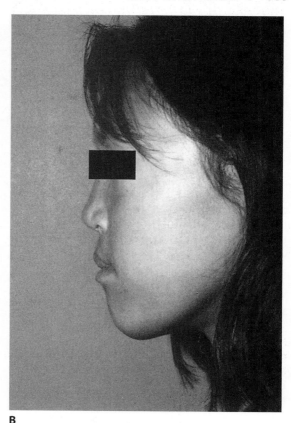

A **B**

Figure 19–21. Le Fort I maxillary advancement. **(A)** Profile prior to advancement. This patient had a cleft palate only. **(B)** Profile after maxillary Le Fort I procedure with rigid fixation.

these procedures are done near skeletal maturity, since the mandible is one of the last bones to stop growing—in early teens for girls, later for boys. It is important to monitor the patient's speech after maxillary advancement because the palate may come forward enough to produce nasal air escape where none was present previously (Figure 19–21).

American Cleft Palate Association. Parameters for evaluation and treatment of patients with cleft lip/palate or other craniofacial anomalies. *Cleft Palate Craniofac J.* 1993;30:S1. [PMID: 8457579] (Consensus paper from the American Cleft Palate Association that summarizes their recommendations for team care of patients with cleft lip and palate.)

Furlow LT Jr. *Operative Techniques in Plastic Surgery.* Philadelphia: WB Saunders, 1995. (Collection of contributions by the best in the field, describing numerous procedures for cleft lip and nose repairs.)

Millard R. *Cleft Craft: The Evolution of Its Surgery.* Boston, MA: Little, Brown, 1976. (Classic text on cleft repairs. Even if dated, it is encyclopedic in scope, covering both history and technical aspects of cleft lip and palate surgery.)

Randall P, LaRossa D. *Operative Techniques in Plastic and Reconstructive Surgery: Cleft Lip Repair.* Philadelphia: WB Saunders. 1995. (Collection of contributions by the best in the field, describing numerous procedures for cleft lip and nose repairs.)

Management of Adenotonsillar Disease

Yelizaveta Shnayder, MD, Kelvin C. Lee, MD,[†] & Joseph M. Bernstein, MD

The tonsils and adenoids can be a source of infection and obstruction for both adults and children and are responsible for a significant proportion of childhood illnesses. Tonsillectomy and adenoidectomy remain two of the most commonly performed procedures by otolaryngologists.

■ ANATOMY & PHYSIOLOGY

Although often thought of as distinct and separate structures, the tonsils and the adenoids are both components of **Waldeyer tonsillar ring.** The tissues comprising this lymphoid ring have similar histology and probably similar overall function. In addition to the palatine tonsils and the adenoids or pharyngeal tonsils, there are readily identifiable lingual tonsils.

The lymphoid tissue of Waldeyer tonsillar ring contains B-cell lymphocytes, T-cell lymphocytes, and a few mature plasma cells. This tissue is primarily involved in inducing secretory immunity and regulating immunoglobulin production. The cells are organized in lymphoid follicles similar to lymph nodes, but have specialized endothelium-covered channels that facilitate antigen uptake directly into the tissue, similar to Peyer patches in the colon. The independence of this system from lymphatic drainage is a unique advantage for antigen acquisition. The location of Waldeyer tonsillar ring and its design allow direct exposure of the immunologically active cells to foreign antigens entering the upper aerodigestive tract, which maximizes the development of immunologic memory. These tissues are most active from the ages of 4 to 10 and tend to involute after puberty. After their involution, the secretory immune function of these tissues remains, but not at the same level as previously.

The palatine tonsils are the largest component of the ring and have the most specialized structures. The lymphoid tissue itself is more compact in its normal state, with clearly identifiable crypts. These crypts are lined with stratified squamous epithelium and extend deeply into the tonsillar tissue. Though they maximize the exposure of tissue to surface antigen, they can also harbor debris and bacteria and may be the reason that tonsils are so commonly infected. A specialized portion of the pharyngobasilar fascia, forming a distinct fibrous capsule, binds the deep surface of the tonsil. The lymphoid tissue is very adherent to the capsule, thus making it difficult to separate, but there is loose connective tissue between the capsule and the muscles of the tonsillar fossa. With the inflammation resulting from either acute or chronic infection, which is limited by this capsule, tonsillar tissue swelling usually extends medially into the oropharyngeal airway. The potential space between the tonsil and the pharyngeal muscles is the usual site of a peritonsillar abscess.

Three thin pharyngeal muscles form the **tonsillar fossa.** The palatoglossus muscle forms the anterior tonsillar pillar whereas the palatopharyngeal muscle forms the posterior tonsillar pillar. The base of the tonsillar fossa is formed by the pharyngeal constrictors (primarily the superior constrictor). Under this thin muscle lies the glossopharyngeal nerve; the neurovascular structures of the carotid sheath are found more deeply beneath. With deep dissection or with sutures placed beyond the tonsillar capsule, these vital structures can be damaged inadvertently.

The arterial blood supply and innervation of the tonsil is primarily based at the inferior pole. The tonsillar branch of the dorsal lingual artery, the ascending branch of the palatine artery, and the tonsillar branch of the facial artery enter the inferior pole of the tonsil. The superior pole receives its blood supply from the ascending pharyngeal artery and anteriorly, from the lesser palatine artery. Venous drainage is more diffuse, with a venous peritonsillar plexus about the capsule. This plexus drains into the lingual and pharyngeal veins, which feed into the internal jugular vein. Lymphatic drainage is usually to the tonsillar lymph node

---

(just behind the angle of the mandible), or to the jugulodigastric or other upper cervical lymph nodes. The nerve supply of the tonsil is primarily from the tonsillar branch of the glossopharyngeal nerve, but also has contributions from the descending branches of the lesser palatine nerve. Because the glossopharyngeal nerve also has a tympanic branch, severe tonsillitis frequently presents with referred pain to the ear.

The adenoids or pharyngeal tonsils and the lingual tonsils are not as well defined or specialized as the palatine tonsils. These structures consist of lymphoid tissue covered by a specialized, pseudostratified, ciliated columnar epithelium that forms redundant surface folds to maximize the surface area of the tissue. The adenoids are located over the surface of the superior and posterior wall of the nasopharynx, and often demonstrate dramatic growth in the first years of life. Though they can be obstructive in this confined space, by approximately age 5 the adenoids start to regress and, combined with continued skull base growth, are rarely problematic beyond this period. The blood supply to the adenoids includes numerous branches of the palate and pharynx. Venous drainage is to the pharyngeal plexus, and the lymphatics drain into the retropharyngeal and pharyngomaxillary lymph nodes.

Nave H, Gebert A, Pabst R. Morphology and immunology of the human palatine tonsil. *Anat Embryol.* 2001;204:367. [PMID: 11789984] (Review summarizing current data on anatomy, histology, pathology, and immunology of palatine tonsils.)

■ INFECTIONS

To most patients, tonsillitis and "strep throat" are the same process, but many other organisms can infect the tonsils. The oropharynx and Waldeyer tonsillar ring are normally colonized by many different species of aerobic and anaerobic bacteria, including *Staphylococcus,* nonhemolytic streptococci, *Lactobacillus, Bacteroides,* and *Actinomyces.* These organisms, as well as many other pathogenic bacteria, viruses, fungi, and parasites, can cause infections of tonsillar and adenoid tissue. Oropharyngeal cultures obtained during the infection are not always useful in distinguishing the offending pathogen as they often yield multiple organisms, reflecting the normal flora of the oral mucosa.

VIRAL INFECTIONS

Patients presenting with viral tonsillitis, usually simultaneously with viral pharyngitis, commonly complain of sore throat and difficulty swallowing. Upon examination, there is often fever and oropharyngeal erythema, usually without a tonsillar exudate. Viruses such as adenovirus, rhinovirus, reovirus, respiratory syncytial virus (RSV), and the influenza and parainfluenza viruses have all been shown to be possible pathogens. Most of these infections are self-limited and require only symptomatic treatment.

The Epstein-Barr virus (EBV) causes acute pharyngitis as a part of infectious mononucleosis syndrome. It is common in children and young adults, is transmitted by oral contact, and manifests as fever, generalized malaise, lymphadenopathy, hepatosplenomegaly, and pharyngitis. Upon examination, petechiae may be present at the junction of the soft and hard palates. The tonsils are severely enlarged, sometimes to the point of compromising the airway, and classically are covered with an extensive grayish-white exudate. A complete blood count may be significant for lymphocytosis with atypical lymphocytes (activated T cells). A Monospot test is more sensitive and specific than a heterophil antibody test, which can be negative in 10–15% of patients in the first week of illness. Treatment is largely supportive, with intravenous fluids and rest. In the case of progressive airway obstruction due to obstructive tonsillar swelling, a short course of systemic steroids can be very helpful. Rarely, a nasopharyngeal airway, nasotracheal intubation, or tracheotomy may be required to secure the airway.

Tonsillar infections with the coxsackie virus result in herpangina, which presents as ulcerative vesicles over the tonsils, posterior pharynx, and palate. The disease commonly occurs in children under the age of 16. Patients present with generalized symptoms of headache, high fever, anorexia, and odynophagia.

Treatment for viral infections is mostly supportive, but the tonsils can have a bacterial superinfection that results in more severe symptoms. These patients can benefit from systemic antibiotics.

FUNGAL INFECTIONS

Oropharyngeal candidiasis (ie, thrush) often presents in immunocompromised patients or in patients who have undergone prolonged treatment with antibiotics. On exam, there are white cottage-cheese-like plaques over the pharyngeal mucosa, which bleed if removed with a tongue depressor. Treatment consists of topical nystatin or clotrimazole (eg, Mycelex) troches.

BACTERIAL INFECTIONS

1. Acute Streptococcal Pharyngotonsillitis

Group A beta-hemolytic *Streptococcus* is the most common and important pathogen causing acute bacterial pharyngotonsillitis. This infection most commonly presents in children aged 5–6 and is characterized by fever, dry sore throat, cervical adenopathy, dysphagia, and odynophagia. The tonsils and pharyngeal mucosa are erythematous and may be covered with purulent exudate; the tongue may also become red ("strawberry tongue"). The major consideration in diagnosing and treating pharyngitis caused by group A beta-hemolytic *Streptococcus* is in preventing its sequelae: acute rheumatic fever and poststreptococcal glomerulonephritis. In cases of strongly suspected pharyngitis caused by group A beta-hemolytic *Streptococcus,* the combination of rapid strep tests based on ELISA (enzyme-linked immunosorbent assay) or latex agglutination, with a throat culture if negative, increases the sensitivity and specificity of either test alone. The primary antibiotic treatment for streptococcal pharyngotonsillitis consists of penicillin. However, if no response is evident within 48 hours of therapy or another resistant organism is suspected, amoxicillin with clavulanate is indicated. Therapy should be continued for 10 days to decrease the recurrence rates.

2. Other Acute Bacterial Infections

Numerous other pathogenic bacteria can cause acute bacterial pharyngotonsillitis. **Vincent angina** is caused by *Treponema vincentii* and *Spirochaeta denticulata* and arises most often in conditions of overcrowding. Patients present with fever, unilateral pain on swallowing, and ipsilateral cervical lymphadenopathy; physical examination is significant for a unilateral deep ulcer on the upper pole of the tonsil, which is covered by a white exudative membrane. This ulcer heals in approximately 7–10 days. Treatment is usually with penicillin and oral hygiene.

Despite the widespread use of childhood immunization, 200–300 cases of tonsillar infection caused by *Corynebacterium diphtheriae* are still seen annually in the United States, mostly in nonimmunized persons. In addition to the usual symptoms of acute pharyngitis, this disease is characterized by a gray, velvety, firmly adherent pseudomembrane that covers the tonsils. When wiped off, with difficulty, the underlying surface usually bleeds. Sixty percent of cases are localized to the pharynx; in 8% of cases, the disease spreads to the larynx, potentially compromising the airway. Toxigenic strains can produce lethal diphtheriae exotoxin. A gram stain of the pseudomembrane reveals gram-positive aerobic bacillus within 1 hour. The disease is reportable and treatment should be started immediately, even before confirmation with the culture. It should be treated with antitoxin, which should be administered within 48 hours of the onset of symptoms, and high-dose penicillin.

Patients with exposure to sexually transmitted diseases can develop tonsillar infections with *Neisseria gonorrhoeae* or *Treponema pallidum.* Gonococcal infections present as an exudative pharyngitis; syphilitic infections result in oral chancres with primary infections and patchy exudative lesions with secondary disease.

3. Recurrent Acute Tonsillitis

Many patients experience episodes of acute tonsillitis with complete recovery between episodes. The tonsils, because of their location and numerous crypts and crevices, seem to harbor bacteria. Aggressive medical therapy for acute tonsillitis may not be sufficient to prevent additional infections. Otolaryngologists and primary care providers have debated the role of surgery for these patients for many years. Most surgeons now agree that tonsillectomy is indicated in patients with recurrent acute tonsillitis involving 6–7 episodes of acute tonsillitis in 1 year, 5 episodes/y for 2 consecutive years, or 3 episodes/y for 3 consecutive years.

4. Chronic Tonsillitis

Chronic tonsillitis is defined by persistent sore throat, anorexia, dysphagia, and pharyngotonsillar erythema. It is also characterized by the presence of malodorous tonsillar concretions and the enlargement of jugulodigastric lymph nodes. The organisms involved are usually both aerobic and anaerobic mixed flora, with a predominance of streptococci.

5. Tonsilloliths

Normally, the content of tonsillar crypts is drained into the oral cavity. However, in deep or stenotic crypts, food and secretions may stagnate, leading to bacterial overgrowth and a localized infection. In certain patients, a sensation of a foreign body in the throat and expressible, hard white material coming from the tonsils may occur; these latter are called tonsilloliths. The treatment for these tonsillar concretions or chronic tonsillitis is aggressive mouth care, which includes irrigation of the tonsils or cleaning them with a cotton swab soaked in 3% hydrogen peroxide. With time, the cellular debris is often retained in the branching crypts and with recurrent formation of focal bacterial abscesses in the tonsillar parenchyma, which later undergoes fibrosis and scarring; local care may not control these symptoms. Tonsillar surgery and elimination of these cryptic structures may be needed to control these infections.

Complications of Acute Adenotonsillitis

The historic focus on diagnosis and treatment of acute streptococcal adenotonsillitis or "strep throat" has been due to the morbidity of the nonsuppurative complications of these bacterial infections. The emphasis on rapid diagnosis and the widespread use of antibiotics have markedly decreased the incidence of these complications. In contrast, suppurative complications of acute bacterial tonsillitis are still commonly encountered.

A. NONSUPPURATIVE COMPLICATIONS

1. Scarlet fever—Scarlet fever is associated with fever, severe dysphagia, a yellow membranous exudate covering the tonsils and the pharynx, and a diffuse erythematous rash, which usually follows pharyngeal symptoms. The tongue may also become red, with desquamation of the papillae ("strawberry tongue"); facial flush and petechiae in body folds may be present. The eruptions, followed by desquamation, occur because of the erythrogenic exotoxin produced by the *Streptococcus* and are pathognomonic for this organism. Though scarlet fever is not itself a morbid complication, symptom identification and treatment planning are important to prevent the other complications related to streptococcal infection. The traditional treatment is with penicillin.

2. Acute rheumatic fever—Acute rheumatic fever usually occurs 18 days after an infection caused by group A beta-hemolytic *Streptococcus,* when the throat culture is no longer positive. Streptococcal infection results in production of cross-reactive antibodies, leading to damage of the heart tissues with subsequent endocarditis, myocarditis, or pericarditis. Once heart tissue damage occurs, little can be done to reverse the process. Patients should be placed on a penicillin prophylaxis or undergo tonsillectomy to eliminate the reservoir of streptococcal infection; preventing rheumatic fever requires eradicating the *Streptococcus* from the pharynx in addition to resolving the episode of pharyngitis.

3. Poststreptococcal glomerulonephritis—Poststreptococcal glomerulonephritis typically occurs as an acute nephritic syndrome about 10 days after a pharyngotonsillar infection (12–25% incidence) or as skin infections with a nephrogenic strain caused by group A beta-hemolytic *Streptococcus* (10% incidence), depending on the genetic host susceptibility factors. Acute poststreptococcal glomerulonephritis is on the decline in developed countries, whereas it continues to occur in developing countries. The pathogenic mechanism of the disease involves injury to the glomerulus by deposition of the immune complexes as well as circulating autoantibodies of the streptococcal antigen. Antibiotic treatment has not been shown to affect the incidence of the disease.

4. Other nonsuppurative complications—Recently, a temporal association between pharyngotonsillitis induced by group A beta-hemolytic *Streptococcus* and a new onset of obsessive compulsive disorders (OCDs) and other tics has been recognized in a subset of the pediatric population. The disease has been identified as **PANDAS** (pediatric autoimmune neuropsychiatric disorders associated with streptococcal infections). The symptoms include obsessive thoughts and fears, ritualistic compulsions, tics, and anxiety disorders. The abrupt onset of the disease is clearly within a few weeks of the pharyngotonsillitis caused by group A beta-hemolytic *Streptococcus,* as opposed to **Sydenham chorea**, which is characterized by psychological disturbances and abnormal choreiform motor activity that develop many months later. The proposed cause is a cross-reactivity of antistreptococcal antibodies with basal ganglia neurons. The exacerbations of the disease can be monitored by measuring antistreptolysin-O titers. Treatment with either antibiotics or a tonsillectomy has been correlated with a decrease in OCD symptoms.

B. SUPPURATIVE COMPLICATIONS

1. Peritonsillar abscess—With each episode of acute adenotonsillitis, the bacterial infection can extend beyond the tonsillar capsule and into the surrounding tissues. When this occurs, the most common manifestation is a peritonsillar abscess. The abscess usually lies in the potential space between the tonsillar capsule and the surrounding pharyngeal muscle bed and is most frequently found in patients with recurrent infections. These patients can present with an initial acute infection and may have some initial improvement if administered medication. When the abscess develops, patient symptoms intensify, with marked malaise, and they can have severe enough odynophagia to be dehydrated and have significant trismus. Examination reveals a bulging palate with the corresponding tonsil displaced to the midline or beyond. Needle aspiration confirms the diagnosis and helps to locate the abscess. Even with the aspiration of a significant quantity of purulent fluid, definitive incision and drainage are usually performed with an incision near the tonsil edge adjacent to the abscess. Some physicians have reported their experience with needle aspiration alone, but careful follow-up and possible reaspiration are essential because of the significant recurrent accumulation of infection, despite the start of systemic antibiotics. Appropriate patient selection for needle aspiration alone is extremely important.

In patients who have a peritonsillar abscess and recurrent tonsillitis, the possibility of recurrence of another peritonsillar abscess in the future is significant enough to warrant a tonsillectomy. Certain surgeons favor a **"Quincy tonsillectomy,"** which is a tonsillectomy that is performed while the patient is acutely infected. However, most surgeons prefer either to perform surgery after all the acute infection has resolved or to perform an interval tonsillectomy. There appears to be no significant difference in perioperative complications or pain after surgery in these patients.

2. Deep neck infections—Deep neck infections as a complication of bacterial tonsillitis or pharyngitis continue to occur at a significant rate in most regions. In decades past, the most common cause of parapharyngeal abscesses was bacterial pharyngitis or tonsillitis. With the widespread use of antibiotics, the incidence of these complications has dramatically decreased. However, patients who present with severe symptoms of odynophagia, trismus, and shortness of breath need careful evaluation to rule out this serious complication. Examination may reveal asymmetric pharyngeal swelling, including the palate, but this swelling extends more inferiorly than the tonsil into the hypopharynx. Classically, these patients also have "woody," diffuse neck swelling, but in some cases this phenomenon appears only as the infection progresses. Though ultrasound may be helpful, a definitive diagnosis requires a computed tomography (CT) scan of the neck. In most cases, management includes control of the airway, intravenous antibiotics, and surgical drainage of the abscess.

3. Chronic adenotonsillar hypertrophy—Lymphoid tissue of the Waldeyer ring is very small in infants. It increases in size by the time the child is 4 years of age in association with immunologic activity, since tonsils and adenoids are the first lymphoid organs in the body to encounter ingested and inhaled pathogens. Tonsillar and adenoid tissue has many specialized immunologic compartments responsible for humoral and cellular immune response, such as crypt epithelium, lymphoid follicles, and extrafollicular regions. Therefore, hypertrophy of the lymphoid tissue as a whole occurs in response to colonization with normal flora as well as with pathogenic microorganisms. Second-hand smoke exposure in the home environment has also been linked to adenotonsillar hypertrophy.

Nasal obstruction, rhinorrhea, and a hyponasal voice are the usual presenting symptoms of adenoid hypertrophy, whereas tonsillar enlargement can cause snoring, dysphagia, and either a hypernasal or a muffled voice. Chronic adenotonsillar hypertrophy is the most common cause of sleep-disordered breathing in children, with symptoms ranging from upper airway obstruction to obstructive sleep apnea syndrome (OSAS). Upper airway obstruction can manifest as loud snoring, chronic mouth breathing, and secondary enuresis. A history of witnessed apneic episodes, hypersomnolence or hyperactivity, frequent nighttime awakenings, poor school performance, and a general failure to thrive are common manifestations of obstructive sleep apnea. Over time, more severe cases of OSAS can lead to pulmonary hypertension, cor pulmonale, and alveolar hypoventilation resulting in chronic CO_2 retention, which can be slow to resolve even after relieving the obstruction with adenotonsillectomy.

Adenotonsillar hypertrophy and chronic mouth breathing due to nasal obstruction are associated with craniofacial growth abnormalities in children and can lead to the development of an increased anterior facial height and a retrognathic mandible, with subsequent malocclusion. The diagnosis of adenotonsillar hypertrophy is based on the clinical history and physical examination. Craniofacial abnormalities, other causes of nasal obstruction, and the degree and symmetry of tonsillar hypertrophy should be assessed. The hard and soft palates should be examined carefully to rule out a submucous cleft palate, which would predispose the patient to the postoperative development of velopharyngeal insufficiency.

Flexible endoscopy is helpful in diagnosing adenoid hypertrophy, adenoid infections, and velopharyngeal insufficiency (VPI), as well as ruling out other causes of nasal obstruction. Lateral neck soft tissue radiography can be helpful in documenting hypertrophic adenoids if endoscopy is not performed. Because of the difficulties in performing sleep studies in young children, the use of polysomnography to document obstructive sleep apnea in these patients remains controversial. This test is usually reserved for patients without a clear history whose examination is consistent with obstruction or for patients with craniofacial anomalies and neurologic disorders.

Brook I, Shah K. Bacteriology of adenoids and tonsils in children with recurrent adenotonsillitis. *Ann Otol Rhinol Laryngol.* 2001;110(9):844. [PMID: 11558761] (Adenoids may serve as a potential source of tonsillitis caused by group A beta-hemolytic *Streptococcus.*)

Kawashima S. Craniofacial morphology in preschool children with sleep-related breathing disorder and hypertrophy of tonsils. *Acta Paediatr.* 2002;91(1):71. [PMID: 11883823] (Thirty-eight preschool children with sleep-related breathing disorders had characteristic craniofacial growth abnormalities compared with the control subjects.)

Li AM. Use of tonsil size in evaluation of obstructive sleep apnea. *Arch Dis Child.* 2002;87(2):156. [PMID: 12138072] (Tonsillar-pharyngeal ratio, determined on lateral neck radiographs, but not clinical tonsil size, correlated with the apnea-hypopnea index.)

Orvidas LJ, Slattery MJ. Pediatric autoimmune neuropsychiatric disorders and streptococcal infections: role of otolaryngologist. *Laryngoscope.* 2001;111(9):1515. [PMID: 11568599] (Discusses two cases of siblings diagnosed with PANDAS who improved after tonsillectomies; includes literature review on PANDAS.)

TONSILLAR NEOPLASMS

Asymmetric tonsillar hypertrophy is a physical finding that should prompt the physician to include neoplasms in the differential diagnosis. When this finding is accompanied by a suspicious clinical course or history, a tonsillectomy should be performed for biopsy. Lymphoma and squamous cell carcinoma are the most common primary tonsillar neoplasms, but other malignant tumors may also present. Many primary malignant neoplasms (eg, melanoma and renal cell, lung, breast, gastric, and colon carcinomas) have been reported to metastasize to the tonsil. Benign tumors of the tonsil are rare and they include lipomas, fibromas, and schwannomas. Parapharyngeal space tumors are important to consider as a diagnosis, since they may present with signs and symptoms mimicking an asymmetric tonsillar hypertrophy or a tonsillar abscess.

The predictive value of a malignant process is increased when tonsillar asymmetry is associated with rapid enlargement, constitutional symptoms, atypical tonsillar appearance, ipsilateral cervical lymphadenopathy, and a history of previous malignant growths. In the absence of these risk factors, the likelihood of a malignant neoplasm is small. Unilateral tonsillar enlargement in asymptomatic children is rarely of neoplastic etiology, and a true asymmetry of the tonsillar specimen is confirmed in fewer than half of cases. However, the diagnosis of tonsillar lymphoma should be considered when unilateral tonsillar enlargement is present either in an immunocompromised child or when acute tonsillitis is asymmetric and unresponsive to medical therapy.

Harley EH. Asymmetric tonsil size in children. *Arch Otolaryngol Head Neck Surg.* 2002;128(7):767. [PMID: 12117331] (Prospective controlled study of the implication of pediatric tonsillar asymmetry.)

Syms MJ, Birkmire-Peters DP, Holtel MR. Incidence of carcinoma in incidental tonsil asymmetry. *Laryngoscope.* 2000;110(11):1807. [PMID: 11081589] (Retrospective review examining the incidence of malignant neoplasms in incidentally discovered unilateral tonsillar enlargement.)

POST-TRANSPLANT LYMPHOPROLIFERATIVE DISORDER

Post-transplant lymphoproliferative disorder is not a true neoplasm but is a neoplastic-like disorder. It must be considered in the appropriate clinical setting. This disorder is a life-threatening complication of immunosuppression that may develop after solid organ and bone marrow transplantation. Post-transplant lymphoproliferative disorder is a proliferative B-cell disorder that is associated with the Epstein-Barr virus in an immunocompromised host. High clinical suspicion is important. Tonsillectomy is needed for airway relief and diagnosis followed by a reduction of immunosuppression and antiviral therapy.

Huang RY, Shapiro NL. Adenotonsillar enlargement in pediatric patients following solid organ transplantation. *Arch Otolaryngol Head Neck Surg.* 2000;126(2):159. [PMID: 10680866] (Retrospective review of the management of post-transplant lymphoproliferative disorder as it relates to adenotonsillectomy.)

Indications for Tonsillectomy & Adenoidectomy

In the last several decades, when the fear of complications resulting from streptococcal infections was strong and the complication rate for tonsillectomy was not well known, tonsillectomy was widely performed as a public health measure. Entire families of children had tonsillectomies performed all on the same day. As the rate of complications after tonsillectomy became better established, the need for tonsillectomy came under scrutiny, and some pediatricians questioned whether tonsillectomy should be performed for any child. This debate sparked clinical studies that focused on the need for tonsillectomy and its efficacy in reducing infections in children. Investigators showed a significant improvement with tonsillectomy, and guidelines were established for performing this procedure. In addition, over the last decade, there has been an increasing recognition of the impact of obstructive sleep apnea on the development of children. Adenotonsillar hypertrophy is the primary cause of OSAS in children and increasing numbers of children are having adenotonsillectomy for this indication.

The current indications for tonsillectomy are listed in Table 20–1. In all cases, the potential benefits of tonsillectomy should be weighed against the significant morbidity of the procedure and the potential postoperative complications. The adenoids or pharyngeal tonsils

Table 20–1. Surgical indications for tonsillectomy and adenoidectomy.

Infectious Disease
Recurrent, acute tonsillitis, with more than 6–7 episodes in one year, 5 episodes per year for two years, or 3 episodes per year for three years
Recurrent, acute tonsillitis, with recurrent febrile seizures, or cardiac valvular disease
Chronic tonsillitis, unresponsive to medical therapy or local measures
Peritonsillar abscess with history of tonsillar infections
Obstructive Disease
Heroic snoring with chronic mouth breathing
Obstructive sleep apnea or sleep disturbances
Adenotonsillar hypertrophy with dysphagia or speech abnormalities
Adenotonsillar hypertrophy with craniofacial growth or occlusive abnormalities
Mononucleosis with obstructive tonsillar hypertrophy, unresponsive to steroids
Other
Asymmetric growth or tonsillar lesion suspicious for neoplasm (without adenoidectomy)

Table 20–2. Surgical indications for adenoidectomy alone.

Infectious Disease
  Adenoid hypertrophy with eustachian tube dysfunction and persistent ear infection or middle ear effusion
  Adenoid hypertrophy associated with chronic sinusitis, unresponsive to medical therapy
  Obstructive adenoid hypertrophy
  Heroic snoring with chronic mouth breathing
  Obstructive sleep apnea or sleep disturbances
  Craniofacial growth or occlusive abnormalities
Other
  Adenoid mass or lesion or asymmetric enlargement

are often involved in the primary process affecting the tonsils and should be included in any discussion of tonsillar disease management. Because adenoidectomy has minimal additional morbidity when compared with tonsillectomy, it is often performed simultaneously with tonsillar surgery if the surgeon feels it will benefit the patient. The indications for adenoidectomy without tonsillectomy are listed in Table 20–2.

A. Tonsillectomy

At present, traditional tonsillectomy usually consists of a subcapsular dissection and total removal of the tonsils. The procedure usually involves an incision of the mucosa adjacent to the tonsil along the anterior and posterior tonsillar pillars. The dissection is initiated to find the tonsillar capsule, and it is then dissected free from the underlying muscle bed. Blood vessels are usually seen extending from the muscle bed into the tonsillar capsule, particularly at the superior and inferior poles, which are carefully cauterized. This dissection is continued until the entire tonsil with the tonsillar capsule is removed from the operative field. The muscle-lined tonsillar bed is then carefully examined and any additional bleeding sites are cauterized. Some of the blood vessels encountered may be quite large and need isolation and control with suture ties. Suture ligatures with needles should be avoided, if possible, given the real potential for inadvertent damage to larger vascular structures that can result in massive delayed hemorrhage.

Tonsillectomy has a postoperative course with significant morbidity and potential complications. After surgery, patients usually have considerable odynophagia, a change of diet, and decreased activity. The recovery period for children is usually 4 days to 1 week, whereas adults may have symptoms for up to 2 weeks. The odynophagia can be severe enough to limit oral intake, and children and adults on occasion may become dehydrated and require admission for intrave-

nous fluids. Despite a multitude of studies performed using numerous perioperative medications and different surgical modalities, none has undisputedly improved this postoperative course. The use of high-dose steroids, antibiotics, and local anesthesia have all shown some benefit in certain studies, but not all studies have reliably shown a reduction of pain or a more rapid recovery. New surgical modalities, such as laser, ionized field ablation, and the ultrasonic scalpel, have also shown some benefit in reducing the morbidity of this surgery, but, currently, none is widely used.

As increasing numbers of patients have tonsillectomies performed for obstructive tonsillar hypertrophy, some physicians have performed subtotal (ie, intracapsular) tonsillectomy for these patients. In this procedure, the tonsillar capsule as well as some minor percentage of the tonsillar tissue lining the capsule is preserved. Initially, the carbon dioxide (CO_2) laser was used for a subtotal reduction of the hypertrophic tonsils in children with obstructive symptoms. The postoperative course was significantly better than with traditional total tonsillectomy and appeared to have similar efficacy after a 1-year follow-up. Other surgical modalities, such as ionized field ablation and powered tissue debriders, have been used to perform subtotal tonsillectomy with similar results.

A recent study reviewed the postoperative complications in patients who had undergone subtotal intracapsular tonsillectomy using ionized field ablation. The rate of postoperative bleeding and other complications of this procedure compared favorably with reports of other patients who underwent a total tonsillectomy. The study concluded that subtotal intracapsular tonsillectomy may offer a decreased rate of postoperative bleeding and should be considered for patients undergoing tonsillar surgery for obstructive tonsillar hypertrophy. Further study of these novel approaches to tonsillar disease is needed, but they may offer a significant decrease in the morbidity long associated with traditional tonsillar surgery.

B. Adenoidectomy

Traditional adenoidectomy has been performed under general anesthesia, using the blade of an adenotome or adenoid curette. Given that there is no adenoid capsule, the precise removal of the adenoids has always been difficult to achieve with any surgical technique. With a nasopharyngeal mirror, removal involves a specially designed curette that is used to incise the adenoids near their base at the junction of the nose and nasopharynx. The blade of the curette passes deep within the tissue, at a sharp angle, exiting the mucosa at the level of the palate. This gross removal of tissue is usually followed by electrocautery for hemostasis. The morbidity of this procedure is fairly low, with minimal pain and a low incidence of postoperative bleeding, halitosis, or neck pain. Though a few case reports of nasopharyngeal stenosis and velopharyngeal insufficiency after surgery have been reported in the literature, the significant incidence of specific complications has not been established, probably because so few occur.

Surgeons have reported the use of other surgical modalities to manage obstructive adenoid hypertrophy. Powered tissue debriders have been used to rapidly remove adenoid tissue and allowed surgeons to sculpt the tissue as they desire, with minimal bleeding and similar efficacy. Others physicians have used suction electrocautery devices to thermally ablate the tissue layer by layer. These surgeons contend that the controlled removal of the adenoids makes both nasopharyngeal stenosis and velopharyngeal insufficiency less likely to occur.

Darrow DH, Siemens C. Indications for tonsillectomy and adenoidectomy. *Laryngoscope*. 2002;112:6. [PMID: 12172229] (A thorough review of the indications for tonsillectomy and adenoidectomy based on evidence in the medical literature.)

Krisha P, Lee D. Post-tonsillectomy bleeding: a meta-analysis, *Laryngoscope*. 2001;111:1358. [PMID: 11568568] (A review of reports on post-tonsillectomy bleeding, the major complication of tonsillectomy.)

Paradise JL, Bluestone CD, Bachman RZ et al. Efficacy of tonsillectomy for recurrent throat infection in severely affected children: results of parallel randomized and nonrandomized clinical trials. *N Engl J Med*. 1984;310:674. [PMID: 6700642] (Landmark report of controlled clinical trial showing efficacy of tonsillectomy for recurrent tonsillitis.

Parapharyngeal Space Neoplasms & Deep Neck Space Infections

21

Demetrio J. Aguila III, MD, & Edward J. Shin, MD

ANATOMY OF THE PARAPHARYNGEAL SPACE

The parapharyngeal space forms an inverted pyramid with its base at the skull and its apex at the greater cornu of the hyoid bone. The fascial margins of the parapharyngeal space are complex, comprising different layers of the deep cervical fascia. As it curves around the lateral side of the pharyngeal mucosal space, the middle layer of the deep cervical fascia forms the medial fascial margin. The lateral fascial margin is formed by the medial slip of the superficial layer of the deep cervical fascia as it curves around the deep border of the masticator and parotid spaces. Posteriorly, the parapharyngeal space fascia is made up of the anterior part of the carotid sheath, formed by the fusion of all three layers of the deep cervical fascia.

Extending from the medial pterygoid plate to the styloid process, the tensor veli palatini and its fascia divide the parapharyngeal space into pre- and post-styloid spaces. The post-styloid compartment contains cranial nerves IX–XII: the glossopharyngeal nerve (CN IX), the vagus nerve (CN X), the accessory or spinal nerve (CN XI), and the hypoglossal nerve (CN XII), as well as the carotid artery, the jugular vein, the cervical sympathetic chain, and glomus bodies. The prestyloid compartment, bound anteriorly by both the medial pterygoid muscle and the mandible, contains fat, minor or ectopic salivary glands, the internal maxillary artery, and the branches of V3 (ie, the mandibular branch of the trigeminal nerve). Understanding these fascial compartments and spaces facilitates the accurate interpretation of images and preoperative diagnosis.

■ PARAPHARYNGEAL SPACE NEOPLASMS

 ESSENTIALS OF DIAGNOSIS

- Neck mass, snoring, possible sleep apnea, mild dysphagia.
- Medial displacement of oropharyngeal wall without erythema.
- Prestyloid or post-styloid mass as determined by computed tomography (CT) scanning or magnetic resonance imaging (MRI).
- Cytologic findings diagnostic of benign or malignant tumor.

General Considerations

A wide spectrum of benign and malignant neoplasms may be encountered in the parapharyngeal space, synonymous with the pterygomaxillary space, the pterygopharyngeal space, the pharyngomaxillary space, and the lateral pharyngeal space. These masses include primary neoplasms, masses extending from adjacent regions, and metastatic tumors. Modern imaging has advanced the understanding of this complex anatomic area, aiding in the diagnosis and management of tumors within the parapharyngeal space. Several large series of retrospective and single institution studies have contributed to the rational management of these tumors.

Clinical Findings

A. SYMPTOMS AND SIGNS

Parapharyngeal space tumors may present with a number of symptoms; the most common are neck mass, pain, and dysphagia (Table 21–1). Mass effect may result in symptoms of pressure, characterized by dysphagia, dysarthria, and airway obstruction that may manifest as sleep apnea or snoring. Trismus suggests infiltration into the pterygoid muscles or a mechanical obstruction of the coronoid process. Otologic symptoms most commonly relate to eustachian tube dysfunction, resulting from compression of the cartilaginous portion of the eustachian tube by a tumor. Pulsatile tinnitus, hearing loss, and otalgia have also been noted.

The need for a thorough head and neck evaluation cannot be overemphasized. A surprising number of asymptomatic benign tumors are detected on a routine clinical examination or on an imaging study performed

Table 21–1. Symptoms of parapharyngeal space neoplasms.

Neck mass	46%
Pain	20%
Dysphagia	13%
Pharyngeal mass	9%
Hoarseness	7%
Foreign body sensation	6%
Parotid mass	4%
Otalgia	4%
Trismus	2%

Data from Carrau RL et al. Management of tumors arising in the parapharyngeal space. *Laryngoscope* 1990;100:583.

Table 21–2. Imaging characteristics of prestyloid versus poststyloid masses.

Prestyloid space
Intraparotid mass
    Fat planes between tumor and parotid gland lost
    Parapharyngeal fat displaced anteriorly and laterally
    Carotid artery displaced posteriorly
Extraparotid mass
    Fat planes between tumor and parotid gland preserved
    Parapharyngeal fat displaced anteriorly and laterally
    Carotid artery displaced posteriorly
Poststyloid space
Schwannoma
    Fat planes between tumor and parotid gland preserved
    Parapharyngeal fat displaced anteriorly and laterally
    Carotid artery displaced anteriorly and/or medially*
    Smooth enlargement of involved skull base foramen
Paraganglioma
    Fat planes between tumor and parotid gland preserved
    Parapharyngeal fat displaced anteriorly and laterally
    Carotid artery displaced anteriorly and/or medially†
    Ragged, irregular enlargement of involved skull base foramen

*Sympathetic chain schwannomas may displace the carotid artery posteriorly *or* anteriorly.
†Carotid body paragangliomas typically splay the internal and external carotid arteries.

for unrelated symptoms. Displacement of the medial wall of the oropharynx and tonsil is usually the first sign of a parapharyngeal space lesion. Alternately, the mass may be found posterior or inferior to the angle of the mandible, as one would see with a mass in the neck or in the parotid gland. A careful cervical and bimanual intraoral evaluation allows the clinician to formulate an impression of the extent of tumor.

Because cranial nerves IX–XII pass through the post-styloid compartment, each nerve may be affected. The tumor may arise from a nerve, or it may cause compression of the adjacent neural structures. Patients with schwannoma or paraganglioma of the vagus nerve may present with vocal cord paralysis. Tumors of the skull base and jugular foramen may produce neuropathy of the glossopharyngeal nerve (CN IX), the vagus nerve (CN X), or the accessory nerve (CN XI), presenting as (1) a reduction or absence of the gag reflex, (2) vocal cord paralysis, and (3) trapezius weakness with shoulder drop, respectively.

B. LABORATORY FINDINGS

If imaging studies suggest a paraganglioma, urine screening for vanillylmandelic acid (VMA), metanephrine, and normetanephrine should be performed. It is important to ask specifically for a history of hypertension, hypertensive episodes, facial flushing, or tachyarrhythmia.

C. IMAGING STUDIES

MRI or CT imaging allows localization of the tumor within one of the fascial compartments, relying on the relationship of the neoplasm both to surrounding fat planes and to structures such as the styloid process or skull base foramina (Table 21–2).The fatty triangle of the parapharyngeal space is easily identified on routine axial CT scans and MRI. Only when a mass is very large is the parapharyngeal space fat completely obscured. Tumors in the post-styloid parapharyngeal space, presumed to be nerve sheath lesions or paragangliomas, dis-

place the parapharyngeal fat anteriorly and laterally. Tumors of the prestyloid space are most commonly salivary gland neoplasms. The preservation of the fat plane between the mass and the deep lobe of the parotid gland strongly suggests a neoplasm with an extraparotid origin, whereas the loss of a fat line between the mass and the parotid gland suggests a tumor that arises from the deep lobe of the parotid gland (Figures 21–1 and 21–2). Tumors originating from the deep lobe of the parotid gland may occasionally pass through the stylomandibular tunnel and have a dumbbell-like appearance.

Radiographic visualization of carotid artery displacement is highly correlated with tumor groupings. Salivary gland tumors tend to displace the carotid artery in a posterior direction, whereas neuromas and glomus tumors distort the carotid sheath compartment in an anterior direction. The advantages of CT scans include lower cost, evidence of osseous invasion, and the demonstration of calcification within tumors. In contrast, MRI provides better soft tissue visualization of neural and vascular structures. By analyzing the inherent signal characteristics in combination with the surrounding fat plane distortion and the internal carotid artery displacement on MRI, the most common parapharyngeal masses may be distinguished.

Angiography should be considered if the initial CT scan or MRI suggests a vascular tumor or if carotid

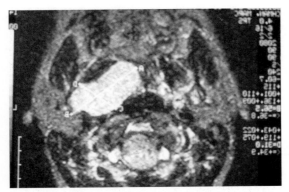

Figure 21–1. MRI of pleomorphic adenoma. Note continuity of tumor with deep parotid gland. (Photo courtesy of Dr. Mark Urken.)

artery involvement is suspected. The precise blood vessels supplying the tumor can be determined and occluded before surgery. A carotid occlusion study may be necessary to determine whether a patient can tolerate the loss of the carotid artery.

D. FINE-NEEDLE ASPIRATION BIOPSY

Fine-needle aspiration (FNA) biopsy may contribute to the preoperative evaluation of parapharyngeal space tumors. Aspiration may be undertaken transcutaneously with tumors that are palpable in the neck or transorally with tumors that displace the pharyngeal wall significantly. CT-

guided FNA may be appropriate in deeply seated parapharyngeal masses. FNA may be especially useful when clinical and radiographic findings suggest a malignant neoplasm, affording the surgeon an opportunity to better counsel the patient and family preoperatively.

FNA results that do not correlate with other clinical findings suggest that a sampling error may have occurred. In addition, FNA is best avoided when a paraganglioma is suspected because of the potential for bleeding.

Cramer H, Lampe H, Downing P. Intraoral and transoral fine-needle aspiration. *Acta Cytol.* 1995;39:340. [PMID: 7543234] (Eight out of nine parapharyngeal space masses correctly diagnosed with FNA, with one third representing a malignant growth.)

Shin JH, Lee HK, Kim SY, Choi CG, Suh DC. Imaging of parapharyngeal space lesions: focus on the prestyloid compartment. *AJR Am J Roentgenol.* 2001;177:1465. [PMID: 11717108] (Multiple MRI images of the prestyloid space with a review of the differential diagnosis and imaging characteristics.)

Differential Diagnosis

Tumors of the parapharyngeal space include primary neoplasms, tumors with direct extension from adjacent regions, and metastatic tumors (Tables 21–3 and 21–4).

A. SALIVARY GLAND NEOPLASMS

Pleomorphic adenoma is the most common salivary gland neoplasm arising in the parapharyngeal space. It can arise from any portion of the parotid gland or from extraparotid salivary tissue. Other benign salivary gland tumors have been reported in the parapharyngeal space, including Warthin tumors, oncocyto-

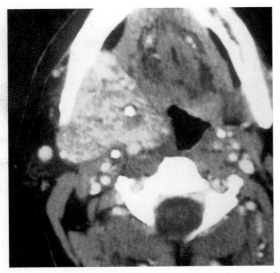

Figure 21–2. Venous malformation of parapharyngeal space. (Photo courtesy of Dr. Mark Urken.)

Table 21–3. Benign parapharyngeal space neoplasms.

Salivary gland
Benign lymphoepithelial disease
Monomorphic adenoma
Oncocytoma
Pleomorphic adenoma
Warthin's tumor
Neurogenic
Ganglioneuroma
Neurilemoma
Neurofibroma
Paraganglioma
Miscellaneous
Arteriovenous malformation
Branchial cleft cyst
Lipoma
Meningioma

Data from Olsen KD. Tumors and surgery of the parapharyngeal space. *Laryngoscope* 1994;104(63):1.

Table 21–4. Malignant parapharyngeal space neoplasms.

Salivary gland
Acinic cell carcinoma
Adenocarcinoma
Adenoid cystic carcinoma
Mucoepidermoid carcinoma
Neurogenic
Malignant paraganglioma
Neurofibrosarcoma
Miscellaneous
Chondrosarcoma
Fibrosarcoma
Liposarcoma
Lymphoma
Metastatic disease

Data from Olsen KD. Tumors and surgery of the parapharyngeal space. *Laryngoscope* 1994;104(63):1.

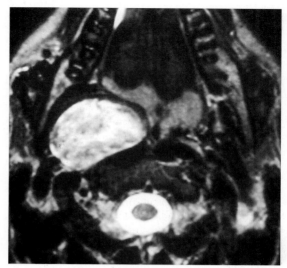

Figure 21–3. Schwannoma of cervical sympathetic chain. (Photo Courtesy of Dr. Mark Urken.)

mas, and benign lymphoepithelial lesions. These tumors are commonly found in the prestyloid compartment. Rarely, mucoepidermoid carcinomas, malignant mixed tumors, adenoid cystic carcinomas, or adenocarcinomas may be encountered.

B. NEUROGENIC NEOPLASMS

1. Neurilemomas—Neurilemomas or benign schwannomas are the most common neurogenic neoplasm of the parapharyngeal space. The tumors typically present as slow-growing neck masses arising from any nerve with a Schwann cell sheath, including cranial nerves V3, IX, X, XI, and XII; the sympathetic nerve trunk; and the upper cervical nerves. Neurologic deficits do not always correlate with the nerve from which the neoplasm arises, and many patients are asymptomatic. The treatment of schwannomas is enucleation or tumor removal with preservation of the involved nerve. However, the large size of many of these tumors often precludes nerve preservation (Figure 21–3).

2. Paragangliomas—Chemodectomas or paragangliomas of the head and neck are rare and comprise 0.6% of head and neck tumors. They are usually slow growing and 2–3 times more common in women than in men. Paragangliomas involving the parapharyngeal space originate from either vagal or carotid bodies. Paraganglia develop from neuroectodermal tissue and are thought to function as part of the autonomic nervous system that monitors changes in the levels of pH, oxygen, and carbon dioxide. Ten percent of patients have a family history of these tumors, representing an inherited familial form. Multicentric neoplasms occur in 10–20% of sporadic cases and in up to 80% of

familial cases. Thus, these patients should undergo routine preoperative screening for urinary catecholamines as well as abdominal and carotid scanning to rule out clinically unrecognized tumors. In addition, a metastatic workup is warranted when imaging or clinical exam yield suspicious lesions; the therapeutic plan should address possible metastasis.

Overall, less than 10% of paragangliomas are malignant. Approximately 6% of carotid body tumors and 16–17% of vagal paragangliomas may be malignant. It is generally accepted that a paraganglioma is malignant only when metastasis to non-neuroendocrine tissue is demonstrated. Most commonly, paragangliomas spread regionally to the cervical lymph nodes or distantly to the lung, the liver, or the skin.

The most common presenting symptom of a vagal paraganglioma is a mass in the neck, often associated with hoarseness. The most common presenting symptom of a carotid paraganglioma is a mass located at the carotid bifurcation that is horizontally mobile, but vertically immobile.

Surgical removal of paragangliomas is the treatment of choice. Angiography with preoperative embolization minimizes bleeding as well as injury to the adjacent cranial nerves. Timing of surgical intervention is controversial. The patient and the surgeon must consider that these tumors are often benign and slow growing. Surgical resection may convert an asymptomatic patient to a patient with significant impairments of speech and deglutition. Observation may be warranted unless there is an increased suspicion for malignancy. For example, in cases of vagal paresis, surgical intervention may be delayed until the vagus nerve is completely nonfunctional. Patients fare better when given time to accommodate to a slowly progressive loss rather than to an acute iatrogenic paralysis.

Radiation therapy is another therapeutic option. To avoid debilitating bilateral paralyses to cranial nerves X and XII in multicentric tumors (eg, bilateral vagal or carotid paragangliomas), careful consideration should be given to which tumor should be resected initially and whether radiation therapy should be used in the management of one of these tumors. Radiation therapy can prevent further growth in many patients; however, late tumor progression can occur. Radiation does not reduce paraganglioma volume by the destruction of tissue; rather it induces fibrosis and decreases the fine vasculature of the tumor. In addition, poor surgical candidates (based on comorbidities, tumor size, tumor recurrence, or any combination of these factors) may elect radiation therapy for local control or symptomatic relief.

Carrau RL, Myers EN, Johnson JT. Management of tumors arising in the parapharyngeal space. *Laryngoscope.* 1990;100:583. [PMID: 2348735] (A review of 54 patients undergoing evaluation and the treatment of parapharyngeal space tumors.)

Hamza A, Fagan JJ, Weissman JL, Myers EN. Neurilemomas of the parapharyngeal space. *Arch Otolaryngol.* 1997;123:622. [PMID: 9193224] (Reviews the surgical management of neurilemomas of the parapharyngeal space in 26 patients.)

Lee JH, Barich F, Karnell LH et al. National cancer database report on malignant paragangliomas of the head and neck. *Cancer.* 2002;94:730. [PMID: 11857306] (A review of 59 cases of patients with malignant paraganglioma, including their symptoms. Presents a treatment algorithm.)

Olsen KD. Tumors and surgery of the parapharyngeal space. *Laryngoscope.* 1994;104(63):1. [PMID: 8189998] (An excellent review of the anatomy, presentation, and treatment of tumors affecting the parapharyngeal space.)

Pensak ML, Gluckman JL, Shumrick KA. Parapharyngeal space tumors: an algorithm for evaluation and management. *Laryngoscope.* 1994;104:1170. [PMID: 8072368] (A review of 123 patients, including their symptoms. Presents a treatment algorithm.)

Surgical Treatment

Surgery is the mainstay of treatment. Intraoral biopsy and excision are generally contraindicated for all tumors.

A. TRANSCERVICAL APPROACH

The transcervical approach is used for excising post-styloid space neoplasms. After flap elevation and identification of the ramus mandibularis, direct access to the post-styloid space is gained without dissecting the submandibular triangle. This approach has the distinct advantage of excellent cosmesis.

B. TRANSCERVICAL-SUBMANDIBULAR APPROACH

The prestyloid parapharyngeal space may be satisfactorily approached through this method. A transverse incision is made in the most superior major skin fold, and then the superior portion of the cervical skin flap is elevated. The mandibular branch of the facial nerve must be identified and preserved. Retraction of the posterior belly of the digastric muscle permits the division and ligation of the facial artery, allowing the submandibular gland to be retracted anteriorly. The submandibular gland may be removed and the digastric tendon divided if additional exposure is required.

C. TRANSPAROTID-SUBMANDIBULAR APPROACH

The excision of tumors arising from the deep lobe of the parotid gland and extending into the parapharyngeal space require a transparotid-submandibular approach, including dissection of the facial nerve. A superficial parotidectomy is performed and then the deep lobe of the parotid gland is dissected free from the facial nerve. The mandibular branch of the facial nerve must be identified and preserved. Retraction of the posterior belly of the digastric muscle permits the division and ligation of the facial artery, allowing the submandibular gland to be retracted anteriorly. Lysis of the stylomandibular ligament enhances exposure; the neoplasm is then mobilized from the wound in a three-dimensional fashion.

D. TRANSMANDIBULAR APPROACH

The lateral mandibulotomy approach, commonly called the transmandibular approach, is best used for a pharyngeal malignant neoplasm that extends to the parapharyngeal space. This approach provides exposure and vessel control for vascular tumors extending to the skull base.

E. OTHER APPROACHES

Infratemporal fossa dissection and craniofacial approaches are reserved for malignant tumors, tumors involving the skull base, or tumors with intracranial extension.

Malone JP, Agrawal A, Schuller DE. Safety and efficacy of transcervical resection of parapharyngeal space neoplasms. *Ann Otol Rhinol Laryngol.* 2001;110:1093. [PMID: 11768696] (33 patients undergoing the transcervical approach for parapharyngeal space neoplasms with excellent local control.)

Complications

Paragangliomas account for most of the surgical morbidity (Table 21–5). There is a significant incidence of permanent deficits when operating on these neoplasms. A rehabilitation plan should be outlined with the patient and with family members who will aid in the support of the patient. The rehabilitation of speech and deglutition is facilitated if the patient understands (1) the function of cranial nerves IX, X, and XII and (2) the deficits that result with the functional loss of each nerve. The rehabilitation of a vagal paraganglioma may consist initially of augmentation by vocal fold injection with subsequent

Table 21–5. Complications of parapharyngeal space surgery.

Hematoma
Seroma
Airway obstruction
Infection
Tumor recurrence
First bite pain
Frey's syndrome
Cerebrospinal fluid leak
Meningitis
  Nerve injury (greater auricular, facial, glossopharyngeal, vagus, spinal accessory, hypoglossal, cervical, or sympathetic)
Vessel injury (stroke, hemorrhage, or death)

Data from Olsen KD. Tumors and surgery of the parapharyngeal space. *Laryngoscope* 1994;104(63):1.

medialization laryngoplasty. Persistent velopharyngeal insufficiency may require palatoplasty.

Benign neurilemomas, soft tissue tumors, and salivary gland neoplasms are typically associated with less morbidity and rare recurrence compared with paragangliomas. Recurrence of pleomorphic adenomas may be re-resected, followed by postoperative radiation therapy to improve local control. Alternately, neutron beam therapy for multiply recurrent pleomorphic adenoma may be considered.

Carew JF, Spiro RH, Singh B, Shah JP. Treatment of recurrent pleomorphic adenomas of the parotid gland. *Otolaryngol Head Neck Surg.* 1999;121:539. [PMID: 10547466] (31 patients with recurrent pleomorphic adenoma treated by surgical excision and radiation therapy.)

Douglas JG, Einck J, Austin-Seymour M, Koh WJ, Laramore GE. Neutron radiotherapy for recurrent pleomorphic adenomas of major salivary glands. *Head Neck.* 2001;23:1037. [PMID: 11774388] (Excellent local control rates in 16 patients with multiply recurrent pleomorphic adenomas treated with neutron radiation therapy.)

Elshaikh MA, Mahmoud-Ahmed AS, Kinney SE. Recurrent head-and-neck chemodectomas: a comparison of surgical and radiotherapeutic results. *Int J Radiat Oncol.* 2002;52:943. [PMID: 11958888] (Salvage radiation for patients with recurrent glomus jugulare and glomus tympanicum tumors. Surgical resection for recurrent carotid body tumors produced excellent local control.)

■ DEEP NECK SPACE INFECTIONS

ANATOMY OF FASCIAL NECK PLANES & SPACES

The spatial compartments within the neck are defined by fascial planes. An understanding of this complex anatomy aids the clinician in diagnosing the cause of an infection and its likely routes of spread. Commonly affected spatial compartments are the retropharyngeal, parapharyngeal, and submandibular spaces.

The fascia of the neck comprises the superficial and the deep layers. The deep layer of cervical fascia is further divided into three layers: superficial, middle, and deep. The superficial portion of the deep cervical fascia envelops the sternocleidomastoid and trapezius muscles. It extends superiorly to the hyoid bone where it surrounds the submandibular gland and the mandible. Inferiorly, it attaches to the clavicle and, medially, it forms the floor of the submandibular space as it covers the muscles of the floor of mouth. The middle layer of deep cervical fascia, also known as the visceral or pretracheal fascia, surrounds the infrahyoid strap muscles, the thyroid, the larynx, the trachea, and the esophagus. Below the hyoid, this layer continues inferiorly to fuse with the pericardium. Above the hyoid, this layer continues on the posterior pharyngeal wall as the buccopharyngeal fascia. Between the middle and deep layers of deep cervical fascia is the retropharyngeal space.

The deep layer of cervical fascia, also known as the prevertebral fascia, surrounds the prevertebral muscle. Anteriorly, the deep layer of cervical fascia divides to form a thin alar layer and a thicker prevertebral layer. Between these two layers is the "danger space," extending from the skull base to the diaphragm.

The submandibular space is bound in four ways: (1) anteriorly by the mandible, (2) superiorly by the mucosa of the floor of mouth, (3) inferiorly by the superficial layer of the deep cervical fascia, and (4) posteriorly by the parapharyngeal space. The mylohyoid muscle further divides this space into the submaxillary space (below the mylohyoid muscle) and sublingual space (above the mylohyoid muscle).

 ESSENTIALS OF DIAGNOSIS

- *Sore throat, dysphagia, odynophagia, neck pain.*
- *Fever, trismus, neck mass.*
- *CT scan with contrast, ring enhancement, scalloping of the abscess wall, or any combination of these findings.*

General Considerations

Deep space infections of the head and neck are problems encountered by both primary care physicians and otolaryngologists. Despite the wide use of antibiotics to treat early infections of the head and neck, infectious organisms still cause abscesses. These infections tend to follow the fascial planes of the neck. Controversy exists concerning the choices of empiric antimicrobial therapy, imaging modalities, and medical versus surgical treatment. The successful management of these potentially life-threatening infections depends on an understanding of the anatomy of the cervical fascial planes and spaces, bacteriology, and the potential complications that may arise.

Clinical Findings

A. SYMPTOMS AND SIGNS

A thorough history and physical exam help to localize the etiology and the extent of infection. Patients should be asked about a history of tonsillitis and peritonsillar abscess. A history of trauma to the retropharynx, either by intubation or the swallowing of a chicken or a fish bone, may lead the clinician to suspect a retropharyngeal abscess. Sialadenitis, dental caries and abscess, or localized cutaneous infections may lead to infections afflicting the submandibular space. An upper respiratory tract infection in the absence of other symptoms may be the only source of a necrotic parapharyngeal or retropharyngeal node. Diabetes, immunodeficiencies, or immunosuppression may contribute to the severity and the progression of disease. Generally, these patients tend to present with fever and leukocytosis, as well as signs and symptoms affecting the aerodigestive tract, including odynophagia, dysphagia, trismus, and dyspnea. On the physical exam, a parapharyngeal space abscess pushes medially to the tonsil and the lateral pharyngeal wall. Alternately, posterior wall swelling may be noted with a retropharyngeal space abscess.

B. LABORATORY FINDINGS

Laboratory tests should include a complete blood count, a measure of electrolytes with creatinine, and blood cultures. Leukocytosis is common and an increased hematocrit count may be suggestive of dehydration. Renal function should be checked before administration of intravenous contrast during the CT scan. Blood cultures should be drawn and sent before administering the first dose of antibiotics, especially if the imaging is suggestive of cellulitis rather than abscess.

C. IMAGING

Although the history and physical exam generally are sufficient to suggest deep neck abscesses, a variety of imaging studies may be useful both to confirm clinical suspicion and to delineate the extent of the infection. In the past, lateral plain radiographs aided in diagnosing retropharyngeal abscess; however, CT scans with intravenous contrast have become the cornerstone of diagnosis. Features of ring enhancement around a hypodense center have yielded a sensitivity of 87–95% and a specificity of 60–92% in

larger series. Furthermore, an irregular enhancing border around a hypodense region on a CT scan is associated with an increased specificity (94%) for purulence at the time of surgery. However, given that it is a late finding associated with the breakdown of the lymph node or abscess wall, its sensitivity is only 60%.

Ultrasound may be a more effective means of distinguishing an abscess from cellulitis. However, CT scans provide additional information about the extent of the infection, its relation to the great vessels, and, in the case of prevertebral and retropharyngeal space infections, CT scans can rule out mediastinal extension. This combination of information is important in determining the safest surgical approach to ensure complete drainage.

Although MRI gives overall better soft tissue detail, it has not been used extensively in the evaluation of deep neck abscesses. The clinician is often limited by its availability, but it is of obvious benefit in patients with renal dysfunction or contrast allergies.

Lazor JB, Cunningham MJ, Eavey RD, Weber AL. Comparison of computed tomography and surgical findings in deep neck infections. *Otolaryngol Head Neck Surg*. 1994;111(6):746. [PMID: 7991254] (Assesses the accuracy of CT scans in patients manifesting signs and symptoms of deep neck infection. The false-positive rate was 13.2% and the false-negative rate was 10.5%.)

Wetmore RF, Mahboubi S, Soyupak SK. Computed tomography in the evaluation of pediatric neck infections. *Otolaryngol Head Surg*. 1998;119:624. [PMID: 9852537] (Evaluates the efficacy of CT scans in superficial and deep neck infections; there is a 92% correlation between surgical and CT scan findings for deep neck infection.)

Differential Diagnosis

The differential diagnosis of a patient with fever, sore throat, and neck mass includes a broad spectrum of disorders. The diagnoses include pharyngitis with lymphadenopathy, suppurative lymphadenopathy, infected branchial cleft cyst, and deep neck abscess. A CT scan with contrast may help distinguish these various entities. Patients who present without fever or tenderness but with evidence of centrally hypodense lymph nodes should alert the physician to consider other less common entities such as mycobacterial infection, undiagnosed metastatic thyroid malignancy, and squamous cell carcinoma.

Treatment

The airway should be assessed on initial evaluation. If compromised, plans should be made for an immediate local tracheotomy or a fiberoptic intubation. Although fine-needle aspiration and intravenous antibiotics have demonstrated efficacy for superficial neck abscesses, the treatment of deep neck abscess is generally incision and drainage. Patients with equivocal radiographic findings (low or heterogeneous lesions without ring enhancement) may initially be treated with antibiotics alone. Common organisms from deep neck infections include *Staphylococcus, Streptococcus,* and *Bacteroides melaninogenicus.* Because of the increased incidence of penicillin resistance, antibiotics should cover gram-positive and anaerobic bacteria. If there is no clinical improvement on intravenous antibiotics within 48–72 hours, a repeat CT scan may document the evolution to abscess, therefore dictating the need for surgical intervention.

The surgical approach taken depends on the cause and the anatomic involvement of the infection. For example, in the retropharynx, lymph nodes generally involute with age. Thus, an abscess in the retropharyngeal space of an adult typically results from either trauma or the secondary spread of infection from a separately infected space. This infection is usually free to track vertically along fascial planes. In contrast, most pediatric abscesses result from suppurative adenitis. Because these pediatric abscesses typically originate in a lymph node, they are usually well contained in an inflammatory rind. Most pediatric otolaryngologists advocate transoral drainage for a patient with an infection of a retropharyngeal space abscess medial to the great vessels when it represents a confined process with no evidence of spread along the fascial planes. Abscesses with extension lateral to the great vessels may require transcervical or combined approaches for adequate drainage; these approaches may also be necessary in treating deep neck abscesses in adult patients.

Gidley PW, Ghorayeb BY, Stiernberg CM. Contemporary management of deep neck space infections. *Otolaryngol Head Neck Surg.* 1997;116(1):16. [PMID: 9018251] (Evaluation and treatment of infections of cervical neck spaces with a discussion of complications of deep neck space infections.)

Kirse DJ, Roberson DW. Surgical management of retropharyngeal space infections in children. *Laryngoscope.* 2001;111(8):1413. [PMID: 11568578] (Management of 73 retropharyngeal space tumors discussing the approach to and clinical significance of scalloping on a CT scan with contrast.)

Lalakea M, Messner AH. Retropharyngeal abscess management in children: current practices. *Otolaryngol Head Neck Surg.* 1999;121:398. [PMID: 10504595] (Pediatric otolaryngologists were surveyed to determine the current standard of care for retropharyngeal abscesses in children.)

Complications

With antibiotics, the incidence of complications of deep neck space infections has greatly diminished. Meningitis and cavernous sinus thrombosis have been reported as rare complications of these infections.

A. CAROTID ARTERY RUPTURE

Carotid artery rupture should be suspected with recurrent small hemorrhages, hematoma of the surrounding tissues, a protracted clinical course, and shock. Radiographic imaging, which allows for an earlier accurate diagnosis and appropriate intervention, has made this a rare sequela.

B. MEDIASTINITIS

Mediastinitis can occur from an infection spreading along the retropharyngeal, "danger," or prevertebral spaces. Patients may have increasing chest pain; a chest radiograph or CT scan may show a widened mediastinum. Adequate drainage may require thoracotomy.

C. INTERNAL JUGULAR VEIN THROMBOPHLEBITIS

The most common vascular complication is Lemierre syndrome (internal jugular vein thrombophlebitis). Sepsis and septic emboli frequently ensue and affect the lungs, the musculoskeletal system, and, occasionally, the liver. The treatment generally consists of β-lactamase-resistant antibiotics with good anaerobic coverage. The role of anticoagulation is controversial. The most common offending organism is *Fusobacterium necrophorum.* Surgical intervention is indicated when there is a lack of improvement after 48–72 hours of intravenous antibiotics.

William A, Nagy M, Wingate J, Bailey L, Wax M et al. Lemierre syndrome: a complication of acute pharyngitis. *Int J Pediatr Otorhinolaryngol.* 1998;45(1):51. [PMID: 9804020] (Case presentation and review of clinical presentation, diagnosis, and management.)

Benign & Malignant Lesions of the Oral Cavity, Oropharynx, & Nasopharynx

22

Nancy Lee, MD, & Kelvin Chan, BA

◼ BENIGN & MALIGNANT LESIONS OF THE ORAL CAVITY & OROPHARYNX

 ESSENTIALS OF DIAGNOSIS

- *Nonhealing ulcer, painful or bleeding lesion.*
- *Lump in oral cavity or oropharynx.*
- *Neck mass.*
- *Dysphagia or dysphonia or otalgia.*
- *Weight loss.*
- *Mass on imaging in primary site or neck.*
- *Positive biopsy of lesion.*

General Considerations

Cancer of the oral cavity includes several subsites: lip, anterior two thirds of the tongue, buccal mucosa, floor of mouth, hard palate, upper and lower gingiva, and retromolar trigone. There is an estimated annual incidence of 30,000 new oral cancers in the United States with approximately 4800 deaths per year. Men are affected 2–4 times more often than women for all racial and ethnic groups. The incidence of oral cancer increases with age.

Tobacco use (both chewing and smoking), alcohol, and poor oral hygiene are well-established causes of oral cavity cancer. Chewing betel nut, a common practice in Southeast Asia, is also a known cause of cancer of the buccal mucosa. Recent studies have identified HSV-1 and HPV-2, 11, and 16 as possible etiologic agents.

The oropharynx is posterior to the oral cavity and includes the posterior third of the tongue, also called base of tongue or lingual tonsil, palatine tonsil, soft palate, and posterior pharyngeal wall. These lesions are often silent in early stages and are frequently advanced at the time of presentation. Cancer of the oropharynx occurs in 8750 patients in the United States each year, resulting in approximately 4250 deaths. Males are afflicted 3–5 times more frequently than females. The incidence is related to tobacco and alcohol use.

Staging

Staging for both lip and oral cavity cancer is determined according to 2002 TNM (tumor, node, metastasis) staging (Table 22–1).

Pathogenesis

The oral cavity and the oropharynx are lined by squamous epithelium. Therefore, most cancers arising from these regions are squamous in origin. Verrucous carcinoma is a type of squamous cell carcinoma that is low grade and rarely metastasizes. Minor salivary glands found throughout the oral cavity and the oropharynx can give rise to adenocarcinoma, adenoid cystic carcinoma, mucoepidermoid carcinoma, and polymorphous low-grade carcinoma. Lymphoma is a particular consideration for tumors of the tonsillar fossa.

Cancers of the oral cavity are often heralded by precancerous lesions. Leukoplakia and erythroplakia are white and red areas, respectively, which are abnormal, but not necessarily neoplastic. The seriousness of these lesions can be determined only by a biopsy with evaluation under the microscope. These areas may be entirely benign, precancerous, or frankly invasive. A precancerous lesion is termed dysplastic and describes malignant cells that have not invaded normal underlying epithelial tissues. Dysplasia is classified by its tendency to progress to cancer as mild, moderate, or severe. Dysplasia, in

Table 22–1. 2002 Cancer staging: lip and oral cavity.

Primary Tumor (T)

T_X:	Primary tumor cannot be assessed
T_0:	No evidence of primary tumor
T_{is}:	Carcinoma *in situ*
T_1:	Tumor ≤ 2 cm in greatest dimension
T_2:	Tumor > 2 cm but not > 4 cm in greatest dimension
T_3:	Tumor > 4 cm in greatest dimension
T_4:	(Lip) Tumor invades through cortical bone, inferior alveolar nerve, floor of mouth, or skin of face, ie, chin or nose[1]
T_{4a}:	(Oral cavity) Tumor invades through cortical bone, into deep (extrinsic) muscle of tongue (genioglossus, hyoglossus, palatoglossus, and styloglossus), maxillary sinus, or skin of face
T_{4b}:	Tumor involves masticator space, pterygoid plates, or skull base and/or encases internal carotid artery

Regional Lymph Nodes (N)

N_X:	Regional lymph nodes cannot be assessed
N_0:	No regional lymph node metastasis
N_1:	Metastasis in a single ipsilateral lymph node ≤ 3 cm in greatest dimension
N_2:	Metastasis in a single ipsilateral lymph node > 3 cm but not > 6 cm in greatest dimension; or in multiple ipsilateral lymph nodes, none > 6 cm in greatest dimension; or in bilateral or contralateral lymph nodes, none > 6 cm in greatest dimension
N_{2a}:	Metastasis in a single ipsilateral lymph node > 3 cm but not > 6 cm in greatest dimension
N_{2b}:	Metastasis in multiple ipsilateral lymph nodes, none > 6 cm in greatest dimension
N_{2c}:	Metastasis in bilateral or contralateral lymph nodes, none > 6 cm in greatest dimension
N_3:	Metastasis in a lymph node > 6 cm in greatest dimension

Distant Metastasis (M)

M_X:	Distant metastasis cannot be assessed
M_0:	No distant metastasis
M_1:	Distant metastasis

Stage Grouping:

0:	T_{is}	N_0	M_0
I:	T_1	N_0	M_0
II:	T_2	N_0	M_0
III:	T_3	N_0	M_0
	T_1	N_1	M_0
	T_2	N_1	M_0
	T_3	N_1	M_0
IVA:	T_{4a}	N_0	M_0
	T_{4a}	N_1	M_0
	T_1	N_2	M_0
	T_2	N_2	M_0
	T_3	N_2	M_0
	T_{4a}	N_2	M_0
IVB:	Any T	N_3	M_0
	T_{4b}	Any N	M_0
IVC:	Any T	Any N	M_1

[1]Superficial erosion alone of bone/tooth socket by gingival primary is not sufficient to classify as T4.

Histology Grade (G)

G_X:	Grade cannot be assessed
G_1:	Well differentiated
G_2:	Moderately differentiated
G_3:	Poorly differentiated

(continued)

Table 22–1. 2002 Cancer staging: lip and oral cavity. (*Continued*)

Residual Tumor (R)

R_x:	Presence of residual tumor cannot be assessed
R_0:	No residual tumor
R_1:	Microscopic residual tumor
R_2:	Macroscopic residual tumor

Additional Descriptors

For identification of special cases of TNM or pTNM classifications, the "m" suffix and "y," "r," and "a" prefixes are used. Although they do not affect the stage grouping, they indicate cases needing separate analysis.

- **m suffix** indicates the presence of multiple primary tumors in a single site and is recorded in parentheses: pT(m)NM.
- **y prefix** indicates those cases in which classification is performed during or following initial multimodality therapy. The cTNM or pTNM category is identified by a "y" prefix. The ycTNM or ypTNM categorizes the extent of tumor actually present at the time of that examination. The "y" categorization is not an estimate of tumor prior to multimodality therapy.
- **r prefix** indicates a recurrent tumor when staged after a disease-free interval, and is identified by the "r" prefix: rTNM.
- **a prefix** designates the stage determined at autopsy: aTNM.

Lymphatic vessel invasion (L)

L_x:	Lymphatic vessel invasion cannot be assessed
L_0:	No lymphatic vessel invasion
L_1:	Lymphatic vessel invasion

Venous invasion (V)

V_x:	Venous invasion cannot be assessed
V_0:	No venous invasion
V_1:	Microscopic venous invasion
V_2:	Macroscopic venous invasion

mild forms, can regress if the carcinogenic agent is removed. Leukoplakia is usually a benign condition that is unlikely to progress into cancer (5%). Erythroplakia is more likely to advance to cancer at the time of the initial biopsy (51%).

Clinically, early mucosal lesions appear as an indurated nodule or shallow ulcer with poorly defined margins. These tumors may become exophytic or infiltrative, expanding rapidly into underlying muscles, which results in difficulty with speech or eating.

The incidence of lymph node involvement from cancers of the oral cavity is related to the site and size of the primary tumor. Cancers of the oral tongue and floor of mouth have a higher incidence of nodal metastases than do cancers of the lip, hard palate, and buccal mucosa. Cancers of the lip most commonly involve the lower lip and rarely proceed to lymphatic spread (5–10%). In the case of nodal spread from lip cancer, it is typically the submental and submandibular nodes that are involved. Lateral tongue, floor of mouth, and buccal cancers drain to the ipsilateral submandibular node as well as to the upper and mid-mandibular jugular nodes. Midline tumors may drain bilaterally.

Oropharyngeal tumors are frequently associated with nodal metastases at the time of diagnosis. The extensive lymphatics in this region drain primarily to the jugulodigastric basin. It is important to remember, however, that the retropharyngeal nodes are also at risk with oropharyngeal cancers.

Lung, liver, and bone are common metastatic sites for oral cavity and oropharyngeal cancers.

Prevention

Tobacco use accounts for 80–90% of oral cavity and oropharynx cancers in the United States. Stopping the use of tobacco products can greatly reduce the risk of oral cancer. Decreasing alcohol intake, particularly in smokers, also decreases the risk of oral cavity cancers. Cancer of the lip can be caused by exposure to the sun. This risk can be avoided with the use of sunscreen or a wide-brimmed hat. Pipe smokers are particularly at risk for cancer of the lower lip. Cessation of pipe smoking reduces this risk significantly.

Clinical Findings

A. SYMPTOMS AND SIGNS

The signs and symptoms of benign and malignant lesions of the oral cavity and the oropharynx include bumps on the lip or mouth and white or red patches in the oral cavity. Other symptoms suggesting a malignant growth include a nonhealing ulcer on the lip or mouth; unusual pain or bleeding in the mouth; difficulty or pain with chewing, swallowing, or speech; a change in the fit of dentures; a change in voice; referred ear pain; and neck masses.

B. LABORATORY FINDINGS

A standard laboratory evaluation should include a complete blood cell count and blood chemistry profile, including liver function tests, to rule out possible metastatic disease.

C. IMAGING STUDIES

A computed tomography (CT) scan, magnetic resonance imaging (MRI), or both types of imaging of the head and neck should be performed to evaluate the primary lesion and lymph node metastases. An MRI is preferred for the evaluation of soft tissue involvement; a CT scan is better to evaluate cortical bone involvement. A chest x-ray should be performed to rule out metastases.

D. SPECIAL TESTS AND EXAMINATIONS

Additional texts and examinations that may be recommended to further establish the correct diagnosis and staging include (1) examination under anesthesia, (2) direct laryngoscopy, (3) tumor mapping with toluidine blue dye and acetic acid, (4) a positron emission tomography (PET) scan to rule out metastatic disease if suspected in advanced-stage disease, (5) a pre-radiation dental evaluation and audiology exam, and (6) Panorex films of the mandible to rule out mandibular invasion.

Differential Diagnosis

When evaluating a patient with any of the above symptoms, the differential diagnosis for a malignant lesion should also include bacterial or viral infection, leukoplakia or erythroplakia, dysplasia, eosinophilic granuloma, fibroma, giant cell tumor, pyogenic granuloma, papilloma, and verruciform xanthoma.

Treatment

Surgery and radiation therapy are the primary treatment modalities for cancers of the oral cavity and the oropharynx. Surgery with or without postoperative radiation therapy is the preferred treatment modality for oral cavity cancer. A variety of surgical techniques are recommended for each of the various subsites within the oral cavity. Combined-modality treatment consisting of concurrent chemotherapy with radiation therapy and reserving surgery for salvage is the preferred treatment modality for cancer of the oropharynx.

Historically, radiation has been used in the postoperative setting for patients with a high risk of locoregional recurrence. Indicators of high risk include advanced T stage, close or positive margins, perineural invasion, multiple positive lymph nodes, and extracapsular lymph node extension. Two recent randomized trials showed that the addition of postoperative chemotherapy to radiation therapy can improve locoregional control and disease-free survival rates in patients with multiple positive lymph nodes, positive margin, and extracapsular extension. One of these studies also showed an improvement in the overall survival rate. A recent randomized trial has suggested that primary treatment with concurrent chemoradiotherapy offers equivalent control to surgery for various oropharyngeal lesions, with the potential advantage of maintaining swallowing and speech function.

In the postoperative setting, radiation is typically delivered through opposed lateral beams (Figure 22–1) with an anteroposterior beam to treat the low neck and supraclavicular fossa with a minimum prophylactic dose. Prophylactic doses are typically 5040–5400 cGy and are administered to regions at risk for micrometastases, but with no pathologic or radiologic evidence of involvement. A boost dose can be given to smaller areas at higher risk for recurrence via a variety of methods, including CT-based treatment planning, brachytherapy (Figure 22–2), or an intraoral cone. Higher doses at 6000–6300 cGy are given to nodal areas of involvement without any remaining gross disease.

For definitive treatment with radiation, higher doses are required because of the increased tumor mass. Areas of known gross or macroscopic disease require doses of 7000–7600 cGy. It is often advantageous to deliver these

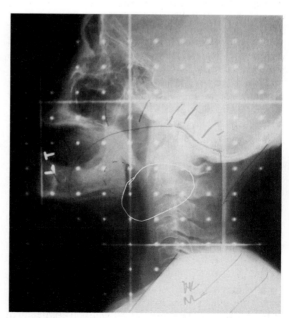

Figure 22–1. Simulation field for base of tongue cancer using parallel opposed beams.

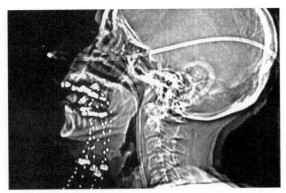

Figure 22–2. Simulation film of brachytherapy implant for oral tongue cancer.

higher doses through more sophisticated CT-based treatment planning techniques owing to the increased risk of toxic side effects with opposed lateral beams. Boosts can also be delivered via brachytherapy or an intraoral cone.

Standard fractionation for radiation is 180–200 cGy per day. This fractionation provides adequate tumor cell kill while allowing for DNA damage repair of normal tissues. Because of the high rate of tumor cell repopulation between fractions in head and neck cancers, a variety of hyperfractionation schedules (in smaller but more frequent doses) have been used. One such technique, the concomitant boost technique, gives a dose of 180 cGy to a larger area, including the tumor and primary nodal drainage, and a dose of 150 cGy 6 hours later to a smaller area of known involvement during the last 12 days of treatment. This regimen has been shown to provide better tumor control compared with standard fractionation.

Recent studies have also found that the use of *cis*-platinum-based chemotherapy during the course of radiation also gives better locoregional control and survival rates compared to radiation alone.

The toxic side effects of both hyperfractionation schemes and concurrent chemotherapy are tolerable, but significantly worse than standard fractionation radiation alone and must be considered when recommending treatment for individual patients.

The advent of intensity-modulated radiation therapy (IMRT) has been shown to decrease the rate of late effects such as xerostomia. Modulation of the intensity of the radiation beams aimed targeting the gross tumor while sparing the surrounding normal structures has resulted in improvement in patients' quality of life.

A. LIP

Small tumors of the lip (< 2 cm) can usually be cured surgically with a "V" excision with excellent functional and cosmetic results. Larger tumors (2–4 cm) are often treated with surgery. However, a reconstructive flap from the uninvolved opposing lip (eg, Abbe-Estlander technique) is often required to maintain cosmesis and function. Postoperative radiation is required for positive margins or perineural invasion. Tumors larger than 4 cm are best treated with a combination of surgery and postoperative radiation.

The lymph nodes are not usually treated for early-stage cancers of the lip unless clinically involved. Larger tumors require neck dissection, prophylactic irradiation of the cervical lymph nodes, or both because of an increased risk of micrometastatic disease.

B. ORAL TONGUE

For early T1 and T2 lesions that are deemed surgically resectable without significant functional morbidity, hemiglossectomy with neck dissection is the primary treatment modality. Postoperative radiation is indicated for high-risk features. For primary treatment with radiation, small lesions can be treated with brachytherapy alone, with neck dissection at the time of implant, whereas larger lesions require external-beam treatment to all nodal regions at risk with a boost to the primary tumor given via brachytherapy, an intraoral cone, or CT-based treatment planning.

Advanced T3 and T4 disease with deep muscle invasion is often associated with lymph node metastases and is typically treated with surgery and postoperative radiation, with or without concurrent chemotherapy. Neck dissection is indicated at the time of primary resection with postoperative radiation therapy to the neck for multiple positive lymph nodes or extracapsular extension.

C. FLOOR OF MOUTH

Small T1 or T2 tumors are highly curable with surgery or radiation alone. Postoperative radiation is indicated for positive margins or perineural invasion. For primary radiation therapy, small lesions may be managed with brachytherapy alone. Lesions in close proximity to the mandible should not be treated with brachytherapy owing to the risk of osteonecrosis. Selective nodal dissection, prophylactic nodal treatment with radiation, or both is warranted for T1 or T2 lesions with a thickness > 4 mm.

Larger infiltrative T3 or T4 lesions are best treated by radical surgery—often a composite resection—followed by postoperative radiation therapy, with or without chemotherapy. Ipsilateral neck dissection is indicated for advanced lesions and bilateral neck dissections for lesions approaching the midline.

D. BUCCAL MUCOSA

Small superficial T1 lesions can be treated with surgical excision alone with good local control. T2 lesions and those lesions approaching the commissure are better treated with radiation because of the better cosmetic and functional outcome. Radiation can be delivered via external beam, brachytherapy, or an oral cone, depending on the clinical situation. For small lesions with clinically negative nodes, the neck can be observed.

T3 and T4 lesions with deep muscle invasion are usually treated with radical surgery followed by postoperative radiation with or without chemotherapy. Ipsilateral neck dissection is indicated in all T3 and T4 disease.

E. ALVEOLAR RIDGE AND RETROMOLAR TRIGONE

T1 lesions with minimal cortical invasion may be treated with surgery or radiation alone, with postoperative radiation for positive margins.

More advanced lesions require radical surgery, with removal of involved bone and neck node dissection followed by postoperative radiation therapy. Primary treatment with irradiation is not recommended for lesions with bone invasion.

Because of the tendency for lymph node metastases (an average of 30%), selective neck dissection of levels I, II, and III is recommended for all tumors with bone invasion. More advanced lesions require full neck dissections with postoperative radiation.

F. HARD PALATE

T1 and T2 disease can be managed surgically with an infrastructure maxillectomy. Elective treatment of the neck is not necessary. If the primary disease extends beyond the hard palate, a limited neck dissection of levels I, II, and III is indicated.

Advanced lesions require radical surgery with total removal of the palate and neck dissection with postoperative radiation for nodal disease, positive margins, or both.

G. BASE OF TONGUE

Early lesions can be treated with equal efficacy with surgery or radiation. Surgery usually entails a hemiglossectomy and regional node dissection. Postoperative radiation is indicated for high-risk features.

Advanced lesions of the base of tongue often require total glossectomy and laryngectomy as well as bilateral neck dissection often followed by postoperative radiation. Because of the severe functional morbidity of this procedure, an increasing number of these patients are being treated with an organ-sparing treatment approach with concurrent chemotherapy and radiation, reserving surgery for salvage with equal efficacy.

H. TONSIL, TONSILLAR FOSSA, AND SOFT PALATE

Early-stage disease, most commonly from the soft palate or tonsillar pillar, can be treated with surgery, including ipsilateral neck dissection. Tumors approaching the midline require bilateral neck dissection. Radiation can be used

postoperatively for high-risk features, such as close or positive margins and positive lymph nodes. Likewise, radiation can be used as a primary treatment for early-stage lesions. The advantages of radiation include a more comprehensive treatment of the regional nodes, including the retropharyngeal nodes, which are often difficult to address surgically.

Advanced lesions are commonly from the tonsillar fossa and have historically been treated with radical surgery followed by postoperative radiation. However, owing to the severe functional morbidity of this treatment, there has been increasing interest in primary treatment with radiation, with or without chemotherapy. For lesions arising from the tonsillar fossa, it is important to rule out a diagnosis of lymphoma before proceeding with the treatment.

I. PHARYNGEAL WALL

Much like tumors of the tonsillar region, early lesions may be treated with surgery or radiation. Surgical resection often entails a transhyoid approach and wide excision with removal of the prevertebral fascia. Bilateral neck dissection is indicated for all early pharyngeal wall lesions. Since a surgical margin is difficult to obtain in this area, postoperative radiation is often indicated. Likewise, radiation therapy fields must include a prophylactic dose to the neck bilaterally with a boost to the primary tumor, being careful to avoid an excessive dose to the spinal cord.

Advanced lesions of the posterior pharyngeal wall usually require combined-modality therapy with radical surgery, followed by postoperative radiation or definitive treatment with radiation, with or without chemotherapy.

Complications

A. SURGICAL COMPLICATIONS

The complications of surgery include infection; weight loss; facial swelling; difficulty with speech, phonation, and swallowing; and loss of speech or swallowing capability.

B. RADIATION-RELATED COMPLICATIONS

The complications of radiation include fatigue and weight loss; mucositis; xerostomia (dryness of mouth) and loss of taste; erythema and moist desquamation of skin; and laryngeal edema, causing hoarseness. Rare, but severe, complications of radiation include possible hearing loss, osteoradionecrosis, trismus, and carotid artery rupture. With the advent of IMRT, the rate of xerostomia has significantly decreased, resulting in improvement in the patient's quality of life.

Prognosis

For T1, T2, T3, and T4 tumors of the oral cavity and the oropharynx, the 5-year survival rates are approximately 80%, 60%, 40%, and 20%, respectively. The presence of nodal metastases halves the prognosis for any given T stage. Survival rates are variable for each individual subsite.

Adelstein DJ, Li Y, Adams GL et al. An intergroup phase III comparison of standard radiation therapy and two schedules of concurrent chemoradiotherapy in patients with unresectable squamous cell head and neck cancer. *J Clin Oncol.* 2003;21(20):3887. [PMID: 12506176] (The use of chemotherapy with radiation for definitive treatment of advanced head and neck cancers gives improved results compared with radiation alone.)

Bernier J, Domenge C, Ozsahin M et al. Postoperative irradiation with or without concomitant chemotherapy for locally advanced head and neck cancer. *N Engl J Med.* 2004;350:1945.

Cooper JS, Pajak TF, Forastiere A et al. Post-operative concurrent radiochemotherapy in high-risk SCCA of the head and neck: Initial Report of RTOG 9501-Intergroup Phase III Trial. *N Engl J Med.* 2004;350:1937.

de Arruda FF, Puri D, Zhung J et al. Intensity-modulated radiation therapy for the treatment of oropharyngeal carcinoma: the Memorial Sloan-Kettering Cancer Center experience. *Int J Radiat Oncol Biol Phys.* 2006, in press. (The use of IMRT in the treatment of oropharyngeal cancer has resulted in excellent locoregional control and improvement in patient quality of life.)

Denis F, Garaud P, Bardet E et al. Final results of the 94-01 French Head and Neck Oncology and Radiotherapy Group randomized trial comparing radiotherapy alone with concomitant radiochemotherapy in advanced-stage oropharynx carcinoma. *J Clin Oncol.* 2004;22(1):19. [PMID: 14657228] (The use of chemotherapy with radiation gives improved results in oropharyngeal cancer patients over radiation alone.)

Fu KK, Patak TF, Trotti A et al. A radiation therapy oncology group phase III randomized study to compare hyperfractionation and two variants of accelerated fractionation to standard fractionation radiotherapy for head and neck squamous cell carcinomas: first report of RTOG 9003. An update of this trial presented in the American Society of Therapeutic Radiation Oncology has shown a 40% Grade 3 or higher late complication. *Int J Radiat Oncol Biol Phys.* 2000;48(1):7. [PMID: 109249666] (Concomitant boost technique gives better control compared with standard fractionation.)

Huang DT, Johnson CR, Schmidt-Ullrick R, Grimes M. Postoperative radiotherapy in head and neck carcinoma with extracapsular lymph node extension and/or positive resection margins: a comparative study. *Int J Radiat Oncol Biol Phys.* 1992; 23:737. [PMID: 1618666] (Indications for postoperative radiotherapy in patients with head and neck cancers.)

Mashburg A, Samit AM. Early detection, diagnosis, and management of oral and oropharyngeal cancer. *Cancer J Physicians.* 1989;39:67. [PMID: 24951159] (Review of diagnosis and management of oral and oropharyngeal cancers.)

WEB SITES

[The Cancer Group Institute]
http://www.cancergroup.com (Background epidemiological information on oral cavity and oropharyngeal cancers.)

[The National Cancer Institute]
http://www.cancer.gov (Treatment and prevention of oral cavity and oropharyngeal cancers.)

[Web MD Corporation]

http://www.webmd.lycos.com (A review of lip and oral cavity cancer, presenting symptoms, staging, and treatment.)

[The American Cancer Society]
http://www.cancer.org (Overview of benign and malignant lesions of the oral cavity and oropharynx.)

■ BENIGN & MALIGNANT LESIONS OF THE NASOPHARYNX

ESSENTIALS OF DIAGNOSIS

- Positive biopsy.
- Mass on CT or MRI.
- Neck mass.
- Epistaxis or nasal discharge.
- Refractory otitis media.
- Ear pain or hearing loss.

General Considerations

The nasopharynx is a roughly cuboidal muscular tube located behind the nose in the upper part of the pharynx. The borders of the nasopharynx include the posterior nasal cavity anteriorly, the sphenoid superiorly, the first and second vertebrae posteriorly, and the soft palate inferiorly. The lateral walls include the eustachian tube, the torus tuberis, and the fossa of Rosenmüller. The most common site of origin within the nasopharynx is the fossa of Rosenmüller.

Lymphatics from the nasopharynx run in an anteroposterior direction toward the base of the skull, where cranial nerves IX (the glossopharyngeal nerve) and XII (the hypoglossal nerve) lie. Other lymphatic pathways include deep drainage to the posterior cervical lymph nodes and to the jugulodigastric nodes. Lymphadenopathy is very common—about 80%—at presentation. Distant metastases, most frequently to the bone, correlate strongly with lymph node involvement (eg, N0 patients have a 17% incidence of metastases, whereas N3 patients have a 73% incidence).

Pathologic subtypes include keratinizing squamous cell carcinoma, nonkeratinizing squamous cell carcinoma, undifferentiated tumors, lymphoepithelioma, and lymphoma. Rare histologic subtypes include sarcoma, adenoid cystic carcinoma, plasmacytoma, melanoma, and rhabdomyosarcoma. Lymphoepithelioma and non-keratinizing tumors are the most common subtype and share the best prognosis due to their high radiosensitivity.

Each year there are approximately 11,000 new cases of nasopharyngeal carcinoma. There is a predominance in males, with a 2.5:1.0 male-to-female ratio, and it is primarily prevalent in individuals from southern China.

Staging

Staging for nasopharyngeal cancer is different from that for the oral cavity and the oropharynx (Table 22–2).

Pathogenesis

There is a suggestion of a genetic predisposition as first-

Table 22–2. Cancer staging: pharynx (including base of tongue, soft palate, and uvula).

Primary Tumor (T)	
T_x:	Primary tumor cannot be assessed
T_0:	No evidence of primary tumor
T_{is}:	Carcinoma *in situ*
Nasopharynx	
T_1:	Tumor confined to the nasopharynx
T_2:	Tumor extends to the soft tissues
T_{2a}:	Tumor extends to the oropharynx and/or nasal cavity without parapharyngeal extension[1]
T_{2b}:	Any tumor with parapharyngeal extension[1]
T_3:	Tumor involves bony structures and/or paranasal sinuses
T_4:	Tumor with intracranial extension and/or involvement of cranial nerves, infratemporal fossa, hypopharynx, orbit, or masticator space
Oropharynx	
T_1:	Tumor ≤ 2 cm in greatest dimension
T_2:	Tumor > 2 cm but not > 4 cm in greatest dimension
T_3:	Tumor > 4 cm in greatest dimension
T_{4a}:	Tumor invades the larynx, deep/extrinsic muscle of tongue, medial pterygoid, hard palate, or mandible
T_{4b}:	Tumor invades lateral pterygoid muscle, pterygoid plates, lateral nasopharynx, or skull base or encases carotid artery
Hypopharynx	
T_1:	Tumor limited to one subsite of hypopharynx and 2 cm or less in greatest dimension
T_2:	Tumor invades more than one subsite of hypopharynx or an adjacent site, or measures > 2 cm but not > 4 cm in greatest dimension without fixation of hemilarynx
T_3:	Tumor measures > 4 cm in greatest dimension or within fixation of hemilarynx
T_{4a}:	Tumor invades thyroid/cricoid cartilage, hyoid bone, thyroid gland, esophagus, or central compartment soft tissue[2]
T_{4b}:	Tumor invades prevertebral fascia, encases carotid artery, or involves mediastinal structures
Regional Lymph Nodes (N)	
Nasopharynx	
N_x:	Regional lymph nodes cannot be assessed
N_0:	No regional lymph node metastasis
N_1:	Unilateral metastasis in lymph node(s) ≤ 6 cm in greatest dimension, above supraclavicular fossa[3]
N_2:	Bilateral metastasis in lymph node(s) ≤ 6 cm in greatest dimension, above supraclavicular fossa[3]
N_3:	Metastasis in lymph node(s) > 6 cm and/or to supraclavicular fossa
N_{3a}:	> 6 cm in greatest dimension
N_{3b}:	Extension to the supraclavicular fossa[3]
Oropharynx and Hypopharynx	
N_x:	Regional lymph nodes cannot be assessed
N_0:	No regional lymph node metastasis
N_1:	Metastasis in a single ipsilateral lymph nodes ≤ 3 cm in greatest dimension
N_2:	Metastasis in a single ipsilateral lymph nodes > 3 cm but not > 6 cm in greatest dimension; or in multiple ipsilateral lymph nodes, none > 6 cm in greatest dimension; or in bilateral or contralateral lymph nodes, none > 6 cm in greatest dimension

(continued)

Table 22–2. Cancer staging: pharynx (including base of tongue, soft palate, and uvula). *(Continued)*

N_{2a}:	Metastasis in a single ipsilateral lymph node > 3 cm but not > 6 cm in greatest dimension
N_{2b}:	Metastasis in multiple ipsilateral lymph nodes, none > 6 cm in greatest dimension
N_{2c}:	Metastasis in bilateral or contralateral lymph nodes, none > 6 cm in greatest dimension
N_3:	Metastasis in a lymph node > 6 cm in greatest dimension

Distant Metastasis (M)

M_x:	Distant metastasis cannot be assessed
M_0:	No distant metastasis
M_1:	Distant metastasis

[1]Parapharyngeal extension denotes posterolateral infiltration of tumor beyond the pharyngobasilar fascia.
[2]Central compartment soft tissue includes prelaryngeal strap muscles and subcutaneous fat.
[3]Midline nodes are considered ipsilateral nodes.

Stage Grouping: Nasopharynx

0:	T_{is}	N_0	M_0
I:	T_1	N_0	M_0
IIA:	T_{2a}	N_0	M_0
IIB:	T_1	N_1	M_0
	T_2	N_1	M_0
	T_{2a}	N_1	M_0
	T_{2b}	N_0	M_0
	T_{2b}	N_1	M_0
III:	T_1	N_2	M_0
	T_{2a}	N_2	M_0
	T_{2b}	N_2	M_0
	T_3	N_0	M_0
	T_3	N_1	M_0
	T_3	N_2	M_0
IVA:	T_4	N_0	M_0
	T_4	N_1	M_0
	T_4	N_2	M_0
IVB:	Any T	N_3	M_0
IVC:	Any T	Any N	M_1

Stage Grouping: Oropharynx and Hypopharynx

0:	T_{is}	N_0	M_0
I:	T_1	N_0	M_0
II:	T_2	N_0	M_0
III:	T_3	N_0	M_0
	T_1	N_1	M_0
	T_2	N_1	M_0
	T_3	N_1	M_0
IVA:	T_{4a}	N_0	M_0
	T_{4a}	N_1	M_0
	T_1	N_2	M_0
	T_2	N_2	M_0
	T_3	N_2	M_0
	T_{4a}	N_2	M_0
IVB:	T_{4b}	Any N	M_0
	Any T	N_3	M_0
IVC:	Any T	Any N	M_1

Histology Grade (G) (Oropharynx, Hypopharynx)

G_x:	Grade cannot be assessed
G_1:	Well differentiated
G_2:	Moderately differentiated

(continued)

Table 22–2. Cancer staging: pharynx (including base of tongue, soft palate, and uvula). (*Continued*)

G$_3$:	Poorly differentiated

Residual Tumor (R)

R$_x$:	Presence of residual tumor cannot be assessed
R$_0$:	No residual tumor
R$_1$:	Microscopic residual tumor
R$_2$:	Macroscopic residual tumor

Additional Descriptors

For identification of special cases of TNM or pTNM classifications, the "m" suffix and "y," "r," and "a" prefixes are used. Although they do not affect the stage grouping, they indicate cases needing separate analysis.

• **m suffix** indicates the presence of multiple primary tumors in a single site and is recorded in parentheses: pT(m)NM.

• **y prefix** indicates those cases in which classification is performed during or following initial multimodality therapy. The cTNM or pTNM category is identified by a "y" prefix. The ycTNM or ypTNM categorizes the extent of tumor actually present at the time of that examination. The "y" categorization is not an estimate of tumor prior to multimodality therapy.

• **r prefix** indicates a recurrent tumor when staged after a disease-free interval, and is identified by the "r" prefix: rTNM.

• **a prefix** designates the stage determined at autopsy: aTNM.

Lymphatic vessel invasion (L)

L$_x$:	Lymphatic vessel invasion cannot be assessed
L$_0$:	No lymphatic vessel invasion
L$_1$:	Lymphatic vessel invasion

Venous invasion (V)

V$_x$:	Venous invasion cannot be assessed
V$_0$:	No venous invasion
V$_1$:	Microscopic venous invasion
V$_2$:	Macroscopic venous invasion

generation Chinese Americans retain a higher incidence rate than Caucasian Americans. Genetic associations to nasopharyngeal carcinoma include HLA-BW46, and HLA-B17. Other causes include viral infection with the Epstein-Barr virus (EBV); dietary factors, including salt-cured fish; and environmental factors such as sawdust and smoke inhalation. As in other head and neck cancers, smoking is associated with a higher incidence, particularly in Caucasian males.

Prevention

Smoking cessation and dietary modification to reduce salt-cured fish intake are factors that may be modified to reduce the risk of nasopharyngeal carcinoma.

Clinical Findings

A. SYMPTOMS AND SIGNS

The signs and symptoms of nasopharyngeal carcinoma include cervical adenopathy, which is the most common presenting symptom; epistaxis; serous otitis media, unilateral hearing impairment, or both; nasal obstruction; cranial nerve paralysis (CN VI, the abducens nerve, which is the most commonly involved); *retrosphenoidal syndrome of Jacod* (ie, difficulty with facial expression, as well as eye and jaw movement problems), *retroparotidian syndrome of Villaret* (ie, trouble swallowing, and tongue and neck movement problems), and referred ear pain.

B. LABORATORY FINDINGS

Complete blood count and liver function tests should be checked to rule out metastatic disease. EBV titers are elevated in patients with undifferentiated nasopharyngeal tumors and should be checked in the case of an unknown primary tumor of the head and neck.

C. IMAGING STUDIES

Standard imaging studies include CT with bone windows to rule out cortical bone involvement and MRI of the head and neck. Unless contraindicated, an MRI scan should be obtained. A chest x-ray should be obtained to rule out metastatic disease.

D. Special Tests and Examinations

Additional tests and examinations should include a pre-treatment dental evaluation and fiberoptic endoscopic examination. A bone scan should be done in the setting of advanced disease to rule out metastatic disease. PET scans have been used to evaluate extent of disease.

Differential Diagnosis

The differential diagnosis for nasopharyngeal carcinoma includes infection, Tornwaldt cyst (a nasopharyngeal cyst, usually midline, which may cause foul discharge), malignant metastasis from another primary site, and lymphoma.

Treatment

Because of the difficulty in obtaining adequate surgical margins, the primary treatment for nasopharyngeal carcinoma is with definitive radiation therapy, even in early-stage lesions. Radiation therapy fields include bilateral neck and supraclavicular nodes, as well as retropharyngeal nodes, owing to the high propensity for nodal metastases. Prophylactic doses of 5040 cGy are given to nodal regions at risk with a boost of 2000–3000 cGy to the primary tumor and involved nodal regions. Several techniques have been used to deliver the boost, including brachytherapy via a Rotterdam applicator, 3-D conformal treatment planning (3D-CRT), as well as inversely planned IMRT. IMRT offers advantages over other treatment modalities in that it allows for the precise delivery of high doses of radiation with relative sparing of essential tissues, such as the parotid glands, optic apparatus, and the brainstem. Recent randomized data from Hong Kong showed an improvement in the rate of xerostomia for patients who undergo IMRT versus conventional radiation therapy.

Advanced lesions are treated preferably with IMRT as brachytherapy boosts are not adequate in these larger lesions. Recent randomized studies have consistently shown an advantage to treating T3 and T4 lesions with concurrent radiation and chemotherapy. Chemotherapy regimens include three cycles of cisplatin (100 mg/m^2) during radiation, and three cycles of cisplatin (80 mg/m^2) and 5-FU (1000 mg/m^2) after the completion of radiation.

Treatment for nasopharyngeal recurrence with radiation has shown some success (40% local control and survival) in patients who received more than 6000 cGy to the site of recurrence.

Complications of Radiation Therapy

Complications of radiation therapy for nasopharyngeal carcinoma include xerostomia, although this has dramatically decreased since the introduction of IMRT, chronic external otitis, otitis media, hearing impairment, dental problems, pituitary dysfunction, trismus (decreased range of jaw motion), and soft tissue or bone necrosis.

Prognosis

Early-stage T1 and T2 nasopharyngeal cancers have very high (> 95%) 5-year locoregional control rates. The 5-year overall survival rates are significantly lower, 70–75%, emphasizing the propensity of these lesions to metastasize. Advanced T3 and T4 lesions have average locoregional control rates of 70% and 50%, respectively. Locoregional control rates of 97% have been reported for all stages when treated with IMRT (50% of patients in one study had T3 or T4 lesions). The 5-year progression-free and overall survival rates for patients with advanced-stage cancers treated with concurrent chemotherapy and radiation therapy are 66% and 76%, respectively. Treatment for recurrent nasopharyngeal carcinoma with radiation doses > 6000 cGy gives a 5-year local control and overall survival rate of 40%.

Al-Sarraf M, Le Blanc M, Giri PG et al. Chemoradiotherapy versus radiotherapy in patients with advanced nasopharyngeal cancer: phase III randomized intergroup study 0099. *J Clin Oncol.* 1998;16(4):1310. [PMID: 9552031] (Chemotherapy with radiation gives improved results over radiation alone for patients with Stages III and IV nasopharyngeal carcinoma.)

Hwang JM, Fu KK, Phillips TL et al. Results and prognostic factors in the retreatment of locally recurrent nasopharyngeal carcinoma. *Int J Radiat Oncol Biol Phys.* 1998;41(5):1099. [PMID: 9719121] (Treatment of recurrent nasopharyngeal cancer with doses to 6000 cGy gives 40% survival and control rates.)

Lee N, Xia P, Quivey JM et al. Intensity-modulated radiotherapy in the treatment of nasopharyngeal carcinoma: an update of the UCSF experience. *Int J Radiat Oncol Biol Phys.* 2002;53(1):12. [PMID: 12007936] (IMRT for nasopharyngeal carcinomas gives 97% local control rates.)

WEB SITES

[The Cancer Group Institute]
http://www.cancergroup.com (Background information on nasopharyngeal cancer.)

[National Cancer Institute]
http://www.cancer.gov (Description of treatment for nasopharyngeal cancer.)

Mandibular Reconstruction

23

Jeffrey H. Spiegel, MD, FACS, & Jaimie DeRosa, MD

ESSENTIALS OF DIAGNOSIS

- *Mandibular reconstruction may be indicated for the following:*
- *Segmental defect of mandible following tumor ablation.*
- *Chronic osteomyelitis of the mandible or comminuted nonhealing mandible fracture.*
- *Acquired or congenital malformation of the mandible.*

General Considerations

Among the most exciting advances in modern surgery has been an improved ability to reconstruct surgical defects and areas of tissue loss. Reconstruction of an area implies recreating not only the shape and appearance of the missing or injured tissues, but also the function. That is, ideally, the reconstructed region would look, move, feel, and sense precisely the way the native tissues once did when they were in good health.

It is in the head and neck where the need for accuracy in both functional and aesthetic reconstruction becomes the most evident. In general, it is a person's face that identifies him to others and is the interface through which he both detects the feelings and sentiments of others and conveys his own emotions.

Pathogenesis

Several disease processes may result in significant injury to the mandible. Severe trauma (eg, a gunshot wound) can result in a comminuted nonhealing fracture or tissue loss. Similarly, a neoplastic process (most commonly squamous cell carcinoma) can invade the mandible. Regrettably, the current state of medicine is such that the surgical removal of some disease processes (eg, certain malignant conditions) still provides the best chance of curing these otherwise fatally progressive disorders. Thus, the ability to reconstruct the mandible retains significance.

Aesthetically, the mandible provides the shape for the lower third of the face, defines the border between the face and the neck, and positions the mentum and lower lip (with the mandibular dentition). Functionally, the mandible supports the masticatory forces and the mandibular dentition. The mandible helps support the tongue in both position and function—a fact easily remembered when one recognizes the significant role a small mandible with a large tongue can play in creating obstructive sleep disturbance. Masticatory bite forces can be significant, with an average of 726 N and maximal forces at the molar occlusal surfaces of 4346 N. Thus, the mandible must be strong and rigid.

Treatment

To choose an appropriate reconstruction method, the following factors should be considered in reconstructing the mandible: (1) the length and location of the mandibular defect, (2) associated soft tissue loss, (3) the overall health and well-being of the patient, (4) the patient's potential prognosis, (5) potential donor sites, (6) primary versus delayed repair, and (7) the patient's dental health and potential for dental rehabilitation.

A. RECONSTRUCTION OPTIONS

The easiest form of mandibular reconstruction is no reconstruction. That is, when faced with a segmental defect, simply close the surrounding soft tissues over the defect, leaving one or two "free-swinging" mandibular segments. This leaves the patient with a significant cosmetic and functional deficit, although for a small lateral defect in an edentulous patient, the cosmetic and functional deficit may be smaller than expected. Certainly, however, for a person missing a large segment of mandible or the anterior segment of the mandible, this leaves a significant deformity where the lower lip and mentum are extremely retrusive, a situation known as the "Andy Gump deformity" (Figure 23–1).

B. SOFT TISSUE CLOSURES

The earliest soft tissue closures used local tissues, cheek or tongue flaps, or pedicled flaps from the neck, scalp, forehead, or deltopectoral region, many of which required a staged reconstruction. However, without any rigid structural support, neither the form nor function of the mandible was reliably reconstructed with these

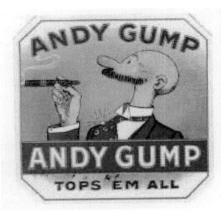

Figure 23–1. An Andy Gump cigar label. Note how the character's face appears to end at the upper lip (absence of the mandible). Ironically, the character is smoking a cigar.

methods. Sometimes, bone fragments pedicled on local flaps were tried, although they had less than desired reliability, particularly in the face of radiation before or after surgery.

C. ALLOPLASTIC IMPLANTS

The advent of alloplastic implants helped correct some of the problems that soft tissue closure alone did not address. These include steel, titanium, and other alloy (eg, Vitallium) implants that are fashioned into either a bar or a tray, which can then be conformed to the shape of the missing mandibular segment. Over time, titanium has become the most common metal with which

to fashion implants as it retains strength, biocompatibility, and rigidity, but can still be contoured using hand-held instruments. All alloplastic implants can eventually suffer metal fatigue and fracture owing to the repetitive stress put on the material through mastication. Unfortunately, materials strong enough to withstand the forces without the risk of fracture are too strong to be contoured in the operating room by the surgeon.

Mandibular replacement with alloplastic implants can provide a rapid, effective mandibular reconstruction without a secondary donor site defect. However, in addition to the risk of plate fracture, there can be a significant risk for plate extrusion and exposure with subsequent infection (Figure 23–2). Experience has demonstrated that a mandibular reconstruction plate, particularly if "wrapped" or otherwise insulated with a muscle pedicle flap (eg, a pectoralis major flap), is an adequate reconstructive option for lateral mandibular defects. Although microvascular free-tissue transfer provides some improvements and benefits, for a lateral defect, a mandibular bar is an acceptable contemporary reconstruction. However, for defects involving the anterior mandible, as well as the symphysis and the parasymphysial regions, mandibular reconstruction with a metal bar has a significantly higher risk of complications than reconstruction with revascularized bone. This may be due to the increased arc of rotation that the bar passes through at the anterior mandible, which causes excessive force on the overlying soft tissue, eventually leading to bar exposure. Also, unfortunately in many cases, metal bars without underlying bone grafting seem to have an increased chance of becoming exposed following radiation treatments. This can create

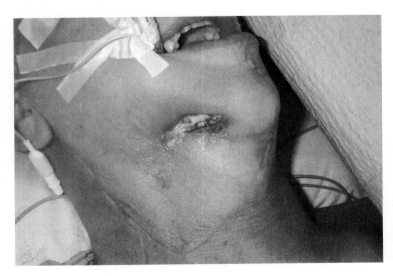

Figure 23–2. Patient after partial mandibulectomy with alloplastic (titanium) implant extruding a year after surgery. Note granulation tissue and purulent drainage.

a very complicated wound-healing challenge, typically requiring removal of the implant.

D. ALLOPLASTIC TRAYS

Alloplastic trays filled with bone chips have been used and in some cases have been successful, although some physicians have noted that 50% or more of their patients end up with an unsatisfactory result using this method. Other times, bone grafts can be used in the form of cancellous bone chips without a tray. In addition, irradiated bone grafts are used. However, in all of these cases, the grafted bone serves as a scaffold for osteoblasts to create new bone, and in the inevitably infected field encountered at the time of ablation, new bone growth is unpredictable and unreliable. Furthermore, irradiated fields create an additional impediment to good bone healing.

E. VASCULARIZED BONE

If bone substitutes (eg, metal bars), and free-bone grafts (in the form of chips or irradiated grafts) are unreliable, the next thing to try would be vascularized bone. Indeed, a variety of pedicled and free-bone flaps have been utilized.

1. Pedicled bone flaps—Initially, pedicled bone flaps were used. Physicians have tried to rotate the clavicle on the sternocleidomastoid muscle, the trapezius muscle, or even on the deltopectoral flap. Regrettably, only mixed success was obtained because the blood supply to the bone in each of these situations was unreliable and random. Somewhat better results were obtained with the pectoralis major muscle with the fifth rib, but again, only unreliable results were achieved. Rib grafts were also pedicled off of the latissimus dorsi muscle, but are not a great choice because, in general, this flap provides an unnecessarily large amount of muscle and soft tissue, with a usually inadequate amount of bone to provide a good reconstruction. Better results have been obtained by transferring the spine of the scapula onto the trapezius muscle. This flap provides approximately 10 cm of bone, and as long as the transverse cervical vessels are not injured during any part of the ablative procedure, the flap has fair reliability.

2. Osteotomies—At various times, a series of sliding osteotomies has been designed for use in the remaining mandible to allow the bone to be advanced to fill in gaps. Though interesting, the nature of the mandibular defect and the subsequent radiation may make these osteotomies unreliable.

F. FREE-TISSUE TRANSFER

To date, the best results have been achieved by free-tissue transfer. This technique provides both vascularized bone and soft tissue and has no restriction on pedicle range or length.

Free-tissue transfer techniques were not widely known even a few years ago, but at this time most academic medical center departments of otolaryngology have at least one surgeon who is trained in microvascular methods. Unfortunately, microvascular transfer remains a relatively long and complex procedure and although certainly valuable for large defects, it is more difficult to decide what to do for small defects. Often the extensive surgery required for a "free flap" seems to be too much when faced with a small anterior defect, however; still, no better alternative is available. Several flaps have been tried, and the four most commonly used osseous free flaps are (1) the radial forearm, (2) the scapula, (3) the iliac crest, and (4) the fibula. Each differs in the amount and nature of the soft tissue and bony components. All of these flaps, except the scapula flap, are sufficiently distant from the head and neck to allow for a second team of surgeons to (conveniently) simultaneously harvest the flap while the ablation is being performed.

1. Radial forearm flaps—The radial forearm flap allows the transfer of a large amount of pliable thin fascia and skin from the ventral surface of the forearm. Arterial supply is through the radial artery; therefore, an Allen test must be carefully performed before harvesting this flap to be certain that the hand has adequate vascular supply from the ulnar artery alone. Venous drainage is through the vena comitans of the radial artery or through the cephalic vein. Approximately 10 cm of bone can be taken. Although the bone is strong cortical bone, it is not thick because only one third of the cross-sectional area of the radial bone can be taken without greatly increasing the risk of stress fractures of the forearm. Tapering the edges of the graft in a "boat tail" fashion further reduces the risk of postoperative fractures, as does a prolonged immobilization of the arm in a splint (3 weeks or longer). Overall, since only a small amount of bone is obtained, this flap is useful for only certain mandibular defects and is probably best suited for reconstruction in which a large amount of soft tissue is required with only a small segmental mandibular defect.

2. Scapular flaps—The scapular flap is among the most versatile of free flaps, since a very large amount of soft tissue is available with the bone. Unfortunately, the usual need to change the position of the patient during surgery from supine to lateral to harvest the flap makes this flap less desirable to harvest than its usefulness might suggest.

The lateral scapula provides 12 cm of bone that can support an osseointegrated implant for dental rehabilitation (unlike the bone of the radial forearm flap). The circumflex scapular system provides the blood supply to the flap and, with dissection, the bone and large skin islands can be harvested off of the subscapular artery.

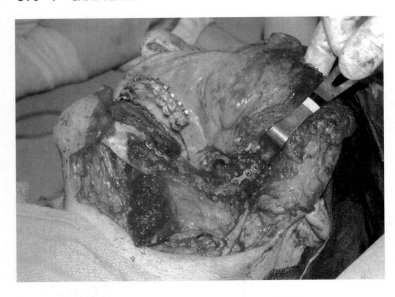

Figure 23–3. Inset iliac crest bone flap at the left mandibular angle. Note how the bone can be contoured without osteotomies due to the large bone stock available at the iliac crest.

Two venae comitantes (veins that travel closely in approximation to the artery) accompany this artery for venous drainage. In general, the scapular system of flaps may be the most versatile of all reconstructive options, providing a good amount of bone and the most independently mobile soft tissue components of any of the osseous composite flaps.

3. Iliac crest flaps—Based off the deep circumflex iliac artery and vein, the iliac crest flap has proved to be quite useful for mandibular reconstruction. Because of the great variety in which the bone can be harvested and contoured, three quarters or more of the mandible can be reconstructed with this flap (Figure 23–3). Furthermore, the natural curvature of the iliac crest bone can be used to help approximate the natural shape of the mandible. The bone is thick and can more than make up for the thickness of the mandible (Figure 23–4). A relatively thick and nonpliable skin flap can be harvested with the iliac crest, although it is often helpful to use a Doppler probe to initially identify perforating vessels to the skin.

The versatility of this flap was greatly enhanced when it was noted that the internal oblique muscle is reliably vascularized by an ascending branch off the deep circumflex

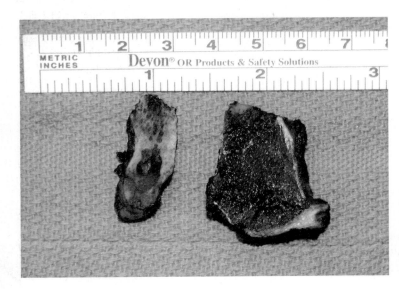

Figure 23–4. Comparison of cross sections of a mandible **(left)** and an iliac crest **(right)**. Note that the iliac crest bone is more than thick enough to recreate the mandible and accept implants for dental reconstruction.

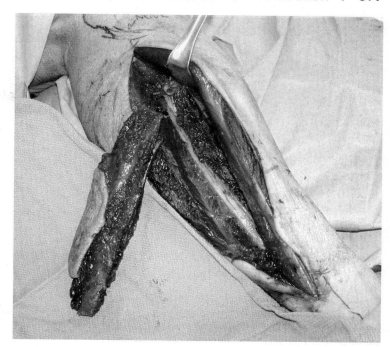

Figure 23–5. Harvesting of the right fibula. The bone and skin have been isolated on the right peroneal vessels.

iliac artery. This provides a thin, pliable muscle flap that can be used to reconstruct a soft tissue defect. For example, with a "through and through" defect of the lateral mandible and cheek, three effects are achieved: (1) the iliac crest bone can replace the mandibular bone, (2) the skin paddle can replace the skin of the external cheek, and (3) the internal oblique muscle can be used to reconstruct the mucosal surface defect and then left either to have mucosa grow over it or be covered with a skin graft. Removing the internal oblique muscle necessitates great care in closure to prevent an abdominal hernia.

Another excellent use for the iliac crest flap is for the reconstruction of a near-total glossectomy with mandibulectomy. In this situation, the iliac crest bone can be positioned transversely so that the bone forms the floor of the mouth. This then elevates the soft tissue skin flap of the iliac crest flap into good position to assist with swallowing once it is fashioned into a "neo-tongue."

4. Fibular flaps—Probably the most commonly used free-tissue flap for mandibular reconstruction, the fibular flap has several advantages. A very long segment of bone is available (approximately 25 cm), since the entire fibula can be harvested except for 8 cm, which should be preserved at the proximal and distal ends for joint stability (Figure 23–5). In addition, a reliable skin paddle is obtained and additional vascular soft tissue is

available as the flexor hallucis longus muscle can be harvested with the flap (Figure 23–6).

The fibular flap is based on the peroneal artery and veins. Preoperative vascular imaging is helpful to protect vascularity to the foot because vascular disease and anatomic irregularities can eliminate the normal three vessels that supply blood to the leg. Angiograms were once routinely ordered, although magnetic resonance imaging can be modified in protocol to provide adequate imaging of vascular anatomy. In addition, if desired, this flap can have sensory reinnervation through the lateral cutaneous branch of the peroneal nerve. Blood supply to the bone is through the periosteum; therefore, as long as most of the periosteum is not disturbed, numerous osteotomies can be made into the harvested fibula bone to allow for good custom contouring of the bone in recreating the mandible (Figure 23–7).

G. DISTRACTION OSTEOGENESIS

Distraction osteogenesis is a new technique that has some value in mandibular reconstruction. In this technique, an appliance is attached to the mandible, and a thin piece of the end of the mandibular segment is cut free from the rest of the mandible. This thin segment is slowly advanced through the use of a "key" attached to the appliance. As it is advanced, the space between the advancing segment and the bulk of the mandible is filled in with new bone. Once enough new bone has been made, the free ends are

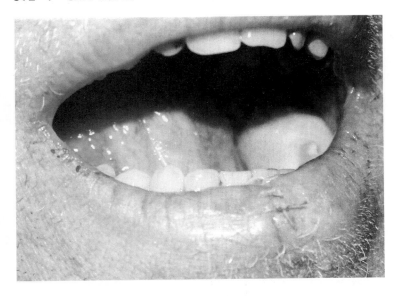

Figure 23–6. Postoperative photograph of viable skin from the fibula flap reconstructing the mucosa of the left "alveolar ridge" over the fibula bone.

"roughened" and then the remaining segments of mandible are plated, as for a mandibular fracture. Though exciting in concept, this technique does not allow for primary reconstruction because the distraction process takes time. Plus, at least one additional procedure is required. Thus far, the technique has been used primarily in cases of congenital mandibular insufficiency.

H. BONE GENERATION

Of current interest is the possibility of creating new bone through the use of growth factors and hydroxyapatite mixtures. The nature of the expression of the various bone morphogenic proteins is becoming increasingly understood, and soon it may be likely to bridge a

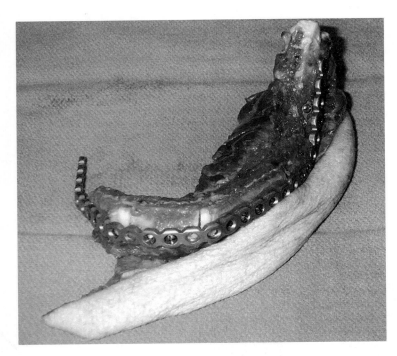

Figure 23–7. Fibular flap contoured to reconstruct the missing segments of the mandible. This tissue will then be inset and microvascular anastomoses will be performed to recreate a vascular supply.

bone gap with a bone-like powder that is mixed with bone growth factors, resulting in new, strong bone within a predictable period. Certainly, the ability to generate bone is far closer than the ability to generate good soft tissue coverage; therefore, the use of the osseous microvascular flap may be limited.

Complications

The most common complications of mandibular reconstruction include flap failure, fistulas, donor site morbidity, and the extrusion of alloplastic materials. A compromised vascular supply can lead to an ischemic flap and the need to either urgently revascularize or débride the tissue. In addition, small areas of dehiscence can lead to a salivary fistula, with the associated vascular risks. Sensory and motor nerves to the hand and foot are at risk during flap harvests, which can lead to donor site morbidity; gait abnormalities can result. Finally, alloplastic materials can extrude, even when placed onto a revascularized bone flap.

Mandpe AH, Singer MI, Kaplan MJ, Greene D. Alloplastic and microvascular restoration of the mandible: a comparison study. *Laryngoscope.* 1998;108(2):224. [PMID: 9473072] (Reviews indications for microvascular repair and when there are true benefits over a reconstruction bar.)

Urken ML, Buchbinder D, Costantino PD et al. Oromandibular reconstruction using microvascular composite flaps: report of 210 cases. *Arch Otolaryngol Head Neck Surg.* 1998;124(1):46. [PMID: 9440780] (Leaders and innovators in microvascular reconstruction review their results.)

Verdaguer J, Soler F, Fernandez-Alba J, Concejo J, Acero J. Sliding osteotomies in mandibular reconstruction. *Plast Reconstr Surg.* 2001;107(5)1107. [PMID: 11373549] (A description of alternatives to microvascular reconstruction or reconstruction bars.)

Jaw Cysts

Richard A. Smith, DDS

Cysts of the maxilla and mandible are common occurrences. Bone cysts occur more frequently in the jawbones than in any other bone because of the presence of epithelium from odontogenic elements (eg, teeth) and nonodontogenic epithelial remnants of embryonic structures.

A cyst is defined as an epithelial-lined pathologic cavity that may contain fluid or a semisolid material. A group of cystic lesions devoid of an epithelial lining is classified as pseudocysts. A jaw cyst is usually located deep within the jawbone, but it may occur on a bony surface, producing a saucerization.

 ESSENTIALS OF DIAGNOSIS

- Well-defined, totally or predominantly radiolucent, and sometimes expansile lesions.
- Usually slow growing and benign.
- Initially asymptomatic unless long-standing with significant enlargement or secondary infection.
- Usually initially discovered on routine dental x-rays.
- Requires histopathologic examination for diagnosis.

General Considerations

Jaw cysts encompass a group of lesions that are variable in their incidence, etiology, location, clinical behavior, and treatment. The most common jaw cyst is the radicular cyst, which is odontogenic and inflammatory in nature. The odontogenic developmental cyst is the second most common jaw cyst. Nonodontogenic cysts, pseudocysts, and ganglionic cysts of the temporomandibular joint (TMJ) are much less common. Cysts occur in both the mandible and the maxilla: inflammatory radicular cysts occur around the roots of nonvital teeth; odontogenic developmental dentigerous cysts and keratocysts occur in the common regions of impacted and unerupted teeth; nonodontogenic developmental cysts are found in regions of epithelial embryonic remnants; pseudocysts usually present in site-specific regions; and ganglionic cysts develop in the TMJ. Each

type of jaw cyst usually has a specific behavior pattern, ranging from small 5–6 mm osteolytic defects to massive involvement of the jaw and contiguous structures.

Classification of Jaw Cysts

The classification of jaw cysts includes (1) odontogenic cysts, (2) nonodontogenic cysts, and (3) pseudocysts. The ganglion cyst, which presents in the TMJ, has been added to this conventional classification for completeness; it is significant to clinicians managing the pathology of the head and neck region.

Pathogenesis

The pathogenesis of jaws cysts varies according to the specific cyst type. Inflammatory cysts derive their epithelial lining from the proliferation of odontogenic epithelium within the periodontal ligament; dentigerous developmental cysts result from the proliferation of reduced enamel epithelium. Figure 24–1 illustrates the development of dentigerous and radicular cysts. Cystic lesions may also result from cortical bone defects or trauma, they may represent reactive lesions, or they may have an unknown pathogenesis. It has been shown that there is an osmotic pressure gradient that produces fluid accumulation within the cyst lumen and generates pressure, creating cyst expansion.

Prevention

It may be possible to prevent odontogenic jaw cyst formation through the immediate treatment of nonvital teeth and the removal of impacted or unerupted teeth. Strategies should include preventing the progression of jaw cysts to large, destructive lesions that require aggressive management. Prevention is aided by routine and regular dental and oral examinations with appropriate imaging.

Clinical Findings

A. SYMPTOMS AND SIGNS

The patient with a small cyst is usually asymptomatic. Symptoms such as pain and swelling occur when the cyst becomes secondarily infected. The patient may report an

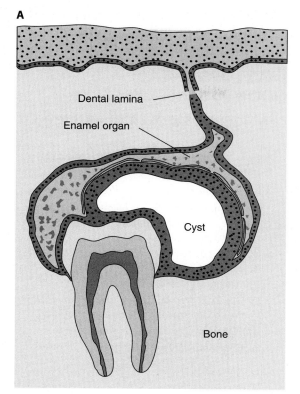

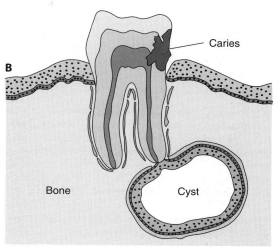

Figure 24–1. **(A)** Development of the dentigerous cyst around the crown of an unerupted tooth. **(B)** Development of a radicular cyst around the root apex of a nonvital tooth.

unpleasant or even foul taste if the cyst has discharged into the mouth through a sinus tract. Teeth contiguous to all cysts, except radicular cysts, have vital pulps, unless coincidental disease of these teeth exists. Tooth vitality can be assessed with electrical pulp testers or ice. Erupted teeth contiguous to a large cyst may maintain their vitality, despite the loss of a significant amount of supporting alveolar bone. Benign jaw cysts rarely produce loosening of adjacent teeth unless the cyst becomes very large. Large cysts can displace the roots of teeth that can be evident clinically, on an x-ray, or both. The clinical absence of one or more teeth, as seen on routine dental x-rays, may suggest the presence of a developing dentigerous cyst.

Extensive cysts in the anterior maxilla may extend under the nasal floor, creating nostril distortion. An infected maxillary cyst may involve the maxillary sinus, producing maxillary sinusitis. Large mandibular cysts may involve the mandibular canal and its contents, the inferior alveolar neurovascular bundle. The mandibular canal and its contents can be deflected inferiorly without producing a neurosensory deficit. However, if

an acute infection develops with pus accumulation, a decrease in lower lip sensibility may be observed.

B. Imaging Studies

The typical radiographic appearance of a jaw cyst is that of a well-defined, round-to-oval, unilocular or multilocular radiolucent cyst that is circumscribed by a dense periphery of reactive bone. Periapical and panoramic x-rays usually suffice for imaging small- to medium-sized cystic lesions, but computed tomography (CT) scans are indicated for large, expansile lesions. Anatomic structures such as the mental foramen, the incisive foramen, and the maxillary sinus may be misinterpreted as pathologic cystic lesions.

C. Special Tests

Needle aspiration of a suspected jaw cyst can reveal valuable diagnostic information. Aspiration of blood from the lesion may indicate the presence of a vascular lesion or an aneurysmal bone cyst. If aspiration of a solid lesion (eg, a tumor) is attempted, no fluid can be aspirated and withdrawing the plunger of the syringe is difficult. Aspiration of a light, straw-colored fluid containing cholesterol crystals (known by their characteristic "shimmering" effect in light) is consistent with a benign odontogenic cyst. Aspiration of a whitish to pale yellow material that appears similar to pus usually reveals an odontogenic keratocyst that contains desquamated cells and keratin. A cyst that has been present for a long time and has become infected may contain a thick yellow or brown material that is difficult to aspirate.

A histopathologic examination is essential for establishing a definitive diagnosis. For small lesions, excisional biopsy is appropriate; for large lesions, an incisional biopsy is indicated to establish a diagnosis, develop a treatment plan, and obtain appropriate informed consent.

Differential Diagnosis

An orderly approach to a differential diagnosis of a jaw lesion can be accomplished by grouping possible lesions into six main categories: (1) cysts, (2) odontogenic tumors, (3) benign nonodontogenic tumors, (4) inflammatory jaw lesions, (5) malignant nonodontogenic neoplasms of the jaw, and (6) metabolic and genetic jaw diseases. An assessment of the radiographic appearance, patient age, and location of the lesion enables the clinician to establish a reasonable differential diagnosis that should ultimately be confirmed by histopathologic examination. A definitive histopathologic diagnosis may rule out more serious lesions (eg, cystic ameloblastoma).

Complications

Complications related to the destruction caused by a jaw cyst and the surgical treatment required include loss of teeth and bone; infection; cyst recurrence; neurosensory deficits; oral or facial sinuses; oral, antral, or nasal fistulas, or a combination of these three complications; and pathologic jaw fracture. Carcinoma arising in an odontogenic cyst is a rare occurrence and requires aggressive treatment.

Treatment

Because contiguous structures—including displaced teeth, resorbed roots, bony supports, the maxillary sinus, and the mandibular canal—may be involved or encroached upon, jaw cysts usually require surgical management. However, jaw cysts that demonstrate slow or no progression or growth may be managed by observation in the elderly or severely medically compromised individuals. The exact nature of the surgery depends on the size, location, and clinical behavior of the specific type of cyst. Treatment is necessary because (1) cysts usually increase in size, causing local tissue destruction and usually becoming infected; and (2) extensive involvement of the mandible is capable of creating a potential pathologic fracture.

■ SPECIFIC TYPES OF JAW CYSTS

DEVELOPMENTAL ODONTOGENIC CYSTS

DENTIGEROUS (FOLLICULAR) CYSTS

 ESSENTIALS OF DIAGNOSIS

- Epithelial-lined, developmental, odontogenic cysts.
- Second most common type of jaw cyst associated with the crown of an impacted, unerupted, or developing tooth.
- Well-defined, radiolucent, sometimes expansile lesion.
- Usually slow growing and benign.
- Initially asymptomatic unless long-standing with significant enlargement or secondary infection.
- Usually discovered on routine dental x-rays.
- Requires histopathologic examination for diagnosis.

General Considerations

Fifteen to eighteen percent of jaws cysts are dentigerous, surround the crowns, and attach at the cementoenamel junction of unerupted teeth. The lower third molars and the upper canines are the most commonly involved teeth.

Pathogenesis

Dentigerous cysts derive their epithelium from the proliferation of the reduced enamel epithelium after the tooth enamel is formed. The cyst develops subsequent to an accumulation of fluid between the remnants of the enamel organ and the contiguous tooth crown. The expansion of this intrabony cyst is associated with an increase in the osmolality of the cyst fluid secondary to the migration of inflammatory cells into the cyst lumen. Epithelial proliferation may also occur simultaneously.

Prevention

Regular dental and oral examinations with appropriate imaging can identify developing cystic jaw lesions before any significant bony destruction can occur. The removal of impacted teeth, when indicated, serves as a preventive measure.

Clinical Findings

A. SYMPTOMS AND SIGNS

Small dentigerous cysts rarely produce clinical symptoms. Larger cysts can produce a bony expansion, which creates an intraoral swelling, an extraoral swelling, or both. They also can result in facial asymmetries or can become secondarily infected, which results in pain.

B. IMAGING STUDIES

The most common radiographic appearance of a dentigerous cyst is that of a well-delineated round-to-oval mass that is associated with an unerupted tooth, which may possibly be displaced. Figure 24–2 demonstrates a typical dentigerous cyst as observed on a panoramic x-ray. Periapical and panoramic x-rays can illustrate the extent of the cyst and contiguous anatomic structures. With large lesions, CT scanning is helpful in assessing the degree of expansion perforation and the involvement of adjacent structures.

C. SPECIAL TESTS

Needle aspiration with possible biopsy of the lumen of a suspected cystic lesion can give confirmatory diagnostic information and rule out a vascular lesion. If there has not been significant expansion of the cyst, with thinning of the bony cortex, it will not be possible to penetrate the bone using a needle and syringe technique. In these cases, if aspiration is desired, a small mucosal incision, followed by drilling a small hole through the buccal cortex, enables needle aspiration. Aspiration of a light, straw-colored fluid is characteristic of a dentigerous cyst (Figure 24–3). Histopathologic examination reveals a thin, nonkeratinized cyst lining. Inflammatory changes may produce epithelial hyperpla-

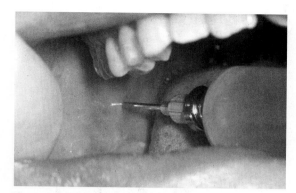

Figure 24–3. Aspiration of a straw-colored fluid from the lumen of a dentigerous cyst.

sia. Mural hemorrhage can result in cholesterol clefts, giant cells, and hemosiderin in the wall of the cyst. Hyaline bodies (eg, Rushton or hyaline bodies) may be present in the epithelium.

Differential Diagnosis

The differential diagnosis should include odontogenic keratocysts, ameloblastomas, cystic ameloblastomas, ameloblastic fibromas, and nonodontogenic tumors.

Complications

Complications related to the damage created by an expanding jaw cyst include bony destruction, infection, oral or facial sinuses, weakening of the jaw, displacement of teeth, resorption of adjacent tooth roots, encroachment on the maxillary sinus floor, and deflection of the inferior alveolar canal. The transformation of the epithelial lining of a dentigerous cyst into an ameloblastoma is also possible. Dysplasia or the carcinomatous transformation of the epithelial lining is possible, but rare. Complications related to the surgical management of cysts include devitalization of adjacent teeth, postoperative infection, neurosensory deficits, oral-antral fistulas, jaw fracture, and cyst recurrence.

Treatment

The treatment of choice consists of enucleation of the cyst and removal of the associated tooth. The surgical exposure is observed in Figure 24–4. The surgical flap can be repositioned and sutured with primary closure. Even large, bony cavities can regenerate new bone over several months' time. If the tissue breaks down, the cavity can be packed with $1/4$-inch gauze and gradually advanced over 7–10 days, followed by frequent saline irrigations to allow healing by secondary intention. For

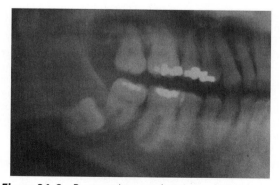

Figure 24–2. Panoramic x-ray showing a dentigerous cyst appearing as a well-defined radiolucency around the crown of an unerupted mandibular third molar.

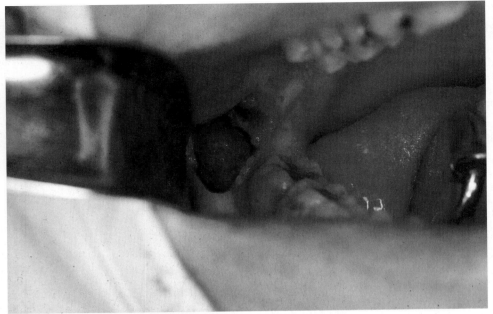

Figure 24–4. Surgical exposure of a dentigerous cyst in preparation for enucleation, in the mandibular third molar region.

extremely large surgical defects, primary bone grafting with autogenous cancellous chips can accelerate the healing process. Marsupialization of the cyst may be considered.

Prognosis

The prognosis after treatment of the cyst is excellent, with the expectation that the surgical defect will heal. The recurrence rate for the cyst is very low.

Rosenstein T, Pogrel MA, Smith RA, Regezi JA. Cystic ameloblastoma: behavior and treatment of 21 cases. *J Oral Maxillofacial Surg.* 2001;59:1311. [PMID: 11688034] (Cystic ameloblastomas have unexpected capacity for bony destruction and recurrence.)

Shimoyama T, Ide F, Horie N et al. Primary intraosseous carcinoma associated with impacted third molar of the mandible: review of the literature and report of a new case. *J Oral Sci.* 2001;43(4):287. [PMID: 11848197] (A primary intraosseous carcinoma occurred in a dentigerous cyst associated with an impacted third molar—mean patient age 73 years.)

ERUPTION CYSTS

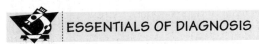

ESSENTIALS OF DIAGNOSIS

- *A variant of the dentigerous cyst.*

- *Presents as a bluish swelling on the alveolar ridge crest at the site of an erupting tooth.*

An eruption cyst occurs most commonly in the molar regions of the jaws in children less than 10 years of age. This cyst results from hemorrhage or fluid accumulation in the space between the crown and the reduced enamel epithelium. A dome-shaped, sometimes painful, frequently bluish swelling of the gingiva overlies an erupting tooth. A periapical or panoramic x-ray confirms the presence of an erupting tooth. The clinical presentation is pathognomonic for an eruption cyst. There may be trauma to the cyst, producing hemorrhage, which results in discoloration and pain. Most eruption cysts rupture spontaneously, and no treatment is required. However, excision of the overlying mucosa yields relief and facilitates eruption of the underlying tooth. The prognosis is excellent, and there should not be any detrimental effect to the associated erupting tooth.

Bodner L, Goldstein J, Sarnat H. Eruption cysts: a clinical report of 24 new cases. *J Clin Pediatr Dent.* 2004;28(2):183. [PMID: 14969381] (The eruption cyst occurs within the mucosa overlying a tooth that is about to erupt, has a raised, bluish appearance on the alveolar ridge, and should be managed conservatively.)

ODONTOGENIC KERATOCYSTS

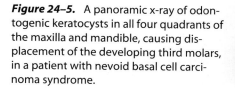

ESSENTIAL OF DIAGNOSIS

- *A developmental odontogenic cyst occurring in the tooth-bearing areas of the jaws or posterior to the mandibular third molar.*
- *Has a parakeratinized epithelial lining.*
- *May be a component of basal cell nevus syndrome (ie, Gorlin-Goltz syndrome).*
- *Has an aggressive clinical behavior with a high recurrence rate after treatment.*

General Considerations

Three to ten percent of odontogenic cysts are keratocysts and can occur at any age; however, 60% of patients are between 10 and 40 years of age. Odontogenic keratocysts may be part of Gorlin-Goltz syndrome, which includes multiple odontogenic keratocysts (Figure 24–5), multiple basal cell carcinomas, cutaneous abnormalities, skeletal anomalies, and cranial calcifications. This syndrome is a genetic disorder with autosomal dominant inheritance (ie, with mutation of the "PATCHED" tumor suppressor gene), high penetration, and variable expression.

Pathogenesis

The epithelium arises from cell rests of the dental lamina. However, it has been suggested that the cyst originates from extension of the basal cell components of the overlying oral epithelium. It also has been suggested that the growth of a keratocyst may be related to epithelial activity or enzymatic action in the fibrous cyst wall.

Prevention

Regular dental and oral examinations with appropriate imaging can assist both in identifying cystic lesions early in their course and preventing the development of large, destructive lesions.

Clinical Findings

A. Symptoms and Signs

The mandible is involved in 60–80% of odontogenic keratocysts, with a tendency to involve the posterior mandible and ascending ramus (Figures 24–6, 24–7, and 24–8). These cysts have a locally aggressive clinical behavior. Small odontogenic keratocysts usually are asymptomatic and are identified during routine dental examination and imaging. Larger odontogenic keratocysts may produce pain, drainage, swelling from secondary infection, and asymmetries from bony expansion. The adjacent teeth are vital, but can be displaced.

The features associated with Gorlin-Goltz syndrome include (1) odontogenic keratocysts of the jaws, (2) multiple basal cell carcinomas, (3) an enlarged occipitofrontal circumference, (4) mild ocular hypertelorism, (5) epidermal cysts, (6) palmar or plantar pits, (7) calcified ovarian cysts, (8) calcified falx cerebri, (9) rib abnormalities, (10) spina bifida, (11) short fourth metacarpals, (12) vertebral anomalies, and (13) pectus excavatum.

B. Imaging Studies

Panoramic x-rays and CT scans for large, expansile lesions reveal a locally destructive, multilocular lesion that can displace teeth, resorb tooth roots, deflect the mandibular canal inferiorly, and displace the floor of the maxillary sinus superiorly.

C. Special Tests

Aspiration of an odontogenic keratocyst produces a whitish or pale yellow, inspissated, cheese-like material

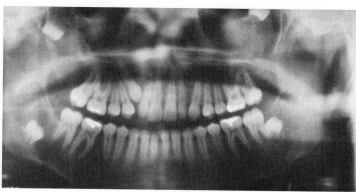

Figure 24–5. A panoramic x-ray of odontogenic keratocysts in all four quadrants of the maxilla and mandible, causing displacement of the developing third molars, in a patient with nevoid basal cell carcinoma syndrome.

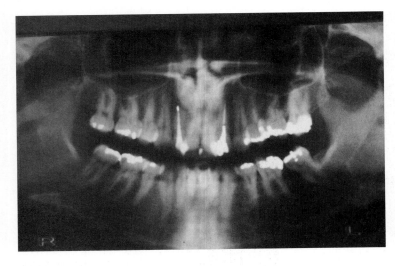

Figure 24–6. Preoperative panoramic x-ray of a left mandibular keratocyst in the premolar and molar regions that extends down to the inferior border of the mandible.

that may appear similar to purulent exudates, but is actually liquid-containing masses of desquamated keratinized cells. The combination of fine-needle aspiration biopsy with immunocytochemical testing for cytokeratin-10 in sampled epithelial cells has been shown to be accurate in distinguishing odontogenic keratocysts from nonodontogenic cysts.

Histopathologic examination of the cyst reveals an epithelial lining with a wavy or "corrugated" appearance and a thickness of 6–10 cell layers. The epithelium demonstrates basal palisading and a thin, refractile, parakeratinized lining. Any budding of the basal layer may produce "daughter cysts," which may be related to the high recurrence rate. A protein level > 4 mg/100 mL is highly suggestive of a keratocyst.

Differential Diagnosis

The differential diagnosis should include dentigerous cysts, ameloblastomas, cystic ameloblastomas, ameloblastic fibromas, and nonodontogenic neoplasms.

Complications

Complications are related to the aggressive clinical behavior of the keratocyst, which results in bony destruction. They are also related to a high recurrence rate, which may be due to the thin, friable cyst wall that is difficult to enucleate intact from the bone. Squamous cell carcinoma has been reported to occur in maxillary odontogenic keratocysts.

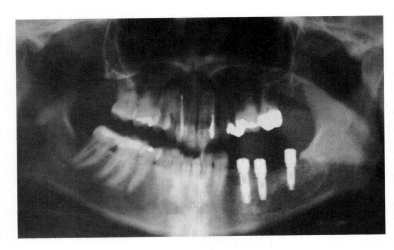

Figure 24–7. Postoperative panoramic x-ray after cyst enucleation, cryotherapy, and placement of a composite bone graft of cancellous bone from the iliac crest and bovine hydroxyapatite. Three endosseous dental implants were placed approximately 6 months later.

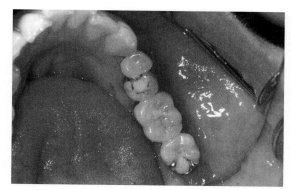

Figure 24–8. Clinical view of prosthetic crowns constructed on the dental implants, replacing the three posterior teeth.

Treatment

Enucleation (Figure 24–9), or decompression and marsupialization are the treatments of choice.

Pogrel MA. Treatment of keratocysts: the case for decompression and marsupialization. *J Oral Maxillofac Surg.* 2005;63:1667. [PMID: 16243185] (Decompression can be performed by making a small opening in the cyst and maintaining its patency with some type of drain.)

Small cysts (approximately 1 cm) may be managed with enucleation, curettage, and peripheral ostectomy. For larger cysts, enucleation followed by cryotherapy with liquid nitrogen may reduce recurrence rates. There have been reports of the effective use of the "Carnoy solution" to eliminate satellite cysts; these cysts are eliminated by the use of a chemical lavage that causes tissue fixation. The

potential for keratocysts to involve the overlying soft tissue through cortical perforation may necessitate a supraperiosteal dissection and excision of the overlying mucosa.

Prognosis

Long-term follow-up is essential because of the high recurrence rate. Most recurrences become evident within 5 years of the initial treatment.

Diaz-Fernandez JM, Infante-Cossio P, Belmonte-Caro R, Ruiz-Laza L, Garcia-Perla-Garcia A, Gutierrez-Perez JL. Basal cell nevus syndrome. Presentation of six cases and literature review. *Med Oral Patol Oral Cir Buccal.* 2005;1;10 (Suppl 1):E57. [PMID: 15800468] (Basal cell nevus syndrome may be associated with aggressive basal cell carcinomas and malignant neoplasias, for which early diagnosis and treatment are essential.)

Makowski GJ. Squamous cell carcinoma in a maxillary odontogenic keratocyst. *J Oral Maxillofac Surg.* 2001;59(1):76. [PMID: 11152194] (Description of a case of a malignant growth that developed in an odontogenic keratocyst.)

Myoung H, Hong SP, Hong SD et al. Odontogenic keratocyst: review of 256 cases for recurrence and clinicopathologic parameters. *Oral Surg Oral Med Oral Pathol Oral Radiol Endod.* 2001;91(3):328. [PMID: 11458242] (Report of a large series of case reviewing the age at diagnosis, gender of the patient, cyst location, radiographic findings, histopathologic findings, and recurrence rates.)

Schmidt BL. The use of enucleation and liquid nitrogen cryotherapy in the management of odontogenic keratocysts. *J Oral Maxillofac Surg.* 2001:59(7):720. [PMID: 11429726] (The combination of enucleation and liquid nitrogen therapy may offer patients improved treatment in the management of odontogenic keratocysts.)

Stoelinga PJ. Long-term follow-up on keratocysts treated according to a defined protocol. *Int J Oral Maxillofac Surg.* 2001;30(1):14. [PMID: 11289615] (Brief discussion of the etiology and pathogenesis of odontogenic keratocysts and a treatment protocol for effective management.)

Stoll C, Stollenwerk C, Riediger D, Mittermayer C, Alfer J. Cytokeratin expression patterns for distinction of odontogenic keratocysts from dentigerous and radicular cysts. *J Oral Pathol Med.* 2005;34(9):558. [PMID: 16138895] (Immunochemical detection of cytokeratin 17 and 19 seems to be a valuable additional parameter differentiating odontogenic keratocysts from other odontogenic cysts.)

GINGIVAL (ALVEOLAR) CYSTS OF NEWBORNS

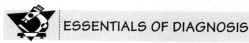 ESSENTIALS OF DIAGNOSIS

- *Superficial, keratin-filled cyst found on the alveolar mucosa of infants.*
- *Present at birth.*

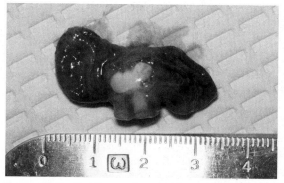

Figure 24–9. Specimen of an enucleated, odontogenic keratocyst and an associated unerupted tooth in a patient with nevoid basal cell carcinoma syndrome.

Gingival cysts are fairly common in newborns but are rarely identified because they have a tendency to rupture and disappear. Similar inclusion cysts, such as Epstein pearls and Bohn nodules, are found on the palates of newborns. These cysts form from remnants of the dental lamina. They are asymptomatic, small (usually 1–2 mm in diameter), whitish papules on the mucosa of the alveolar process of neonates. The appearance of these lesions is pathognomonic. No treatment is required since these lesions spontaneously involute as a result of cyst rupture. The prognosis is excellent and there is usually no recurrence.

LATERAL PERIODONTAL CYSTS AND VARIANT, THE BOTYROID ODONTOGENIC CYST

 ESSENTIALS OF DIAGNOSIS

- *A rare type of odontogenic developmental cyst.*
- *Occurs lateral to a tooth root, most commonly in the premolar region of the mandible (a common location of supernumerary teeth).*

Lateral periodontal cysts are uncommon and are usually discovered on routine dental x-rays. The origin of this cyst may be related epithelial rests in the periodontal membrane. These lesions are usually asymptomatic, with possible expansion of the buccal plate of bone. The adjacent teeth are usually vital and there may be evidence of root divergence caused by expansion of the cyst. Lateral periodontal cysts are characterized by a round to ovoid radiolucency that is lateral to or between the roots of teeth. These cysts are lined by nonkeratinized epithelium and, unless secondarily infected, do not have an inflammatory component. The differential diagnosis includes odontogenic keratocysts and lateral radicular cysts. Complications include local bone destruction, divergence of adjacent tooth roots, and recurrence. Cyst enucleation is the treatment of choice. The prognosis is very good, although cyst recurrence is possible. A more aggressive variant of the lateral periodontal cyst is the botyroid odontogenic cyst.

Ucok O, Yaman Z, Gunhan O, Ucok C, Dogan N, Baykul T. Botryoid odontogenic cyst: report of a case with extensive epithelial proliferation. *Int J Oral Maxillofac Surg.* 2005;34(6):693. [PMID: 16053898] (Botryoid odontogenic cyst is considered a rare multilocular variant of the lateral periodontal cyst, can be aggressive, and can extend beyond the typical inter-radicular location.)

CALCIFYING ODONTOGENIC CYSTS (GORLIN CYSTS)

 ESSENTIALS OF DIAGNOSIS

- *A rare odontogenic, developmental cyst with occasionally aggressive behavior.*
- *Occurs equally frequently in the maxilla and the mandible; most cases are reported in the incisor or canine regions.*

The mean reported age of onset is 33 years, with most cases presenting in the second and third decades. The epithelium is derived from odontogenic sources within the jaw or gingiva. This lesion is considered by some clinicians to be a neoplasm rather than a cyst. It is usually painless and occurs in the tooth-bearing areas of the jaws, but it may be peripheral to the bone in about 25% of cases. Lesions that are extraosseous appear as localized sessile or pedunculated gingival masses. The calcifying odontogenic cyst usually appears as a unilocular or multilocular and well-delineated radiolucency. Radiopacities may appear in the lesion as irregular calcifications or toothlike structures in approximately 50% of cases. The distinctive histopathologic feature of this lesion is "ghost cell" keratinization of the epithelial lining. The keratin may undergo dystrophic calcification. A differential diagnosis should include adenomatoid odontogenic tumors, cystic odontomas, calcifying epithelial odontogenic tumors, and ameloblastic fibro-odontomas. Complications include local bony destruction and the potential for loss of contiguous teeth in aggressive cases. The cyst should be removed by enucleation. The prognosis is good, and only a few cases of recurrences have been reported.

GLANDULAR ODONTOGENIC CYSTS

 ESSENTIALS OF DIAGNOSIS

- *This recently described odontogenic developmental lesion is uncommon.*
- *Occurs in the tooth-bearing areas of the jaws.*

This lesion can occur in any jaw site in adults but is more common in the anterior regions. Most cases of glandular odontogenic cysts reported have been in the adult mandible, and they can be locally aggressive. This cyst usually presents as a multilocular radiolucency of the jaw. Glandular odontogenic cysts are lined by a nonkeratinized epithelium, with localized areas of mucus and clear cells in a pseudoglandular pattern. The differential diagnosis should include odontogenic keratocysts. Local bone destruction can result from the growth of this lesion. Surgical management should be based on the extent and aggressiveness of the lesion. The prognosis is good based on relatively few reported cases, but the potential for recurrence exists.

ODONTOGENIC INFLAMMATORY CYSTS

RADICULAR CYSTS (PERIAPICAL CYSTS)

 ESSENTIALS OF DIAGNOSIS

- *The most common type of jaw cyst.*
- *Associated with a nonvital tooth subsequent to dental caries entering the tooth pulp, trauma, or surgical devitalization.*
- *Usually presents as a radiolucent lesion around the apex of a tooth root.*

General Considerations

This odontogenic inflammatory cyst represents 65–70% of all jaw cysts and can occur around the apex of any tooth (Figure 24–10). If a tooth associated with a radicular cyst is extracted and the cyst is not removed, it may remain and continue to expand, producing a residual cyst.

Pathogenesis

The radicular cyst is the result of dental pulp inflammation that progresses to the periapical area through the apical foramen of the tooth or through a lateral root canal. The epithelium is derived from the epithelial rest of Malassez. This cyst develops within a periapical granuloma at the tooth apex.

Prevention

The prevention of radicular cyst formation can be accomplished by regular dental examination and imaging to identify nonvital teeth. Once these nonvital teeth are identified, they are treated with endodontics (eg, root canal therapy) or extraction to prevent potential cyst development.

Clinical Findings

A. SYMPTOMS AND SIGNS

Small radicular cysts do not usually become acutely infected, are frequently asymptomatic, and can be identified on routine dental x-rays. Larger cysts may produce expansion of the bone, displacement of tooth roots, and crepitus when palpating the expanded alveolar plate. The discoloration of nonvital teeth and a negative response of the affected tooth to electric pulp testing or ice are the presenting signs. In addition, infected radicular cysts are painful, the involved tooth is sensitive to percussion, and there may be swelling of the overlying soft tissues and lymphadenopathy.

B. IMAGING STUDIES

Dental x-rays (periapical, occlusal, and panoramic) show a cyst around the end of the root (most commonly, the maxillary anterior teeth) that can extend beyond the boundaries of the involved tooth (Figure 24–11).

C. SPECIAL EXAMINATIONS

Histopathologic examination reveals a cystic lesion with a nonkeratinized epithelial lining. Remnants of cellular debris and fluid containing proteins predominantly derived from the plasma are usually found within the lumen of the cyst.

Differential Diagnosis

The differential diagnosis should include periapical granulomas, periapical scars (ie, fibrous healing defect), the early stage of periapical cemental dysplasia, giant cell lesions, bone neoplasms, traumatic bone cysts, and metastatic disease.

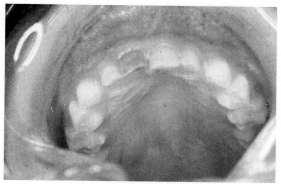

Figure 24–10. Discolored right maxillary deciduous central incisor associated with a radicular cyst.

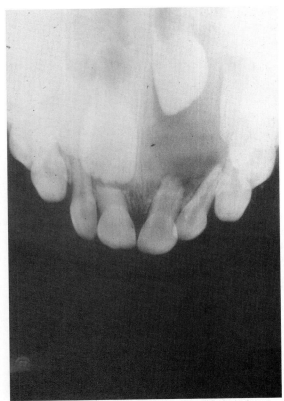

Figure 24–11. Occlusal x-ray demonstrating a radicular cyst associated with a nonvital deciduous maxillary central incisor, causing displacement of the succedaneous permanent central incisor tooth.

Complications

Complications include the loss of supportive alveolar bone and the loss of teeth.

Treatment & Prognosis

Treatment of radicular cysts involves endodontic therapy for small cysts (ie, < 5 mm), endodontic therapy plus periapical surgery and cyst enucleation for larger lesions, or, if the tooth is not restorable, tooth extraction combined with cyst enucleation. The prognosis is excellent following the appropriate treatment and recurrences are rare unless the cyst is left in situ.

Caliskan MK. Prognosis of large cyst-like periapical lesions following nonsurgical root canal treatment: a clinical review. *Int Endod J.* 2004;37(6):408. [PMID: 15186249] (Root canal treatment using calcium hydroxide as an antibacterial dressing in healing large, cyst-like periapical lesions.)

NONODONTOGENIC CYSTS

NASOLABIAL CYSTS (NASOALVEOLAR CYSTS)

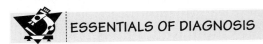 ESSENTIALS OF DIAGNOSIS

- *Rare nonodontogenic developmental cyst.*
- *Occurs as a unilateral swelling (10% incidence of bilateral occurrence) of the upper lip lateral to the midline, superficial to the maxilla.*

The nasolabial cyst is observed most often in adults in the fourth to sixth decades of life with a 3:1 female-to-male predilection. It is believed that the epithelium is derived from remnants of the nasolacrimal duct. A swelling appears in the lateral aspect of the upper lip and is generally painless unless secondarily infected (Figure 24–12). The swelling may elevate the nasal vestibule mucosa and cause obliteration of the nasolabial fold. It may cause nasal obstruction or interfere with the flange of an upper denture. There are no radiographic signs, except for a possible saucerization of the underlying labial surface of the maxilla. The nasolabial cyst is lined by pseudostratified columnar epithelium, which frequently demonstrates cilia and goblet cells. The differential diagnosis should include odontogenic developmental cysts, salivary gland neoplasms, inclusion cysts, and sebaceous cysts. Secondary infection is a potential complicating factor. Transoral surgical excision is the treatment of choice, as observed in Figure 24–13. The prognosis is excellent and recurrence is rare.

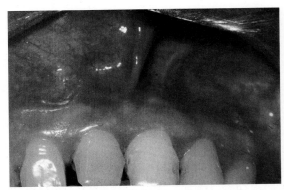

Figure 24–12. Nasolabial cyst obliterating the right mucolabial vestibule in the right maxillary incisor region.

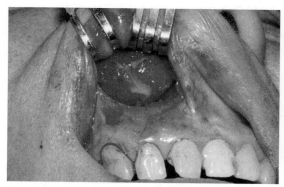

Figure 24–13. Surgical exposure of an infected nasolabial cyst in preparation for enucleation.

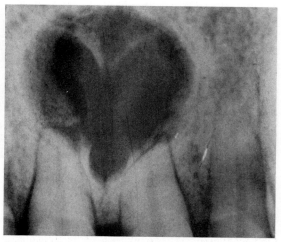

Figure 24–14. Occlusal x-ray of a nasopalatine cyst in the midline contiguous to the maxillary central incisors with apical root resorption.

NASOPALATINE CYSTS (INCISIVE CANAL CYSTS)

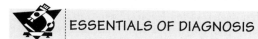 **ESSENTIALS OF DIAGNOSIS**

- *Relatively common nonodontogenic, developmental cyst.*
- *Occurs in the palatal midline behind the maxillary central incisors in the region of the incisive canal.*

Nasopalatine cysts occur in 2–5% of jaw cysts. This cyst derives its epithelium from the embryonic remnants of the nasopalatine duct. The lesion is usually asymptomatic unless secondarily infected. The maxillary central incisors are vital. There may be palatal bone expansion or palatal mucosal swelling. The patient may complain of a salty taste, which results from drainage. This cyst presents as a well-defined, oval- or heart-shaped mass that is created by the anterior nasal spine; it occurs between and apical to the maxillary central incisors. Periapical and occlusal radiographs demonstrate the lesion very clearly (Figure 24–14). It is difficult to determine at times whether the mass is a large incisive foramen or whether it represents a nasopalatine cyst. If the affected area is asymptomatic, if the cyst is less than approximately 7 mm, and if there is a question of the existence of pathology, it is reasonable to follow up the patient clinically and radiographically. The epithelial lining varies from stratified squamous presentation to one that is pseudostratified and ciliated. A differential diagnosis should include periapical cysts, granulomas, and keratocysts. Complications include the loss of bony support for the adjacent incisor teeth, root divergence, root resorption, as well as neurosensory deficit of the anterior palatal mucosa after cyst excision. Surgical enucleation via a pala-

tal flap is the treatment of choice. The prognosis is excellent and recurrence is rare.

Elliott KA, Franzese CB, Pitman KT. Diagnosis and surgical management of nasopalatine cysts. *Laryngoscope.* 2004;114(8):1336. [PMID: 15280704] (Nasopalatine duct cysts are the most common cystic lesion of nonodontogenic origin of the maxilla with enucleation as the preferred treatment and low recurrence rates.)

PSEUDOCYSTS

ANEURYSMAL BONE CYSTS

 ESSENTIALS OF DIAGNOSIS

- *Rare intraosseous jaw lesion characterized by blood-filled spaces associated with a fibroblastic tissue containing multinucleated giant cells and osteoid and woven bone.*
- *Appears more frequently in the mandible than in the maxilla.*

This lesion is typically observed in patients under 30 years of age. Aneurysmal bone cysts are considered reactive rather than neoplastic or cystic lesions. The pathogenesis is unknown, but it is believed that a vascular malformation occurs, producing an alteration of hemodynamic forces that create the cyst. Smaller lesions may be asymptomatic

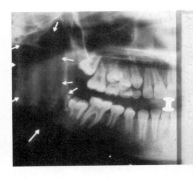
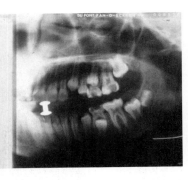

Figure 24–15. Panoramic x-ray of a large aneurysmal bone cyst of the mandible. Arrows show the borders of the lesion with extension into the mandibular condyle.

and are identified on routine x-rays; larger lesions present as occasionally painful, nonpulsatile swellings over the jaw. A multilocular jaw mass with cortical expansion is characteristic, as illustrated in Figure 24–15. Histopathologic examination reveals a fibrous connective tissue stroma containing variable numbers of multinucleated cells in relation to sinusoidal blood spaces. The differential diagnosis should include ameloblastomas, developmental odontogenic cysts, central giant cell granulomas, and central vascular lesions. Complications include a destructive osteolytic process of the involved jaw. Complete excision is the treatment of choice. The prognosis is generally good, provided the lesion is completely removed. Curettage procedures yield high recurrence rates.

Sanchez AP, Diaz-Lopez EO, Rojas SK et al. Aneurysmal bone cyst of the maxilla. *J Craniofac Surg.* 2004;15(6):1029. [PMID: 15547399] (An aneurysmal bone cyst is a nonneoplastic, uncommon solitary bone lesion recognized by distinct radiographic and histopathologic characteristics that can reach a considerable size and is treated by surgical excision.)

TRAUMATIC BONE CYSTS

 ESSENTIALS OF DIAGNOSIS

- *An empty or possibly fluid-filled bone cavity that appears to scallop the roots of vital teeth.*
- *Rather than an epithelial lining, there is a fibrous or granulation tissue component, or no identifiable lining.*
- *Usually identified on routine dental radiographic examination.*

General Considerations

A traumatic bone cyst is usually observed during the second decade of life and is seen in the mandibular body and symphysis. It is a relatively uncommon lesion that can occur in the humerus and other long bones. This cyst is sometimes referred to as a solitary, simple, hemorrhagic cyst.

Pathogenesis

The pathogenesis of this lesion is unknown; theories suggest that its pathology results from a traumatic episode that causes a hematoma to form within the intramedullary bone. Rather than forming a blood clot, it breaks down, producing osteolysis and an empty bone cavity.

Prevention

There are no known preventive measures. Regular dental visits with appropriate imaging are recommended.

Clinical Findings

A. SYMPTOMS AND SIGNS

The traumatic bone cyst is usually asymptomatic and rarely presents with pain or bony expansion. Although the lesion is around the root apices, tooth vitality is maintained. Traumatic bone cysts that occur in association with florid osseous dysplasia have been reported. Percussion of the teeth contiguous to this cyst may produce a dull percussion sound compared with the more high-pitched sound that is heard when percussing teeth not involved with a hollow bone cavity.

B. IMAGING STUDIES

Radiographically, the traumatic bone cyst appears as a well-defined lesion around the roots of contiguous teeth, usually in the mandible (Figure 24–16). Adjacent tooth roots may be displaced.

C. SPECIAL EXAMINATIONS

Histopathologic examination of surgical specimens usually reveals fragments of fibrous or granulation tissue and bone fragments.

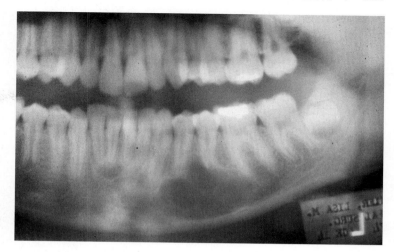

Figure 24–16. Panoramic x-ray of a mandibular traumatic bone cyst in the left mandibular body. The radiolucency scallops the roots of vital premolars and the first molar.

Differential Diagnosis

The differential diagnosis includes odontogenic keratocysts, central giant cell granulomas, or odontogenic tumors.

Complications

Complications include local bone destruction and the displacement of tooth roots.

Treatment

Surgical exploration is the treatment modality most commonly used to rule out the existence of other more aggressive and significant lesions. The aspiration or surgical curettage of the cavity frequently induces hemorrhage, with subsequent healing of the bony cavity.

Prognosis

Traumatic bone cysts may heal spontaneously without surgical intervention, but with surgical exploration, the healing may be accelerated, with bone fill expected in 6–12 months. The prognosis is excellent and recurrence is not expected.

STATIC BONE CYSTS

 ESSENTIALS OF DIAGNOSIS

- A mandibular anatomic defect that has a cyst-like appearance on x-ray.
- May occur in the incisor or in the cuspid or premolar regions of the lingual aspect of the mandible.
- Usually a unilateral phenomenon but may occur bilaterally.

A static bone cyst is an anatomic defect in the mandible (Figures 24–17, 24–18, and 24–19). These cysts are also known as Stafne bone cysts, lingual mandibular salivary gland depressions, latent bone cysts, and lingual cortical mandibular defects. It is believed to be developmental in nature but does not appear at birth and is not seen in children. Most cases are seen in middle-aged or older adults. Eighty to ninety percent of these defects are seen in males. They are stable in size (ie, static) and have been reported to occur in 0.3% of panoramic x-rays. This entity is asymptomatic and nonpalpable and is discovered during routine radiographic examination. A

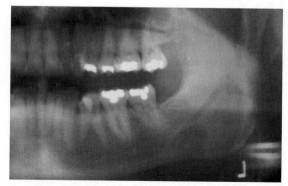

Figure 24–17. Panoramic x-ray of a static bone cyst, illustrating an oval radiolucency of the mandible, posterior to the second molar and inferior to the mandibular canal.

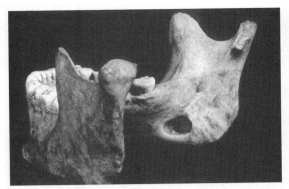

Figure 24–18. Cadaveric mandible with a static bone cyst.

static bone cyst appears as a well-circumscribed, round to oval mass that is located near the angle of the mandible and below the level of the mandibular canal, with no involvement of the tooth roots (Figure 24–20).

Surgical exploration is not indicated, but these defects contain salivary gland or adipose tissue from the floor of the mouth. The radiographic and clinical findings are pathognomonic for this entity. There has been a report of a salivary gland neoplasm developing in the lingual mandibular salivary gland depression. A static bone cyst does not require biopsy or excision unless a mass can be identified or imaged or there are clinical findings. The prognosis is excellent and no treatment is required.

Katz J, Chaushu G, Rotstein I. Stafne's bone cavity in the anterior mandible: a possible diagnostic challenge. *J Endod.* 2001;27(4):304. [PMID: 11485274] (Most Stafne bone cavities occur in the angle of the mandible in the area between the mandibular first molar and the mandibular angle, but some may appear in the anterior mandible, which may be more difficult to diagnose.)

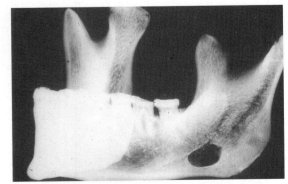

Figure 24–19. X-ray of a cadaveric mandible with a static bone cyst.

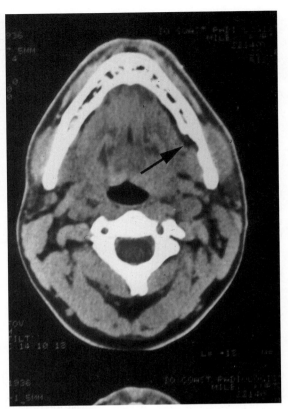

Figure 24–20. CT scan, axial view, of a mandible, revealing a lingual mandibular defect consistent with the diagnosis of a static bone cyst.

GANGLION CYSTS

Ganglions are cystic lesions that develop near joints, including the TMJ. These cystic lesions are not classically described in discussions of cystic lesions of the jaw, but, because of their presentation, they may be confused with parotid tumors.

There are two types of ganglion cysts: (1) those with walls that consist of fibrous connective tissue and (2) those with walls that are lined by synovial cells. Ganglions should be considered when evaluating preauricular swellings. The surgical removal with histopathologic examination of the excised tissue is the treatment of choice for jaw cysts in most cases.

Kim SG, Cho BO, Lee YC et al. Ganglion cyst in the temporomandibular joint. *J Oral Pathol Med.* 2003;32(5):310. [PMID: 12694356] (The ganglion cyst of the temporomandibular joint should be considered in the differential diagnosis of preauricular masses.)

Temporomandibular Disorders

25

Greg Goddard, DDS

General Considerations

Temporomandibular disorders (TMDs) are a set of musculoskeletal disorders affecting the temporomandibular joint (TMJ), the masticatory muscles, or both. TMDs comprise many diverse diagnoses with similar signs and symptoms affecting the masticatory system, which can be acute, recurrent, or chronic. TMDs are rarely life threatening, but can impact heavily on an individual's quality of life.

TMDs occur disproportionately in women of child-bearing age in a ratio of 4:1 to 6:1. The prevalence drops off dramatically for both men and women after age 55.

Etiology

The cause of TMD is variable and uncertain, and it is thought to be multifactorial in most cases. Most factors are not proven causal factors, but they are associated with TMDs. Predisposing factors increase the risk of TMDs. Predisposing factors are trauma, both direct (eg, blows to the jaw) and indirect (eg, whiplash injuries), and stress. Microtrauma is caused by clenching and grinding of the teeth. Stress can be a predisposing factor owing to the disruption of restorative sleep and the increase of nocturnal bruxism. Trauma and stress are also precipitating factors.

Perpetuating factors that sustain a TMD are stress, poor coping skills, harmful habits such as clenching and grinding, and poor posture. Nonrestorative sleep also may be a major factor in the perpetuation of chronic jaw pain.

Controversial Causes

A. BRUXISM

Bruxism, or grinding the teeth during sleep, has been thought to be a predisposing, precipitating, and perpetuating factor. Bruxism can involve excessive activation of the masticatory muscles and excessive loading of TMJs, which can be a factor in the recovery of some patients, whereas in others bruxism does not seem to be a factor. In studies, bruxism has not been clearly demonstrated as a cause of TMD. Some individuals who severely grind their teeth do not have any signs or symptoms of TMD.

Dental and occlusal origins are not generally accepted and the scientific evidence does not support their causal relationship. Experimental occlusal interferences have been placed with no evidence of TMD symptoms. There is no evidence of a higher incidence of TMD with any type of malocclusion, and significant proportions of the population have occlusal discrepancies without any TMD pain.

Pergamalian A, Rudy TE, Zaki HS, Greco CM. The association between wear facets, bruxism, and severity of facial pain in patients with temporomandibular disorders. *J Prosthet Dent.* 2003;90(2):194. [PMID: 12886214] (The amount of bruxism activity was not associated with more severe muscle pain.)

B. WHIPLASH

Whiplash has been thought to be a precipitating factor in the development of TMD. There is very little evidence that a noncontact injury can cause damage to the TMJ. However, many patients claim muscle and joint pain after a whiplash injury. The pain may be referred from the strained sternocleidomastoid muscle, which often refers pain to the ear, or it may be due to injuries to other cervical muscles and ligaments.

C. DISC DISPLACEMENT

Disc displacement has been considered a pathologic condition, but many studies have shown that from 30% to 50% of populations have reducing discs. Most of these individuals have no history of TMJ pain or dysfunction. Disc displacement may be a normal biological variation. Clicking joints are not necessarily painful or pathologic. Studies reporting on the long-term follow-up of patients with disc displacement show the majority are asymptomatic 30 years later (Figure 25–1).

Clinical Findings

A. SYMPTOMS AND SIGNS

The most common TMD complaints are jaw, face, and head pain of moderate intensity. Limited opening, catching or sticking, and locking of the mandible are common functional complaints. Patients often have complaints of

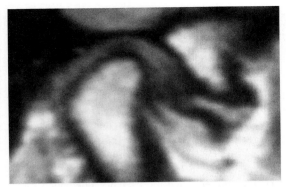

Figure 25–1. MRI showing anterior displaced disc that does not reduce on opening.

joint noises, such as clicking, popping, and grating when the mandible is opened or closed. Patients also have perceived complaints of global headache and neck and shoulder pain that are not related to jaw function. Some patients present with unexplained complaints of tinnitus, ear fullness, hearing loss, and dizziness. Complaints of abnormal tooth wear, tooth sensitivity, and teeth not meeting correctly are often expressed.

B. IMAGING STUDIES

Magnetic resonance imaging (MRI) reveals hard bony tissue as well as soft tissue abnormalities. Computed tomography (CT) scans are useful in showing degenerative changes of the hard tissues. Imaging should be reserved for patients whose abnormal pain, dysfunction, or both does not respond to conservative short-term treatments such as nonsteroidal anti-inflammatory drugs (NSAIDs) and physical therapy. Imaging is also warranted in patients who have a sudden change in the bite or asymmetry of the mandible.

Differential Diagnosis

Temporomandibular disorders are divided into articular disorders and muscle disorders. The diagnosis is largely based on the specific system(s) that is affected. However, many patients have both muscle and articular disorders.

Treatment

The management of TMDs is based on the elimination of pain and the restoration of function and normal activities of daily living. Each specific diagnosis has its own set of management goals based on addressing the problems that affect that patient. Most management plans use conservative, noninvasive treatments; in less than 5% of cases, surgery is used.

The key elements of any conservative management plan are self-care, medication, and physical therapy.

Acupuncture is often helpful, as are biofeedback and orthotic splint therapy.

A. SELF-CARE

Patients with TMD can be more successfully treated by healthcare practitioners who educate patients about their disorder and involve them in their own treatment. Self-care is an essential part of patient treatment. It should be designed to meet each patient's treatment objectives. Self-care should be thoroughly explained to patients in language meaningful to them, and it should be reinforced at each visit. This self-care results in better patient compliance and understanding and in better outcomes. The following are 20 self-care tips that have been effective in helping patients manage their TMD:

> The rest of the muscles and joints allow healing.
> Soft food enables muscles and joints to heal.
> Not chewing gum lessens muscle fatigue and joint pain.
> Relax your facial muscles: "Lips relaxed, teeth apart."
> No clenching; it irritates joints and muscles.
> Yawning against pressure prevents locking open and jaw pain.
> Moist heat for 20 minutes promotes healing and relaxation.
> Ice is for severe pain and new injuries (less than 72 hours).
> Heat and ice—5 seconds of heat, 5 seconds of ice—for pain relief.
> Good posture; avoid head-forward position.
> Sleeping position: Side lying, with good pillow support.
> Jaw exercise: Open and close against finger pressure.
> Exercise: 20–30 minutes at least 3 times a week.
> Acupressure massage between thumb and forefinger.
> Over-the-counter medications: ibuprofen or aspirin.
> Yoga and meditation for stress reduction.
> Massage promotes healing and relaxation.
> An athletic mouthguard can give temporary relief.
> Avoid long dental appointments.
> Do not cradle the telephone; it **aggravates** the neck and jaw.

B. MEDICATION

The most common medications for TMD are (1) NSAIDs; (2) muscle relaxants such as cyclobenzaprine; and (3) low doses (10–50 mg) of tricyclic antidepressants such as amitriptyline, desipramine, or nortriptyline. In patients with TMJ synovitis who have a poor response to NSAIDs, a course of an oral steroid such as methylprednisolone (eg, a Depo-Medrol dose pack) for 6 days can be effective. When chronic pain is moderate to severe and does not respond to other treatments, opioid analgesics are often beneficial. Short-acting opioids such as hydrocodone should be avoided in favor of longer-acting codeine or oxycodone. Newer opioids such as tramadol have shown some promise.

Rizzatti-Barbosa CM et al. Clinical evaluation of amitryptyline for the control of chronic pain caused by temporomandibular joint disorders. *Cranio.* 2003;21(3):221. [PMID: 12889679] (Amitriptyline was an efficient alternative treatment for chronic pain in TMD patients.)

C. Physical Therapy

Physical therapy has been shown to be helpful for many patients with TMD pain and dysfunction. Heat and ice have beneficial effects on reducing pain in some patients. Jaw exercises can be prescribed for increasing mobility, decreasing hypermobility, strengthening and coordinating muscles, and improving muscle endurance. Massage can be helpful because it promotes increased blood flow through the tissue in addition to inducing muscle relaxation. The evaluation of patient posture is important, and patients should be taught proper posture. A forward-head position can exacerbate neck pain and a tense jaw posture can increase jaw and muscle pain.

D. Ultrasound

Ultrasound can provide deep and relaxing heat to muscles and joints, helping to relieve pain and restore function. Transcutaneous electrical nerve stimulation (TENS) can be helpful in controlling pain. Joint manipulation can help improve joint mobility in cases of TMJ disc displacement without reduction.

E. Acupuncture

Acupuncture has been used for the treatment of TMDs, as well as for other musculoskeletal pains. The National Institutes of Health (NIH), in their consensus statement on acupuncture in 1997, stated that acupuncture shows promising results for postoperative dental pain, and in other situations (such as myofascial pain), acupuncture may be useful as an adjunct treatment or an acceptable alternative treatment. A number of studies of acupuncture and chronic pain found positive results in 41% of them and concluded that there is limited evidence that acupuncture is more effective than no treatment for chronic pain.

Goddard G. Short-term pain reduction with acupuncture treatment for chronic orofacial pain patients. *Med Sci Monit.* 2005;11(20):CR71. [PMID: 15668635] (Acupuncture provided short-term pain relief.)

F. Injection of Local Anesthesia

The injection of trigger points in painful muscles with a local anesthetic has been used for over 40 years and is still a popular treatment. Studies have shown that dry needling works just as well, and the difference between dry needling and acupuncture is minimal to none.

G. Splint Therapy

Splints (orthotics) are removable appliances, usually made of acrylic plastic, which fit over the teeth of either the mandible or the maxilla. Splints are the most often prescribed treatment for TMD; more than 3 million splints are made each year.

Despite the extensive use of oral splints in the treatment of TMD and bruxism, their mechanisms of action remain controversial. Oral splints should be used as an adjunct for pain management rather than a definitive treatment.

Treatment with intraoral splints has been shown to have varying levels of efficacy for the treatment of TMD and bruxism. Splints reduce the role of occlusal factors, reduce loading on the joints, and have a strong placebo effect. Splints can reduce tooth damage in patients who grind their teeth and can increase awareness of these detrimental oral habits. Not all patients get relief and some experience a worsening of symptoms with splints. There are possible complications to wearing splints, such as irreversible changes in occlusion that will necessitate either orthodontics or surgery to correct. Therefore, splints should be worn for a short to moderate time period and should be regularly monitored. Nighttime wear is typical and full-time use is contraindicated.

H. Arthrocentesis

Arthrocentesis is the insertion of one or more needles into the superior joint space and irrigation with saline, with or without corticosteroids. It has been reported to be effective in cases of synovitis and limited opening due to anterior displaced disc without reduction.

I. Arthroscopy

Arthroscopy is the insertion of a cannula with fiberoptics that allows visualization of the joint space. Another cannula is then inserted with microtools that allow for débridement, the removal of adhesions, and biopsies.

J. Surgery

Surgery is reserved for those few patients (less than 5%) who do not respond to conservative treatment and in whom an identifiable structural defect can be corrected by surgery. These patients should undergo comprehensive nonsurgical rehabilitation, and surgery should be considered only after all of the contributing factors have been addressed and controlled. Many of the pain symptoms come from the muscular components of TMD, so these muscle diagnoses must be addressed and controlled. Failure to address these issues will likewise result in failed surgical treatment. Pre- and postoperative physical therapy is important for the successful outcome of any surgery. The less invasive surgical techniques seem to be just as efficacious as the more invasive open joint procedures, so arthrocentesis and arthroscopy should be considered as a first step.

Dworkin SF, Huggins KH, Wilson L et al. A randomized clinical trial using research diagnostic criteria for temporomandibular disorders-axis II to target clinic cases for a tailored self-care TMD treatment program. *J Orofac Pain.* 2002;16(1):48. [PMID: 11889659] (At 1 year, patients in the tailored self-care treatment program, compared with the usual TMD treatment, showed significantly decreased TMD pain.)

■ ARTICULAR DISORDERS

The TMJ is a paired synovial joint that is capable of both gliding and hinge movements. It articulates the mandibular condyle and the squamous portion of the temporal bone, with the articular disc of dense fibrous connective tissue interposed between the two bones. Unlike most other synovial joints, the TMJ is lined with dense fibrous connective tissue (Figure 25–2).

TMJ SYNOVITIS

This disorder is an inflammation of the synovial lining of the TMJ; it is characterized by localized pain that is increased by the functioning and loading of the joint. Sometimes patients complain about posterior teeth not meeting on the same side, presumably because of swelling in the joint.

Patients often present with a history of pain in the preauricular region, which is aggravated by chewing or other mandibular movement. Pain on palpation over

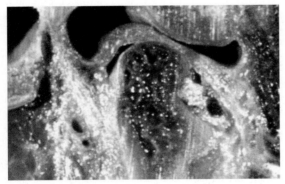

Figure 25–2. Sagittal section through the temporomandibular joint showing good condyle and disc relationship.

the lateral pole of the condyle is evident. Pain is elicited on loading of the TMJ, or on distraction or compression. Range of motion is often limited (< 35 mm). No radiographic changes are found; however, evidence of joint effusion is seen on MRI. Treatment indications can be found in Table 25–1.

DISC DISPLACEMENT DISORDERS

DISC DISPLACEMENT WITH REDUCTION

Disc displacement with reduction is characterized by a clicking jaw joint; an audible or palpable click is heard or felt on opening the mandible and in lateral movements of the mandible. This condition is most often painless and requires no treatment. Up to 50% of people have been shown to have displaced discs and most do not have any pain or dysfunction. When pain accompanies the click, it is most often the result of inflammation in the joint owing to the condyle pressing on the retrodiscal tissues, synovitis, or capsulitis. Symptomatic clicking, in which there is pain on clicking and pain on loading, needs to be treated. MRI shows the anterior position of the disc in a closed position and in a normal position on opening. X-rays may show a decreased joint space, but this is not diagnostic of a displaced disc.

ACUTE DISC DISPLACEMENT

Acute disc displacement without reduction (closed lock) is characterized by a marked limitation in opening (< 35 mm). It is also distinguished by a deflection of the mandible to the affected side on opening. It occurs with a sudden onset and can be painless or painful. No clicking is felt or heard, although the patient usually has a history of clicking at one time. The disc is usually anterior to the condyle and blocks the translation of the condyle, preventing normal opening and causing the mandible to deflect to the affected side. MRI shows the disc anterior to the condyle in the closed position, and it remains anterior on opening. Radiographs can show a decreased joint space that might be an indication of a displaced disc.

CHRONIC DISC DISPLACEMENT

Chronic disc displacement without reduction (closed lock) is a long-standing condition characterized by a slightly limited opening (< 40 mm) which usually improves after the initial onset. The patient has no clicking, either felt or heard, although he or she usually has a history of a previously clicking joint. Pain is not usually a complaint and patients may or may not present with

Table 25–1. Treatment indications for articular disorders.

Articular Disorder	Self-Care	NSAIDs	Physical Therapy	Splint	Acupuncture	Arthrocentesis	Surgery
TMJ synovitis	X	X	X	X	X	X	
Disc displacement with reduction	X	X	X	X	X	X	
Acute disc without reduction	X	X	X	X	X	X	
Chronic disc displacement without reduction	X	X	X	X	X	X	
Osteoarthritis	X	X	X	X	X	X	
Polyarthritides	X	X	X	X	X	X	
Condylar dislocation	X	X	X				
Fibrous ankylosis			X			X	X
Bony ankylosis			X			X	X
Condylar fracture			X				X
Neoplasia			X				X

it. The mandible deflects to the affected side on opening. The disc is anterior to the condyle and is either pushed further anterior on opening or is folded on itself. MRI shows the disc far anterior, often folded on itself, and pushed further forward on opening.

OSTEOARTHRITIS

Osteoarthritis is a noninflammatory arthritic condition that is characterized by deterioration and abrasion of the articular tissues. It is accompanied by remodeling of the underlying subchondral bone. Joint pain is present with function, and crepitus is often heard over the affected joint. Joint stiffness, often worse on awakening or at the beginning of a meal, can be a problem, and the patient may have a limited range of motion. Radiographic evidence of degeneration of the condyles can be seen. Synovitis often is present and accounts for pain, when present. The long-term prognosis is good because osteoarthritis tends to be self-limiting as the joint remodels.

POLYARTHRITIDES

Systemic polyarthritic disorders can affect the TMJ as well as other joints in the body. Various systemic diseases such as rheumatoid arthritis, juvenile rheumatoid arthritis, ankylosing spondylitis, psoriatic arthritis, infectious arthritis, Reiter syndrome, gout, and Lyme disease can involve the TMJ. A common finding is pain to palpation over the TMJ. Pain is usually elicited with function, and the patient may experience a limited range of motion. Crepitus can be heard over the affected joint and degeneration of the condyles may be seen on x-rays.

CONDYLAR DISLOCATION

Condylar dislocation is characterized by a patient who is unable to close his or her mouth. The patient's mouth is fully open upon presentation, and he or she is usually in great distress, with pain and anxiety. This condition occurs after yawning, after eating an apple or other food that requires wide opening, or with prolonged opening, as during a dental appointment. The condyle remains positioned anterior to eminence. There can be joint pain at the time of dislocation and for up to several days afterward. There is usually a history of a self-reducing dislocation.

The condyle can be reduced by manually pushing the mandible both downward and backward into the fossa. This reduction can often be done in the office by placing gloved hands, with the thumbs outside the patient's teeth, on the lateral border of the mandible and distracting the mandible in a downward direction, placing the condyles back into the fossa. If the muscles have gone into spasm, it may be necessary to administer a muscle relaxant such as diazepam; in more severe cases, the patient may need to be placed under general anesthesia before enough muscle relaxation can take place to reduce the condyles. Postoperative pain is managed with NSAIDs and physical therapy is indicated. Self-care can assist in preventing recurrences.

FIBROUS ANKYLOSIS

Fibrous ankylosis is restricted mandibular movement with deviation to the affected side on opening. This condition results from fibrous adhesions that attach the condyle to the disc and the disc to the articular fossa. It may be caused by bleeding in the joint, but the exact mechanism is not known. A history of trauma to the TMJ usually exists. There is a marked limited opening, usually < 20 mm, but the condition is not painful. The mandible deflects to the affected side on opening, and there is a marked limited lateral movement of the mandible to the contralateral side. Radiographs show an absence of condylar translation, but they do show a joint space.

BONY ANKYLOSIS

Bony ankylosis is the union of the bones of the mandibular condyle and the temporal fossa by proliferation of bone cells, which results in the complete immobility of the joint. It is usually secondary to trauma and probably due to bleeding in the joint. A history of trauma to the TMJ usually exists. There is a marked limited opening, usually < 10 mm, although the condition is generally not painful. The mandible deflects to the affected side on opening, and there is a marked limited lateral movement of the mandible to the contralateral side. CT scanning or MRI shows a connection between bony articulating surfaces; x-rays show an absence of condylar translation and bone proliferation in the joint space.

CONDYLAR FRACTURE

Fractures can occur in any of the bony components of the TMJ; however, fracture of the mandibular condyle is the most common. It is often caused by a direct trauma to the jaw, usually by a blow to the chin. This condition is marked by a limited opening (< 25 mm), swelling over the affected joint, and pain with function. There is often bleeding in the joint, and sequelae can include adhesions, ankylosis, and joint degeneration. The mandible deflects to the affected side and the fracture is evident on an x-ray.

Condylar fractures are managed with immobilization, a soft diet, and physical therapy to regain the range of motion. Open joint surgery is required to reduce the fracture only in rare cases.

■ NEOPLASIA

Neoplasms of the TMJ can be benign, malignant, or metastatic. One percent of malignant breast tumors metastasize to the mandible.

BENIGN NEOPLASMS

Benign TMJ neoplasms include osteomas, osteoblastomas, chondromas, benign giant cell tumors, ossifying fibromas, fibrous dysplasias, myxomas, and synovial chondromatosis.

MALIGNANT NEOPLASMS

Malignant TMJ neoplasms are rare and include chondrosarcomas, fibrosarcomas, and synovial sarcomas.

METASTATIC NEOPLASMS

Metastatic TMJ neoplasms are more common than primary tumors; 1% of malignant neoplasms metastasize to the jaws. Squamous cell carcinomas of the maxillofacial region and nasopharyngeal tumors are the tumors that most commonly extend into the TMJ. Neoplasms from the parotid gland, such as adenocystic carcinomas and mucoepidermoid carcinomas, have been reported to involve the TMJ. These neoplasms often present with swelling and pain. Pain is elicited on palpation and with function. There can be an open bite on the affected side where the back teeth do not meet. Imaging shows a lesion.

NEOPLASMS OF THE MASTICATORY MUSCLES

Neoplasms of the masticatory muscles are very rare. They can be malignant or benign, are associated with swelling, and may or may not present with pain, although pain usually accompanies swelling. There is a positive finding of tumor with imaging, and both imaging and biopsy help confirm the diagnosis.

■ MUSCLE DISORDERS

The muscles of mastication are the masseter, temporalis, medial pterygoid, and lateral pterygoid muscles. In addition to neoplasms, which are rarely seen, more common muscle disorders may result in pain, redness, swelling, cramping, and contracture. Treatment indications can be found in Table 25–2.

MYOFASCIAL PAIN

Myofascial pain is characterized by a regional, dull, aching muscle pain, usually of mild to moderate intensity. The pain is aggravated by mandibular function when the muscles of mastication are involved. TMJ pain may result in painful masticatory muscles due to the reflex splinting of these muscles. Often, localized tender areas (ie, trigger points) in the muscle or tendon exist. When the muscle is palpated, the trigger points that elicit pain

Table 25–2. Treatment indications for muscular disorders.

Muscular Disorder	Self-Care	NSAIDs	Physical Therapy	Muscle Relaxant Medication	Splint	Acupuncture	Surgery
Myofascial pain	X	X	X	X	X	X	
Myositis	X	X	X	X	X	X	
Myospasm	X	X	X	X	X	X	
Muscle contracture	X		X		X	X	
Neoplasia			X				X
Fibromyalgia	X		X	X		X	

often refer the pain to distant areas. This referred pain is often felt as a headache, and myofascial pain has been associated with tension-type headaches; it is also associated with ear symptoms, tinnitus, vertigo, and toothache. Patients may also present with a sensation of muscle stiffness or tightness and a sensation of their teeth not meeting correctly. Inactivating the trigger points with a local anesthetic injection, acupuncture, or a vapocoolant spray and muscle stretch often relieves the larger area of referred pain. The pathogenesis is now thought to be due to changes in the central nervous system that are responsible for hyperalgesia of the muscles.

Ekberg E, Nilner M. Treatment outcome of appliance therapy in temporomandibular disorder patients with myofascial pain after 6 and 12 months. *Acta Odontol Scand.* 2004;62(6):343.

[PMID: 15848979] (A stabilization appliance reduced patient pain.)

MYOSITIS

Myositis is characterized by moderate to severe pain, redness, and swelling associated with tissue injury. This condition can result from direct trauma or infection, often secondary to oral surgery or an intramuscular injection. Pain is usually continuous in a localized muscle area following injury or infection, and diffuse tenderness is present over the entire muscle. Pain increases with movement, and a moderate to severe limitation of opening due to pain and swelling is common. A limited range of mandibular motion is often present. Elevated serum levels indicative of inflammation, infection, or both may be present.

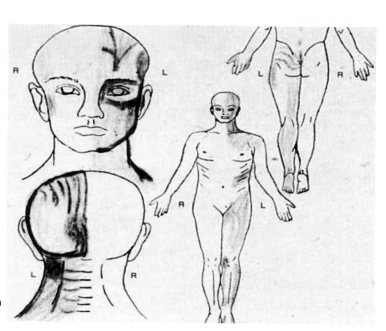

Figure 25–3. Typical pain diagram by a patient with fibromyalgia.

MYOSPASM (TRISMUS)

Myospasm, or muscle cramp, is characterized by a continuous involuntary muscle contraction with severe pain. The patient experiences an acute onset of pain at rest as well as with function. Myospasm is not a common finding in TMDs; when it does occur, it usually resolves within hours.

CONTRACTURE

Muscle contracture is the painless shortening of a muscle, usually secondary to a period of limited range of motion. It is characterized by an unyielding firmness on passive stretch and is usually associated with minimal or no pain unless the muscle is forced to lengthen. Muscle contracture can occur after wiring the jaws following fracture, after jaw surgery, after a prolonged infection, or with an anterior displaced disc without reduction that grossly limits the range of motion for a long period of time. The muscle undergoes fibrotic changes and becomes hard.

FIBROMYALGIA

Fibromyalgia is a generalized whole body muscle pain mostly affecting women between 25 and 50 years of age. It is often accompanied by fatigue, irritable bowel syndrome, muscle stiffness, and sleeping difficulties. The diagnosis is based on the presence of pain to palpation in 11 out of 18 predefined sites and pain in 3 of the 4 quadrants of the body.

Because problems with the masticatory and cervical muscles are typically painful, fibromyalgia is often misdiagnosed as myofascial pain. Studies have shown that up to 20% of patients with TMD are really fibromyalgia patients (Figure 25–3).

Forseth K, Gran JT. Management of fibromyalgia: what are the best treatment choices? *Drugs.* 2002;62(4):577. [PMID: 11893227] (The management of patients with fibromyalgia is mostly based on empirical research, and only a few controlled studies have been performed. Basic drug therapy rests on the administration of amitriptyline and conventional analgesics.)

SECTION VII
Neck

Neck Masses

26

Derrick T. Lin, MD, & Daniel G. Deschler, MD

■ ANATOMY

Knowledge of the anatomy of the neck is essential for both the diagnosis and the treatment of disease processes in the region. Contained within the neck are several triangles, defined anatomically (Figure 26–1). Familiarity with these specific areas assists in generating a differential diagnosis of neck masses by the exact anatomic location.

The sternocleidomastoid muscle divides the neck into two major compartments, anterior and lateral.

ANTERIOR NECK

The following anatomic points define the anterior compartment of the neck: (1) the inferior border of the mandible superiorly, (2) the anterior border of the sternocleidomastoid muscle laterally, (3) the clavicle inferiorly, and (4) the vertical midline from mental symphysis to suprasternal notch medially. The structures that make up the anterior neck include the larynx, trachea, esophagus, thyroid and parathyroid glands, carotid sheath, and suprahyoid and infrahyoid strap muscles.

Triangular regions also define the anterior neck anatomically.

The **submandibular triangle** is a region contained in the anterior neck bordered by the inferior margin of the mandible and the digastric, stylohyoid, and mylohyoid muscles. This region contains the submandibular gland and the marginal mandibular branch of the facial nerve. The **submental triangle** defines a region bordered by the hyoid bone, the paired anterior bellies of the digastric muscles, and the mylohyoid muscle. The upper belly of the omohyoid muscle in the anterior neck further divides the anterior neck into an **upper carotid triangle** and a **lower muscular triangle.**

LATERAL NECK

The lateral neck, also referred to as the **posterior triangle,** is defined by the posterior aspects of the sternocleidomastoid muscle medially, the trapezius muscle laterally, and the middle third of the clavicle inferiorly. The lateral neck contains lymph node–bearing tissue, the spinal accessory nerve, and the cervical plexus. The inferior belly of the omohyoid muscle further defines a **lower subclavian triangle** in the lateral neck that contains the brachial plexus and subclavian vessels.

■ DIAGNOSIS

The differential diagnosis in a patient presenting with a neck mass is broad and extensive. Therefore, a thorough history and physical examination make up the critical first step in the evaluation of a neck mass. Information gathered from a detailed history and physical examination alone often narrows the differential diagnosis to a more manageable level (Figure 26–2).

PATIENT HISTORY

The most important element in the evaluation of a neck mass is the age of the patient. Most pediatric neck masses are inflammatory or congenital and resolve

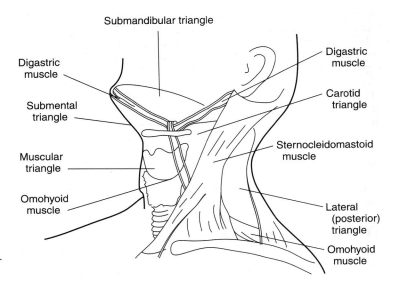

Figure 26–1. Anatomic compartments of the neck.

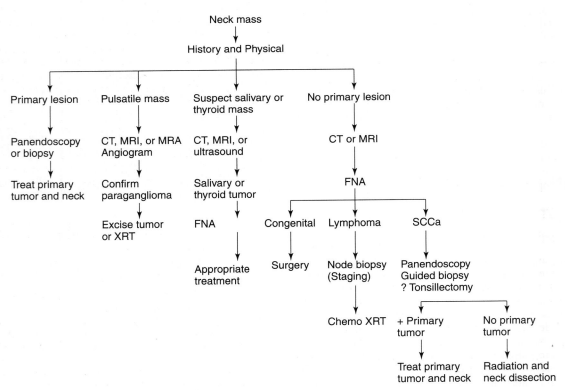

Figure 26–2. Evaluation of the neck mass in the adult.

spontaneously or after appropriate medical therapy. In contrast, a neck mass in an adult over the age of 40 should be considered neoplastic in origin unless proven otherwise. The probability of a benign neck mass in this age group is low, particularly in the setting of tobacco or alcohol use.

The duration, growth pattern, and absence or presence of pain are all critical aspects of the history. A region-specific review of systems, such as a change in voice, hoarseness, difficulty with swallowing, and ear pain are important symptoms to note in addition to generalized complaints such as fever, night sweats, and weight loss. Questions related to a patient's social history, such as alcohol and drug use, smoking, and recent travel, should also be included.

PHYSICAL EXAMINATION

The physical examination should include a systematic investigation of all mucosal and submucosal areas of the head and neck. The mobility, consistency, and tenderness of the mass should be assessed carefully. The location of the neck mass is particularly important in congenital and developmental masses because these masses typically appear in consistent locations. For example, a lateral neck mass in a child is suggestive of a branchial cleft cyst or laryngocele, whereas a midline neck mass is more suggestive of a thyroglossal duct cyst. The location also may be helpful in assessing adult patients. A neck mass located in the supraclavicular region of an older adult should focus the physician's attention to metastasis from a primary lesion located in a site other than the upper aerodigestive tract (eg, a gastrointestinal or pulmonary source). An isolated posterior triangle lymph node in an Asian adult should raise suspicion for a nasopharyngeal carcinoma.

TESTS & STUDIES

Imaging Studies

Imaging studies provide useful information in diagnosing the etiology of a neck mass. Computed tomography (CT) and magnetic resonance imaging (MRI) can (1) differentiate solid, cystic, and vascular masses; (2) localize a mass in relation to the vital structures of the neck; and (3) identify a potential head and neck source for the neck mass. Ultrasonography may be helpful in distinguishing solid from cystic masses, especially in the setting of a suspected thyroid lesion. Chest x-rays may be helpful if there is a high index of suspicion for granulomatous diseases such as sarcoidosis or tuberculosis. A chest film is also able to detect a metastasis from a head and neck cancer or a primary malignant neoplasm within the lungs. Positron emission tomography (PET), which detects increased metabolic activity, is now often used in the detection and surveillance of head and neck cancer.

Serologic Testing

Serologic testing can be used in looking for systemic diseases. For example, antinuclear antibody may be positive in Sjögren syndrome, which can present with parotid enlargement and lymphadenopathy. Serologic testing is also important in the diagnosis of many infectious diseases that may present as a neck mass, including tuberculosis, atypical mycobacteria, mononucleosis, toxoplasmosis, and cat-scratch disease. Patients with lymphoma may also have abnormalities on serologic testing.

Fine-Needle Aspiration Biopsy

Fine-needle aspiration (FNA) biopsy has become a critical step in the evaluation of neck masses. The timing of the FNA biopsy in relation to imaging studies is debatable. Advocates of obtaining imaging studies prior to the FNA biopsy believe that the FNA distorts the architecture of the mass, thus making imaging more difficult to interpret. The procedure for a FNA entails the use of a 23- or 25-gauge needle in obtaining multiple aspirations of the neck mass. FNA biopsies can differentiate a cystic mass from an inflammatory mass and malignant tissue from benign tissue. It is important to know that FNA can differentiate lymphoma from carcinoma, a distinction that is critical in directing further workup and treatment. With the recent advances in molecular biology, polymerase chain reaction (PCR) can be conducted on FNA samples to identify disease processes such as Epstein-Barr virus (EBV), which will guide the physician to the diagnosis of primary nasopharyngeal carcinoma.

Alvi A, Johnson JT. The neck mass: a challenging differential diagnosis. *Postgrad Med.* 1995;97(5):87. [PMID: 8780950] (Outlines the workup of neck masses.)

Amedee RG, Dhurandhar NR. Fine-needle aspiration biopsy. *Laryngoscope.* 2001;111(9):1551. [PMID: 11568593] (Fine-needle aspiration biopsy has a high overall diagnostic accuracy of 95% for all head and neck masses, 95% for benign lesions, and 87% for malignant ones.)

Brown RL, Azizkhan RG. Pediatric head and neck lesions. *Pediatr Clin North Am.* 1998;45(4):889. [PMID: 9728193] (Outlines the workup and differential diagnosis of pediatric neck masses.)

Chang DB, Yang PC, Luh KT et al. Ultrasonic evaluation of cervical lymphadenopathy. *J Formos Med Assoc.* 1990;89(4):548. [PMID: 1976745] (Study of 75 patients with cervical lymphadenopathy who underwent real-time ultrasonographic study of the neck. The study concluded that ultrasonography is a valuable tool to evaluate cervical adenopathy and to clarify the histopathologic features of the affected lymph node with the aid of aspiration cytology.)

Enepekides DJ. Management of congenital anomalies of the neck. *Facial Plast Surg Clin North Am.* 2001;9(1):131. [PMID: 11465000] (Outlines a standardized and complete approach to the evaluation of congenital neck masses.)

Gritzmann N, Hollerweger A, Macheiner P, Rettenbacher T. Sonography of soft tissue masses of the neck. *J Clin Ultrasound.* 2002;30(6):356. [PMID: 12116098] (Review of the uses of ultrasound in the management of neck masses.)

McGuirt WF, Greven K, Williams D, et al. PET scanning in head and neck oncology: a review. *Head Neck.* 1998;20(3):208. [PMID: 9570626] (Review of the uses of positron emission tomography in the diagnosis and treatment of head and neck cancer.)

Nguyen C, Shenouda G, Black MJ, Vuong T, Donath D, Yassa M. Metastatic squamous cell carcinoma to cervical lymph nodes from unknown primary mucosal sites. *Head Neck.* 1994; 16(1):58. [PMID: 8125789] (Outlines the workup for metastatic neck masses.)

Otto RA, Bowes AK. Neck masses: benign or malignant? Sorting out the causes by age group. *Postgrad Med.* 1990;88(1):199. [PMID: 2367255] (Discusses the fact that the differential diagnosis of cervical masses varies with the age of the patient.)

Wetmore RF, Mahboubi S, Soyupak SK. Computed tomography in the evaluation of pediatric neck infections. *Otolaryngol Head Neck Surg.* 1998;119(6):624. [PMID: 9852537] (Study of 66 pediatric patients with neck infections. CT scanning was not particularly helpful in superficial neck infections with regard to the decision to perform surgical drainage; however, it did localize and demonstrate the extent of infection. In deep neck infections, they found a 92% correlation between CT evidence of an abscess and the surgical confirmation of one.)

Weymuller EA Jr. Evaluation of neck masses. *J Fam Pract.* 1980; 11(7):1099. [PMID: 7452169] (Provides an algorithm for the diagnosis of neck masses.)

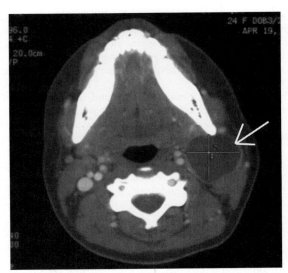

Figure 26–3. Axial CT scan of branchial cleft cyst (arrow).

■ CONGENITAL NECK MASSES

BRANCHIAL CLEFT CYSTS

Branchial cleft cysts arise from the failure of the pharyngobranchial ducts to obliterate during fetal development. They most frequently present in late childhood or early adulthood, when the cysts become infected—usually after an upper respiratory tract infection. A branchial cleft cyst appears as a tender, inflammatory mass located at the anterior border of the sternocleidomastoid muscle (Figure 26–3).

Classification

Branchial cleft cysts fall into three categories: first, second, and third branchial cleft anomalies.

A. FIRST BRANCHIAL CLEFT ANOMALIES

First branchial cleft anomalies make up less than 1% of all branchiogenic anomalies and usually appear on the face or near the auricle. There are two types of first branchial anomalies, Type I and Type II.

1. Type I—Type I first branchial cleft cysts are duplication anomalies of the external canal and are composed of ectodermally derived tissue. They may pass into the parotid gland and close to the facial nerve.

2. Type II—Type II anomalies may comprise ectodermally and mesodermally derived tissues. These lesions typically present below the angle of the mandible, pass through the parotid gland in close proximity to the facial nerve, and end either inferior to the external auditory canal or into the canal at the bony cartilaginous junction.

B. SECOND BRANCHIAL CLEFT ANOMALIES

Second branchial cleft anomalies are the most common of the three types. They present as discrete, rounded masses below the angle of the mandible and at the anterior border of the sternocleidomastoid muscle. The potential tract of an associated sinus passes deep to the second arch structures (eg, the external carotid artery and the stylohyoid and digastric muscles) and superficial to the third arch derivatives (eg, the internal carotid artery), opening into the tonsillar fossa.

C. THIRD BRANCHIAL CLEFT ANOMALIES

Third branchial cleft cysts present anterior to the sternocleidomastoid muscle and lower in the neck than either first or second branchial cleft anomalies. Third branchial cleft cysts are deep to the third arch derivatives (eg, the glossopharyngeal nerve and the internal carotid artery) and superficial to fourth arch derivatives (eg, the vagus nerve). These anomalies end in the pharynx at the thyrohyoid membrane or pyriform sinus.

Treatment

The management of branchial cleft anomalies is initial control of the infection followed by surgical excision of the cyst and tract. As a general rule, incision and drainage procedures should be avoided; however, they may be necessary for acute abscess treatment before definitive excision. Needle aspiration and decompression can be beneficial in preventing incision and drainage, which increases the difficulty of definitive excision.

THYROGLOSSAL DUCT CYSTS

Thyroglossal duct cysts present as midline masses of the anterior neck (Figure 26–4). Like branchial cleft cysts, they may be asymptomatic and appear only when they become infected in the setting of an upper respiratory tract infection. Thyroglossal duct cysts make up approximately one third of all congenital neck masses. Their location may be variable at times, with some cysts presenting more laterally (ie, superior to the hyoid) or as low as the level of the thyroid gland. Thyroglossal duct cysts that occur off the midline may be difficult to differentiate from branchial cleft cysts. A pathognomonic sign on physical examination is vertical motion of the mass with swallowing and tongue protrusion, demonstrating the intimate relation to the hyoid bone.

The **Sistrunk operation** is the standard method of thyroglossal duct cyst excision. The cyst is excised with

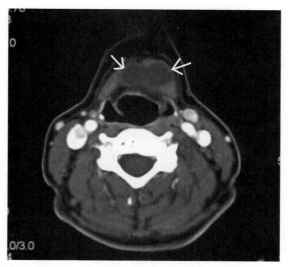

Figure 26–4. Axial CT scan of thyroglossal duct cyst (area between the arrows).

a cuff of tissue, including the center portion of the hyoid bone. During the resection of the hyoid bone, care is taken not to injure the hypoglossal nerves; making the hyoid bone cuts just medial to the lesser cornu assists in safeguarding these nerves. Since thyroid carcinomas can be present in a small percentage of thyroglossal duct cysts, all thyroglossal cysts and tracts should undergo a careful histologic examination.

LARYNGOCELES

A laryngocele is defined as an abnormal dilation or herniation of the saccule of the larynx. Secondary infection of a laryngocele is termed a **laryngopyocele.** Laryngoceles can be classified into three types: internal, external, and combined. A laryngocele is defined as internal if the dilation lies within the limits of the thyroid cartilage. If the laryngocele extends beyond the thyroid cartilage and protrudes through the thyrohyoid membrane producing a lateral neck mass, it is considered external.

Patients with laryngoceles present with hoarseness, cough, dyspnea, dysphagia, a foreign body sensation, or any combination of these symptoms. Laryngoscopy may reveal a smooth dilation at the level of the false cord involving both the false cord and the aryepiglottic fold. A CT scan is helpful in confirming the diagnosis and delineating the extent of the lesion. If symptomatic, the management of laryngoceles consists of (1) laryngoscopic decompression for small lesions, (2) surgical excision through an external approach for larger lesions, or laser endoscopy. If an external approach is done, care must be taken to avoid injury to the superior laryngeal nerve.

PLUNGING RANULAS

Plunging ranulas are mucoceles or retention cysts of the floor of mouth that usually present as slow-growing, painless, submental masses. They arise from the sublingual gland and are defined as plunging when they extend through the mylohyoid muscle into the neck. Treatment for plunging ranulas includes excision of the mass in continuity with the sublingual gland.

LYMPHANGIOMAS

Lymphangiomas are congenital malformations of the lymphatic channels. They arise owing to failure of the lymph spaces to connect to the remaining lymphatic system. The mass is usually soft, doughy, smooth, nontender, and compressible. These masses can characteristically be transilluminated. CT scanning and MRI are important studies both to delineate the extent of the disease and to define any potential associated abnormalities (eg, hemangiomas).

Surgical excision is the mainstay of therapy. Because of the infiltrative nature of these lesions, complete surgical resection may be impossible without damaging vital structures. In such cases, debulking the mass is appropriate and accomplishes the goals of improving cosmetic appearance and symptomatic relief while preserving critical normal anatomic structures.

HEMANGIOMAS

Hemangiomas are malformations of vascular tissue. They can be classified as capillary, cavernous, or juvenile. These lesions usually present in the first few months of life, grow rapidly during the first year, and then begin to slowly involute at 18–24 months of age. In 90% of cases, involution occurs without the need for any therapy.

Hemangiomas present as a red or bluish soft mass that is compressible and increases in size with straining or crying. Bruits may sometimes be auscultated over the lesion. CT scans, MRI, or both are valuable tools in making the diagnosis of this vascular lesion while defining the full extent of the lesion.

Because most hemangiomas involute spontaneously, these lesions can be managed conservatively with observation alone. Consideration should be given to the presence of these lesions in other not readily recognized regions, such as the subglottis, gastrointestinal tract, and spine. Intervention is indicated if the lesion is causing any of the following symptoms: airway compromise, skin ulceration, dysphagia, thrombocytopenia, or cardiac failure. Systemic corticosteroids or surgical laser excision may be warranted in such cases.

TERATOMAS

Teratomas of the head and neck make up approximately 3.5% of all teratomas. Their origin is from pluripotential cells and, by definition, they contain elements from all three germ layers. Teratomas usually present as firm neck masses and are most commonly noted at birth or within the first year of life. There is a 20% associated incidence of maternal polyhydramnios. When large enough, teratomas can cause either respiratory compromise due to tracheal compression or dysphagia secondary to compression of the esophagus and disruption of deglutition. In addition to appearing heterogeneous, calcifications may be seen on CT and MRI scans of teratomas. The most successful treatment method is surgical excision.

DERMOID CYSTS

Dermoid cysts arise from epithelium that has been entrapped in deeper tissue either during embryogenesis or by traumatic implantation. They contain a variety of tissues from all three germ layers and most often form along lines of embryologic fusion. They typically present as midline, nontender, mobile neck masses in the submental region. Surgical excision is the mainstay of treatment.

THYMIC CYSTS

The third branchial pouch gives rise to the thymus during the sixth week of fetal life, elongates in the pharynx, and then descends into the mediastinum. Thymic cysts arise when there is implantation of this thymic tissue along this descent. These cysts present as slow-growing, asymptomatic masses that may be painful if infected. On rare occasions, they grow rapidly and cause dyspnea or dysphagia. CT scanning and MRI are useful in the differential diagnosis. A definitive diagnosis is made histologically by the presence of Hassall corpuscles. Thymic cysts are treated by surgical excision.

STERNOCLEIDOMASTOID TUMORS OF INFANCY

Sternocleidomastoid tumors of infancy present as neck masses that are characterized histologically by dense fibrous tissue and the absence of normal striated muscle. This disorder is intimately related to congenital torticollis. Sternocleidomastoid tumors of infancy typically present as firm, painless, discrete masses within the sternocleidomastoid muscle; they slowly increase in size for 2–3 months and then regress for 4–8 months. Eighty percent of cases resolve spontaneously and do not need any intervention other than physical therapy to prevent restrictive torticollis. Surgical resection is reserved for persistent cases.

Ang AH, Pang KP, Tan LK. Complete branchial fistula: case report and review of the literature. *Ann Otol Rhinol Laryngol.* 2001; 110(11):1077. [PMID: 11713922] (Discusses the diagnosis and management of branchial cleft cysts.)

Brown RL, Azizkhan RG. Pediatric head and neck lesions. *Pediatr Clin North Am.* 1998;45(4):889. [PMID: 9728193] (Outlines the workup and differential diagnosis of pediatric neck masses.)

Cassano L, Lombardo P, Marchese-Ragona R, Pastore A, Marchese Ragona R. Laryngopyocele: three new clinical cases and review of the literature. *Eur Arch Otorhinolaryngol.* 2000;257 (9):507. [PMID: 11131379] (Discusses the diagnosis and treatment of laryngoceles.)

De Caluwe D, Ahmed M, Puri P. Cervical thymic cysts. *Pediatr Surg Int.* 2002;18(5–6):477. Epub 2002 Aug 23. [PMID: 12415385] (Retrospective review of two cases of cervical thymic cysts and review of the literature.)

Enepekides DJ. Management of congenital anomalies of the neck. *Facial Plast Surg Clin North Am.* 2001;9(1):131. [PMID: 11465000] (Outlines a standardized and complete approach to the evaluation of congenital neck masses.)

Forte V, Triglia JM, Zalzal G. Hemangioma. *Head Neck.* 1998; 20(1):69. [PMID: 9464955] (Reviews the diagnosis and management of hemangiomas.)

Hamoir M, Bernheim N, Vander Poorten V et al. Initial assessment of a neck mass in children. *B-ENT.* 2005;Suppl 1:126. [PMID: 16363273] (Review of the management of neck masses in children.)

Ichimura K, Ohta Y, Tayama N. Surgical management of the plunging ranula: a review of seven cases. *J Laryngol Otol.* 1996;110(6):554. [PMID: 8763376] (Reviews the surgical management of plunging ranulas.)

Kennedy TL, Whitaker M, Pellitteri P, Wood WE. Cystic hygroma and lymphangioma: a rational approach to management. *Laryngoscope.* 2001;111:1929. [PMID: 11801972] (Retrospective review of 74 patients with cystic hygroma, outlining a rational approach to the management of cystic hygroma based on the authors' experiences, the natural history of the disease, and the results of surgical treatment.)

Koch BL. Cystic malformations of the neck in children. *Pediatr Radiol.* 2005;35(5):463. [PMID: 15785931] (Review of the diagnosis and management of cystic neck masses in children.)

Maddalozzo J, Venkatesan TK, Gupta P. Complications associated with the Sistrunk procedure. *Laryngoscope.* 2001;111(1):119. [PMID: 11192879] (Reviews the potential complications of the Sistrunk procedure.)

Newman JG, Namdar I, Ward RF. Case report of an anterior neck thymic cyst. *Otolaryngol Head Neck Surg.* 2001;125(6):656. [PMID: 11743473] (Case report of an anterior neck thymic cyst with discussion of the diagnosis and management.)

Paczona R, Jori J, Czigner J. Pharyngeal localizations of branchial cysts. *Eur Arch Otorhinolaryngol.* 1998;255(7):379. [PMID: 9783138] (Reviews the location and development of branchial cysts.)

Sistrunk WE. Technique of removal of cysts and sinuses of the thyroglossal duct. *Surg Gynecol Obstet.* 1928;46:109. (The original paper that discusses the Sistrunk procedure.)

Wetmore RF, Mahboubi S, Soyupak SK. Computed tomography in the evaluation of pediatric neck infections. *Otolaryngol Head Neck Surg.* 1998;119(6):624. [PMID: 9852537] (Discusses the value of CT scanning in pediatric neck infections.)

■ INFLAMMATORY NECK MASSES

INFECTIOUS INFLAMMATORY DISORDERS

REACTIVE VIRAL LYMPHADENOPATHY

Reactive viral lymphadenopathy is the most common cause of cervical adenopathy in children. These neck masses are usually associated with symptoms of an underlying upper respiratory tract infection. The most common viral agents include adenovirus, rhinovirus, and enterovirus. These reactive lymph nodes tend to regress in 1–2 weeks.

The management of reactive viral lymphadenopathy is usually observation; however, a neck mass larger than 1 cm should be considered abnormal and warrant further investigation if it remains for more than 4–6 weeks or increases in size. If the suspected adenopathy persists, biopsies can be taken to search for other causes, such as fungal, granulomatous, or neoplastic processes.

EBV or mononucleosis can also present with lymphadenopathy, although it is usually accompanied by the enlargement of other lymphoid tissues such as the adenoids or tonsils. Patients with the EBV also have accompanying symptoms of fever and pharyngitis. Adenopathy associated with mononucleosis may last as long as 4–6 weeks. The treatment is limited to supportive management.

HIV-ASSOCIATED INFLAMMATORY DISORDERS

1. Cervical Adenopathy

Cervical adenopathy is present in 12–45% of patients with human immunodeficiency virus (HIV). Idiopathic follicular hyperplasia is the most common cause of adenopathy in these patients, although other infectious or neoplastic etiologies must be ruled out, including *Mycobacterium tuberculosis, Pneumocystis carinii,* lymphoma, and Kaposi sarcoma. The treatment of cervical adenopathy in the setting of HIV disease requires treatment of the underlying HIV infection, which is beyond the scope of this chapter.

2. Persistent Generalized Lymphadenopathy

Persistent generalized lymphadenopathy is lymphadenopathy without an identifiable infectious or neoplastic cause; it is commonly seen in patients with HIV infection. The neck is the most common site of persistent generalized lymphadenopathy. Once the diagnosis is made, the treatment of persistent generalized lymphadenopathy secondary to HIV infection requires treatment of the underlying HIV disease.

BACTERIAL LYMPHADENOPATHY

1. Suppurative Lymphadenopathy

Suppurative lymphadenopathy is most frequently caused by *Staphylococcus aureus* and group A *B-Streptococcus.* These neck masses usually develop in the submandibular or jugulodigastric region and are often accompanied by sore throat, skin lesions, and symptoms of upper respiratory tract infection. Empirical antibiotic therapy against anaerobic and gram-positive organisms is recommended as the first line of management. If this fails, either FNA or incision and drainage may be indicated.

2. Toxoplasmosis

Toxoplasmosis is caused by *Toxoplasma gondii* and is contracted through the consumption of poorly cooked meat or the ingestion of oocytes excreted in cat feces. Patients present with fever, malaise, sore throat, and myalgias. The diagnosis is made by serologic testing. Medical management is with sulfonamides or pyrimethamine.

3. Tularemia

Tularemia is caused by the organism *Francisella tularensis* and is transmitted by rabbits, ticks, or contaminated water. Patients present with tonsillitis and painful adenopathy with systemic symptoms of fever, chills, headache, and fatigue. Serologic testing and culture confirm the diagnosis. Streptomycin is the antibiotic of choice.

4. Brucellosis

Brucellosis is caused by a species of gram-negative bacilli, *Brucella*. It is transmitted most commonly to children by the ingestion of unpasteurized milk. Patients present with total body lymphadenopathy, fever, fatigue, and malaise. Serology and culture are mainstays of diagnosis, and treatment is with trimethoprim-sulfamethoxazole or tetracycline.

GRANULOMATOUS DISEASES

The differential diagnoses for granulomatous adenopathy of the neck include cat-scratch disease, actinomycosis, atypical mycobacteria, tuberculosis, atypical tuberculosis, and sarcoidosis.

1. Cat-Scratch Disease

Cat-scratch disease is caused by the bacterium *Rochalimaea henselae*. A history of contact with cats can be elicited in 90% of cases. This disease is more commonly seen in patients younger than 20 years. They present with tender lymphadenopathy, fever, and malaise. The lymphadenopathy is typically preauricular and submandibular in location. The diagnosis is made by serologic testing with indirect fluorescent antibodies. Histologically, the cat-scratch bacillus can often be demonstrated by Warthin-Starry staining. Cat-scratch disease is generally benign and self-limited.

2. Actinomycosis

Actinomycosis is a gram-positive bacillus. Studies have reported that from 50% to 96% of cases of actinomycosis affect the head and neck regions. Patients present with a painless, fluctuant, neck mass in the submandibular or upper digastric regions. The diagnosis is made by clinical suspicion and biopsy; it is confirmed histologically by the presence of granulomas with sulfur granules. Penicillin is the treatment of choice.

3. Atypical Mycobacteria

Atypical mycobacteria typically presents in the pediatric population as a unilateral neck mass located in the anterior triangle of the neck or parotid region. These patients have brawny skin, induration, and pain. The diagnosis is made by culture and skin testing. Surgical excision offers definitive treatment, although incision and curettage along with antibiotic therapy constitute an alternative management strategy.

4. Tuberculosis

Tuberculosis is seen more commonly in adults than in children. The causative organism is *M tuberculosis*. The presenting lymphadenopathy tends to be more diffuse and bilateral in contrast to atypical mycobacteria. Tuberculin skin tests are strongly positive. Cervical tuberculosis is also known as **scrofula** and is responsive to antituberculous medications.

5. Sarcoidosis

Sarcoidosis presents most commonly in the second decade of life with lymph node enlargement, fatigue, and weight loss. Chest radiography shows hilar adenopathy. An elevated angiotensin-converting enzyme (ACE) level is seen in 60–90% of patients with sarcoidosis. The diagnosis is confirmed histologically by the presence of noncaseating granulomas on biopsy specimens. Corticosteroids may be used, depending on the severity of the disease.

FUNGAL INFECTIONS

Immunocompromised patients are particularly susceptible to fungal infections. The most common organisms include *Candida, Histoplasma,* and *Aspergillus.* Serology and fungal cultures are imperative for the diagnosis. Aggressive, systemic antifungal therapy with agents such as amphotericin B is the treatment of choice.

Alvi A, Johnson JT. The neck mass: a challenging differential diagnosis. *Postgrad Med.* 1995;97(5):87. [PMID: 8780950] (Outlines the workup of neck masses.)

Barzan L, Tavio M, Tirelli U, Comoretto R. Head and neck manifestations during HIV infection. *J Laryngol Otol.* 1993; 107(2):133. [PMID: 8496646] (Reviewed 210 HIV-positive patients. Overall, 84% of the observed patients had head and neck manifestations.)

Emery MT, Newburg JA, Waters RC. Evaluation of the neck mass. *J S C Med Assoc.* 1998;94(12):548. [PMID: 9885480] (Outlines the diagnosis and treatment of neck masses.)

Hazra R, Robson CD, Perez-Atayde AR, Husson RN. Lymphadenitis due to nontuberculous mycobacteria in children: presentation and response to therapy. *Clin Infect Dis.* 1999; 28(1): 123. [PMID: 10028082] (Discusses the treatment of nontuberculous mycobacteria.)

NONINFECTIOUS INFLAMMATORY DISORDERS

ROSAI-DORFMAN DISEASE (SINUS HISTIOCYTOSIS)

Rosai-Dorfman disease typically presents in children with massive nontender cervical lymphadenopathy, fever, and skin nodules. It is characterized by benign, self-limited lymphadenopathy. Biopsy shows classically dilated sinuses, plasma cells, and the proliferation of histiocytes.

KAWASAKI DISEASE

Kawasaki disease is an acute multisystem vasculitis in children. Patients present with a number of symptoms: acute, nonpurulent cervical lymphadenopathy; erythema, edema, and desquamation of the hands and feet; polymorphous exanthem; conjunctival injection; and erythema of the lips and oral cavity. The diagnosis is made by clinical judgment. Early identification and treatment with aspirin and γ-globulin are imperative in avoiding serious cardiac complications.

CASTLEMAN DISEASE

Castleman disease is a rare, benign lymphoepithelial disease with the potential for development of Kaposi sarcoma and lymphoma. This disease affects both sexes equally and can occur at any age with its peak incidence in the second to fourth decades. This disease occurs most commonly in thoracic lymph nodes (70%), followed by the pelvis, abdomen, retroperitoneum, skeletal muscle, and head and neck. The diagnosis is made by tissue biopsy with histologic subclassification to the **hyaline-vascular variant** and the **plasma cell variant.** Ninety percent of cases are of the hyaline-vascular variant, which typically presents as an asymptomatic mass. In contrast, of patients who present with the plasma cell variant, 50% have associated symptoms of fever, fatigue, arthralgia, anemia, hypogammaglobulinemia, and thrombocytosis. Furthermore, unlike the hyaline-vascular variant, the plasma cell variant often presents with multicentric disease.

The treatment of this disorder is unrelated to histologic subtype. Isolated Castleman disease is managed by surgical resection with excellent prognosis. Constitutional symptoms resolve after the surgical resection of isolated disease. Multicentric disease is treated with chemotherapy and has a more guarded prognosis.

Ahsan SF, Madgy DN, Poulik J. Otolaryngologic manifestations of Rosai-Dorfman disease. *Int J Pediatr Otorhinolaryngol.* 2001; 59(3):221. [PMID: 11397505] (Discusses the diagnosis and treatment of Rosai-Dorfman disease.)

Gedalia A. Kawasaki disease: an update. *Curr Rheumatol Rep.* 2002; 4(1):25. [PMID: 11798979] (Discusses the diagnosis and management of Kawasaki disease.)

Kumar BN, Jones TJ, Skinner DW. Castleman disease: an unusual cause of a neck mass. *ORL J Otorhinolaryngol Relat Spec.* 1997;59(6):339. [PMID: 9364552] (Reviews the management of Castleman disease.)

Patel U, Forte V, Taylor G, Sirkin W. Castleman disease as a rare cause of a neck mass in a child. *J Otolaryngol.* 1998;27(3): 171. [PMID: 9664249] (A case presentation and review of Castleman disease in the neck.)

Saraf S, Singh RK. Kawasaki disease. *Indian J Pediatr.* 2001;68 (10):987. [PMID: 11758140] (A review of the diagnosis and management of Kawasaki disease.)

◼ NEOPLASTIC DISORDERS

METASTATIC SQUAMOUS CELL CARCINOMAS

A newly discovered neck mass in an adult patient must be presumed malignant until proven otherwise. These metastatic malignant masses tend to present as asymptomatic lesions that progress slowly and are firm to palpation. The associated symptoms are often related to the primary site of the malignant mass and include odynophagia, dysphagia, dysphonia, otalgia, and weight loss. The most common metastatic lesion to the neck is squamous cell carcinoma.

The diagnosis of metastatic squamous cell carcinoma to the neck can be diagnosed accurately by FNA biopsy. FNA is preferred to excisional biopsy of a metastatic cervical lymph node. Some studies report that distant metastases and late regional recurrences are more frequently encountered in patients who have had pretreatment of excisional biopsies than in those patients with the same stage of disease who have not. The pretreatment excisional biopsy group also had a higher incidence of local wound complications.

When the diagnosis of metastatic squamous cell carcinoma is made in a neck mass, the physician should conduct a thorough examination of the following sites: all mucosal surfaces of the head and neck, the thyroid gland, the salivary glands, and the skin of the head and neck. Studies have reported that 50–67% of patients with metastatic squamous cell carcinoma will have their primary tumor site identified in the office examination.

Imaging studies, such as CT scans and MRI, may be helpful in the search for the primary tumor (Figure 26–5).

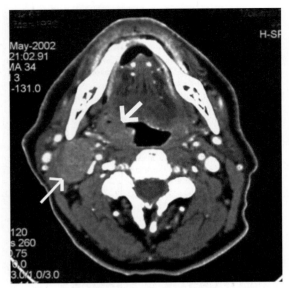

Figure 26–5. Axial CT scan of neck metastasis (thin arrow) from tonsillar squamous cell cancer (large arrow).

If the initial examination and imaging fail, a direct endoscopic examination under general anesthesia should be done. If endoscopy provides no evidence of a primary lesion, then the sites most likely to contain an occult tumor should be biopsied. Knowing the location of the node assists in guiding the surgeon to suspicious areas. Enlarged nodes high in the neck or in the posterior triangle suggest a nasopharyngeal lesion, whereas enlarged jugulodigastric nodes point to a lesion in the tonsils, the base of tongue, or the supraglottic larynx. When the enlarged nodes are in the supraclavicular area, the digestive tract, the tracheobronchial tree, the breast, the genitourinary tract, and the thyroid gland should be considered as lesion sites. The most common sites of an occult primary lesion are the nasopharynx, the tonsils, and the base of the tongue. Some clinicians advocate biopsies of these regions in patients with negative direct endoscopic examinations.

Cystic neck masses in the adult require special attention. Although the benign congenital lesions listed above can present in the adult, consideration must be given to the cystic variants of metastatic disease. Squamous cell carcinoma, metastatic from tonsillar primary lesions, often presents as a cystic mass in the jugulodigastric region. FNA can be diagnostic. Cystic masses in the lower neck, central neck, and mid-jugular lymph node chains should raise the consideration of metastatic papillary thyroid cancer. FNA is often nondiagnostic, but the fluid removed has a dark-brown color indicative of metastatic papillary thyroid cancer. Thyroid ultrasound should be included in the evaluation.

THYROID MASSES

A primary thyroid tumor manifests in the anterior compartment of the neck. A thyroid mass in a patient with hoarseness and a history of neck irradiation should be considered malignant. Ultrasound, thyroid scans, and thyroid function tests should be considered when allowing for the possibility of a thyroid lesion. FNA provides the most diagnostic information in the evaluation of a thyroid mass. The treatment is based on histologic findings.

LYMPHOMAS

Lymphomas can occur in all age groups but are much more common in children and young adults. Among children with Hodgkin disease, up to 80% will have at least one neck mass. A suspicion of lymphoma should arise when a young patient presents with fever, chills, and diffuse lymphadenopathy. The results of an FNA may be suggestive for lymphoma, but this biopsy may not provide sufficient tissue for classification. Therefore, in a patient with an FNA highly suggestive of lymphoma, an open biopsy may be necessary to obtain sufficient tissue for histopathologic classification. Once the diagnosis is made, staging workup should be conducted that includes CT scanning of the head, neck, chest, and abdomen.

SALIVARY NEOPLASMS

Parotid gland neoplasms may present either in front of or below the ear, or they may present at the angle of the mandible. Submandibular gland tumors are found in the submandibular triangle. Most parotid lesions are found to be benign. Submandibular gland tumors, in contrast, although consisting of a similar spectrum of pathology as parotid neoplasms, have an increased incidence of malignant pathology compared with parotid lesions. Benign salivary lesions typically present as asymptomatic masses. Symptoms such as pain, cranial nerve involvement, rapid growth, or overlying skin involvement are highly suggestive of malignant growths. Diagnostic tests include CT scanning, MRI, nuclear scans, and sialography. FNA is the diagnostic test of choice.

PARAGANGLIOMAS

Paragangliomas are neoplasms that arise from extraadrenal paraganglia. Carotid body tumors and glomus tumors are paragangliomas that present as neck masses in the upper jugulodigastric region in close proximity to the carotid bifurcation. They are pulsatile and bruits can usually be heard on auscultation. They are mobile from side to side but not up and down. Histologically, they consist of clusters of epithelioid cells (Zellballen) separated by highly vascular, fibrous stroma.

Ten percent of patients with paragangliomas have a positive family history. Ten to twenty percent of patients present with multiple paragangliomas; 5–10% of all paragangliomas are malignant. The gold standard of diagnosis has been angiography in the past, but it has been supplanted by magnetic resonance angiography (MRA). Carotid body tumors demonstrate a splaying of the internal and external carotid arteries or "lyre" signs on both angiography and MRA. The treatment is surgical excision. Radiation therapy can arrest growth and is reserved for elderly patients, patients with extensive tumors who have a high risk of cranial nerve damage during resection, or patients with multiple paragangliomas. Preoperative embolization may aid in the surgical resection.

LIPOMAS

Lipomas occur most frequently in patients over 35 years of age. They are ill-defined soft masses that can occur in various neck locations. Lipomas are asymptomatic and can be diagnosed on CT scans as having fat-air density or by their bright appearance on T1-weighted MRI. The treatment is surgical excision if symptomatic. Liposarcoma can have a similar imaging appearance but demonstrates a more progressive and locally infiltrative course. Biopsy can be considered in such cases.

SOLITARY FIBROUS TUMOR

Solitary fibrous tumors are rare spindle cell neoplasms of mesenchymal origin. Most solitary fibrous tumors are located in the thorax. An estimated 5–20% of thoracic solitary fibrous tumors have been reported as malignant, but malignant extrathoracic tumors are rare. In the head and neck, the oral cavity is the most common site, but there have been case reports involving all head and neck sites. They often present as asymptomatic slow-growing masses. Treatment is by local resection. Factors that predispose to local recurrence in non–head and neck solitary fibrous tumors are diameter larger than 10 cm, the presence of a malignancy, and microscopically positive surgical margins.

Coleman SC, Smith JC, Burkey BB, Day TA, Page RN, Netterville JL. Long-standing lateral neck mass as the initial manifestation of well-differentiated thyroid carcinoma. *Laryngoscope.* 2000;110:204. [PMID: 10680917] (Reports a case of a thyroid cancer presenting as a lateral neck mass.)

Dailey SH, Sataloff RT. Lymphoma: an update on evolving trends in staging and management. *Ear Nose Throat J.* 2001; 80(3):164. [PMID: 11269220] (Reviews the current management of lymphoma of the head and neck.)

Ganly I, Patel SG, Stambuk HE et al. Solitary fibrous tumors of the head and neck: a clinicopathologic and radiologic review. *Arch Otolaryngol Head Neck Surg.* 2006;132(5):517. [PMID: 16702568] (Review of 12 patients with head and neck solitary fibrous tumors.)

Gluckman JL, Robbins KT, Fried MP. Cervical metastatic squamous carcinoma of unknown or occult primary source. *Head Neck.* 1990;12(5):440. [PMID: 2211107] (Discusses the diagnosis and treatment of unknown primary head and neck squamous cell carcinoma.)

Hamoir M, Bernheim N, Vander Poorten V et al. Initial assessment of a neck mass in children. *B-ENT.* 2005;Suppl 1:126. [PMID: 16363273] (Review of the management of neck masses in children.)

Koch BL. Cystic malformations of the neck in children. *Pediatr Radiol.* 2005;35(5):463. [PMID: 15785931] (Review of the diagnosis and management of cystic neck masses in children.)

Mendenhall WM, Mancuso AA, Amdur RJ, Stringer SP, Villaret DB, Cassisi NJ. Squamous cell carcinoma metastatic to the neck from an unknown head and neck primary site. *Am J Otolaryngol.* 2001;22(4):261. [PMID: 11464323] (Discusses the diagnosis and treatment of unknown primary head and neck squamous cell carcinoma.)

Pellitteri PK, Rinaldo A, Myssiorek D et al. Paragangliomas of the head and neck. *Oral Oncol.* 2004;40(6):563. [PMID: 15063383] (Review of the diagnosis and management of paragangliomas.)

Randall DA, Johnstone PA, Foss RD, Martin PJ. Tonsillectomy in diagnosis of the unknown primary tumor of the head and neck. *Otolaryngol Head Neck Surg.* 2000;122(1):52. [PMID: 10629482] (Reviews the role of tonsillectomy in unknown primary head and neck squamous cell carcinoma.)

Ridge BA, Brewster DC, Darling RC, Cambria RP, LaMuraglia GM, Abbott WM. Familial carotid body tumors: incidence and implications. *Ann Vasc Surg.* 1993;7(2):190. [PMID: 8518138] (Case report and discussion of a patient with bilateral carotid body tumors and a strong family history of such tumors.)

Talmi YP, Hoffman HT, Horowitz Z et al. Patterns of metastases to the upper jugular lymph nodes (the "submuscular recess"). *Head Neck.* 1998;20(8):682. [PMID: 9790288] (Discusses patterns of metastasis to the upper jugular lymph nodes and specifically addresses the issue of whether dissection of the submuscular recess is necessary in elective neck dissections.)

Neck Neoplasms & Neck Dissection

27

Aditi H. Mandpe, MD

◼ NECK NEOPLASMS

ESSENTIALS OF DIAGNOSIS

- *Primary neoplasms of the soft tissue in the head and neck are rare.*
- *The most common benign tumors are paragangliomas and nerve cell tumors.*
- *The most common malignant neoplasm is metastatic squamous cell carcinoma from the upper aerodigestive tract.*
- *The evaluation of a metastatic squamous cell carcinoma without an easily identifiable primary site is extensive, and treatment is controversial.*
- *Neck dissections are performed to treat metastatic neoplasms and to determine the presence of occult metastasis.*

General Considerations

Neck neoplasms include not only metastatic squamous cell carcinoma but also a number of other primary neck tumors. Metastatic squamous cell carcinoma arises from the upper aerodigestive tract and is present in the lymph nodes in the neck; other primary tumors arise from the soft tissue in the neck, such as fat, fibrous tissue, muscle, blood vessels, lymphatic vessels, nerves, and paraganglia. These primary tumors are fairly uncommon, often making a pathologic diagnosis difficult. The evaluation of all neck masses consists of obtaining a complete history and conducting a physical exam.

Clinical Findings

A. SYMPTOMS AND SIGNS

The presenting symptom of a neck neoplasm is a painless enlarging neck mass, which may grow extremely slowly or very rapidly. The location of the mass sometimes suggests its cause.

B. IMAGING STUDIES

Imaging with computed tomography (CT) or magnetic resonance imaging (MRI) is critical for these lesions, especially if these studies are performed before a biopsy is obtained. A preoperative study can better assess both the size and the extent of the lesion without confounding factors such as bleeding and edema. An MRI is often the study of choice because it allows a greater differentiation of soft tissue. A positron emission tomography (PET) scan has been crucial in evaluating patients with metastatic disease to identify additional tumor masses. Additional studies such as angiography and, recently, magnetic resonance angiography (MRA) add valuable information to the diagnosis of vascular lesions (eg, carotid body tumors and vascular malformations).

C. SPECIAL TESTS

1. Fine-needle aspiration (FNA) biopsy—A tissue specimen is vital for the diagnosis of neck neoplasms and can be obtained with a fine-needle aspiration biopsy (FNAB). Metastatic squamous cell carcinoma has an excellent specificity and sensitivity for FNAB. Additional studies such as flow studies, immunohistochemistry techniques, or electron microscopy may be required for an accurate diagnosis of these specimens.

2. Open biopsy—Open biopsies consist of incisional and excisional biopsies. **Excisional biopsy** with sufficient normal surrounding tissue for adequate, clear margins should be used for a small superficial lesion or any lesion smaller than 3 cm. An **incisional biopsy** should be entertained only if the mass is larger than 3 cm. If metastatic squamous cell carcinoma is suspected, an open biopsy should not be considered unless all other avenues have been exhausted including at least two inconclusive FNABs.

3. Other tests—After either an FNAB or open biopsy is performed, the specimen then undergoes evaluation with light microscopy. Immunohistochemistry techniques can stain for cytokeratin, leukocyte common antigen, S-100, and myoglobin to differentiate sarcomas, melanomas, and epithelial carcinomas. Electron microscopy is used to aid in the diagnosis in patients in whom light microscopy and immunohistochemistry techniques prove ineffective.

BENIGN NEOPLASMS

The most common benign masses in the neck are inflammatory lymph nodes and masses of salivary and thyroid gland origins. True soft tissue benign tumors in the neck are relatively uncommon.

PARAGANGLIOMAS

Paragangliomas arise from paraganglia, which are islands of cells derived from neural crest cells, associated with arteries and cranial nerves at the carotid body, vagal body, along laryngeal nerves, and in the jugulotympanic region. The tumors derived from these regions are carotid body tumors, intravagal paragangliomas, and glomus tympanicum and glomus jugulare. Although paraganglia cells are capable of producing catecholamines, the incidence of catecholamine-producing head and neck paragangliomas is exceedingly rare.

1. Carotid Body Tumors

Carotid body tumors are the most common head and neck paragangliomas. The carotid body is found at the bifurcation of the common carotid artery and responds to changes in arterial pH, oxygen, and carbon dioxide.

Clinical Findings

A. SYMPTOMS AND SIGNS

Symptoms are present only with large tumors and include pressure, dysphagia, cough, and hoarseness. On examination, the mass is palpated at the anterior border of the sternocleidomastoid muscle. It is typically mobile laterally but not vertically.

B. LABORATORY FINDINGS

The diagnosis requires a high index of suspicion, because the location is similar to that of many other masses (eg, branchial cleft cysts and enlarged lymph nodes). FNA of these lesions often yields only blood; however, if cells are obtained, FNA can offer a definitive diagnosis.

C. IMAGING STUDIES

The angiogram in Figure 27–1 shows the typical findings of a splayed bifurcation of the carotid artery with a vascular blush. An MRI often proves useful in identifying other paragangliomas as synchronous and metachronous lesions occur in 25–48% of cases. Familial paragangliomas occur in 7–9% of cases.

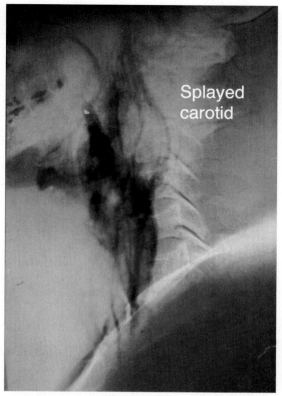

Figure 27–1. Angiogram of a patient with a carotid body tumor showing the classic splaying of the carotid bifurcation.

Treatment

A. SURGICAL MEASURES

The treatment of carotid body tumors is predominantly surgical. Preoperative embolization is useful to minimize blood loss in order to allow for a cleaner dissection. Surgical excision requires the following measures: (1) identification of the proximal and distal carotid artery and (2) identification and preservation of the vagus, hypoglossal, and spinal accessory nerves. Patients with large or recurrent tumors often require vascular reconstruction, which should be planned preoperatively.

B. RADIATION THERAPY

Radiation therapy is not the primary mode of therapy for carotid body tumors, but it has been used as the sole method of treatment in some individuals such as elderly patients who are poor surgical candidates. In patients with carotid body and vagale tumors, radiation therapy alone has been shown to provide a local control rate of as much as 96%. Control rates with surgery alone range from 88% to 100%. Treatment decisions are based on surgical risks and complications; therefore, small tumors should usually be treated surgically, with radiation therapy reserved for large tumors.

2. Intravagal Paragangliomas

Intravagal paragangliomas typically occur in association with one of the vagal ganglia, most commonly the ganglion nodosum. Intravagal paragangliomas account for approximately 3% of all head and neck paragangliomas. Symptoms can include hoarseness, dysphagia, aspiration, tongue weakness, and Horner syndrome. Angiographic imaging shows a mass located above the carotid bifurcation, with lateral and medial displacement of the external and internal carotid arteries. FNA has been useful in the diagnosis of these tumors.

The treatment involves surgical resection, with radiation therapy reserved for patients with high surgical risk, incomplete resection, recurrent disease, and bilateral tumors. Most intravagal paragangliomas can be resected via a cervical approach. If there is intracranial extension, a middle or posterior fossa approach may be needed.

PERIPHERAL NERVE CELL TUMORS

Tumors arising from peripheral nerves typically arise from the Schwann cells in the nerve sheath. Of the many names used to describe these tumors, two in particular—schwannomas and neurofibromas—have significant clinical differences that warrant discussion. As a group, neurogenous tumors occur most commonly in the head and neck regions. They are often asymptomatic and present as lateral neck masses.

1. Schwannomas

Peripheral nerve schwannomas, more appropriately termed neurilemomas, are solitary, well-encapsulated tumors. Histologically, these tumors have characteristic Antoni A and Antoni B tissues. **Antoni A** tissue consists of palisading nuclei around central cytoplasm, and **Antoni B** tissue is composed of a loose edematous matrix. These tumors can arise from cranial nerves, peripheral motor and sensory nerves, and the sympathetic chain. They can sometimes present with a displaced tonsil or a lateral pharyngeal wall when the mass is located in the parapharyngeal space.

2. Neurofibromas

Neurofibromas differ from neurilemomas in that they are not encapsulated. The nerves in neurofibromas tend to traverse the tumors and are integral to them. Solitary neurofibromas are very rare, but multiple neurofibromas are common, especially in patients with **von Recklinghausen disease.** Von Recklinghausen disease is an autosomal dominant disease with clinical findings of café-au-lait spots and neurofibromas.

The treatment of both neurilemomas and neurofibromas consists of simple surgical resection. The function of the affected nerve can typically be preserved with neurilemomas unless the neoplasms are intimately involved with some cranial nerves. These tumors rarely recur and malignant transformation is exceedingly rare.

LIPOMAS

Lipomas are the most common benign soft tissue neoplasms. They arise from the subcutaneous tissue and present as painless, smooth, encapsulated, round masses. Fifteen to twenty percent of all lipomas occur in the head and neck. Most of these neoplasms are solitary lesions and are easily treated with excision. Recurrences are very rare.

MALIGNANT NEOPLASMS

The most common malignant neoplasm in the neck is a cervical metastasis from a primary tumor in the upper aerodigestive tract. In most cases, when a lymph node metastasis in the neck is identified, the primary tumor also can be identified and the treatment proceeds according to the principles dictated by the stage of the primary disease. In less than 10% of cases, the primary site is not located and further evaluation is required. Malignant neoplasms of the salivary, thyroid, and parathyroid glands also can present as malignant cervical masses or with metastases to cervical lymph nodes. (See the following chapters for information on these neoplasms: Chapter 18, Malignant Diseases of the Salivary Glands; Chapter 42, Malignant Thyroid Disorders; and Chapter 43, Parathyroid Disorders.) Other common primary malignant neoplasms of the head and neck are lymphomas. Rarely are sarcomas seen in the head and neck.

UNKNOWN PRIMARY SQUAMOUS CELL CARCINOMA

Clinical Findings

A. SYMPTOMS AND SIGNS

A common problem with an unknown primary squamous cell carcinoma is determining the site of the primary tumor when a known metastatic node has been identified. The incidence of an unknown primary tumor is between 2% and 8% of all patients with head and neck squamous cell carcinoma. The patient examination shows a mass in the neck with no masses or

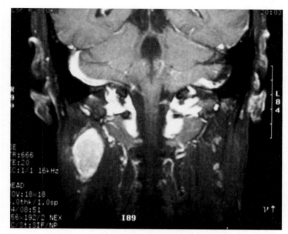

Figure 27–2. Coronal T1-weighted MRI showing a cervical metastasis from an unknown primary site.

abnormalities in the upper aerodigestive tract. It is often on an FNAB that the diagnosis of squamous cell carcinoma is made.

B. IMAGING STUDIES

1. MRI—The evaluation should consist of a thorough examination followed by an MRI scan, if possible. MRI allows for better soft tissue distinction than does a CT scan; therefore, it can better assess the location of small tumors while clearly showing the cervical metastasis (Figure 27–2).

2. Positron emission tomography (PET)—The PET scan shows increased glycolytic activity of tumor cells, identifying a potential tumor site. PET scans can identify small tumors, typically in the base of the tongue and in the tonsil, which would have otherwise escaped detection. PET scans and PET/CT combination scans have been used to follow up patients after treatment to evaluate for recurrence.

C. DIAGNOSTIC TESTS

All patients with unknown primary tumors should undergo an exhaustive search for the primary site so that (1) site-specific treatment can be used; (2) the area can be closely monitored for recurrence; and (3) treatment morbidity, especially with radiation therapy, is markedly reduced.

The next step in the site search is a direct laryngoscopy with biopsy, esophagoscopy, bronchoscopy, and tonsillectomy. If studies suggest a primary site that can be confirmed on direct laryngoscopy, a directed biopsy is often sufficient for the diagnosis. It

is more likely that no abnormalities are noted, and blind biopsies are obtained. The typical sites harboring a primary cancer are in the nasopharynx, the palatine tonsil, the base of tongue, and the pyriform sinus. The mucosa can be easily biopsied from the nasopharynx, the base of tongue, and the pyriform sinus. A tonsillectomy should be performed rather than only a biopsy because 18–26% of patients can harbor a primary tumor in the tonsil.

Staging

The staging of neck tumors is based on the system created by the American Joint Committee on Cancer. This system takes into account the number and size of lymph nodes in the neck; a portion of this staging system is shown in Table 27–1.

Treatment

The treatment of patients with an unknown primary tumor has been controversial. Although the necessity of treating the neck is undisputed, the order of surgery and radiation therapy is debated, as is the extent of the surgery needed. Some clinicians advocate primary radiation therapy with surgery to follow, whereas others promote primary neck dissection with postoperative radiation therapy. The advantage of primary radiation therapy is that all potential tumor sites can be treated and the neck mass may decrease in size to facilitate or, in some cases, prevent the neck dissection. The advantage of primary surgery is that a lower total dose of radiation may be given to the neck to prevent some complications of radiation therapy.

Table 27–1. Staging of regional lymph node metastasis.

Stage	Affected Lymph Nodes
N_X	Regional lymph nodes cannot be assessed
N_0	No regional lymph nodes
N_1	Single ipsilateral lymph node, < 3 cm
N_{2a}	Single ipsilateral lymph node, 3–6 cm
N_{2b}	Multiple ipsilateral lymph nodes, none > 6 cm
N_{2c}	Multiple bilateral or contralateral lymph nodes, none > 6 cm
N_3	Lymph node > 6 cm

The need to treat all potential primary sites also is debated. Wide-field radiation therapy to encompass all potential mucosal sites carries significant morbidity. Proponents of this treatment maintain that wide-field radiation therapy decreases the risk of future tumor emergence. The emergence rates of primary tumors are estimated to be 3–8% a year in patients with primary sites treated with radiation, compared with 32–44% in patients who do not undergo this treatment modality.

The complications of radiation treatment can be severe and include xerostomia, mucositis, and persistent dysphagia. For large, unresectable tumors, palliation is an option.

Hinerman RW, Mendenhall WM, Amdur RJ, Stringer SP, Antonelli PJ, Cassisi NJ. Definitive radiotherapy in the management of chemodectomas arising in the temporal bone, carotid body, and glomus vagale. *Head Neck.* 2001;23:363. [PMID: 11295809] (Provides information on good results with radiation therapy.)

Koch WM, Bhatti N, Williams MF, Eisele DW. Oncologic rationale for bilateral tonsillectomy in the head and neck: squamous cell carcinoma of unknown primary source. *Otolaryngol Head Neck Surg.* 2001;124:331. [PMID: 11241001] (Delineates the importance of tonsillectomy in the evaluation of an unknown primary tumor.)

Nieder C, Gregoire V, Ang KK. Cervical lymph node metastases from occult squamous cell carcinoma: cut down a tree to get an apple? *Int J Radiat Oncol Biol Phys.* 2001;50:727. [PMID: 11395241] (Reviews a diagnostic workup of an unknown primary tumor.)

■ NECK DISSECTION

General Considerations

A neck dissection is a systematic removal of lymph nodes in the neck. It serves to eradicate cancer of the cervical lymph nodes and can help determine the need for additional therapy when no lymph nodes are clinically identified. The indications for a neck dissection in the setting of no clinically palpable nodes are based on the propensity of metastasis from the primary site and the size of the primary tumor.

Classification of Neck Zones

The evaluation of the drainage pattern from the primary tumor sites in the upper aerodigestive tract has led to the understanding and identification of nodal groups at risk for cervical metastasis. The neck has been divided into five such groups called zones (Figure 27–3).

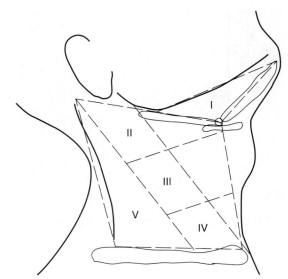

Figure 27–3. Zones of the neck used in classifying the location of a cervical metastasis.

A. Zone I: The Submandibular and Submental Triangles

Zone I consists of the submandibular triangle and the submental triangle. The submandibular triangle is bordered by the mandible superiorly, the posterior belly of the digastric muscle posteroinferiorly, and the anterior belly of the digastric muscle anteroinferiorly. The submental triangle is the region between the bilateral anterior bellies of the digastric muscle and the hyoid bone.

B. Zone II: The Upper Jugular Region

Zone II is known as the upper jugular region. Its boundaries are (1) the skull base superiorly, (2) the carotid bifurcation inferiorly, (3) the posterior border of the sternocleidomastoid muscle laterally, and (4) the lateral border of the sternohyoid and stylohyoid muscles medially. The tissue encompassed within these boundaries includes the upper portion of the internal jugular vein and the spinal accessory nerve. A subsection of Zone II, the **submuscular triangle,** includes the most superior aspect of this zone and lies laterally to the spinal accessory nerve at the skull base.

C. Zone III: The Middle Jugular Region

Zone III is the middle jugular region. It is bordered by (1) the carotid bifurcation superiorly, (2) the junction of the omohyoid muscle and the internal jugular vein inferiorly, (3) the posterior border of the sternocleidomastoid laterally, and (4) the lateral border of the sternohyoid muscle medially.

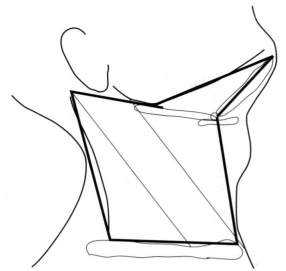

Figure 27–4. Surgical margins of a radical neck dissection.

D. Zone IV: The Lower Jugular Region

Zone IV is the lower jugular region and extends from the omohyoid superiorly to the clavicle inferiorly; it also extends to the posterior border of the sternocleidomastoid muscle laterally and the lateral border of the sternohyoid muscle medially.

E. Zone V: The Posterior Triangle

Zone V is the posterior triangle and includes all of the lymph nodes between the posterior border of the sternocleidomastoid medially and the anterior border of the trapezius muscle laterally; it extends to the clavicle inferiorly. This triangle encompasses the course of the spinal accessory nerve. The supraclavicular region is part of Zone V.

F. Zone VI: The Anterior Compartment

Zone VI is the anterior compartment and includes midline lymph nodes. The borders of this region are the hyoid bone superiorly, the suprasternal notch inferiorly, and the carotid sheaths laterally. This region is typically dissected *only* in conjunction with laryngectomy and thyroidectomy.

Treatment

The current classification of neck dissections includes radical neck dissection, modified radical neck dissection, selective neck dissection, and extended radical neck dissection.

A. Radical Neck Dissection

Radical neck dissection is defined as an en bloc removal of all nodal groups between the mandible and the clavicle; this removal includes the sternocleidomastoid mus-

cle, the internal jugular vein, and the spinal accessory nerve inclusive of Zones I–V. Since this dissection was first classified, many modifications have been proposed, especially in staging neck dissections when no palpable nodes are present (Figure 27–4).

B. Modified Radical Neck Dissection

A modified radical neck dissection involves sparing of at least one of these three structures—the sternocleidomastoid muscle, the internal jugular vein, or the spinal accessory nerve—while still dissecting Zones I–V. The indications for a modified radical neck dissection include definitive treatment of the neck in the presence of metastatic disease. Because the spinal accessory nerve is rarely directly involved with disease, it tends to be preserved to decrease the pain associated with shoulder dysfunction. On occasion, all three structures can be preserved if they are not directly involved with pathologic nodes.

C. Selective Neck Dissection

A selective neck dissection involves the preservation of one or more zones that are typically removed in a radical neck dissection. This procedure is performed when both the treatment of the primary lesion is surgical and the risk of occult metastasis to the cervical lymph nodes is greater than 20%.

1. Supraomohyoid neck dissection—A supraomohyoid neck dissection involves Zones I–III and is usually performed in conjunction with oral cavity tumors and N0 neck disease (Figure 27–5; also refer to Table 27–1). Its most common role is in the dissection of the

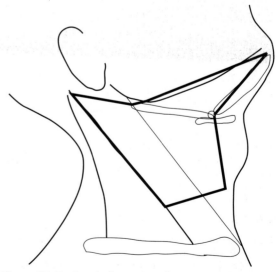

Figure 27–5. Surgical margins of a supraomohyoid neck dissection.

contralateral neck at high risk for cervical metastasis in order to avoid postoperative radiation therapy.

2. Lateral compartment neck dissection—A lateral compartment dissection includes Zones II–IV (Figure 27–6); it is used in conjunction with the surgical resection of tumors of the larynx, hypopharynx, and pharynx. When lateral compartment dissections are needed, they are usually performed bilaterally as the lesions are fairly midline.

3. Posterolateral neck dissection—Posterolateral neck dissections include Zones II–V and include nodes in the retroauricular and suboccipital regions (Figure 27–7). These dissections are often performed when cutaneous malignant tumors metastasize to the neck.

4. Anterior compartment neck dissection—The anterior compartment neck dissection includes Zone VI and is used for tumors found in the larynx, hypopharynx, subglottis, cervical esophagus, and thyroid. It includes the removal of the thyroid lobe and necessitates both the identification and the preservation of the parathyroid glands, with reimplantation as needed.

D. Extended Radical Neck Dissection

Extended neck dissections involve the additional removal of muscle, nerves, vessels, and lymph node groups as dictated by the primary disease and the presence of metastasis. Patients with disease extensive enough to warrant the consideration of a carotid resection should be evaluated preoperatively for carotid reconstruction.

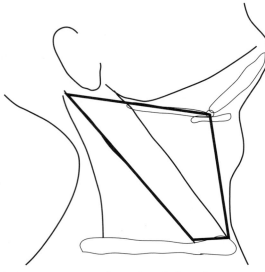

Figure 27–6. Surgical margins of a lateral compartment neck dissection.

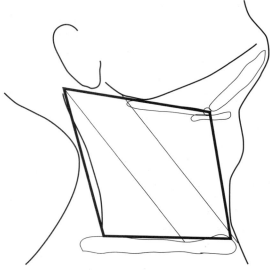

Figure 27–7. Surgical margins of a posterolateral neck dissection.

Complications

The complications associated with neck dissections can occur either intraoperatively owing to poor technique or postoperatively owing to poor nutritional status, alcoholism, or underlying medical conditions such as diabetes.

A. Intraoperative Complications

Surgical complications usually stem from injury to the nerves present in the field. The mandibular branch of the facial nerve can be injured in a submandibular dissection, as can the lingual and the hypoglossal nerves. Injury to the vagus nerve is uncommon but it can lead to vocal cord paralysis, a decreased sensation of the hemipharynx, and dysphagia with a risk of aspiration. Dissection in the neck, below the deep layer of the deep cervical fascia, can cause inadvertent injury to the phrenic nerve, which becomes symptomatic only in patients with significant pulmonary disease.

B. Postoperative Complications

1. Hematomas—A hematoma is a common postoperative complication. The immediate evacuation of a hematoma either by milking the drains (if small) or by exploration is necessary to both prevent wound infections and protect skin flaps.

2. Wound infections—The incidence of wound infections in neck dissections without concomitant pharyngeal surgery and with the use of perioperative antibiotics is 2–5% but increases when performed in conjunction with pharyngeal or laryngeal surgery. The use of perioperative antibiotics in the latter group has decreased the incidence of wound infections as well.

3. Chylous fistulas—A relatively uncommon complication is a chylous fistula, which is caused by injury to the thoracic duct. Even with meticulous surgical technique, the incidence of a chylous leak is between 1% and 2%. This leak often becomes evident after the resumption of enteral feeds. The drain output tends to increase and is of a milky quality. The initial management includes pressure dressings and placing the patient on a medium-chain fatty acid diet. Most leaks resolve with this conservative therapy. However, if the drainage persists, is > 600 mL/d, or is noted immediately postoperatively, surgical exploration with ligation of the stump may be necessary.

4. Carotid artery exposure and rupture—The most feared complication after neck surgery is carotid artery exposure with carotid rupture. Improved surgical techniques and the use of a pedicled and free musculocutaneous flap have minimized this risk. However, patient factors such as preoperative radiation therapy, poor nutritional status, infection, and diabetes continue to be risk factors. If the carotid artery becomes exposed and a sentinel bleed occurs, it is advisable to electively ligate the carotid artery both proximal and distal to the rupture. The carotid artery can sometimes be managed with embolization by highly experienced neurointerventional radiologists.

Erkal HS, Mendenhall WM, Amdur RJ, Villaret DB, Stringer SP. Squamous cell carcinomas metastatic to cervical nodes from an unknown head and neck mucosal site treated with radiation therapy with palliative intent. *Radiother Oncol.* 2001;59:319. [PMID: 11369074] (Palliation of neck metastasis with radiation therapy can be successful.)

Iganej S, Kagan R, Anderson P. Metastatic squamous cell carcinoma of the neck from an unknown primary site: management options and patterns of relapse. *Head Neck.* 2002;24:236. [PMID: 11891955] (Radiation therapy decreases the appearance of primary tumors after the treatment of the neck. However, it is not sufficient for N2–3 disease.)

Randall DA, Johnstone PA, Foss RD, Martin PJ. Tonsillectomy in diagnosis of the unknown primary tumor of the head and neck. *Otolaryngol Head Neck Surg.* 2000;122:52. [PMID: 10629482] (Supports tonsillectomy for the evaluation of an unknown primary tumor.)

Schechter NR, Gillenwater AM, Byers RM et al. Can positron emission tomography improve the quality of care for head-and-neck cancer patients? *Int J Radiat Oncol Biol Phys.* 2001;51:4. [PMID: 11516844] (Study supporting the use of PET imaging in detecting recurrences.)

SECTION VIII
Larynx & Hypopharynx

Clinical Voice Assessment: The Role & Value of the Phonatory Function Studies

28

Krzysztof Izdebski, PhD, CCC-SLP, FASHA

The purpose of a clinical voice evaluation is to provide the referring laryngologist with patient-specific, clinically relevant pathophysiologic information of the actual voice production process used by the dysphonic patient, the nature of the dysphonic sound generated by a patient, and the physiologic conditions responsible for the sound. The generated report must be clear and explanatory enough to aid the referring laryngologist with differential diagnosis and treatment planning. Moreover, the generated information must be capable of predicting treatment outcomes and powerful enough to warn the treating physician of any possible complications to the voice that may result from the proposed or planned treatment—whether medical, surgical, therapeutic, or a combination. Clinical voice evaluation is not a quick procedure. It may take up to 1 hour to conduct phonatory function studies (PhFS) on a noncomplicated patient, whereas it may take a substantially longer time to evaluate a patient who is a professional voice user.

The clinical exam comprises a battery of PhFS composed of at least of two primary parts: (1) an acoustic portion that examines the nature of the generated sound (CPT 92520 and 92506), and (2) a visual portion that examines via stroboscopic transoral or transnasal approach the glottis and surrounding area including the subglottis. Visualization of the subglottis is of paramount clinical value when examining papilloma, trauma, and/or subglottic stenosis patients. The exam must result in a clinically relevant description of the parameters that specify and reg-

ulate the vibratory patterns of the vocal cords and/or the other vocal tract elements that are causative of dysphonia. This portion of the exam is coded as 35812 using CPT code. (*Note:* When examining alaryngeal patient, additional CPT codes apply.)

PHONATORY FUNCTION STUDIES

PhFS consist of acoustic and physiologic components. These studies are considered a standard of modern voice care because they provide information beyond subjective clinical impressions; they also provide objective descriptions of normal and pathologic phonatory processes. These processes include (1) mapping acoustic voice characteristics, (2) correlating voice with physiologic findings, (3) providing guidelines for the development of efficacious treatment plans, (4) predicting the progress and outcomes of treatment plans, (5) providing preoperative-postoperative lesion mappings, and (6) providing documentation for medicolegal purposes. PhFS are reproducible and allow a contrast of individual results to a database specific to the patient's age and gender. The information these studies provide also allows for a frank discussion with the patient and education of the patient, including discussion of the risks and alternatives associated with various treatments.

The acoustic portion (92520, and various modifiers can be used) records and analyzes the voice of the patient. This portion is of paramount value, specifically when a surgical intervention is planned and when the patient uses voice as a tool of labor. Not having a voice recording of a patient as a chart record is simply inexcusable and must be treated as a serious error on the part of the practicing laryngologist. Having a voice recording is a must even if a litigation is not pending. *Do not ignore* this part of the exam. Acoustic recordings—if possible video recordings—should encompass content (vocal-text) relevant to the work needs and work conditions of the patient.

The physiologic portion visualizes via stroboscopic exam (phonoscopy) the mechanics of phonation and also maps the location, the extent, and the effects of phonatory lesions (when present), and their contribution to dysphonia. Keep in mind that a mismatch may be present between the acoustic and visual data (ie, large lesion but a relatively good voice, or a small lesion and a very poor voice), that not all glottic lesions require an immediate surgical procedure, and that not having an organic finding warrants a diagnosis of a functional dysphonia or even worse, a finding of malingering. In today's clinical practice, it is necessary to have at your disposal a comprehensive documentation of the phonatory mechanism. Documentation that shows objectively the location of the lesion or the mechanism of dysphonia is a necessity when postoperative dispute occurs. When operating on a patient, one must have preoperative stroboscopic mapping and voice recordings. Once visualization is conducted, the relevant videographs should be taken to the operating room (OR), placed in OR records, and compared with the visualization obtained during direct laryngoscopy.

In addition to these two primary components, special tests may also be a part of the PhFS battery. These include delayed auditory feedback, voice load tests, nerve blocks, manual compression tests, and so on.

In addition to the goals discussed, the information derived through PhFS is crucial in providing pre- postsurgical documentation, in mapping acoustic and visual lesion(s), and in matching the presence or absence of lesions to the voice quality produced. PhFS are also crucial in documenting follow-up and when considering treatment revision in patient education; moreover, they are a must in medicolegal proceedings.

Izdebski K. Magnetic sound recording in laryngology. *Am J Oto-laryngol.* 1981;2:48.

Izdebski K, Manace ED, Skiljo-Haris J. The challenge of determining work-related voice/speech disabilities in California. In: Dejonkere PH, ed. *Occupational Voice—Care and Cure.* The Hague: Kugler Publishing, 2001:149–154.

Izdebski K, Ross JC, Klein JC. Transoral rigid laryngovideostroboscopy (phonoscopy). *Semin Speech Lang.* 1990;1:16.

Leonnard R, Izdebski K. Laryngeal imaging with stroboscopy: its value in therapeutic assessment. In Pais Clemente M, ed. *Voice Update,* International Congress Series 1997, The Hague, Netherlands: Elsevier, 1997.

VOICE PRODUCTION

Voice is an acoustic product resulting from the semicyclical vibrations of the two vocal cords (VC) (ie, vocal folds) that are located in the larynx, commonly referred to as the *voice box.* Therefore, abnormal voice is a consequence of the underlying phonatory pathophysiology, reflecting the physical conditions of the vocal cords and the rest of the vocal tract, comprising the subglottic and supraglottic structures.

The vibration of the vocal cords is age and gender dependent and is controlled by myoelastic properties and aerodynamic forces; the vibration is generated as the air expelled under pressure from the lungs passes between the vocal cords and sets the cords into an oscillatory motion.

The myoelastic properties consist of the paired intrinsic laryngeal muscles, which are responsible for the size, shape, length, mass, stiffness, and tension characteristics of the vocal cords. The intrinsic laryngeal muscles include the thyroarytenoid muscles, the pairs of lateral cricoarytenoid muscles, the posterior cricoarytenoid muscles, and the interarytenoid muscle, which consists of both transverse and oblique portions. The intrinsic laryngeal muscles are innervated by the recurrent laryngeal nerves and all muscles, with the exception of the posterior cricoarytenoid muscles (the only vocal cord abductor), are responsible for vocal cord adduction and vocal cord approximation needed for the voice to take place. The bilateral cricothyroid musculature is responsible for the thyroid cartilage downward tilt that elongates the vocal cords. These muscles are principally responsible for pitch elevation. The nonmuscular myoelastic properties include membranes (mucosa), ligaments, glandular elements, a blood supply, and nerves, all of which are located within the articulating cartilaginous housing that comprises the thyroid, the cricoid, and the two arytenoid cartilages.

Normal voice is actually generated by the vibratory wave-generating oscillations of the membranous portion of the vocal cords (the mucosa), which slides/glides in an undulating manner over the underlying muscle. When the mucosa, the submucosal space, the muscles, the vascular elements, the cartilages, or the compression of the glottis are affected, including the subglottic and supraglottic structures, pathologic voice quality results, and voice may not be a product only of the true vocal cords, but may be produced in alternative ways. Therefore, PhFS must be capable of revealing altered phonation and of describing the glottic and the nonglottic mechanism that either generates, confuses, or co-produces the sound of the patient. This description is of paramount importance in differential diagnosis of dysphonia in patients in whom no visible VC pathology is noted, but in whom a dysphonic output is present.

The entire voice box rests on the trachea and is suspended above from the hyoid bone, which communicates with the base of the tongue. When this connection is affected by as little as minor lingual tension or inappropriate vertical larynx positioning, the result may include altered voice production.

In addition to the intrinsic articulation accomplished at the cricoarytenoid and cricothyroid (ie, synovial type) joints, the entire larynx is subject to vertical motions produced by the action of the paired extrinsic laryngeal musculature. These vertical laryngeal motions are crucial in phonation (singing), swallowing, respiration, and yawning, and in speech articulation. When this vertical movement is affected, voice production may be severely compromised even if the glottis looks "normal" on a routine ear, nose, and throat exam.

Izdebski K, Dedo HH. Non-glottic phonation in non-laryngectomized patients. A review of compensatory mechanism for alternative phonation sources in humans. In preparation, 2007.

Shipp T, Izdebski K. Vocal frequency and vertical larynx positioning by singers and non-singers. *J Acoust Soc Am.* 19975;58: 1104.

Titze I. *Principles of Voice Production.* Englewood Cliffs, NJ: Prentice Hall, 1994.

MOTOR & SENSORY CONTROL

Both voluntary and involuntary phonation occurs after the efferent signals generated in the motor cortex proceed via the brainstem nuclei and the left and right branches of the vagus nerve (CN X) to reach the two vocal cords. Signals terminate in the motor end plates of the intrinsic laryngeal muscles via the left and right recurrent laryngeal nerves, resulting in vocal cord contractions. The entire efferent process can be accomplished within 90 milliseconds, and it requires coordination of all vocal tract and respiratory laryngeal musculature via the central nervous system motor neurons. The coordination of these movements is achieved by a complex neural network with access to phonatory motor neuron pools that receive proprioceptive input from the various receptors associated with these three systems and by control of voluntary vocalization rather than involuntary vocalization involving different brain regions.

The recurrent laryngeal nerve is a mixed nerve containing an average of 1200 myelinated axons and thousands of unmyelinated axons, including some specialized endoneural organs.

The left recurrent laryngeal nerve is longer than the right nerve, but because of the differential axonal com-

position of both nerves, the efferent impulses manage to arrive at the two vocal cords almost simultaneously, causing the vocal cord vibration to be semi-periodic. This type of vibration makes the sound of the voice "human."

The vagus nerve also branches into the left and right superior laryngeal nerves (SLNs), which mediate the afferent signals from the larynx via their internal branches. The external branches of the SLNs are the motor branches innervating the paired cricothyroid muscles, which function as the primary pitch elevators. This specific vagus nerve branching explains why combined recurrent and superior laryngeal nerve injuries (eg, paralysis) are rare. The action of the cricothyroid musculature is also responsible for the motion of the vocal cords seen in paralysis of the vocal cords due to recurrent laryngeal nerve (RLN) involvement. When some motion of the vocal cord is observed on the paralyzed side, it must be interpreted with caution as a sign of recovery, but rather as motion secondary to the ipsilateral SLN-mediated impulses. When the SLN is out in addition to the RLN, the posterior glottis will not approximate, a wider posterior gap will be present, and the arytenoids will not touch on phonation. Observing and documenting these conditions during clinical PhFS are of paramount importance for treatment planning.

Because of the contra- and ipsilateral innervation of the corticobulbar tract, a unilateral corticobulbar tract lesion will not cause unilateral vocal cord paralysis.

Carlsoo B, Domeij S, Hellstrom S, Dedo HH, Izdebski K. An endoneural microglomus of the recurrent laryngeal nerve. *Acta Otolaryngol Suppl.* 1982;386:184.

Dedo HH, Townsend JJ, Izdebski K. Current evidence for the organic etiology of spastic dysphonia. *Otolaryngology.* 1978; 86:87. [PMID: 225708] (Histologic examination of segments of the recurrent laryngeal nerve removed from patients with adductor spasmodic dysphoria revealed myelin abnormalities in 30% of the nerves examined, while neurologic examination indicated brain stem or basal ganglia disturbances.)

Jurgens U. Neural pathways underlying vocal control. *Neurosci Biobehav Rev.* 2002;26(2):235.

VOCAL CORDS

With regard to phonation, the vocal cords are subdivided into muscular components (the so-called "body") and nonmuscular components (the so-called "cover"). The body of the vocal cords is formed by the two thyroarytenoid muscles, which contain fast (adductive) and slow (eg, phonatory) fibers that determine the length, contour, and glottic closure shape of the vocal cords and that regulate the tension of the cover that slides over the body of the vocal cords to create the mucosal vibratory wave. The mucosal vibratory wave cannot be

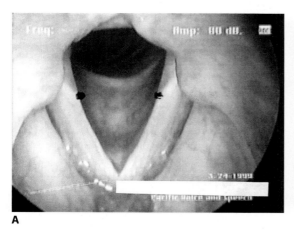
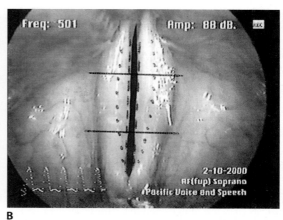

A   **B**

Figure 28–1. **(A)** The vocal cords at rest, forming a V-shaped space (the glottis), divided into the vibratory (membranous) and nonvibratory (cartilaginous) portions. **(B)** The vocal cords during phonatory approximation. The vocal cords are divided into anterior, mid, and posterior thirds. With regard to phonation, the vocal cords are divided into the upper vibratory lips (*dotted line*) and the lower vibratory lips (*dashed lines*).

observed with simple visualization, but under stroboscopic illumination or super-fast filming, where it is seen to undulate, proceeding from the inferior (ie, lower lip) to the superior surface (ie, upper lip) of the vocal cords (Figure 28–1).

The area between the upper and lower lips adjusts as pitch and loudness change; therefore, when a phonatory lesion is located within this space, its location and size determine the area of pitch and loudness dysfunction. Typically, more severe symptoms are caused by small but anteriorly located lesions than by larger lesions located toward the upper lip or on the superior phonatory surfaces. Typically, an anterior commissure lesion located ± 3 mm above the lower lip profoundly affects the voice, whereas even a large inferiorly located web (< 3 mm below the lower lip) does not affect the voice. This is crucial to both treatment and diagnosis. To secure this observation, PhFS are needed.

The cover is subdivided into the outer and the inner layers and the lamina propria; the latter consists of three layers: superficial (the Reinke space), intermediate, and deep. The vocal ligament is the free edge of the conus elasticus, belonging to the deep and intermediate layers of the lamina propria. Obliteration of the Reinke space retards or prevents the mucosal vibratory wave, resulting in dysphonia of varying severity. However, if one vocal cord is stiff but straight (nonvibratory) and the other vibrates and approximates well against the nonvibrating vocal cord, the voice may be remarkably good despite the insufficiency of one cord. Therefore, it is important at times not to "repair" the stiff vocal cord, but to leave it alone or even make it stiffer to improve the overall voice quality. Most benign phonatory mucosal lesions are typically found within the superficial

layer. If the lesion is located on the superior surface of the vocal cord away from the vibratory edge, the voice may not be affected at all, even if the lesion is large. These findings are crucial in determining the extent of surgical interventions. A common sense real estate rule of "location, location, location" should prevail. In other words, it is often the location and not the size of the lesion that determines its value to the voice quality.

From the clinical point of view, vocal cords are also subdivided into the vibratory (membranous) and nonvibratory (cartilaginous) portions. At rest, they outline a V-shaped space called the glottis (see Figure 28–1). The front of this V forms the anterior glottic commissure, and the back of the V forms the posterior glottic commissure. The posterior end of each vocal cord (the thyroarytenoid muscle) inserts into the muscular process of each of the arytenoid cartilages. The maximum width of the posterior commissure occurs during inspiration or cough and measures approximately 9–12 mm, or three times the most posterior width of the muscular portion of the vocal cord at rest.

After puberty, the length of the vibratory portions of the vocal cords at rest is approximately 13 mm for women and 16 mm for men. When the vocal cords approximate for phonation, the entire glottis is closed in a male, whereas a small posterior chink is often present in a female, giving the female voice quality a slightly softer and airy tone. The specific shapes of glottic phonatory closure allow variations in normal voice qualities.

Furthermore, the vocal cords are clinically subdivided into anterior, middle, and posterior thirds, with nodular lesions usually located at the anterior third juncture and opposite each other if bilateral. An asymmetric location of mucosal lesions is found in mixed-type organic dysphonias.

Dworkin JP, Meleca RJ. *Vocal Pathologies: Diagnosis, Treatment and Case Studies.* San Diego: Singular Publishing Group, 1997.

Hirano M. Structure and vibratory behavior of the vocal folds. In: Sawashima T, Cooper F, eds. *Dynamic Aspects of Speech Production.* Tokyo: Tokyo University Press, 1977:3.

Schonharl E. *Die Stroboskopie in der Praktischen Laryngologie.* Stuttgart: Thieme, 1960.

THE VIBRATORY PROCESS

The two thyroarytenoid muscles, together with the other intrinsic laryngeal muscles and the extrinsic laryngeal muscles, control the relative elasticity and stiffness of the vocal cords. They also determine the shape of the mucosal vibratory wave, which in turn determines the pitch, loudness, and tone of the voice. The amplitude of the mucosal vibratory wave is wider at the lower pitches, whereas reduced mucosal vibratory wave amplitude predominates at high pitches or at any pitch level when the cover is stiff.

The duration and shape of the mucosal vibratory wave cycle form specific opening and closing phases that determine specific vibratory modes or vocal qualities (eg, fry, normal, overpressured, breathy, or falsetto). The time interval between cycles is called the **fundamental period** (F_0), whereas in perceptual terms it is referred to as a pitch period.

THE AERODYNAMIC PROPERTIES OF PHONATION

The aerodynamic properties of phonation include the subglottic air pressure (P_s), the airflow, the supraglottic pressure (P_s), the intraoral pressure (P_{io}), and the glottal resistance, all of which are responsible for the Bernoulli effect, which separates the approximated vocal cords during phonation.

To generate sound, P_s must reach at least 5 cm H_2O, but P_s can exceed 50 cm H_2O in loud or overly pressured (ie, pathologic) phonation. Typically, a normal conversational voice is produced between 6–10 cm H_2O P_s at approximately 65–70 dB, whereas a loud voice can reach 85–95 dB.

The mean airflow in normal phonation ranges from 89 to 141 mL/s and increases as the fundamental period and the loudness are elevated. The glottal resistance cannot be measured directly, but is estimated to vary from 20 to 150 dyne/s/cm³ depending on the pitch and sound intensity.

Izdebski K. Overpressure and breathiness in spastic dysphonia. An acoustic (LTAS) and perceptual study. *Acta Otolaryngol Scand.* 1984;97:122. [PMID: 6720314] (Pre- and post-recur-rent laryngeal nerve section speech segments spoken by adductor spasmodic dysphoria patients were analyzed by long-time-average-spectrum (LTAS) analysis and perceptually for breathiness and overpressure. Breathy phonation corresponded to a steep fall in the LTAS, whereas overpressured phonation produced higher spectral levels and a less steep fall. Correlation with perceptual assessment of weak and strangled voice was shown to be valid.)

Shipp T, Izdebski K, Schutte H. Subglottic air pressure in adductor spasmodic dysphonia. *Folia Phoniatrica.* 1985;43:114. [PMID: 3220337] (Article explaining the physiologic reasons and the techniques of subglottic pressure measurements and their application in examining pathologic voices.)

RESONATION

When the voice (F_0) resonates within the entire vocal tract (ie, the larynx, trachea, pharynx, and oral and nasal cavities) and when the vocal tract articulates, speech, singing, or other forms of communication are formed. Because of specific vocal tract configuration, in the voices of opera singers, specific sound regions are amplified; these areas are referred to as formants (F1–F5), and their combination determines the characteristic of each vowel. Opera singers form unique vocal tract shapes to allow noninjurious and efficient singing, and they show a unique clustering of powerful spectral peaks (the so-called singing formants) at about 3 kHz. This clustering results in an acoustic boost that helps a singer to compete with the sound of an orchestra. The production of singers' formants is possible when the entire larynx is lowered in the neck, but not when the larynx goes up as pitch elevates. Other acoustic features are emphasized in different singing styles. Because inappropriate larynx tracking can be potentially injurious to the voice, an examination of the vertical larynx position (VLP) is advised when evaluating the vocal problems of individuals who use their voices professionally. Ornamentation in voice can result from specific vocal tract configurations and specific time-locked acoustic events, with rate approximating 5–6 Hz for vibrato or vocal tremor. It is interesting to note that tremor-like vocal oscillations having similar rate may be present in deception.

Shipp, T, Izdebski K. Letter: Vocal frequency and vertical larynx positioning by singers and nonsingers. *J Acoust Soc Am.* 1975;58(5):1104. [PMID 11945621] (This article explains the reasons singers and nonsingers adjust their vocal tracts to produce acoustically advantageous effects.)

Shipp T, Izdebski K. Current evidence for the existence of laryngeal macrotremor and microtremor. *J Forensic Sci.* 1981;26:501. [PMID: 7252466] (The existence of laryngeal microtremors was tested using vocal vibrato in normal singers and in vocal tremor.)

Stone RE Jr, Cleveland T, Sundberg J. Formant frequencies in country singers' speech and singing. *J Voice.* 1999;13:161. [PMID: 10442747] (The study describes acoustic differences in voice quality in the same singer when the singer speaks and sings.)

LARYNGOLOGIC CONDITIONS

A multitude of laryngologic conditions can cause voice problems. Some of these conditions demonstrate a visible organic pathology on an initial routine ear, nose, and throat (ENT) exam, either with a mirror or fiberoptics. Other conditions do not. Therefore, it is extremely important not to dismiss a patient's claim of "hoarseness," specifically in the absence of a visible pathology. Any voice condition, but specifically when hoarseness is present and the larynx looks normal, calls for PhFS to be performed as soon as possible. Delays in arriving at a diagnosis can result in medical complications (including potential legal consequences), as well as delays in treatment and a potential loss of income to the patient. Unfortunately, the concerns of many patients with dysphonia, especially patients who use their voices professionally, are often dismissed. These patients may be accused of "wrong" singing or poor training because no visible pathology was noted at the initial routine medical or ENT exam and because referrals for in-depth voice evaluations are not always initiated.

The specific conditions that can affect voice production are numerous and include the following: (1) congenital anomalies that can cause dysphonia by changing the shape and form of the mucosal vibratory wave; (2) benign vocal cord lesions that affect the mucosal vibratory wave, resulting in air loss, noise, vocal cord stiffness, and pitch restrictions; (3) premalignant and malignant lesions that restrict or obliterate the mucosal vibratory wave; (4) infectious and inflammatory disorders of the larynx, which can cause a variety of vibratory and approximation changes, depending on the severity and extent of the disease; (5) acquired voice disorders; (6) neurologic disorders that can affect all aspects of phonatory processes; (7) blunt or penetrating trauma to the larynx that causes injury (eg, fractures, dislocations, or crushes) to the laryngeal housing and the neural or vascular supplies; (8) pharmacologic agents that have either adverse effects (eg, antihistamines, virilizing drugs) or positive effects (eg, hydrating agents, asthma inhalers, corticosteroids, and bronchodilators); (9) iatrogenic dysphonia caused by (a) a clinical intervention in a nondysphonic patient (eg, vocal cord paralysis that results from an unintentional injury to the recurrent laryngeal nerve), (b) the planned treatment (eg, an overinjection of polytef [ie, Teflon] during attempts to correct breathy paralytic dysphonia or irradiation), or (c) a change to the underlying nature of the primary dysphonia as a function of treatment (eg, denervation of the vocal cord to combat vocal spasticity, Botox, and vagal stimulation); (10) functional dysphonia (eg, persistent prepubertal voice in a postpubertal male, elective aphonia, ventricular dysphonia, and inhalational dysphonia); (11) gender euphoria; (12) emotional causes; and (13) environmental-occupational causes.

Gastroesophageal reflux disease (GERD) has been recently linked to a multitude of voice disorders. However, this association is controversial, and cause-effect correlation is far from being established unequivocally. Some clinicians, however, believe that GERD is the primary cause of many voice problems, whereas others minimize its role in the formation of dysphonia. When GERD is perceived as the cause of voice disorders, it is cited as causing changes that range from alterations of vocal cord mucosa to more general supraglottic tissue changes. GERD may cause a chronic or intermittent dysphonia that is characterized by vocal fatigue, voice breaks, cough, globus syndrome, and, occasionally, dysphagia.

Flower RM, Izdebski K. *Common Speech Disorders in Otolaryngologic Practice*. Rochester, Minnesota: American Academy of Otolaryngology Press, 1979.

Izdebski K, ed. *Emotions in the Human Voice*. Volumes 1–3. San Diego: Plural Publishing, 2007.

Izdebski K, Dedo HH, Wenokur R, Johnson J. Voice and vocal cord findings in asthma inhaler (Advair) users. Western Section: Triological Society. San Diego, California. February 3, 2006. In press (2007).

Koufman JA. Gastroesophageal reflux and voice disorders. In: Rubin JS, Sataloff RT, Korovin GS, Gould WJ, eds. *Diagnosis and Treatment of Voice Disorders*. New York: Ikagu-Shoin, 1995:161.

Rubin JS, Sataloff RT, Korovin GS, Gould WJ. *Diagnosis and Treatment of Voice Disorders*. New York: Ikagu-Shoin, 1995.

Ylitalo R, Lindestad PA, Ramel S. Symptoms, laryngeal findings, and 24-hour pH monitoring in patients with suspected gastroesophageal-pharyngeal reflux. *Laryngoscope*. 2001;111(10):1735. [PMID: 11801936] (Discussion of controversies of GERD on voice and its role in formation of various dysphonias.)

ACOUSTICS

An acoustic voice assessment provides information on the nature of the generated sound and should include physical voice recordings (analog, digital, or video) and an objective acoustic analysis; it should also include a subjective psychoacoustic analysis, a psychometric analysis, a phonometric analysis, or all of the above. The psychoacoustic and psychometric analyses require a trained ear and longstanding expertise, not unlike what is needed to assess auscultatory noises. However, the problems with these analyses result from the potential for loose terminology and a non-uniform interpretation. A subjective description of one type of dysphonia used over 350 different clinical terms. Therefore, using numerical perceptual rating scales is preferred when subjectively assessing voice problems. Attempts to use acoustic objective analysis to detect voice quality correlations with underlying pathology continue, but solutions are far from being reached.

Godino-Llorente JI, Gomez-Vilda P, Blanco-Velasco M. Dimensionality reduction of a pathological voice quality assessment system based on Gaussian mixture models and short-term cepstral parameters. *IEEE Trans Biomed Eng.* 2006;53(10):1943. [PMID: 17019858] (Paper demonstrates promising acoustic technique in detecting voice pathologies.)

Izdebski K. Spastic dysphonia. In: Darby J, ed. *Speech Evaluation in Medicine and Psychiatry,* Vol. II: *Medicine.* New York: Grune & Stratton, 1981.

Izdebski K, Shipp T, Dedo HH. Predicting postoperative voice characteristics of spastic dysphonia patients. *Otolaryngol Head Neck Surg.* 1979;87:428. [PMID 503503] (Describes techniques of predicting surgical voice outcomes of selected dysphonic patients based on presurgical phonatory function studies.)

SUBJECTIVE ASSESSMENT

The subjective assessment often uses a mixture of perceptual and musical terms to describe the patient's voice quality, pitch, loudness, the duration and rate of phonation, prosody, registration, tessitura, and respiratory characteristics.

Common Assessment Findings

Below is a review of terms used to clinically describe the various dysphonic qualities. These semantic descriptors can be quite accurate, but when the voice is abnormal the term *hoarseness* is a generic word used by most clinicians (and lay people) when referring to or describing many kinds of dysphonia. Hoarseness is frequently used as a wastebasket term and leads to a wrong impression or diagnosis. It is especially used in error when one is attempting to define a rough or harsh voice quality, since this is typically associated with vocal cord stiffness and possibly cancer.

Breathy or **soft** voice is used to describe a voice that is generated by incomplete glottic closure (eg, in unilateral vocal cord paralysis, vocal cord bowing, neurologic disorders, benign mucosal lesions, and psychogenic voice disorders).

A **tight, strangled,** or **strained voice** represents an overclosed glottis and is found in dystonias and pseudobulbar palsies, including psychogenic disorders.

A **diplophonic** or **multiphonic voice** is present when the vibratory pattern between the vocal cords or within a single vocal cord is unequal. This condition can be caused by a myriad of benign and malignant mucosal lesions, neurologic complications, laryngeal fractures, or psychosomatic problems.

A **wet, gargling voice,** also referred to as **hydrophonia,** describes phonation that is produced by excessive mucus within the glottic space.

A **rough voice** may describe a true vocal cord vibration that is mixed with a ventricular vibration. This may be present when mucosal lesions are found between the lower and upper phonatory lips and when mucosal wave is partially obliterated.

A **harsh, rough, and stiff voice quality** with a short maximum phonation time should be used to refer to voices that are produced with adynamic "cover." This can be found in invasive carcinoma or in Teflon overinjection, or when mucosa is prevented from vibration by lesions pressing on the vocal cord from above.

A **shrill, metallic voice** with abrupt onset can be associated with muscular tension dysphonia, a benign phonatory lesion, and hyperfunctional dysphonia.

Sudden pitch or **loudness breaks** in the absence of clearly visible phonatory mucosal lesions may be an indicator of functional problems, postpubertal dysphonia, or virilization of the female voice.

A **limited upper pitch range** with soft breathy phonation, no mucosal lesions, and rotation of the posterior larynx can indicate **superior** laryngeal nerve involvement.

Rapid pitch (at about 5–6 Hz) and intensity oscillations reflect vocal tremor, whereas pitch-dependent oscillations or vocal arrests reflect specific movement disorders, while in muscular tension dysphonia, or functional (psychosomatic) dysphonia oscillations my be random.

Odynophonia describes a sensation rather than voice quality and is associated with pain or discomfort when speaking or vocalizing.

Total aphonia, or lack of voice in the absence of a phonatory cough, can indicate severe separation of the glottis either caused by organic and functional origins or following total laryngectomy. Ankylosis of the arytenoid cartilages can be suspected, but when a phonatory cough is present, total aphonia should arouse suspicion of a psychosomatic conversion dysphonia.

Stridor should be reserved to describe uncontrollable vocal production ("voicing") during inhalation, when the glottis is not abducting. Asthmalike wheezing happens only on exhalation when the vocal cords are open. When female patients inhale asthma medications, vocal cord mucosa can be affected and severe dysphonia can occur. Typically, stopping medication is enough to reverse the condition.

No matter how the voice sounds, the sound of the pathologic voice may evoke negative emotions that are noncongruent with the emotions intended by the patient. This incongruence can be very frustrating and may cause a patient to react as if the condition has a functional cause, when it clearly does not. An understanding of these factors by the examining clinician goes a long way toward enhancing bedside manners.

ACOUSTIC ANALYSIS

Acoustic analysis provides an objective and quantitative description of the generated sound in a reliable and noninvasive way. The purpose is to map out phonatory characteristics, demonstrate phonatory deficits, and correlate findings with visual (ie, physiologic) data. Barring minor technical problems, either dedicated instrumentation or a computerized approach can be used for a fast, reliable, and reproducible acoustic analysis. Acoustic analysis provides information on sound duration, loudness, pitch, and spectral context, including static and dynamic pitch changes of the voice during speech.

Izdebski K. Pathologic voice evokes wrong emotions. In: Izdebski K, ed. *Emotions in the Human Voice*. San Diego: Plural Publishing, to be published in 2007.

Shipp T, Izdebski K. Current evidence for the existence of laryngeal macrotremor and microtremor. *J Forensic Sci*. 1981;26:501. [PMID 7252466] (Analyzes the existence of laryngeal microtremors detected during deception versus the macrotremors found in the voice of singers and also found in vibrato and subjects with pathologic vocal tremor, using electromyographic and acoustic signals from laryngeal muscles.)

Wheeler KM, Collins SP, Sapienza CM. The relationship between VHI scores and specific acoustic measures of mildly disordered voice production. *J Voice*. 2006;20(2):308. [PMID: 16126368] (Elucidates the relation between the Voice Handicap Index and laboratory measurements and shows that these two methods give independent information and essentially correlate poorly.)

PITCH ASSESSMENT

Pitch expressed in musical intervals is a perceptual and therefore subjective measure. However, in objective acoustic terms, pitch refers to the fundamental frequency of the voice or the speaking fundamental frequency, both of which are recorded in vocal cycles per second or hertz (Hz). Deviations in the fundamental frequency are expressed by jitter measures, or a pitch perturbation factor. Jitter is defined as a fundamental frequency value that is obtained by subtracting the duration of the pitch period from the duration of the period immediately preceding it. Because pitch changes over time, serial correlation coefficients may be used to more accurately represent these changes. The pitch pattern is related to the intensity profile as shown in Figure 28–2.

Fundamental frequency is age and gender dependent. The average level of fundamental frequency for a child is approximately 250 Hz; it is 200 Hz for an adult female, and for an adult male, it is approximately 120 Hz. The maximum fundamental frequency range for

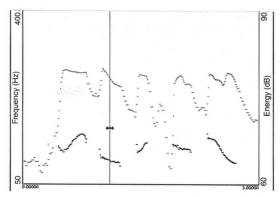

Figure 28–2. Intonation pattern of a sentence spoken by a male speaker showing pitch (lower tracing) and intensity (upper tracing) contours. (Reproduced with permission of KayPENTAX, Lincoln Park, NJ.)

both genders is from 36 Hz to 1760 Hz, or roughly the distance from D1 to A6 on a piano. Vocal training can develop an individual's voice to be an exquisite instrument; an extreme vocal span can range over four octaves (eg, from E3, which is approximately 164 Hz, up to F6, which is approximately 1760 Hz).

The speaking fundamental frequency of males typically drops with the termination of a spoken sentence without constituting a pathologic condition. In contrast, the fundamental frequency of females is often elevated at the end of a spoken sentence. This distinction is of import when examining patients with gender reassignment, patients on psychotropic medications, or those with a history of using virilizing drugs. The speaking fundamental frequency of females drops over the life span, whereas this frequency becomes elevated in male geriatric populations.

When assessing patients who sing professionally, their vocal registration should be included in the evaluation. Using a musical scale notation is a preferred method of communicating clinical findings to these patients.

Baken RJ. *Clinical Measurements of Speech and Voice*. San Diego: College Hill Press, 1997.

Izdebski K, Ross JC, Klein JC. Rigid transoral laryngovideostroboscopy (phonoscopy). *Semin Speech Lang*. 1990;1:16.

LOUDNESS ASSESSMENT

Loudness represents acoustic intensity that is measured in decibels and is dependent on both the subglottic air pressure and the airflow exiting the glottis. Obtaining the absolute phonatory intensity is difficult; therefore, it is typically reported in relative rather than in absolute decibels. Moreover, because the acoustic intensity is affected by the fundamental frequency, normal loudness is actually greatest at mid-frequency ranges and lowest at both the low and high levels of fundamental frequency. As with fundamental frequency, means, medians, standard deviations, coefficients of variation, and loudness perturbation factors (known as "shimmer") are used to describe acoustic intensity variation and dispersion. The typical loudness level of speaking is approximately 65–75 dB. Values below or above this measure are considered pathologic.

PHONETOGRAM

To make a more orderly representation of pitch and loudness, a profile of the fundamental frequency, measured in decibels and referred to as a phonetogram, has been developed. The phonetogram, which is a voice range profile, represents the minimums and the maximums of vocal loudness at selected levels of fundamental frequency within the total frequency range of a speaker (Figure 28–3). Clinically, a phonetogram is a reflection of the vocal capacities rather than the measurement of the glottic function. Vocal intensity profiles are used to assess vocal cord paralysis, vocal cord bowing, presbyphonia, odynophonia, functional disorders, and patients who use their voices professionally.

SPECTRAL ANALYSIS

Spectrography

Spectrography (Figure 28–4) provides a three-dimensional representation of sound: time, intensity, and frequency. Narrow-filter spectrography shows the har-

monic structure (partials) of the sound, from which values of fundamental frequency can be derived. Wide-filter spectrography shows vocal tract resonation, represented by the formants (ie, F1–F5).

Spectrography provides information on (1) noise; (2) phonatory breaks; (3) vocal discontinuity; (4) diplophonia; (5) the size and speed of fluctuations in the fundamental frequency; (6) the size and speed of amplitude fluctuations; (7) the richness of harmonics; (8) the relative noise level; (9) an analysis of rising and falling tones, as well as voice efficiency over time; and (10) glottic air transfer. These features are critical when analyzing vocal cord stiffness, vibratory irregularity due to lesions that are benign, mucosal, iatrogenic (eg, with the use of Teflon or thyroplasty), or that cause adynamic vibration. These features are also significant when evaluating patients who use their voices professionally, have neurologic or functional dysphonias, have carcinoma, or experience stridor, noise, wheezing, or obstructive airway problems (eg, snoring).

Long-Time Average Spectrum

The long-time average spectrum technique is used to plot compressed speech spectrum levels over time. This technique relates the acoustic parameters to perceptual observations and has been used successfully to describe various dysphonias.

Izdebski K. Overpressure and breathiness in spastic dysphonia: an acoustic and perceptual study. *Acta Otolaryngol.* 1984;97:373. [PMID: 6720314] (Pre- and post-recurrent laryngeal nerve section speech segments spoken by adductor spasmodic dysphoria patients were analyzed by long-time-average-spectrum (LTAS) analysis and perceptually for breathiness and overpressure. Breathy phonation corresponded to a steep fall in the LTAS, whereas overpressured phonation produced higher spectral levels and a less steep fall. Correlation with perceptual assessment of weak and strangled voice was shown to be valid.)

Multidimensional Voice Profile

The multidimensional voice profile displays, in a graphic form, multiple vocal parameters all at one time (Figure 28–5). The use of the multidimensional voice profile is advantageous in comparing pretreatment and post-treatment results. It also provides an overall description of dysphonia, because single acoustic parameters alone are insufficient in delineating the complexity of phonatory pathologies. The multidimensional voice profile can compare individual clinical data with a built-in database adjusted to age and gender. Therefore, this profile is very useful in analyzing changes over time.

Rate Analysis

Instrumentally based rate analyses are used to define the rate and extent of specific acoustic variations (ie, vocal

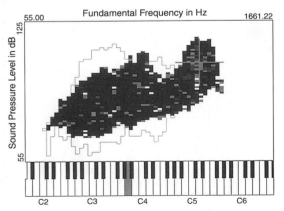

Figure 28–3. A phonetogram (a voice range profile). A thin line outside the "map" corresponds to previous measurements. (Reproduced with permission of KayPENTAX, Lincoln Park, NJ.)

Figure 28–4. A sound spectrograph. **(A)** Representation of vocal tract resonation, referred to as formants (F1–F5); the transitions are shown here as heavy, dark semihorizontal bars. **(B)** A narrow-filter spectrograph displaying the harmonic structure (partials) of the sound, shown here as narrow horizontal lines. Fundamental frequency values can be derived from the position of the tenth harmonic. The fuzzy dark portions of the spectrograph represent the noise present in voiceless consonants. (Reproduced with permission of KayPENTAX., Lincoln Park, NJ.)

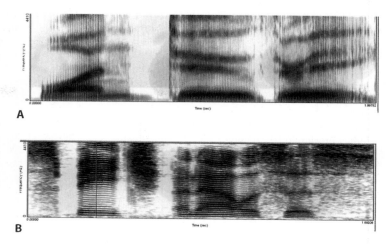

tremor, vocal arrests, or vibrato). Rate analysis is used in the differential diagnosis of vocal movement disorders and in assessing the vocal problems of singers. Pathologic vocal rates are between 5 Hz and 6 Hz, a rate similar to the vibrato rate.

Dejonckere PH, Hirano M, Sundberg J. *Vibrato.* San Diego: Singular Publishing Group, 1995.

Shipp T, Izdebski K. Current evidence for the existence of laryngeal macrotremor and microtremor. *J Forensic Sci.* 1981;26: 501. [PMID: 7252466] (The existence of laryngeal microtremors was tested using vocal vibrato in normal singers and in vocal tremor.)

Vocal Cord Contact Area

A normal voice is produced when the glottic approximation is normal during sustained phonation. The percentage of vocal cord contact area loss can be derived from acoustic measures. When a voice is hoarse, the

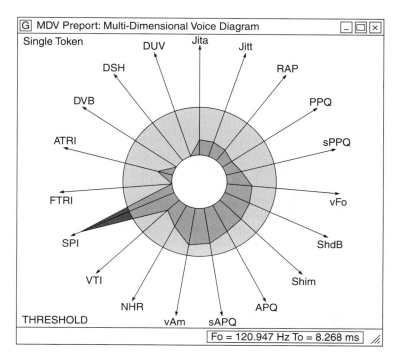

Figure 28–5. A multidimensional voice profile. A soft, breathy voice is shown by severe SPI (soft phonatory index). (Reproduced with permission of KayPENTAX, Lincoln Park, NJ.)

percentage of phonatory contact (ie, perturbations) goes down. Values below 90% are considered abnormal.

Vowel Space

Vowel quality is affected by the fundamental frequency and loudness. Therefore, substantial difficulties in maintaining vowels on target are encountered when singers must sing loudly. These elevated levels make for the poor intelligibility of sung text. Therefore, vowel production should be examined when studying patients who sing professionally.

Maximum Phonation Time

The maximum phonation time corresponds to the time an individual can phonate per each inhalation. Normal maximum phonation time values are between 17 and 35 seconds for adult males and between 12 and 26 seconds for adult females. A reduction of the maximum phonation time is expected in a hypofunctional glottis, whereas prolonging this time is characteristic for an overapproximated glottis. Although the maximum phonation time lacks diagnostic capabilities, it is useful in the preoperative and postoperative assessments of unilateral vocal cord paralysis and bowing, in monitoring medialization (eg, thyroplasty or various intracordal injections), and in lateralization procedures (eg, Botox injections, as well as nerve resections, blocks, or stimulation).

Baken RJ. *Clinical Measurements of Speech and Voice.* San Diego: College Hill Press, 1997.

Hirano M. *Clinical Examination of Voice.* New York: Springer-Verlag, 1981.

■ PHYSIOLOGIC VOICE EVALUATION

Physiologic voice evaluation comprises rigid or flexible stroboscopic visualization, aerodynamics, glottography, electromyography, and special studies.

PHONOSCOPY

Phonoscopy refers to stroboscopic (or laryngovideostroboscopic) visualization of the vocal cords during vibration (Figure 28–6). It is considered to be a principal procedure among PhFS studies. The technique is based on the principle of illuminating a vibrating object with light flashes just below or above the frequency at which it vibrates, therefore making the vibrating object appear at a standstill or as if it is vibrating in slow motion. Laryngovideostroboscopy or digital stroboscopy provides an image of the vocal cord vibrations averaged

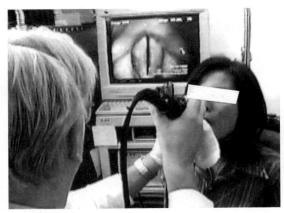

Figure 28–6. Phonoscopic transoral rigid procedure showing the on-line visualization of the vibratory process of the vocal cords. The image obtained is displayed immediately on a VCR monitor. The glottographic signal and pitch and intensity values are displayed for analysis.

over many vibratory cycles while newly introduced high speed stroboscopy shows consective cycles and not averages it can only show short sign duration. The most detailed images are obtained either via a 90° or a 70° rigid transoral scope. The images are captured on videotape or in digital form and are displayed on a monitor for either immediate or subsequent viewing and analysis.

Phonoscopy provides the clinician with a wealth of information. Among the large amount of information it provides, phonoscopy (1) maps the location of the phonatory lesion in relationship to the acoustic findings, (2) gives fundamental frequency values, (3) shows the symmetry of vocal cord vibrations, (4) reveals the configuration of the glottic closure, (5) shows the horizontal excursion of the vocal cords (ie, their amplitude), (6) reveals the appearance and the workings of the upper and lower phonatory lips, (7) shows the type and the nature of the glottic closure, and (8) demonstrates the nature of the mucosal vibratory wave (including the presence or absence of adynamic segments). Compared with traditional exams, a phonoscopic exam significantly increases the diagnostic accuracy and therefore provides for more effective treatment options.

Colton R, Casper JK. *Understanding Voice Problems: A Physiological Perspective for Diagnosis and Treatment.* Baltimore: Williams & Wilkins, 1996.

Dworkin JP, Meleca RJ. *Vocal Pathologies: Diagnosis, Treatment and Case Studies.* San Diego: Singular Publishing Group, 1997.

Hertegard S, Larsson H, Wittenberg T. High-speed imaging: applications and development. Logopedics Phoniactrics Vocology 2003;28:3,133–139.

Hirano M. *Clinical Examination of Voice.* New York: Springer-Verlag, 1981.

Izdebski K, Ross JC, Klein JC. Rigid transoral laryngovideostroboscopy (phonoscopy). *Semin Speech Lang.* 1990;1:16.

Remacle M. The contribution of videostroboscopy in daily ENT practice. *Acta Oto Rhino Laryngologica Belg.* 1996;50:265. [PMID: 9001636]

ELECTROGLOTTOGRAPHY

Electroglottography is another method of evaluating vocal cord vibration. This technology uses the principle of electrical impedance across tissue and open space. Electrodes are placed on the neck over the lamina of the thyroid cartilages; a weak current is passed between the electrodes, which generate an impedance curve that corresponds to the shape and nature of the vibratory cycle.

Other forms of glottographic technology include photoelectric and ultrasound glottography. A new technique of assessing vocal cord cycles based on the kymography principle has been recently introduced; however, its clinical value remains questionable at this time.

Guimaraes I, Abberton E. Fundamental frequency in speakers of Portuguese for different voice samples. *J Voice.* 2005; 19(4):592. [PMID: 16301105] (This article shows usage of electroglottography to assess voice qualities across gender and age.)

Larsson H, Hertegard S, Lindestad PA, Hammarberg B. Vocal fold vibrations: high-speed imaging, kymography, and acoustic analysis: a preliminary report. *Laryngoscope.* 2000;110 (12): 2117. [PMID: 11129033] (This article suggests that combined high-speed acoustic-kymographic analysis package can be helpful for specification of the terminology of voice qualities.)

Yan Y, Ahmad K, Kunduk M, Bless D. Analysis of vocal-fold vibrations from high-speed laryngeal images using a Hilbert transform-based methodology. *J Voice.* 2005;19(2):161. [PMID: 15907431] (This article assesses potential use of this tool for voice pathology analysis.)

Zagolski O, Carlson E. Electroglottographic measurements of glottal function in vocal fold paralysis in women. *Clin Otolaryngol Allied Sci.* 2002;27(4):246. [PMID: 12169125] (This article suggests that electroglottography is a suitable noninvasive tool for tracking the patients' long-term progress.)

AERODYNAMIC TESTS

The purpose of aerodynamic tests is to evaluate how air—"the voice fuel"—behaves during phonation. Aerodynamics measure subglottic and supraglottic (ie, intraoral) air pressures as well as the glottic air impedance and the type of airflow at the glottis, including the volume velocity.

Aerodynamics is important when assessing vocal cord paralysis, stenosis, webs, or patients who use their voices professionally (ie, singers). Aerodynamic tests are important when examining a voice that may have been affected by the inhalation of noxious gases or stage smoke. They are also useful when the volume of gas

expired during the first second (the forced expiratory volume in the first second, or FEV_1) from the beginning of the forced vital capacity (FVC) shows deficits (eg, methacholine challenge).

Measurements of phonatory airflow are performed via pneumotachography on vocalic segments; they differ from pulmonary function studies in that airflow is measured as a function of phonation. The individual values can be fitted against expected age and gender values, with critical values for a normal population ranging from 40 to 200 mL/s. The interpretation of aerodynamic tests should be conducted with caution because these tests are subject to voluntary motor responses and are affected by variations in vocal intensity and vocal register.

Granqvist S, Hertegard S, Larsson H, Sundberg J. Simultaneous analysis of vocal fold vibration and transglottal airflow: exploring a new experimental setup. *J Voice.* 2003;17(3):319. [PMID: 14513955] (This article critically reviews airflow across the glottis. The article points that relationships between these two entities is complex specifically with respect to phonation modes.)

ELECTROMYOGRAPHY

An electromyogram (EMG) examines the neuromuscular integrity of a striated muscle by recording in a visual form, an auditory form, or both, the electrophysiologic properties (ie, discharges) of the muscle. These discharges provide information on the characteristics of single motor unit potential as well as on the interference pattern representing serial muscle discharges over time (Figure 28–7).

Specialized equipment is needed to conduct an EMG. Typically, either needle or hooked-wire electrodes are used. Surface electrodes can only be used to sample muscles that are close to the skin's surface (ie, the cricothyroid muscle or the extrinsic laryngeal muscles). When examining the motor unit potential, needle electrodes, preferably bipolar, should be used.

The usefulness of laryngeal EMG in diagnosing dysphonia has not been well established, including assessing unilateral or bilateral vocal cord paralysis. It is difficult at times to conclude whether the muscle is undergoing denervation or reinnervation; in this circumstance, the clinical experience of the examiner plays an important role.

Blitzer A. Laryngeal electromyography. In: Rubin JS, Sataloff RT, Korovin GS, Gould WJ, eds. *Diagnosis and Treatment of Voice Disorders.* New York, Tokyo: Ikagu-Shoin, 1995.

Dedo HH, Hall WN. Electrodes in laryngeal electromyography: reliability comparison. *Ann Otol Rhinol Laryngol.* 1969;78: 172. [PMID: 5763185] (Article discusses that using unipolar electrodes will provide word information.)

Jacobs IN, Finkel RS. Laryngeal electromyography in the management of vocal cord mobility problems in children. *Laryngo-*

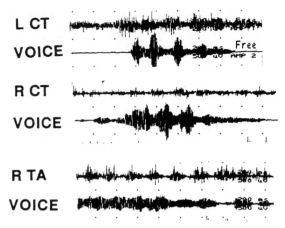

L CT

VOICE

R CT

VOICE

R TA

VOICE

Figure 28–7. Electromyograph (EMG) tracing. This figure shows the interference pattern representing the left cricothyroid muscle, the right cricothyroid muscle, and the right thyroarytenoid muscle. These muscles discharge over time during phonation. The EMG signals are displayed simultaneously with the acoustic signal (voice) showing a 5.5-Hz vocal tremor.

scope. 2002;112:1243. [PMID: 12169907] (Evaluates the efficacy and usefulness of electromyography, with a specific focus on the pediatric patient as well as in determining the differential diagnosis of vocal cord paralysis versus vocal cord fixation.)

Shipp T, Izdebski K, Reed C, Morrisey P. Intrinsic laryngeal muscle activity in a spastic dysphonia patient. *J Speech Hearing Dis.* 1985;50:54. [PMID: 3974213] (Description of electromyography activity from intrinsic laryngeal muscles in adductor spasmodic dysphoria demonstrated normal morphology of recurrent laryngeal nerves and intrinsic laryngeal muscles and suggested a neurologic cause for this disorder.)

Sittel C, Stennert E, Thrumfart WF, Dapunt U, Eckel HE. Prognostic value of laryngeal electromyography in vocal fold paralysis. *Arch Otolaryngol Head Neck Surg.* 2001; 127:155. [PMID: 11177032] (This article analyzes the value of electromyography in predicting vocal function recovery from acute neurogenic injuries [ie, paralysis] of the vocal cords.)

Woo P. Laryngeal electromyography is a cost-effective clinically useful tool in the evaluation of vocal fold function. *Arch Otolaryngol Head Neck Surg.* 1998;124:471. [PMID: 9559701] (Outlines the clinical usefulness of electromyography in evaluating various vocal cord dysfunctions in the absence of visible organic mucosal lesions.)

Yin SS, Quu WW, Stucker FJ. Major patterns of laryngeal electromyography and their clinical applications. *Laryngoscope.* 1997;107:126. [PMID: 9001277] (Presents detailed electromyographic [EMG] techniques and describes physiologic tasks needed to study the actions of the intrinsic laryngeal muscles by EMG in various groups of dysphonic patterns.)

■ SPECIAL STUDIES

When studying complex voice problems, specially tailored voice tests often need to be designed or conducted. These special tests include acoustic, physiologic, and radiographic studies.

ACOUSTIC TESTS

Special acoustic tests include the voice load test, auditory masking, voice performance tests, phonetically balanced tests, delayed auditory feedback, and the use of an electrolarynx. These tests are useful when determining the differential diagnoses of psychogenic dysphonias.

Izdebski K. The voice load test: an objective acoustic test to assess voice quality as a factor of voice usage over time. In Proceedings of the 2nd World Voice Congress and 5th International Symposium on Phonosurgery. Sao Paulo, Brazil. 1999.

PHYSIOLOGIC TESTS

Special physiologic tests include aerodynamic tests, manual pressure tests, and temporary denervation procedures. An upper esophageal insufflation test is used to test failures in acquiring voice after tracheal puncture procedures. Because sudden change in aerodynamics affects the glottic biomechanics, as does inhaling gases of other density than air (eg, helium), such tests are useful when examining a suspected psychogenic voice disorder.

The manual pressure test, also known as the laryngeal circumference pressure test, is useful in testing for muscular tension dysphonia as well as psychogenic dysphonia. It is also useful in assessing the viability of medialization procedures. Similarly, the head-positioning test, which can cause changes in vocal cord approximation, can be used as a predictor of the correction potential (therapeutic, surgical, or both) of breathy dysphonia. A neck pressure test can also be used to test failures in acquiring voice after esophageal injection (eg, following total laryngectomy).

An array of nerve blocks, as well as the so-called oral lidocaine bath, can be very useful in the differential diagnosis of psychogenic dysphonia. In addition, a recurrent laryngeal nerve block is often crucial in testing for adductor spasmodic dysphonia and vocal tremor. A temporary block of the superior laryngeal nerves can be used in testing for abductor spasmodic dysphonia and in persistent postpubertal infantile dysphonia. The neural block test can also be used to test problems with air insufflation in patients after a total laryngectomy.

Radiologic PhFS include a videofluoroscopic exam of a nonfunctional phonatory segment after total laryngectomy. It also appears that neuroradiographic studies that use enhanced viewing to reveal fat deposits in vocal cords may be useful in studying nonmobile vocal cords. With additional testing, this technique may prove to be excellent in the differential diagnosis of voice disorders due to vocal cord paralysis or due to mechanical problems (eg, arytenoid joint dislocation or vocal cord fixation, or ankylosis).

Izdebski K, Dedo HH. Selecting the side of the RLN section for spastic dysphonia. *Otolaryngol Head Neck Surg.* 1981;89:423.

Izdebski K, Manace ED, Skiljo-Haris J. The challenge of determining work-related voice and speech disabilities in California. In: Dejonkere PH, ed. *Occupational Voice: Care and Cure.* Hague, Netherlands: Kugler Publishers, 2001.

Izdebski K, Ward R. Differential diagnosis of ADD-ABDuctor spasmodic dysphonia, vocal tremor and ventricular dysphonia by auditory and phonoscopic observations. In: Clemente M, ed. *Voice Update, International Congress Series.* The Hague, Netherlands: Elsevier, 1997.

Shipp T, Izdebski K, Morrisey P. Physiologic stages of vocal reaction times. *J Speech Hear Res.* 1984;27:14. [PMID: 6330455] (Describes the cortical and mechanical muscular speeds with which humans process and execute sensory motor processes to initiate phonation.)

Benign Laryngeal Lesions

Michael Wareing, FRCS (ORL-HNS), & Rupert Obholzer, MRCS

The human larynx plays a pivotal role in airway protection, respiration, and phonation. Most patients with benign laryngeal disorders present with dysphonia. These disorders are particularly prevalent in individuals who use their voices professionally. Malignant neoplastic disease should be excluded as an underlying cause of voice problems: Every patient who presents with dysphonia should undergo a thorough head and neck examination. Once it is established that there is no evidence of malignancy, patients can be treated appropriately, ideally within a voice clinic. A properly equipped voice clinic must have access to video-laryngeo-stroboscopy and be conducted with a suitably qualified speech therapist.

The diagnosis should include a thorough appreciation of the patient's lifestyle and occupational habits as well as a detailed examination of the vocal folds including stroboscopy. Most benign laryngeal lesions are treatable with a combination of surgery and speech therapy, but measures to prevent the recurrence of disease by instigating and maintaining lifestyle changes are also necessary.

ANATOMY & PHYSIOLOGY

The larynx consists of a cartilaginous framework comprising the single thyroid, cricoid, and epiglottic cartilages and the paired arytenoid, corniculate, and cuneiform cartilages. The larynx is suspended from the hyoid bone by the thyrohyoid membrane. The vocal folds run from the angle formed by the thyroid lamina anteriorly to the vocal process of the arytenoid cartilages posteriorly. Alteration in the position and length of the vocal folds is primarily the result of movement of the synovial cricoarytenoid joints, with a contribution from movement of the cricothyroid joints. Above the vocal folds run the false cords, formed by the medial border of the aryepiglottic folds. These are separated from the vocal folds by horizontal sinus known as the laryngeal ventricle, which contains numerous mucin-secreting glands.

The vocal folds are covered with a stratified squamous epithelium that has up to 20 layers; this epithelium covers the lamina propria, which has three layers, beneath which

lies the vocal ligament and vocalis muscle. Loose collagen cross-linkages between the epithelium and the superior layer of the lamina propria (ie, Reinke space) allow oscillation of the mucosal wave during phonation, as the epithelium is able to glide over Reinke space.

Sound is produced following creation of subglottic pressure as expiration occurs against a closed glottis. As air passes between the adducted vocal folds, the Bernoulli effect causes vibration of the mucosa of the vocal folds, producing sound. Abnormalities preventing full adduction of the vocal folds or directly interfering in vibration of the mucosa produce dysphonia.

Rosen AC, Murray T. Nomenclature of voice disorders and vocal pathology. *Otolaryngol Clin North Am.* 2000;33:1035. [PMID: 10986070] (Classification of the pathology of vocal cord lesions and voice disorders.)

CLINICAL ASSESSMENT

PATIENT HISTORY

The onset, duration, and progression of any voice change should be ascertained. Any preceding upper respiratory tract infections, direct or vocal trauma, or endotracheal intubation should be noted. Persistent, progressive dysphonia in a smoker must always raise the possibility of malignant disease, particularly if associated with dysphagia or odynophagia.

A key consideration is the patient's age. Adults have a greater incidence of malignant disease, whereas in children who are hoarse the chief differential diagnosis is between vocal cord nodules and juvenile papillomatosis. An occupational history is of particular relevance, because the voice disorder may be secondary to the pattern of voice use or working conditions. A history of previous surgery is essential, as is documenting any previous laryngeal treatment or speech therapy. Additional patient history questions should include (1) smoking habits; (2) fluid intake, including caffeine and alcohol intake; and (3) symptoms of nasal allergy or sinusitis. Direct questioning should assess the presence of symp-

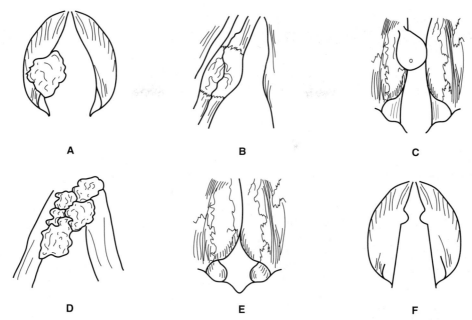

Figure 29–1. Benign laryngeal lesions. **(A)** Vocal cord granuloma, **(B)** intracordal cyst, **(C)** pedunculated vocal cord polyp, **(D)** laryngeal papillomatosis, **(E)** Reinke edema, and **(F)** vocal cord nodules.

toms suggestive of gastroesophageal (or laryngopharyngeal) reflux, and hypothyroidism.

PATIENT EXAMINATION

The patient examination should include a full ear, nose, and throat exam, including a conventional inspection of the larynx followed by a more detailed evaluation of vocal fold movement using video stroboscopy.

A full ENT examination is performed, including mirror indirect laryngoscopy. This guides the chances of successfully performing rigid laryngoscopy and often makes the diagnosis. The two alternative methods, which allow photodocumentation and a more leisurely view, are flexible nasolaryngoscopy, or rigid endoscopy, using a 70° or a 90° endoscope. In both techniques, stroboscopic light may be used to identify defects of the mucosal wave.

Nasolaryngoscopy allows thorough inspection of the nose, postnasal space, pharynx, and larynx in a physiologic position. Rigid endoscopy, conducted via the oropharynx, offers the most detailed view of the larynx in the compliant patient. Both methods can use video systems for photodocumentation: Visualization of the larynx by patients significantly improves understanding and compliance with speech therapy.

Figure 29–1 illustrates the characteristic appearances of some common benign laryngeal lesions.

VIDEOSTROBOSCOPY

Videostroboscopy is an important tool in monitoring rehabilitation and providing feedback during speech therapy. It is also useful in the diagnosis of lesions such as intracordal cysts and in differentiating these lesions from vocal cord nodules.

Stroboscopic examination allows visualization of the mucosal wave occurring at the medial edge of the vocal fold, the appearance being one of a 'slow motion' film. This appearance is created by the flickering stroboscopic light illuminating consecutive mucosal waves at a similar point in the wave form. The frequency of stroboscopic illumination differs slightly from the frequency of the mucosal wave, creating the perception of a slowly moving mucosal wave. This effect is lost if pathology results in a mucosal wave lacking a consistent periodicity. High-speed video recording now allows direct visualization of the mucosal wave, rather than the perception of visualizing the wave created by stroboscopy. This technique has some advantages; however, it requires greatly slowed playback and therefore does not allow "live" images, which are particularly helpful in patients' understanding of their pathology.

Hertegård-Stellan. What have we learned about laryngeal physiology from high-speed digital videoendoscopy? *Curr Opin Otolaryngol Head Neck Surg.* 2005;13:152. [PMID: 15908812]

Sataloff RT. Evaluation of professional singers. *Otolaryngol Clin North Am.* 2000;33:923. [PMID: 10984762] (Summary article of ENT history and examination in singers.)

Simpson CB, Fleming DJ. Medical and vocal history in the evaluation of dysphonia. *Otolaryngol Clin North Am.* 2000;33:719. [PMID: 10918656] (Review of history taking in voice disorders.)

COMMON LARYNGEAL LESIONS

PHONOTRAUMA

Pathogenesis

Most vocal cord nodules, polyps, and the condition known as Reinke edema arise as a result of repetitive trauma to the vocal cords, which is known as *phonotrauma*, and is associated with a local inflammatory response. Shear forces occur during phonation at the area of maximal wave amplitude, which is the border of the anterior and midde third of the vocal fold. Hence vocal pathology secondary to phonotrauma tends to occur at this site.

Dikkers FG, Nikkels PG. Lamina propria of the mucosa of benign lesions of the vocal cords. *Laryngoscope.* 1999;109:1684. [PMID: 10522943] (Study demonstrating correlation between duration and pattern of phonotrauma and the histopathology of benign vocal cord lesions.)

Verdolini K, Rosen CA, Branski RC, Hebda PA. Shifts in biochemical markers associated with wound healing in laryngeal secretions following phonotrauma: a preliminary study. *Ann Otol Rhinol Laryngol.* 2003;112(12):1021. [PMID: 14703104] (Study demonstrating elevation of markers of acute inflammation in the vocal folds following prolonged voice use.)

VOCAL CORD NODULES

 ESSENTIALS OF DIAGNOSIS

- *Usually affects children or individuals who use their voices professionally.*
- *History of voice abuse common, such as frequent shouting in a young child.*
- *Bilateral, pale lesions at the junction of the anterior one third and posterior two thirds of the vocal cords.*

General Considerations

Vocal cord nodules are the most common cause of persistent dysphonia in children. They are also a frequent cause of deterioration in the voice quality of individuals who use their voices professionally, particularly singers;

these nodules are commonly referred to as "singers' nodules." Treatment strategies should be conservative; speech therapy is the primary treatment. The patient is taught how to use the voice appropriately, which often promotes regression of the vocal cord nodules.

Clinical Findings

Laryngoscopy clearly shows the presence of small, well-defined vocal cord lesions. These lesions are distinguishable from the normal vocal fold by their whitish hue and are most commonly found at the junction of the anterior third and posterior two thirds of the vocal fold. They are bilateral, though often asymmetric.

Treatment

A. SPEECH THERAPY

Speech therapy should be used as a first-line treatment. It is the mainstay of treatment in both children and adults. Photodocumentation of the nodules in voice clinic indicates the treatment progress and aids patient compliance during speech therapy.

B. MICROLARYNGOSCOPY

Microlaryngoscopy should be performed under the following circumstances: (1) vocal cord nodules are suspected in a child, but the age or noncompliance of the patient prevents examination; and (2) in adults, either when microsurgical excision of the nodules is considered or when the diagnosis is not clear. Nodules may be excised using appropriate microsurgical instruments, or vaporized using a pulsed CO_2 laser.

Benninger MS. Microdissection or microspot CO_2 laser for limited vocal fold benign lesions: a prospective randomized trial. *Laryngoscope.* 2000;110:1. [PMID: 10678578] (Study establishing the efficacy of the CO_2 laser in the treatment of superficial benign vocal fold lesions.)

VOCAL CORD POLYPS

 ESSENTIALS OF DIAGNOSIS

- *Usually unilateral, pedunculated lesions.*
- *Associated with smoking and voice abuse.*
- *Located throughout the glottis, particularly between the anterior and middle thirds of the vocal folds.*

General Considerations

Vocal cord polyps are most commonly found in men with a history of voice abuse and heavy smoking. The treatment is most often surgical to confirm the diagnosis, exclude any coexisting malignant neoplasms, and provide resolution. Conservative voice therapy is often not successful.

Clinical Findings

Polyps are pedunculated, unilateral lesions that are morphologically similar to the laryngeal epithelium. They often occur on the true vocal folds and may have noticeable vascular markings. They generally occur at the point of maximal vibration, the middle of the true junction of the anterior and middle thirds of the vocal fold, in contrast to vocal process granulomas.

Treatment

The treatment involves a microlaryngoscopic examination of the larynx plus excision of the polyp both to confirm the diagnosis and exclude any other coexistent pathology. A large polyp may conceal an occult, early laryngeal squamous cell carcinoma. Excision is performed using appropriate microsurgical instruments, or laser. Smoking and vocal abuse should also be addressed.

VOCAL PROCESS GRANULOMAS (INTUBATION GRANULOMA)

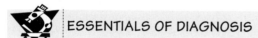 ESSENTIALS OF DIAGNOSIS

- *Arise posteriorly, adjacent to the vocal process.*
- *Frequent history of intubation trauma.*

General Considerations

Vocal process granulomas are often associated with endotracheal intubation. There is an association with gastroesophageal reflux.

Clinical Findings

Patients present with dysphonia and a combination of other symptoms, including odynophagia, cough, and globus symptoms. Vocal process granulomas are usually unilateral and are related to the vocal processes of arytenoid cartilage with an underlying perichondritis. Forceful glottic closure further traumatizes the lesion and is likely to be a factor in its failure to resolve.

Treatment

The initial focus of treatment should be on conservative voice therapy, combined with aggressive antireflux therapy. Antibiotics and systemic steroids may be of use.

Microlaryngoscopy is rarely required to exclude malignancy. Recurrence after surgical excision is common; the incidence may be reduced by the concomitant use of botulinum toxin to paralyze the affected hemilarynx and hence prevent further vocal process trauma.

REINKE EDEMA

 ESSENTIALS OF DIAGNOSIS

- *Strong association with cigarette smoking and heavy voice use.*
- *Diffuse edematous changes of the vocal cords.*
- *Usually bilateral.*

General Considerations

Although a definite mechanism of injury has not been identified, there is a very strong association of cigarette smoking with the development of Reinke edema. The distinguishing feature of this condition is the diffuse nature of the swelling, which is an accumulation of fluid in the superficial layer of the lamina propria of the vocal fold.

Clinical Findings

Patients present with diffuse swelling of the vocal cords, which is usually bilateral. The cords feel boggy when manipulated during microlaryngoscopy, and the swelling can be rolled beneath the instruments.

Treatment

Smoking cessation is the key to resolving Reinke edema. In mild cases, speech therapy may also prevent the need for surgical treatment. However, severe Reinke edema, which is intractable to speech therapy, may have to be treated surgically. Surgical measures involve making a lateral incision on the superior aspect of the vocal fold and extravasating the fluid before carefully replacing the mucosa. Trimming the excess mucosa may be required, but care must be taken not to injure the underlying vocal ligament.

LARYNGEAL CYSTS

Mucous glands are found throughout the larynx, with the exception of the medial edge of the vocal cord, and associated cysts may therefore occur also throughout the larynx. Their presentation and treatment are dictated primarily by their site; therefore, they are dealt with here on this basis.

1. Intracordal Cysts

 ESSENTIALS OF DIAGNOSIS

- *Often found within the middle third of the vocal cords.*
- *Unilateral, associated small area of hyperkeratosis on opposite cord.*
- *Do not respond to speech therapy.*

General Considerations

Intracordal cysts may be simple mucous retention cysts or epidermoid cysts containing keratin.

Clinical Findings

Laryngoscopy reveals a unilateral cyst, usually of the middle third of the vocal cord with a corresponding area of hyperkeratosis on the opposite cord. Stroboscopy reveals loss of the mucosal wave at the site of the lesion.

Treatment

Intracordal cysts do not respond to voice therapy and should be excised with phonosurgical instruments, using a local flap technique.

2. Saccular Cysts

 ESSENTIALS OF DIAGNOSIS

- *May be congenital or acquired.*
- *Adults generally present with voice change.*
- *Children commonly present with airway compromise.*
- *Unilateral supraglottic mass, overlying mucosa unremarkable.*

General Considerations

The laryngeal saccule arises as a diverticulum from the anterior end of the laryngeal ventricle. It extends upward between the false vocal fold and the inner surface of the thyroid cartilage and contains mucus-secreting glands. A saccular cyst occurs as a result of obstruction of these glands, which may be secondary to a congenital anomaly or acquired.

Clinical Findings

Examination reveals expansion of the aryepiglottic fold by the cyst within it, which may extend into the neck through the thyrohyoid membrane. Computed tomography (CT) imaging demonstrates a cyst expanding the supraglottis; the absence of air within the lesion distinguishes it from a laryngocele. Mesodermal tissue may be apparent in the wall of congenital saccular cysts and may influence the surgical approach.

Treatment

Most saccular cysts may be managed endoscopically, either by marsupialization or excision, generally with the aid of a CO_2 laser. Lesions extending beyond the larynx and congenital cysts containing mesodermal elements are optimally managed by a transcervical approach. The excised cyst should undergo histologic examination. Cysts displaying oncocytic metaplasia (oncocytic cysts) are more often multiple and more prone to recurrence.

LARYNGOCELE

 ESSENTIALS OF DIAGNOSIS

- *Generally present as an anterior triangle neck mass.*
- *Increase in size with elevated intralaryngeal pressure.*
- *Associated with malignancy in the laryngeal ventricle.*

General Considerations

A laryngocele is an abnormal expansion of the laryngeal ventricle, which may be confined by the thyroid cartilage (internal laryngocele) or extend through the cricothyroid membrane into the neck (external laryngocele). Their development is often associated with activities leading to raised intralaryngeal pressure—classically trumpet playing—but may occur secondary to a malignancy within the laryngeal ventricle, which must be excluded.

Clinical Findings

Laryngoscopy demonstrates a smooth swelling of the affected supraglottis; external laryngoceles are also palpable as a smooth, relatively soft anterior triangle mass. CT imaging demonstrates the characteristic finding of air within the lesion, which may be partially fluid filled.

Treatment

Internal laryngocele may be managed by endoscopic laser surgery; external laryngocele requires a transcervical approach.

PAPILLOMATOSIS

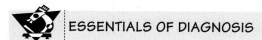

ESSENTIALS OF DIAGNOSIS

- *Patient age at onset is usually 2–4 years.*
- *Rare after age 40.*
- *Multiple warty lesions of "true" and "false" vocal cords.*

General Considerations

Recurrent respiratory papillomatosis (RRP) is characterized by the development of exophytic warty lesions, primarily within the larynx, but which may be found in the nose, pharynx, and trachea. The condition is benign but associated with significant morbidity and mortality.

There is a bimodal distribution; juvenile-onset RRP is generally diagnosed between the ages of 2 and 4 years and is more aggressive than adult-onset disease, which peaks in the third decade.

Pathogenesis

RRP is caused by human papilloma virus (HPV), subtypes 6 and 11, and less commonly by subtypes 16 and 18. HPV 6 and 11 are also the most common causes of genital papillomatosis, and transmission from the genital tract is believed to be the primary cause of RRP.

Vertical transmission of the virus from mother to child occurs either as ascending uterine infection or through direct contact in the birth canal. However, the risk of a child developing RRP after vaginal delivery in the presence of a condyloma acuminatum is estimated at only 1 in 400. The factors dictating susceptibility remain under investigation.

Clinical Findings

Papillomas typically appear as multiple, friable, irregular warty growths in the larynx. These lesions particularly affect the "true" and "false" vocal cords, but they are also found in other parts of the larynx and upper aerodigestive tract.

Presentation depends on the site of the lesion. Patients with glottic lesions present with dysphonia; those with supraglottic lesions may present with stridor.

Treatment

HPV cannot be eradicated from the larynx. Even after spontaneous remission, HPV DNA can be detected in otherwise normal mucosa. The aim of treatment is therefore to remove symptomatic lesions with minimal morbidity. Suitable techniques include CO_2 laser resection, cold steel dissection, or use of the laryngeal microdebrider. Tracheostomy should be avoided and is associated with distal airway involvement. Adjuvant treatments include intralaryngeal injection of cidofovir (Vistide), which is an off-label use with no conclusive evidence of efficacy, although an excellent response has been noted in some patients.

A vaccine for HPV 6, 11, 16, and 18 is currently undergoing trials, and its introduction could significantly reduce the incidence of RRP.

Prognosis

Spontaneous remission does occur, but recurrence can arise many years later. There is a small risk of malignant change.

Derkay CS, Darrow DH. Recurrent respiratory papillomatosis. *Ann Otol Rhinol Laryngol.* 2006;115:1. [PMID: 16466093] (Summary of the current management of respiratory papillomatosis.)

Forte V, Fuoco G, James A. A new classification system for congenital laryngeal cysts. *Laryngoscope.* 2004;114:1123. [PMID: 15179225] (Classification for laryngeal cysts that correlates with management.)

Hogikyan ND, Bastian RW. Endoscopic CO_2 laser excision of large or recurrent laryngeal saccular cysts in adults. *Layngoscope.* 1997;107(2):260. [PMID: 9023253] (Review of laser excision of saccular cysts.)

Orloff LA, Goldman SN. Vocal fold granuloma: successful treatment with botulinum toxin. *Otolaryngol Head Neck Surg.* 1999;121(4):410. [PMID: 10504597]

Shehab N, Sweet BV, Hogikyan ND. Cidofovir for the treatment of recurrent respiratory papillomatosis: a review of the literature. *Pharmacotherapy.* 2005;25:977. [PMID: 16006276] (Review of cidofovir in recurrent respiratory papillomatosis.)

Steinbrook R. The potential of human papillomavirus vaccines. *N Engl J Med.* 2006;354:1109. [PMID: 16540608] (Review of human papilloma virus vaccination.)

RARE LARYNGEAL LESIONS

CHONDROMAS

Chondromas are benign tumors of the laryngeal cartilages that predominantly affect men in the fourth to sixth decades. Patients present with a slowly progressive dysphonia, dyspnea, and dysphagia; therefore, these benign growths can mimic malignant neoplasms in their presentation. Chondromas commonly appear as smooth, firm lesions of the subglottic larynx or any of the other cartilages. Occasionally, they present as a lump in the neck.

CT scanning is useful in delineating the extent of the neoplasm whereas CO_2 laser is useful in performing a biopsy. However, the definitive treatment relies on total surgical excision of the tumor through an open approach. Endoscopic excision is reserved for small tumors.

NEUROGENIC NEOPLASMS

Neurogenic neoplasms are rare tumors and are usually either schwannomas or neurofibromas. It has now been confirmed that granular cell neoplasms are also of nerve sheath origin.

Schwannomas originate from Schwann cells that cover the nerve fibers outside the central nervous system. These lesions are solitary, encapsulated neoplasms that are benign and slow growing, although they can undergo sarcomatous change. **Neurofibromas** are benign proliferations of nerve fibers and are often multiple (eg, in von Recklinghausen disease). In contrast to schwannomas, they are not encapsulated.

Because neurogenic neoplasms are slow growing, patients present with voice change, throat clearing, and the sensation of a lump in the throat. Cough and respiratory compromise follow.

Neurogenic neoplasms are submucosal and smooth and are often located in the aryepiglottic folds. CT scans can accurately define the extent of the lesion prior to treatment. Small tumors may be resected endoscopically, but larger tumors require an open approach.

AMYLOIDOSIS

The larynx is the most common site in the respiratory tract for amyloid deposition. Patient presentation is characterized by the presence of a submucosal mass, which may arise anywhere in the larynx and may impair vocal cord mobility.

The diagnosis is confirmed by the presence of "apple green" birefringence seen with a polarizing microscope after staining with Congo red dye. Treatment involves local resection, usually accomplished endoscopically. Laryngeal amyloid is usually primary and localized, but

has been associated with cardiac involvement and thorough systemic evaluation is essential.

SARCOIDOSIS

One to five percent of patients with sarcoidosis present with lesions within the larynx. The epiglottis is the most common site of involvement. Small, noncaseating granulomas are present on histology, but other granulomatous conditions such as fungal or mycobacterial infections should be ruled out. Spontaneous remission occurs, and treatment is therefore symptomatic, with endoscopic resection when required and systemic steroids in certain cases.

WEGENER GRANULOMATOSIS

Wegener granulomatosis is a multisystem autoimmune disease that may involve necrotizing granulomata of the respiratory tract, disseminated vasculitis, and glomerulonephritis. Focal disease may arise throughout the laryngotracheobronchial tree, but is particularly associated with the immediate subglottic region. Presentation is usually with obstructive symptoms, although dysphonia may be present. Systemic disease is treated with immunosuppressive agents. Local disease without systemic involvement is optimally managed with local treatment, including intralesional corticosteroids.

Dean CM, Sataloff RT, Hawkshaw MJ, Pritikin E. Laryngeal sarcoidosis. *J Voice.* 2002;16:283. [PMID: 12150382] (Etiology, presentation, and management of laryngeal sarcoidosis.)

Franco RAJ, Singh B, Har-El G. Laryngeal chondroma. *J Voice.* 2002;16:92. [PMID: 12008653] (Summary of presentation, investigation, and management of laryngeal chondroma.)

Hoffman GS, Thomas-Golbanov CK, Chan J, Akst LM, Eliachar I. Treatment of subglottic stenosis, due to Wegener's granulomatosis, with intralesional corticosteroids and dilation. *J Rheumatol.* 2003;30:1017. [PMID: 12734898] (Discussion of intralesional corticosteroid in Wegener granulomatosis.)

Pribitkin E, Friedman O, O'Hara B et al. Amyloidosis of the upper aerodigestive tract. *Laryngoscope.* 2003;113:2095. [PMID: 14660909] (Review of laryngeal amyloidosis.)

Malignant Laryngeal Lesions

30

Adriane P. Concus, MD, Tuyet-Phuong N. Tran, MD, Nicholas J. Sanfilippo, MD, & Mark D. DeLacure, MD

General Considerations

Each year, 11,000 new cases of larynx cancer will be diagnosed in the United States (1% of new cancer diagnoses), and approximately one third of these patients will die of their disease. The current male-to-female ratio for larynx cancer is 4:1, but the relative percentage of women with this, as with other smoking-related illness, has been on the rise. Larynx cancer is most prevalent in the sixth and seventh decades of life and is more prevalent among lower socioeconomic groups, for whom it is often not diagnosed until more advanced stages. More than 90% of larynx cancer is squamous cell carcinoma (SCC) and is directly linked to tobacco and excessive alcohol use. Because of the complex and multifaceted nature of this disease, treatment planning is best delivered through a multidisciplinary tumor board format.

Anatomy

The larynx functions not only to produce voice, but also to divide and protect the respiratory from the digestive tracts. It acts as a sphincter during deglutition, protecting against the penetration of bypassing food by closing off the trachea at two sites: the epiglottic flap and the closure of the vocal cords. The larynx consists of a framework of cartilages connected by ligaments, membranes, and muscles covered by a respiratory and stratified squamous mucosal epithelium (Figure 30–1).

The larynx can be divided into three parts: the supraglottis, the glottis, and the subglottis (Figure 30–2). The supraglottic larynx extends from the tip of the epiglottis and vallecula superiorly to the ventricle and undersurface of the "false" cords inferiorly; it includes the arytenoid cartilages, the aryepiglottic folds, the false vocal cords, and the epiglottis. The glottic larynx encompasses the "true" vocal cords, extending from the ventricle between the true and false cords to 0.5 cm below the free edge of the true cords, including the anterior commissure and interarytenoid area. The subglottic larynx extends from the inferior extent of the glottis to the inferior edge of the cricoid cartilage.

Understanding the embryologic origin of these regions of the larynx helps to explain the difference in clinical behavior between cancers arising from these laryngeal subsites. The supraglottis derives from the midline buccopharyngeal primordium and branchial arches 3 and 4 with rich bilateral lymphatics. The glottis, on the other hand, forms from the midline fusion of lateral structures derived from the tracheobronchial primordium and arches 4, 5, and 6. There is a paucity of lymphatics and, compared with supraglottic primary neoplasms, malignant glottic tumors have less of a tendency for bilateral regional lymphatic spread and remain confined to the glottis for longer periods of time.

Fibroelastic membranes and ligaments further divide the larynx into the pre-epiglottic and paraglottic spaces. These structures, including the conus elasticus, the quadrangular and thyrohyoid membranes, and the hyoepiglottic ligament, act as barriers to spread of tumor (Figure 30–3). The thyroid and cricoid cartilages and their perichondrium are further barriers to tumor spread. The anterior commissure tendon (Broyle's ligament) and thyroepiglottic ligaments are not effective barriers to tumor spread, and tumors involving the anterior commissure are more likely to have direct regional spread.

The muscles of the larynx are divided into intrinsic and extrinsic groups. The intrinsic muscles are those of the vocal cords and cartilages contained within the larynx itself. The extrinsic muscles, the strap muscles and constrictors, help with laryngeal elevation and pharyngeal constriction. Innervation of the intrinsic muscles is from the recurrent laryngeal branches of the vagus nerve on both sides. Arterial blood supply is from the external carotid artery and off the thyrocervical trunk via the superior and inferior thyroid arteries. Venous drainage is into the internal jugular vein. Lymphatic drainage is to levels II, III, and IV, as well as sometimes to level VI of the neck.

Kirchner JA. One hundred laryngeal cancers studied by serial section. *Ann Otol.* 1969;78:689. [PMID: 5799397] (Classic paper studying anatomic and histologic cross section of larynx cancers.)

Pathogenesis

More than 90% of patients with larynx cancer have a history of heavy tobacco and alcohol use. Cigarette smoke,

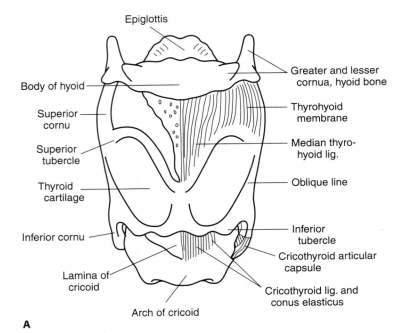

Epiglottis

Body of hyoid

Superior cornu

Superior tubercle

Thyroid cartilage

Inferior cornu

Lamina of cricoid

Arch of cricoid

Greater and lesser cornua, hyoid bone

Thyrohyoid membrane

Median thyro-hyoid lig.

Oblique line

Inferior tubercle

Cricothyroid articular capsule

Cricothyroid lig. and conus elasticus

A

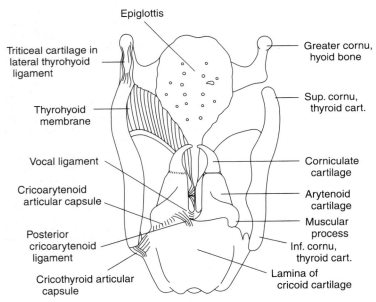

Epiglottis

Triticeal cartilage in lateral thyrohyoid ligament

Thyrohyoid membrane

Vocal ligament

Cricoarytenoid articular capsule

Posterior cricoarytenoid ligament

Cricothyroid articular capsule

Greater cornu, hyoid bone

Sup. cornu, thyroid cart.

Corniculate cartilage

Arytenoid cartilage

Muscular process

Inf. cornu, thyroid cart.

Lamina of cricoid cartilage

B

Figure 30–1. Cartilages and ligaments of the larynx. **(A)** Frontal view and **(B)** posterior view. (Adapted, with permission, from Hollinshead WH. *Anatomy for Surgeons: The Head and Neck,* 3rd ed. Philadelphia: JB Lippincott, 1982.)

in particular, is a risk factor for cancer of the larynx. The combination of smoking and alcohol use has a more than additive carcinogenic effect on the larynx.

Other risk factors have been identified. Laryngeal infection with the human papillomavirus (HPV) results in laryngeal papillomatosis, which is usually benign, but sub-

types 16 and 18 are known to degenerate into SCC. Gastroesophageal reflux has been implicated; however, a causal relationship with laryngeal cancer is still uncertain, although therapies directed at suppressing acid appear to decrease the recurrence of laryngeal cancer. Various occupational exposures and toxic inhalations (such as asbestos and

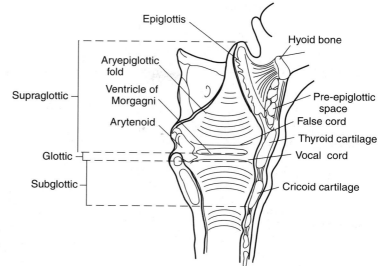

Figure 30–2. The supraglottic, glottic, and subglottic anatomic subdivisions of the larynx. (Adapted, with permission, from Bailey BJ (ed). *Head and Neck Surgery—Otolaryngology,* 3rd ed. Philadelphia: Lippincott Williams & Wilkins, 2001.)

mustard gas), nutritional deficiencies, and previous neck irradiation have all been linked to larynx cancer as well.

Increasingly, molecular and genetic markers of malignant potential, degeneration, and metastasis are being identified, unlocking the genetic causes of larynx cancer. Attention is being paid to predictors of clinical outcome and the response to specific therapy. Once these pathways are understood, gene therapy and other novel therapeutic approaches can be developed. Genes and gene products being investigated for their link to larynx cancer include p53, the Bcl-2 family of genes and other markers of apoptosis, proliferating cell nuclear antigen (PCNA), Ki67, cyclin D1, the ras gene and other oncogenes, tumor suppressor genes, and the loss of heterozygosity and changes in the DNA content of tumors.

Bradford CR. Predictive factors in head and neck cancer. *Hematol Oncol Clin North Am.* 1999;13(4):777. [PMID: 10494513] (Review of molecular and genetic predictive factors for head and neck cancer, with a focus on selecting patients for specific or adjuvant therapies.)

Bradford CR, Wolf GT, Carey TE et al. Predictive markers for response to chemotherapy, organ preservation, and survival in patients with advanced laryngeal carcinoma. *Otolaryngol Head Neck Surg.* 1999;121(5):534. [PMID: 10547465] (The overexpression of p53 and elevated PCNA as well as the T-stage predicted successful organ preservation in the VA Larynx Trial.)

Kreimer AR, et al. Human papillomavirus types in head and neck squamous cell carcinomas worldwide: a systemic review. *Cancer Epidemiol Biomarkers Prev.* 2005;14(2):467. [PMID: 15734974] (Review of the relationship between the different subtypes of human papillomavirus and head and neck cancers.)

Qadeer MA, Colablanchi N, Strome M et al. Gastroesophageal reflux and laryngeal cancer: causation or association? A critical review. *Am J Otolaryngol.* 2006;27(2):119. [PMID: 16500476] (A look at the literature on the relationship between gastroesophageal reflux disease and laryngeal cancer.)

Qadeer MA, Lopez R, Wood BG et al. Does acid suppressive therapy reduce the risk of laryngeal cancer recurrence? *Laryngoscope.* 2005;115(10):1877. [PMID: 16222214] (Study to determine the effects of gastroesophageal reflux disease and acid-suppressive therapy on recurrence of laryngeal cancers after larynx-preserving therapies.)

Staton J et al. Factors predictive of poor functional outcome after chemoradiation for advanced laryngeal cancer. *Otolaryngol Head Neck Surg.* 2002;127(1):43. [PMID: 12161729] (Study to determine the pre-treatment parameters that predict poor outcomes related to laryngeal function in patients who survived larynx-preservation therapies for advanced laryngeal cancers.)

Syrjanen S. Human papillomavirus (HPV) in head and neck cancer. *J Clin Virol.* 2005;32(Suppl 1):S59. [PMID: 15753013] (Review of the data on relationship of human papillomavirus to head and neck cancers.)

Torrente MC et al. Molecular detection and typing of human papillomavirus in laryngeal carcinoma specimens. *Acta Otolaryngol.* 2005;125(8):888. [PMID: 16158538] (Evidence for human papillomavirus infection as an etiologic factor in some laryngeal carcinomas.)

Epidemiology

Malignant disorders of the glottic larynx outnumber those of the supraglottis 1.5:1.0 in the United States (Table 30–1). This ratio does not hold worldwide. In Finland, for example, supraglottic cancers outnumber glottic cancers. The worldwide variation in the epidemiology of larynx cancer may reflect local tobacco and alcohol use customs, other environmental factors, or also the genetic makeup of the populations affected.

Malignant disorders arising in the subglottis are universally rare. For this reason, data on the incidence of nodal

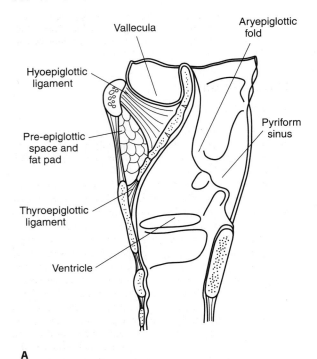

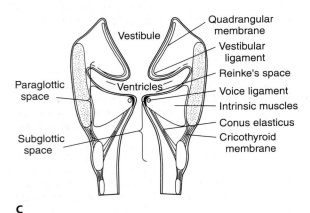

A

C

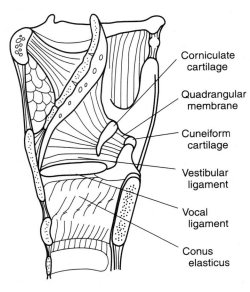

B

Figure 30–3. Laryngeal membranes and ligaments act as barriers to tumor spread and define the paraglottic and pre-epiglottic spaces. **(A)** Sagittal view, with mucosa intact and mucosa removed and **(B)** coronal view. (Reprinted with permission, from Tucker HM. *The Larynx.* New York: Thieme Medical Publishers, 1987.)

metastases and prognosis are scant, and the discussion of the diagnosis and management of larynx cancers that follows focuses on primary supraglottic and glottic cancers. Most larynx cancers involving the subglottis are extensions of primary cancers arising in the glottis or supralglottis.

As explained above, cancers arising in the supraglottic larynx have a richer lymphatic drainage and are more often diagnosed with nodal metastases and, therefore, at a higher clinical stage (Table 30–2).

Jemal A, Thomas A, Murray T et al. Cancer statistics, 2002. *CA Cancer J Clin.* 2002;52(1):23. [PMID: 11814064] (American Cancer Society statistics.)

Table 30–1. Incidence of larynx cancer by site.

Supraglottic—40%
Glottic—59%
Subglottic—1%

Prevention

Many studies address the protective effect of retinoids, beta-carotene, and other antioxidants against the development of

Table 30–2. Larynx cancer: incidence of neck metastases by site.

	T1	T2	T3	T4	All T
Supraglottis	15–40%	35–42%	50–65%	>65%	25–50%
Glottis	<5%	5–10%	10–20%	25–40%	
Subglottis					50%

larynx cancer. A reversal of laryngeal leukoplakia after treatment with retinyl-palmitate has been demonstrated.

Issing WJ, Struck R, Naumann A. Impact of retinyl palmitate in leukoplakia of the larynx. *Eur Arch Otorhinolaryngol.* 1997; 254;S105. [PMID: 9065641] (Study showing the reversal of laryngeal leukoplakia with this antioxidant therapy.)

Staging

Cancers of the larynx are staged according to the TNM (tumor, node, metastasis) system of the American Joint Committee on Cancer (Table 30–3). For staging purposes, positive neck nodes are considered locoregional metastases; metastases to other parts of the body (such as lung, mediastinum, liver, and bone) are considered distant. For the first time, T4 tumors are divided into resectable (T4a) and unresectable (T4b) tumors; accordingly, Stage IV tumors are now subdivided into IVA, IVB, and IVC (distant metastases present) staging. Studies before this date, however, are based on the 1998 or earlier systems in which there was a single umbrella T4 and Stage IV designation. Accordingly, the discussion in the rest of this chapter refers to the older system.

A shortcoming of the TNM staging system, which the subdivision of the T4 and Stage IV categories is starting to address, is that tumors of varying size and prognosis are frequently categorized together. Other indicators of the prognosis in laryngeal carcinoma have been identified and proposals exist to incorporate these into staging systems. These indicators include (1) the histologic characteristics of the tumor, such as extracapsular spread in nodal metastases, angiolymphatic invasion, perineural spread, and a high histologic grade; (2) various chromosomal and molecular markers, such as p53 mutations, Ki67 or PCNA overexpression, DNA content, and loss of heterozygosity; and (3) the presence of patient comorbidities.

Greene FL, Page DL, Fleming ID et al (eds.). American Joint Committee on Cancer: *AJCC Cancer Staging Manual,* 6th ed. New York, Berlin, Heidelberg: Springer Verlag, 2002. (The definitive reference for the currently used American Joint Committee on Cancer staging system.)

Piccirillo JF. Importance of comorbidity in head and neck cancer. *Laryngoscope.* 2000;110(4):593. [PMID: 10764003]

(Prospective study, including 341 head and neck cancer patients, demonstrating the prognostic value of comorbidity and providing data in support of incorporating comorbidity into accepted staging systems.)

Clinical Findings

A. Symptoms and Signs

Signs and symptoms of malignant laryngeal lesions include hoarseness, dysphagia, hemoptysis, a mass in the neck, throat pain, ear pain, airway compromise, and aspiration.

Because only the slightest change in contour, thickness, or vibratory characteristics of the vocal cord results in perceived changes in the voice (namely, hoarseness), glottic larynx cancers often come to medical attention while still at an early stage. Patients with supraglottic cancers, however, typically present at a more advanced stage because tumors are bulkier (ie, at a higher T stage) before voice changes, dysphagia, airway compromise, or aspiration become apparent. Furthermore, because the supraglottis has a richer lymphatic supply, supraglottic primary lesions tend to metastasize earlier and are more often diagnosed at the advanced N stage. Clinical cervical adenopathy at the time of diagnosis portends a poor prognosis and advances the overall stage. Significant weight loss often accompanies the diagnosis of an advanced larynx cancer because of swallowing difficulties. Of note, throat and ear pain are usually symptoms of advanced-stage tumors.

B. Physical Examination

When a larynx cancer is suspected, complete head and neck examination is performed, focusing on the larynx and the neck. The quality of the voice is noted. A breathy voice may indicate a vocal cord paralysis and a muffled voice, a supraglottic lesion.

1. Laryngoscopy—Laryngoscopy (or visualization of the larynx) is done in the office setting using either a laryngeal mirror (indirect laryngoscopy) or a fiberoptic endoscope. Irregularities in the contour, color, vibratory characteristics, and mobility of the vocal cords are noted. Malignant laryngeal lesions can appear to be fungating, friable, nodular, or ulcerative, or simply as changes in mucosal color (Figure 30–4). A stroboscopic video laryngoscopy can highlight subtle irregularities in the mucosal vibration, periodicity, and closure of the vocal cords. Careful attention must be paid to the airway status. Some large, bulky lesions require urgent airway intervention with either intubation, tumor debulking, or tracheotomy. Direct laryngoscopy is performed under general anesthesia and provides the definitive examination of tumor extent.

2. Neck examination—The neck is examined by palpation for enlarged lymph nodes and by noting their

Table 30–3. T (tumor), N (nodes), M (metastases), staging for malignant laryngeal disorders.

Supraglottis	
T_1	Tumor limited to one subsite of supraglottis
T_2	Tumor involving more than one adjacent subsite of supraglottis, glottis, or region outside the supraglottis (vallecula, tongue base, medial wall of pyriform sinus)
T_3	Tumor causes vocal cord fixation and/or invades pre-epiglottic space, postcricoid area
T_{4a}	Tumor invades through thyroid cartilage, and/or extends to nonlaryngeal soft tissues of neck
T_{4b}	Tumor invades prevertebral space or mediastinum, or encases carotid artery
Glottis	
T_1	Tumor limited to vocal cord; may involve anterior or posterior commissure
T_2	Tumor extends to supraglottis, glottis, and/or impaired vocal cord mobility
T_3	Vocal cord fixation
T_{4a}	Tumor invades through thyroid cartilage, and/or extends to nonlaryngeal soft tissues of neck
T_{4b}	Tumor invades prevertebral space or mediastinum, or encases carotid artery
Subglottis	
T_1	Tumor limited to the subglottis
T_2	Tumor extends to vocal cord with normal or impaired mobility
T_3	Vocal cord fixation
T_{4a}	Tumor invades through cricoid or thyroid cartilage, and/or extends to nonlaryngeal soft tissues of neck
T_{4b}	Tumor invades prevertebral space or mediastinum, or encases carotid artery
N_0	No cervical lymph nodes positive
N_1	Single ipsilateral lymph node ≤ 3 cm
N_{2a}	Single ipsilateral lymph node > 3 cm and ≤ 6 cm
N_{2b}	Multiple ipsilateral lymph nodes, each ≤ 6 cm
N_{2c}	Bilateral or contralateral lymph nodes, each ≤ 6 cm
N_3	Single or multiple lymph nodes > 6 cm
M_0	No distant metastases
M_1	Distant metastases present

Stage	T	N	M
I	T_1	N_0	M_0
II	T_2	N_0	M_0
III	T_3	N_0	M_0
	T_{1-3}	N_1	M_0
IVA	T_{4a}	N_{0-2}	M_0
	T_{1-4a}	N_0	M_0
IVB	T_{4b}	any N	M_0
	any T	N_3	M_0
IVC	any T	any N	M_1

location, size, firmness, and mobility. Restricted laryngeal crepitus (the "clicking" movement from side to side across the pharynx and prevertebral fascia) can reveal postcricoid or even retropharyngeal invasion.

3. Assessment of nutritional status—Nutritional status should also be assessed and supplementation discussed, if indicated. Caloric dietary supplements may suffice in some cases; others may require gastrostomy or other feeding tube placement.

C. LABORATORY FINDINGS AND SPECIAL TESTS

Squamous cell carcinoma of the head and neck can spread to virtually any site of the body, but it is rare in the absence of lung, mediastinal, or liver metastases. Therefore, routine metastatic survey consists of the following tests.

1. Biopsy—Biopsy of a laryngeal lesion is necessary to establish the diagnosis of malignancy. Biopsy of the lar-

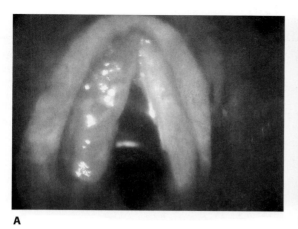
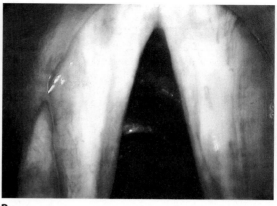

A   **B**

Figure 30–4. Stage I, T1 squamous cell carcinoma of the left true vocal cord, endoscopic view. **(A)** At diagnosis and **(B)** a complete response, 8 months after the completion of radiation therapy.

ynx is best accomplished in the operating room with the patient under general anesthesia and neuromuscular paralysis. Direct laryngoscopy is performed. A variety of laryngoscopes are available designed to enhance visualization of the endolarynx in a range of anatomic and clinical situations. The suspected lesion is mapped and possibly photographed/videotaped. The lesion can be palpated to assess the depth of invasion, and passive mobility of both vocal cords can be checked. Biopsies of suspected malignant sites are done with cup forceps.

With the patient anesthetized and paralyzed, a thorough neck examination is obtained. Esophagoscopy and bronchoscopy can also be performed at this setting as part of a cancer staging workup.

For patients who cannot tolerate a general anesthetic, the biopsy of laryngeal lesions can be performed as an office procedure. Under fiberoptic guidance, with generous topical anesthesia (typically using lidocaine or Cetacaine), a flexible biopsy forceps passed through the fiberoptic scope is used.

2. Chest imaging—Cancer of the larynx spreads first to the regional cervical nodes. The next most common site of spread is the lungs. For this reason, patients with head and neck cancer should have a chest x-ray as part of a routine metastatic evaluation. This test should be repeated once or twice yearly to screen for metastases. If there are any significant abnormalities noted on the chest x-ray, a computed tomography (CT) scan of the chest should be performed to confirm the lesions. Bronchoscopy with cytologic evaluation of bronchial washings or transbronchial biopsy should be done if there are suspicious lesions. Alternately, thoracoscopy, mediastinoscopy, and biopsy are done if lesions are more amenable to these approaches. Chest and lung lesions may represent either metastases from the lar-

ynx primary neoplasm or second primary tumors, because the risk factor of smoking is common to both tumors.

D. IMAGING STUDIES

Radiologic imaging of the larynx and neck is not necessary for an early-stage glottic cancer with a clinically N0 neck. Because the risk of occult nodal disease is high even for early-stage supraglottic cancer, it is sometimes recommended to obtain neck imaging in these cases. If there is any suspicion of impaired vocal cord mobility, a scan should be obtained. Radiologic imaging is generally performed for clinically advanced larynx cancers to aid with staging and treatment planning. CT scanning (Figure 30–5) or magnetic resonance imaging (MRI) is useful in identifying preepiglottic or paraglottic space invasion, laryngeal cartilage erosion, and cervical nodal metastases. Larynx cancers are clinically upstaged as frequently as 25–40% on the basis of CT scanning or MRI. Both imaging modalities are useful to assess the above characteristics. MRI is more sensitive for soft tissue abnormalities, whereas CT scan is better for bony and cartilaginous defects.

Other imaging modalities are being investigated for their role in larynx cancer, but at this time they are not the standard of care. Positron emission tomography (PET) scanning uses fluorescence-tagged glucose and the increased metabolic rate of malignant tissues to identify cancers. Application of PET in the head and neck has focused on (1) identifying occult nodal metastases, (2) distinguishing the recurrence of malignant growth from radionecrosis and other sequelae of prior treatment, and (3) identifying the location of an unknown primary cancer. Some evidence suggests that PET scan may be able to detect superficial laryngeal cancers that CT scan cannot. Nonethe-

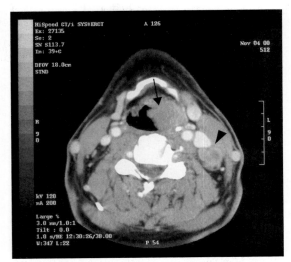

Figure 30–5. Contrast CT scan showing bulky left supraglottic tumor (arrow) with ipsilateral lymph node metastasis (arrowhead).

less, PET scan information does not replace the accuracy of direct visualization and biopsy of the larynx and is not superior to CT or MRI in identifying the additional staging criteria of pre-epiglottic or paraglottic space invasion, cartilage erosion, soft tissue extension into the neck, and cervical metastasis.

If there is a question of distant metastases, then bone scanning may be of use.

Ultrasound of the neck can be useful in the diagnosis of larynx cancer. In Europe, this noninvasive imaging modality is used to identify cervical metastases and even to characterize laryngeal abnormalities, but it is not typically used in North America for these purposes.

Anzai Y, Carroll WR, Qunit DJ et al. Recurrence of head and neck cancer after surgery or irradiation: prospective comparison of 2-deoxy-2-[F-18]fluoro-D-glucose PET and MR imaging diagnoses. *Radiology.* 1996;200(1):135.[PMID: 8657901] (Study of patients with recurrent head and neck cancer, demonstrating the improved sensitivity and specificity of PET over MRI and CT scans in detecting the recurrence.)

Gordin A et al. Fluorodeoxyglucose-positron emission tomography/computed tomography imaging in patients with carcinoma of larynx: diagnostic accuracy and impact on clinical management. *Laryngoscope.* 2006;116(2):273. [PMID: 1646778] (Study to assess the value of PET/CT on patients with laryngeal cancer compared with PET or CT alone and the impact that PET/CT had on clinical management.)

McGuirt WF, Greven KM, Keyes JW et al. Laryngeal radionecrosis versus recurrent cancer: a clinical approach. *Ann Otol Rhinol Laryngol.* 1998;107:293. [PMID: 9557763] (Study showing the usefulness of the PET scan to distinguish recurrent laryngeal cancer from laryngeal radionecrosis.)

Differential Diagnosis

Definitive tissue diagnosis must be obtained before starting treatment for a laryngeal cancer because lesions that appear malignant may, in fact, be benign. These benign conditions include infectious, inflammatory, and granulomatous diseases such as tuberculosis, sarcoidosis, blastomycosis, papillomatosis, and granular cell tumors. The next section provides a discussion of malignant laryngeal lesions.

Histologic Types

A. SQUAMOUS CELL CARCINOMA

SCC represents > 90% of larynx cancers and is linked to tobacco and excessive alcohol use. Histologically, the carcinogenesis of SCC is viewed as a continuum of change from normal phenotype, to hyperplasia, to dysplasia, to carcinoma in situ, to invasive carcinoma. Invasive SCC can be well, moderately, or poorly differentiated and is characterized by nests of malignant epithelial cells in a surrounding desmoplastic, inflammatory stroma (Figure 30–6). Varying degrees of mitoses and necrosis are seen. Keratin pearls are a pathognomonic feature seen in well- and moderately differentiated SCC. SCC can invade blood and lymphatic vessels as well as nerves. Immunohistochemical staining is positive for keratin proteins.

Variants of SCC include verrucous carcinoma, spindle cell carcinoma, basaloid SCC, and adenosquamous carcinoma. Verrucous carcinoma, which is characterized grossly by a warty, exophytic tumor that is highly differentiated with bulbous "rete pegs" pushing into the underlying stroma and low metastatic potential, is typically treated surgically because many physicians view this tumor as being radiation-resistant. Spindle cell carcinoma presents as malignant spindle cells seen in the

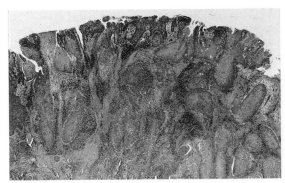

Figure 30–6. Moderately well-differentiated laryngeal squamous cell carcinoma. Note nests of tumor extending deep into the stroma.

stroma usually predominating over foci of conventional SCC and is often confused with sarcoma. The spindle cells typically stain positive for keratin on immunohistochemistry. Basaloid SCC presents as compact nests of subepithelial basaloid cells associated with SCC in situ or invasive SCC. Adenosquamous carcinoma is a high-grade malignant neoplasm with features of both SCC with epithelial differentiation and adenocarcinoma with glandular differentiation.

B. Salivary Gland Cancers

Malignant disorders can arise from the minor salivary glands that line the mucosa of the larynx. Adenoid cystic carcinoma (ACC) and mucoepidermoid carcinoma (MEC) are the most common, although other histologic types have been reported as well. Women and men are affected equally by ACC of the larynx. The histology resembles that of the major salivary gland counterparts, with cribriform, tubular, and solid architectural patterns for ACC and low-grade cystic patterns to high-grade solid patterns for MEC. The clinical behavior is also similar to that of the corresponding major salivary gland neoplasms. ACC has an indolent clinical course and tendency for perineural spread. Low-grade MEC has a better prognosis than high-grade MEC. Surgery is the preferred treatment for both, with guidelines for adjuvant radiation similar to those for malignant disorders of the major salivary glands.

C. Sarcomas

Malignant growths of mesenchymal origin are rarely seen in the larynx. The most common is chondrosarcoma. Chondrosarcoma of the larynx arises most often from the cricoid cartilage and is characterized by a submucosal mass of the posterior glottis with stippled calcification on CT scan (Figure 30–7). The diagnosis can be difficult both because an adequate biopsy may be challenging and because the histologic differentiation from a benign chondroma may be difficult. Chondrosarcomas have a nonaggressive clinical behavior, and, for this reason, partial laryngeal surgery with preservation of some laryngeal function is often attempted. Radiation is generally viewed as ineffective in treating laryngeal chondrosarcoma.

Other types of laryngeal sarcoma include malignant fibrous histiocytoma, angiosarcoma, and synovial sarcoma.

D. Other Neoplasms

Other tumors that can occur in the larynx include neuroendocrine tumors such as carcinoid tumors, lymphoma, and metastases from other primary sites. Malignant tumors of the thyroid can invade into the larynx with or without vocal cord paralysis.

Gripp S, Pape H, Schmitt G. Chondrosarcoma of the larynx: the role of radiotherapy revisited—a case report and review of the literature. *Cancer.* 1998;82:108. [PMID: 9428486] (Review of the literature and existing case reports on larynx chondrosarcoma, revisiting the idea of radiation as a treatment for this type of cancer.)

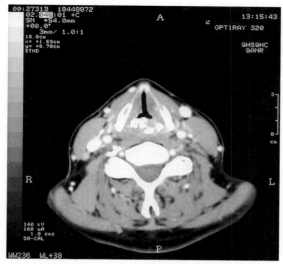

Figure 30–7. Contrast CT scan demonstrating calcified stippling in a mass arising from the cricoid cartilage; this finding is characteristic of chondrosarcoma.

Treatment

A. Treatment of Early-Stage Larynx Cancer

Early-stage larynx cancer (Stages I and II) can be treated with either surgery or radiation in single-modality therapy. Current recommendations by the American Society of Clinical Oncology are that all patients with T1 or T2 laryngeal cancer, with rare exceptions, should be treated initially with the intent to preserve the larynx. The advantages of surgery compared with radiation are a shorter treatment period (compared with 6–7 weeks for radiation) and the option of saving radiation for recurrence. Specific surgical procedures used in the treatment of early larynx cancer are discussed in the following section. In addition to the risks inherent in any surgical procedure, surgery often results in a poorer voice quality and, for external surgical approaches, a worse cosmetic outcome.

The chief advantage of radiation therapy is better voice quality. Specific radiation therapy techniques for larynx cancer are discussed under "Nonsurgical Measures." For early-stage lesions, short-term complications of radiation include odynophagia and laryngeal edema. The long-term complications include a remote possibility of laryngeal fibrosis, radionecrosis, or hypothyroidism. Delayed development of sarcoma (radiation-induced), though possible, is exceedingly rare, with an incidence of 0.03–0.3%.

B. TREATMENT OF ADVANCED-STAGE LARYNX CANCER

Advanced-stage larynx cancer (Stages III and IV) was historically treated by dual-modality therapy with surgery and radiation. For most T3 and T4 tumors, where total laryngectomy is required for the complete removal of the tumor with amply clear margins, organ preservation treatment with combined chemotherapy and radiation therapy is preferred in most centers because there is no difference in overall survival and a superior quality of life. Still, extirpative surgery may be used in selected patients, such as those with bone or cartilage destruction in which reasonable organ function is unlikely after conservation therapy. Voice rehabilitation after total laryngectomy is discussed below. For T1, T2, and some T3 lesions, partial laryngectomy procedures with preservation of the voice may be considered (see "D. Surgical Treatment of Larynx Cancer"). Patient selection is critical with the goal of rendering the patient disease free with surgery alone because postoperative radiation after partial laryngectomy may result in significant functional impairment. The type of neck dissection chosen is guided by the extent of the neck disease, also discussed below.

Adjuvant radiation should start within 6 weeks of surgery and, on once-daily protocols, lasts 6–7 weeks. The primary site is treated with external-beam irradiation with doses of 55–66 Gy whereas draining nodal basins typically receive a slightly lower dose, depending on the extent of neck disease. Complications of radiation therapy include those described for radiation given as single-modality treatment for early-stage larynx cancer; however, since the treated area is more extensive, side effects also include mucositis during therapy and chronic xerostomia after treatment. Less common complications include hypothyroidism, radionecrosis, and esophageal stricture.

Organ-preserving protocols have evolved over the past decade. The landmark work study of the Veterans Administration Larynx Cancer Study Group randomized 332 patients to receive neoadjuvant chemotherapy followed by radiation, compared with traditional total laryngectomy with postoperative radiation. The study found that two thirds of patients responded favorably to chemotherapy after just one or two cycles. In two thirds of these cases, larynges were preserved, and survival was similar to the traditional approach of laryngectomy with postoperative radiation. As a subgroup, patients with larger T4 tumors did not fare as well and, for this reason, organ-preserving protocols sometimes are not offered to patients in this category, particularly if cartilaginous invasion is present. The VA study was followed by a three-arm randomized study comparing induction chemotherapy (cisplatin plus 5-fluorouracil) followed by radiation, concurrent chemoradiation with cisplatin, and once-daily radiation alone in 547 patients. At 2 years, superior organ preservation was achieved with the concurrent chemoradiation group; therefore, this treatment strategy has become the standard of care in most centers. Ongoing studies of combined-modality treatment include radiation with different systemic therapies and systemic therapy with altered radiation schedules, including twice-daily treatment.

C. TREATMENT OF THE NECK IN LARYNX CANCER

A neck without clinically apparent nodal metastases should be treated in larynx cancer if the risk of nodal metastasis exceeds 20–30% (see Table 30–2). The treatment of both the ipsilateral and contralateral necks should be considered, therefore, for early-stage, primary cancers of the supraglottis in general and for all advanced laryngeal cancers. Neck disease staged as N0 or N1 can be treated with a single modality—surgery or radiation. Neck disease staged as N2 or N3 requires a combined-modality treatment.

Neck dissection is tailored to the extent of neck disease. Selective neck dissection (preserving the sternocleidomastoid muscle, internal jugular vein, and spinal accessory nerve) can be performed for clinically N0 necks. For N1 necks, dissection is usually limited to levels II–IV, as metastasis to levels I or V is rare in this condition. Radical or extended radical neck dissection, sacrificing the sternocleidomastoid muscle, the internal jugular vein, and the spinal accessory nerve, and addressing neck levels I–V or more, is performed for extensive neck disease with the involvement of vessels, nerves, muscles, or any combination of these structures. A modified radical neck dissection preserves some of these structures, according to feasibility.

D. SURGICAL TREATMENT OF LARYNX CANCER

Surgical options for treating larynx cancer include a variety of partial laryngectomy procedures in addition to total laryngectomy. Understanding the lymphatic drainage patterns of the laryngeal subsites permits the surgeon to resect more closely than the 1- to 2-cm margins that typically are recommended at other head and neck sites. This helps preserve functional voice, respiration, and deglutition in partial laryngectomy procedures.

A preoperative consultation with a speech therapist is appropriate if significant voice or swallowing changes are anticipated. These sessions help educate patients about the speech and swallowing functions of the larynx and prepare the patient for postoperative rehabilitation and therapy.

1. Microlaryngeal surgery—The endoscopic removal of selected larynx cancers can be achieved safely and effectively with use of the operating microscope and microlaryngeal dissection instruments. The carbon dioxide laser, used with direct laryngoscopy and microscope guidance, is

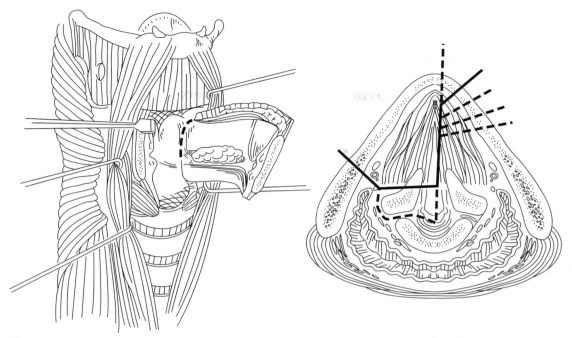

Figure 30–8. Schematic of the anatomic resection for a vertical hemilaryngectomy. (Modified and reprinted, with permission of Myers EN, Suen JY. *Cancer of the Head and Neck*, 3rd ed. Philadelphia: WB Saunders, 1996.)

also a useful dissection tool, especially for supraglottic lesions. Laser cordectomy has been shown to provide excellent local control and laryngeal preservation of early-stage glottic cancer; it offers low morbidity and excellent retreatment options in case of local failure.

2. Hemilaryngectomy—Hemilaryngectomy is the removal of one vertical half of the larynx (or a part thereof; Figure 30–8). Appropriate tumors for this surgery are those with (1) subglottic extension no more than 1 cm below the true vocal cords; (2) a mobile affected cord; (3) unilateral involvement (involvement of the anterior commissure and anterior extent of the contralateral true cord can, in certain cases, also be treated with an extended vertical hemilaryngectomy); (4) no cartilage invasion; and (5) no extralaryngeal soft tissue involvement.

Vocal cord reconstruction is most often done by transposing a flap of strap muscle or microvascular free flap to provide bulk against which the remaining unaffected vocal cord can vibrate (Figure 30–9). Vertical hemilaryngectomy can be done in appropriate surgical candidates who have failed radiation therapy.

3. Supraglottic laryngectomy—A supraglottic laryngectomy entails removal of the supraglottis or the upper part of the larynx (or a part thereof). This surgery may be considered when the following conditions are met: (1) for tumors with a T stage of T1, T2, or T3 by pre-epiglottic space involvement only; (2) the vocal cords are mobile; (3) cartilage is not involved; (4) the anterior commissure is not involved; (5) the patient has good pulmonary status/reserve; (6) the base of the tongue is not involved past the circumvallate papillae; (7) the

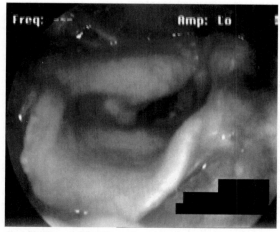

Figure 30–9. Vertical right hemilaryngectomy, postoperative endoscopic view. Note the absence of arytenoid, but the presence of the "pseudocord."

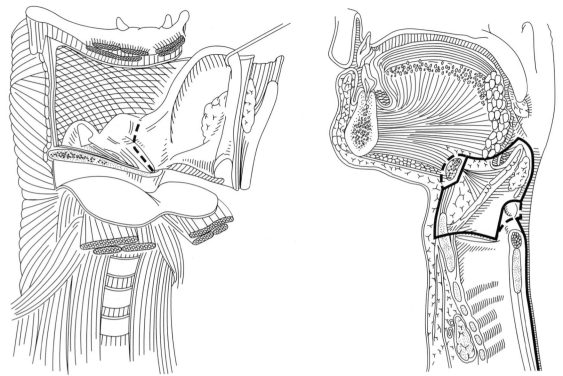

Figure 30–10. Schematic of the anatomic resection for a supraglottic laryngectomy. (Modified and reprinted, with permission of Myers EN, Suen JY. *Cancer of the Head and Neck,* 3rd ed. Philadelphia: WB Saunders, 1996.)

apex of the pyriform sinus is not involved; and (8) the FEV_1 (the forced expiratory volume in the first second) is predicted to be > 50%.

A supraglottic laryngectomy can be performed endoscopically using a carbon dioxide laser or with a more standard open, external approach. Endoscopic surgery typically removes just the involved portion of the supraglottis. The traditional supraglottic laryngectomy removes the entire supraglottis from the apex of the laryngeal ventricle, including the false cords, the epiglottis, and the pre-epiglottic space; the arytenoids and part of the thyroid cartilage are preserved (Figure 30–10). Closure in an open supraglottic laryngectomy is done by collapsing the remaining glottic part of the larynx to the base of tongue (Figure 30–11).

Although the patient's voice is generally normal in quality, some degree of aspiration is an expected side effect of this operation. For this reason, patients with borderline pulmonary function (FEV_1 predicted to be < 50%) who cannot tolerate chronic aspiration are generally not considered good candidates for supraglottic laryngectomy. Patients must learn a double-swallow technique called the supraglottic swallow to minimize aspiration with oral intake. Regular visits with a speech therapist are critical to properly learn this technique.

4. Supracricoid laryngectomy—This is a newer surgical technique, which expands on the traditional supraglottic laryngectomy procedure to preserve voice for those with cancers located at the anterior glolttis,

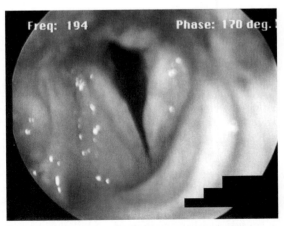

Figure 30–11. Supraglottic laryngectomy, postoperative endoscopic view. Note the absence of the epiglottis.

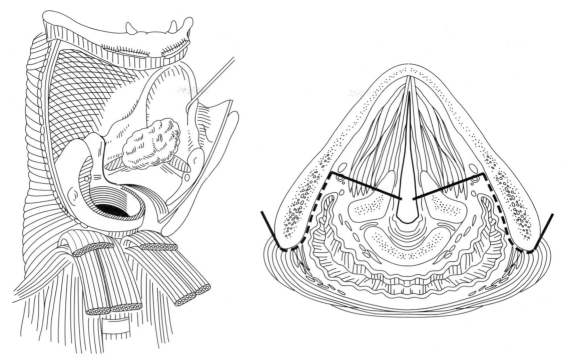

Figure 30–12. Schematic of the anatomic resection for a supracricoid laryngectomy. (Modified and reprinted, with permission of Myers EN, Suen JY. *Cancer of the Head and Neck,* 3rd ed. Philadelphia: WB Saunders, 1996.)

including the commissure, or those with more extensive pre-epiglottic space involvement. The true vocal cords, the supraglottis, and thyroid cartilage are taken, preserving the cricoid and arytenoid cartilages (Figure 30–12). Half of the patients remain dependent on their tracheotomy. Pulmonary function and prior radiation candidacy criteria for supraglottic laryngectomy apply for supracricoid laryngectomy as well. Voice results are reported as adequate. Supraglottic swallow techniques must be used.

5. Near-total laryngectomy—A near-total laryngectomy is a more extended partial laryngectomy procedure in which only one arytenoid is preserved and a tracheoesophageal conduit is constructed for speech (Figure 30–13). Voice is generated by the lungs, but has a more limited range of pitch. Oral intake and swallowing are in the usual fashion, with some aspiration concerns. Patients remain dependent on a tracheotomy for breathing. This procedure is not offered to patients whose radiation treatments have failed, those with poor pulmonary reserve, or those with tumor invovement below the cricoid ring. Candidates are patients with large T3 and T4 lesions with one uninvolved arytenoid, or with unilateral transglottic tumors with cord fixation.

6. Total laryngectomy—A total laryngectomy entails the removal of the entire larynx, including the thyroid and cricoid cartilages, possibly some upper tracheal rings, and the hyoid bone (Figure 30–14). The proximal tracheal stump is anastomosed to an opening at the root of the neck anteriorly in a permanent tracheostoma; this results in the complete anatomic separation of the respiratory and digestive tracts. Indications for total laryngectomy are (1) T3 and T4 cancers not amenable to the above partial laryngectomy procedures or organ preservation therapy with chemoradiation, (2) extensive involvement of thyroid or cricoid cartilage, (3) the direct invasion of surrounding soft tissues of the neck, and (4) tongue base involvement beyond the circumvallate papillae. Closure is done by reapproximating the pharyngeal mucosa. If a partial or total pharyngectomy is also required because of the size of the tumor, then free flap or regional flap aids the closure and prevents pharyngoesophageal stricture. The goal is for patients to ingest nutrients by mouth and swallow in the usual manner.

Voice rehabilitation after a total laryngectomy is best accomplished with tracheoesophageal speech, using a tracheostomal device that is a one-way valve directing air into the neopharynx during exhalation when the tracheostoma

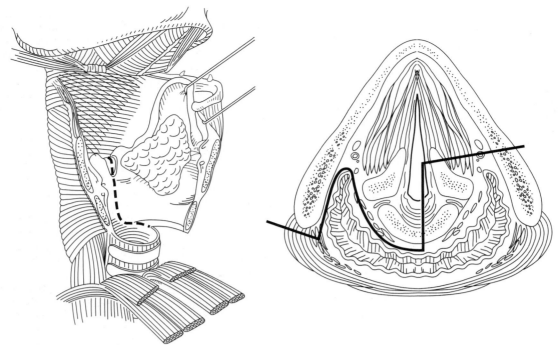

Figure 30–13. Schematic of the anatomic resection for a near-total laryngectomy. (Modified and reprinted, with permission of Myers EN, Suen JY. *Cancer of the Head and Neck,* 3rd ed. Philadelphia: WB Saunders, 1996.)

is occluded (Figure 30–15). The individual accomplishes this with digital occlusion, but foam buttons and hands-free techniques also exist. There are several models of the electrolarynx, which achieves its sound by external vibration. Learning to use the device to optimize comprehensibility is a challenge to most patients; those listening to an individual using an electrolarynx must also be familiar with the sound to understand the speech. Some patients learn pure esophageal speech by forcing air into the esophagus and releasing the air while using the tongue, teeth, cheeks, and lips to produce speech. A speech therapist familiar with postlaryngectomy voice rehabilitation is an essential member of the patient care team for patients undergoing a partial or total laryngectomy.

E. NONSURGICAL MEASURES

1. Photodynamic therapy—Photodynamic therapy is an emerging modality of treating early larynx cancer, as well as cancer arising from other primary mucosal sites of the head and neck. A photosensitizing agent (a chemical preferentially taken up by tumor tissue and sensitive to specific wavelengths of light) is administered intravenously. A laser is then used to activate the photosensitizing agent and induce the destruction of tumor tissue. This treatment has been shown to be effective in treating cancers as deep as 5 mm, with local control and survival rates similar to traditional treatment modalities. The side effects of photodynamic therapy include light sensitivity that can linger for several weeks after the administration of the photosensitizing agent. For this reason, patients must wear sun-protective clothing during this period of time and avoid being outside during the hours of maximal sun intensity.

2. Radiation treatment techniques for larynx cancer—Radiation given as the primary treatment for larynx cancer or as an adjuvant treatment after surgery is most often done using an external-beam technique; a dose of 6000–7000 cGy is administered to the primary site. When the risk of locoregional nodal metastasis in a clinically negative neck exceeds 15–20%, 5000 cGy is delivered prophylactically to the neck as well. The indications for postoperative adjuvant radiation include advanced-stage disease, close or positive margins, extracapsular spread of tumor in a lymph node, perineural or angiolymphatic spread, subglottic extension, and the involvement of nodes in multiple neck levels (in particular, levels IV or V, or the mediastinum). Although conventional adjuvant radiation treatment consisted of radiation alone, two recent randomized trials have shown improved local control with concurrent radiation and cisplatin for certain risk factors. Patient selection for such treatment continues to be debated, but patients with good performance status and adverse tumor features should be seriously considered for postoperative adjuvant

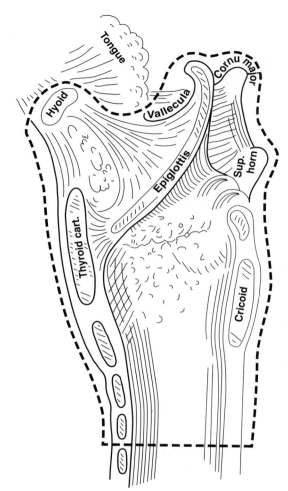

Figure 30–14. Schematic of the anatomic resection for a total laryngectomy. (Modified and reprinted, with permission of Cummings CW, Sessions DG, Weymuller EA, Wood P. *Atlas of Laryngeal Surgery.* St. Louis: CV Mosby, 1984.)

concurrent chemoradiation. As noted previously, newer protocols are using various combinations of radiation with systemic therapies for tumor sensitization and eradication of micrometastatic disease. Altered radiation schedules are also being studied—both with and without systemic agents. Advances in treatment delivery with intensity-modulated radiation therapy (IMRT) have allowed for more accurate tumor dose delivery with greater sparing of normal tissue, including salivary gland preservation with reduced xerostomia. Before undergoing radiation, patients should have a thorough dental examination. When the field will encompass the oral cavity, carious teeth are extracted before starting radiation owing to the radiation-induced dental decay and increased risk of osteoradionecrosis.

Short-term side effects of radiation, lasting up to 6 weeks after the conclusion of therapy, include mucositis, odynophagia, dysphagia, skin and erythema, altered taste, and edema. Common long-term side effects include varying degrees of xerostomia, fibrosis, and edema. Uncommon side effects include hypothyroidism, chondroradionecrosis, and osteoradionecrosis. As noted previously, an exceedingly rare complication is radiation-induced sarcoma.

3. Chemotherapy for larynx cancer—Chemotherapy had not traditionally been part of larynx cancer primary treatment protocols. Starting in the 1980s, organ-preserving protocols using chemotherapy in conjunction with radiation for advanced-stage laryngeal cancer have been compared with standard surgery and radiation treatment. Comparable survival rates have been shown with differing treatment morbidities. In general, lowered rates of distant metastasis are seen, although questionably higher rates of local recurrence are also cited in comparison with surgery and locoregional radiation protocols.

Cisplatin and 5-fluorouracil are the two agents found to be the most effective against larynx cancer. Recently, paclitaxel (Taxol) and docetaxel (Taxotere) have demonstrated activity without the side effects of cisplatin, which include neurotoxicity, ototoxicity, and renal toxicity. Chemotherapy has been given in the neoadjuvant (induction) setting concurrent with radiation and also in the adjuvant setting. Even though successes have been reported for all three approaches, concurrent chemoradiation has generally been deemed the most successful. Trials with neoadjuvant and concurrent intra-arterial chemotherapy have shown excellent local tumor response in selected cases, but with enhanced local toxicity.

Cisplatin is the most commonly used agent in concurrent protocols. Agents, such as amifostine, are being used to mitigate side effects and preserve salivary function in the setting of radiation.

Chemotherapy may also be used for the palliation of advanced larynx cancer. Once again, cisplatin is the preferred agent, but methotrexate was historically used with some benefit.

Chemotherapy is not considered a first-line treatment or standard of care for early-stage (Stages I and II) larynx cancer.

F. COMPLICATIONS OF TREATMENT

The complications of larynx cancer reflect the treatment modality (or modalities) used.

1. Vocal problems—Hoarseness may complicate any treatment of larynx cancer, even the smallest larynx cancer. Voice changes can be as subtle as the loss of vocal range, vocal fatigue, and lowered threshold for bouts of laryngitis. Deepening of the voice or a raspy, rough quality of the voice is common. Failure to achieve tracheoesophageal

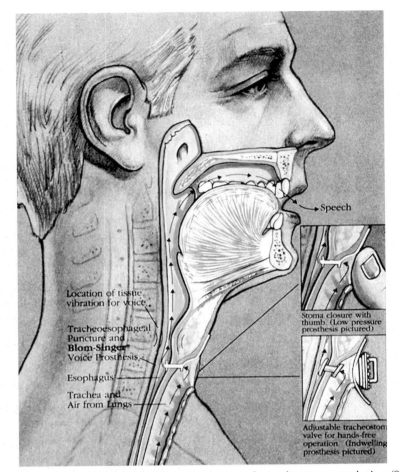

Figure 30–15. Tracheoesophageal speech requires a prosthesis and a tracheostoma occlusion. (Reprinted, with permission, InHealth Technologies, Carpinteria, CA.)

speech after a total laryngectomy can be due to hypertonicity or stricture of the neopharyngeal segment, an inappropriately positioned voice prosthesis, problems with digital occlusion of the stoma, or other neurologic impairment.

2. Swallowing problems—After partial laryngectomy procedures, aspiration risk is significant. This can be due to surgical removal or to denervation, in whole or in part, of the protective mechanisms of the larynx. Acute side effects of radiation include mucositis, thick secretions, odynophagia, and edema, which all contribute to swallowing difficulties in the immediate peri-radiation period. Xerostomia is a long-term side effect of radiation that also contributes to dysphagia. Stricture, stenosis, or fibrosis of the pharyngoesophageal segment as a result of surgical scarring or as a residual effect of radiation can lead to intolerance of solid foods or an inability to take adequate nutrition by mouth.

3. Loss of taste and smell—Radiation can permanently damage taste buds, although this side effect is often transient. After total laryngectomy, anatomic changes result in a lack of airflow through the nose and mouth. This severely changes the patient's sense of smell and, therefore, the sense of taste.

4. Fistula development—A fistula, or connection between the pharynx and skin of the neck, reflects the failure of the pharyngeal surgical closure to seal after laryngectomy. This results in the leakage of saliva and pharyngeal contents (including food) into the neck. When this initial fluid collection ruptures, leakage of mucoid and fluid material occurs onto the skin. Fistulas are more prone to occur in patients who have undergone previous radiation (up to 35% more likely) or surgery, and in those in whom the pharyngeal closure is tight. A fistula is more likely to occur if the nutritional status of the patient is poor (common) and may reflect a residual underlying cancer. Most fistulas close by secondary intention with conservative management, including feeding through a nasogastric or gastrostomy tube. Occasionally, surgical closure with a flap is advisable for vascular protection, for control of infection, or for facilitation of the delivery of indicated postoperative adjuvant therapy.

5. Airway problems—Some patients undergoing partial laryngectomy procedures are left with either an inadequate laryngeal airway or significant aspiration; for these reasons, they remain dependent on tracheotomy tubes. Excessive laryngeal edema can also happen as a sequela of radiation treatment alone. For patients who undergo a total laryngectomy, excessive secretions and crusting mucus can occlude the tracheostoma. Patients who undergo total laryngectomy often have an increased air temperature sensitivity, which manifests by cough; the lack of airway protection may also result in increased risk of aspiration and drowning.

6. Cranial nerve injury—During the surgical dissection for a partial or total laryngectomy with neck dissection, cranial nerves VII (the marginal mandibular branch), IX, X, XI, and XII are encountered and are therefore at risk for potential injury. Injury can be temporary or permanent. Preoperatively, patients need to be counseled about the following potential postoperative complications: asymmetric smile and mouth closure, swallowing difficulties, hoarseness and aspiration, shoulder drop and range-of-motion limitation, hoarseness, and the impairment of tongue mobility. Similarly, patients with aggressive larynx tumors with neck extension or locoregional metastases may present with or develop these cranial nerve deficits because of tumor involvement of the nerve.

7. Vascular injuries and events—Stroke is a risk of laryngectomy and neck dissection, but occurs surprisingly infrequently. A long-term sequela of radiation to the neck is acceleration of carotid atherosclerosis, and patients who have undergone radiation to the neck have a greater risk for stroke because of this.

In advanced tumors with necrosis and the resulting exposure of the carotid artery or the internal jugular vein, rupture (a carotid or jugular "blowout") is a risk. In cases of sentinel bleeds, angiographic embolization or stenting can prevent or stave off further bleeding. Flap coverage with vascularized tissue, when feasible, can protect against further bleeding. For patients who do experience a carotid blowout, the incidence of major debilitating stroke is > 50% in attempts at surgical salvage. Surgical salvage consists of ligating the carotid artery or more rarely attempting bypass. Major vessel rupture is otherwise a commonly fatal event.

8. Dropped shoulder—Injury to the spinal accessory nerve during neck dissection results in a loss of trapezius muscle function, an inability to abduct the arm past 90°, and downward and inward rotation of the shoulder. These limitations can also occur as a result of

primary tumor or neck metastases involving the spinal accessory nerve. Patients complain of a loss of shoulder function and pain. With intensive physical therapy, these deficits and pain can be overcome by increasing the strength of the other muscles of the shoulder girdle.

9. Tissue fibrosis—Because of radiation and surgery, which are augmented by the loss of the function of cranial nerve XI (when it occurs), larynx cancer patients often experience significant fibrosis of neck tissues. This manifests by stiffening, loss of range of motion, and pain. Fibrosis of the larynx and ankylosis of the cricoarytenoid joint have also been observed as a result of radiation treatment, leading to bilateral vocal cord immobility many years after the treatment.

10. Hypothyroidism—A loss of thyroid function can occur as a result of radiation to the lower anterior neck from a thyroidectomy done as part of laryngectomy, devascularization, or as a combined result of both. Hypothyroidism may not become apparent clinically or by serum tests until 6–12 months (or longer) after the completion of treatment for larynx cancer. Severe hypofunction may be responsible for poor healing of flaps and fistulas. For this reason, thyroid function tests should be performed periodically. Replacing the thyroid hormone with appropriately titrated doses of enteral thyroxin is curative, but requires periodic monitoring.

11. Other complications—Other risks of laryngectomy include hematoma and infection.

G. Long-Term Clinical Follow-Up

Patients with larynx cancer should be followed up clinically in the same manner in which patients with cancer of the head and neck are generally followed up. After treatment is completed, routine office visits are scheduled at 4- to 6-week intervals. During these visits, a complete head and neck examination is performed, focusing on the primary site for signs of recurrence, but also screening for metachronous primary malignant lesions. So-called "second" primary lesions have an annual incidence of 4–7%. After the first year, visits can extend to every 2 months during the second year, every 3 months during the third and fourth years, and every 6–12 months thereafter. Most recurrences of head and neck cancer occur within the first 2 years after treatment. Individuals are considered to be cured of their index primary after 5 years of disease-free status. The signs and symptoms of recurrence are the same as those of the initial presentation, including hoarseness, dysphagia, otalgia, hemorrhage, cervical adenopathy, and pain. The findings of the physical examination, the evaluation for metastases, and the diagnostic tests are the same for recurrences as they were for the original occurrence.

Ambrosch P, Kron M, Steiner W. Carbon dioxide laser microsurgery for early supraglottic carcinoma. *Ann Otol Rhinol Laryngol.* 1998;107(8):680. [PMID: 9716871] (Results of patients treated with laser microsurgery for early-stage supraglottic carcinoma showing comparable results to open supraglottic laryngectomy and superior functional results.)

Back G, Sood S. The management of early laryngeal cancer: options for patients and therapists. *Curr Opin Otolaryngol Head Neck Surg.* 2005;13(2):85. [PMID: 15761281] (Study to evaluate the different treatment modalities for early laryngeal cancer.)

Bernier J, Domenge C et al. Postoperative irradiation with or without concomitant chemotherapy for locally advanced head and neck cancer. *N Engl J Med.* 2004;350:1945. [PMID: 15128894] (Study showing that the addition of concurrent chemotherapy to adjuvant radiation improves local control in selected patients with high-risk squamous cell carcinoma who have primary surgical treatment.)

Chao KS, Majhail N, Huang CJ et al. Intensity modulated radiation therapy reduces late salivary toxicity without compromising tumor control in patients with oropharyngeal carcinoma: a comparison with conventional techniques. *Radiother Oncol.* 2001;61(3):275. [PMID: 11730977] (Series illustrating the efficacy of intensity-modulated radiation therapy in sparing salivary flow in patients with head and neck cancer without compromising tumor control.)

Cooper JS, Pajak TF et al. Postoperative concurrent radiotherapy and chemotherapy for high risk squamous cell carcinoma of the head and neck. *N Engl J Med.* 2004;350:1937. [PMID: 15128893] (Study showing that the addition of concurrent chemotherapy to adjuvant radiation improves local control in selected patients with high-risk squamous cell carcinoma who have primary surgical treatment.)

Dilkes MG et al. Treatment of primary mucosal head and neck squamous cell cancer using photodynamic therapy: results after 25 treated cases. *J Laryngol Otol.* 2003;117(9):713. [PMID: 14561360] (Study demonstrating the efficacy of Foscan, a photosensitizer, in the treatment of a variety of primary mucosal head and neck cancers.)

Forastiere A, Goepfert H, Maor M et al. Concurrent chemotherapy and radiotherapy for organ preservation in laryngeal cancer. *N Engl J Med.* 2003;349(22):2091. [PMID: 14645636] (Trial establishing concurrent chemoradiation as the superior to sequential chemoradiation for locally advanced larynx cancer. Concurrent therapy is now the mainstay of treatment.)

Galli J, De Corso E, Volante M et al. Postlaryngectomy pharyngocutaneous fistula: incidence, predisposing factors, and therapy. *Otolaryng Head Neck Surg.* 2005;133(5):689. [PMID: 16274794] (Study evaluating the predisposing factors, incidence, and management of pharyngocutaneous fistula.)

Gallo A, Manciocco V, Simonelli M et al. Supracricoid partial laryngectomy in the treatment of laryngeal cancer: univariate and multivariate analysis of prognostic factors. *Arch Otolaryngol Head Neck Surg.* 2005;131(7):620. [PMID: 16027286] (Study evaluating the results of supracricoid laryngectomy in the treatment of glottic and supraglottic cancers, showing that it is effective in maintaining laryngeal functions while achieving a high rate of local control.)

Krengli M, Policarpio, Manfredda I et al. Voice quality after T1a glottic carcinoma. *Acta Oncologica.* 2004;33(3):284. [PMID: 15244235] (Study examining the functional outcome of patients treated with radiation or CO_2 laser excision and shows that radiation results in superior voice quality.)

Laccourreye O, Hans S, Borzog-Grayeli A, Maulard-Durdux C, Brasnu D, Housset M. Complications of postoperative radiation therapy after partial laryngectomy in supraglottic cancer: a long term evaluation. *Otolaryngol Head Neck Surg.* 2000;122(5):752. [PMID: 10793360] (Series examining complications and functional status of patients treated with partial laryngectomy and postoperative radiation therapy.)

Mortuaire G, Francois J, Wiel E, Chevalier D. Local recurrence after CO_2 laser cordectomy for early glottic carcinoma. *Laryngoscope.* 2006;116(1):101. [PMID: 16481819] (Study evaluating the prognostic factors of local recurrence after endoscopic cordectomies.)

Patel S, See A, Williamson P et al. Radiation induced sarcoma of the head and neck. *Head Neck.* 1999;21(4):346. [PMID: 10376755] (Series illustrating the incidence of delayed sarcoma development in patients treated with definitive radiation therapy for cancer of the head and neck.)

Paydarfar JA, Birkmeyer NJ. Complications in head and neck surgery: a meta-analysis of postlaryngectomy pharyngocutaneous fistula. *Arch Otolaryngol Head Neck Surg.* 2006;132(1):67. [PMID: 16415432] (Paper summarizing the risk factors for postlaryngectomy pharyngocutaneous fistula.)

Peretti G, Piazza C, Bolzoni A. Endoscopic management for early glottic cancer: indications and oncologic outcome. *Otolaryngol Clin North Am.* 2006;39(1):173. [PMID: 16469662] (Review of the indications and outcome for endoscopic management of early glottic cancer.)

Pfister DG, Laurie SA, Weinstein GS et al. American Society of Clinical Oncology Clinical Practice Guideline for the Use of Larynx-Preservation Strategies in the Treatment of Laryngeal Cancer. *J Clin Oncol.* 2006. [PMID: 16832122] (American Society of Clinical Oncology guidelines for treatment of laryngeal cancer.)

Prepageran N, Raman R. Delayed complication of radiotherapy: Laryngeal fibrosis and bilateral vocal cord immobility. *Med J Malaysia.* 2005;60(3):377. [PMID: 16379198] (Case report of bilateral vocal cord immobility many years after treatment with radiation.)

Schweitzer VG. Photofrin-mediated photodynamic therapy for treatment of early stage oral cavity and laryngeal malignancies. *Lasers Surg Med.* 2001;29(4):305. [PMID: 11746107] (Review of larynx and oral cavity carcinomas either not amenable to or failing conventional treatment in which photodynamic therapy demonstrated high rates of complete response and cure with minimal side effects.)

Sessions DG, Lenox J, Spector GJ. Supraglottic laryngeal cancer: analysis of treatment results. *Laryngoscope.* 2005;115(8):1402. [PMID: 16094113] (Study analyzing the results of different management strategies for supraglottic laryngeal cancer.)

Sigston E, de Mones E, Babin E et al. Early stage glottic cancer: oncological results and margins in laser cordectomy. *Arch Otolaryngol Head Neck Surg.* 2006;132(2):147. [PMID: 16490871] (Study assessing the local control of laser cordectomies compared with external partial laryngectomy procedures in the treatment of early-stage glottic cancers.)

Strome SE, Weinman EC. Advanced larynx cancer. *Curr Treat Options Oncol.* 2002;3(1):11. [PMID: 12057083] (Review of treatment philosophy and options for advanced larynx cancer.)

Terrell J, Fisher S, Wolf G. Long term quality of life after treatment of laryngeal cancer. *Arch Otolaryngol Head Neck Surg.* 1998;124: 964. [PMID: 9738814] (Study examining the quality of life in patients who enrolled in the VA larynx study with findings of superior results in those who had preserved larynges.)

Table 30–4A. Larynx cancer: 5-year survival rates by stage.

Stage I – > 95%
Stage II – 85–90%
Stage III – 70–80%
Stage IV – 50–60%
All Stages – 68%

Urba S, Wolf G, Eisbruch A et al. Single-cycle induction chemotherapy selects patients with advanced laryngeal cancer for combined chemoradiation: a new treatment paradigm. *J Clin Oncol.* 2006;24(4):593. [PMID: 16380415] (Study comparing primary chemoradiation with radiation alone or conventional laryngectomy in the treatment of advanced laryngeal cancer.)

Wolf GT. Induction chemotherapy plus radiation compared with surgery plus radiation in patients with advanced laryngeal cancer: The Department of Veterans Affairs Laryngeal Cancer Study Group. *N Engl J Med.* 1991;324:1685. [PMID: 2034244] (Study showing that survival with chemotherapy and radiation was equivalent to surgery in lo-

Table 30–4B. Larynx cancer: 5-year survival rates by site and stage.

Supraglottis	Glottis	Subglottis
Stage I – 53–82%	Stage I – 74–100%	All Stages – 36–42%
Stage II – 50–64%	Stage II – 64–76%	
Stage III – 50–60%	Stage III – 50–60%	
Stage IV – < 50%	Stage IV – 30–57%	

cally advanced larynx cancer, thus establishing the organ preservation as the mainstay of treatment.)

Zacharek MA, Pasha R, Meleca RJ et al. Functional outcomes after supracricoid laryngectomy. *Laryngoscope.* 2001;111(9):1558. [PMID: 11568604] (Report of adequate voice and swallowing at 5-year follow-up on 10 patients who underwent supracricoid laryngectomy.)

Zhang B, Xu ZG, Tang PZ. Elective neck dissection for laryngeal cancer in the clinically negative neck. *J Surg Oncol.* 2006;93(6):464. [PMID: 16615158] (Study evaluating the efficacy of a lateral neck dissection in the elective treatment of the clinically negative necks in patients with laryngeal cancer.)

Prognosis

Cure for larynx cancer, defined as 5-year disease-free survival, is generally better than for other primary site tumors of the upper aerodigestive tract (Table 30–4). This reflects the prevalence of primary glottic tumors over primary supraglottic tumors and the early stage at which glottic tumors are diagnosed. Persistent hoarseness is one indication for which an individual will seek clinical care usually before the emergence of nodal metastasis. Nonetheless, 5-year survival rates have not improved over the last three decades despite advances in surgical technique, the expansion of treatment options, and decrease in morbidity.

Ganly I, Patel SG, Matsuo J et al. Results of surgical salvage after failure of definitive radiation therapy for early-stage squamous cell carcinoma of the glottic larynx. *Arch Otolaryngol Head Neck Surg.* 2006;132(1):59. [PMID: 16415431] (Study reporting the results of partial or total laryngectomy for recurrent or persistent laryngeal cancer after definitive radiotherapeutic treatment.)

Vocal Cord Paralysis

31

Michael Wareing, FRCS (ORL-HNS), & Rupert Obholzer, MRCS

True vocal cord paralysis signifies loss of active movement of the "true" vocal cord, or vocal fold, secondary to disruption of the motor innervation of the larynx. Disruption of innervation may occur along the length of the recurrent laryngeal nerves and the vagi and may include damage to the motor nuclei of the vagus. It should be differentiated from fixation of the vocal cord secondary to direct infiltration of the vocal fold, larynx, or laryngeal muscles. It should also be distinguished from fixation at the cricoarytenoid joint, encountered with rheumatoid arthritis or following traumatic intubation.

The site of disruption of the nerve supply leads to a characteristic pattern in the position of the vocal cords. However, distinguishing between recurrent laryngeal nerve paralysis and vocal cord paralysis secondary to disruption of the vagus nerve can be difficult.

Table 31–1 summarizes the main causes of vocal cord paralysis in adults. Once the cause of the vocal cord paralysis is ascertained, the next stage is to consider the rehabilitation and treatment of the patient depending on his or her symptoms.

■ ANATOMY

The relevant anatomy of the larynx is best understood in terms of the muscles producing abduction and adduction of the vocal cords and their nerve supply. All of the intrinsic laryngeal muscles, except the cricothyroid muscle, which is supplied by the external branch of the superior laryngeal nerve, are supplied by the recurrent laryngeal nerve. The sole abductor of the vocal cords is the posterior cricoarytenoid muscle. Table 31–2 provides a summary of the relevant laryngeal musculature and their innervation.

To understand the causes of vocal cord paralysis, it is important to understand the pathways of the vagus and recurrent laryngeal nerves. The course of the vagi in both sides of the head and neck are identical, but the recurrent laryngeal nerves differ significantly in their course once they leave the vagus.

The nuclei lie in the upper medulla and give rise to 8–10 rootlets that lie between the glossopharyngeal nerve superiorly and the spinal root of the accessory nerve inferiorly. The muscles of the pharynx, upper esophagus, larynx, and palate are all supplied by motor fibers originating in the nucleus ambiguus. Most of these fibers join the vagus at the inferior cervical ganglion below the jugular foramen, from the cranial root of the accessory nerve.

The vagus leaves the cranial cavity via the jugular foramen with the glossopharyngeal and hypoglossal nerves. It then descends vertically in the neck within the carotid sheath, adherent to the internal carotid artery, lying deep between the internal jugular vein and the artery itself.

The right vagus enters the thorax crossing superficial to the right subclavian artery. The right recurrent laryngeal nerve then leaves the vagus, curling underneath the artery to run superiorly in the tracheoesophageal groove and pass under the inferior constrictor of the pharynx, into the larynx.

The left vagus enters the thorax deep to the left brachiocephalic vein, between the carotid and subclavian arteries. The left recurrent laryngeal nerve leaves the vagus as it crosses the aortic arch, and then passes under the ligamentum arteriosum before taking a similar course to the right recurrent laryngeal nerve.

■ PATIENT EVALUATION

The initial evaluation of any patient presenting with dysphonia must include a systemic voice assessment (see Chapter 29). A thorough history must be taken, noting the onset and duration of the dysphonia. A detailed medical and surgical history is particularly important. The examination must include a full ear, nose, and throat examination as well as a detailed inspection of the vocal cords and larynx (see Chapter 29) to rule out an associated infiltrating lesion. This lesion can produce fixation of the vocal fold, which may be missed with a mirror examination. Although difficult to distinguish clinically, if unilateral or bilateral vocal cord paralysis secondary to high disruption of the vagus nerve can be ascertained

Table 31–1. Etiology of vocal cord paralysis in adults.

Type of Paralysis	Etiology
Unilateral recurrent	Neoplasia
Laryngeal	Iatrogenic causes
	Trauma
	Aneurysms
	Idiopathic causes
Bilateral recurrent	Post-thyroid surgery
Laryngeal	Thyroid neoplasia
Unilateral vagal	Iatrogenic causes
	Neoplasia
	Neurologic causes
	Brainstem infarction
	Skull base
	Osteomyelitis
	Idiopathic causes
Bilateral vagal	Neurologic causes

Table 31–2. Summary of innervation of the vocal cord.

Muscle	Nerve
Adductors (lateral cricoarytenoid, thyroarytenoid, interarytenoids)	Recurrent laryngeal (adductor branch)
Posterior cricoarytenoid	Recurrent laryngeal (abductor branch)
Cricothyroid	External laryngeal

- *Unilateral paramedian vocal fold paralysis.*
- *Voice may tire with use.*

General Considerations

The initial stage in evaluating a unilateral vocal cord paralysis is to establish whether the paralysis is secondary to a recurrent laryngeal nerve injury or to disruption of the vagus nerve. Lesions producing the characteristic paramedian vocal cord palsy are found below the origin of the superior laryngeal nerve. The paralyzed vocal cord is found in the paramedian position owing to the unopposed action of the cricothyroid muscle (Figure 31–1). Left vocal cord paralysis is more common than paralysis of the right vocal cord because of the longer and more convoluted course of the left recurrent laryngeal nerve. The right vocal cord is involved in 3–30% of cases.

Most unilateral vocal cord paralyses are secondary to surgery; therefore, the relative timing of the onset of the dysphonia to any relevant surgery is crucial.

Etiology

The causes of unilateral recurrent laryngeal paralysis can be iatrogenic (eg, following thyroid, esophageal, cervical spine, and thoracic surgery). It can also be caused by a primary and secondary lung carcinoma or a malignant

after inspecting the vocal cords, a full examination of the other cranial nerves should be instituted.

Laryngeal electromyography may be helpful in distinguishing between denervation of the intrinsic muscles and vocal cord fixation. It may also estimate the prognosis relative to reinnervation.

Koufman JA, Postma GW, Whang CS et al. Diagnostic laryngeal electromyography: the Wake Forest experience 1995-1999. *Otolaryngol Head Neck Surg.* 2001;124:603. [PMID: 11391248] (Evaluation of laryngeal electromyography in the management of vocal cord paralysis.)

Simpson CB, Fleming DJ. Medical and vocal history in the evaluation of dysphonia. *Otolaryngol Clin North Am.* 2000;33:719. [PMID: 10918656] (Review of history taking in voice disorders.)

Sulica L, Blitzer A. Electromyography and the immobile vocal fold. *Otolaryngol Clin North Am.* 2004;3759. ISSN: 0030-6665.

■ UNILATERAL VOCAL CORD PARALYSIS

UNILATERAL RECURRENT LARYNGEAL PARALYSIS

 ESSENTIALS OF DIAGNOSIS

- *Dysphonia.*
- *"Bovine" cough.*

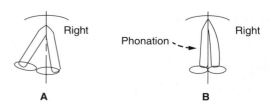

Figure 31–1. Right recurrent laryngeal nerve paralysis (dotted line = midline). **(A)** At rest, the paralyzed cord takes up a paramedian position. **(B)** On phonation.

tumor of the esophagus or thyroid. Aneurysms of the aorta or left atrial dilation (Ortner syndrome) and trauma may also contribute to the development of this palsy. The etiology may also be idiopathic.

Clinical Findings

A. SYMPTOMS AND SIGNS

The presenting symptoms associated with the dysphonia as well as the position of the vocal cords are the key to the underlying diagnosis. Patients present with dysphonia; their voices may become weak with use. It is important to question patients regarding respiratory symptoms such as cough, hemoptysis, and dyspnea, particularly in patients who smoke as these symptoms may indicate an underlying malignant chest neoplasm. Signs suggestive of underlying chest malignancy include evidence of clubbing, which is seen in patients with bronchogenic carcinoma; Horner syndrome; and a pleural effusion.

Vocal cord paralysis secondary to recurrent laryngeal nerve paralysis classically produces an immobile vocal cord in the paramedian position. Depending on the time of patient presentation after the development of dysphonia, the other vocal fold may compensate for the immobile one, thus limiting the degree of hoarseness experienced.

B. IMAGING STUDIES

For patients with recurrent laryngeal nerve palsy, accurate imaging of the neck and chest must be performed; the first sign of a malignant chest neoplasm may be recurrent laryngeal nerve palsy. A chest CT should identify an intrathoracic cause. If negative, an MRI of the neck and posterior fossa should be performed (as in practice it is often difficult to distinguish between vagal and recurrent laryngeal nerve palsy). If still negative, an endoscopy including bronchoscopy should be considered.

Treatment

A. NONSURGICAL MEASURES

Expectant treatment is recommended when there is no underlying malignant growth. Most unilateral cord palsies compensate within 6–18 months. Patient age, occupation, and preference as to how aggressively the vocal cord paralysis should be treated should all influence the treatment plan.

B. SURGICAL MEASURES

Among the surgical treatments available, the two primary surgical measures are injection laryngoplasty and laryngeal framework surgery.

1. Injection laryngoplasty—Injection laryngoplasty uses calcium hydroxylapatite, absorbable gelatin paste

(ie, Gelfoam paste), Bioplastique, or fat. The substance is injected laterally into the vocal fold to displace it medially. The use of calcium hydroxylapatite in this context is a recent development and appears to generate minimal tissue reaction and produce a long-lasting result. Gelfoam paste is useful in restoring vocal function in patients whose recovery is expected and who use their voices on a professional basis. Gelfoam injection can be repeated, if necessary. Fat is a useful alternative to Gelfoam and can also be repeated. Teflon has gone out of fashion.

Hughes RGM, Morrison M. Vocal cord medialization by transcutaneous injection of calcium hydroxylapatite. *J-Voice.* 2005; 19:674. ISSN: 0892-1997.

2. Laryngeal framework surgery—Laryngeal framework surgery (in the form of thyroplasty) involves the placement of a Silastic implant lateral to the vocal fold via a window cut in the thyroid cartilage. The Silastic displaces the vocal fold medially, ensuring adequate glottic closure.

UNILATERAL COMPLETE VAGAL PARALYSIS

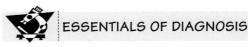 **ESSENTIALS OF DIAGNOSIS**

- *Weak, breathy hoarseness.*
- *Possible history of aspiration.*
- *Site of injury above the origin of the superior laryngeal nerve.*
- *Vocal cord in lateralized intermediate position.*

General Considerations

During the evaluation of a unilateral high vagal palsy, it is important to establish whether the site of damage to the nerve is at the skull base, the brainstem, or the cerebrum. Because of the inevitable loss of superior laryngeal nerve function, there is a decreased sensation of the larynx above the vocal cords on the affected side and a loss of cricothyroid muscle function. This loss of vagal nerve function leads to the paralyzed cord lying more laterally in the intermediate, or cadaveric, position (Figure 31–2).

Etiology

The origins of unilateral complete vagal paralysis include (1) iatrogenic causes (eg, skull base surgery), (2) neurologic causes (eg, multiple sclerosis, syringomyelia, and

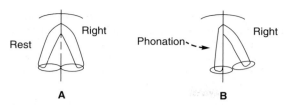

Figure 31–2. Right vagal nerve paralysis. **(A)** At rest, the paralyzed cord takes up an intermediate position. **(B)** On phonation.

encephalitis), (3) a brainstem infarction (eg, Wallenberg syndrome), (4) a malignant growth (primary or secondary), and (5) inflammation (eg, skull base osteomyelitis).

Clinical Findings

A. SYMPTOMS AND SIGNS

Disruption of the vagus nerve at the skull base or at the motor nucleus of the vagus inevitably results in the loss of unilateral supraglottic sensation; a history of aspiration may therefore be obtained. Compensation of the contralateral vocal cord is often inadequate, and consequently the patient's voice remains weak and breathy.

Lesions of the skull base or brainstem may involve other cranial nerves (eg, the hypoglossal or glossopharyngeal nerves). Unilateral brainstem involvement is uncommon.

B. LABORATORY FINDINGS

Depending on the history and pattern of cranial nerve involvement, it may be worthwhile to obtain inflammatory markers such as a C-reactive protein or ESR (erythrocyte sedimentation rate), particularly if the patient has no history of surgery.

C. IMAGING STUDIES

Imaging studies should adequately identify lesions of the skull base. MRI is the imaging modality of choice for the skull base because inflammatory changes on CT scans tend to present late and CT scanning does not image the brainstem satisfactorily.

Isotope bone scans may have use in patients who present with jugular foramen syndrome secondary to skull base osteomyelitis.

Treatment

Injection laryngoplasty is often unsuccessful in cases of complete vagal nerve paralysis because the relatively abducted position of the vocal cord leads to failure of injected materials to adequately displace the cord medially.

Medialization laryngoplasty, using silicone implants, is the optimal treatment method. Laryngoplasty may be combined with arytenoid adduction when the posterior glottic aperture is still not satisfactorily approximated. Most procedures are performed both to prevent aspiration and improve voice quality.

Anderson TD, Mirza N. Immediate percutaneous medialization for acute vocal fold immobility with aspiration. *Laryngoscope.* 2001;111:1318. [PMID: 11568562] (Efficacy of Gelfoam injection laryngoplasty.)

Carrau RL. Laryngeal framework surgery for the management of aspiration. *Head Neck.* 1999;21:139. [PMID: 10091982] (Medialization laryngoplasty with silicone, with or without arytenoid adduction.)

Hughes CA. Unilateral true vocal cord paralysis: cause of right-sided lesions. *Otolaryngol Head Neck Surg.* 2000;122:678. [PMID:10793345] (Etiology of right vocal cord palsy.)

Kriskovich MD. Vocal fold paralysis after anterior cervical spine surgery: incidence, mechanism, and prevention of injury. *Laryngoscope.* 2000;110:1467. [PMID: 10983944] (Incidence of 2–6%; mechanism due to compression of the nerve during retraction.)

Lo CY. A prospective evaluation of recurrent laryngeal nerve paralysis during thyroidectomy. *Arch Surg.* 2000;135:204. [PMID: 10668882] (0.9% of patients developed permanent unilateral vocal cord palsy.)

Msiung MW. Fat augmentation for glottic insufficiency. *Laryngoscope.* 2000;110:1026. [PMID: 10852525] (Fat injection laryngoplasty as an alternative to Gelfoam.)

Ramadan HH. Outcome and changing cause of unilateral vocal cord paralysis. *Otolaryngol Head Neck Surg.* 1998;118:199. [PMID: 9482553] (Surgical and neoplastic causes underlying the majority of vocal cord paralyses.)

■ BILATERAL VOCAL CORD PARALYSIS

BILATERAL RECURRENT LARYNGEAL NERVE PARALYSIS

 ESSENTIALS OF DIAGNOSIS

- *Often presents with stridor.*
- *Voice may be normal.*
- *Usually a history of thyroid surgery.*
- *Vocal cords fixed in median to paramedian position.*

General Considerations

The patient may have a recent history of thyroid surgery—usually total thyroidectomy. Rarely, an advanced

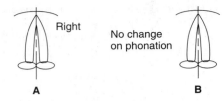

Figure 31–3. Bilateral recurrent laryngeal nerve paralysis (dotted line = midline). **(A)** At rest and **(B)** on phonation.

malignant thyroid tumor may be an underlying cause. If unrecognized, presentation may be late as normal voice production is possible because of the close approximation of the vocal cords (Figure 31–3).

Clinical Findings

A patient who presents with a bilateral recurrent laryngeal nerve palsy usually does so in an emergency situation, following the development of stridor. The patient may have been well previously, with an apparently normal voice, but developed airway decompensation after an upper respiratory tract infection. Because the vocal folds are adducted, minimal swelling may precipitate stridor.

Treatment

In an emergency situation, tracheostomy is often the only viable option. It is important to discuss with the patient the possible options for long-term treatment if decannulation is to be considered, since any operation to improve the airway may make the voice worse and increase the risk of aspiration. Some patients are happy maintaining their tracheostomy tube on a long-term basis and a fenestrated, cuffless tube is suitable in most cases.

Stitch lateralization of the vocal cord is an effective option during the recovery of nerve function because it prevents the need for a long-term tracheostomy. Partial or full recovery may occur in more than 50% of patients. The main operative procedure currently in practice is laser arytenoidectomy or unilateral or bilateral cordectomy.

Other lateralization procedures exist; however, though improving the airway, they carry the risk of increasing vocal impairment and aspiration.

BILATERAL COMPLETE VAGAL NERVE PARALYSIS

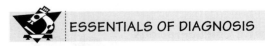

ESSENTIALS OF DIAGNOSIS

- *Weak voice.*
- *History of aspiration and choking.*
- *Vocal cords in intermediate position.*
- *Satisfactory glottic aperture at rest.*

General Considerations

Bilateral, high vagal, or brainstem involvement is unusual and often secondary to a neurologic cause. The complete loss of supraglottic sensation results in a significant risk of aspiration. Vagal paralysis is often accompanied by the involvement of other cranial nerves, typically the glossopharyngeal and hypoglossal nerves.

Etiology

Neurologic causes of bilateral complete vagal nerve paralysis include brainstem infarction, multiple sclerosis, and motor neuron disease (eg, amyotrophic lateral sclerosis [ALS]).

Clinical Findings

A. SYMPTOMS AND SIGNS

Patients present with either an acute or progressive onset of a weak, breathy voice associated with a history of choking and dysphagia. There may be a history of nasopharyngeal regurgitation. Patients are short of breath on exertion and may develop stridor in the presence of respiratory tract infection. The patient may be dysarthric and have signs of other cranial nerve involvement, such as paralysis of the tongue and loss of a gag reflex. Bilateral vagal nerve paralysis produces immobile vocal cords located in an intermediate position with a widened glottic aperture (Figure 31–4). There may be passive glottic closure on forced inspiration; therefore, it is important to correlate cord movement with the phase of respiration.

B. IMAGING STUDIES

Brainstem disease is best visualized with the aid of MRI scans.

Treatment

Treatment is directed at preventing aspiration and ensuring adequate nutrition. If stridor develops, which is often in the

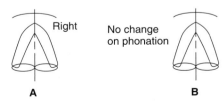

Figure 31–4. Bilateral vagal nerve paralysis. **(A)** At rest and **(B)** on phonation.

presence of an underlying pneumonia or upper respiratory tract infection, then a tracheostomy is usually required. A cuffed tracheostomy tube also helps to diminish aspiration. Long-term enteral nutrition via a percutaneous gastrostomy tube is often necessary. If the vocal cord paralysis is stable, then medialization techniques may be used.

Miyamoto RC, Parikh SR, Gellad W, Licameli GR. Bilateral congenital vocal cord paralysis: a 16-year institutional review. *Otolaryngol Head Neck Surg.* 2005;133:241. ISSN: 0194-5998.

Rovo L, Jori J, Brzozha M, Caigner J. Airway complications after thyroid surgery: minimally invasive management of bilateral recurrent nerve injury. *Laryngoscope.* 2000;110:140. [PMID: 10646730] (Stitch lateralization as an alternative treatment for bilateral recurrent laryngeal nerve palsy.)

Segas J, Stavroulakis P, Manolopoulos L, Yiotakis J, Adamopoulos G. Management of bilateral vocal cord paralysis: experience at the University of Athens. *Otolaryngol Head Neck Surg.* 2001;124:68. [PMID: 11228456] (Laser-assisted posterior cordectomy.)

Stridor in Children

32

Philip D. Yates, MB ChB, FRCS, & Shahram Anari, MD, MRCS

Stridor is a harsh noise produced by turbulent airflow through a partially obstructed airway. It may be inspiratory, expiratory, or both (biphasic). The term **stertor** is used to describe airway noise originating in the nose, nasopharynx, and oropharynx; therefore, stridor is generally of laryngeal or tracheal origin. As a general rule, **inspiratory stridor** originates from the supraglottis and glottis, **expiratory stridor** from the trachea, and **biphasic stridor** from the subglottis. There is a wide variety of causes of airway obstruction in children (Table 32–1). This chapter describes the more common laryngeal abnormalities that can cause stridor.

LARYNGOMALACIA

 ESSENTIALS OF DIAGNOSIS

- Intermittent, positional inspiratory stridor (usually mild).
- Gradual worsening of stridor followed by spontaneous resolution.
- Supraglottic collapse on inspiration.

General Considerations

Laryngomalacia is the most common cause of stridor in infants and is also the most common congenital laryngeal abnormality, accounting for approximately 60% of cases. Stridor occurs as a result of prolapse of the supraglottic structures into the laryngeal inlet on inspiration. The exact mechanism by which laryngomalacia develops is not completely understood. The epiglottis is classically described as being omega shaped and folded in upon itself so that the lateral margins lie close to each other (Figure 32–1). The aryepiglottic folds are tall, foreshortened, and thin, and the arytenoids are large with redundant mucosa. Mucosal edema resulting from repeated vibratory trauma to the supraglottis exacerbates the symptoms. Other factors that have been implicated in the etiology of laryngomalacia include abnormally pliable supraglottic cartilage, neuromuscular abnormalities, and gastroesophageal reflux.

Although most cases of laryngomalacia have a benign course without any long-term sequelae, the most severe cases, in which significant desaturation occurs, can result in significant morbidity, such as pulmonary hypertension and cor pulmonale.

The incidence of synchronous airway lesions associated with laryngomalacia has been reported in 12–45% of cases, although less than 5% of these cases require intervention.

Clinical Findings

A. SYMPTOMS AND SIGNS

Infants with laryngomalacia usually have no sign of respiratory abnormality at birth. Inspiratory stridor typically develops after a few days or weeks and is initially mild, but over the ensuing months becomes gradually more pronounced, usually peaking at the age of 6–9 months. Spontaneous improvement then occurs and symptoms usually completely resolve by the age of 18 months to 2 years of age, although persistent cases beyond age 5 have been reported. Stridor is not constantly present; rather, it is intermittent and variable in intensity. Typically, symptoms are worse during sleep, and positional variations occur; stridor is worse when the patient is in the supine position and is improved when the patient is prone. Both feeding and exertion tend to result in more pronounced stridor. Although an infant with laryngomalacia usually has a normal cry, stridor may be exacerbated by crying owing to a more forceful inspiratory effort. In most cases, symptoms are mild and self-limiting, but a small proportion of cases have severe stridor, apneic episodes, feeding difficulties, and failure to thrive.

Clinical examination of the patient may reveal no abnormality. If the infant is sleeping or crying, then stridor is more likely to be observed and its associated signs, such as tachypnea and intercostal and subcostal recessions, should be sought. Cyanosis is extremely unusual in laryngomalacia and should raise the suspicion of some other pathology.

B. EVALUATION

1. Endoscopy—The use of a flexible fiberoptic endoscope under local anesthesia has been suggested. This

Table 32–1. Causes of airway obstruction in infants and children.

	Congenital	Acquired
Supralaryngeal	Choanal atresia Craniofacial abnormalities Retrognathia Macroglossia	Adenotonsillar hypertrophy Foreign body Retropharyngeal abscess Ludwig's angina

Laryngeal	Laryngomalacia
	Laryngeal cysts
	Laryngeal webs
	Posterior laryngeal cleft
	Vocal cord paralysis
	Cricoarytenoid joint fixation
	Subglottic hemangioma
		Iatrogenic (surgical and intubation traumas)
		   Laryngeal webs
		   Subglottic stenosis
		Vocal cord paralysis
		Inflammatory
		   Epiglottitis
		   Laryngotracheobronchitis
		   Hereditary angioedema
		Neoplasms
		   Respiratory papillomatosis
		   Rhabdomyosarcoma
		External compression
		   Thyroid
		   Cystic hygroma
		Foreign bodies
		Burns (caustic and thermal)
		External trauma

Tracheal	Tracheobronchomalacia
	Stenosis
	Vascular compression
	   Aberrant innominate artery
	   Double aortic arch
	   Pulmonary artery sling
	Tracheal cysts
		Laryngotracheobronchitis
		Bacterial tracheitis
		Foreign bodies
		External compression
		   Thyroid
		   Cystic hygromas
		   Mediastinal tumors

procedure is safe and allows a dynamic assessment of the glottis and supraglottis and avoids the risks associated with general anesthesia.

2. Laryngotracheobronchoscopy—Laryngotracheobronchoscopy is often considered an essential study before a definitive diagnosis can be made in order to rule out any synchronous airway pathology.

3. Polysomnography—In severe cases, polysomnography can be performed to detect episodes of hypoxia or hypercapnia. The results of this study can influence the decision to undertake surgical management of the condition.

Treatment

In most patients, laryngomalacia is a self-limiting condition that does not result in any harm to the patient; therefore, observation is all that is required. In the most severe cases of laryngomalacia, which is encountered in a small percentage of patients, a temporary tracheotomy may be unavoidable.

Surgical intervention is indicated for approximately 10% of patients. The main indications for surgery are severe stridor, apnea, failure to thrive, pulmonary hypertension, and cor pulmonale. A variety of procedures have

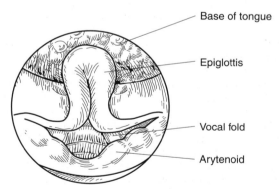

Figure 32–1. Appearance of the infantile larynx in laryngomalacia.

been described for the treatment of laryngomalacia (referred to as supraglottoplasty), which are largely aimed at reduction of the redundant laryngeal mucosa. These procedures include (1) division of the aryepiglottic folds, (2) excision of a wedge of the aryepiglottic fold with or without trimming the arytenoids or the lateral border of the epiglottis, and (3) suturing of the epiglottis to the base of the tongue. There is disagreement as to whether microdissection or laser surgery is the optimum treatment modality. Physicians who favor laser surgery contend that bleeding is less of a problem compared with microdissection; physicians who favor microdissection maintain that the risk of postoperative scarring is greater with the use of laser.

Complications of supraglottoplasty include bleeding, aspiration, and supraglottic scarring. The risk of supraglottic stenosis is lessened by excising the least amount of supraglottic mucosa to produce an improvement in symptoms. Scarring is particularly problematic in the interarytenoid region; therefore, an island of mucosa must be left in this area.

High rates of reflux have been demonstrated in patients with laryngomalacia, and it has therefore been implicated as a causative factor. However, the relationship remains unproven; hence the controversy in the antireflux medication for laryngomalacia.

Loke D, Ghosh S, Panarese A, Bull PD. Endoscopic division of the aryepiglottic folds in severe laryngomalacia. *Int J Pediatr Otorhinolaryngol.* 2001;60:59. [PMID: 11434955] (Presents results of simple division of the aryepiglottic folds for laryngomalacia, concluding that this is sufficient in all but the most severe cases.)

Masters IB, Chang AB, Patterson L et al. Series of laryngomalacia, tracheomalacia, and bronchomalacia disorders and their associations with other conditions in children. *Pediatr Pulmonol.* 2002;34(3):189. [PMID: 12203847] (Describes the association of respiratory malacia with other anomalies.)

Rosbe KW, Kenna MA, Auerbach AD. Extraesophageal reflux in pediatric patients with upper respiratory symptoms. *Arch Otolaryngol Head Neck Surg.* 2003;129(11):1213. [PMID: 14623753] (Review of the evidence for reflux in pediatric airway pathologies.)

LARYNGEAL CYSTS

Laryngeal cysts are a rare cause of stridor in infants. The two main types of laryngeal cysts are ductal and saccular cysts. **Ductal cysts** are more common and are thought to originate from obstruction of the submucous glands. They can arise anywhere in the larynx, but are most commonly found in the supraglottis. **Saccular cysts** arise in the laryngeal ventricle and are usually congenital in infants. Unlike laryngoceles, which usually present in adults, saccular cysts do not communicate with the laryngeal lumen.

The most common symptoms arising from laryngeal cysts are stridor, feeding difficulties, and cyanotic episodes. Laryngeal cysts can usually be managed by endoscopic de-roofing or excision.

VOCAL CORD PARALYSIS

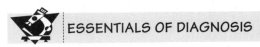

ESSENTIALS OF DIAGNOSIS

(1) Unilateral Vocal Cord Paralysis
- *Hoarse or breathy voice/cry.*
- *± Mild dyspnea, stridor, or both.*
- *± Aspiration.*
- *Spontaneous improvement or resolution.*

(2) Bilateral Vocal Cord Paralysis
- *Severe stridor.*
- *± Aspiration.*
- *Usually requires tracheotomy.*

General Considerations

Vocal cord paralysis in infants and children can be either congenital or acquired and either unilateral or bilateral. It is the second most common congenital abnormality of the larynx, accounting for approximately 10% of cases. Congenital vocal cord palsy is slightly more common in males and is more commonly bilateral.

There are many causes of acquired vocal cord palsy (Table 32–2), although most commonly the paralysis is idiopathic. Central nervous system (CNS) abnormalities usually result in bilateral vocal cord palsy. The most common congenital CNS abnormality resulting in vocal cord palsy is the Arnold-Chiari malformation. Acquired CNS causes of vocal cord paralysis are rare in infants and children, as are acquired peripheral neuropathies. Congenital abnormalities of the heart and great vessels may lead to vocal cord palsy, or the paralysis may result from surgery to correct these abnormalities. In this situation, the left side is more commonly affected because of the longer course of the left recurrent laryngeal nerve through the mediastinum. Rarely, esophageal surgery, such as repair of a tracheoesophageal fistula, can result in a bilateral palsy. Other traumatic causes of vocal cord paralysis include birth trauma, intubation, and head injury. Inflammatory conditions such as encephalopathies and Guillain-Barré usually produce bilateral vocal cord paralysis. Neoplastic causes of vocal cord palsy are rare in infants and children. Familial X-linked vocal cord paralysis has been reported, but is extremely rare.

Clinical Findings

A. SYMPTOMS AND SIGNS

The symptoms arising from vocal cord palsy vary widely. Patients may be asymptomatic, or they may have an acute

Table 32–2. Etiology of acquired vocal cord paralysis.

Idiopathic
Central nervous system
  Arnold-Chiari malformation
  Hydrocephalus
  Encephalocele
  Syringomyelia or syringobulbia
Peripheral nervous system
  Myasthenia gravis
  Myotonic dystrophy
  Charcot-Marie-Tooth disease
Trauma
  Surgical
  Head injury
  Endotracheal intubation
  Birth trauma
Neoplasia
  Thyroid carcinoma
Inflammatory
  Viral
  Bacterial
  Granulomatous
Cardiovascular anomalies
  Tetralogy of Fallot
  Cardiomegaly
  Patent ductus arteriosus
  Vascular rings

airway obstruction that requires emergency intervention. Patients with unilateral vocal cord palsy do not usually have signs of airway obstruction; therefore, stridor is not a common feature, although dyspnea may occur. More often the presenting features are a hoarse, breathy voice or cry and a weak cough. Feeding problems and aspiration are more likely to occur if the lesion is proximal to the superior laryngeal nerve since this nerve supplies sensation to the supraglottis. Bilateral vocal cord paralysis tends to have more pronounced symptoms such as stridor, apnea, and cyanosis; however, if the vocal cords lie in the intermediate position, then airway obstruction does not occur and aspiration is the primary problem.

B. Evaluation

If any doubt about the stability of the airway exists, then the patient should be evaluated in the operating room and the airway secured before further investigation is considered.

Although fiberoptic endoscopy can reliably demonstrate a vocal cord palsy, the airway needs to be assessed by laryngotracheobronchoscopy for two reasons: (1) The arytenoid cartilage must be palpated to exclude the rare finding of a fixed cricoarytenoid joint. (2) The possibility of synchronous pathology in the airway must be excluded.

If a cause is not apparent, then a magnetic resonance imaging (MRI) scan including the brain, brainstem, neck, and chest (the course of the vagus and recurrent laryngeal nerves) should be performed. In patients in whom aspiration is suspected, a contrast swallow or videofluoroscopy can provide information on deglutition and laryngeal penetration. Functional endoscopy evaluation of swallowing (FEES) is also used in the pediatric group.

Treatment

The function of the glottis is to protect the lungs from the aspiration of food while providing an adequate airway. A secondary, though important, function is to provide a voice. Management decisions are influenced by the underlying cause (if known), the severity of symptoms, and the likelihood of spontaneous recovery. Spontaneous recovery occurs more frequently in acquired than in congenital vocal cord palsy, and it is also more likely in unilateral than bilateral vocal cord palsy.

A. Unilateral Vocal Cord Paralysis

Most children with unilateral vocal cord paralysis have minimal symptoms because the normal vocal cord adopts a more medial position to compensate for the paralyzed vocal cord. If poor voice quality is persistent, then speech therapy is the preferred treatment. In the rare instance in which the airway is significantly compromised, tracheotomy is indicated. Successful decannulation without the need for further laryngeal surgery is usually possible as the larynx develops.

B. Bilateral Vocal Cord Paralysis

In children with bilateral vocal cord palsy, the vocal cords usually lie in the adducted position, which results in a compromised airway. This circumstance indicates that the majority of cases of bilateral vocal cord palsy will require a tracheotomy to maintain the airway. Once a tracheotomy has been performed, serial endoscopy should be planned to monitor any spontaneous recovery of vocal cord function. It is recommended that irreversible surgical procedures on the larynx are not considered for at least 1 year after a tracheotomy. Some otolaryngologists prefer to wait until the child is old enough to make his or her own decision about further surgery. The aim of surgery for permanent bilateral vocal cord palsy is to produce an airway of sufficient size to allow decannulation without compromising the protective function of the larynx or producing an unacceptable voice quality. Various surgical techniques have been described to accomplish this goal. Excisional techniques simply remove tissue from the glottis to produce an improved airway. Lateralization techniques mechanically fix the vocal cord in a more abducted position. Neuromuscular techniques partially reinnervate the intrinsic muscles of the larynx, particularly the posterior cricoarytenoid muscle, thereby restoring a degree of active abduction.

Brigger MT, Hartnick CJ. Surgery for pediatric vocal cord paralysis: a meta-analysis. *Otolaryngol Head Neck Surg.* 2002; 126(4):349. [PMID: 11997772] (Meta-analysis of current surgical treatments for bilateral vocal cord paralysis.)

Friedman EM, De Jong AL, Sulek M. Pediatric vocal fold immobility: the role of the carbon dioxide laser posterior transverse partial cordotomy. *Ann Otol Rhinol Laryngol.* 2001;110:723. [PMID: 11510728] (Describes an excisional surgical technique modified for use in pediatric patients with bilateral vocal cord palsy.)

Parikh SR. Pediatric unilateral vocal fold immobility. *Otolaryngol Clin North Am.* 2004;37(1):203. [PMID: 15062694] (General review of unilateral vocal cord palsy including the diagnosis and the management.)

CONGENITAL LARYNGEAL WEBS

Laryngeal webs are thought to arise from a failure of complete recanalization of the larynx in the embryo. Although webbing can occur at all levels in the larynx, it is most commonly seen in the anterior glottis. When webbing is severe, it is often associated with subglottic stenosis. Complete atresia of the larynx is extremely rare and requires immediate tracheotomy at birth.

The most common presenting symptoms are an abnormal cry and stridor. The diagnosis is made at endoscopy, and other airway abnormalities should be excluded. Small, thin webs usually respond to simple incision. More severe webbing may require an excision via a laryngofissure approach, with insertion of a stent.

POSTERIOR LARYNGEAL CLEFTS

A posterior laryngeal cleft is a rare congenital abnormality that occurs as a result of the failure of fusion of the posterior larynx and, in some cases, the trachea. The abnormality is classified according to the extent of the cleft (Figure 32–2). The predominant symptoms are hoarseness and aspiration; stridor is a rare feature. The severity of symptoms varies and depends on the extent of the abnormality. Type I clefts often have minimal symptoms, whereas Type IV clefts produce severe aspiration pneumonia and carry a poor prognosis even if surgical closure is attempted.

The diagnosis of posterior laryngeal clefts is made by demonstrating penetration of the larynx on contrast swallow, and the presence of a cleft is confirmed at endoscopy. Mild clefts may require no treatment other than the thickening of feeds; however, if aspiration persists, then endoscopic closure should be considered. More extensive clefts require surgical closure using either a lateral pharyngotomy or laryngofissure approach.

LARYNGEAL FOREIGN BODIES

Most inhaled foreign bodies pass through the larynx and trachea and become lodged distally. There is often a history of the child having something in the mouth, commonly a peanut, before the onset of symptoms. If a

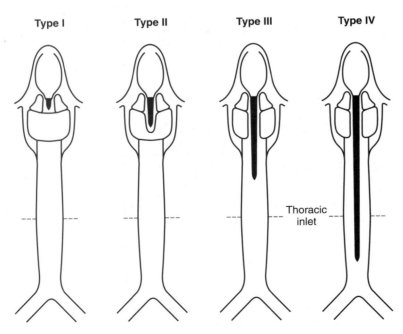

Figure 32–2. Classification of posterior laryngeal clefts. **Type I:** Interarytenoid cleft; superior to the glottis. **Type II:** Partial cricoid cleft; extends inferior to the glottis and partially through the posterior lamina of the cricoid. **Type III:** Total cricoid cleft, with or without extension into the cervical tracheoesophageal wall. **Type IV:** Laryngotracheoesophageal cleft extending beyond the thoracic inlet.

foreign body becomes lodged in the larynx and causes complete obstruction, it will cause sudden death unless removed immediately. If the airway is only partially obstructed, then stridor, hoarseness, and cough are the predominant symptoms. If the object is radiopaque, its site of impaction can be confirmed by x-ray. Removal under general anesthesia is generally required.

SUBGLOTTIC STENOSIS

 ESSENTIALS OF DIAGNOSIS

(1) Congenital Subglottic Stenosis
- *Stridor at birth, if moderate to severe stenosis.*
- *Intermittent stridor, associated with respiratory tract infections, if mild stenosis.*

(2) Acquired Subglottic Stenosis
- *Commonly as a consequence of prolonged endotracheal intubation.*

- *Presents with repeated failure of attempted extubation, or with gradual onset of stridor following extubation.*

General Considerations

The subglottis is the narrowest portion of the airway in children, and the cricoid cartilage is the only complete cartilaginous ring in the airway. Because airflow in a cylinder is directly proportional to the fourth power of the radius, even a slight reduction in the area of the subglottis can lead to significant obstruction.

The Myer-Cotton grading system describes the severity of stenosis according to the percentage of subglottic stenosis present (Figure 32–3). The percentage is calculated by measuring the largest sized endotracheal tube that can be passed through the subglottis and comparing this with the age-appropriate tube size for

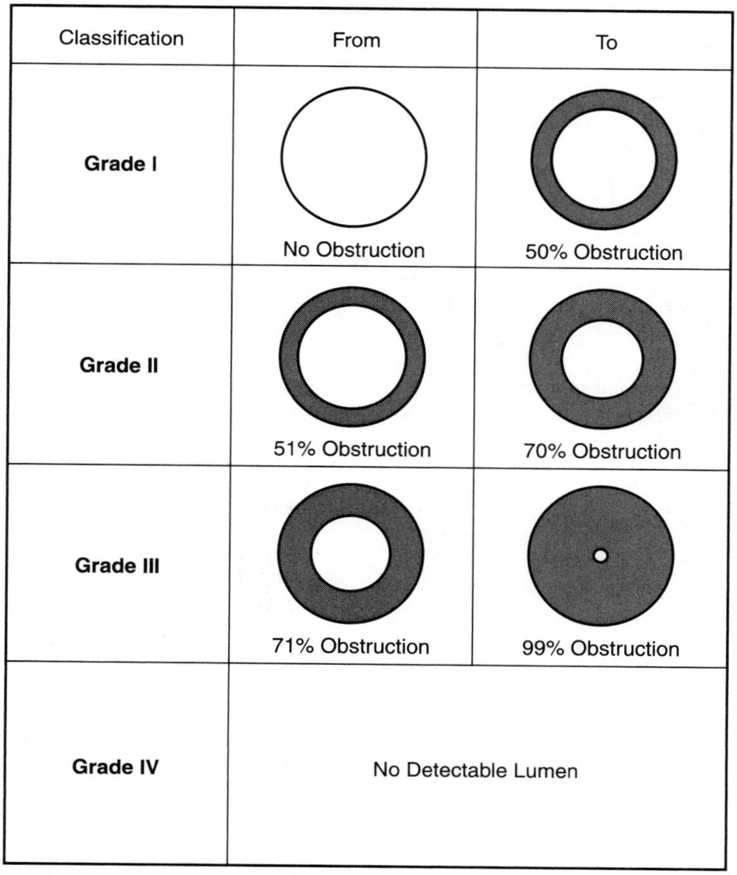

Classification	From	To
Grade I	No Obstruction	50% Obstruction
Grade II	51% Obstruction	70% Obstruction
Grade III	71% Obstruction	99% Obstruction
Grade IV	No Detectable Lumen	

Figure 32–3. Myer-Cotton grading system for subglottic stenosis.

the child. A subglottic diameter of ≤ 4 mm in a full-term neonate is considered to be abnormal.

Classification of Subglottic Stenosis

Subglottic stenosis can be either congenital or acquired. A diagnosis of congenital stenosis is made when there is absence of any factors that are known to lead to acquired stenosis and there is no previous documentation of a normal airway.

A. CONGENITAL SUBGLOTTIC STENOSIS

Congenital subglottic stenosis is considered to be the third most common congenital abnormality of the larynx. Its true incidence is not known since some patients diagnosed with acquired stenosis after endotracheal intubation may have had a mild preexisting congenital stenosis.

B. ACQUIRED SUBGLOTTIC STENOSIS

Acquired subglottic stenosis is much more common than congenital subglottic stenosis and is generally more severe and difficult to manage. The most common cause of acquired subglottic stenosis in children is endotracheal intubation trauma, accounting for approximately 90% of cases, although it can also occur as a result of surgical trauma, inflammation, external trauma, and thermal or chemical burns.

Pathogenesis

Subglottic stenosis secondary to endotracheal intubation is a result of pressure necrosis of the subglottic mucosa. The duration of intubation is the most important factor in the development of subglottic stenosis. Edema and ulceration occur followed by secondary infection and perichondritis. Granulation tissue then forms over the areas of perichondritis and the deposition of fibrous tissue results in stenosis. The role of gastroesophageal reflux in the pathogenesis of subglottic stenosis is not clear yet.

Prevention

The reported incidence of subglottic stenosis in children following endotracheal intubation ranges from 1% to 9%. This rate has fallen because of the introduction of preventive measures by pediatric intensive care units, although the reduction in incidence is somewhat offset by the increased survival of low birth weight infants requiring prolonged intubation. Factors that have reduced the incidence of subglottic stenosis include (1) the use of uncuffed, polyvinylchloride tubes; (2) the use of smaller tubes to reduce pressure on the subglottic mucosa; and (3) nasotracheal intubation, which produces better tube fixation and less frictional trauma.

Clinical Findings

A. SYMPTOMS AND SIGNS

The degree of stenosis dictates the severity of stridor. Severe congenital subglottic stenosis presents at birth with stridor and respiratory distress. Less severe stenosis is likely to present in the first few months of life when increased activity requires increased respiratory efforts. The subglottic edema produced by upper respiratory tract infections often precipitates stridor, which leads to misdiagnosis of recurrent laryngotracheobronchitis. In the case of acquired subglottic stenosis in neonates, the first indication may be a failed trial of extubation. Older children who sustain subglottic trauma may be successfully extubated, but gradually develop symptoms of respiratory distress over a period of weeks, as the fibrosis progresses.

B. EVALUATION

Lateral neck and chest x-rays may show a stenosis of the airway in the subglottic region; however, confirmation of the diagnosis requires laryngotracheobronchoscopy under general anesthesia. At this point, staging of the stenosis can be performed.

Treatment

The management of subglottic stenosis is dictated by the type of stenosis, the grade of stenosis, and the age and general condition of the patient. Surgical reconstruction is indicated when conservative efforts to establish a satisfactory airway are inappropriate or have failed.

A. OBSERVATION

In patients with minimal symptoms (Grade I or II), it may be possible to avoid surgical intervention with close observation and repeated endoscopies. This conservative approach ensures that the airway is increasing in dimension with the growth of the child.

B. TRACHEOTOMY

A tracheotomy is frequently performed in patients with symptomatic subglottic stenosis to ensure that the airway is safe until laryngeal reconstruction is planned. It allows time for weight gain and recovery from pulmonary disorders in preterm neonates.

C. ENDOSCOPIC TREATMENT

Endoscopic use of the laser is useful in the treatment of early intubation injuries, particularly for the removal of granulation tissue and mild stenosis. The disadvantage of laser use is that thermal damage can result in scarring and possible worsening of the stenosis in the long term.

D. ANTERIOR CRICOID SPLIT

This procedure is used primarily as an alternative to tracheotomy in premature infants with an acquired subglottic stenosis who have failed multiple extubation attempts. By dividing the cricoid cartilage and the first two tracheal rings anteriorly, the cricoid is able to expand, thereby improving the airway.

E. LARYNGOTRACHEAL RECONSTRUCTION

A variety of surgical techniques aimed at achieving an adequate airway have been described. Following laryngofissure, a cartilage graft can be inserted anteriorly, or both anteriorly and posteriorly. Conventionally, a stent is left in the larynx for a prolonged period until healing occurs; a tracheotomy is also required to maintain airway patency. Once a satisfactory laryngeal airway is achieved, decannulation can be considered. Single-stage laryngotracheal reconstruction has been introduced. Cartilage grafts are inserted, but endotracheal intubation is maintained for 7–10 days to stent the larynx, and a tracheotomy is not required. This technique avoids the complication of long-term stenting, but there is an increased potential risk to the airway in the perioperative period.

F. CRICOTRACHEAL RESECTION

In contrast to laryngotracheal reconstruction, which is designed to enlarge the stenosed portion of the larynx, cricotracheal resection excises the stenotic region. This procedure carries a higher rate of success, but a possible favorable outcome must be weighed against the potential complications of recurrent laryngeal nerve damage and dehiscence of the anastomosis.

Cotton RT. Management of subglottic stenosis. *Otolaryngol Clin North Am.* 2000;33:111. [PMID: 10637347] (Detailed review of the management of subglottic stenosis including a discussion on the role of gastroesophageal reflux.)

Hartley BEJ, Cotton RT. Pediatric airway stenosis: laryngotracheal reconstruction or cricotracheal reconstruction? *Clin Otolaryngol Allied Sci.* 2000;25:342. [PMID: 11012644] (Discussion of surgical procedures for subglottic stenosis with a description of the operative technique for cricotracheal resection.)

SUBGLOTTIC HEMANGIOMAS

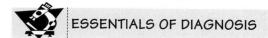 ESSENTIALS OF DIAGNOSIS

- Stridor in first 6 months of life.
- Commonly associated with cutaneous hemangioma.
- Progression of symptoms from intermittent to persistent.
- Vascular mass in subglottis.
- Spontaneous resolution over several years.

General Considerations

Hemangiomas can occur in any part of the larynx, but the subglottis is the most common site. Subglottic hemangiomas are typically unilateral, but they can also be circumferential or can arise from multiple sites. They are vascular hamartomas that are most commonly capillary in nature on histologic examination; however, cavernous or mixed types can also occur. Subglottic hemangiomas are rare, accounting for approximately 1.5% of all congenital laryngeal anomalies. **Cutaneous hemangiomas**, a relatively common congenital abnormality, are found in about half of patients with a subglottic hemangioma and are frequently found in the head and neck region. There is a female preponderance, being twice as common in females.

The natural progression of hemangiomas is from an initial proliferative phase to an involutional phase. The proliferative phase starts soon after birth and usually continues for 12 months, after which gradual involution occurs over a period of years. Most hemangiomas will have resolved by the age of 5 years.

Clinical Findings

A. SYMPTOMS AND SIGNS

Because hemangiomas do not start to proliferate until after birth, they rarely present in the first weeks of life, but 80–90% will have presented by the age of 6 months. Initially, when the lesion is small, inspiratory stridor is intermittently present. At this stage, symptoms may be exacerbated by upper respiratory tract infections, which may lead to an initial diagnosis of recurrent laryngotracheobronchitis. As the lesion enlarges, the stridor becomes biphasic, and dyspnea and cyanosis may occur. The cry is usually normal unless the hemangioma extends onto the vocal folds.

B. EVALUATION

The diagnosis of subglottic hemangioma may be suspected from the clinical presentation and reinforced by the finding of an asymmetric narrowing of the subglottis on lateral neck and chest x-rays. However, confirmation of the diagnosis requires laryngotracheobronchoscopy under general anesthesia. The typical finding on endoscopy is a unilateral, sessile, submucosal, compressible vascular lesion in the subglottis. The role of biopsy for histopathologic confirmation of the diagnosis is controversial, since it carries the risk of significant hemorrhage, although biopsy without associated bleeding is widely reported. Biopsy is generally reserved for those in which the diagnosis is uncertain.

In cases of a large cutaneous hemangioma in the neck associated with a hemangioma of the airway, further investigation with MRI is indicated since the lesions may be contiguous.

Treatment

Observation may be appropriate if the lesion is small and the symptoms are minimal. Most patients require a multimodality treatment. The aims of treatment are to overcome the airway obstruction while avoiding complications and long-term sequelae, particularly subglottic stenosis. A variety of treatment modalities are currently in use.

A. Tracheotomy

When tracheotomy is used as the sole treatment, decannulation is the ultimate aim. Decannulation can be attempted only when the airway is no longer compromised (as a result of the increased dimensions of the growing larynx and spontaneous involution of the hemangioma). Tracheotomy, however, is not without complications. Subglottic stenosis, in particular, is a recognized complication of tracheotomy and may require surgical intervention before decannulation can be achieved. If the hemangioma is large, there is a risk of complete airway obstruction if the tracheotomy tube becomes dislodged; therefore, skilled home care is required. There is also a significant effect on speech and language development, and multiple endoscopies are required to assess the stage of the airway. In view of these problems, treatment modalities have been developed to either expedite the possibility of decannulation or to avoid tracheotomy altogether.

B. Steroids

For the treatment of subglottic hemangiomas, steroids can be administered either systemically or by intralesional injection. It is not known how steroids accelerate the involution of hemangiomas, but it may be as a result of estrogen receptor blockade. Systemic steroids need to be used over a prolonged period, which may result in growth retardation, hypertension, and cushingoid appearance. The use of intralesional steroid injection aims to avoid these systemic side effects. However, local edema often results in an initial worsening of the airway, and if tracheotomy is to be avoided, then long-term intubation may be required until resolution of the edema has occurred. Repeated injections may be required before a satisfactory result is achieved.

C. Laser Therapy

Both the carbon dioxide (CO_2) and potassium titanyl phosphate (KTP) lasers have been used for the treatment of subglottic hemangioma. The advantage of using the laser is its hemostatic properties. This is par-

ticularly true of the KTP laser because the wavelength of light is better absorbed by vascular tissue. It may be possible to avoid tracheotomy with repeated laser treatment, but equally repeated treatment increases the risk of scarring and subsequent subglottic stenosis.

D. Surgical Excision

The surgical excision of subglottic hemangiomas has been reserved for the most severe cases or cases that do not respond to more conventional therapy. However, with the development of the single-stage laryngotracheoplasty in the management of subglottic stenosis, primary excision is likely to become more commonplace as the need for a tracheotomy is avoided.

E. Interferon

Interferon alfa-2a has antiangiogenic activity and is therefore effective as a treatment for hemangiomas in their proliferative phase. Its use is generally reserved for patients with multiple airway sites or extensive cervical disease with external compression of the airway. The early withdrawal of treatment during the proliferative phase may result in rapid rebound growth; therefore, treatment must be prolonged. Because of the unknown side effects of long-term treatment in children, interferon remains an option only in the most severe unresponsive cases.

Kacker A, April M, Ward RF. Use of potassium titanyl phosphate (KTP) laser in management of subglottic hemangioma. *Int J Pediatr Otorhinolaryngol.* 2001;59:15. [PMID: 11177013] (Discusses the results of KTP laser use for subglottic hemangiomas and compares the relative merits of CO_2 and KTP lasers.)

Rahbar R, Nicollas R, Roger G et al. The biology and management of subglottic hemangioma: past, present, future. *Laryngoscope.* 2004;114(11):1880. [PMID: 15510009] (Review of the natural history and management of the subglottic hemangioma.)

Sie CY, Tampakopoulou DA. Hemangiomas and vascular malformation of the airway. *Otolaryngol Clin North Am.* 2000; 33:209. [PMID: 10637353] (Review of subglottic hemangiomas and other congenital vascular lesions of the pediatric airway.)

RESPIRATORY PAPILLOMATOSIS

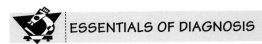 ESSENTIALS OF DIAGNOSIS

- *Hoarse voice.*
- *Gradual onset of stridor.*
- *Recurrent disease requiring multiple surgical procedures.*
- *Viral etiology.*

General Considerations

Although juvenile-onset recurrent respiratory papillomatosis is a rare disease, it is the most common neoplasm of the larynx in children. Diagnosis is most commonly made between the ages of 2 and 5 years, but papillomas can present in any age group. There is no difference in incidence between males and females. The first-born, vaginally delivered child of a teenage mother is associated with an increased chance of developing respiratory papillomatosis.

Papillomatosis is caused by infection with human papillomavirus (HPV), the most commonly identified subtypes being HPV-6 and HPV-11 (HPV-11 is more aggressive and more prone to malignant changes). The same HPV subtypes are responsible for genital warts, and there is a recognized association between maternal genital warts and respiratory papillomatosis. The precise mode of transmission is not clearly understood, although the aspiration of amniotic fluid during vaginal delivery and viremia leading to hematogenous infection of the fetus are the commonly accepted modes. The larynx is the most commonly affected site in respiratory papillomatosis, particularly the glottis and the anterior commissure, but the mouth, the pharynx, the tracheobronchial tree, and the esophagus can all be affected. Pulmonary papillomatosis is rare but carries high morbidity and mortality. The malignant transformation from benign nonkeratinizing squamous papillomas to squamous cell carcinoma can occur in children, but is rarely seen. Malignant transformation most commonly occurs in the distal bronchopulmonary tree, and the prognosis is universally poor.

Juvenile-onset respiratory papillomatosis has a more severe clinical course than that of adult-onset papillomatosis. Characteristically, multiple foci of papilloma recur frequently after treatment and usually require multiple surgical interventions. Spontaneous remission does occur but is unpredictable, and recurrence has been reported after prolonged disease-free periods.

Clinical Findings

A. Symptoms and Signs

Hoarseness, abnormal cry, or both are the most common presenting symptoms of respiratory papillomatosis. If the disease is untreated, then a gradual progression to dyspnea, stridor, and eventually, complete airway obstruction can occur. Stridor and airway obstruction are rarely the first symptoms. Examination may reveal a papilloma in the mouth or pharynx, although this finding is unusual. In a cooperative child, the diagnosis can be made by inspecting the larynx with either a laryngeal mirror or a flexible fiberoptic endoscope.

B. Evaluation

If the diagnosis of respiratory papillomatosis is suspected, then a histopathologic confirmation is required. At microlaryngoscopy, the papillomas are seen to be firm, irregular, exophytic lesions that bleed easily on manipulation. Examination should include tracheobronchoscopy to determine whether distal spread has occurred.

Treatment

The primary treatment modality for respiratory papillomatosis is surgery. The aims of treatment are to maintain an adequate airway while avoiding tracheotomy, preserving the voice, and controlling the papilloma. The most widely accepted means of surgical ablation of respiratory papilloma is with the CO_2 laser. Because respiratory papillomatosis typically requires multiple procedures to maintain the airway, there is a significant risk of scarring and web formation due to repeated thermal damage caused by the laser. For this reason, it is advisable to leave small amounts of the papilloma in sites where scarring is likely to occur, such as the anterior commissure. Other disadvantages of using the laser include destruction of the papilloma, which both precludes histologic examination and exposes the operating room staff to virus particles in the laser plume. Removal of laryngeal papilloma has been reported using a powered shaver developed for use in the larynx. Although this system reduces the risks associated with the laser, it carries the potential disadvantage of poor hemostatic control. This finding does not appear to be problematic in preliminary reports.

Up to 20% of reported cases of respiratory papillomatosis are severe enough to require tracheotomy, although, if possible, a tracheotomy should be avoided because of the increased risk of distal spread.

Several adjuvant systemic therapies are available. The risks and benefits of adjuvant therapy should be carefully considered before use. Adjuvant therapies in use or under investigation include indole 3-carbinol, diindolymethane, alfa interferons, acyclovir, photodynamic therapy, ribavirin, retinoic acid, mumps vaccine injections, and cidofovir. There is still insufficient evidence on the effectiveness of antiviral therapy. The ideal dose, frequency, and duration of cidofovir therapy are yet to be known.

Dekay CS. Recurrent respiratory papillomatosis. *Laryngoscope.* 2001; 111(1):57. [PMID: 11192901] (General review of the condition and the practice guidelines.)

Shehab N, Sweet BV, Hogikyan ND. Cidofovir for the treatment of recurrent respiratory papillomatosis: a review of the literature. *Pharmacotherapy.* 2005;25(7):977. [PMID: 16006276] (Review of the safety and efficacy of cidofovir therapy in respiratory papillomatosis.)

■ INFLAMMATORY CAUSES OF STRIDOR

The major causes of inflammatory stridor in children are laryngotracheobronchitis, epiglottitis, and, rarely, bacterial tracheitis. The major features of laryngotracheobronchitis and epiglottitis are compared in Table 32–3.

LARYNGOTRACHEOBRONCHITIS (CROUP)

ESSENTIALS OF DIAGNOSIS

- *Gradual onset of symptoms.*
- *Barking cough.*
- *Stridor.*

General Considerations

Laryngotracheobronchitis is the most common infectious cause of airway obstruction in children, usually occurring between the ages of 6 months and 3 years. It is a viral infection most commonly caused by the parainfluenza virus, although numerous other organisms have been reported. Symptoms occur as a result of mucosal edema in the larynx, trachea, and bronchi.

Recurrent episodes of laryngotracheobronchitis should raise the suspicion of underlying abnormalities; therefore, further investigation is indicated.

Table 32–3. A comparison of the main features of epiglottitis and laryngotracheobronchitis.

	Epiglottitis	Laryngotracheobronchitis
Microbiology	*Haemophilus influenzae* type b	Parainfluenza virus
Age group	2–6 years	< 3 years
Onset	Rapid (hours)	Slow (usually days)
Cough	Absent	Barking cough
Dysphagia	Severe	None
Stridor	Inspiratory	Biphasic
Temperature	Elevated	Elevated
Posture	Sitting forward	Lying back
Drooling	Marked	None
Voice	Muffled	Hoarse
X-ray	Thumbprint sign	Steeple sign

Clinical Findings

A. SYMPTOMS AND SIGNS

Characteristically, the symptoms of laryngotracheobronchitis are gradual in onset and are often preceded by an upper respiratory tract infection. A barking cough is invariably present along with hoarseness and stridor. If stridor is present, it is usually inspiratory in nature, and the onset of biphasic stridor and other signs of respiratory distress are indicative of severe airway obstruction. Symptoms typically last between 3 and 5 days, although the child may be infectious for 2 weeks.

B. EVALUATION

Although the diagnosis of laryngotracheobronchitis is mainly based on clinical findings, plain-film x-rays of the neck and chest can be useful. The upper trachea and subglottis may be narrowed (steeple sign) in laryngotracheobronchitis, and other diagnoses, such as foreign body, can be excluded. A blood film reveals a leukocytosis in some cases. If the child has significant symptoms of airway obstruction, then the management should be as described for epiglottitis.

Treatment

Over 85% of cases of laryngotracheobronchitis are mild and can be managed in the community. Parents are typically advised to nurse their child in a humidified room and it seems to be effective anecdotally.

In patients with more severe symptoms, nebulized racemic epinephrine produces a rapid improvement in symptoms by vasoconstriction and reduction in mucosal edema. Heliox has also proved to be beneficial in the acute phase. Both nebulized and systemic steroids have been demonstrated to produce an improvement in the symptoms and the length of time spent in the hospital as well as a decreased need for other interventions such as intubation. Because the beneficial effects of steroids require several hours before onset, the simultaneous administration of racemic epinephrine and steroids results in both immediate and lasting symptom relief. A small number of cases of laryngotracheobronchitis (1.5%) do not respond to medical therapy and airway obstruction worsens. In this situation, endotracheal intubation and ventilation is indicated until the edema resolves.

SUPRAGLOTTITIS (EPIGLOTTITIS)

ESSENTIALS OF DIAGNOSIS

- *Rapid progression of symptoms.*
- *Severe odynophagia with drooling.*

- Irritability, fever, toxicity, or any combination of these symptoms.
- Stridor (late sign).

General Considerations

In *epiglottitis,* or more correctly, *supraglottitis,* the cellulitis involves multiple areas of the supraglottis. Typically, acute supraglottitis presents in children between the ages of 2 and 6 years, although any age group, including adults, can be affected. *Haemophilus influenzae* type B (HIB) is the responsible pathogen in most cases, and, as a result of the introduction of the HIB vaccine, the incidence of supraglottitis has been reduced by more than 90%. Although supraglottitis is a rare infection, awareness of the disease is important because of its high mortality rate (if not promptly diagnosed and treated) and the changing trends of the disease in the HIB vaccination era (eg, an increase in the presenting age in children).

Clinical Findings

A. SYMPTOMS AND SIGNS

Symptoms of acute supraglottitis progress rapidly over a matter of hours. The typical features are fever, difficulty in breathing, and severe odynophagia, which results in drooling. The child is usually irritable sitting or leaning forward, and if the child can speak, the voice is typically muffled. Inspiratory stridor is a late feature occurring when the airway is almost completely obstructed.

B. EVALUATION

Once the diagnosis of supraglottitis is suspected, further investigations should not be undertaken since any procedures that induce anxiety in the patient, including intraoral examination and venipuncture, may precipitate complete airway obstruction. In mild cases without respiratory distress, the most useful diagnostic tool is a lateral neck x-ray, which classically demonstrates a swollen epiglottis (the "thumb print" sign) and can help exclude other diagnoses, such as a foreign body or a retropharyngeal abscess. Also, transnasal flexible fiberoptic laryngoscopy can be judiciously used in the evaluation of the stridulous patients with no respiratory distress, based on the patient's age, condition, and cooperation.

Treatment

The management of a child with suspected supraglottitis requires close cooperation among the otolaryngologist, the anesthesiologist, and the pediatrician. The child should be directly transferred to the operating room where equip-

ment for emergency tracheotomy must be available. After inhalational anesthesia, the supraglottis can be inspected and the presence of erythema and edema confirms the diagnosis. The airway is then secured by endotracheal intubation. Once the airway is safe, blood cultures and swabs of the supraglottis can be obtained and an intravenous cannula inserted. Parenteral antibiotic therapy (eg, ceftriaxone or cefotaxime) should then be started. Supraglottitis usually responds rapidly to treatment and extubation is often possible after 48–72 hours.

BACTERIAL TRACHEITIS

Bacterial tracheitis is a rare infection that is thought to occur as a secondary bacterial colonization following a viral respiratory tract infection. Involvement of the subglottis and main bronchi is not uncommon. The age at presentation is much more diverse than that seen with croup and has been reported from infancy to adulthood, although the seasonal variation in incidence mirrors that of viral infections of the respiratory tract. The most commonly isolated bacterial pathogen is *Staphylococcus aureus.*

The initial clinical course of bacterial tracheitis is often similar to that seen with croup and is followed by an acute exacerbation of airway obstruction with associated high fever and toxicity. This rapid onset of symptoms is similar to that of supraglottitis, but drooling and dysphagia are absent.

Plain-film x-rays of the neck may demonstrate narrowing of the tracheal lumen, but endoscopy is required to confirm the diagnosis. The typical appearance is a diffusely ulcerated tracheal mucosa with copious purulent secretions partially obstructing the lumen of the trachea. Specimens should be sent for culture at the time of endoscopy, and the tracheal and bronchial secretions should be suctioned. Most patients require endotracheal intubation and ventilation, which secures the airway and allows repeated tracheal suction. Broad-spectrum parenteral antibiotics should be initiated and adjusted accordingly when the causative organism is identified.

Ausejo Segura M, Saenz A, Pham B et al. Glucocorticoids for croup (Cochrane review). *The Cochrane Library.* Issue 4, 2001. Oxford: Update Software. [PMID: 10796674] (Meta-analysis to determine the effectiveness of glucocorticoids in the management of croup.)

Shah RK, Roberson DW, Jones DT. Epiglottitis in the *Haemophilus influenzae* type B vaccine era: changing trends. *Laryngoscope.* 2004;114(3):557. [PMID: 15091234] (A 10-year retrospective study to evaluate the changing trends in the demographics, causative organisms and natural history of epiglottitis after the introduction of the HIB vaccine.)

Stroud RH, Friedman NR. An update on inflammatory disorders of the pediatric airway: epiglottitis, croup, and tracheitis. *Am J Otolaryngol.* 2001;22(4):268. [PMID: 11464324] (Discusses the pathogenesis, clinical presentation, and management of the common pediatric inflammatory airway diseases.)

Laryngeal Trauma

33

Andrew H. Murr, MD, FACS, & Milan R. Amin, MD

ESSENTIALS OF DIAGNOSIS

- *Hoarseness, neck pain, crepitus, loss of normal midline neck landmarks.*
- *Fiberoptic examination is key to the diagnosis; computed tomography scans are extremely helpful.*
- *Consider concomitant injuries with penetrating trauma.*

General Considerations

The larynx serves three important functions: airway protection, regulation of respiration, and phonation. Injury to the larynx resulting from trauma can therefore be devastating. Fortunately, laryngeal trauma is rare and occurs in only a small percentage of trauma victims. Standardized protocols have been developed to help guide the accurate evaluation and identification of injuries requiring operative intervention. Early diagnosis and treatment are critical to prevent dire consequences, including death.

Pathogenesis

A. EXTERNAL LARYNGEAL TRAUMA

The relatively low incidence of laryngotracheal injuries results from the natural defenses that the body has to protect the vital structures that allow us to breathe. The relative high position of the sternum and low position of the mandible along with the thick musculature of the lateral neck allows only a relatively short segment of the airway to be exposed.

Furthermore, there is a naturally protective reflex that causes the head to be flexed downward when startled, allowing for further protection of this region. Injury typically occurs when the body cannot protect this area. This generally occurs in motor or recreational vehicle accidents, assaults (including domestic violence), sports injuries, or strangulation. In motor vehicle accidents, the laryngeal skeleton may be shattered between the steering wheel and the cervical spine.

Clothesline injuries, although rare, may result classically in cricotracheal separation and bilateral recurrent laryngeal nerve injuries.

The pediatric age group deserves special mention because children have anatomic differences that make the management of laryngeal injuries a distinct entity when compared with the management of similar injuries in adults. Although children are less prone to laryngeal fracture owing to the high position of the larynx in the neck and the increased pliability of the laryngeal cartilage, their diminutive anatomy makes them more vulnerable to life-threatening complications from the injury.

B. PENETRATING NECK TRAUMA

Penetrating trauma to the neck is challenging because up to 30% of patients have multiple structures injured. Penetrating neck trauma usually results from stabbings or gunshot wounds. The severity of a penetrating injury is determined by the mass and velocity of the missile. Therefore, generally, high-velocity, large-caliber bullets will create more damage. However, a variety of bullet types are available that can increase local tissue damage, either by breaking up or exploding on contact or by spiraling in the tissues.

C. INTUBATION INJURY

Because of sophisticated intensive care units, critically ill patients are being sustained longer on ventilatory support with the potential long-term consequences of affected speech and airway patency. Such complications may include scarring of the laryngeal structures, subglottic or tracheal stenosis, formation of granulation tissue, and vocal fold paralysis/paresis. Although the true incidence is unknown, complication rates of 4–19% have been reported after prolonged intubation; therefore, converting an intubated patient to a tracheotomy is often contemplated after 5–7 days. The benefits of tracheotomy as a management strategy for the prolonged intubation patient include the ability to (1) decrease dead space, (2) improve pulmonary toilet, (3) increase comfort and decrease the need for sedation, (4) ease the process of weaning, and (5) lessen the risk of long-term complications.

Many factors determine the severity of intubation injury. Anatomic variations predispose some patients to a difficult or traumatic intubation. Underlying illness, infection, and reflux laryngitis all may exacerbate the injury. Although glottic edema and superficial ulceration may be seen within just hours of intubation, the use of large-diameter endotracheal tubes, excessive patient movement, repeated self-extubation, overinflated endotracheal tube cuffs, and prolonged intubation increase the risk of long-term damage.

Intubation-related injuries may be reduced by eliminating or controlling the above-listed factors. We routinely ensure that cuff pressures are kept below 20 mm Hg, and patients are maintained on antireflux medications while intubated.

Arytenoid dislocation is a special consideration that has been reported as a result of intubation problems. The cause is likely either extreme force applied directly to the arytenoids by a laryngoscope or endotracheal tube or careless extubation with an inflated cuff. The diagnosis is controversial. Some clinicians propose that it is often misdiagnosed and may actually represent the appearance of new onset vocal fold paralysis.

Benjamin B. Prolonged intubation injuries of the larynx: endoscopic diagnosis, classification, and treatment. *Ann Otol Rhinol Laryngol Suppl.* 1993;160:1. [PMID: 8470867] (Management and preservation of the common intubation injury are based on the sequential progression of superficial ulcerations and granulation tissue to various degrees of stenosis.)

Kuttenberger JJ, Hardt N, Schlegel C. Diagnosis and initial management of laryngotracheal injuries associated with facial fractures. *J Cranio-Maxillofac Surg.* 2004;32:80. (The key to proper management of laryngotracheal trauma associated with other injuries is early recognition and evaluation.)

Merritt RM, Bent JP, Porubsky ES. Acute laryngeal trauma in the pediatric patient. *Ann Otol Rhinol Laryngol.* 1998;107(2):104. (Children with laryngeal trauma usually are managed conservatively but also require increased vigilance for airway complications.)

Sataloff RT, Bough DB Jr, Spiegel JR. Arytenoids dislocation: diagnosis and treatment. *Laryngoscope.* 1994;104:1353. [PMID: 7968164] (Arytenoid dislocation is diagnosed by history and findings on ancillary testing; best results are obtained when reduced early.)

Clinical Findings

A. Symptoms and Signs

1. Patient history—The evaluation of a patient with a suspected laryngeal injury begins with a detailed history (when possible) that specifically addresses the following items: (1) the development of symptoms, (2) the mechanism of injury, and (3) the trajectory of any involved weapons. This information is often difficult to elicit in a patient with multiple traumas because the ability to provide information is compromised by the severity of the injuries. These injuries can include communication

deficits caused by concomitant head injuries or illicit substance abuse. Common symptoms include hoarseness, pain, dysphagia, odynophagia, and dyspnea. The failure to elicit these symptoms, however, does not ensure the integrity of the airway. Therefore, a high index of suspicion is mandatory in any patient with neck trauma.

2. Physical examination—The physical examination begins with careful attention to the voice and breathing. The presence of hemoptysis, stridor, or crepitus should alert the physician to a high probability of airway injury. Stridor may help localize the injury. Inspiratory stridor is classically seen with an extrathoracic injury, whereas expiratory stridor results from an injury that is intrathoracic. Biphasic stridor may be a sign of injury at the level of the glottis. Point tenderness or flattening of the thyroid cartilage prominence is suggestive of an acute laryngeal fracture. Penetrating trauma may involve multiple vital structures such as the esophagus or the carotid neurovascular bundle. An expanding hematoma, a pulse deficit, or the presence of **bruit** and thrill all are signs of vascular injury. The prompt diagnosis of these life-threatening injuries requires a methodical investigation. Further evaluation is directed by careful attention to subtle signs and symptoms (Figure 33–1).

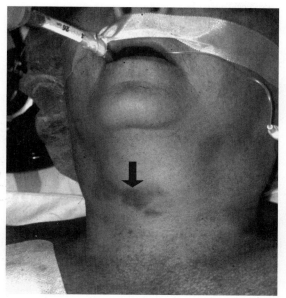

Figure 33–1. Anterior neck bruise (see arrow) in a middle-aged woman involved in a motor vehicle accident. (Courtesy of Andrew N. Goldberg, MD, University of California, San Francisco.)

One of the most important instruments in diagnosing laryngeal trauma is the fiberoptic nasopharyngoscope. It is well tolerated in a patient who is awake and is a quick diagnostic test that allows a complete upper airway and laryngeal evaluation. In using this device, the larynx should be evaluated carefully for vocal cord mobility and arytenoid symmetry. Notation should also be made regarding findings of edema, hematoma, soft tissue tears, and exposed cartilage. If available, stroboscopy may be helpful as well to aid in diagnosing injury. An attempt should also be made to evaluate the upper trachea by direct examination if the patient tolerates the exam.

B. Imaging Studies

1. Conventional x-rays and soft tissue films— Plain-film x-rays of the chest and soft tissue neck films continue to be essential components in patient evaluation. Any abnormal air surrounding the trachea, mediastinum, or thorax may be the first sign of impending tension pneumothorax and airway embarrassment.

2. Computed tomography (CT)—High-resolution fine-cut CT of the larynx is the best radiographic tool available to evaluate laryngeal trauma (Figure 33–2). It is especially helpful when the examination is normal but there is a high index of suspicion for occult laryngeal injury. It may reveal a subtle fracture that requires fixation or it may obviate the need for rigid endoscopy if the scanned image is completely normal. A CT scan is not mandatory in patients with injuries that obviously require operative intervention or in asymptomatic patients with an unremarkable physi-

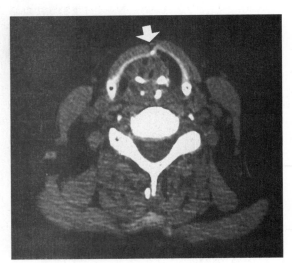

Figure 33–2. CT scan revealing a paramedian fracture (see arrow) from an acute blunt laryngeal trauma. (Courtesy of Andrew N. Goldberg, MD, University of California, San Francisco.)

cal examination. However, CT scanning may be valuable in helping to plan the operative procedure in a patient with a controlled and stable airway.

3. Rigid esophagoscopy and contrast swallow studies—Rigid esophagoscopy or contrast swallow studies are used often to rule out concomitant esophageal perforation in penetrating trauma. When used together, the sensitivity of these tests is approximately 90%. A water-soluble contrast may be preferred to barium because it is less inflammatory to soft tissues, especially if an injury is present or suspected. A negative study then may be repeated with barium, which provides more mucosal detail. A useful adjunct when not dealing with esophageal perforation is flexible esophagoscopy, either in the operating room or at the bedside using a transnasal esophagoscope. These instruments may offer more detail than is available with a barium swallow or rigid esophagoscopy.

4. Angiography—Angiography is often used in the diagnostic evaluation of penetrating neck trauma, especially when the injury involves Zones I and III. (See zone definitions in the section on Definitive Treatment.) Angiography is the gold standard for evaluating vascular injury and is therapeutic when used with interventional neuroradiology embolization. In some centers, duplex ultrasound or noninvasive angiography (CT or magnetic resonance angiography) has replaced conventional angiography for the evaluation of vascular injuries because of its lower cost and risk.

Kennedy TL, Gilroy PA, Millman B, Greene JS, Pellitteri PK, Harlor M. Strobovideolaryngoscopy in the management of acute laryngeal trauma. *J Voice.* 2004;18(1):130. (Videostroboscopy may improve clinical assessment of patients with laryngotracheal injury.)

Miller PR, Fabian TC, Croce MA et al. Prospective screening for blunt cerebrovascular injuries: analysis of diagnostic modalities and outcomes. *Ann Surg.* 2002;236(3):386. (Conventional angiography remains more sensitive than less invasive techniques and is an important part of the diagnostic workup in patients with neck trauma.)

Mokhashi MS, Wildi SM, Glenn TF et al. A prospective, blinded study of diagnostic esophagoscopy with a superthin, standalone, battery-powered esophagoscope. *Am J Gastroenterol.* 2003;98(11):2383. (Ultrathin endoscopy is accurate in detecting esophageal pathologies when compared to traditional esophagoscopy.)

Treatment

A. Emergent Management (for Unstable Patients)

The initial resuscitation begins with three steps: (1) securing the airway, (2) obtaining hemodynamic stability while controlling the bleeding, and (3) immobilizing the cervical spine. The optimal choice of airway control is often debated. Intubation may be performed safely if

Table 33–1. Classification of laryngeal injury.

Group	Characteristics
I	Minor endolaryngeal hematoma; minimal airway compromise, if any; no detectable fractures
II	Endolaryngeal hematoma or edema associated with compromised airway; minor mucosal lacerations without exposed cartilage; nondisplaced fracture shown on computed tomographic scan
III	Massive endolaryngeal edema with airway obstruction; mucosal tears with exposed cartilage; immobile vocal cord(s)
IV	Same as group III with more than 2 fracture lines on imaging studies; massive derangement of endolarynx
V	Laryngotracheal separation

Reproduced, with permission, from Gold SM, Gerber ME, Shott SR, Myer CM III. Blunt laryngeal trauma in children. *Arch Otolaryngol Head Neck Surg* 1997;123:83.

the vocal folds are easily seen, there are no visible injuries, and the smallest tube possible is used. However, endotracheal intubation can cause further injury to an already tenuous airway, resulting in an emergent need for airway control. Surgical airway control such as an awake tracheotomy (performed under local anesthetic) or a cricothyroidotomy may be necessary. If a cricothyroidotomy is performed, it should be converted to a formal tracheotomy as soon as possible to prevent long-term sequelae (eg, subglottic stenosis).

In contrast to adults, pediatric patients are unlikely to cooperate with a tracheotomy while awake. In addition, their neck anatomy is often more challenging owing to a high laryngeal position and soft cartilage. Therefore, a pediatric airway is preferably secured with a rigid bronchoscope while maintaining spontaneous respiration before a tracheotomy is performed.

After stabilization of the airway, the patient should be examined and the injury stratified to help guide further management.

B. DEFINITIVE TREATMENT

1. External laryngeal trauma—Laryngeal injuries are grouped according to increasing severity (Table 33–1; Figure 33–3). Patients with Group I injuries have minor endolaryngeal hematomas or lacerations. These patients are treated successfully with medical management alone, typically. Group II injuries demonstrate airway compromise, more severe soft tissue injury, or single nondisplaced laryngeal fractures. These patients are usually managed with a tracheotomy followed by direct laryngoscopy and esophagoscopy. If an arytenoid dislocation is discovered, then closed reduction should be attempted. Group III injuries include patients with massive edema, mucosal tears with exposed cartilage, displaced fractures, or vocal cord immobility. Group IV describes the unstable larynx with comminuted fractures. A Group V classification is the most severe type of injury; these patients present with complete laryngotracheal separation. Injuries within Groups III–V require immediate operative repair. The ability to restore the integrity of the larynx impacts a patient's long-term outcome with regard to voice, airway, and the quality of life.

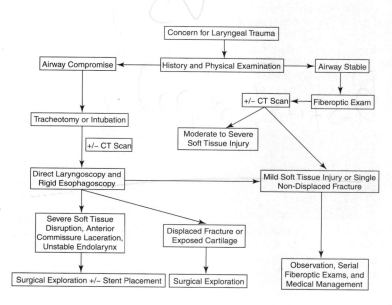

Figure 33–3. Treatment algorithm for the acute management of external laryngeal trauma. (Modified and reproduced, with permission, from Schaefer SD: The acute management of external laryngeal trauma: a 27-year experience. *Arch Otolaryngol Head Neck Surg.* 1992;118:598.)

a. Nonsurgical measures—Group I and II injuries often heal spontaneously and have excellent outcomes. These injuries are usually managed nonsurgically with humidified air, head of bed elevation, and voice rest. To prevent complications from an undetected or progressive injury, the patient should be closely observed with serial fiberoptic examinations and continuous pulse oximetry for 24–48 hours. Antibiotics are often prescribed when there is observable mucosal injury. The use of steroids is controversial. Steroids probably decrease edema if given within the first few hours after injury. The prophylactic treatment of laryngopharyngeal reflux is also recommended to prevent exposure of an injured larynx to acidic gastric contents.

b. Surgical measures—In more severe injuries, the careful approximation of mucosal tears and the reduction of fracture segments are required to prevent long-term voice disturbance or airway compromise. Findings that tend to lead to a recommendation for surgery include (1) lacerations involving the anterior commissure, injury to the free edge of the true vocal fold, or the finding of exposed cartilage; (2) displaced or comminuted fractures; (3) vocal fold immobility; or (4) arytenoid dislocation.

Some data indicate that patients with treatment delays of 48 hours have inferior outcomes when compared with patients whose injuries are repaired soon after the initial trauma. Early intervention is generally preferable since it allows an accurate identification of the injury, less scarring, and superior long-term results.

Fractures can affect the voice by changing the geometry of the larynx and glottal configuration. Therefore, the precise reduction and fixation of even minimally displaced or angulated fractures is often advocated. Fractures traditionally have been repaired with stainless-steel wires or absorbable sutures. Miniplates (titanium or absorbable) provide immediate stability and good results, although the lack of rigidity in the cartilage may limit their efficacy (Figure 33–4).

When there is disruption of the endolaryngeal soft tissue, a midline thyrotomy to the level of the cricothyroid membrane is performed through a horizontal anterior neck incision. The arytenoids are palpated and reduced if dislocated or avulsed. Only obvious devitalized tissue is débrided. Mucosal lacerations are repaired with primary closure or local flaps to cover any exposed cartilage with the goal of preventing perichondritis, the formation of granulation tissue, and scarring. Grafts are rarely needed.

The use of stents is controversial because of the increased risk of infection and granulation formation. Stents provide structural stability and are indicated in patients with laryngeal instability following inadequate fracture fixation. In the presence of severe soft tissue disruption or lacerations involving the anterior commissure, stents may help prevent synechiae. After 1 or 2 weeks, they are typically removed endoscopically.

2. Penetrating neck trauma—Penetrating neck trauma is classified by the level of injury based on the clinical features and the ease of surgical access: (1) Zone I extends from the sternal notch to the cricoid; (2) Zone II extends from the cricoid to the angle of the mandible; (3) Zone III extends cranially from the mandible to the skull base. This classification system directs the diagnostic evaluation and treatment.

With sophisticated ancillary tests and the accurate identification of localizing signs and symptoms, the surgical exploration of penetrating neck trauma is being used increasingly on a selective basis. Immediate operative exploration including triple endoscopy (direct laryngoscopy, bronchoscopy, and esophagoscopy) is used for all patients with hemodynamic instability or airway compromise. The hypopharynx should be closely inspected for injury. Injuries above the level of the arytenoids often heal spontaneously and may be expectantly managed. Lower hypopharyngeal and cervical esophageal injuries require open exploration, primary closure, and drainage due to the higher incidence of salivary leak, infection, and subsequent fistula.

The stable patient is stratified depending on the presence of other signs or symptoms such as expanding hematoma, dysphonia, hemoptysis, hematemesis, or dysphagia. This group of symptoms is explored more selectively.

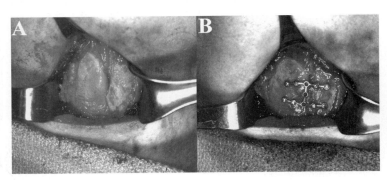

Figure 33–4. Intraoperative photographs of the patient from Figures 33–1 and 33–2. The first photograph **(A)** was taken before rigid fixation using a plating system; the second photograph **(B)** was taken after the plate was inserted. Note that the plate is carefully bent to restore the proper anterior commissure angle. (Courtesy of Andrew N. Goldberg, MD, University of California, San Francisco.)

Injuries crossing into Zones I and III of the neck are more difficult to examine clinically and approach surgically; therefore, imaging—including angiography—is often performed. Zone I injuries are studied with preoperative arteriography and often gastrograffin swallow studies because of the risk of occult injuries reported by some clinicians. Because of difficult surgical access to the vasculature at the base of the skull, patients with Zone III injuries are also studied with arteriography, with the therapeutic option of embolization should an injury be found. Patients with isolated Zone II injuries, however, are usually explored surgically, often without imaging.

The management of asymptomatic patients is controversial. With these patients, some evidence supports observation alone because the physical examination is extremely sensitive in detecting injuries that require operative intervention. In these patients, imaging and adjunctive testing are very helpful in guiding further management.

3. Intubation injury—Intubation injuries may cause a wide variety of acute and chronic conditions. High endotracheal tube cuff pressures may cause progressive hoarseness or airway obstruction from glottic or subglottic edema. Compressive neuropathies caused by direct pressure of the cuff may lead to vocal fold paralysis. Mucosal injury is commonly seen, particularly in the posterior larynx and subglottis and usually results from pressure necrosis due to the presence of the tube and/or cuff or from traumatic intubation. These injuries may progress and lead to granuloma formation, fixation of the cricoarytenoid joint, web formation, or stenosis. The incidence of posterior glottic stenosis increases with the length of intubation and may occur in up to 14% of patients intubated for more than 10 days. Differentiating glottic stenosis from vocal fold paralysis can often be difficult, since both result in partial or complete vocal fold immobility. Typically, the cause of the immobility can be elucidated either by manual assessment of arytenoid mobility or by the use of laryngeal electromyography (LEMG).

Most cases of granulation tissue formation seen after intubation trauma resolve spontaneously after some time. However, further treatment may be necessary in certain cases. This treatment typically involves a combination of voice therapy and antireflux medication. This combination reduces the impact of behavioral and local inflammatory factors that are presumed to cause ongoing laryngeal irritation. In certain refractory cases, botulinum toxin injections can be used to forcibly reduce the impact of ongoing phonotrauma. Pulsed-dye laser treatment has also been successful in certain cases. Operative removal of the granuloma is rarely necessary except in cases of partial airway obstruction. It should be noted that surgical removal does not obviate the need for voice therapy and antireflux medications. Without controlling these factors, granulomas may recur after surgical excision alone.

The management of stenosis depends on its location and severity. It may be detected weeks or months after extubation, when a patient presents for the evaluation of recent exercise intolerance or stridor. Thin webs that tether the anterior glottis can be surgically divided. A keel may then be placed to prevent the web from reforming between apposed denuded mucosa. Posterior laryngeal stenosis and cricoarytenoid joint fixation are typically treated with repeated dilation through an endoscopic approach. However, occasionally, an open approach through a laryngofissure or the use of a stent is required. Other techniques utilized to treat failures or more severe cases include arytenoidectomy or partial posterior cordotomy.

Subglottic or tracheal stenoses may be initially approached with endoscopic laser incision and dilation. More severe stenoses may require laryngotracheal reconstruction or segmental resection with primary anastomosis. Tracheal segments 4–5 cm in length may be removed if performed with release maneuvers.

In unilateral vocal fold paralysis, patients with persistent dysphonia or significant aspiration—despite therapy—may benefit from vocal fold augmentation with a temporary injection material while awaiting the spontaneous return of function. A medialization laryngoplasty with or without arytenoid adduction or injection augmentation with a more permanent substance is typically recommended if the paralysis is likely to be permanent.

Patients with bilateral vocal fold immobility often present with stridor. Relieving the airway obstruction may require a partial posterior cordectomy, arytenoidectomy or arytenoid lateralization procedure. In more pressing cases, airway relief is often provided via a tracheostomy.

The finding of arytenoid dislocation is suggested by an uneven vocal cord level seen on laryngoscopy. However, this appearance can also be seen with vocal fold paralysis, which occurs much more commonly. Laryngeal EMG and CT scanning can be used to clarify the diagnosis.

Benninger MS, Gillen JB, Altman JS. Changing etiology of vocal fold immobility. *Laryngoscope.* 1998;108:1346. [PMID: 9738754] (Vocal fold immobility is most commonly a result of a malignant disorder and surgical trauma, while intubation injuries still account for a significant number of cases.)

Butler AP, Wood BP, O'Rourke AK, Porubsky ES. Acute external laryngeal trauma: experience with 112 patients. *Ann Otol Rhinol Laryngol.* 2005;114:5. (Outcome may be predicted by the initial severity of injury and is improved with earlier intervention.)

Clyne SB, Halum SL, Koufman JA, Postma GN. Pulsed dye laser treatment of laryngeal granulomas. *Ann Otol Rhinol Laryngol.* 2005;114(3):198. (In-office use of the pulsed dye laser is a relatively safe and effective method for treating laryngeal granulomas that do not respond to antireflux therapy and speech therapy.)

De Mello-Filho FV, Carrau RL. Management of laryngeal fractures using internal fixation. *Laryngoscope.* 2000;110:2143. [PMID:

11129037] (Adaptation plating systems are well tolerated and effective, and provide immediate stabilization of laryngeal fractures.)

Gold SM, Gerber ME, Shott SR, Myer CM. Blunt laryngotracheal trauma in children. *Arch Otol Head Neck Surg.* 1997;123(1):83. (Review of pediatric laryngotracheal injuries, which combines the classification systems proposed by Fuhrman et al and Schaefer and Brown for laryngotracheal injuries.)

Schweinfurth JM. Endoscopic treatment of severe tracheal stenosis. *Ann Otol Rhinol Laryngol.* 2006;115(1):30. (Severe and complete tracheal stenoses may be successfully treated endoscopically, which is associated with few complications, low morbidity, a short operative time, and a short length of hospitalization when compared with tracheal resection.)

Sekharan J, Dennis JS, Veldenz HC, Miranda F, Frykberg ER. Continued experience with physical examination alone for evaluation and management of penetrating Zone II neck injuries: results of 145 cases. *J Vasc Surg.* 2000;32:483. [PMID: 10957654] (Penetrating neck trauma of Zone II may be safely and accurately managed based on the findings of the physical examination of vascular injury.)

Stanley RB Jr, Armstrong WB, Fetterman BL, Shindo ML. Management of external penetrating injuries into the hypopharyngeal-cervical esophageal funnel. *J Trauma.* 1997;42:675. [PMID: 9137257] (The severity of injuries increases as they descend from the upper hypopharynx to the cervical esophagus, with the former being amenable to expectant treatment.)

Thompson EC, Porter JM, Fernandez LG. Penetrating neck trauma: an overview of management. *J Oral Maxillofacial Surg.* 2002;60(8):918. (Review of management of penetrating trauma to the neck.)

Yin SS, Qiu WW, Stucker FJ. Value of electromyography in differential diagnosis of laryngeal joint injuries after intubation. *Ann of Otol Rhinol Laryngol.* 1996;105(6):446. (Laryngeal electromyography can help in the diagnosis of cricoarytenoid joint fixation.)

Complications

The initial goal in managing laryngeal trauma is to preserve life; the secondary goal is to prevent long-term sequelae to the voice and airway. Although the injuries to the larynx and trachea can be life-altering, it has to be remembered that early aggressive intervention may also lead to long-term complications. In many instances of more minor injury, the best course is conservative observation, particularly with asymptomatic airway stenosis. Complications of more aggressive treatments, such as laryngofissure, laryngotracheal reconstruction, and tracheal resection may include worsening voice, restenosis, airway loss, pneumothorax, infection, vocal fold paralysis, and fistula formation.

Prevention

Seatbelts, traffic safety devices, speed limits, and technologic advances in automotive safety (eg, airbags) continue to be the mainstay of accident prevention. These safety measures have resulted in a decrease in the incidence of blunt trauma. The adherence to careful intubation techniques, the early identification of patients who require tracheotomy for prolonged intubation, and the development of softer and relatively inert endotracheal tubes have also contributed to a decrease in the incidence of iatrogenic intubation-related injuries.

Prognosis

Postintubation injury occurs more frequently than is brought to clinical attention. Most injuries heal spontaneously and never require further intervention. As more factors that may contribute to these injuries are elucidated, the severity and incidence of complications may be minimized.

Penetrating neck trauma is associated with a 3–6% fatality rate. Management strategies are evolving toward the selective exploration of these injuries.

The outcomes of laryngeal trauma in patients managed according to the protocols discussed earlier have been consistently satisfactory. Group I or II injuries heal almost uniformly with excellent results. However, some select injuries (eg, displaced cricoid cartilage, arytenoid subluxation, or recurrent laryngeal nerve injury) carry a more unfavorable prognosis. Study findings indicate that suboptimal results are only seen in patients with more severe injuries.

Biffl WL, Moore EE, Rehse DH, Offner PJ, Franciose RJ, Burch JM. Selective management of penetrating neck trauma based on cervical level of injury. *Am J Surg.* 1997;174:678. [PMID: 9409596] (Selective management with selective utilization of adjunctive testing in penetrating neck trauma of Zones II and III may be performed safely in asymptomatic patients.)

Schaefer SD. The acute management of external laryngeal trauma: a 27-year experience. *Arch Otolaryngol Head Neck Surg.* 1992;118:598. [PMID: 1637537] (Lessons learned from the largest series of patients with external laryngeal trauma managed by a consistent protocol.)

SECTION IX
Trachea & Esophagus

Congenital Disorders of the Trachea & Esophagus

Steven F. Fowler, MD, & Hanmin Lee, MD

ESOPHAGEAL ATRESIA & TRACHEOESOPHAGEAL FISTULA

 ESSENTIALS OF DIAGNOSIS

- Coughing, cyanosis, or vomiting with onset of feeds.
- Association with VACTERL.
- Inability to pass feeding tube.
- Orogastric tube curled up in upper chest or neck on chest x-ray.
- Intestinal gas indicates esophageal atresia with a tracheoesophageal fistula; no gas represents isolated esophageal atresia.

General Considerations

Esophageal atresia and tracheoesophageal fistula have a prevalence of 1 in 3000 live births. The male-to-female ratio is equal. Infants with these conditions are often premature, and polyhydramnios is commonly diagnosed prenatally.

Classification

Esophageal atresia and tracheoesophageal fistula are classified based on the presence of atresia and the rela-

tion of the fistula location to the atresia. Older classification methods have been replaced with anatomical descriptions (Figure 34–1). The incidence of these two conditions is found in Table 34–1.

A. TYPE 1

Esophageal atresia with a distal tracheoesophageal fistula is the most common anomaly, comprising 85.4% of cases. The lower esophageal segment begins as a fistula that arises from the distal trachea near the carina. The proximal esophageal pouch is found as a blind-ending segment near the thoracic inlet. The blood supply to the superior esophageal segment is via the thyrocervical trunk, whereas branches of the gastric arteries supply the distal esophageal segment.

B. TYPE 2

Isolated esophageal atresia comprises 7.3% of cases. The lower pouch is usually only 1–2 cm above the diaphragm, whereas the upper pouch ends near the thoracic inlet, creating a long gap between the two ends that can complicate repair. This anomaly does not allow amniotic fluid to pass to the remainder of the developing gut, explaining the finding of polyhydramnios prenatally. However, esophageal atresia with a relatively narrow distal tracheoesophageal fistula can produce similar findings.

C. TYPE 3

Isolated tracheoesophageal fistula is the third most common anomaly, comprising 2.8% of cases. The loca-

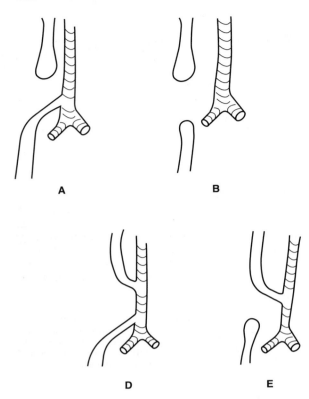

A   **B**   **C**

D   **E**

Figure 34–1. Types of esophageal atresia and tracheoesophageal fistula: **(A)** Type 1, esophageal atresia with distal tracheo-esophageal fistula; **(B)** Type 2, esophageal atresia without tracheoesophageal fistula; **(C)** Type 3, tracheoesophageal fistula with-out esophageal atresia; **(D)** Type 4, esoph-ageal atresia with proximal and distal tra-cheoesophageal fistula; and **(E)** Type 5, esophageal atresia with proximal tracheo-esophageal fistula.

tion of the fistula is variable, occurring between the cri-coid cartilage and carina. More than one fistula can occur. The fistula angles downward from the trachea to the esophagus.

D. TYPE 4

Esophageal atresia with proximal and distal tracheoesopha-geal fistula is less common and comprises 2.1% of cases.

E. TYPE 5

Esophageal atresia with proximal tracheoesophageal fis-tula is the least commonly encountered anomaly, com-

Table 34–1. Incidence of esophageal atresia and tracheoesophageal fistula (TEF).

Atresia with distal TEF	85.4%
Atresia without TEF	7.3%
TEF without atresia	2.8%
Atresia with proximal & distal TEF	2.1%
Atresia with proximal TEF	< 1.0%

prising < 1% of cases. The fistula angles downward from the trachea to the esophagus. The space between the two esophageal ends is pronounced.

Pathogenesis

By the 26th day of embryologic development, the dorsal foregut has separated from the ventral trachea. A primary mechanism of esophageal atresia develops by an unknown etiology. Animal models demonstrate a branch of a tra-cheal trifurcation growing caudally, which connects to the stomach, creating the fistula. Esophageal atresia and tracheoesophageal fistula, seen in association with other embryologic abnormalities, is referred to by the acronym **VACTERL** (**v**ertebral, **a**nal, **c**ardiac, **t**racheoesophageal, **r**enal, and **l**imb anomalies). Patients with esophageal atresia and tracheoesophageal fistula have approximately a 50% chance of having one of these associated anoma-lies, prompting the physician to rule out these other pro-cesses. Cardiac anomalies are the most commonly associ-ated defects.

The esophagus of patients with esophageal atresia and tracheoesophageal fistula has a decreased number of Auer-bach plexuses, explaining the neuronal element of altered esophageal motor function and partly explaining the chronic nature of dysmotility seen with these patients.

Pulmonary development may be impeded via two pathways. Direct pressure on the trachea by a distended proximal esophagus can contribute to tracheomalacia. Secondly, a fistula drains amniotic fluid out of the pulmonary tree. This fluid pressure has been implicated in playing a part in parenchymal lung development.

Crisera CA, Connelly PR, Marmureanu AR et al. Esophageal atresia with tracheoesophageal fistula: suggested mechanism in faulty organogenesis. *J Pediatr Surg.* 1999;34:204. [PMID: 10022173] (Animal model demonstrating a primary atresia of the esophagus with a secondary phenomenon of tracheoesophageal fistula development.)

Clinical Findings

A. SYMPTOMS AND SIGNS

1. Respiratory symptoms—Patients are often asymptomatic at birth. They can present with excessive drooling because of an inability to swallow. Upon feeding, the infant may cough, choke, regurgitate, or become cyanotic. The prevention of saliva from traveling to the stomach leads to aspiration, which can present as respiratory distress, atelectasis, and pneumonia.

Patients with the rare tracheoesophageal fistula without esophageal atresia are often diagnosed at a later stage because of a less pronounced symptom complex. Presentation can be subtle, with chronic upper respiratory symptoms and choking, repeated pneumonias, or asthmatic symptoms.

2. Gastrointestinal symptoms—Patients with a distal tracheoesophageal fistula can have gastric distention resulting from the passage of air from the trachea to the distal esophagus. This situation may result in either gastric reflux into the trachea, causing a chemical tracheobronchitis, or compromised respiratory status by abdominal distention and pulmonary compression.

B. IMAGING STUDIES

1. Esophageal catheter and esophagram—Gentle placement of a catheter into the esophagus that will not pass into the stomach is often the first study suggestive of esophageal atresia. The catheter position should be noted on a plain radiograph. A standard barium swallow is not recommended because of possible spillage into the pulmonary tree. An esophagram may be useful in diagnosing an isolated tracheoesophageal fistula.

2. Abdominal x-ray—An abdominal radiograph can suggest which type of anomaly is present. In patients with a fistula connecting the distal esophagus, x-rays show gas in the stomach and small bowel. A gasless abdomen suggests either esophageal atresia without a tracheoesophageal fistula or a proximal fistula.

C. SPECIAL TESTS

1. Bronchoscopy and esophagoscopy—With high clinical suspicion and a negative barium study, isolated tracheoesophageal fistulas can be demonstrated with concurrent bronchoscopy and esophagoscopy.

2. Echocardiogram—An echocardiogram should be performed for two reasons: (1) to rule out the presence of cardiac anomalies and (2) to determine the side of the aortic arch. A right-sided aortic arch dictates repair through a left thoracotomy, as opposed to standard repair via a right thoracotomy.

D. SPECIAL EXAMINATIONS

Prenatal sonography can suggest esophageal atresia with the findings of polyhydramnios and no visible stomach. Because of the association of VACTERL, any findings suggestive of these anomalies should promote an evaluation for esophageal atresia and tracheoesophageal fistula. Prenatal MRI may be helpful to further delineate anomalies.

Langer JC, Hussain H, Khan A et al. Prenatal diagnosis of esophageal atresia using sonography and magnetic resonance imaging. *J Pediatr Surg.* 2001;36:804. [PMID: 11329594] (MRI increases the accuracy of diagnosis of patients suspected of having esophageal atresia on prenatal ultrasound.)

Differential Diagnosis

A. LARYNGOTRACHEOESOPHAGEAL CLEFT

Laryngotracheoesophageal cleft is a rare defect related to esophageal atresia and tracheoesophageal fistula. It occurs in the midline between the trachea and the esophagus. The defect can be minimal, or it can extend down past the carina. Symptoms range from chronic cough to respiratory distress. The diagnosis is made by rigid bronchoscopy. Severe cases require operative repair involving a right anterolateral cervical approach with lateral pharyngotomy to expose the defect.

B. ESOPHAGEAL STENOSIS

Esophageal stenosis is a rare congenital anomaly. Anatomically, there can be tracheal elements in the wall of the esophagus or a mucosal web. Patients present later in life with difficulty swallowing solids. The diagnosis is made by barium swallow and esophagoscopy. Dilatation is effective for patients with only muscular stenosis, but segmental resection may be required for rigid defects as is found with cartilaginous remnants.

C. TRACHEAL STENOSIS

Congenital tracheal stenosis is a rare disease ranging from an isolated defect to pulmonary agenesis. It is often fatal. The diagnosis is made by bronchoscopy.

Individual reports of successful segmental resection or alternative grafts have been noted.

Treatment

A. PRETREATMENT RISK EVALUATION

The **Waterston classification** has been used as a risk evaluation to predict the outcome and determine the surgical timing. Historically, patients in **Category A,** which is defined as a birth weight > 5.5 pounds, receive prompt surgical correction. A patient in **Category B,** with a birth weight of 4.0–5.5 pounds or an infant who presents with pneumonia and congenital anomaly, has short-term delay of surgical intervention. Patients receive a gastrostomy and are stabilized before surgical repair. Very ill infants with significant respiratory compromise due to a wide-open fistula may require ligation of the fistula, stabilization, and then subsequent esophageal reconstruction. A **Category C** classification, which is characterized by a patient birth weight of < 4.0 pounds or an infant who presents with severe pneumonia and congenital anomaly, classically receives a staged repair. Infants traditionally had improved outcomes with a staged procedure. However, the addition of total parenteral nutrition (TPN) to maintain the newborn's nutritional status and the fact that newborn mortality is attributed mostly to associated congenital anomalies have allowed patients in Category C to be treated with a delayed primary closure. In addition, low birth weight may not be an absolute contraindication to early repair. Currently, most children, with the exception of the most ill infants, undergo early complete repair.

B. PREOPERATIVE CARE

Before surgery, patients are kept in a head-up position with an oroesophageal tube for continuous suction and frequent pharyngeal aspiration. Broad-spectrum antibiotics are instituted, such as ampicillin and gentamicin. Parenteral nutrition is started if repair is delayed. Associated VACTERL anomalies are ruled out. In patients with a distal fistula, a gastrostomy tube for decompression may be necessary if patients present with severe abdominal distention and respiratory compromise.

C. SURGICAL MEASURES

Operative repair is performed through a right posterior lateral thoracotomy at the fourth intercostal space. A left-sided approach, which is the exception, is often used for an anomalous right-sided aortic arch. The procedure is usually performed extrapleurally. The dissection proceeds posteriorly, with the lung reflected anteriorly. The azygos vein overlies the fistula and is either reflected superiorly or divided. The vagus is identified lying over the two esophageal segments. The fistula is divided and the trachea is closed with interrupted non-

absorbable sutures followed by coverage with adjacent tissue. The proximal esophagus is dissected freely up to the thoracic inlet to provide adequate length; it is also approximated to the distal esophageal segment.

Care must be taken when dissecting the esophagus from the membranous portion of the trachea, since the two structures are usually adherent. Single-layer, full-thickness interrupted sutures create the anastomosis. A drainage catheter is placed in the retropleural space. Difficult repairs that are due to a long gap between the proximal and distal esophageal ends have been approached by serial stretching of the proximal segment with twice-daily bougie catheter dilations. Intraoperatively, either proximal circumferential or proximal spiral esophagomyotomies can provide the extra length needed. If insufficient length to perform the anastomosis is encountered, a staged repair with a cervical esophagotomy with serial stretching followed by anastomotic construction can be performed. Another method of repairing a long-gap esophageal atresia is lengthening the esophageal ends by placing sutures on the ends of the esophagus, exteriorizing them, and then putting them on tension. The anastomosis is then completed within 10 days.

Alternately, an esophageal replacement can be performed with a colon interposition or gastric tube graft. If a long-gap atresia is expected, particularly with isolated esophageal atresia, then a gastrostomy should be performed initially, with a subsequent esophageal reconstruction or replacement. Increasingly, repair of esophageal atresia and tracheoesophageal fistula is being repaired using a thoracoscopic technique.

Bax KM, van Der Zee DC. Feasibility of thoracoscopic repair of esophageal atresia with distal fistula. *J Pediatr Surg.* 2002;37:192. [PMID: 11819197] (Case series report on thoracoscopic repair examining outcomes in addition to complications of anastomotic leak and stenosis.)

Foker JE, Linden BC, Boyle EM Jr, Marquardt C. Development of a true primary repair for the full spectrum of esophageal atresia. *Ann Surg.* 1997;226(4):533. [PMID: 9351721] (Case series report on elongation of esophageal ends using traction with sutures.)

Kimura K, Nishijima E, Tsugawa C et al. Multistaged extrathoracic esophageal elongation procedure for long-gap esophageal atresia: experience with 12 patients. *J Pediatr Surg.* 2001;36:1725. [PMID: 11685713] (Case series with follow-up of a multistaged procedure for repair of long-gap esophageal atresia.)

Complications

A. ANASTOMOTIC LEAK

Anastomotic leak occurs in 10–20% of patients. Most reports implicate anastomotic tension and esophagomyotomy as factors increasing the chance for leak. This condition can be diagnosed with saliva in the postoperative chest tube aspirate. Barium swallow diagnoses the location and the extent of the leak. Most small leaks close spontaneously with nonoperative management.

B. Anastomotic Stricture

Anastomotic stricture presents in approximately 25% of cases. Patients can present with aspiration, malnutrition, and food obstruction. Strictures are diagnosed by barium swallow and usually treated successfully with one or more esophageal dilatations. Occasionally, a segmental esophageal resection is required for refractory strictures.

C. Gastroesophageal Reflux Disease (GERD)

Gastroesophageal reflux can contribute to anastomotic stricture. It occurs in about 50% of patients. Intrinsic poor esophageal motility allows for the reflux of gastric acids, leading to aspiration, esophagitis, and scarring. The diagnosis is made by 24-hour esophageal pH monitoring. The treatment is aggressive medical therapy; however, about 30% of patients require antireflux fundoplication.

D. Tracheomalacia

Tracheomalacia is diagnosed by bronchoscopy. Some studies report a 25% incidence. This disorder can result from poor development of the cartilaginous rings at the level of the fistula. It should be suspected in any patient with respiratory symptoms. Mild cases usually improve by age 1 or 2; however, severe cases are treated with aortopexy.

Dutta HK, Gover VP, Dwivedi SN, Bhatnagar V. Manometric evaluation of postoperative patients of esophageal atresia and tracheoesophageal fistula. *Eur J Pediatr Surg.* 2001;11:371. [PMID: 11807665] (Manometry of patients who received repair for esophageal atresia and tracheoesophageal fistula demonstrating altered pressure and contractility profile of the esophagus.)

Prognosis

Esophageal atresia is lethal if not corrected. Patients with the VACTERL association have a poorer prognosis owing to the presence of the other anomalies. In fact, the mortality risk is greater for the associated anomalies than for esophageal atresia and tracheoesophageal fistula. The current survival rate of postsurgical repair is reported to be > 90%.

Driver CP, Shankar KR, Jones MO et al. Phenotypic presentation and outcome of esophageal atresia in the era of the Spitz classification. *J Pediatr Surg.* 2001;36:1419. [PMID: 11528619] (Cohort study over a 12-year period. Patients with increasing incidence of cardiac anomalies.)

Benign & Malignant Disorders of the Esophagus

35

Marco G. Patti, MD, Fernando A. Herbella, MD, & Michael Korn, MD

ANATOMY

The esophagus is a muscular tube that extends from the level of the sixth cervical vertebra to the 11th thoracic vertebra, spanning three anatomic regions. The cervical esophagus lies left of the midline and posterior to the larynx and trachea. This portion receives its blood supply from branches of the inferior thyroid arteries and drains into the inferior thyroid veins. The upper portion of the thoracic esophagus passes behind the tracheal bifurcation and the left mainstem bronchus. The lower portion of the thoracic esophagus passes behind the left atrium and then enters the abdomen through the esophageal hiatus of the diaphragm.

The thoracic esophagus is supplied by the bronchial arteries (upper portion) and the branches of the thoracic aorta (midportion) and drains into the hemiazygos and azygos veins. The abdominal esophagus ends at the level of the junction with the stomach. The lowermost thoracic esophagus and the abdominal esophagus are nourished by the branches of the left gastric and inferior phrenic arteries and drain into the left gastric veins. Abundant lymphatics form a dense submucosal plexus. Lymph from the upper esophagus drains mostly in the cervical and paratracheal lymph nodes, whereas the lower thoracic and abdominal esophagus drains preferentially into the retrocardiac and celiac nodes.

The architecture of the esophageal wall consists of three layers. The mucosa is made of squamous epithelium overlying a lamina propria and a muscularis mucosa. The submucosa is made of elastic and fibrous tissue and is the strongest layer of the esophageal wall. The esophageal muscle is composed of an inner circular and an outer longitudinal layer. The upper third of the esophageal musculature consists of skeletal muscle and the lower two thirds consist of smooth muscle. The upper esophageal sphincter is formed by the cricopharyngeus muscle along with the inferior constrictors of the pharynx and fibers of the esophageal wall.

The lower esophageal sphincter is not a distinct anatomic structure. The esophagus does not have a serosal layer.

PHYSIOLOGY

The coordinated activity of the upper esophageal sphincter (UES), the esophageal body, and the lower esophageal sphincter (LES) is responsible for the motor function of the esophagus.

UPPER ESOPHAGEAL SPHINCTER

The UES receives motor innervation directly from the brain (ie, the nucleus ambiguus). The sphincter is continuously in a state of tonic contraction, with a resting pressure of approximately 60–100 mm Hg. The sphincter prevents both the passage of air from the pharynx into the esophagus and the reflux of esophageal contents into the pharynx. During swallowing, a food bolus is moved by the tongue into the pharynx, which contracts while the UES relaxes. After the food bolus has reached the esophagus, the UES regains its resting tone (Figure 35–1).

ESOPHAGEAL BODY

When food passes through the UES, a contraction is initiated in the upper esophagus, which progresses distally toward the stomach. The wave initiated by swallowing is referred to as *primary peristalsis*. It travels at a speed of 3–4 cm/s and reaches peak amplitudes of 60–140 mm Hg in the distal esophagus.

LOWER ESOPHAGEAL SPHINCTER

The LES measures 3–4 cm in length and its resting pressure ranges between 15 and 24 mm Hg. At the time of swallowing, the LES relaxes for 5–10 seconds to allow the food bolus to enter the stomach, and then it regains its rest-

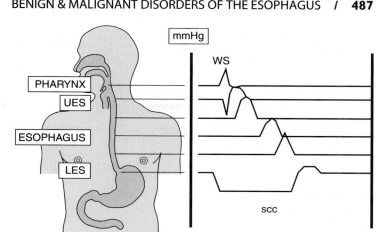

Figure 35–1. The swallowing process. LES, lower esophageal sphincter; SCC, squamous cell carcinoma; UES, upper esophageal sphincter; WS, wet swallow.

ing tone (see Figure 35–1). The LES relaxation is mediated by vasoactive intestinal polypeptide and nitric oxide, both nonadrenergic and noncholinergic neurotransmitters. The resting tone depends mainly on intrinsic myogenic activity. The LES has a tendency to relax periodically at times, independent from swallowing. These periodic relaxations are called *transient lower esophageal sphincter relaxations* to distinguish them from relaxations triggered by swallows. The cause of these transient relaxations is not known, but gastric distention probably plays a role.

Transient LES relaxations account for the small amount of physiologic gastroesophageal reflux present in any individual and are also the most common cause of reflux in patients with gastroesophageal reflux disease (GERD). A decrease in the length or the pressure (or both) of the LES is responsible for abnormal reflux in the remaining patients. Overall, it is thought that although transient LES relaxation is the most common mechanism of reflux in patients with either absent or mild esophagi-

tis, the prevalence of a mechanically defective sphincter (ie, hypotensive, short, or both) increases in patients with more severe esophagitis. The crus of the esophageal hiatus of the diaphragm contributes to the resting pressure of the LES. The pinchcock action of the diaphragm is particularly important because it protects against reflux caused by sudden increases of intraabdominal pressure, such as with coughing or bending. This synergistic action of the diaphragm is lost when a sliding hiatal hernia is present, since the gastroesophageal junction is displaced above the diaphragm (Figure 35–2).

Lang IM, Shaker R. Anatomy and physiology of the upper esophageal sphincter. *Am J Med.* 1997;103:50. [PMID: 9422624] (Review of the anatomy and physiology of the upper esophageal sphincter.)

Mittal RK, Balaban DH. The esophagogastric junction. *N Engl J Med.* 1997;336:924. [PMID: 9070474] (Review of the anatomy and physiology of the esophagogastric junction.)

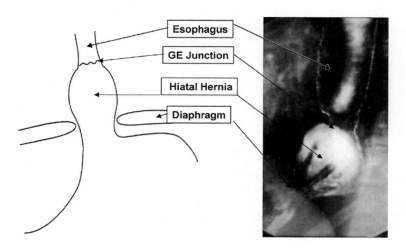

Figure 35–2. Hiatal hernia.

Patti MG, Gantert W, Way LW. Surgery of the esophagus: anatomy and physiology. *Surg Clin North Am.* 1997;77:959. [PMID: 9347826] (Review of the esophageal anatomy and physiology.)

BENIGN DISORDERS OF THE ESOPHAGUS

ACHALASIA

 ESSENTIALS OF DIAGNOSIS

- *Dysphagia.*
- *Regurgitation.*
- *Radiologic evidence of distal esophageal narrowing.*
- *Absence of esophageal peristalsis on manometry.*

General Considerations

Esophageal achalasia is a primary esophageal motility disorder characterized by the absence of esophageal peristalsis and increased pressure of the LES, which fails to relax completely in response to swallowing. The disease is rare, with an incidence of about 1 in 100,000 individuals. It affects men more than women, and it can occur at any age.

Pathogenesis

The cause of esophageal achalasia in unknown. A degeneration of the myenteric plexus of Auerbach has been documented, with loss of the postganglionic inhibitory neurons. These neurons contain nitric oxide and vasoactive intestinal polypeptide, which mediate LES relaxation. Because the postganglionic cholinergic neurons are spared, there is unopposed cholinergic stimulation with an increased LES resting pressure and insufficient relaxation.

Clinical Findings

A. SYMPTOMS AND SIGNS

Dysphagia, for solids and liquids, is the most common symptom. Most patients adapt to this symptom by changing their diet and are able to maintain a stable weight, whereas others experience a progressive increase in dysphagia that eventually leads to weight loss. Regurgitation is the second most common symptom and it is present in about 60% of patients. It occurs more often in the supine position and may lead to the aspiration of undigested food. Heartburn is present in about 40% of patients, and it is caused by stasis and fermentation of undigested food in the distal esophagus. Chest pain also occurs in 40% of patients.

B. IMAGING STUDIES

In evaluating a patient with dysphagia, a barium swallow should be the first test performed. It usually shows a narrowing at the level of the gastroesophageal junction (Figure 35–3A). A dilated, sigmoid esophagus may be present in patients with long-standing achalasia (Figure 35–3B). An endoscopy should be performed to rule out a tumor of the esophagogastric junction and gastroduodenal pathology.

C. SPECIAL TESTS

1. Esophageal manometry—Esophageal manometry is the key test for establishing the diagnosis of esophageal achalasia. The classic manometric findings are (1) absence of esophageal peristalsis and (2) a hypertensive LES that relaxes only partially in response to swallowing.

2. Ambulatory pH monitoring—In patients who have undergone pneumatic dilatation or a myotomy, ambulatory pH monitoring should always be performed to rule out abnormal gastroesophageal reflux; if present, it should be treated with acid-reducing medications.

Differential Diagnosis

Benign strictures caused by gastroesophageal reflux and esophageal carcinoma may mimic the clinical presentation of achalasia. Sometimes an infiltrating tumor of the cardia can mimic not only the clinical and radiologic presentation of achalasia, but also the manometric profile. This condition is known as **secondary achalasia** or **pseudoachalasia** and should be suspected in patients older than 60 years of age who present with a recent onset of dysphagia and excessive weight loss. An endoscopic ultrasound or a computed tomography (CT) scan can help to establish the diagnosis.

Complications

The aspiration of retained and undigested food can cause repeated episodes of pneumonia. Achalasia is also a risk factor for esophageal cancer. Squamous cell carcinoma is probably due to the continuous irritation of the mucosa by the retained and fermenting food. However, adenocarcinoma can occur in patients who develop gastroesophageal reflux after either pneumatic dilatation or myotomy.

Treatment

Therapy is palliative and is directed toward relieving symptoms by decreasing the outflow resistance caused

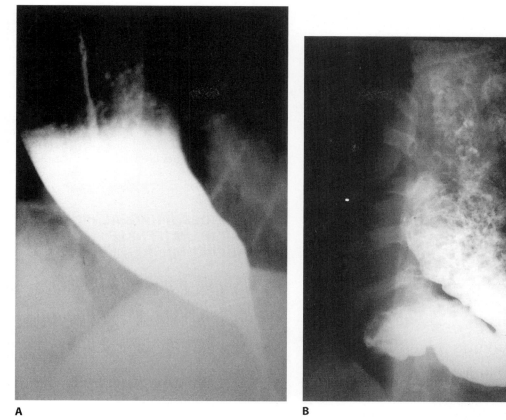

A   **B**

Figure 35–3. Achalasia. **(A)** "Bird-beak." **(B)** Dilated and sigmoid esophagus.

by the dysfunctional LES. Because peristalsis is absent, gravity becomes the key factor that allows the emptying of food from the esophagus into the stomach. Several treatment modalities are available to achieve this goal.

A. NONSURGICAL MEASURES

1. Calcium channel blockers—Calcium channel blockers are used to decrease LES pressure. However, only 10% of patients benefit from this treatment. It should be used primarily in elderly patients who have contraindications to either pneumatic dilatation or surgery.

2. Endoscopy—An intrasphincteric injection of botulinum toxin is used to block the release of acetylcholine at the level of the LES, therefore restoring the balance between excitatory and inhibitory neurotransmitters. This treatment, however, is of limited value since only 30% of treated patients still experience a relief of dysphagia 2.5 years later. It should be used primarily in elderly patients who are poor candidates for dilatation or surgery.

3. Pneumatic dilatation—Pneumatic dilatation has been the main form of treatment for many years. The initial success rate is between 70% and 80%, but it decreases to 50% 10 years later, even after multiple dilatations. The perforation rate is approximately 5%. If a perforation occurs, patients are taken emergently to the operating room, where closure of the perforation and a myotomy are performed through a left thoracotomy. The incidence of abnormal gastroesophageal reflux is about 25%. Patients who fail pneumatic dilatation are usually treated by a Heller myotomy.

B. SURGICAL MEASURES

A **laparoscopic Heller myotomy** and partial fundoplication is the procedure of choice for esophageal achalasia. The operation consists of a controlled division of the muscle fibers (ie, a myotomy) of the lower esophagus (5 cm) and proximal stomach (2 cm), followed by a partial fundoplication to prevent reflux (Figure 35–4). Patients remain in the hospital for 24–48 hours, and return to regular activities in about 2 weeks. The opera-

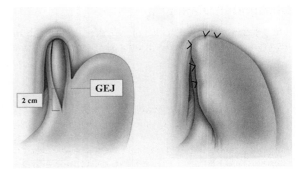

Figure 35–4. Heller myotomy **(left)** and Dor fundoplication **(right)**. GEJ, gastroesophageal junction.

tion effectively relieves symptoms in 85–95% of patients, and the incidence of postoperative reflux is between 10% and 15%. Because of the excellent results, short hospital stay, and fast recovery time, a laparoscopic Heller myotomy and partial fundoplication is considered today to be the primary treatment modality for esophageal achalasia.

Prognosis

A laparoscopic Heller myotomy allows for the excellent relief of symptoms in the majority of patients and should be preferred to pneumatic dilatation whenever surgical expertise is available. Botulinum toxin and medications should be used only in patients who are not candidates for pneumatic dilatation or laparoscopic Heller myotomy. Periodic follow-up by endoscopy is recommended to rule out the development of esophageal cancer.

Khajanchee YS, Kanneganti S, Leatherwood A et al. Laparoscopic Heller myotomy with Toupet fundoplication: outcomes predictors in 121 consecutive patients. *Arch Surg.* 2005;140:827. (Heller myotomy relieves symptoms in more than 90% of patients.)

Moonka R, Patti MG, Feo CV et al. Clinical presentation and evaluation of malignant pseudoachalasia. *J Gastrointest Surg.* 1999;3:456. [PMID: 10482700] (Esophageal tumors can mimic the clinical and manometric picture of achalasia.)

Patti MG, Gorodner MV, Galvani C et al. Spectrum of esophageal motility disorders: implications for diagnosis and treatment. *Arch Surg.* 2005;140:442. (Largest published series of diagnosis and treatment of esophageal motility disorders).

Patti MG, Molena D, Fisichella PM et al. Laparoscopic Heller myotomy and Dor fundoplication for achalasia. *Arch Surg.* 2001;136:870. [PMID: 11485521] (Heller myotomy relieves symptoms in more than 90% of patients.)

Vaezi MF, Richter JE, Wilcox CM et al. Botulinum toxin versus pneumatic dilatation in the treatment of achalasia: a randomized trial. *Gut.* 1999;44:231. [PMID: 9895383] (Pneumatic dilatation is superior to botulinum toxin for the treatment of achalasia.)

West RL, Hirsch DP, Bartelsman JF et al. Long-term results of pneumatic dilatation in achalasia followed more than 5 years. *Am J Gastroenterol.* 2002;97:1346. [PMID: 12094848] (Long-term follow-up of patients after pneumatic dilatation.)

ESOPHAGEAL DIVERTICULA

Diverticula of the esophagus are mainly located above the LES (epiphrenic diverticulum) or the UES (pharyngoesophageal—or Zenker—diverticulum). They are both caused by abnormalities involving the LES or the UES, which result in protrusion of the mucosa and submucosa through the muscular layers.

PHARYNGOESOPHAGEAL DIVERTICULUM (ZENKER DIVERTICULUM)

 ESSENTIALS OF DIAGNOSIS

- *Dysphagia.*
- *Regurgitation of undigested food (with risk of aspiration).*
- *Gurgling sounds in the neck.*
- *Halitosis.*

General Considerations

Zenker diverticulum originates from the posterior wall of the esophagus in a triangular area of weakness, limited inferiorly by the cricopharyngeus muscle and superiorly by the inferior constrictor muscles (ie, the Killian triangle). As the diverticulum enlarges, it tends to deviate from the midline, mostly to the left (Figure 35–5).

Pathogenesis

Zenker diverticulum results from either a lack of coordination between the pharyngeal contraction and the opening of the UES or a hypertensive UES. Because of the increased intraluminal pressure, there is progressive herniation of mucosa and submucosa through the Killian triangle.

Clinical Findings

A. Symptoms and Signs

Dysphagia is the most common symptom. The regurgitation of undigested food from the diverticulum often occurs and can lead to both aspiration into the tracheobronchial tree and pneumonia. Patients frequently have

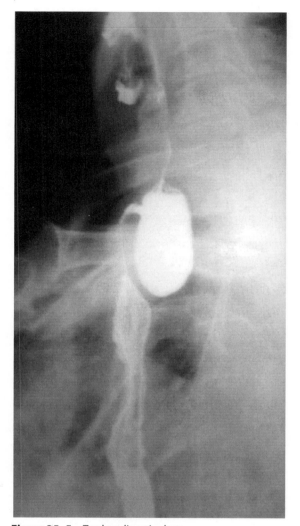

Figure 35–5. Zenker diverticulum.

halitosis and can hear gurgling sounds in the neck. About 30–50% of patients have associated GERD.

B. IMAGING STUDIES

A barium swallow can clearly show the position and size of the diverticulum. It can also show a hiatal hernia.

C. SPECIAL TESTS

Esophageal manometry can demonstrate a lack of coordination between the pharynx and the cricopharyngeus muscle, as well as a hypertensive UES. In addition, it can show a hypotensive LES and abnormal esophageal peristalsis. Ambulatory pH monitoring can determine whether abnormal esophageal acid exposure is present.

Differential Diagnosis

The differential diagnosis of Zenker diverticulum includes esophageal stricture, achalasia, esophageal cancer, and pneumonia.

Treatment

The standard treatment consists of excision of the diverticulum and myotomy of the cricopharyngeus muscle, including the upper 3 cm of the posterior esophageal wall. For small diverticula (ie, < 2 cm), myotomy alone is sufficient. As an alternative to the conventional treatment, a transoral endoscopic approach, using an endoscopic stapling instrument, can be used for diverticula between 3 cm and 6 cm. If GERD is present, it should be treated aggressively with either proton pump inhibitors or fundoplication in order to avoid aspiration into the tracheobronchial tree.

Prognosis

The prognosis is excellent in about 90% of cases.

Aly A, Devitt PG, Jamieson GG. Evolution of surgical treatment for pharyngeal pouch. *Br J Surg.* 2004;91:657. [PMID: 15164432] (Review article describing the evolution of treatment of Zenker's diverticulum.)

Counter PR, Hilton ML, Baldwin DL. Long-term follow-up of endoscopic stapled diverticulotomy. *Ann R Coll Surg Engl.* 2002;84:89. [PMID: 11995771] (Endoscopic, stapled diverticulotomy.)

Smith SR, Gendene M, Urken ML. Endoscopic stapling technique for the treatment of Zenker diverticulum vs standard open-neck technique: a direct comparison and charge analysis. *Arch Otolaryngol Head Neck Surg.* 2002;128:141. [PMID: 11843721] (Endoscopic stapled diverticulotomy is more cost effective than open surgery.)

EPIPHRENIC DIVERTICULUM

 ESSENTIALS OF DIAGNOSIS

- *Dysphagia.*
- *Regurgitation.*
- *Diverticulum evident on barium swallow.*
- *Esophageal motility disorder shown by esophageal manometry.*

General Considerations

Epiphrenic diverticula are located just above the diaphragm (Figure 35–6). The diverticulum is not a primary anatomic abnormality but rather the consequence

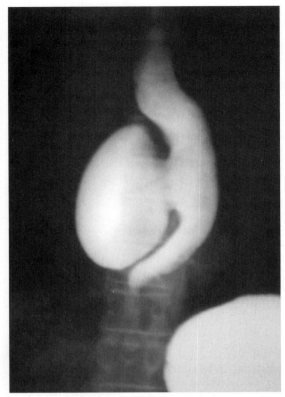

Figure 35–6. Epiphrenic diverticulum.

of an underlying motility disorder of the esophagus; achalasia is the most common, followed by diffuse esophageal spasm. The disorder causes an outflow obstruction at the level of the gastroesophageal junction, with a consequent increase in intraluminal pressure as well as progressive herniation of mucosa and submucosa through the esophageal muscle wall.

Clinical Findings

A. SYMPTOMS AND SIGNS

The symptoms experienced by patients with epiphrenic diverticulum are in part due to the underlying motility disorder (eg, dysphagia or chest pain) and in part due to the diverticulum per se (ie, regurgitation with the risk of aspiration). Some diverticula, however, can be asymptomatic.

B. IMAGING STUDIES

A chest radiograph can show an air-fluid level in the posterior mediastinum. A barium swallow clearly shows the position and size of the diverticulum (see Figure 35–6).

C. SPECIAL TESTS

In most cases, esophageal manometry identifies the underlying motility disorder.

Differential Diagnosis

A paraesophageal hernia can be confused with an epiphrenic diverticulum. Barium swallow and endoscopy help in establishing the diagnosis.

Treatment

The treatment is surgical and the laparoscopic approach is currently preferred. This procedure consists of (1) resection of the diverticulum, (2) a long myotomy, and (3) a partial fundoplication to prevent gastroesophageal reflux. The myotomy is performed in the side of the esophagus opposite to where the diverticulum is located. It should extend proximally to the upper border of the neck of the diverticulum and distally for 2 cm onto the gastric wall; a partial fundoplication is then performed.

Prognosis

A laparoscopic diverticulectomy, with myotomy and fundoplication, is successful in 80–90% of cases.

Klaus A, Hinder RA, Swain J, Achem SR. Management of epiphrenic diverticula. *J Gastrointest Surg.* 2003;7:906. [PMID: 14592666] (Laparoscopic treatment of epiphrenic diverticula.)

Nehra D, Fumagulli W, Bona S et al. Physiologic basis for the treatment of epiphrenic diverticulum. *Ann Surg.* 2002;235:346. [PMID: 11882756] (A physiologic approach to the treatment of epiphrenic diverticulum.)

Tedesco P, Fisichella PM, Way LW, Patti MG. Cause and treatment of epiphrenic diverticula. *Am J Surg.* 2005;190(6):891.

GASTROESOPHAGEAL REFLUX DISEASE

 ESSENTIALS OF DIAGNOSIS

- *Heartburn.*
- *Regurgitation.*
- *Sliding hiatal hernia on barium swallow.*
- *Esophagitis on endoscopy.*
- *Abnormal esophageal exposure on ambulatory pH monitoring.*

General Considerations

GERD is the most common upper gastrointestinal disorder in the Western world and accounts for approximately 75% of esophageal diseases. Heartburn, usually considered synonymous with the presence of abnormal gastroesophageal reflux, is experienced by 20–40% of the adult population of Western countries. The incidence of reflux symptoms increases with age, and both sexes seem to be equally affected. Symptoms are more common during pregnancy, probably because of hormonal effects on the LES and the increased intra-abdominal pressure of the enlarging uterus.

Pathogenesis

GERD is caused by the abnormal retrograde flow of gastric contents into the esophagus, resulting in symptoms, mucosal damage, or both. A defective LES is the most common cause of GERD. Transient LES relaxations account for most reflux episodes in patients either without mucosal damage or with mild esophagitis, whereas a short and hypotensive LES is more frequently found in patients with more severe esophagitis. In 40–60% of patients with GERD, abnormalities of esophageal peristalsis are also present. Because esophageal peristalsis is the main determinant of esophageal acid clearance (ie, the ability of the esophagus to clear gastric contents refluxed through the LES), patients with abnormal esophageal peristalsis have more severe reflux and slower clearance. Therefore, these patients often have more severe mucosal injury and more frequent atypical symptoms such as cough or hoarseness. A hiatal hernia also contributes to the incompetence of the gastroesophageal junction by altering the anatomic relationship between the LES and the esophageal crus. In patients with large hiatal hernias, the LES is usually shorter and weaker and the amount of reflux is greater.

Clinical Findings

A. Symptoms and Signs

Heartburn, regurgitation, and dysphagia are considered typical symptoms of GERD. However, a clinical diagnosis of GERD, based on typical symptoms such as heartburn and regurgitation, is correct in only 70% of patients when compared with the results of pH monitoring. A good response to therapy with proton pump inhibitors is instead a better predictor of the presence of abnormal reflux. In addition to the typical symptoms, patients with GERD can present with atypical symptoms such as cough, wheezing, chest pain, hoarseness, and dental erosions. These symptoms represent extra-esophageal presentations of the disease, including respiratory disorders such as asthma, as well as ear, nose, and throat abnormalities such as laryngitis (Table 35–1). Two mechanisms have been postulated for GERD-induced respiratory symptoms: (1) a vagal reflux arc resulting in bronchoconstriction and (2) microaspira-

Table 35–1. Typical and atypical symptoms of GERD.

Typical symptoms
Heartburn
Regurgitation
Dysphagia
Atypical symptoms
Hoarseness
Chronic laryngitis and sore throat
Globus sensation
Otitis media
Dental erosions
Noncardiac chest pain
Chronic cough
Aspiration pneumonia
Asthma

tion into the tracheobronchial tree. Ear, nose and throat symptoms such as hoarseness or dental erosions are instead secondary to the upward extent of the acid with direct damage.

B. Imaging Studies

1. Barium swallow—A barium swallow provides information about the presence and size of a hiatal hernia, the presence and length of a stricture, and the length of the esophagus. This test, however, is not diagnostic of GERD since a hiatal hernia or reflux of barium can be present in patients who do not have GERD.

2. Endoscopy—The value of endoscopy is mostly limited to the detection of the complications of GERD (eg, esophagitis, Barrett esophagus, and stricture) and to the exclusion of other pathology (esophageal, gastric, or duodenal). The value of endoscopy in diagnosing GERD is limited because only 50% of patients with GERD have esophagitis. In addition, there is major inter-observer variation among endoscopists for the low grades of esophagitis.

C. Specials Tests

1. Esophageal manometry—Esophageal manometry provides information about the LES, including the resting pressure, length, and relaxation, as well as about the quality of esophageal peristalsis. In about 40% of patients with GERD, the pressure of the LES and the peristalsis are normal. In addition, manometry is essential for proper placement of the pH probe for ambulatory pH monitoring (5 cm above the upper border of the LES).

2. Ambulatory pH monitoring—Ambulatory pH monitoring is the most reliable test in the diagnosis of GERD, with a sensitivity and specificity of about 92%. Acid-suppressing medications must be stopped 3 days (eg, H_2-blocking agents) to 14 days (eg, proton pump inhibitors)

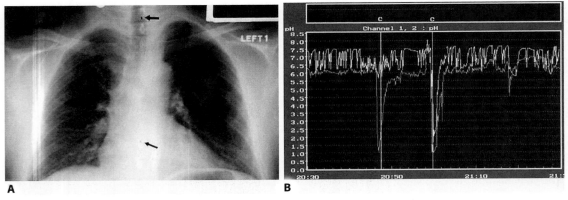

Figure 35–7. Ambulatory pH monitoring. **(A)** Two sensors located 5 and 20 cm above the lower esophageal sphincter. **(B)** Correlation between episodes of reflux and cough (c).

prior to the study. Diet and exercise are unrestricted during the test in order to mimic a typical day of the patient's life. This test should always be performed (1) in patients who do not respond to medical therapy; (2) in patients who relapse after the discontinuation of medical therapy; (3) before antireflux surgery; and (4) when atypical symptoms are present. In patients with atypical symptoms a pH probe with two sensors (5 and 20 cm above the LES) is used to determine the upward extent of the reflux. The tracing should be analyzed for a temporal correlation between symptoms and episodes of reflux (Figure 35–7).

Differential Diagnosis

Irritable bowel syndrome, achalasia, cholelithiasis, and coronary artery disease can present with heartburn. Esophageal manometry and pH monitoring are essential to determine with certainty whether GERD is present.

Complications

Esophagitis is the most common complication. Barrett esophagus (ie, metaplastic changes from squamous to columnar epithelium) is found in about 12% of patients with reflux documented by pH monitoring. This complication may lead to the development of adenocarcinoma. Asthma, aspiration pneumonia, laryngitis, chronic sinusitis, and dental erosions can also occur.

Treatment

A. NONSURGICAL MEASURES

1. Life-style modifications—Patients should eat frequent, small meals during the day to avoid gastric distention. They should also avoid fatty foods, spicy foods, and chocolate, because these foods lower the LES pressure. The last meal of the day should be no less than 2 hours before going to bed.

To increase the effect of gravity, the head of the bed should be elevated over 4- to 6-inch blocks.

2. Other nonsurgical measures—Antacids are useful for patients with mild intermittent heartburn. Acid-suppressing medications are the mainstay of medical therapy. H_2 blocking agents are usually prescribed for patients with mild symptoms or mild esophagitis. Proton pump inhibitors are superior to H_2 blocking agents because they exert a more profound control of acid secretion—healing of the esophagitis occurs in 80–90% of these patients. However, both the symptoms and esophagitis tend to recur in most patients after therapy is discontinued so that most patients need chronic maintenance therapy. In addition, about 50% of patients on maintenance proton pump inhibitors require increasing doses to maintain healing of the esophagitis. Medical therapy is largely ineffective for the treatment of the extra-esophageal manifestations of GERD due to the upward extension of the gastric contents. In these patients, acid-suppressing medications only alter the pH of the gastric refluxate, but reflux and aspiration still occur because of an incompetent LES and an ineffective esophageal peristalsis.

B. SURGICAL MEASURES

1. Laparoscopic fundoplication—The goal of surgical therapy is to restore the competence of the LES. A laparoscopic total fundoplication (360°) is considered the procedure of choice because it increases the resting pressure and length of the LES and decreases the number of transient LES relaxations (Figure 35–8).

2. Indications for surgery—A laparoscopic fundoplication provides the same excellent results of open surgery, with symptom resolution in more than 90% of patients. It now requires a 1- to 2-day hospital stay and results in both minimal postoperative discomfort and a fast return to regular activity.

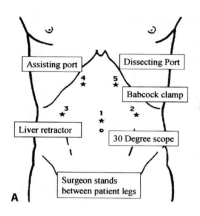

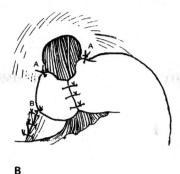

Figure 35–8. Laparoscopic Nissen fundoplication. **(A)** Position of the trocars. **(B)** Completed fundoplication.

The ideal patient is one who has a good response to proton pump inhibitors. A patient who is nonresponsive to medical therapy requires a thorough work-up to elucidate the cause of the foregut symptoms, and an alternative diagnosis ranging from irritable bowel syndrome to gallbladder disease is frequently found. Young patients might also choose an operation early in the course of their disease to avoid a life-long commitment to life-style changes and medications.

Patients who have regurgitation with respiratory symptoms or hoarseness are also ideal candidates for a fundoplication. Even the complete elimination of gastric acid secretion by proton pump inhibitors frequently fails to control these symptoms, since it only alters the pH of the gastric refluxate but does not prevent the regurgitation and upward extent of the reflux. Analyzing the pH tracing for a correlation between the symptoms and the episodes of reflux helps to predict the surgical outcome (see Figure 35–7).

Many surgeons also consider the presence of Barrett esophagus as an indication for surgical rather than medical treatment, based on the following considerations: (1) Proton pump inhibitors, although effective in controlling the acid component of refluxate, do not eliminate the reflux of bile, which is a major contributor to the pathogenesis of Barrett epithelium. (2) Patients with Barrett esophagus have a lower LES pressure and a defective peristalsis more often than patients without Barrett esophagus. As a consequence, their mucosa is exposed to larger amounts of gastric refluxate. (3) Evidence suggests that an effective antireflux operation can prevent the progression from metaplasia to dysplasia. The definite answer, however, awaits the results of further randomized control studies; therefore, endoscopic surveillance after laparoscopic fundoplication is recommended.

Prognosis

After a fundoplication, the control of typical symptoms is obtained in about 90% of patients. The success rate is in the range of 70–90% for patients with atypical symptoms, since it is often more difficult to establish, preoperatively, a strong correlation between gastroesophageal reflux and symptoms.

Campos GM, Peters JH, DeMeester TR et al. Multivariate analysis of factors predicting outcome after laparoscopic Nissen fundoplication. *J Gastrointest Surg.* 1999;3:292. [PMID: 10481122] (Preoperative factors that predict a good outcome after laparoscopic fundoplication.)

Diener U, Patti MG, Molena D, Fisichella PM, Way LW. Esophageal dysmotility and gastroesophageal reflux disease. *J Gastrointest Surg.* 2001;5:260. [PMID: 11360049] (Patients with abnormal esophageal peristalsis have more acid reflux, slower clearance, and worse mucosal injury.)

Gaynor EB. Laryngeal complications of GERD. *J Clin Gastroenterol.* 2000;30:31. [PMID: 10777169] (Ear, nose, and throat manifestations of gastroesophageal reflux disease.)

Jailwala JA, Shaker R. Oral and pharyngeal complications of gastroesophageal reflux disease: globus, dental erosions, chronic sinusitis. *J Clin Gastroenterol.* 2000;30:35. [PMID: 10777170] (Ear, nose, and throat manifestations of gastroesophageal reflux disease.)

Patti MG, Arecerito M, Tamburini A et al. Effect of laparoscopic fundoplication on gastroesophageal reflux disease-induced respiratory symptoms. *J Gastrointest Surg.* 2000;4:143. [PMID: 10675237] (Laparoscopic fundoplication is an effective treatment for GERD-induced respiratory symptoms.)

Patti MG, Diener U, Tamburini A, Molena D, Way LW. Role of esophageal function tests in the diagnosis of gastroesophageal reflux disease. *Dig Dis Sci.* 2001;46:597. [PMID: 11318538] (Esophageal manometry and pH monitoring are necessary to establish the diagnosis of gastroesophageal reflux disease.)

Patti MG, Robinson T, Galvani C et al. Total fundoplication is superior to partial fundoplication even when esophageal peristalsis is weak. *J Am Coll Surg.* 2004;198:863. [PMID: 15194064] (Study comparing total and partial fundoplication for gastroesophageal reflux disease.)

Patti MG, Tedesco P, Golden J et al. Idiopathic pulmonary fibrosis. How often is it really idiopathic? *J Gastrointest Surg.* 2005;9:1053. [PMID: 16269375] (Gastroesophageal reflux disease has probably a cause-and-effect relationship with idiopathic pulmonary fibrosis.)

Richter JE. Extraesophageal presentations of gastroesophageal reflux disease: an overview. *Am J Gastroenterol.* 2000;95:1. [PMID: 10950098] (Atypical symptoms of gastroesophageal reflux disease.)

Wetscher GJ, Glaser K, Hinder RA et al. Respiratory symptoms in patients with gastroesophageal reflux disease following medical therapy and following antireflux surgery. *Am J Surg.* 1997;174:639. [PMID: 9409589] (Surgical therapy is more effective than medical therapy for GERD-induced respiratory symptoms.)

■ MALIGNANT DISORDERS OF THE ESOPHAGUS

BARRETT ESOPHAGUS

ESSENTIALS OF DIAGNOSIS

- *GERD symptoms (typical and atypical).*
- *Endoscopic evidence of "salmon pink" epithelium above gastroesophageal junction.*
- *Specialized columnar epithelium on esophageal biopsy.*

General Considerations

Barrett esophagus is a metaplasia of the esophageal mucosa caused by the replacement of the squamous epithelium with columnar epithelium. About 10–12% of patients who undergo endoscopy for symptoms of GERD are found to have Barrett esophagus. It occurs more frequently in white men older than 50 years of age. This metaplasia may progress to high-grade dysplasia and eventually to adenocarcinoma. Thus, adenocarcinoma represents the final step of a sequence of events in which a benign disease (GERD) evolves into a preneoplastic disease and eventually into cancer (Figure 35–9).

Pathogenesis

Barrett esophagus is due to reflux of gastric acid and duodenal juice into the esophagus. Barrett metaplasia is considered an advanced stage of GERD characterized by a panesophageal motor disorder. When compared with patients with GERD with no mucosal injury or less severe esophagitis, patients with Barrett esophagus have a shorter and weaker LES and a decreased amplitude of esophageal peristalsis. As a consequence, the amount of reflux is greater and esophageal clearance is slower. In addition, hiatal hernia is more common in patients with Barrett metaplasia.

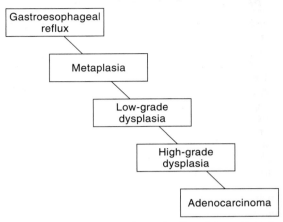

GER - Barrett's esophagus - Adenocarcinoma sequence.

Figure 35–9. Gastroesophageal reflux disease, Barrett esophagus, and adenocarcinoma sequence.

Clinical Findings

A. SYMPTOMS AND SIGNS

Patients with Barrett esophagus typically have a long history of GERD. Although most patients experience both typical and atypical symptoms of GERD, other patients may become asymptomatic over time because of the decreased sensitivity of the metaplastic epithelium.

B. IMAGING STUDIES

Barium swallow may show ulcerations, a hiatal hernia, or a stricture. Endoscopy shows a "salmon pink" epithelium above the gastroesophageal junction, which replaces the whitish squamous epithelium. The diagnosis is confirmed by pathologic examination of the esophageal mucosa and requires the identification of intestinal type epithelium, characterized by the presence of goblet cells.

C. SPECIAL TESTS

Esophageal manometry often shows a short and hypotensive LES and abnormal esophageal peristalsis. Ambulatory pH monitoring usually shows a severe amount of acid reflux. Esophageal exposure to duodenal juice can be quantified by a fiberoptic probe that measures intraluminal bilirubin (as a marker for duodenal juice). In patients with GERD, the prevalence of esophageal bilirubin exposure parallels the degree of mucosal injury; the bilirubin exposure is higher in patients with Barrett esophagus.

Treatment

A. BARRETT ESOPHAGUS: METAPLASIA

The treatment options for patients with Barrett esophagus are similar to those of patients with GERD without metaplasia; they consist of either proton pump inhibitors or a fundoplication. A surgical approach might offer an advantage over medical therapy for the following reasons: (1) The successful elimination of reflux symptoms with proton pump inhibitors does not guarantee the control of acid reflux. When pH monitoring is performed in patients with asymptomatic Barrett esophagus who are treated with these medications, up to 80% of them still experience abnormal reflux. (2) Proton pump inhibitors do not eliminate the reflux of bile, a major contributor to the pathogenesis of Barrett epithelium. An antireflux operation prevents both acid and bile refluxate by restoring the competence of the gastroesophageal junction. (3) Recent studies have shown regression of short-segment Barrett's epithelium (< 3 cm) in 15–50% of patients. However, because there is no definitive evidence that treatment (medical or surgical) prevents disease progression to cancer, regular follow-up should be performed with endoscopic examination and biopsy.

B. BARRETT ESOPHAGUS: HIGH-GRADE DYSPLASIA

When high-grade dysplasia is found (and confirmed by two experienced pathologists), two treatment options are available. (1) Patients can enroll in a program of strict endoscopic surveillance, with endoscopy performed every 3 months and four quadrant biopsies obtained for every centimeter of Barrett esophagus. The goal is to detect cancer before it becomes invasive and spreads to lymph nodes. (2) Alternately, for young and medically fit patients, an esophagectomy can be performed. Invasive cancer is already present in about 30% of patients thought to have high-grade dysplasia at the time of the operation. The prognosis depends on the pathologic staging.

New treatment modalities have been devised for endoscopic ablation of the columnar lining. The rationale for this treatment modality is to ablate the columnar epithelium, allowing regeneration of the squamous mucosa. Different techniques can be used, such as photodynamic therapy, thermal ablation, argon-beam plasma coagulation, and radiofrequency. These forms of therapy are still considered experimental.

Bowers SP, Mattar SG, Smith CD et al. Clinical and histologic follow-up after antireflux surgery for Barrett's esophagus. *J Gastrointest Surg*. 2002;6:532. [PMID: 12127118] (Effect of antireflux surgery on Barrett's epithelium.)

Castell DO. Medical, surgical, and endoscopic treatment of gastroesophageal reflux disease and Barrett esophagus. *J Clin Gastroenterol*. 2001;33:262. [PMID: 11588538] (Review of medical and surgical therapy for Barrett esophagus.)

Gerson LB, Shetler K, Triadafilopoulos G. Prevalence of Barrett esophagus in asymptomatic individuals. *Gastroenterology*. 2002;123:461. [PMID: 12145799] (Barrett esophagus can be found in patients without symptoms of gastroesophageal reflux disease.)

Lagergren J, Bergstrom R, Lindgren A, Nyren O. Symptomatic gastroesophageal reflux as a risk factor for esophageal adenocarcinoma. *N Engl J Med*. 1999;340:825. [PMID: 10080844] (Gastroesophageal reflux disease is a risk factor for adenocarcinoma.)

Oelschlager BK, Barreca M, Chang L et al. Clinical and pathologic response of Barrett's esophagus to laparoscopic antireflux surgery. *Ann Surg*. 2003;238:458. [PMID: 14530718] (Antireflux surgery determines regression of short segment columnar epithelium in up to 56% of patients.)

Schnell T, Sontag SJ, Chejfec G et al. Long-term nonsurgical management of Barrett esophagus with high-grade dysplasia. *Gastroenterology*. 2001;120:1607. [PMID: 11375943] (Nonsurgical treatment of patients with high-grade dysplasia.)

ESOPHAGEAL CANCER

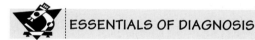 ESSENTIALS OF DIAGNOSIS

- *Progressive dysphagia, initially for solids and later for liquids.*
- *Progressive weight loss.*
- *Diagnosis confirmed by endoscopy and biopsies.*

General Considerations

In the United States, esophageal carcinoma accounts for 10,000 to 11,000 deaths per year. The last 30 years have seen a major change in the epidemiology of esophageal cancer in the United States. Until the 1970s, squamous cell carcinoma was the most common type of esophageal cancer, accounting for approximately 90% of the total incidence. It commonly occurred in the thoracic esophagus and mostly affected black men. Over the last three decades, the incidence of adenocarcinoma of the distal esophagus and gastroesophageal junction has progressively increased; currently, it accounts for more than 50% of all new cases of esophageal cancer. Squamous cell cancer is still the most common type worldwide. Esophageal cancer occurs mostly during the sixth and seventh decades of life and is more common in men than in women.

Pathogenesis

The most common contributing factors for squamous cell carcinoma are cigarette smoking and chronic alcohol exposure. Chronic ingestion of hot liquids or foods, poor oral hygiene, and nutritional deficiencies may play a role. Certain medical conditions such as achalasia, caustic injuries of the esophagus, and Plummer-Vinson syndrome are associated with an increased incidence of squamous cell cancer. GERD is the most common predisposing factor for adenocarcinoma of the esophagus. In these cases, adenocarcinoma represents the last event of a sequence that starts with GERD and progresses to metaplasia, high-grade dysplasia, and adenocarcinoma (see Figure 35–9).

Esophageal cancer arises in the mucosa and subsequently tends to invade the submucosa and the muscle layers. Eventually, structures located next to the esophagus may be infiltrated (eg, the tracheobronchial tree, the aorta, and the recurrent laryngeal nerve). At the same time, the tumor tends to metastasize to the periesophageal lymph nodes (mediastinal, celiac, and cervical) and eventually to the liver and the lungs.

Clinical Findings

A. Symptoms and Signs

Dysphagia is the most common presenting symptom. Dysphagia initially manifests with the ingestion of solids, but eventually it is experienced with the consumption of liquids. As a result, weight loss occurs in more than 50% of patients. Patients may have pain when swallowing. Pain over bony structures may be due to metastases. Hoarseness is usually due to invasion of the right or left recurrent laryngeal nerve, with paralysis of the ipsilateral vocal cord. Respiratory symptoms may be due to the regurgitation and aspiration of undigested food or to invasion of the tracheobronchial tree, with development of a tracheoesophageal fistula.

B. Imaging Studies

1. Barium swallow—Barium swallow can show both the location and the extent of the tumor. Esophageal cancer usually presents as an irregular intraluminal mass or a stricture (Figure 35–10).

2. Endoscopy—Endoscopy allows for the direct visualization and biopsy of the tumor. For tumors of the upper and mid-esophagus, bronchoscopy is indicated to rule out invasion of the tracheobronchial tree.

C. Special Tests

After the diagnosis is established, it is important to determine the staging of the cancer (Table 35–2). Abdominal and chest CT scans are used to rule out metastases and the invasion of structures next to the esophagus. Alternately, positron emission tomography (PET) scanning can be used. Endoscopic ultrasound is the most sensitive test to determine the penetration of

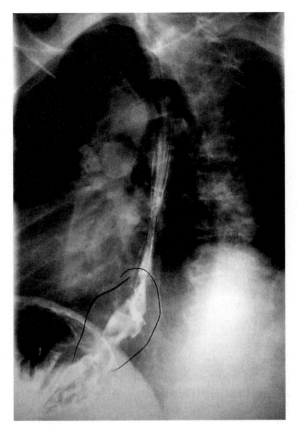

Figure 35–10. Adenocarcinoma of the distal esophagus.

the tumor, the presence of enlarged periesophageal lymph nodes, and the invasion of structures next to the esophagus. A bone scan is indicated in patients who present with a new onset of bone pain.

Table 35–2. TNM staging for esophageal cancer.

TNM	Stage
$T_{is}\,N_0\,M_0$	0
$T_1\,N_0\,M_0$	I
$T_2\,N_0\,M_0$	IIA
$T_3\,N_0\,M_0$	
$T_1\,N_1\,M_0$	IIB
$T_2\,N_1\,M_0$	
$T_3\,N_1\,M_0$	III
T_4 any N M_0	
Any T any N M_1	IV

Differential Diagnosis

Differential diagnoses include peptic strictures due to reflux, achalasia, and benign esophageal tumors.

Treatment

A. SURGICAL MEASURES

Patients with esophageal cancer are considered candidates for esophageal resection if the following criteria are met: (1) there is no evidence of the spread of the tumor to structures next to the esophagus, such as the tracheobronchial tree, the aorta, or the recurrent laryngeal nerve; (2) there is no evidence of distant metastases; and (3) the patient is fit from a cardiac and respiratory point of view.

An esophagectomy can be performed by using (1) an abdominal and a cervical incision with blunt dissection of the thoracic esophagus through the esophageal hiatus (**transhiatal esophagectomy**) or (2) an incision into the abdomen and the right side of the chest (**transthoracic esophagectomy**). After removing the esophagus, continuity of the gastrointestinal tract is reestablished by using either the stomach or the colon. Many retrospective and prospective randomized studies have shown no difference in the survival rate between the two operations, suggesting that it is not the *type* of operation that influences survival but the *stage of the disease* at the time the operation is performed. The morbidity rate of the operation is approximately 30% and is mostly due to cardiac complications (eg, arrhythmias), respiratory complications (eg, atelectasis or pleural effusion), and septic complications (eg, anastomotic leak or pneumonia). The mortality rate in specialized centers is less than 5%. As with other complex operations (cardiac surgery, as well as liver and pancreatic resections), a lower mortality rate is obtained in "high-volume centers" because of the presence of an experienced team composed of surgeons, anesthesiologists, cardiologists, radiologists, and nurses.

B. NONSURGICAL MEASURES

Neoadjuvant therapy based on a combination of radiation therapy and chemotherapy has been attempted to improve both the local control, via radiation therapy, and the distant control of the disease, via chemotherapy. Unfortunately, with the exception of one study, all the randomized trials have failed to show a survival benefit in patients treated by neoadjuvant therapy followed by surgery compared with patients who had surgery alone. Nonoperative therapy is reserved for patients who are not candidates for surgery because of local invasion of the tumor, metastases, or a poor functional status. The goal of therapy in these patients is palliation of the dysphagia, which will allow them to eat. The following treatment modalities are available to achieve this goal: (1) Expandable, coated, metallic stents can be deployed by endoscopy under fluoroscopic guidance to keep the esophageal lumen open. They are particularly useful when a tracheoesophageal fistula is present. (2) Laser therapy (Nd:YAG laser) relieves dysphagia in up to 70% of patients. However, multiple sessions are usually required to keep the esophageal lumen open. (3) Radiation therapy is successful in relieving dysphagia in about 50% of patients.

Prognosis

The stage of the disease is the most important prognostic factor. The overall 5-year survival rate for esophageal cancer remains approximately 25–30%. Patients without lymph node metastases have a significantly better 5-year survival rate than patients with lymph node involvement.

Burmeister BH, Smithers BM, Gebski V et al. Surgery alone versus chemoradiotherapy followed by surgery for resectable cancer of the oesophagus: a randomised controlled phase III trial. *Lancet Oncol.* 2005;6:659. [PMID: 16129366] (Neoadjuvant therapy does not improve survival.)

Devesa SS, Blot WJ, Fraumeni JF. Changing patterns in incidence of esophageal and gastric carcinoma in the United States. *Cancer.* 1998;83:2049. [PMID: 9827707] (Increased incidence of adenocarcinoma over the last three decades.)

Ferguson MK, Durkin A. Long-term survival after esophagectomy for Barrett adenocarcinoma in endoscopically surveyed and nonsurveyed patients. *J Gastrointest Surg.* 2002;6:29. [PMID: 11986015] (Surveillance endoscopy allows early diagnosis of cancer in patients with Barrett esophagus.)

Dimick JB, Wainess RM, Upchurch GR Jr et al. National trends in outcomes for esophageal resection. *Ann Thorac Surg.* 2005; 79:212. [PMID: 15620945] (Lower mortality rate for esophageal resection is obtained in high-volume centers.)

Law S, Wong J. Current management of esophageal cancer. *J Gastrointest Surg.* 2005;9:291. [PMID: 15694827] (Experience from the University of Hong Kong.)

Patti MG, Corvera C, Glasgow RE, Way KW. A hospital's annual rate of esophagectomy influences the operative mortality rate. *J Gastrointest Surg.* 1998;2:186. [PMID: 9834415] (Study that shows that high-volume centers have better results because of a team approach.)

Visser BC, Venook AP, Patti MG. Adjuvant and neoadjuvant therapy for esophageal cancer: a critical reappraisal. *Surg Oncol.* 2003;12:1. [PMID: 12689665] (Review article on the value of adjuvant and neoadjuvant therapy for esophageal cancer.)

Benign & Malignant Disorders of the Trachea

36

Andrew J. Schreffler, MD, & David M. Jablons, MD

◼ ANATOMY OF THE TRACHEA

ANATOMIC RELATIONSHIPS

The trachea is a fibromuscular tube supported by cartilaginous rings that extends from the inferior border of the cricoid cartilage to the carinal bifurcation. It measures 10–13 cm in length and 2.0–2.5 cm in lateral diameter. In infants and children, the proximal half of the trachea is extrathoracic, beginning at the level of the fourth cervical vertebra. In adults, it begins around the sixth cervical vertebra, leaving only the proximal third extrathoracic. The carina occurs at the level of the sternomanubrial junction anteriorly, and at the fourth or fifth thoracic vertebra posteriorly. The trachea slides freely within its anatomic plane, and cervical flexion or kyphosis may transfer the entire trachea into the thorax.

As the trachea courses inferiorly, it migrates from an anterior, subcutaneous position in the neck to a deep, posterior position near the vertebral column at the carina. Throughout its course, the posterior wall of the trachea is applied to the esophagus, which lies just left of the tracheal midline, passing behind the origin of the left main bronchus.

In the neck, the trachea is flanked by the carotid sheaths bilaterally. The thyroid gland is adherent to the anterior and lateral aspects of the trachea at its most superior limits. More inferiorly, the lateral margins of the trachea are bounded by lymph nodes and loose connective tissue. The right recurrent laryngeal nerve loops around the origin of the right subclavian artery and ascends to the larynx, lying within the tracheoesophageal groove only as it approaches the thyroid gland. A right, nonrecurrent laryngeal nerve occurs in 1% of patients and is associated with an anomalous subclavian artery. The left nerve recurs around the aortic arch and ascends the length of the trachea within the tracheoesophageal groove.

The aorta arches over the left main bronchus at its origin and slightly indents the anterolateral wall of the distal trachea on that side. It gives rise to the brachiocephalic trunk, which courses obliquely across the anterior trachea and divides into the right carotid and subclavian arteries at the thoracic inlet. In children and occasionally in adults, the brachiocephalic artery crosses the trachea more superiorly and is found at the base of the neck.

The left brachiocephalic vein crosses the trachea anterior to the aortic arch vessels and receives a variable network of descending inferior thyroidal and thymic veins. The azygous vein joins the superior vena cava after looping over the right main bronchus near its origin at the carina. Just anterior and inferior to the carina, the right pulmonary artery courses toward the right hilum.

STRUCTURE

The tracheal rings, derived from splanchnic mesoderm, occupy the anterior two thirds of the tracheal circumference. The rings are incomplete posteriorly, resulting in a flattened, membranous portion of tracheal wall that consists of fibromuscular tissue. There are approximately two cartilaginous rings per centimeter of tracheal length, with the intervening spaces composed of an investing fibroelastic membrane. The first ring is attached to the inferior boarder of the cricoid cartilage by the cricotracheal ligament and is generally broader than the rest. The tracheal rings are highly elastic but may ossify with advanced age or after trauma.

Tracheal muscle fibers of mesodermal origin are contained in scattered, longitudinal bundles and in a thin, transverse layer of the membranous wall, the trachealis muscle. The respiratory epithelium arises from foregut endoderm and in the trachea consists of pseudostratified, ciliated columnar cells and mucous glands.

Anomalies of tracheal development give rise to a number of clinically important anatomic lesions. Failure of tracheoesophageal septation may result in agenesis of the trachea (fatal at birth), stenosis of the trachea or esophagus, or a tracheoesophageal fistula. Tracheal stenosis also may be caused by compression from anomalous mediastinal vasculature or the presence of complete tracheal rings. Numerous variations of aberrant tracheal bronchi have been described, including unilateral, bilateral, and double ipsilateral configurations.

BLOOD SUPPLY

The blood supply of the trachea is derived from multiple sources and is shared with the esophagus. The inferior thyroid artery and tracheoesophageal branches of the subclavian artery supply the upper trachea, whereas the lower third is supplied by the bronchial arteries and branches from the intercostal and internal mammary arteries. The vessels approach the tracheoesophageal groove laterally and divide to send branches to each organ. Intercartilaginous branches traverse the tracheal circumference and interconnect via longitudinal arcades and a rich, submucosal plexus. Circumferential dissection with disruption of the lateral vascular pedicles should be limited to 1–2 cm of any portion of the trachea that is to remain in situ.

Allen MS. Surgical anatomy of the trachea. *Chest Surg Clin North Am.* 2003;13(2):191. [PMID: 12755308] (A thorough review of the surgical anatomy of the trachea.)

Cauldwell EW, Siskert RG, Linninger RE, Anson BJ. The bronchial arteries: an anatomic study of 150 human cadavers. *Surg Gynecol Obstet.* 1948;86:395. (Definitive study of tracheal blood supply.)

Salassa JR, Pearson BW, Payne WS. Gross and microscopical blood supply of the trachea. *Ann Thorac Surg.* 1977;24:100. [PMID: 327958] (Classic study of the tracheal blood supply, particularly as related to tracheal resection.)

Watanabe A, Kawabori S, Osanai H, Taniguchi M, Hosokawa M. Preoperative computed tomography diagnosis of non-recurrent inferior laryngeal nerve. *Laryngoscope.* 2001;111:1756. [PMID: 11801940] (Documents association of nonrecurrent laryngeal nerve with aberrant right subclavian artery.)

■ TRACHEAL INJURIES

TRAUMA

ESSENTIALS OF DIAGNOSIS

- *History of trauma to head, neck, or chest.*
- *Pain, dyspnea, stridor, hemoptysis, dysphonia.*
- *Subcutaneous or deep cervical emphysema.*
- *Pneumomediastinum, pneumothorax despite chest tube drainage.*

General Considerations

Injuries to the trachea from blunt or penetrating trauma are rare, with an incidence of 0.5–2.0% in blunt trauma patients and 3–6% in patients with penetrating cervical wounds. The mechanisms of injury most commonly reported include gunshot and stab wounds, hanging, and deceleration injuries. Penetrating tracheal wounds, which most commonly involve the cervical airway, result in focal tissue loss and are frequently associated with serious injuries to adjacent organs, such as blood vessels or the esophagus. Blunt trauma typically produces avulsion-type injuries at the laryngotracheal junction or at branch points in the tracheobronchial tree, most within 2.5 cm of the carina. Blunt tracheal injuries are rarely isolated, occurring most frequently in patients with multisystem trauma.

Clinical Findings

A. SYMPTOMS AND SIGNS

The examination of any trauma patient should occur in the setting of a coordinated, comprehensive trauma evaluation. Tracheal injury may be suspected based on the likely trajectory of a penetrating object or on the patient's presenting history and physical examination. Signs and symptoms of laryngotracheal trauma include pain, hoarseness, dyspnea, stridor, dysphonia, subcutaneous emphysema, and hemoptysis. Plain chest radiographs and cervical films may reveal subcutaneous air, tracheal deviation, pneumomediastinum, or pneumothorax.

Further assessment of tracheal wounds is individualized based on the patient's associated injuries. The definitive diagnosis (and repair) of airway trauma may be facilitated in patients undergoing operative exploration, usually for associated vascular injuries.

B. IMAGING STUDIES

1. Angiography—In stable patients, the evaluation of potential tracheal injuries should be coordinated with the assessment of adjacent structures, with angiography of the aortic arch and thoracic outlet vessels usually taking precedence.

2. Computed tomography (CT) scanning—CT scanning readily demonstrates the manifestations of tracheal trauma, including pneumomediastinum, pneumothorax, and air within the tissue planes of the neck. However, it is rarely able to define the exact location or extent of the injury.

3. Bronchoscopy—Bronchoscopy remains the gold standard for defining the precise location and extent of tracheal injuries. At bronchoscopy, a thorough evaluation is essential and requires the meticulous evacuation of secretions and aspirated blood in order to allow adequate inspection of the tracheal mucosa. Careful manipulation of the endotracheal tube is required in intubated patients to visualize the proximal trachea.

Treatment

The treatment of tracheal injuries is not standardized, but the first priority in all cases is to establish an adequate, reliable airway. Insertion of an endotracheal tube, often difficult in the presence of upper airway trauma, may be facilitated by flexible bronchoscopy. Tracheostomy, when required, should be performed at the level of the injury in order to minimize the amount of tracheal damage.

A. Nonsurgical Measures

In stable patients, minor or occult injuries may be successfully treated with conservative measures. If the patient is not intubated, antibiotic coverage and close observation are often sufficient. If mechanical ventilation is necessary, treatment should also include placement of the endotracheal cuff beyond the injury and avoidance of high airway pressures. Such conservative measures should also be initiated for larger tracheal wounds and may allow for an elective repair rather than an urgent exploration.

B. Surgical Measures

Patient instability or worsening pneumomediastinum, persistent pneumothorax despite chest tube drainage, evidence of mediastinitis, or inadequate ventilation or oxygenation mandates operative intervention. The operative approach to tracheal repair is dictated by the location of the wound and associated injuries. A low collar incision provides exposure of all but the most distal trachea and may be extended into a partial or complete median sternotomy, if needed. The distal trachea is best approached through a right, fourth intercostal thoracotomy, which allows access to the trachea, the carina, the right and proximal left main bronchi, and the entire intrathoracic esophagus. Injuries to the thoracic trachea, however, are usually associated with injuries to the heart and great vessels, which are best approached by a median sternotomy. In such cases, the trachea may be exposed by transpericardial dissection between the superior vena cava and the ascending aorta.

Simple tracheal injuries may be débrided and repaired primarily, with care taken to preserve the lateral vascular pedicles and the recurrent laryngeal nerves. Wounds causing significant damage require circumferential tracheal resection and end-to-end anastomosis. An anterior longitudinal tracheotomy via a cervical incision allows for the repair of injuries to the membranous trachea without lateral or posterior dissection.

Prognosis

Results of both repaired and conservatively managed tracheal injuries are generally good and are related more to the patient's associated injuries than to tracheal healing.

A delay in the diagnosis of tracheal or associated injuries increases mortality significantly. Minor injuries and primarily repaired wounds heal well with minimal formation of granulation tissue or stenosis. Severe tracheal injuries managed conservatively eventually require repair to achieve decannulation, since they typically heal with significant stenosis.

Cassada DC, Munyikwa MP, Moniz MP, Dieter RA Jr, Schuchmann GF, Enderson BL. Acute injuries of the trachea and major bronchi: importance of early diagnosis. *Ann Thorac Surg.* 2000;69:1563. [PMID: 10881842] (Retrospective review of single center experience managing tracheal trauma.)

Francis S, Gaspard DJ, Rogers N, Stain SC. Diagnosis and management of laryngotracheal trauma. *J Nat Med Assoc.* 2002;94:21. [PMID: 11837348] (Review and discussion of the management of laryngotracheal injuries in a series of trauma patients.)

Granholm T, Farmer DL. The surgical airway. *Respir Care Clin North Am.* 2001;7:13. [PMID: 11584802] (Review of diagnosis, management, and outcome of pediatric tracheal injuries.)

Huh J. Management of tracheobronchial injuries following blunt and penetrating trauma. *Am Surg.* 1997;63:896. [PMID: 9322668] (Retrospective review of an urban trauma center's experience managing tracheal trauma.)

Lee RB. Traumatic injury to the cervicothoracic trachea and major bronchi. *Chest Surg Clin North Am.* 1997;7:285. [PMID: 9156293] (Comprehensive review.)

Rossbach MM, Johnson SB, Gomez MA, Sako EY, Miller OL, Calhoon JH. Management of major tracheobronchial injuries: a 28-year experience. *Ann Thorac Surg.* 1998;65:182. [PMID: 9456114] (Large review of an urban trauma center's experience managing tracheal injuries.)

Shrager JB. Tracheal trauma. *Chest Surg Clin North Am.* 2003;13(2):291. [PMID: 12755314] (Review of the incidence, diagnosis, and management of tracheal injuries.)

IATROGENIC & OTHER TRACHEAL INJURIES

Iatrogenic injury of the trachea is infrequent, occurring almost exclusively in relation to endotracheal intubation. Less common iatrogenic causes include percutaneous tracheostomy, transhiatal esophageal mobilization, median sternotomy, and laser-associated endotracheal fire. Tracheoesophageal and tracheoinnominate artery fistulas, as well as tracheomalacia, are rare complications of airway manipulation and a variety of other conditions. Paroxysmal coughing and severe vomiting may cause spontaneous tracheal tears.

INTUBATION INJURIES

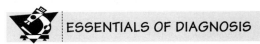

ESSENTIALS OF DIAGNOSIS

• *History of difficult or urgent intubation.*

- *Difficulty achieving adequate ventilation or oxygenation.*
- *Pneumomediastinum or pneumothorax.*
- *More common in women.*

General Considerations

Trauma due to endotracheal intubation may occur at any level of the airway, from the posterior pharynx to the mainstem bronchi. A history of multiple attempts at a difficult or emergent intubation is typical, although injuries may follow seemingly routine intubations as well. Women are affected far more frequently than men are.

Clinical Findings

Intubation injuries are typically limited to the posterior membranous trachea, but may extend its entire length and even involve the carina and mainstem bronchi. Extensive injuries usually compromise airway management and are diagnosed at the time of their occurrence. Minor lacerations may go unrecognized until signs such as pneumomediastinum or pneumothorax are seen on chest x-ray.

Treatment & Prognosis

Stable patients may be successfully managed conservatively, as outlined above for minor tracheal trauma. Unstable patients and those failing conservative management require operative repair. Most lacerations may be approached through a cervical anterior longitudinal tracheotomy, avoiding lateral and posterior dissection. Extensive and very distal lesions require a right thoracotomy for repair. Healing of intubation injuries is excellent, and patient survival is related to the underlying illness that necessitated intubation.

Borasio P, Ardissone F, Chiampo G. Post-intubation tracheal rupture: a report of ten cases. *Eur J Cardiothorac Surg.* 1997; 12:98. [PMID: 9262088] (Retrospective review of surgical and conservative management.)

Hofmann HS, Rettig G, Radke J, Neef H, Silber RE. Iatrogenic ruptures of the tracheobronchial tree. *Eur J Cardiothorac Surg.* 2002;21:649. [PMID: 11932162] (Retrospective review of 19 patients with iatrogenic trauma.)

Kaloud H, Smolle-Juettner FM, Prause G, List WF. Iatrogenic ruptures of the tracheobronchial tree. *Chest.* 1997;112:774. [PMID: 9315814] (Retrospective review of 12 patients with iatrogenic tracheal injuries.)

Mussi A, Ambrogi MC, Menconi G, Ribechini A, Angeletti CA. Surgical approaches to membranous tracheal wall lacerations. *J Thorac Cardiovasc Surg.* 2000;120:115. [PMID: 10884663] (Retrospective review of surgical and conservative management of intubation injuries that emphasizes cervical exposure technique.)

TRACHEOINNOMINATE ARTERY FISTULA

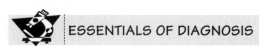 **ESSENTIALS OF DIAGNOSIS**

- *Presence of endotracheal or tracheostomy tube.*
- *Premonitory or exsanguinating hemorrhage around or through the endotracheal or tracheostomy tube.*

Pathogenesis

A tracheoinnominate artery fistula is a rare complication of tracheal intubation in which erosion into the innominate artery causes massive bleeding. The innominate artery, which arises from the aortic arch, courses obliquely across the anterior surface of the fifth or sixth tracheal ring to supply the right subclavian and common carotid arteries. In children and occasionally in adults, it crosses the trachea at the base of the neck. The most common cause of a tracheoinnominate artery fistula is erosion through the tracheal wall into the artery by the tip, balloon, or shaft of a tracheostomy or endotracheal tube. The placement of a tracheostomy too low or near an unusually high artery increases the risk. Rarely, a tracheoinnominate artery fistula occurs after tracheal resection.

Clinical Findings

Mortality from tracheoinnominate artery fistulas is approximately 90%, and patient survival depends on timely diagnosis and treatment. Premonitory bleeding around or through the tracheostomy tube commonly precedes an exsanguinating hemorrhage and should be considered a true surgical emergency. Any such bleeding should be rigorously investigated to exclude arterial injury as the source. The diagnosis may require bronchoscopy and wound exploration, which are best performed in the operating room.

Treatment

A. NONSURGICAL MEASURES

The diagnosis becomes self-evident in patients with massive bleeding, and only rapid control of both the artery and the airway will save the patient's life. The initial control of the artery should be attempted by overdistention of the tracheostomy (or endotracheal tube) cuff. If this is unsuccessful, the artery should be compressed against the manubrium anteriorly with a finger introduced through the tracheostomy wound. While these maneuvers are performed, an oral endotracheal tube should be placed, resuscitation instituted, and the operating room readied. Control of the artery is maintained during transport to the operating room and during prepping and draping of the patient.

B. SURGICAL MEASURES

The tracheostomy incision should be developed to include a partial median sternotomy with extension into the right third or fourth intercostal space. The innominate vein should be carefully avoided. After proximal and distal control of the artery is achieved, the damaged portion should be resected and the ends oversewn. Primary repair of the artery should not be attempted because it invariably fails, leading to recurrent bleeding and increased mortality. The need for vascular reconstruction is controversial. The tracheal defect may be débrided and repaired or packed and allowed to heal secondarily.

Jones JW, Reynolds M, Hewitt RL, Drapanas T. Tracheo-innominate artery erosion: successful surgical management of a devastating complication. *Ann Surg.* 1976;184:194. [PMID: 782389] (Extensive retrospective study and literature review discusses causation, predisposing factors, management, and outcomes of tracheoinnominate artery fistula.)

Allan JS, Wright CD. Tracheoinnominate fistula: diagnosis and management. *Chest Surg Clin North Am.* 2003;13(2):331. [PMID: 12755317] (A comprehensive review of the pathogenesis, diagnosis, and management of tracheoinnominate artery fistulas.)

TRACHEOESOPHAGEAL FISTULA

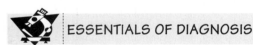

ESSENTIALS OF DIAGNOSIS

- *History of prolonged mechanical ventilation or a neoplasm of the upper aerodigestive tract, especially if irradiated.*
- *Increased tracheal secretions containing gastric contents, aspiration with pulmonary sequela, gastric distention.*

General Considerations

An acquired tracheoesophageal fistula is an abnormal communication between the trachea and the esophagus. It is an infrequent complication of a variety of conditions, occurring most commonly in relation to prolonged mechanical ventilation, upper aerodigestive tract tumors, and trauma. Other causes include mediastinal inflammation and operative manipulation, particularly esophagectomy with involvement of the gastric neoesophagus.

Pathogenesis

In the case of patients requiring prolonged ventilation, fistula formation typically is caused by pressure necrosis of the tissues interposed between the endotracheal or tracheostomy tube cuff and a nasogastric tube in the esophagus. The process often is associated with a circumferential tracheal injury and may involve the entire membranous trachea.

Clinical Findings

Signs of a tracheoesophageal fistula include persistent aspiration and its pulmonary sequelae (eg, pneumonia), as well as increased tracheal secretions and gastric distention. The diagnosis of a suspected tracheoesophageal fistula may be confirmed by direct visualization through the tracheostoma or via bronchoscopy. Esophagoscopy is rarely needed unless an esophageal process underlies the fistula. Contrast studies are usually unnecessary.

Treatment

The treatment of a tracheoesophageal fistula is dictated by its cause, its location, and the need for continued mechanical ventilation. Patients with incurable malignant disorders ideally are treated with stenting of the esophagus, the trachea, or both. Benign fistulas are best managed surgically; however, the repair of a tracheoesophageal fistula in patients requiring prolonged ventilation should not be attempted while the patient remains intubated because such efforts invariably fail.

A. NONSURGICAL MEASURES

Until the patient can be weaned from the ventilator, conservative measures should be used to optimize the patient's condition. The nasogastric tube should be removed to prevent further injury and because some spontaneous healing may occur. Gastric and jejunal tubes should be placed for drainage and alimentation, respectively. The tracheal cuff should be positioned distal to the fistula to minimize further pulmonary soilage, and aggressive suctioning and pulmonary toilet instituted. If the fistula is too distal to control with the cuffed tube, esophageal diversion may be required.

B. SURGICAL MEASURES

The definitive repair of most tracheoesophageal fistulas may be performed through a cervical incision, with a partial upper sternotomy, if needed. More distal or extensive fistulas may require a right thoracotomy. Once identified, the fistula is divided and the esophagus is débrided and repaired in two layers. If the injury to the trachea is limited, primary repair of the defect may be sufficient. Larger areas of damage to the trachea, including circumferential injuries and stenosis, require segmental resection and primary anastomosis. A pedicle of strap muscle should be interposed between the tracheal and esophageal repairs.

Prognosis

Surgical repair achieves closure of tracheoesophageal fistulas in more than 90% of cases. Segmental resection of the involved trachea may improve results, even in the absence of circumferential injury. Complications include recurrent fistula in 10% of patients and esophageal stricture in 15%. The former is treated by reoperation and the latter by endoscopic dilatation.

Baisi A, Bonavina L, Narne S, Peracchia A. Benign tracheoesophageal fistula: results of surgical therapy. *Dis Esophagus.* 1999;12:209. [PMID: 10631915] (Retrospective review of a single center's experience managing tracheoesophageal fistula.)

Dartevelle P, Macchiarini P. Management of acquired tracheoesophageal fistula. *Chest Surg Clin North Am.* 1996;6:819. [PMID: 8934011] (Comprehensive review.)

Macchiarini P, Verhoye JP, Chapelier A, Fadel E, Dartevelle P. Evaluation and outcome of different surgical techniques for postintubation tracheoesophageal fistulas. *J Thorac Cardiovasc Surg.* 2000;119:268. [PMID: 10649202] (Reports retrospective results of various techniques for management of tracheoesophageal fistulas.)

Mathisen DJ, Grillo HC, Wain JC, Hilgenberg AD. Management of acquired nonmalignant tracheoesophageal fistula. *Ann Thorac Surg.* 1991;52:759. [PMID: 1929626] (Report of the largest American experience managing tracheoesophageal fistulas.)

Reed MF, Mathisen DJ. Tracheoesophageal fistula. *Chest Surg Clin North Am.* 2003;13(2):271. [PMID: 12755313] (A thorough review of the management of a wide variety of tracheoesophageal fistulas.)

ACQUIRED TRACHEOMALACIA

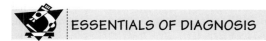 **ESSENTIALS OF DIAGNOSIS**

- *History of emphysema or polychondritis, or tracheal intubation, injury, compression.*
- *Brassy cough, impaired clearance of secretions.*
- *Dyspnea on exertion, expiratory wheeze, stridor.*
- *Plateau in expiratory spirogram.*

Pathogenesis

Tracheomalacia refers to a derangement in the structural integrity of the trachea, resulting in a fixed or dynamic obstruction of airflow. Typically, the decreased rigidity and elasticity of damaged tracheal rings cause the collapse of malacic segments during exhalation. Redundancy of the membranous trachea seen in tracheomegaly and emphysema may also cause a functional airway obstruction.

Congenital disorders, discussed elsewhere within this book, that are associated with tracheomalacia include vascular anomalies, tracheoesophageal fistulas, and tracheobronchomegaly related to Mounier-Kuhn syndrome. The causes of acquired tracheomalacia include trauma (particularly postintubation injuries), chronic external compression, emphysema, and relapsing polychondritis. Diffuse, pathologic pliability of the tracheal cartilage develops in the latter two conditions, while in cases of trauma or compression, malacic collapse is limited to the damaged segments alone.

Clinical Findings

The signs and symptoms of tracheomalacia include impaired exhalation manifest by wheezing, stridor, and a barking cough. Exercise tolerance and clearance of respiratory secretions are impaired. Pulmonary function testing demonstrates a plateau in the expiratory spirogram. The diagnosis may be confirmed on CT scan with the comparison of inspiratory and endexpiratory measurements of tracheal cross-sectional area and diameter, as well as cineradiographic studies. The collapse of malacic segments may be visualized during bronchoscopy.

Treatment & Prognosis

The treatment of acquired tracheomalacia is not standardized owing to its rarity. The external support of a diffusely diseased membranous or cartilaginous trachea with prosthetic materials, such as Marlex mesh, may stabilize the airway, but a potentially fatal erosion into adjacent structures is a recognized complication. Functionally significant tracheomalacia is only rarely present after the relief of extrinsic tracheal compression. The exceptional patient with respiratory difficulty should be managed conservatively with a short course of endoluminal stenting. Segmental resection and end-to-end anastomosis of limited tracheomalacia resulting from prolonged intubation and other trauma is curative.

Amedee R, Mann WJ, Lyons GD. Tracheomalacia repair using ceramic rings. *Otolaryngol Head Neck Surg.* 1992;106:270. [PMID: 1589219] (Surgical series describes the indications, technique, and results of using ceramic rings for the treatment of tracheomalacia.)

Heussel CP, Hafner B, Lill J, Schreiber W, Thelen M, Kauczor HU. Paired inspiratory and expiratory spiral CT and continuous respiration cine CT in the diagnosis of tracheal instability. *Eur Radiol.* 2001;11:982. [PMID: 11419175] (Demonstrates utility of cine CT in diagnosis of tracheomalacia.)

Jokinen K, Palva T, Sutinen S, Nuutinen J. Acquired tracheobron-chomalacia. *Ann Clin Res.* 1977;9:52. [PMID: 883758] (Review of the clinical features of acquired tracheomalacia in a series of 94 patients. Follow-up study reported by Nuutinen [see below].)

Nuutinen J. Acquired tracheobronchomalacia: a bronchologic follow-up study. *Ann Clin Res.* 1977;9:359. [PMID: 616225] (Reports the long-term follow-up, including repeat bronchoscopy, of 94 patients with acquired tracheobronchomalacia, providing insights into the natural history of the condition.)

Rainer WG, Newby JP, Kelble DL. Long-term results of tracheal support surgery for emphysema. *Dis Chest.* 1968;53:765. [PMID: 5653753] (Reports the results of patients undergoing prosthetic splinting of membranous trachea.)

Wright CD. Tracheomalacia. *Chest Surg Clin North Am.* 2003; 13(2):349. [PMID: 12755319] (Review of tracheomalacia and its management.)

■ TRACHEAL STENOSIS

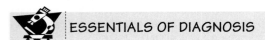

ESSENTIALS OF DIAGNOSIS

- *History of tracheal injury, intubation, mediastinal process.*
- *Worsening wheeze, cough, stridor, and dyspnea on exertion.*
- *Difficulty raising secretions, recurrent pulmonary infections.*

Benign stenosis of the trachea has a diverse causality that comprises congenital, idiopathic, and acquired conditions. Most acquired stenoses develop as a result of the fibrous maturation of healed tracheal injuries. Postintubation injury to the trachea represents the most common cause of benign tracheal stenosis.

Symptoms of stenotic tracheal obstruction usually develop insidiously with stridor, wheezing, cough, and dyspnea on exertion. The severity of symptoms and their progression correlates with the degree of stenosis. Stridor and wheezing are usually inspiratory, but with intrathoracic stenosis or malacia, are worse on expiration. The cough is typically brassy and nonproductive, and recurrent infections may occur as a result of the inability to clear secretions across the stenosis. Dyspnea at rest occurs when the cross-sectional area of the trachea is decreased by 75%. Patients with underlying pulmonary disease may develop significant dyspnea at lesser degrees of stenosis.

Frequently, the diagnosis is delayed since symptoms are attributed to asthma or, in the case of patients with postintubation stenosis, to the process that necessitated

mechanical ventilation. High-resolution spiral CT scanning with sagittal and coronal reconstructions provides detailed information regarding the extent and geometry of the stenotic segment and extratracheal anatomy. Bronchoscopy allows for the direct visualization of the entire airway and permits a thorough assessment of the lesion and any associated mucosal damage. The use of a rigid bronchoscope ensures control of even very difficult airways and allows for therapeutic dilatation and clearance of secretions distal to the obstruction.

Gluecker T, Lang F, Bessler S et al. 2D and 3D CT imaging correlated to rigid endoscopy in complex laryngo-tracheal stenoses. *Eur Radiol.* 2001;11:50. [PMID: 11194917] (Discusses the accuracy of CT scanning in the diagnosis and characterization of benign tracheal stenosis.)

CONGENITAL ANOMALIES

Congenital anomalies that may present with tracheal stenosis or obstruction include tracheal agenesis or atresia, tracheoesophageal fistula, complete tracheal rings, vascular rings, aberrant bronchi, and tracheomalacia. These entities usually come to attention immediately, but occasionally do not cause symptoms until later in life. Surgical correction is required in most cases.

IDIOPATHIC TRACHEAL STENOSIS

General Considerations

Idiopathic stenosis of the trachea is a rare condition in which dense fibrous stenosis of the proximal trachea occurs in the absence of any inciting event, including infection, mediastinal mass or inflammation, gastroesophageal reflux disease, trauma, inhalational injury, or intubation. The process affects women primarily and involves the subglottic larynx and the proximal 2–4 cm of the trachea circumferentially.

Clinical Findings

In addition to the typical symptoms of tracheal stenosis, a small percentage of patients may have systemic findings suggestive of autoimmune dysfunction, including hypocomplementemia, polyarteritis, vasculitis, polyarthritis, and valvular heart disease.

Treatment & Prognosis

The proximity of the process to the vocal cords should be established by radiographic studies and endoscopy because this information guides treatment options. Laser ablation effectively relieves symptoms and is occasionally curative; however, in most cases, stenosis recurs. The use of topical mitomycin-C as an adjuvant therapy to laser resection may improve results. In nearly all cases, laryngotracheal resection is curative. Resolution of the stenosis has been reported in patients with systemic autoimmune findings treated with azathioprine and steroids.

Ashiku SK, Mathisen DJ. Idiopathic laryngotracheal stenosis. *Chest Surg Clin North Am.* 2003;13(2):257. [PMID: 12755312] (A comprehensive review of idiopathic tracheal stenosis.)

Dedo HH, Catten MD. Idiopathic progressive subglottic stenosis: findings and treatment in 52 patients. *Ann Otol Rhinol Laryngol.* 2001;110:305. [PMID: 11307904] (Review of a single institution's experience managing idiopathic subglottic stenosis.)

Grillo HC. Management of idiopathic tracheal stenosis. *Chest Surg Clin North Am.* 1996;6:811. [PMID: 8934010] (Review of the author's extensive experience managing idiopathic stenosis.)

Valdez TA, Shapshay SM. Idiopathic subglottic stenosis revisited. *Ann Otol Rhinol Laryngol.* 2002;111:690. [PMID: 12184589] (Retrospective review discusses results of laser ablation and adjuvant mitomycin-C for treatment of idiopathic stenosis.)

EXTRINSIC TRACHEAL COMPRESSION

General Considerations

Tracheal obstruction may result from extrinsic compression of the cervical or mediastinal trachea by a variety of lesions. In addition to congenital vascular rings, aneurysms of the innominate artery and distortion of the aorta also may produce vascular compression of the trachea. The latter, known as postpneumonectomy syndrome, is a rare complication of pneumonectomy, in which mediastinal structures shift toward the operated side, causing a horizontal rotation of the aortic arch.

Symptoms of tracheal compression are also frequently the presenting complaints of patients with mediastinal tumors, large goiters, and extensive lymphoma. Sarcoidosis, histoplasmosis, and tuberculosis may also cause tracheal stenosis due to lymphadenopathy and mediastinal fibrosis.

Treatment

The treatment of tracheal stenosis due to extrinsic compression is directed at the causative process. If the appropriate treatment does not alleviate symptoms, endotracheal stenting may provide satisfactory palliation.

Valji AM, Maziak DE, Shamji FM, Matzinger FR. Postpneumonectomy syndrome: recognition and management. *Chest.* 1998;114:1766. [PMID: 9872215] (Review of a series.)

POST-TRAUMATIC TRACHEAL STENOSIS

Injuries to the trachea, whether iatrogenic or traumatic, generally heal with some degree of tracheal stenosis. The obstruction may be mechanical in nature, owing to stricture or granuloma formation, or it may be functional, owing to tracheomalacia. More than one type of lesion may be present.

Granulation tissue may proliferate at the site of tracheal injuries managed conservatively or repaired primarily. Laser ablation provides satisfactory treatment but is rarely required. Severe tracheal injuries, unrecognized or managed conservatively, heal with significant stricture formation. Such lesions produce marked obstructive symptoms that require operative repair—usually segmental resection and end-to-end anastomosis.

POSTINTUBATION TRACHEAL STENOSIS

General Considerations

With the refinement and widespread use of mechanical ventilatory support, postintubation tracheal injury has become the most important cause of benign tracheal stenosis. Historically, such injuries were associated with the high-pressure, low-volume cuffs of early endotracheal and tracheostomy tubes. Yet, despite the adoption of low-pressure, high-volume cuffs and an increased attentiveness to preventive measures, postintubation stenosis remains a common complication of assisted ventilation, occurring in 8–13% of ventilated patients.

Tracheal damage resulting in stenosis is seen with the use of both endotracheal and tracheostomy tubes, including tubes placed by percutaneous dilatational methods. Each type of tube most commonly causes injury at the level of the inflatable cuff, but each may cause damage at other levels of the airway as well. In addition to tracheal stenosis, symptoms may be caused by granulations, tracheal pseudomembrane, subglottic stenosis, tracheomalacia, or tracheoesophageal fistula. More than one lesion may be present.

Classification

Postintubation tracheal stenoses may be classified according to the site of tracheal injury and include cuff-level, tracheostoma-level, and subglottic stenoses.

A. CUFF-LEVEL STENOSIS

Tracheal injury at the level of the inflatable cuff is a direct result of mucosal ischemia from pressure exerted by the cuff. High-volume, low-pressure cuffs are designed to conform to the tracheal lumen across a broad area and provide an adequate seal at cuff pressures below that of mucosal perfusion, which is 20–30 mm Hg. Unfortunately, in the ICU setting, unless cuff pressures are systematically measured, they are almost uniformly inflated above 40 mm Hg, even by experienced intensivists.

Injury to the tracheal mucosa may occur after even brief periods of intubation. In patients who require prolonged assisted ventilation, the incidence of tracheal damage correlates roughly with the length of intubation. Superficial erosion develops initially, followed by full-thickness mucosal ulceration. Exposure of the underlying tracheal cartilage, which receives its blood supply from the mucosa, results in ischemia.

1. Circumferential damage—Circumferential damage from the cuff is common and results in a greater degree of stenosis than less extensive wounds. As healing occurs, deposition of fibrous scar tissue leads to tracheal stenosis. Symptoms are rarely present soon after extubation, but develop over several weeks to months as the scar matures. The administration of steroids can occasionally minimize the degree of eventual stenosis; however, it may predispose the area to tracheomalacia instead.

2. Tracheal pseudomembrane and granulation tissue formation—Other lesions that occur at the level of the inflatable cuff include tracheal pseudomembrane and the formation of granulation tissue. The latter responds well to endoscopic laser ablation, although repetitive treatments may be necessary.

Obstructive fibrinous tracheal pseudomembrane is a rare but potentially fatal cause of cuff-level postintubation stenosis. Acute airway obstruction is caused by a tubular, fibrinous pseudomembrane, which remains in the trachea following extubation. The tissue, which molds to the tube at the level of the cuff, develops within days of intubation and likely represents an early response to tracheal injury. It contains inflamed and necrotic tracheal epithelium and is associated with hemorrhagic ulceration of the submucosa.

Obstructive symptoms that progress to acute respiratory distress develop within hours to days of extubation. Stridor and wheezing may not be present if the patient is too weak to generate sufficient airflow, and obstruction may be positional if the membrane is partially dislodged. Because obstructive fibrinous tracheal pseudomembrane has only recently been characterized and because its presentation may not be typical of tracheal stenosis, symptoms are usually attributed to other causes of postextubation respiratory distress.

An accurate diagnosis requires bronchoscopy, which may also aid in reintubation, if necessary. Treatment consists of aggressive respiratory support and the mechanical debridement of the pseudomembrane via rigid bronchoscopy. Recurrence has not developed following this approach in the only reported series.

B. Tracheostoma-Level Stenosis

Postintubation tracheal stenosis may develop at the tracheostomy site as a result of granulations or scar formation. Upon decannulation, closure of the tracheal defect is effected by collapse and reapproximation of the stomal margins. Further wound maturation and scar-

ring result in an anterolateral area of stenosis that spares the posterior membranous trachea, creating a triangular-shaped, stenotic lumen.

Several factors affect the eventual degree of stenosis at the stoma site, including the operative technique, pressure necrosis, and infection. At tracheostomy, the smallest size tube that still provides an adequate airway should be used, and the tracheal incision should be just large enough to allow its passage. During the patient's term of assisted ventilation, the ventilator and tracheostomy tubing should be positioned in such a way as to prevent leverage against the stomal margins, which can lead to pressure necrosis and extension of the defect. Secretions, which usually are infected, should not be allowed to accumulate around the stoma or the cuff as localized infection exacerbates tracheal injury and subsequent stenosis.

C. Subglottic Stenosis

Injury to the larynx and subglottis may occur after transoral intubation, cricothyroidotomy, or an inappropriately high tracheostomy. In the latter case, a tracheotomy at the first or second tracheal ring causes a stoma-level injury, as described above, which encroaches on the cricoid cartilage and subglottic larynx. Direct pressure and erosion by the tube at the proximal margin may result in loss of the anterior cricoid arch.

Translaryngeal tubes typically cause trauma to the posterior larynx, particularly the interarytenoid area, which may result in glottic stenosis upon healing. The extension of damage to the cricoarytenoid joint impairs vocal cord abduction. Obstructing granulation tissue may also develop at this level.

Treatment

A. Pretreatment Considerations

Most cases of postintubation tracheal stenosis can be treated electively. As previously described, symptoms usually develop and progress over weeks to months, allowing adequate time for an accurate diagnosis and subsequent evaluation. Lesions that have not fully matured should be managed conservatively to allow acute inflammation to subside.

B. Emergent Treatment

Obstructive fibrinous tracheal pseudomembrane presents acutely with respiratory distress, requiring emergent treatment. Other types of postintubation stenosis occasionally present emergently as well, because of an acute exacerbation of symptoms. A prolonged misdiagnosis or expectant treatment may allow for the development of a tight stenosis that is tolerated by the patient until factors such as poor underlying lung function, infection due to retained secretions, irritation from cigarette smoke, or superimposed illness result in significant impairment.

The emergent management of tracheal stenosis should secure the airway and stabilize the patient, allowing definitive treatment to proceed electively. Initial measures should include the use of humidified oxygen, bronchodilators, inhaled or systemic steroids, inhaled racemic epinephrine, and heliox. The latter, a mixture of oxygen and helium, improves oxygen delivery across the obstruction by decreasing turbulent flow. Patients who do not respond to the above measures require emergent rigid bronchoscopy, which is almost uniformly successful in securing the airway.

Dilatation of the lesion may be performed as a temporizing step to allow the postponement of definitive treatment, which should never be attempted emergently. Every effort should be made to avoid tracheostomy, but if absolutely required, it should be placed through the area of stenosis to avoid further damaging the trachea.

C. Definitive Treatment

The successful definitive treatment of postintubation tracheal stenosis requires meticulous planning, which should include a thorough evaluation of the lesion using radiographic imaging and bronchoscopic visualization as described previously. Patient conditions such as nutritional status, steroid use, previous exposure to tracheal irradiation, propensity for aspiration, medical fitness for surgery, and the potential need for assisted ventilation in the future should be carefully considered. Segmental resection provides optimal treatment for the majority of lesions, although other methods such as dilatation, laser ablation, stenting, and plastic reconstruction may be appropriate in certain situations.

1. Dilatation and laser ablation—Dilatation or laser ablation of very short postintubation strictures (< 0.5 cm) may be curative, but in most cases results in gradual restenosis. Though temporary, such procedures may benefit patients who are unfit or unwilling to undergo resection; they may also be useful before stent placement or while waiting for lesions to mature. Laser resection should not be attempted for subglottic lesions.

2. Stenting—The stenting of symptomatic tracheal strictures may be used to ensure an adequate airway during wound maturation or while waiting for the patient's condition to improve prior to resection. Tracheal stents may also provide definitive treatment when the patient's condition, or characteristics of the lesion, prevent resection. When used in such a manner, endoluminal stents reliably provide symptomatic relief, but may not address the underlying lesion. In addition, they are prone to complications such as obstruction by granulations or secretions, infection due to the retention of secretions, migration, and erosion. Silastic T-tubes permit better

hygiene, are not prone to obstructing granulations, and can also be used to treat subglottic lesions. Depending on variables such as the patient's overall condition and the nature of the stricture, stent removal may be possible after 1–2 years with good results.

3. Segmental resection and reconstruction—Segmental resection and reconstruction should be considered the ideal treatment for most postintubation tracheal strictures, including those of the subglottis. Most lesions can be exposed through a cervical incision and do not require specialized techniques of tracheal mobilization to achieve a primary end-to-end anastomosis. Strictures involving the subglottis are best managed by laryngotracheal resection and thyrotracheal anastomosis, though occasionally, complex lesions may require plastic reconstruction for which a variety of autologous grafts have been used.

Prognosis

The results of segmental resection for both tracheal and subglottic stenoses are excellent, with a 90–95% success rate at experienced centers. Perioperative mortality is approximately 2–4%. Most patients enjoy a normal voice and minor or no dyspnea on exertion. Symptomatic restenosis at the anastomotic site occurs in 5–10% of cases and is usually related to problems of anastomotic tension or perfusion.

Patients with recurrent stenosis develop symptoms within weeks of the initial operation and frequently require intervention such as dilatation or stenting. These patients should be managed just as those presenting with an initial postintubation stricture using conservative, temporizing measures to maintain the airway until postoperative inflammation subsides. The lesion should be fully characterized with imaging studies and bronchoscopy and the patient considered for repeat segmental resection. The results of resection and primary anastomosis of postoperative strictures are nearly as good as for primary lesions. Specialized techniques of tracheal mobilization are often required, however, and a slightly larger proportion of patients experience aspiration, weakness of the voice, and dyspnea on exertion postoperatively.

Braz JR, Navarro LH, Takata IH, Nascimento JP. Endotracheal tube cuff pressure: need for precise measurement. *Sao Paulo Med J.* 1999;117:243. [PMID: 10625887] (Cross-sectional study of cuff pressures in ICU and recovery room settings demonstrates widespread cuff hyperinflation.)

Deslee G, Brichet A, Lebuffe G, Copin MC, Ramon P, Marquette CH. Obstructive fibrinous tracheal pseudomembrane: a potentially fatal complication of tracheal intubation. *Am J Respir Crit Care Med.* 2000;162:1169. [PMID: 10988148] (First report identifying obstructive fibrinous tracheal pseudomembrane as a distinct clinical entity; discusses pathology, presentation, diagnosis, and management in a series of patients.)

Donahue DM, Grillo HC, Wain JC, Wright CD, Mathisen DJ. Reoperative tracheal resection and reconstruction for unsuccessful repair of postintubation stenosis. *J Thorac Cardiovasc Surg.* 1997;114:934. [PMID: 9434688] (Retrospective review of largest reported series in the world examining management of failed initial repair of postintubation tracheal stenosis.)

Donahue DM. Reoperative tracheal surgery. *Chest Surg Clin North Am.* 2003;13(2):375. [PMID: 12755322] (Review of perhaps the world's largest experience in reoperative tracheal surgery.)

Grillo HC, Donahue DM. Postintubation tracheal stenosis. *Semin Thorac Cardiovasc Surg.* 1996;8:370. [PMID: 8899924] (Comprehensive treatment of postintubation tracheal stenosis including the authors' review of their series of 503 patients, the largest reported in the world.)

Heitmiller RF. Tracheal release maneuvers. *Chest Surg Clin North Am.* 2003;13:201. [PMID: 12755309] (Review of techniques used to mobilize the trachea for anastomosis following extensive tracheal resection.)

Liu HC, Lee KS, Huang CJ, Cheng CR, Hsu WH, Huang MH. Silicone T-tube for complex laryngotracheal problems. *Eur J Cardiothorac Surg.* 2002;21:326. [PMID: 11825744] (Retrospective review reports results of using T-tube for treatment of a variety of benign obstructing tracheal lesions.)

Pearson FG, Gullane P. Subglottic resection with primary tracheal anastomosis: including synchronous laryngotracheal reconstructions. *Semin Thorac Cardiovasc Surg.* 1996;8:381. [PMID: 8899925] (Comprehensive treatment of subglottic stenosis includes review of an 80 patient series.)

Schmidt B, Olze H, Borges AC et al. Endotracheal balloon dilatation and stent implantation in benign stenoses. *Ann Thorac Surg.* 2001;71:1630. [PMID: 11383812] (Retrospective review reports the results of stenting after balloon dilatation of benign tracheal stenosis.)

Wain JC. Postintubation tracheal stenosis. *Chest Surg Clin North Am.* 2003;13(2):231. [PMID: 12755310] (Authoritative review of the management of tracheal stenosis.)

Wolf M, Shapira Y, Talmi YP, Novikov I, Kronenberg J, Yellin A. Laryngotracheal anastomosis: primary and revised procedures. *Laryngoscope.* 2001;111:622. [PMID: 11359130] (Cohort study compares the results of reoperation for failed repair of laryngotracheal stenosis with those for initial repair.)

■ TRACHEAL NEOPLASMS

PRIMARY TRACHEAL NEOPLASMS

 ESSENTIALS OF DIAGNOSIS

- *Males.*
- *A history of cigarette smoking.*
- *Worsening wheeze, cough, stridor, and dyspnea on exertion.*
- *Difficulty raising secretions, recurrent pulmonary infections.*
- *Hemoptysis, hoarseness of voice.*
- *Constitutional features of malignancy (eg, fatigue, weight loss).*

General Considerations

Primary tracheal tumors are exceedingly rare, with an estimated incidence of only 2–3 cases per 1 million persons per year. In adults, 80–90% of tumors are malignant, whereas in children, 90% are benign. Of malignant lesions, more than 75% are either squamous cell or adenoid cystic carcinoma. Tracheal tumors are slightly more prevalent in males and smokers.

Pathogenesis

Tumors of the trachea may be classified as primary or secondary. Primary neoplasms include a wide variety of both benign and malignant neoplasms (Table 36–1), whereas secondary neoplasms (discussed below) are, by definition, malignant.

Clinical Findings

A. SYMPTOMS AND SIGNS

Tracheal tumors cause signs and symptoms of upper airway obstruction as described previously for tracheal

Table 36–1. Tumors of the trachea.

Benign Neoplasms	Malignant Neoplasms
Inflammatory pseudotumor	Squamous cell carcinoma
Hamartoma	Adenoid cystic carcinoma
Squamous cell papilloma	Mucoepidermoid carcinoma
Papillomatosis	Small cell carcinoma
Chondroma	Chondrosarcoma
Chondroblastoma	Spindle cell sarcoma
Hemangioma	Adenocarcinoma
Hemangioendothelioma	Adenosquamous carcinoma
Carcinoid	Carcinoid
Leiomyoma	Leiomyosarcoma
Granular cell	Rhabdomyosarcoma
Fibrous histiocytoma	Malignant histiocytoma
Glomus	Melanoma
Fibroma	Lymphoma
Neurofibroma	*Secondary tracheal neoplasms*
Schwannoma	Direct invasion
Lipoma	Metastatic involvement
Pleomorphic adenoma	
Pseudosarcoma	

stenosis. In addition, patients may present with hemoptysis, features of recurrent laryngeal nerve involvement such as hoarseness, or signs of a malignant process such as weight loss and weakness. The onset and progression of findings correlate with the rate of tumor growth and in many cases is very slow. Stridor and dyspnea at rest occur when the tracheal lumen is reduced to 25% of its normal cross-sectional area, but patients with poor underlying lung function may become symptomatic sooner.

The initial symptoms of cough, wheezing, and dyspnea on exertion are common features of pulmonary dysfunction, and patients often are treated inappropriately for asthma or other respiratory conditions. The rarity of tracheal tumors, the paucity of clues on physical exam, and the absence of obvious signs on chest x-ray also confuse the diagnosis, which is typically delayed for more than a year after the onset of symptoms. Occasionally, subtle features such as changes in the patient's strength or quality of voice, a primarily inspiratory wheeze, and positional changes in symptoms are recognized and lead to an earlier diagnosis.

B. Laboratory Findings

Bronchoscopy is essential in the diagnosis, examination, and management of tracheal tumors. It allows for a direct visualization of the tumor and its relationship to the rest of the airway. The tracheobronchial tree distal to the lesion can also be evaluated. Bronchoscopic biopsies provide a tissue diagnosis and, when taken above and below the lesion, identify occult tumor spread, which is important in determining the potential extent of resection.

Facilities for rigid bronchoscopy should be readily available if flexible bronchoscopy is to be performed, because manipulation or biopsy may result in bleeding or complete airway collapse. Bronchoscopic examination, therefore, is often performed in the operating room and may be delayed until the time of resection. If obstructive symptoms require intervention either before resection or in patients who are not operative candidates, rigid bronchoscopy can be used to secure the airway and core open the lumen with biopsy forceps, coagulation, or laser ablation. The subsequent palliation of unresectable tumors with stent placement provides a satisfactory airway in most cases.

C. Imaging Studies

Plain chest x-rays demonstrate tracheal tumors in less than half of cases and the findings, which may be subtle, are often overlooked without a high index of suspicion. Spiral CT scanning with sagittal and coronal reconstruction provides detailed information regarding the extent of the tumor and its relationship to the larynx and carina. It also demonstrates extratracheal involvement and metastatic disease. Contrast esophagography may be added to exclude esophageal involvement.

The radiographic features of tracheal tumors that suggest benignity include smooth, sharply demarcated lesions < 2 cm in size that are completely intraluminal with limited tracheal involvement. Calcifications are present in 80% of chondromas. If fat is also seen within the lesion, a hamartoma is likely. Carcinoid tumors often demonstrate marked enhancement with IV contrast. Malignant lesions are generally larger, with indistinct margins that extend circumferentially and longitudinally within the trachea and invade the wall.

Treatment

A. Initial Measures

Emergent management of respiratory distress due to partial airway occlusion has been discussed previously and is applicable to symptomatic tracheal tumors as well. The availability of rigid bronchoscopy is essential for managing bleeding, distal secretions, or complete airway collapse. Most patients with tracheal tumors do not present acutely, which allows for elective treatment.

Patients with unresectable tumors, or those unfit or unwilling to undergo resection, may be managed with a combination of endoscopic ablation, stenting, and radiation therapy. Irradiation of most malignant tracheal neoplasms provides excellent local control; however, without resection, most tumors recur and long-term survival is rare.

B. Resection and Reconstruction

Most tracheal tumors are best managed by circumferential resection and primary reconstruction, although some (eg, lymphoma and small cell tumors) are treated with chemoradiotherapy alone. Although tracheal tumors usually are advanced by the time of diagnosis, every patient should undergo a thorough evaluation to determine operability. Approximately half of the trachea can be safely resected, and specialized techniques of laryngotracheal and carinal reconstruction allow for the resection of tumors in those locations. The presence of lymph node or pulmonary metastases in patients with indolent neoplasms (eg, adenoid cystic carcinoma) does not preclude meaningful survival with resection of the primary lesion.

Tumors involving the upper two thirds of the trachea can be approached through a cervical incision extended to include a partial or complete median sternotomy, if needed. Neoplasms of the distal third of the trachea and carina are approached through a sternotomy or a high, right thoracotomy. The operative field should allow extension of a sternotomy incision into the fourth intercostal space, if needed, and for cervical or hilar tracheal mobilization maneuvers.

For benign tumors, the plane of dissection is kept close to the trachea, and identification of the recurrent nerves is not performed. The resection of malignant tumors, however, should include as much adjacent tissue as possible. Mediastinal lymph nodes should be sampled, but extensive nodal dissection should be avoided because it results in tracheal devascularization. The recurrent laryngeal nerves should be identified distant from the tumor and traced throughout their course. The sacrifice of an involved nerve is acceptable, but the resection of both recurrent laryngeal nerves should not be performed unless the implications of such a step are discussed with the patient preoperatively.

Care should be taken during exposure of the involved trachea to preserve the lateral vascular pedicles of any portion that will not be resected. The anterior and posterior planes may be bluntly mobilized to the level of the main bronchi. After resection of the tumor, the proximal and distal tracheal margins should be submitted for frozen-section examination to determine the adequacy of resection.

Four to five centimeters of trachea can be removed and safely reconstructed with a primary anastomosis. If the extent of the tumor requires further resection, additional tracheal mobilization can be performed using either laryngeal release procedures proximally or a hilar release distally. With these techniques, about half of the trachea can be safely resected.

Occasionally, the limits of tracheal mobilization and reconstruction preclude complete resection. Histologically positive margins should be accepted rather than compromising the success of the tracheal reconstruction. Involved margins do not affect healing and in some lesions, such as adenoid cystic tumors, may still be associated with long-term survival.

C. POSTOPERATIVE CONSIDERATIONS

Postoperatively, the prevention of anastomotic tension is paramount to the success of the operation. At the conclusion of the procedure, as well as for the first postoperative week, the patient's chin should be sutured to the chest, with head supported to maintain maximal cervical flexion. An aggressive regimen of pulmonary toilet and optimal nutrition should be observed throughout the patient's recovery. The identification and management of aspiration or swallowing difficulties are important, especially in patients who have undergone laryngeal release maneuvers.

D. ADJUVANT RADIATION THERAPY

Adjuvant radiation therapy has been shown to prolong survival in patients with squamous cell and adenoid cystic carcinomas of the trachea who have undergone incomplete resection due to involved margins. The survival of patients with residual carcinoma in situ is better than that of patients with invasive cancer at the resection margin. Adjuvant radiation therapy does not appear to change the survival rate in patients with positive mediastinal lymph nodes or after complete resection. However, given the narrow margins typically accepted in tracheal surgery, the potential benefits, and the lack of significant side effects, adjuvant radiation therapy is recommended—to a dose of 50–60 Gy—for all patients undergoing resection of squamous cell or adenoid cystic tumors of the trachea.

Complications

The mortality rate for resection of malignant tracheal neoplasms is 5–15% and is usually due to anastomotic dehiscence, pneumonia, pulmonary embolism, or erosion into the innominate or pulmonary artery. Complications such as anastomotic leak, aspiration, vocal cord dysfunction, pneumonia, and wound infection occur in 20–40% of cases. Anastomotic stenosis requiring dilatation, laser ablation, or reoperation develops in about 5–14% of patients and is more frequent if postoperative complications occur. Factors that increase morbidity and mortality include extensive tracheal resection, the use of tracheal mobilization procedures, laryngotracheal or carinal reconstruction, and squamous cell histology.

BENIGN TRACHEAL NEOPLASMS

Benign primary tracheal neoplasms may arise from any element of the airway. Inflammatory pseudotumors and tracheal foreign bodies can mimic truly neoplastic lesions. Benign tumors account for 10–20% of adult tracheal neoplasms but comprise nearly all pediatric lesions.

1. Squamous Cell Papillomas

Squamous cell papilloma is a superficial sessile or papillary tumor with a connective tissue core covered by squamous epithelium. In adults, it is usually solitary and associated with heavy smoking. In children, it is frequently multifocal and is known as *juvenile laryngotracheal papillomatosis*. It is the most common pediatric laryngotracheal neoplasm, and its association with human papillomaviruses (HPV) 6 and 11 is well established. Laryngeal involvement usually regresses spontaneously at puberty, but tracheobronchial lesions may not, and malignant degeneration and metastasis can occur. Symptomatic lesions may be treated with endoscopic resection or laser ablation, but recurrence is common.

2. Chondromas

Chondromas are the most common tracheal neoplasms of mesenchymal origin and may arise from any of the cartilaginous elements of the upper airway—most frequently from the posterior cricoid lamina. They are typically hard tumors covered by intact mucosa. Chondromas are well known for malignant degeneration to chondrosarcomas, and histologic differentiation between the two may be difficult. Because incomplete resection invariably leads to recurrence, resection rather than endoscopic ablation is the treatment of choice.

3. Hemangiomas

Hemangiomas of the upper airway occur in adults as well as children and are one of the most common causes of subglottic obstruction in the pediatric population. In adults, they tend to occur in the larynx and proximal trachea. Hemangiomas develop in the submucosa and appear as sessile lesions with a blue tint beneath a normal mucosa. Fifty percent of children with tracheal involvement also have a cutaneous hemangioma. Obstructive symptoms can usually be managed conservatively, but occasionally endoscopic laser ablation is required. Most tracheal hemangiomas resolve spontaneously by 3 years of age.

MALIGNANT TRACHEAL NEOPLASMS

Eighty to ninety percent of primary tracheal tumors in adults are malignant. Of these, 70–80% are either squamous cell or adenoid cystic carcinoma. Other malignant tumors (see Table 36–1) include carcinoid, mucoepidermoid, and small cell neoplasms.

1. Squamous Cell Carcinoma

Squamous cell carcinoma is the most common malignant neoplasm of the trachea. It is tightly associated with cigarette smoking and nearly every patient presents with such a history. Squamous cell tumors of the trachea occur 3–4 times more frequently in men than in women and typically develop in the sixth to seventh decades of life. Forty percent of patients have either a synchronous or a metachronous squamous cell cancer of the respiratory tract.

Squamous cell neoplasms may occur at any level of the airway and in the trachea may be single or multiple. Lesions may demonstrate exophytic or sessile growth and ulceration is common. Nearly 50% of patients with squamous cell cancer of the trachea have tumors that are unresectable at the time of presentation owing to the extent of the primary lesion or the presence of metastatic disease. Of patients undergoing resection, one fourth will have nodal metastases.

2. Adenoid Cystic Carcinoma

Adenoid cystic carcinoma is the most frequently resected malignant tumor of the trachea and the second

most common overall. In contradistinction to squamous cell tumors, adenoid cystic cancers are not related to cigarette smoking, occur in both sexes with equal frequency, and may develop at any age throughout adult life, most often in the fourth decade.

In addition, adenoid cystic cancers are remarkable for their extremely slow progression and relatively favorable prognosis. Metastatic disease, which ultimately occurs in about 50% of patients, does not preclude long-term survival and should not be considered an absolute contraindication for resection of the tracheal lesion.

Adenoid cystic carcinoma arises from cells within the mucosal glands of the trachea and spreads in the submucosal plane both longitudinally and circumferentially. The tracheal wall is typically invaded and a significant amount of extratracheal tumor may be present. Adenoid cystic tumors rarely invade other mediastinal structures, but rather push them away. Extensive submucosal growth beyond the visible lesion is nearly uniform and intraoperative frozen section evaluation is required to ensure uninvolved resection margins. Local recurrence can develop decades after incomplete resection.

Prognosis

The survival of patients following the resection of adenoid cystic carcinoma of the trachea is good, with 5- and 10-year survival rates of 70–75% and 50–55%, respectively. Patients with uninvolved mediastinal lymph nodes and negative resection margins tend to survive longer than those with positive lymph nodes or margins. The local recurrence of adenoid cystic carcinoma may develop as much as 25–30 years after resection. Metastatic disease usually manifests 5–10 years after the diagnosis and may remain asymptomatic for years.

Long-term survival after the resection of squamous cell cancers of the trachea is poor, with a 5-year survival rate of approximately 15–50%. Histologically involved resection margins significantly decrease the survival time. The effect on survival of mediastinal nodal metastases in the surgical specimen is unclear.

Chao MW, Smith JG, Laidlaw C, Joon DL, Ball D. Results of treating primary tumors of the trachea with radiotherapy. *Int J Radiat Oncol Biol Phys.* 1998;41:779. [PMID: 9652838] (Review of a single center's experience; discusses prognostic factors.)

D'Cunha J, Maddaus MA. Surgical treatment of tracheal and carinal tumors. *Chest Surg Clin North Am.* 2003;13(1):95. [PMID: 12698640] (Review of the management of tracheal and carinal neoplasms.)

Gaissert HA. Primary tracheal tumors. *Chest Surg Clin North Am.* 2003;13(2):247. [PMID: 12755311] (Review of the types, diagnosis, and management of tracheal neoplasms.)

Grillo HC, Mathisen DJ, Wain JC. Management of tumors of the trachea. *Oncology.* 1992;6:61. [PMID: 1313276] (Overview of tracheal tumors discusses the authors' series of 198 patients, the largest experience in the world.)

Heitmiller RF. Tracheal release maneuvers. *Chest Surg Clin North Am.* 2003;13(2):201. [PMID: 12755309] (Review of techniques used to mobilize the trachea for anastomosis after extensive tracheal resection.)

Maziak DE, Todd TR, Keshavjee SH, Winton TL, van Nostrand P, Pearson FG. Adenoid cystic carcinoma of the airway: thirty-two year experience. *J Thorac Cardiovasc Surg.* 1996; 112:1522. [PMID: 8975844] (Large review of a single center's experience managing adenoid cystic cancers.)

Regnard JF, Rourquier P, Levasseur P. Results and prognostic factors in resections of primary tracheal tumors: a multicenter retrospective study. The French Society of Cardiovascular Surgery. *J Thorac Cardiovasc Surg.* 1996;111:808. [PMID: 8614141] (European retrospective multicenter review of 208 patients undergoing resection.)

SECONDARY TRACHEAL NEOPLASMS

Secondary tracheal tumors are, by definition, malignant, and occur most commonly as a result of direct invasion from adjacent organs. A variety of neoplasms can metastasize to the trachea, but this is exceedingly rare. Invasion of the trachea by thyroid, esophageal, and bronchogenic tumors accounts for the majority of secondary tumors.

Resection of invasive thyroid tumors with en bloc segmental tracheal resection prevents the morbidity and possible mortality associated with tracheal obstruction and may result in long-term survival. Ideally, tracheal involvement is identified preoperatively so that a combined resection can be planned. Typically, however, airway involvement is identified intraoperatively, and the tumor is simply dissected off the trachea, resulting in incomplete resection. Referral for subsequent tracheal resection in such cases prevents recurrence and improves survival.

Upper lobe lung cancer and esophageal tumors that invade the trachea are usually too widespread to justify tracheal resection. Palliation of these and other inoperable secondary tracheal tumors can be achieved using a combination of endoscopic ablation, stenting, and radiation therapy.

Hammoud ZT, Mathisen DJ. Surgical management of thyroid carcinoma invading the trachea. *Chest Surg Clin North Am.* 2003;13(2):359. [PMID: 12755320] (Review of the management of thyroid carcinoma invading the trachea.)

Koike E, Yamashita H, Noguchi S et al. Bronchoscopic diagnosis of thyroid cancer with laryngotracheal invasion. *Arch Surg.* 2001;136:1185. [PMID: 11585513] (Prospective study reports the use of preoperative bronchoscopy to determine the need for airway resection.)

Nakao K, Kurozumi K, Fukushima S, Nakahara M, Tsujimoto M, Nishida T. Merits and demerits of operative procedure to the trachea in patients with differentiated thyroid cancer. *World J Surg.* 2001;25:723. [PMID: 11376406] (Retrospective review reports results of tracheal resection, en bloc, for invasive thyroid tumors.)

Nishida T, Nakao K, Hamaji M. Differentiated thyroid carcinoma with airway invasion: indication for tracheal resection based on the extent of cancer invasion. *J Thorac Cardiovasc Surg.* 1997;114(1):84. [PMID: 9240297] (Retrospective review examining the indications for tracheal resection in the management of invasive thyroid cancer.)

Wang JC, Takashima S, Takayama F et al. Tracheal invasion by thyroid carcinoma: prediction using MRI imaging. *AJR Am J Roentgenol.* 2001;177:929. [PMID: 11566708] (Demonstrates the viability of using combination of MRI findings to predict tracheal invasion.)

Airway Management & Tracheotomy

Kenneth C.Y. Yu, MD

With airway obstruction, trauma, or elective surgery, control of the airway is the first priority that must be accomplished before any other intervention can proceed. In cases of a rapidly decompensating airway, particularly in pediatric patients or patients with airways that are difficult to manage, the otolaryngologist is frequently consulted to assist in patient airway management.

Patient Evaluation

Successful airway management must begin with a careful, thorough, and rapid evaluation of the airway. Healthy patients presenting with normal head and neck anatomy who undergo elective surgery represent relatively straightforward cases in which standard endotracheal intubation can provide an easy and secure airway. Patients presenting with upper airway obstruction must be evaluated quickly, efficiently, and accurately.

Physical examination is a key element in diagnosing upper airway obstruction. Stridor, or noisy respiration, is a hallmark symptom of upper airway obstruction. The timing of the stridor with respiration can frequently indicate where the obstruction lies. **Inspiratory stridor** normally results when the obstruction is at the larynx or above. **Expiratory stridor** usually indicates a more distal obstruction (eg, a tracheal obstruction). **Biphasic stridor** (ie, noise on both inspiration and expiration) may indicate a subglottic obstruction. The quality of the voice is also important. A muffled voice may reflect supraglottic obstruction, such as from the epiglottitis. A hoarse voice may indicate laryngeal involvement (eg, papillomas or tumors). A breathy or weak voice or cry may suggest vocal cord paralysis. Other signs of upper airway obstruction include suprasternal or substernal retractions, tachypnea, and cyanosis.

An accurate history is also critical in evaluating the airway and formulating the best plan to manage it. The physician should determine whether the obstruction occurred acutely or chronically. The age of the patient also helps in distinguishing the cause of the obstruction. Congenital airway anomalies (eg, laryngomalacia, choanal atresia, hemangioma, and tracheomalacia) and acute inflammatory causes (eg, croup and epiglottitis) are more common in children. In adults, tumors are a more common cause of obstruction. Trauma can cause airway obstruction, and this circumstance is usually easy to diagnose. However, it is important to carefully ascertain the mechanism and type of injury. Suspicion of laryngeal trauma may make conventional endotracheal intubation perilous because it can potentially result in a more compromised airway due to laryngotracheal separation. In these circumstances, the physician should consider performing a tracheotomy while the patient is awake. Similarly, massive maxillofacial trauma may preclude normal translaryngeal intubation; a flexible fiberoptic intubation or a tracheotomy while the patient is awake should be considered in these situations.

Treatment

A. NONSURGICAL MEASURES

Patients with difficult airways should be identified before the induction of anesthesia and intubation so that proper planning and communication between the anesthesiologist and the surgeon can be coordinated. A difficult airway is defined as a situation in which a conventionally trained anesthesiologist experiences difficulty with mask ventilation, endotracheal intubation, or both. In addition, the physician should be prepared for a potentially difficult airway or possible airway loss if both anesthesia induction and intubation are difficult. Both of these situations can be managed with a number of nonsurgical airway management techniques.

1. Oxygen administration—The first and most important task in nonsurgical airway management is to administer oxygen to relieve hypoxia. As the airway obstruction worsens, the physician may have to mask, ventilate, and provide a chin lift and jaw thrust to maintain a patent airway until a more definitive airway can be established. A helium-oxygen mixture of 80% helium to 20% oxygen can be used in some cases to improve ventilation temporarily until definitive control of the airway can be achieved. This mixture, known as heliox, depends on the decreased density of helium to deliver oxygen past the obstructing airway lesions.

2. Topical decongestants and steroids—Adjunctive medical therapy can be used to decrease upper airway obstruction if there is a component of soft tissue edema. Racemic epinephrine and epinephrine aerosols act as topical decongestants and can be given to try to decrease the edema. However, the effect is short in duration, and they may cause a rebound effect if used repeatedly. Consequently, their use is limited to the inpatient setting. The use of steroids in relieving upper airway obstruction can also be helpful, especially in cases in which edema or inflammation is present (eg, angioedema, croup, and adult supraglottitis). A suggested treatment is to administer methylprednisolone sodium succinate (125 mg IV) as a first dose and then continue with dexamethasone (8 mg IV every 8 h) for several doses; methylprednisolone succinate has a more rapid onset of action than dexamethasone.

3. Oropharyngeal and nasopharyngeal airways—Oropharyngeal and nasopharyngeal airways are adjuncts to airway support that can be helpful in certain cases. For example, patients emerging from anesthesia or suffering from an altered mental state can have their airways supported with these devices until their mental status improves.

Oropharyngeal airways prevent obstruction caused by a relaxed and prolapsed tongue. However, an incorrectly placed oropharyngeal airway can itself cause airway obstruction by pushing the tongue posteriorly into the hypopharynx. If placed in a patient who is still under light anesthesia, coughing and laryngospasm can occur. The traumatic insertion of nasal or nasopharyngeal airways can cause bleeding.

4. Translaryngeal intubation—The definitive nonsurgical control of the airway is via translaryngeal intubation. This procedure should be considered the preferred method of establishing control of the airway in most cases, provided the patient's condition is not so dire that an immediate airway is required, or in situations in which intubation is contraindicated (eg, laryngeal trauma or an obstructing tumor that makes intubation difficult). It is extremely important that a good airway history be obtained and a thorough examination be performed whenever possible before inducing anesthesia and performing an intubation.

5. Jackson sliding laryngoscope—A unique instrument familiar to otolaryngology surgeons is the Jackson sliding laryngoscope (Figure 37–1). This laryngoscope has better leverage and lighting compared with the

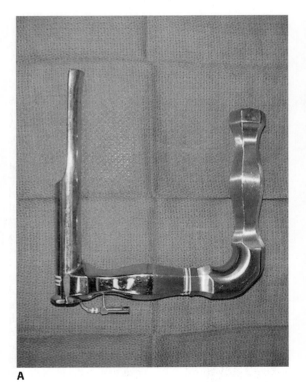

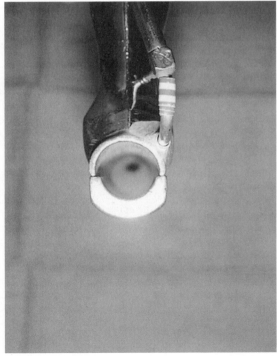

A   B

Figure 37–1. **(A)** Side view of a sliding Jackson laryngoscope. **(B)** View along the aperture. The floor can be slid out after insertion of an endotracheal tube.

anesthesiologist's blades; the design of the laryngoscope makes it easier to manipulate past obstructing lesions or edematous soft tissue and suction can be used concurrently. Once the glottis is identified, an endotracheal tube is passed into the trachea and the laryngoscope's floor can be slid out to facilitate removal of the laryngoscope. Frequently, the difficult airway can be managed with this technique.

6. Guided endotracheal intubation—Guided endotracheal intubation using a flexible fiberscope is an excellent technique for both routine and difficult airways. Placing an endotracheal tube with a fiberscope tube is particularly useful for an intubation in an awake, spontaneously breathing patient with a known or suspected difficult airway. Fiberoptic endotracheal intubations can be performed either via a nasal or an oral route. Once the route is chosen and anesthesia is achieved (topical or general), the endoscope is passed through the endotracheal tube, through the mouth or nose, and through the larynx into the trachea. The endotracheal tube is then advanced over the endoscope and into the trachea, using the endoscope as a "guidewire." The endoscope is withdrawn after confirming the correct positioning of the endotracheal tube. Flexible fiberoptic intubation has limitations as well. Minimal trauma to these endoscopes may damage the delicate optics and distort the visual field. Bleeding and secretions can obscure the view and make visualization of the glottis extremely difficult. This technique may also be difficult in the uncooperative patient or in patients with inadequate topical anesthesia. Finally, introduction of the endoscope may actually cause complete airway obstruction in patients with severe intrinsic or extrinsic compression of the laryngeal or tracheal airways.

7. Laryngeal mask airway—The laryngeal mask airway (LMA) is useful for establishing the airway in both routine elective cases and many emergency situations involving difficult airways. The laryngeal mask airway can be considered a hybrid between an endotracheal tube and a face mask (Figure 37–2). It can easily be inserted blindly into the hypopharynx; insertion is complete when resistance is felt. No neck movement or laryngoscopy is required. Once the mask is inflated, it fills the hypopharynx and covers the laryngeal inlet. Due to the LMA's size and shape, it is not possible to pass it into the esophagus.

Several series report excellent success rates of 95–99%. Other advantages of the laryngeal mask airway include its simplicity in learning and use, fewer postoperative sore throats and coughing, and less potential for laryngeal injuries. These features also make the laryngeal mask airway an excellent instrument to use in many emergency situations involving the airway. Because this device can be inserted quickly and blindly, it has the potential to provide lifesaving ventilation while a more definitive airway is established. A flexible fiberoptic endoscope can also be passed through the mask's open slit

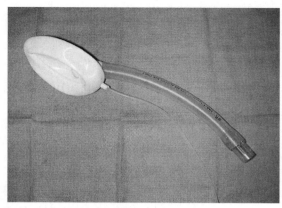

Figure 37–2. Laryngeal mask airway.

into the trachea, and an endotracheal tube can be passed over the endoscope. Since the laryngeal mask airway does not completely separate the airway from the esophagus, the greatest risk in using this device is pulmonary aspiration of regurgitated stomach contents. Contraindications to using this airway include patients with full stomachs or hiatal hernias, obesity, and emergency and abdominal surgeries. The need for controlled ventilation and prone or lateral positions are strong relative contraindications for elective use of this device. Understandably, if the mouth cannot be opened, the laryngeal mask airway is not useful.

8. Other nonsurgical measures—Less common instruments and techniques used in difficult airway situations include the esophageal Combitube, light wand, and the Bullard laryngoscope. The esophagotracheal Combitube is an emergency airway management device for patients requiring rapid airway control. In many cases, this device can provide lifesaving emergency ventilation and oxygenation until a surgical airway can be established. The esophagotracheal Combitube is a double-lumen tube with an open "tracheal" cannula and a blocked distal "esophageal" end, which has ventilating side holes located proximally (Figure 37–3). This device is also blindly inserted, and the upper and lower balloons inflated. Because of its design, the esophagotracheal Combitube can effectively ventilate the upper airway regardless of whether it is placed into the trachea or into the esophagus. If the Combitube tip is in the esophagus, ventilation is achieved through the proximal side ventilation holes of the esophageal port. If this device is inserted into the trachea during the blind intubation, ventilation is accomplished conventionally through the tracheal port. Because of its relatively large size, this Combitube is contraindicated in pediatric and very small adult patients. It should be used with caution in patients with upper esophageal pathology, upper air-

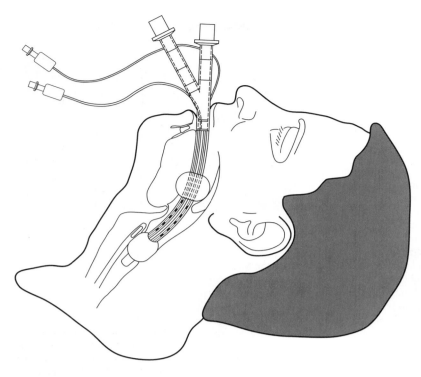

Figure 37–3. Esophagotracheal Combitube. The diagram depicts the esophagotracheal Combitube in the esophagus. Ventilation is accomplished via the proximal side ports. (Combitube is a registered trademark of Kendall/Tyco Healthcare, Mansfield, MA.)

way tumors, or other compressive lesions of the hypopharynx, larynx, or trachea. Finally, laryngospasm and laryngotracheal foreign bodies can impair ventilation if this device is inserted into the esophagus.

B. Surgical Measures

When endotracheal intubation is not feasible, a surgical airway must be obtained. The two basic surgical techniques to obtain an airway are cricothyroidotomy and tracheotomy. The terms *tracheotomy* and *tracheostomy* are often used interchangeably in error. A **tracheotomy** is generally described as a procedure that involves opening the trachea. A **tracheostomy** is a procedure that exteriorizes the trachea to the cervical skin, resulting in a more permanent tracheal cutaneous fistula; therefore, the term tracheostomy should be reserved for these particular procedures.

The indications for establishing an urgent surgical airway include the following: (1) severe maxillofacial trauma in which injuries make the airway inaccessible for translaryngeal intubation, (2) significant laryngeal trauma in which intubation may potentially cause more damage, (3) excessive hemorrhage or emesis obscuring landmarks required for successful intubation, (4) cervical spine injury with vocal cords that are difficult to visualize, and (5) failed translaryngeal intubation. In emergency situations, cricothyroidotomy is generally considered the pro-

cedure of choice because it is fast and simple to perform and it requires very few instruments. However, a tracheotomy can also be performed urgently. It is technically more difficult, bloody, and dangerous compared with elective tracheotomy or cricothyroidotomy. There are rare circumstances in which an emergent tracheotomy is preferred over a cricothyroidotomy, such as true subglottic obstruction (eg, subglottic carcinoma or large thyroid tumors). Cricothyroidotomy should also be avoided in children because the cricoid cartilage is the narrowest portion of their airway.

1. Tracheotomy—The primary objective of a tracheotomy is to provide a secure airway. The indications for performing a tracheotomy include (1) bypassing an upper airway obstruction, (2) providing a means for assisting mechanical ventilation (ie, chronic ventilator dependency), (3) enabling more efficient pulmonary hygiene, (4) temporarily securing an airway in patients undergoing major head and neck surgery, (5) relieving obstructive sleep apnea, and (6) eliminating pulmonary "dead space." Ideally, tracheotomies should be performed in a controlled setting—preferably in the operating room—where adequate lighting, instruments, specialized intubation equipment, and assistance are available.

Figure 37–4 depicts the surface anatomy of the neck and the location of the incision for the tracheotomy. The cricothyroid membrane has a relatively superficial

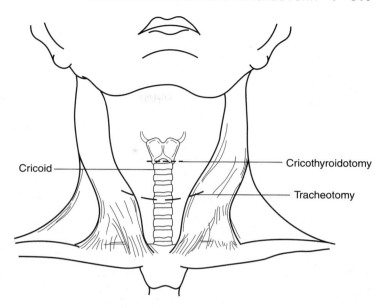

Cricoid

Cricothyroidotomy

Tracheotomy

Figure 37–4. Diagram of the neck, indicating locations of cricothyroidotomy and tracheotomy incisions.

location and is therefore fairly easy to access in an emergency situation. A tracheotomy is most easily performed if the patient is already intubated and general anesthesia has been administered. However, if the patient has a tenuous airway with impaired ventilatory status, the tracheotomy should be performed with local anesthesia and sedation to avoid paralysis. If the patient is anesthetized, he or she is placed in the supine position with a shoulder roll to extend the neck. The patient with a tenuous airway who undergoes a tracheotomy while awake should be placed in a semi-upright position. Landmarks such as the thyroid notch, the cricoid, the sternal notch, and planned incisions are marked. A transverse incision is marked approximately two fingerbreadths above the sternal notch. Alternately, a vertical incision can be used. The incision is then infiltrated with a local anesthetic containing epinephrine to help decrease bleeding. The neck and upper chest are then prepped and draped in a standard sterile fashion.

The skin incision is made with a 15 blade and the platysma is divided. The strap muscles are then separated in the midline at the median raphe. The strap muscles can then be retracted laterally with appropriate retractors. The anterior jugular veins can also be retracted laterally or ligated and divided as needed. Once the strap muscles are retracted laterally, the thyroid isthmus should be visible in the center of the field. The surgeon can then retract the isthmus superiorly or inferiorly as needed to obtain exposure to the planned tracheotomy. Frequently, in order to facilitate exposure, the clinician can divide and ligate the isthmus. A cricoid hood is used to retract the cricoid superiorly and pull the trachea forward. A Kittner sponge dissector is then used to push the fine fascia away from the anterior wall of the trachea and clearly identify the individual rings. An incision is made between the second and third tracheal rings. A **Björk flap** can be made by creating an inferiorly based tracheal ring flap and suturing this flap to the inferior skin margin (Figure 37–5). This technique greatly reduces the incidence of accidental decannulation and makes reinsertion of the tracheotomy tube easier if inadvertent decannulation occurs. Alternately, the surgeon can also resect a single tracheal ring or

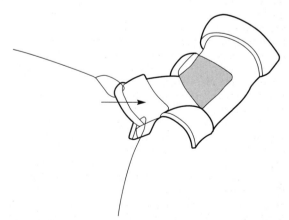

Figure 37–5. Björk flap. The incised tracheal ring (see arrow) is then sutured to the inferior neck skin.

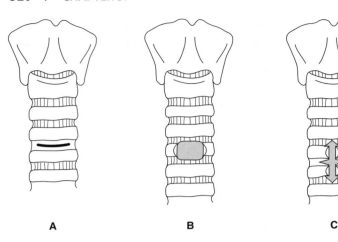

Figure 37–6. Various incisions used in entering the trachea. **(A)** Simple horizontal intercartilaginous incision; **(B)** resection of cartilage ring creating an anterior tracheal window; **(C)** cruciate incision.

make a cruciate incision (Figure 37–6). The Björk flap is contraindicated in children because it carries a high risk of tracheal stenosis and persistent tracheocutaneous fistula. It may also be less desirable in patients requiring tracheotomy for only a few days (eg, after maxillofacial trauma or extensive surgery of the oral cavity). Before making the intended tracheotomy incision, the physician should palpate the wound inferiorly to ensure that a high-riding innominate artery is not present; a higher tracheotomy incision may need to be made. After the trachea is entered, the endotracheal tube is withdrawn just proximal to the tracheotomy. A previously tested and appropriately sized cuffed tracheotomy tube is then inserted into the tracheotomy. The ventilator circuit is then switched to the tracheotomy tube, and satisfactory ventilation and oxygenation are confirmed by the anesthesiologist before the tracheal hook and retractors are removed. The tracheotomy plate is then secured to the neck with tracheotomy ties, sutures to the skin, or both. The endotracheal tube can then be removed.

2. Emergent tracheotomy—The emergent tracheotomy is best performed through a vertical incision, beginning at the level of the cricoid cartilage and extending approximately 1.0–1.5 inches. If the surgeon is right-handed, the left hand stabilizes the larynx and the right hand holds the scalpel. The incision is made through skin, platysma, and subcutaneous tissues in one swift motion. Strap muscles and the thyroid isthmus are rarely identified during the maneuver. The left index finger is used to palpate the trachea. The blade is then used to incise the trachea where the second or third tracheal ring is estimated to be. Once the airway is entered, the endotracheal tube is inserted into the trachea. A tracheal dilator is useful, but not necessary. A tracheal hook is often helpful to pull the trachea forward and stabilize it while the endotracheal tube is passed. This technique is particularly helpful in the patient with an obese neck. During the procedure, signifi-

cant bleeding is ignored until the airway is established; once it is, bleeding in the wound is controlled. If the situation allows, the tracheotomy should be carefully assessed and appropriate revisions made. The vertical skin incision is crucial to the speed of this procedure and can prevent damage to adjacent neck structures.

3. Pediatric tracheotomy—Tracheotomy in the child is carried out in a fashion similar to that of the adult tracheotomy; however, a simple vertical incision in the trachea is used. A Björk flap or the excision of tracheal rings should be avoided in the pediatric patient. Furthermore, tracheotomy in children should be performed with a bronchoscope or endotracheal tube in place to secure the airway. Emergent tracheotomy should be avoided, if possible. At the time of tracheotomy, it is wise to place 4.0 or 5.0 nonabsorbable monofilament guide sutures (one on either side of the vertical tracheal incision) to serve as guides should the tracheotomy tube accidentally come out. By gently pulling the sutures, the trachea can be elevated into the wound and the tracheal incision opened slightly to assist in tube reinsertion.

4. Percutaneous tracheotomy—Interest in percutaneous tracheotomy has increased recently. The procedure entails transcutaneous entry with a needle inserted into the trachea, a guidewire passage into the lumen, and serial dilation. A tracheotomy tube is then passed into the lumen. Initial disastrous outcomes led to debates regarding the safety and efficacy of this procedure. Proponents argue that percutaneous tracheotomy is easy to perform, has a shorter operative time, can be performed at the patient's bedside, is lower in cost, and lacks having to transport the patient to the operating room with the inherent dangers associated with the transport (ie, an unstable patient or line dislodgment). Opponents of percutaneous tracheotomy argue that the potential complications, which may be significant, are associated with blind entry into the trachea. However, many recent studies have demonstrated favorable complication rates with percutaneous tracheotomy when flexible bronchoscopy is performed concurrently. There is more consensus that percutaneous tracheotomy is best avoided in children (higher complication rate, difficulty ventilating with a bronchoscope through the ventilating tube). Excluding children, current literature supports endoscopic percutaneous tracheotomy as a viable alternative to surgical tracheotomy if performed by an experienced surgeon.

C. POSTOPERATIVE CARE

Careful postoperative care is important to the success of tracheotomies. Humidifying inspired air is necessary to prevent crusting and tracheitis. Suctioning the tube and trachea on a frequent basis immediately postoperatively is necessary to clear secretions and prevent plugging. The frequency of suctioning can be decreased as the postoperative time increases and the patient recovers. Stay sutures and Björk flap sutures can be removed in approximately 3–5 days. Also, changing the tracheotomy tube can usually be performed at this time, after an adequate tract has formed.

D. DECANNULATION

Before decannulation can occur, the disease process that resulted in the need for a tracheotomy must be resolved. Good airway patency allows for successful decannulation. Patency can be evaluated either with a mirror exam of the larynx or by direct fiberoptic endoscopy. Another practical approach is to change the tube to a smaller uncuffed tube. This tube can then be occluded and the patient's respiration observed. The patient with an adequate airway after tube occlusion should tolerate decannulation; tube removal is usually performed after 24 hours of tube occlusion.

Complications

The complications of tracheotomy are listed in Table 37–1. Meticulous hemostasis should be achieved before leaving the operating room. Occasionally, **subcutaneous emphysema** results when air is trapped in the subcutaneous tissues from suturing the surgical incision. The treatment involves removing the skin sutures and inflating the cuff. The physician must monitor for the potential development of either pneumomediastinum or pneumothorax if the condition progresses. **Pneumomediastinum** results when air is sucked through the wound or from coughing that forces air into the deep tissue planes of the neck and into the mediastinum. **Pneumothorax** may result from progressive pneumomediastinum or from direct injury to the pleura during tracheotomy. A **tracheoesophageal fistula** can occur if the tracheal incision is made too deep, causing inadvertent injury to the underlying esophagus. **Recurrent laryngeal nerve damage** is possible if

Table 37–1. Complications of tracheotomies.

Early
Infection
Hemorrhage
Subcutaneous emphysema
Pneumomediastinum
Pneumothorax
Tracheoesophageal fistula
Recurrent laryngeal nerve injury
Tube displacement
Delayed
Tracheal-innominate artery fistula
Tracheal stenosis
Delayed tracheoesophageal fistula
Tracheocutaneous fistula

dissection occurs lateral to the trachea. **Tube displacement** is a risk of surgery and can be minimized by the use of stay sutures or the Björk flap.

One of the most dire complications of tracheotomy is a **tracheal-innominate artery fistula,** which occurs when the major vessel is eroded by pressure necrosis from the tracheotomy cuff or directly from the tip of the tube itself. It usually presents within 2 weeks of the tracheotomy and carries a 73% mortality rate. It may be indicated by minor sentinel bleeding. The treatment consists of controlling the hemorrhage by overinflating the tracheotomy tube cuff or inserting an endotracheal tube below the level of bleeding while compressing the innominate artery anteriorly against the sternum, with the index finger inserted through the tracheotomy wound. The patient should then be rushed to the operating room for definitive repair.

Tracheal stenosis is another delayed complication and can occur at the level of the stoma, the tracheotomy tube cuff, or the tube tip. A **tracheoesophageal fistula** can also occur in the delayed setting and is considered to be secondary to pressure necrosis from the tracheotomy tube cuff or the tip of a malpositioned tube. An indwelling nasogastric tube may predispose the patient to postoperative complications. A persistent **tracheocutaneous fistula** can sometimes occur after decannulation of a long-standing tracheotomy. Surgical closure is indicated if the stoma remains patent longer than 2 months. Closure involves excising the fistula tract and closing, in layers, the trachea, strap muscles, platysma, and skin.

Altman KW, Waltonen JD, Kern RC. Urgent surgical airway intervention: a 3-year county hospital experience. *Laryngoscope.* 2005;115:2101. [PMID: 16369150] (Discusses how to manage an urgent surgical airway situation in a controlled manner and provides some excellent pearls for one of the most stressful situations that otolaryngologists can encounter.)

Henderson JJ, Popat MT, Latto IP, Pearce AC. Difficult Airway Society guidelines for management of the unanticipated difficult intubation. *Anaesthesia.* 2004;59:675. [PMID: 15200543] (Thorough discussion of the management of the unexpected difficult airway intubation with an algorithm on managing this situation before a surgical airway must be considered.)

Kost KM. Endoscopic percutaneous dilatational tracheotomy: a prospective evaluation of 500 consecutive cases. *Laryngoscope.* 2005;115(10 Pt 2):1. [PMID: 16227862] (Excellent prospective evaluation of 500 endoscopic-guided percutaneous tracheotomies with thorough review and analysis of current literature. Presents a strong case for this procedure.)

Foreign Bodies

38

Kristina W. Rosbe, MD

 ESSENTIALS OF DIAGNOSIS

- *Patient history.*
- *Witnessed ingestion and history of choking.*
- *High level of clinical suspicion.*
- *Respiratory and swallowing symptoms.*
- *Posteroanterior and lateral neck and chest x-rays are diagnostic.*

General Considerations

Foreign body ingestions are an important cause of morbidity and mortality in the pediatric population. Most of these patients present under age 3. Aerodigestive tract foreign bodies are the cause of approximately 150 pediatric deaths per year in the United States, and choking causes 40% of accidental deaths in children less than 1 year of age. A high level of clinical suspicion can prevent delays in diagnosis and complications related to these delays.

Pathogenesis

Children under 3 years of age have a high propensity for placing objects in their mouths. Increased mobility and the introduction of adult foods add to the risk of ingestion or aspiration. Incomplete dentition and immature swallowing coordination may also play a role. Coins are the most commonly ingested foreign body, whereas food is the most commonly aspirated material. Nuts and seeds are the most likely foods to be aspirated (Figure 38–1). Though fortunately rare, the aspiration of latex balloons is associated with especially high mortality rates. In older children, fish or chicken bones may lodge in the oropharynx.

Damage to the surrounding aerodigestive tract mucosa is proportional to the length of time the foreign body has been present. Granulation tissue formation, erosive lesions, and infections can occur over time and can be minimized with early diagnosis and surgical intervention.

Prevention

The prevention of ingestion is the most important intervention for potential aerodigestive tract foreign body ingestions. The Consumer Products Safety Act was passed in 1979 and includes criteria for the minimum size of objects (> 3.17 cm in diameter and > 5.71 cm in length) allowable for children to play with, but these regulations are not uniformly enforced.

Children older than 5 years have been found to be more likely to aspirate school supplies than food. Children with esophageal motility disorders or neurologic disorders should be encouraged to chew food slowly and completely to avoid esophageal impactions or aspiration.

Clinical Findings

A. SYMPTOMS AND SIGNS

A witnessed ingestion or aspiration episode should be brought to the attention of a physician. Information that is important to elicit from parents includes the approximate time of ingestion, any history of esophageal dysfunction, and both the severity and the duration of swallowing and respiratory symptoms since the time of ingestion. When an unusual foreign body is aspirated or ingested, it may also be helpful to have the parents bring in a similar object from home.

Typical signs and symptoms of esophageal foreign body ingestion include drooling, dysphagia, emesis, and chest pain. Airway foreign bodies may present with cough, wheezing, stridor, cyanosis, or asymmetric breath sounds. Esophageal foreign bodies may also cause respiratory symptoms in a young child. A high index of suspicion should be maintained when evaluating children presenting with recurrent croup, asthma, or pneumonia without the expected response to treatment.

B. IMAGING STUDIES

Posteroanterior and lateral x-rays of the neck and chest are the imaging studies of choice. Radiopaque foreign bodies should be straightforward to diagnose, whereas other foreign bodies may be more difficult. Even if no foreign body is visualized, localized atelectasis or infiltrates, unilateral hyperinflation, or mediastinal shift may be present on plain film x-rays (Figure 38–2). However, high clinical suspicion or historical evidence (ie, witnessed ingestion or aspiration) warrants rigid endoscopy even if x-rays are normal. If plain films are not diagnostic

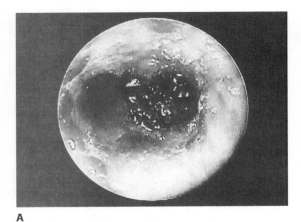
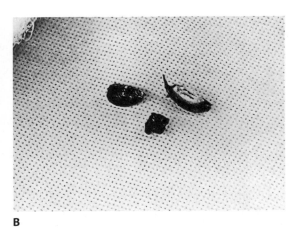

A   B

Figure 38–1. **(A)** Clot and surrounding granulation tissue of the right mainstem bronchus; **(B)** sunflower seed husks pulled from the right mainstem bronchus after removal of clot.

or the patient cannot cooperate for the imaging exam, airway fluoroscopy is sometimes used. This study has the added advantage of demonstrating a dynamic view of the airway; however, it is dependent on the expertise of the radiologist performing the exam. Barium swallow is generally not indicated, and the presence of barium can make esophageal foreign body extraction more difficult.

Differential Diagnosis

The differential diagnosis of aerodigestive tract foreign body is generated in part using presenting symptoms, but

it is more dependent on the history obtained from parents or other caregivers. As previously mentioned, children with esophageal foreign bodies may present with airway symptoms or symptoms mimicking nonspecific gastrointestinal illness. These children may be misdiagnosed with pharyngitis or gastroenteritis.

Bronchial foreign bodies may present with chronic cough or wheezing. Common misdiagnoses include asthma, croup, and pneumonia. In children with these diagnoses who continue to seek medical attention and do not appear to respond to appropriate treatments, the presence of an airway foreign body should be considered.

Complications

The complications of aerodigestive tract foreign body can be classified as early or late. The initial symptoms and signs of a laryngeal or bronchial foreign body can be severe, including cyanosis, respiratory distress, and even respiratory arrest. A ball-valve effect can occur with a partially occluding bronchial foreign body causing hyperexpansion of the affected lung. If complete bronchial occlusion is present, total or partial lung collapse can occur. In the case of esophageal foreign bodies, late complications include granulation tissue formation, mucosal erosions, esophageal perforation, tracheoesophageal fistula, esophageal-aortic fistula, and mediastinitis. With bronchial foreign bodies, late complications include pneumonia, empyema, bronchial fistula, and pneumothorax.

Treatment

The treatment of choice for aerodigestive tract foreign body is rigid endoscopic removal under general anesthesia. Rarely, an oropharyngeal foreign body in an older, cooperative child, such as a fishbone impaling the

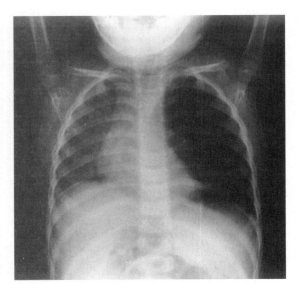

Figure 38–2. Hyperinflated left-lung field secondary to a peanut obstructing the left mainstem bronchus.

tonsil, may be successfully extracted when the patient is awake.

Alternate methods of removal (eg, Fogarty catheters or flexible endoscopes) have been used in the past, but are generally not recommended because of the difficulty in protecting the airway or adequately controlling the foreign body with these methods. Meat tenderizers, muscle relaxants, and promotility agents have been used in the past for esophageal foreign bodies in adults, but no evidence supports their use in pediatric patients. The optimal setting for aerodigestive tract foreign body removal is the operating room with proper pediatric endoscopic equipment and pediatric anesthesiologists.

The timing of removal is a topic of debate for children with esophageal foreign bodies. An asymptomatic older child with a distal or midesophageal coin present for less than 24 hours and no history of esophageal disorders may be observed to see if the coin will pass. Spontaneous coin passage rates range widely from 9–77% in this patient population. In contrast, a child with a suspected disc battery ingestion requires urgent removal in the operating room to avoid mucosal erosion or perforation. Most surgeons agree that an airway foreign body should be addressed at the time of presentation. Rapid sequence techniques may be preferred if aspiration of stomach contents is a concern.

All equipment should be assembled and connected to appropriate light sources and video equipment before the patient enters the operating suite. The operating surgeon should be gloved and in position before induction, and the plan for induction should have already been discussed between the surgeon and the anesthesiologist.

If an esophageal foreign body has been diagnosed or is suspected, intubation can be done prior to rigid esophagoscopy. The esophagoscope may be introduced with the help of a laryngoscope or under direct vision. Once the foreign body has been identified, extraction may require removing the entire telescopic forceps and the esophagoscope complex. Care should be taken to avoid accidental extubation by having the anesthesiologist manually secure the endotracheal tube during removal of the esophagoscope. At least one more pass of the esophagoscope should be performed to check for multiple foreign bodies or mucosal damage. The esophagoscope should never be forced, but should be gently advanced, taking care to have the lumen centered in the field of vision. A notation of the distance from the esophageal inlet to any signs of mucosal damage should be recorded.

During endoscopic removal in the operating room, communication with the pediatric anesthesiologist is paramount. During manipulation, a stable esophageal foreign body can become an unstable tracheobronchial foreign body, or a partially obstructing bronchial foreign body can become an obstructing laryngeal foreign body. The otolaryngologist and anesthesiologist must be in constant communication to anticipate the patient's developing respiratory status.

If the foreign body is removed easily without mucosal trauma, the child can be extubated and discharged from the recovery room if he or she is able to take adequate oral intake. If the foreign body has been present for an unknown length of time and there are signs of mucosal damage, the patient may require a longer period of observation postoperatively. Dexamethasone (ie, Decadron) at a dose of 0.5–1.0 mg/kg intravenous may be given if significant edema is present. A chest x-ray should be performed if there is evidence of a traumatic extraction and any concern of significant mucosal damage to rule out perforation and mediastinal air.

For airway foreign bodies, paralysis should not be induced and the patient should be kept spontaneously breathing. After mask induction with an inhalational agent, topical lidocaine should be used to anesthetize the vocal folds. Direct laryngoscopy should be performed and a rigid bronchoscope introduced under direct vision. Once the bronchoscope has been introduced, the anesthesiologist may connect to the ventilation port. Once the foreign body is identified, removal may require withdrawing, as a unit, the telescopic forceps and bronchoscope (Figure 38–3). Care should be taken to avoid premature release of the foreign body because this can result in an obstructing laryngotracheal foreign body. The surgeon should also communicate with the anesthesiologist to confirm the depth of anesthesia so that laryngospasm is avoided upon withdrawal of the bronchoscope. The bronchoscope should be advanced again to rule out further foreign bodies in the more distal airway.

Nuts and other foods may require multiple passes. Care should be taken to minimize mucosal trauma. Flexible suction catheters can be advanced down the side port to remove secretions and facilitate visualization. Depending on the ease of extraction, the child may require a postoperative chest x-ray and close follow-up to rule out the development of pneumonia.

Prognosis

Most children make a full recovery without permanent sequelae from aerodigestive tract foreign body ingestion. Delays in the diagnosis cause the most severe morbidity. Children who have a delayed or technically difficult extraction should be observed postoperatively in an inpatient setting until they no longer require airway support or can tolerate an age-appropriate diet.

Crysdale WS, Sendi KS, Yoo J. Esophageal foreign bodies in children: 15-year review of 484 cases. *Ann Otol Rhinol Laryngol.* 1991;100:320. [PMID 2018291] (Analysis of esophageal foreign bodies in 426 children revealing that coins are the most commonly ingested foreign body.)

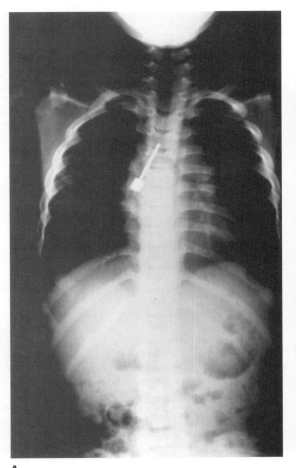

A

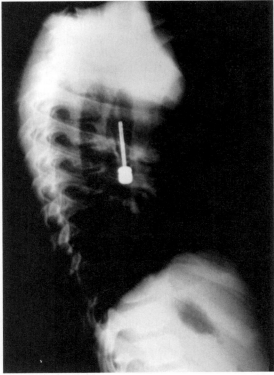

B

C

Figure 38–3. **(A)** Posteroanterior chest x-ray revealing a foreign body in the right mainstem bronchus; **(B)** lateral x-ray of a foreign body in the right mainstem bronchus; **(C)** telescopic removal of the foreign body through a rigid bronchoscope.

Donnelly LF, Frush DP, Bissett GS. The multiple presentations of foreign bodies in children. *AJR AM J Roentgenol.* 1998;170(2):471. [PMID: 9456967] (Multiple interesting radiographs stressing the variety of pediatric foreign body presentation.)

Reilly JS. Prevention of aspiration in infants and young children: federal regulations. *Ann Otol Rhinol Laryngol.* 1990;99:273. [PMID: 2327696] (Analysis of the Consumer Product Safety Commission's current standards for toys and its relation to prevention of aerodigestive tract foreign body aspirations in young children.)

Waltzman ML, Baskin M, Wypij D, Mooney D, Jones D, Fleisher G. A randomized clinical trial of the management of esophageal coins in children. *Pediatrics.* 2005;116(3):614. [PMID: 16140701] (Randomized, prospective study of 80 children with coin ingestion demonstrating that the spontaneous passage rate is associated with older age, male gender, and coins in the distal third of the esophagus.)

Zaytoun GM, Rouadi PW, Baki DHA. Endoscopic management of foreign bodies in the tracheobronchial tree: predictive factors for complications. *Otolaryngol Head Neck Surg.* 2000;123:311. [PMID: 10964313] (Review of 504 bronchoscopic procedures for airway foreign bodies revealing type of foreign body, duration of procedure, and history of previous bronchoscopy as most useful predictors of complications.)

Airway Reconstruction

39

Kristina W. Rosbe, MD

ESSENTIALS OF DIAGNOSIS

- *Patient history, including prematurity, history of intubation, feeding history, prior airway surgery, and other medical conditions.*
- *Physical exam, including weight, stridor, voice quality and cry, craniofacial abnormalities, pulmonary status, and cardiac status.*

The following tests are diagnostic:

Flexible laryngoscopy
Posteroanterior and lateral neck and chest x-rays
Fluoroscopy
CT and MRI imaging
Rigid endoscopy and microlaryngoscopy

General Considerations

Advances in care of premature infants in the last few decades have resulted in increased survival rates and a new population of patients with a history of prolonged intubation. A proportion of these patients developed subglottic stenosis: up to 8% according to some reports. Further advances in endotracheal tube and ventilation management in the last 30 years have decreased the incidence of subglottic stenosis in the neonatal population to < 1%. A second population of infants born with congenital subglottic stenosis has remained stable at approximately 5%. It is these patients who provide some of the greatest diagnostic and management challenges for the otolaryngologist.

Other airway abnormalities—both congenital and iatrogenic—including laryngomalacia, vocal fold paralysis, and supraglottic and glottic stenosis, have prompted otolaryngologists to continue to refine surgical airway reconstruction techniques.

Cotton RT. The problem of pediatric laryngotracheal stenosis: a clinical and experimental study on the efficacy of autogenous cartilaginous grafts placed between the vertically divided halves of the posterior lamina of the cricoid cartilage. *Laryngoscope.* 1991;101:1. [PMID: 1766310] (Comprehensive review of the history of subglottic stenosis diagnosis and management.)

Walner DL, Loewen MS, Kimura RE. Neonatal subglottic stenosis: incidence and trends. *Laryngoscope.* 2001;111:48. [PMID: 11192899] (Review of the incidence trends of neonatal subglottic stenosis revealing improvement over the last 3 decades.)

Pathogenesis

A. SUBGLOTTIC STENOSIS

The incidence of congenital subglottic stenosis is approximately 5%. The cricoid cartilage develops abnormally and may be elliptical or flattened in shape, causing cartilaginous stenosis. The remainder of subglottic stenosis is considered to be iatrogenic; airway instrumentation with both tube size relative to the airway and the duration of intubation plays a role. A linear relationship does not exist, however, because some children intubated for a very short time develop subglottic stenosis, whereas others with a prolonged intubation history do not.

Acquired subglottic stenosis more often involves soft tissue stenosis in contrast to the congenital form, which results in cartilaginous stenosis. Pressure is considered to play a role, causing initial mucosal edema and inflammation with subsequent ulceration and finally fibrosis (Figure 39–1). Other factors may exacerbate stenosis development, such as gastroesophageal reflux disease (GERD) and infection. The characterization of stenosis during diagnostic endoscopy, including the location, severity, and length of the stenosis, is extremely important and helps to direct management options and predict outcomes.

B. LARYNGOMALACIA

Laryngomalacia is the most common cause of neonatal stridor. The supraglottis, which comprises the epiglottis, aryepiglottic folds, and arytenoid cartilages, prolapses into the airway during inspiration. Laryngomalacia is generally classified into three main types based on the anatomic portion of the supraglottic structures that is prolapsing, although any combination can coexist.

Two main theories of etiology exist. The first proposes that immature cartilage lacks the stiff structure of more mature cartilage. The second theory suggests immature neural innervation, which is a form of hypotonia. Laryngomalacia can be exacerbated by other entities such as GERD, with a co-incidence of up to 80%.

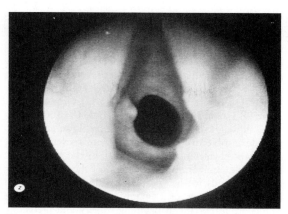

Figure 39–1. Circumferential acquired subglottic stenosis.

C. VOCAL FOLD PARALYSIS

Vocal fold paralysis is the second most common cause of stridor in neonates. This condition may be congenital or secondary to an abnormality along the course of the recurrent laryngeal nerve. The most common etiology is secondary to hydrocephalus from a malformation such as Arnold-Chiari. Once the primary cause has been addressed, the paralysis should resolve. For idiopathic vocal fold paralysis, surgical intervention may be required.

D. GLOTTIC STENOSIS AND SUPRAGLOTTIC STENOSIS

Glottic stenosis is generally iatrogenic, resulting from either traumatic intubation involving a similar pathogenesis as subglottic stenosis or prior laser procedures on the airway such as CO_2 laser excision of a papilloma. The etiology of supraglottic stenosis may also involve prior airway laser surgery or previous open airway procedures involving long-term indwelling stents with subsequent granulation tissue and fibrosis formation. GERD may also play a role in both of these diagnoses.

E. LARYNGEAL WEB

Laryngeal webs can be either congenital or acquired secondary to prior airway procedures (Figure 39–2). The pathogenesis of acquired laryngeal web generally involves development of an inflammatory process in reaction to the initial insult, with subsequent maturation and scar formation.

Daya H, Hosni A, Bejar-Solar I et al. Pediatric vocal fold paralysis: a long-term retrospective study. *Arch Otolaryngol Head Neck Surg.* 2000;126:21. [PMID: 10628706] (Review of 102 patients with vocal fold paralysis including etiologies, treatments, and prognoses.)

Holinger LD. Histopathology of congenital subglottic stenosis. *Ann Otol Rhinol Laryngol.* 1999;108:101. [PMID: 10030225] (Summary of classifications of congenital subglottic stenosis found in 29 specimens.)

Matthews BL, Little JP, McGuirt WF et al. Reflux in infants with laryngomalacia: results of 24-hour double-probe pH monitoring. *Otolaryngol Head Neck Surg.* 1999;120:860. [PMID: 10352440] (Comparison of proximal and distal probe results in 24 patients presenting with laryngomalacia. 100% demonstrated pharyngeal acid exposure.)

Olney DR, Greinwald JH, Smith RJH et al. Laryngomalacia and its treatment. *Laryngoscope.* 1999;109:1770. [PMID: 10569405] (Excellent review of laryngomalacia diagnosis and management.)

Perkins JA, Inglis AF, Richardson MA. Iatrogenic airway stenosis with recurrent respiratory papillomatosis. *Arch Otolaryngol Head Neck Surg.* 1998;124:281. [PMID: 9525512] (Seven of 50 patients treated for recurrent respiratory papillomatosis over a 6-year period were found to have iatrogenic airway stenosis.)

Walner DL, Holinger LD. Supraglottic stenosis in infants and children. *Arch Otolaryngol Head Neck Surg.* 1997;123:337. [PMID: 9076242] (Of 17 patients with supraglottic stenosis, 59% had undergone laryngotracheal reconstruction, and 53% had a history of gastroesophageal reflux disease.)

Walner DL, Stern Y, Gerber ME et al. Gastroesophageal reflux in patients with subglottic stenosis. *Arch Otolaryngol Head Neck Surg.* 1998;124:551. [PMID: 9604982] (A review of esophageal pH probes results in 74 patients with subglottic stenosis, revealing a high incidence of gastroesophageal reflux disease.)

Prevention

Advances in airway management of the premature infant over the last 30 years have brought incidence rates of subglottic stenosis from 8% down to < 1%. Awareness of the dangers of aggressive laser use in the airway has also contributed to decreased rates of iatrogenic airway lesions such as glottic stenosis and laryngeal web formation.

Clinical Findings

A. SYMPTOMS AND SIGNS

Stridor is one of the foremost features of airway pathology. A more typical presentation of acquired subglottic stenosis, however, may be of a premature infant with a

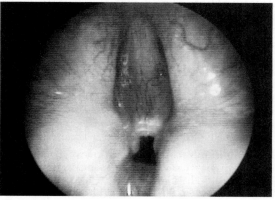

Figure 39–2. Congenital laryngeal web.

history of intubation that failed on several attempts at extubation in the intensive care unit. For an older child with an initially less severe airway lesion, voice changes, feeding difficulties, or progressive respiratory symptoms may develop.

B. Imaging Studies

Posteroanterior neck and chest x-rays can be helpful in diagnosing some airway lesions. Airway fluoroscopy may demonstrate coexisting pathology, such as tracheomalacia, but is dependent on the expertise of the radiologist for the diagnosis. Preoperative barium swallow is recommended if a child has a history of feeding difficulties. Computed tomography (CT) scanning or magnetic resonance imaging (MRI) can provide information on both the severity and the length of the stenoses, but should never replace endoscopic evaluation. Imaging studies may also be helpful in diagnosing tracheal compression secondary to a vascular lesion.

C. Special Tests

The association between airway pathology and GERD has been documented. Most airway surgeons currently recommend a preoperative evaluation for GERD for patients undergoing open airway procedures. The study of choice for diagnosis is a **dual-channel pH probe.** This test involves a probe in the pharynx (above the upper esophageal sphincter) and in the esophagus (above the lower esophageal sphincter) for detection of acid over a 24-hour period. If GERD is found, medical therapy for 3 months is recommended before considering airway surgery. If a repeat pH probe is still found to be positive, antireflux surgery is recommended before considering airway surgery.

D. Special Examinations

1. Flexible endoscopic evaluation of swallowing— Flexible endoscopic evaluation of swallowing (FEES) is a relatively new study being recommended for patients undergoing laryngotracheal reconstruction. The exam can determine whether there is evidence of laryngeal penetration, premature spillage, aspiration, hypopharyngeal clearance, hypopharyngeal pooling, or laryngeal and hypopharyngeal sensation. In a study of 255 patients undergoing FEES, airway reconstruction plans were altered in 15% of patients after identifying poor airway protective mechanisms. This planned alteration resulted in G-tube placement for some patients; for other patients, planned surgical reconstruction was modified with the goal of preventing both compromised postoperative recovery secondary to aspiration and the inability to maintain adequate nutrition.

2. Flexible endoscopy— A preoperative dynamic view of the airway is essential when contemplating airway reconstruction. It is important to rule out possible synchronous lesions such as vocal fold paralysis or laryngomalacia, both of which are difficult to diagnose when the child is under anesthesia, even if allowed to breathe spontaneously.

3. Rigid bronchoscopy and microlaryngoscopy— Preoperative endoscopy is mandatory to assess the characteristics of a patient's airway pathology. A standard grading scale has been devised based on stenosis of the airway lumen: (1) **Grade I:** < 50% stenosis; (2) **Grade II:** 51–70%; (3) **Grade III:** 71–99%; (4) **Grade IV:** 100%. This scale, although still somewhat subjective, is an attempt to provide an objective parameter of stenosis severity. Other important characteristics to consider in the preoperative endoscopic exam include the length of the stenosis, how close it extends to the vocal folds, and whether it is an anterior, a posterior, or a circumferential lesion. All these factors are important in planning surgery and predicting outcomes.

4. Pulmonary function tests— A patient's preoperative pulmonary status is an important indicator of the airway reconstruction technique that should be used. Patients with poor pulmonary reserve are not candidates for certain airway reconstruction procedures. Many of these patients are former premature infants and may have an element of chronic lung disease, the severity of which should be identified before proceeding with open airway reconstruction.

5. Voice evaluation— Although most previous studies have evaluated only postoperative voice quality after airway reconstruction surgery, ideally, a preoperative exam would add value for comparison and, in the future, may be included more routinely in the preoperative evaluation.

Halstead LA. Gastroesophageal reflux: a critical factor in pediatric subglottic stenosis. *Otolaryngol Head Neck Surg.* 1999;120:683. [PMID: 10229593] (Of 25 patients presenting with subglottic stenosis empirically treated for gastroesophageal reflux disease, 9 resolved with medical therapy alone, 16 patients underwent endoscopic repair, and only 1 eventually required tracheotomy.)

Myer CM III, O'Connor DM, Cotton RT. Proposed grading system for subglottic stenosis based on endotracheal tube sizes. *Ann Otol Rhinol Laryngol.* 1994;103:319. [PMID: 8154776] (Revised grading system of subglottic stenosis.)

Smith ME, Marsh JH, Cotton RT et al. Voice problems after pediatric laryngotracheal reconstruction: videolaryngostroboscopic, acoustic, and perceptual assessment. *Int J Pediatr Otorhinolaryngol.* 1993;25:173. [PMID: 8436462] (Summary of voice evaluations in 8 patients who had undergone laryngotracheal reconstructions revealing patient cooperation as a critical factor both in evaluation quality and abnormalities in all patients postoperatively.)

Willging JP. Benefit of feeding assessment before pediatric airway reconstruction. *Laryngoscope.* 2000;110:825. [PMID: 10807361] (Results of feeding assessments of 255 patients with structural abnormalities of the aerodigestive tract; 15% had results that altered further management plans.)

Differential Diagnosis

The differential diagnosis of subglottic stenosis is extensive and reinforces the importance of preoperative endoscopy. It is also important to consider the possibility of synchronous lesions. Diagnoses to consider include laryngomalacia; vocal fold paralysis; laryngeal web, cyst, or cleft; laryngocele; subglottic hemangioma; tracheoesophageal fistula; tracheal stenosis; tracheal compression secondary to a vascular anomaly; and primary tracheomalacia.

Complications

Complications can be grouped into three general categories: intraoperative, early postoperative, and late postoperative. Complications are more likely in patients who have severe initial lesions that require more extensive procedures.

A. INTRAOPERATIVE COMPLICATIONS

Intraoperative complications can include either pneumothorax (usually secondary to costal cartilage graft harvesting with violation of the pleura) or vocal fold paralysis (usually secondary to dissection around the trachea). Extreme care should be taken when dissecting around the pleura or recurrent laryngeal nerve to avoid injury.

B. EARLY POSTOPERATIVE COMPLICATIONS

1. Endotracheal tube and stent displacement— Early postoperative complications can be related to endotracheal tube or stent displacement such as subcutaneous emphysema, pneumothorax, or pneumomediastinum. Care should be taken to secure endotracheal tubes or other stents to avoid these complications. Seroma or wound infection can also occur. Some surgeons recommend empiric or culture-directed antibiotic therapy during the postoperative period.

2. Atelectasis—Atelectasis (with the potential to develop pneumonia) secondary to prolonged intubation, prolonged sedation, and paralysis, as well as narcotic withdrawal, is also a significant postoperative concern. The surgeon and intensive care unit staff must balance the risk of stent dislodgement with the risks of sedation and paralysis. Postoperative care is currently not standardized. After experiences with accidental extubation, some physicians have found alternative airway management methods to avoid reinstrumentation of the airway (eg, the use of BiPAP [bilateral positive airway pressure]). Other physicians have recommended an interrupted schedule of paralysis and narcotics or avoidance of all pharmacologic restraints in order to avoid unwanted side effects. Prolonged nasotracheal intubation can also cause alar necrosis if vigilant daily inspection of the nose and endotracheal tube taping is not performed.

3. Other complications—Patients may also experience dysphagia, aspiration, and even failure to thrive postoperatively secondary to indwelling stents. Adjusting the stent position can sometimes resolve symptoms. Some children may require feeding tube placement until stent removal to allow for adequate nutritional support.

C. LATE POSTOPERATIVE COMPLICATIONS

1. Granulation tissue formation and stenosis—Late complications can include granulation tissue formation at the stent tip, and glottic or supraglottic stenosis. Cartilage grafts can also prolapse into the airway, causing restenosis. These complications may be avoided if routine postoperative endoscopy is performed at regular intervals. Some physicians advocate empiric postoperative GERD therapy to eliminate gastroesophageal reflux as a possible cause of either postoperative granulation tissue formation or stenosis. Posterior glottic stenosis may require expansion surgery with a posterior cartilage graft.

2. Problems with voice quality—Voice quality postoperatively may worsen and can be secondary to anterior commissure asymmetry, formation of a glottic web, or vocal fold scarring. Care should be taken intraoperatively to avoid incision of the anterior commissure. Reconstruction with keel placement can be considered if there is no improvement with conservative measures. Postoperative voice therapy may be indicated since delays in language and communication skills can be a source of significant morbidity for patients and their families.

3. Tracheocutaneous fistula—A persistent tracheocutaneous fistula is another potential complication after a long-standing tracheotomy and may require repair with excision of the epithelial-lined tract.

4. Suprastomal collapse—Suprastomal collapse can occur in patients with long-standing tracheotomies and may require rigid support with cartilage.

5. Arytenoid prolapse and supraglottic collapse—Arytenoid prolapse may occur, most commonly after cricotracheal resection or extensive laryngotracheal expansion procedures. A partial arytenoidectomy may be required, although the potential increased risk of aspiration should also be considered. Postoperative supraglottic collapse can be an extremely challenging problem.

6. Inability to decannulate—An inability to decannulate secondary to restenosis is the most devastating late complication and is more common in Grade III and IV stenoses. Revision airway surgery may increase decannulation rates.

Bauman NM, Oyos TL, Murray DJ et al. Postoperative care following single-stage laryngotracheoplasty. *Ann Otol Rhinol Laryngol.* 1996;105:317. [PMID: 8604897] (Comparison of two protocols for postoperative neuromuscular blockade.)

Cotton RT. Management of subglottic stenosis. *Otolaryngol Clin North Am.* 2000;33(1):111. [PMID: 10637347] (Excellent comprehensive review of diagnosis and management of subglottic stenosis.)

Hertzog JH, Siegel LB, Hauser GJ et al. Noninvasive positive-pressure ventilation facilitates tracheal extubation after laryngotracheal reconstruction in children. *Chest.* 1999;116(1):260. [PMID: 10424540] (Two case reports demonstrating success with BiPAP in maintaining adequate airway parameters as an alternative to reintubation after accidental extubation.)

Ludemann JP, Hughes CA, Noah Z et al. Complications of pediatric laryngotracheal reconstruction: prevention strategies. *Ann Otol Laryngol Rhinol.* 1999;108:1019. [PMID: 10579227] (Review of 82 patients revealing bronchiolitis, wound abscess, ossified cricoid cartilage, Grade IV stenosis, and untreated gastroesophageal reflux disease as indicators of restenosis.)

Treatment

A. SUBGLOTTIC STENOSIS

Historically, the treatment of symptomatic subglottic stenosis has involved three options: (1) tracheotomy, (2) endoscopic management with laser and dilation for mild to moderate lesions, and (3) airway expansion surgery for severe lesions. Observation is reserved for mild lesions with intermittent, nonprogressive symptoms.

1. Tracheotomy—Tracheotomy continues to be a mainstay of treatment, although most surgeons see this treatment option as temporary, with the eventual goal being decannulation either with or without airway expansion surgery. Tracheotomy is not without complications, however, and requires a significant amount of education about and resources for postoperative care, which can sometimes overwhelm parents.

2. Anterior cricoid split—The anterior cricoid split was developed in an effort to avoid tracheotomy in a specific population of patients: premature infants weighing at least 1500 g without significant confounding cardiac or pulmonary compromise and evidence of anterior subglottic stenosis on bronchoscopy. In this procedure, the anterior cricoid cartilage is divided in the midline, and the incision is extended superiorly through the lower third of the thyroid cartilage and inferiorly through the first and second tracheal rings. The existing endotracheal tube is removed and replaced with a larger diameter tube that is used as a stent for 7–10 days. Steroids are given at 1 mg/kg/d 24 hours before extubation and for 5 days postoperatively. The intended outcome is for a fibrous band to form at the incision site, causing the airway to stay expanded even after stent removal. The success rate of the procedure is reported to be between 70% and 80%. There has been concern that the procedure may disrupt future cartilage growth, but this concern has not been demonstrated thus far.

3. Airway expansion surgery—In older children, the mainstay of airway expansion surgery has been to divide the stenotic area with placement of a cartilaginous graft. Although general principles apply to all laryngotracheal reconstruction procedures, the unique characteristics of each patient's lesion and overall health determine the specific procedure appropriate for that patient.

a. Single-stage surgery—The trend has been toward single-stage reconstruction, meaning that the tracheotomy is removed at the time of expansion surgery with short-term postoperative stenting (7–14 days) with an endotracheal tube. Single-stage reconstruction is not appropriate for all patients, however, especially those with more severe stenoses (Grades III and IV) or with poor pulmonary reserve. Single-stage reconstruction also requires prolonged hospitalization in an intensive care unit and immobilizing the endotracheal tube for the entire postoperative healing period. In the case of younger children, this prolonged immobilization may necessitate heavy sedation or paralysis, which can create complications such as atelectasis or narcotic withdrawal. Endotracheal tube air leak has been used as a prognostic indicator for successful extubation. Leak pressures of < 20 cm H_2O are associated with successful extubation.

b. Multistage surgery—Multistage airway expansion procedures are generally reserved for children with more severe lesions or with confounding cardiac, pulmonary, or neurologic compromise. These procedures involve cartilaginous grafting and indwelling stents, but the tracheotomy is retained and not removed until after stent removal. Division of the lateral cricoid walls without graft placement may allow for even greater expansion of the subglottic lumen. Sleep studies using a capped tracheotomy may also be helpful in assessing potential decannulation success.

4. Cartilage grafts—The classic cartilage graft used is costal cartilage, but hyoid, thyroid, and auricular cartilage have also been tried. The initial concern about using cartilage grafts was that they may not survive, but histologic studies have demonstrated excellent survival and growth over time. Important graft properties include that (1) it is of the correct depth so as not to protrude into the airway, (2) the perichondrium is left intact and faces the lumen, and (3) the graft is adequately secured. Traditionally, grafts have been sutured into position, although newer techniques such as fibrin glue and miniplate fixation have also been tried. The classic anterior costal cartilage graft is shaped like a boat with flanges, which, when the graft is inserted into the anterior cricoid incision, are flush with the lateral native cricoid ring. Caution must be taken that the graft does not protrude into the lumen, thereby compromising the lumen diameter. Newer techniques have now been described for endoscopic placement of cartilage grafts to address the posterior component of circumferential subglottic stenosis.

5. Stenting—Patients who undergo posterior cartilage grafting for posterior stenosis generally require a longer period of stenting than patients who undergo anterior grafting alone. Long-term stenting can be associated with significant complications. Many types of stents have been used, leading surgeons to conclude that no one stent necessarily guarantees a complication-free recovery and healing period. The most commonly used stents include rolled silicone sheeting (the "Swiss roll"), polytef tubes (eg, Aboulker or Cotton-Lorenz), and preformed hollow silicone tubes (eg, Montgomery T-tube.)

The optimal stent duration to maximize healing and avoid complications is controversial. For anterior cricoid splits or single-stage laryngotracheal reconstruction with an anterior cartilage graft, a duration of 7–10 days is considered adequate. For posterior cartilage grafts, a stent duration of 2–8 weeks has been recommended. For multistage procedures, stents have been kept in place from several weeks to over a year. Because of the many possible complications of indwelling stents, the most rational approach involves limiting stent duration; ideally, technically adequate expansion surgery should not require long-term stenting. Other medical conditions that may impact healing, such as diabetes and chronic steroid dependence, should also be considered during surgical planning.

6. Decannulation—The decannulation rates of all open airway expansion procedures that include Grades II–IV range from 37% to 100%. Newer techniques are being developed to prevent restenosis, which is the most common reason for decannulation failure. Fibroblast inhibitors have been used with mixed initial results, including mitomycin-C and 5-fluorouracil (5-FU). Other, more extensive procedures designed to remove rather than expand the stenotic segment have also been developed, including cricotracheal resection, slide tracheoplasty, and even tracheal homograft transplantation.

7. Cricotracheal resection—Cricotracheal resection was originally reserved for patients who failed initial laryngotracheal reconstruction with grafting, but it is now being implemented as a first-line treatment for some patients with severe and even moderate stenoses. The procedure involves resection of the entire anterior cricoid arch with preservation of a posterior mucosal flap along the posterior cricoid plate. The normal trachea is then transected and telescoped into the posterior cricoid plate and secured with sutures to the mucosal flap and thyroid cartilage. Involvement of the vocal folds is a contraindication, and generally, a superior margin of 3 mm is recommended for success. Inferior resection margins have extended as low as the second tracheal ring, with the longest reported resection length being 3.0 cm. A tension-free anastomosis is critical for success and a suprahyoid release has been used to achieve this. Care also must be taken to avoid injury to the recurrent laryngeal nerves. A subperichondrial tracheal dissection is recommended to avoid nerve injury.

Stenting may involve a single-stage or multistage procedure, with a duration ranging from 1 week to 3 months. Decannulation rates of 87–88% have been reported in patients with a history of failed decannulation after prior laryngotracheal reconstruction.

8. Slide tracheoplasty—Slide tracheoplasty has been used for congenital long-segment tracheal stenosis, which is often associated with a pulmonary artery sling. The principles of slide tracheoplasty involve tracheal transection at the midpoint of the stenosis with an anterior midline incision of the distal tracheal segment and a posterior midline incision of the proximal tracheal segment. The segments are then telescoped and sutured, ideally doubling the tracheal circumference and quadrupling the cross section of tracheal lumen.

B. Laryngomalacia

The majority of children with laryngomalacia can be managed conservatively. Rarely, a child with significant cardiac or pulmonary compromise or failure to thrive may need surgical treatment. Tracheotomy is the procedure of choice for severe laryngomalacia. Supraglottoplasty may be used in less severe cases. Patients should always be evaluated for GERD before undergoing supraglottoplasty since comorbid rates up to 80% have been demonstrated and GERD compromises postoperative healing.

Supraglottoplasty may be performed with the CO_2 laser or microlaryngeal instruments. The technique is tailored to the type of laryngomalacia that exists in the particular patient. A wide-mouthed laryngoscope (eg, a Lindholm laryngoscope) may be helpful in providing the best view of the supraglottis. The procedure is usually performed under general anesthesia with spontaneous ventilation. The three most common techniques include (1) trimming the lateral edges of the epiglottis, (2) releasing foreshortened aryepiglottic folds, or (3) excising redundant arytenoid mucosa. Care must be taken to avoid lasing adjacent surfaces to prevent scar formation; overly aggressive surgery can also lead to an increased risk of postoperative aspiration. Most patients can be extubated at the end of the procedure, and often a short course of postoperative steroids is given.

C. Posterior Glottic Stenosis and Vocal Fold Paralysis

Posterior glottic stenosis and bilateral vocal fold paralysis may often be difficult to distinguish and can have similar presenting symptoms. Electromyogram (EMG) testing can be included as part of the endoscopic evaluation to confirm vocal fold innervation. Tracheotomy is an option for both diagnoses, but is generally not considered an optimal long-term solution. Endoscopic procedures such as partial or complete arytenoidectomy, cordotomy, and partial cordectomy have been used in small series of pediatric patients with varying success rates. The other functions of the larynx, including airway protection, may worsen with any of these procedures, thereby increasing the risk of aspiration. Open or endoscopic procedures with posterior cartilage graft placement may also be used.

D. LARYNGEAL WEB

Laryngeal webs can be challenging to address surgically. Thin webs may be successfully incised with short-term stent placement. Thicker webs generally require laryngofissure with keel placement and a short-term tracheotomy for definitive repair.

Bean JA, Rutter MJ. Pediatric cricotracheal resection: surgical outcomes and risk factor analysis. *Arch Otolaryngol Head Neck Surg.* 2005;131(10):896. [PMID: 16230593] (Review of outcomes of 100 children undergoing cricotracheal resection with a 71% overall decannulation rate and identification of vocal cord paresis as main risk factor for decannulation failure.)

Carr MM, Poje CP, Kingston L et al. Complications in pediatric tracheotomies. *Laryngoscope.* 2001;111:1925. [PMID: 11801971] (Review of 142 pediatric tracheotomies reveals a 43% incidence of serious complications.)

Cotton RT, Seid AB. Management of the extubation problem in the premature child: anterior cricoid split as an alternative to tracheotomy. *Ann Otol Rhinol Laryngol.* 1980;89:508. [PMID: 7458136] (Introduction of a new technique, the anterior cricoid split, as an alternative to tracheotomy in the management of premature infants who have failed extubation attempts.)

Hartnick CJ, Hartley BEJ, Lacy PD et al. Surgery for pediatric subglottic stenosis: disease-specific outcomes. *Ann Otol Rhinol Laryngol.* 2001;110:1109. [PMID: 11768698] (A valiant attempt to characterize outcomes of airway reconstruction surgery in 199 children with varied lesions and surgical procedures.)

Hartnick CJ, Hartley BEJ, Lacy PD et al. Topical mitomycin application after laryngotracheal reconstruction. *Arch Otolaryngol Head Neck Surg.* 2001;127:1260. [PMID: 11587609] (Randomized, double-blind, placebo-controlled trial of mitomycin application in laryngotracheal reconstruction revealing no difference in restenosis rates.)

Inglis AF, Perkins JA, Manning SC et al. Endoscopic posterior cricoid split and rib grafting in 10 children. *Laryngoscope.* 2003;113(11):2004. [PMID: 14603064] (Review of outcomes of patients undergoing endoscopic management of posterior glottic stenosis.)

Mankarious LA, Goetinck PF. Growth and development of the human cricoid cartilage: an immunohistochemical analysis of the maturation sequence of the chondrocytes and surrounding cartilage matrix. *Otolaryngol Head Neck Surg.* 2000;123:174. [PMID: 10964286] (Immunohistochemical study of cricoid cartilage from various developmental stages revealing a chondrocyte proliferation rate decreasing from ages 1–4.)

Milczuk HA, Smith JD, Everts EC. Congenital laryngeal webs: surgical management and clinical embryology. *Int J Pediatr Otorhinolaryngol.* 2000;52:1. [PMID:10699233] (Comprehensive review of surgical management of laryngeal webs.)

Rutter MJ, Hartley BEJ, Cotton RT. Cricotracheal resection in children. *Arch Otolaryngol Head Neck Surg.* 2001;127:289. [PMID: 11255473] (Review of 44 children undergoing cricotracheal resection with a decannulation rate of 86%.)

Prognosis

The success of airway reconstruction techniques is determined by many factors, including the initial severity of the lesion, other patient comorbidities, and the technical expertise and experience of both the surgeon and intensive care unit staff; however, decannulation rates of 80–90% should be obtainable. A team approach is paramount to success. In managing these cases, patients should be counseled not to expect a one-time "fix," but that multiple procedures will most likely be required, including interval endoscopy.

Sleep Disorders

40

Kevin C. Welch, MD, & Andrew N. Goldberg, MD, MSCE

■ SLEEP DISORDERS IN ADULTS

Sleep disorders are prevalent in American society, and the National Commission on Sleep Disorders Research estimates that almost 20% of adults suffer from chronic sleep disorders and that an additional 10% suffer from intermittent sleep disorders. Sleep disorders have been linked to over 100,000 automobile accidents yearly with nearly 1500 fatalities and 75,000 injuries annually. They may also be responsible for up to 30% of commercial truck driving accidents. It has been estimated that chronic sleep deprivation costs $15 billion annually in direct medical expenses and an estimated $70 billion in lost productivity.

Although there are many disorders of sleep, this chapter deals specifically with sleep-disordered breathing because it is referable to the otolaryngologist.

CLASSIFICATION OF SLEEP & SLEEP DISORDERS

Sleep

Sleep is a reversible physiologic and behavioral state that manifests as decreased awareness and reaction to external stimuli. Normal sleep architecture comprises two distinct phases: **NREM (non-rapid eye movement) sleep** comprises 75–80% of sleep and occurs in four stages (Stages I–IV), whereas **REM (rapid eye movement) sleep** comprises 20–25% of sleep and occurs in two stages. In the normal adult, these two phases of sleep occur in semiregular cycles, which last approximately 90–120 minutes and occur 3–4 times per night.

A. NREM SLEEP

In the normal adult male, **Stage I sleep,** which is considered the transition to sleep, occupies 2–5% of sleep and is characterized by an increase in theta waves and a decrease in alpha waves on an electroencephalogram (EEG). Stage I sleep is also marked by a decrease in awareness and in muscle tone. **Stage II sleep** occupies 45–55% of sleep and is characterized by K-complexes and spindles on EEG as well as decreases in muscle tone

and awareness. Stage II sleep is considered by most authorities to be the "true" onset of sleep. **Stage III and Stage IV sleep** comprise deep sleep, and it occurs predominantly in the first third of the night. The hallmark of deep sleep is the abundance of delta waves on EEG. Stage III sleep occupies 3–8% of sleep, and Stage IV sleep occupies 10–15% of sleep. Stages III and IV are widely considered the most restful stages of sleep. With increasing age, deep sleep progressively occupies less and less of total sleep time.

B. REM SLEEP

The remaining portion of sleep is composed of REM sleep, which is divided into tonic and phasic stages. During the **tonic stage,** the EEG becomes asynchronous and muscles lose tone. The **phasic stage** of REM sleep is characterized by rapid eye movements as well as erratic cardiac and respiratory patterns.

Sleep Disorders

Derangements in sleep are categorized by the American Sleep Disorders Association in the International Classification of Sleep Disorders (ICSD), which arranged sleep disorders into four categories: dyssomnias, parasomnias, sleep disorders associated with medical-psychiatric disorders, and proposed sleep disorders (Table 40–1).

The term **apnea** refers to a period of at least 10 seconds during which air flow is absent by nose or mouth. Apnea may be obstructive or central in origin. A **hypopnea** is a decrease in airflow to 10–70% of baseline for more than 10 seconds, associated with arousals or desaturation by at least 3%. The respiratory disturbance index (RDI) or apnea-hypopnea index (AHI) is the number of apneas and hypopneas per hour of sleep time and is based on a minimum of 2 hours of sleep. Many have debated the significance of this index because it does not reflect the absolute number of apneas and/or hypopneas, the duration of such events, or the distribution of such events during sleep. Some authors use the sleep disturbance index (SDI), which is the RDI + arousal index, to help correlate with patient symptomatology.

Obstructive sleep apnea (OSA) is present when the RDI is ≥ 5 events/h. It is further classified as mild (5–15 events/h), moderate (15–30 events/h), and severe (> 30

535

Table 40–1. Classification of sleep disorders.

Category	Subtype	Examples
Dyssomnia	Intrinsic Extrinsic Circadian rhythm disorder	Insomnia, narcolepsy, obstructive sleep apnea Poor sleep hygiene Advanced or delayed sleep phase disorder
Parasomnia	Disorder of arousal Sleep-wake transition disorder REM-associated Other	Sleep walking, sleep terrors Sleep talking, nocturnal leg cramps Nightmares Bruxism, infant sleep apnea
Medical-psychiatric disorders	Mental disorders Neurologic disorders Other	Psychosis, anxiety disorders Dementia, fatal familial insomnia COPD, sleep-related GERD
Proposed		Sleep hyperhidrosis, sleep-related laryngospasm

COPD, chronic obstructive pulmonary disease; GERD, gastroesophageal reflux disease; REM, rapid eye movement.

events/h). The **obstructive sleep apnea syndrome** (OSAS) is diagnosed when the RDI is > 15 and the patient has nighttime *and* daytime symptoms.

The **obesity hypoventilation syndrome** is the most clinically severe form of sleep-disordered breathing and is characterized by chronic alveolar hypoventilation, obesity, daytime hypercapnia ($PaCO_2$ > 45 mm Hg). It frequently becomes manifest with pulmonary hypertension and right heart failure.

American Sleep Disorders Association. *The International Classification of Sleep Disorders Diagnosis & Coding Manual.* American Sleep Disorders Association, Rochester, MN, 1990. (Lists and explains the various sleep disorders.)

National Commission on Sleep Disorders Research. *Wake up America: A National Sleep Alert.* Washington, DC: Government Printing Office, 1993. (Offers facts and findings regarding sleep deprivation and its effects on citizens.)

SLEEP APNEA

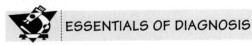 ESSENTIALS OF DIAGNOSIS

- *History of habitual snoring, excessive daytime sleepiness, or witnessed apneas.*
- *Neck size > 17 inches in males or > 15 inches in females and/or body mass index (BMI) > 27 kg/m².*
- *Definitive evidence of OSA by polysomnography.*

General Considerations

Obstructive sleep apnea is a disorder characterized by loud, habitual snoring and the repetitive obstruction of the upper airway during sleep that result in prolonged intervals of hypoxia and fragmented sleep. As a result, patients with OSA suffer from excessive daytime sleepiness, enuresis, poor work performance, and erectile dysfunction. The long-term sequelae are severe and can include accidents, hypertension, ischemic heart disease, cardiac arrhythmias, and stroke.

Large cohort studies have demonstrated that OSA is common: almost 25% of adult men 20–60 years old and 9% of adult women 20–60 years have an RDI > 5 events/h. It was further found that 4% of adult men and 2% of adult women had obstructive sleep apnea syndrome with an RDI > 15 and both daytime and nighttime symptoms. Despite its prevalence, it is estimated that almost 85% of people with OSA remain undiagnosed.

Pathogenesis

The pathogenesis of OSA is multifactorial, and it is widely accepted that OSA lies somewhere on a continuum of sleep-disordered breathing (Figure 40–1) that begins with snoring and ends with obesity hypoventilation syndrome. Determining what causes a person to be susceptible to the conditions on the continuum is one of the goals of treatment.

Air moving through the upper airway encounters resistance in transit to the lungs, and in the apneic person, this resistance is increased. This new resistance increases the load on the respiratory musculature, which is required to overcome upper airway resistance with higher negative inspiratory pressures. The negative inspiratory pressure narrows the upper airway in an incremental fashion until, theoretically, the airway collapses. Soft tissue compliance, redundant upper airway mucosa, and pharyngeal dilator muscle tone are

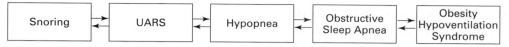

Figure 40–1. The continuum of sleep-disordered breathing. The concept of sleep-disordered breathing is that increasing upper airway resistance (UARS) can cause progressively worsening disease that can manifest with similar as well as new signs and symptoms.

all presumed to play an important role. Clinically, this translates to progressive vibration and collapse of the upper aerodigestive soft tissue structures, causing snoring and obstruction of air flow.

The nose and nasal cavity appear to play less crucial roles in the pathogenesis of OSA. Over half of the normal resistance in the upper airway is generated at the internal nasal valve, and obstruction at this point narrows this inlet and increases upper airway resistance. Septal deviation and other causes of nasal obstruction may play a role in the pathogenesis of sleep-disordered breathing, and patients with allergic rhinitis have an increased risk for developing sleep-disordered breathing because of significant turbinate or mucosal swelling. However, these features are not believed to play significant roles in the average patient with OSA.

Prevention

A number of risk factors for OSA have been identified. Obesity is one. A three-fold increase in the prevalence of OSA occurs with 1 standard deviation increase in BMI above normal. Results from one study demonstrate a positive correlation between RDI severity and both the BMI and the circumference of a patient's neck. Although men represented 47.2% of the study cohort, 71% of the participants with an RDI > 30 were men, indicating that men disproportionately represent those with OSA.

Although whites and blacks appear to be evenly represented as RDI severity increases, Native Americans appear to be disproportionately represented in groups with higher RDI. In addition to weight, neck circumference, sex, and race, other factors such as genetic syndromes (discussed later) and endocrine factors have also been implicated OSA. Patients with growth hormone abnormalities, specifically acromegaly, may develop OSA as a consequence of changes in craniofacial structure and upper airway collapsibility.

Clinical Findings

A. SIGNS AND SYMPTOMS

The most common nighttime symptoms of OSA include loud, habitual snoring, apneas, choking or gasping sounds, and nocturia or enuresis. Vibrations in upper airway soft tissues produce the loud, crescendo snoring and signify increased upper airway resistance. Apneas, which frequently terminate abruptly with gasping noises, represent complete upper airway obstruction. The negative inspiratory pressure generated during apneic events is transmurally delivered to the contracting heart and stretches the right atrium. As a consequence, atrial natriuretic peptide is released, leading to nocturia and enuresis in some patients. The repetitive arousals and frequent awakenings to micturate lead to sleep fragmentation, which may lead to daytime symptoms.

Nearly 30% of adult men and 40% of adult women with an RDI > 5 events/h report not feeling refreshed in the morning when arising. In addition, 25% of adult men and 35% of women with an RDI > 5 events/h complain of excessive daytime sleepiness, which can cause frequent napping or dozing, poor work performance, and automobile accidents.

B. PHYSICAL EXAM

1. Systemic evaluation—All patients should be evaluated for hypertension since it is correlated with OSA severity. Because studies have shown a positive correlation between OSA and BMI > 27.8 kg/m² in men and BMI > 27.3 kg/m² in women as well as neck circumference—measured at the level of the cricothyroid membrane—> 17 inches in men and > 15 inches in women, weight and neck circumference should be recorded.

The outward appearance of thyromegaly or signs of dry skin, coarse hair, or myxedema may lead to a diagnosis of hypothyroidism, and an inattentive or unkempt patient who seems disengaged or speaks with a sad or flat affect may have undiagnosed depression. Both these conditions can cause excessive sleepiness or fatigue and should be considered before diagnosing OSA.

2. Head and neck—The patient is always examined in the Frankfurt plane—a line bisecting the inferior orbital rim and the superior rim of the external auditory meatus that is always parallel with the floor. To assess the patient for maxillary retrusion, a line dropped from the nasion to the subnasale should be perpendicular to the Frankfurt plane. To assess the patient for retrognathia, a line bisecting the vermillion border of the lower lip with the pogonion should be perpendicular to the Frankfurt plane as well. If the pogonion is retroposed more than 2 mm, retrognathia is suspected. A lateral cephalometric x-ray helps evaluate this area with precision.

3. Nose—The nose should be examined for signs of gross deformity, tip ptosis, asymmetry of the nostrils, and internal valve obstruction. The examiner can perform the Cottle maneuver to assess for improvement in breathing. The nasal cavity should be thoroughly examined for turbinate size, signs of polyps, masses, rhinitis, and purulent discharge. The septum should be examined for signs of defects or deviation. Nasopharyngoscopy permits evaluation of the posterior choanae (to evaluate stenosis or atresia), the eustachian tube orifices, the velopharyngeal valve, and the adenoids, and it can provide direct observation of the velopharynx during the Müller maneuver, which some believe to be helpful in identifying the site of obstruction in OSA.

4. Oral cavity—The tongue should be examined for size and for stigmata of OSA. A normal-sized tongue rests below the occlusal plane, and a tongue that extends above this plane is graded as mildly, moderately, or severely enlarged. Tongue crenations, or ridging, if found, may indicate macroglossia. The relationship between the tongue and the soft palate should also be observed, specifically to determine whether an enlarged tongue obscures vision of the palate, whether the palate itself is low-lying or deviated, or whether the posterior pharyngeal wall is obscured by both. The morphology of the soft palate (ie, thick, webbed, posteriorly located, low, and so on) should also be noted. The uvula is also described as normal, long (> 1 cm), thick (> 1 cm), or embedded in the soft palate. The tonsils should be described as being surgically absent or by their size (1, 2, 3, or 4+, respectively, indicating a 0–25%, 25–50%, 50–75%, or > 75% lateral narrowing of the oropharynx). The tonsils should also be examined for any asymmetry or any other pathology. A narrow oropharynx, independent of tonsil size, should also be noted.

5. Hypopharynx—The hypopharynx can be evaluated by means of nasopharyngoscopy to assess the base of tongue and the lingual tonsils and to look for masses obstructing the supraglottic, glottic, or subglottic larynx. Any abnormalities in appearance, symmetry, and movement of the vocal cords should be noted. Many perform the Müller maneuver to assess collapse of the retropalatal and retroglossal areas during inspiration against a closed nose and mouth. Opinions on the clinical usefulness of this maneuver are mixed.

C. IMAGING STUDIES

A host of imaging modalities can play a role in identifying the patient with OSA; however, most of them have limited clinical application, and some remain investigational.

1. Cephalometry and x-rays—Lateral cephalometric studies and plain film x-rays are useful in evalu-

ating the patient with observable craniofacial abnormalities such as midface hypoplasia or mandibular retrusion. These studies are required for precise evaluation of maxillary retrusion, retrognathia, and micrognathia, and they help in planning Phase I and Phase II surgical procedures (discussed later in this chapter). The studies are inexpensive to perform, and the equipment is widely available. However, as a diagnostic tool for OSA in general, they suffer from several limitations including exposure to radiation, absence of supine imaging, and lack of soft tissue resolution.

2. Computed tomography (CT) scanning and magnetic resonance imaging (MRI)—CT scanning and MRI are also commonly available and have facilitated an increased understanding in the differences between the normal and apneic airways (Figure 40–2). Images obtained with both modalities can be used to recreate three-dimensional models of the upper airway and have been used to evaluate apneic airway dynamics during respiration. Both modalities, however, are significantly more expensive than the previously mentioned modalities and have a number of contraindications. Furthermore, CT and MRI have yet to be proved effective in identifying patients with OSA or reliably characterizing OSA severity.

D. SPECIAL TESTS

1. Subjective tests—Subjective tests permit the patient to evaluate his or her drive to sleep. These include the **Epworth Sleepiness Scale (ESS)** and the **Stanford Sleepiness Scale (SSS)**. For the ESS, the examinee is asked to rate the likelihood of falling asleep during particular events; for the SSS, the examinee is asked to rate how sleepy he or she is at the current moment. The ESS offers the advantage of having correlated with multiple sleep latency testing and with RDI.

2. Multiple sleep latency testing—The multiple sleep latency test is an objective test that evaluates sleep drive and consists of a series of naps occurring at 2-hour intervals repeated every 2 hours. Patients are encouraged to sleep while their physiologic parameters are monitored. Normal sleep latency is 10–20 minutes; however, patients with excessive daytime sleepiness often have sleep latencies of 5 minutes or less.

3. Polysomnography—The definitive study to evaluate OSA is overnight polysomnography (PSG) because it permits direct monitoring of the patient's brain activity, respiratory patterns, and muscle activity during sleep. The PSG records the duration of sleep and events (snoring, hypopneas, apneas, thoracoabdominal excursion, limb movement, and so on) occurring during sleep. Its clinical utility lies in its ability to diagnose and characterize the severity of OSA. In addition, PSG can

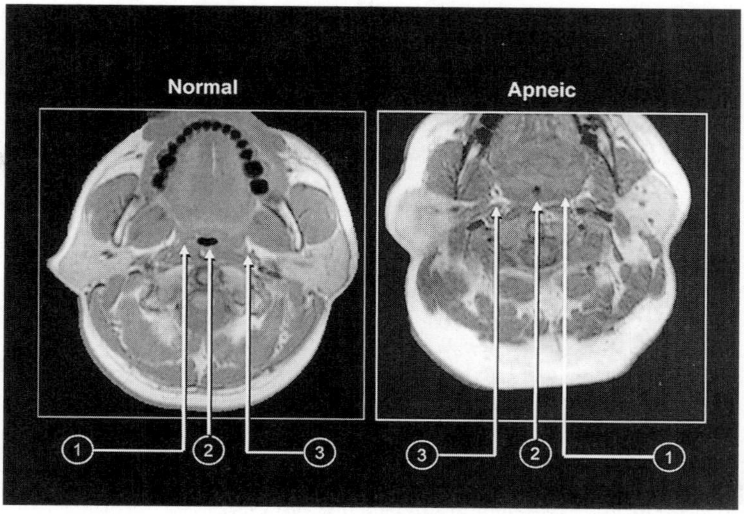

Figure 40–2. Comparative axial anatomy. Axial magnetic resonance images acquired at the retropalatal levels in a normal patient (left) and an apneic patient (right) demonstrating (1) increased lateral pharyngeal wall dimensions, (2) decreased retropalatal airway area, and (3) increased lateral pharyngeal fat pads in a representative apneic patient. (Figure courtesy of Richard J. Schwab, MD, University of Pennsylvania Health System, Philadelphia, PA.)

differentiate among OSA, central sleep apnea, and some other causes of excessive sleepiness.

Complications

Nearly 20% of all drivers report falling asleep behind the wheel at least once in their lives, and patients with OSA have an increased risk. Patients with an RDI > 40 events/h are more than three times more likely to crash an automobile than are controls, and patients with excessive daytime sleepiness can be as incapacitated as intoxicated (blood alcohol level > 0.1%) volunteers on reaction-timed sequences. Predicting who has an increased risk, however, is difficult. Legal standards and obligations of the physician vary from state to state with regard to the issue of reporting patients at risk or with a history of sleep-related accidents.

Establishing a relationship between OSA and hypertension has been confounded by multiple clinical variables; however, one study has demonstrated that men and women with an RDI > 30 events/h have a 1.5 relative risk and a 1.17 relative risk, respectively, for developing hypertension. When studies control for hypertension, patients with OSA have an increased risk of cardiovascular mortality secondary to myocardial ischemia: patients studied overnight with Holter monitors demonstrate myocardial ischemia that is decreased with continuous positive airway pressure (CPAP) therapy. There is strong evidence for the increased incidence of fatal and nonfatal cardiovascular outcomes in patients with severe OSA who have not been treated when compared with normal volunteers in recent studies. An increased prevalence of sleep-disordered breathing has been found in patients with first-time stroke as early as RDI > 5 events/h, and patients with RDI > 11 events/h have 1.5 times the odds-adjusted risk for stroke.

Treatment

A. NONSURGICAL MEASURES

1. CPAP therapy—The most widely deployed treatment for OSA is CPAP, which is the first recommended therapy for patients with OSA. CPAP decreases snoring and apneas and improves symptoms of excessive daytime sleepiness. Moreover, a 3-year study demonstrated that patients with excessive daytime sleepiness who were treated with CPAP significantly decreased their accident rates to levels comparable to normal controls. The American College of Chest Physicians recommends initiating CPAP therapy for all patients with an RDI > 30 events/h and for all patients with an RDI of 5–30 events/h who are symptomatic. Although CPAP is 90–95% effective in eliminating OSA, its continued efficacy relies on patient compliance, with average usage being 4–5 h/night and an 85% compliance at 6 months under the absolute best of circumstances. Despite immediate objective and subjective improvements, no definitive studies establish the duration of regular use necessary to reduce or eliminate long-term sequelae. Patients often complain of claustrophobia, headache, rhinitis, facial or nasal irritation, aerophagia, and inconvenience or social embarrassment while using CPAP, all of which limit its use.

2. Oral appliances—Oral appliances can be used in patients with primary snoring, those with mild-to-moderate OSA, and those refusing CPAP. The more thoroughly tested of the oral appliances are the **titratable mandibular repositioning devices**. In mild-to-moderate OSA, these devices have been shown to decrease RDI to levels comparable to CPAP therapy, to improve symptoms of excessive daytime sleepiness, and to decrease RDI in some patients unsuccessfully treated with uvulopalatopharyngoplasty. Nightly use of oral appliances is typically tolerated better than CPAP. Patients wearing oral appliances may complain of jaw or temporomandibular joint pain (both of which seem to be lessened by the titratable oral appliances), headaches, and excessive salivation. The long-term effects and outcomes of patients with OSA who use oral appliances are incompletely studied.

3. Weight loss—Overweight patients should be encouraged to lose weight because moderate reductions in weight have been demonstrated to increase upper airway size and improve upper airway function. Coordination of weight loss with a dietitian may improve outcome and in many cases is necessary (eg, in diabetics and the morbidly obese). Since many patients with OSA are morbidly obese, bariatric surgery has been evaluated as a treatment for weight loss in this population, but it is not recommended for routine weight loss in patients with OSA.

4. Lifestyle modifications—Patients should also be informed to avoid sedatives, alcohol, nicotine, and caffeine in the evening because these substances can influence upper airway muscle tone and central mechanisms.

5. Positional therapy—Positional therapy has been suggested as an adjunctive therapy for patients who have primarily supine-dependent obstructive events, which are easily identified on PSG. Patients are instructed to sleep in the lateral decubitus position rather than the supine position, and a host of techniques have been used to prevent reversion to the supine, such as sewing tennis balls to the backs of shirts and rearranging pillows.

6. Other treatment—External nasal dilators and ephedra- or ephedrine-based products are also popular treatments for snoring and OSA. Although some have been demonstrated to reduce snoring in patients with chronic rhinitis or nasal obstruction, most of these products have failed to show any consistent benefit in the treatment of primary snoring or OSA. Ephedra-based products are not evaluated by the FDA and are therefore discouraged as treatment.

B. SURGICAL MEASURES

1. Preoperative considerations—One of the most widely accepted protocols for approaching sleep apnea surgery is based on a series of 306 consecutive surgically treated patients with OSA. In this protocol, selecting patients for surgery begins with a thorough physical exam, upper airway endoscopy with the Müller maneuver, cephalometric studies, and overnight PSG.

2. Phase I surgery—Patient treatment is initiated with Phase I surgery: (1) patients with **Type I** upper airway anatomy (ie, oropharyngeal obstruction) undergo uvulopalatopharyngoplasty (UPPP); (2) patients with **Type II** upper airway anatomy (ie, oropharyngeal and hypopharyn-

geal obstruction) undergo UPPP and genioglossus advancement with or without hyoid myotomy; and (3) patients with **Type III** upper airway anatomy (hypopharyngeal obstruction) undergo genioglossus advancement without palatal surgery. Of note, patients with an RDI > 30 events/h have an increased risk for perioperative airway complications and require overnight observation; they also have a decreased threshold for intubation or a temporary tracheotomy.

All patients undergoing Phase I surgery require general anesthesia and must be informed of potential risks related to anesthesia, postoperative pain, infection, bleeding, and short-term and long-term velopharyngeal insufficiency in UPPP patients.

a. Uvulopalatopharyngoplasty—The UPPP procedure entails conservative excision of the inferior margin of the soft palate, including the uvula, as well as excision of redundant mucosa with suture fixation of the pharynx and palate. If the tonsils are present, they are excised. Meta-analysis demonstrates that UPPP significantly reduces RDI, apnea indices, and oxygen desaturations as well as increases REM sleep in postoperative patients. UPPP is effective in eliminating snoring in 90% of selected patients. When "success" is defined as a 50% reduction in RDI, UPPP is 53% successful and has been demonstrated to increase upper airway cross-sectional area and airway volume at the retropalatal level (Figure 40–3). When patients have Type II or Type III upper airway anatomy, as age, BMI, and RDI increase, UPPP becomes less effective.

b. Genioglossus advancement—Performing genioglossus advancement attempts to correct the retroglossal obstruction that occurs in patients with Type II and Type III upper airway anatomy by placing the geniohyoid muscle and genioglossus muscle under increased tension via a mandibular osteotomy. Genioglossal advancement can be achieved by performing a limited osteotomy (Figure 40–4A) or by creating a rectangular window and *sliding* the geniohyoid complex anteriorly (Figure 40–4B). The latter procedure may by performed using various sagittal or circular osteotomy devices with custom or prefabricated plating systems. Suspension of the hyoid bone from the mandible has been largely supplanted by approximating the hyoid bone and the thyroid cartilage (Figure 40–5). (Genioglossus advancement, therefore, increases retroglossal airspace by virtue of drawing the genial tubercle and genioglossus complex anteriorly. Typically, patients with an RDI > 30 events/h require genioglossus advancement for treatment because of base of tongue obstruction. Phase I surgery in patients with Type II upper airway anatomy is approximately 60–65% successful (defined as a 50% reduction in RDI or a postoperative RDI equivalent to preoperative RDI while using CPAP). Phase I surgery in patients with Type III upper airway anatomy who undergo genioglossus advancement alone is 66–85% successful. In these two groups (UPPP with genioglossus advancement

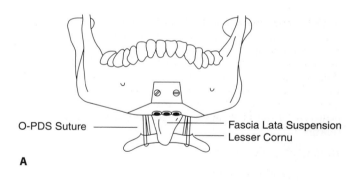

Figure 40–3. Pre- and post-UPPP axial anatomy. Axial magnetic resonance images acquired at the same retropalatal level in a patient before and after UPPP. UPPP, uvulopalatopharyngoplasty. (Figure courtesy of Schwab RJ et al. University of Pennsylvania Health System, Philadelphia, PA.)

and genioglossus advancement alone), the nocturnal oxygen desaturation is significantly improved.

3. Phase II surgery—Patients who do not improve (as evidenced by PSG) by 6 months after Phase I surgery are encouraged to undergo Phase II surgery.

a. Maxillary-mandibular osteotomy—Maxillary-mandibular osteotomy, or advancement of both the maxilla and mandible, is performed in Phase II surgery. Phase II surgery (following Phase I surgery) is 97–100% successful in reducing RDI and in improving blood-oxygen desaturation, as well as increasing Stages III, IV, and REM sleep. For patients adhering to the Phase I and II protocol, the overall success rate is approximately 95% (observed over a 1- to 4-year follow-up period). However, the overall success rate, which includes those dropping out of the protocol, is 77% (observed over an average of 9 months of follow-up).

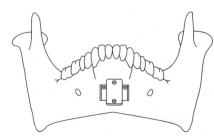

Figure 40–4. Genioglossal advancement. **(A)** Mortise genioplasty. **(B)** Block genioplasty.

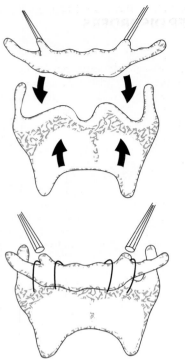

Figure 40–5. Hyoid myotomy. Modified myotomy in which the hyoid bone is advanced anteriorly and inferiorly and approximated to the thyroid cartilage.

4. Laser-assisted uvuloplasty (LAUP)—LAUP is similar to UPPP in that the inferior margin of the soft palate and the uvula are excised. However, LAUP differs from UPPP in that it uses a laser (CO_2, argon, KTP) rather than a knife, is performed with topical and local anesthesia, is not designed to address the tonsils or pharyngeal narrowing, and is performed in 1–3 office sessions. If there is evidence of obstructing tonsils or redundant pharyngeal mucosa, LAUP should not be offered. In addition, LAUP is not typically used in patients with an RDI > 30 events/h. Results of LAUP in selected populations are variable, and the procedure is approximately 50% effective for OSA and 80–90% effective for snoring with fewer complications and less morbidity for patients than UPPP. Side effects of LAUP include moderate pain, bleeding, risk of velopharyngeal insufficiency, and infection.

5. Radiofrequency ablation—Radiofrequency ablation of the palate is also a relatively new procedure that can be used to treat patients with primary snoring or an RDI < 15 events/h who have predominantly palatal obstruction. Radiofrequency ablation delivers approximately 500 Joules to target tissues causes coagulative necrosis, scarring, and eventually tissue contraction.

Initial reports suggest that radiofrequency ablation is approximately 75% effective in eliminating snoring, and despite improvement in ESS scores, it does not change RDI. Radiofrequency ablation of the tongue and tongue base may also be used. Risks of radiofrequency ablation include pain, bleeding, velopharyngeal insufficiency, palatal fistula, and infection.

6. Tracheostomy—The final and gold standard surgical treatment for OSA is tracheostomy, which bypasses the upper airway obstruction completely. Tracheostomy is indicated in patients with cor pulmonale, obesity hypoventilation syndrome, nighttime arrhythmias or disabling excessive daytime sleepiness who refuse CPAP and surgical intervention or in those who have failed previous surgical interventions. Tracheostomy is highly successful in eliminating excessive daytime sleepiness, improving RDI to normal levels, and normalizing sleep architecture. However, it is not 100% effective in eliminating symptoms and sequelae in all patients, and it is associated with complications such as dysphagia, plugging, tracheal stenosis, and granuloma formation. Decannulation and reversal of tracheostomy usually are uncomplicated and result in the return of symptoms.

7. Palatal implants—The placement of soft palate implants has been approved for use in snoring and in mild-to-moderate OSA. When inclusion criteria are met for this procedure, approximately 63.9% of patients experience a reduction in RDI to < 10 events/h. Complications such as implant extrusion and worsening of symptoms have been reported. More clinical studies need to be performed to draw conclusions regarding the efficacy of palatal implants.

8. Postoperative considerations—All patients should be reexamined by repeat PSG 4–6 months after surgery. Continued postoperative follow-up permits the evaluation of subjective and objective improvement as well as the opportunity to address additional sites of obstruction as necessary.

George CF. Reduction in motor vehicle collisions following treatment of sleep apnoea with nasal CPAP. *Thorax.* 2001;56:508. [PMID: 11413347] (A 3-year study evaluating patients with OSA before and after use of CPAP related to incidence of automobile accidents.)

Loube DI et al. Indications for positive airway pressure treatment of adult obstructive sleep apnea patients: a consensus statement. *Chest.* 1999;115:863. [PMID: 10084504] (Reviews the indications for use of CPAP in adult patients with obstructive sleep apnea.)

Lowe AA et al. Treatment, airway and compliance effects of a titratable oral appliance. *Sleep.* 2000;23:S172. [PMID: 10973562] (Evaluates the effect of a titratable oral appliance on airway size and obstructive sleep apnea as well as compliance.)

Nieto FJ et al. Association of sleep-disordered breathing, sleep apnea, and hypertension in a large community-based study. Sleep Heart Health Study. *JAMA.* 2000;283:1829. [PMID:

10770144] (Multicenter, large community study evaluating the association of sleep-disordered breathing and hypertension.)

Peker Y et al. Respiratory disturbance index: an independent predictor of mortality in coronary artery disease. *Am J Respir Crit Care Med.* 2000;162:81. [PMID: 10903224] (Study assessing for increased cardiovascular mortality in patients with obstructive sleep apnea and coronary artery disease.)

Riley RW et al. Obstructive sleep apnea syndrome: a review of 306 consecutively treated surgical patients. *Otolaryngol Head Neck Surg.* 1993;108:117. [PMID: 8441535] (A review of 306 patients with obstructive sleep apnea undergoing Phase I and Phase II surgery protocol.)

Schwab RJ et al. Upper airway assessment: radiographic and other imaging techniques. *Otolaryngol Clin North Am.* 1998;31:931. [PMID: 9838010] (A review of imaging modalities useful in diagnosis and research of obstructive sleep apnea.)

Sher AE et al. The efficacy of surgical modifications of the upper airway in adults with obstructive sleep apnea syndrome. *Sleep.* 1996;19:156. [PMID: 8855039] (Comprehensive review of Phase I and Phase II surgeries, alternative surgeries, and outcomes.)

Wright J et al. The efficacy of nasal continuous positive airway pressure in the treatment of obstructive sleep apnea syndrome is not proven. *Am J Respir Crit Care Med.* 2000;161:1776. [PMID: 10852740] (An editorial reviewing the associations of OSA and daytime symptoms reminds clinicians of the need to continue studying the long-term consequences of CPAP therapy.)

Yaggi HK et al. Obstructive sleep apnea as a risk factor for stroke and death. *N Engl J Med.* 2005;353(19):2034. [PMID: 16282178] (Review of the risk of severe obstructive sleep apnea and fatal and nonfatal cardiovascular events.)

Young T et al. The occurrence of sleep-disordered breathing among middle-aged adults. *N Engl J Med.* 1993;328:1230. [PMID: 8464434] (Cohort study of middle-aged adults determining prevalence, risk factors, and symptoms of sleep-disordered breathing.)

■ SLEEP DISORDERS IN CHILDREN

Sleep disorders in children are common, and the prevalence of these disorders varies with the developmental age of the child. Parents of infants and toddlers bring to routine health care visits disturbance of sleep as their most frequent complaint. Thirty to fifty percent of these parents request specialized care to address their child's perceived sleep problems. Sleep disorders also affect adolescents: More than 50–75% of adolescents report that they desire more sleep than they are currently receiving. Although the emergence of the various sleep disorders occurs at different stages of ontogeny, sleep disorders in children are classified with adult sleep disorders according to the American Sleep Disorders Association International Classification of Sleep Disorders.

CLASSIFICATION OF SLEEP & SLEEP DISORDERS

Sleep

In children, recognizable sleep stages do not arise until they are approximately 6 months of age. Before 6 months, PSG can be used reliably to distinguish only NREM sleep from REM sleep. In the neonate, NREM sleep occupies approximately 50% of total sleep time and NREM-REM cycles occur fairly regularly throughout the night—approximately every 50 minutes. Infants generally spend half of their day asleep and frequently sleep uninterrupted for 3–4 hours punctuated by awakenings for feeding; this cycle tends to decrease in frequency as infants progress in age. By the second year of life, children begin to develop separation anxieties that may inhibit sleep initiation.

The development of preschool-aged children often presents a challenge to parents because this age group desires to stay up later than parents allow. Encouraging preschool-aged children to sleep can be difficult and may become manifest with pleas for continued parental attention (eg, rereading a bedtime story). Concrete dreaming is observed in preschool-aged children, and the appearance of dyssomnias (eg, hypersomnolence or obstructive sleep apnea) is also frequently observed in this group.

Sleep Disorders

Parasomnias appear largely in school-aged children. The most common parasomnias seem to be nightmares, night terrors, somnambulism, and enuresis, all of which occur during Stage IV sleep. School-aged children may also cling to preschool-aged behaviors or habits that interfere with sleep, such as wanting to stay up late, sleeping with parents, or sleeping with the light on or the door open.

The development of normal adult sleep architecture occurs throughout the adolescent period. Adolescents generally require approximately 9 hours of sleep per night, which is more than the 7–8 hours of sleep required by adults. Sleep deficit in adolescents often becomes manifest with excessive sleepiness and poor school performance that can be confused with other psychiatric, medical, or sleep disorders when it is merely due to insufficient sleep time. Disorders such as narcolepsy and advanced/delayed sleep phase syndromes also begin to appear in this age group.

As in adults, the otolaryngologist deals primarily with the diagnosis and treatment of sleep disorders related to sleep-disordered breathing, mainly OSA. As previously stated this dyssomnia usually emerges in preschool-aged children (but can appear at any age) and is often quite different in children than in their adult counterparts.

SLEEP APNEA

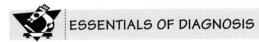 ESSENTIALS OF DIAGNOSIS

- *History of snoring, witnessed apneas, restless sleep, or enuresis.*
- *Evidence of obstructive tonsils and/or adenoids on physical exam.*
- *Evidence of OSA from overnight PSG.*

General Considerations

A number of epidemiologic studies have determined that OSA in children is common. As in adults, OSA in children is characterized by snoring and transient obstruction of the upper airway during sleep that results in sustained periods of hypoxia and a host of nighttime and daytime symptoms. Nighttime symptoms in children are comparable to those in adults; however, the daytime symptoms and sequelae are often not comparable, with children developing agitation or attention deficits (as opposed to excessive sleepiness) and unique long-term health complications such as failure to thrive and poor growth in addition to the usual cardiopulmonary problems.

Studies have shown that primary snoring, which should be distinguished from OSA, is found in approximately 3–12% of preschool-aged children, and OSA occurs in approximately 2–3% of children aged 6 months to 18 years, with peaks in prevalence in preschool-aged children. In this population of children, a number of risk factors are highly predictive of sleep-disordered breathing.

Pathogenesis

The most common cause of upper airway obstruction in children is adenotonsillar hypertrophy. Specifically, the pathology underlying adenotonsillar hypertrophy and upper airway obstruction is related to the disproportionate growth in adenotonsillar tissue and in the pharynx itself during development. Many, but not all, studies have demonstrated adenotonsillar hypertrophy as the primary etiology in childhood sleep-disordered breathing; others not finding a relationship between adenotonsillar hypertrophy and upper airway obstruction implicate muscle tone, upper airway narrowing, as well as adenotonsillar hypertrophy as the critical factors. Tonsillar hypertrophy has been well described as a cause of upper airway obstruction, and studies have demonstrated that children with OSA are more likely to have 3+ and 4+ tonsils (75% of children with OSA studied) than children without OSA.

Other less common causes of OSA in children are attributed to genetic disorders that cause nasopharyngeal or oropharyngeal obstruction early in life, such as Down syndrome, Crouzon syndrome, Apert syndrome, and bilateral choanal stenosis or atresia. Syndromes with micrognathia or retrognathia, such as Pierre Robin sequence, mandibulofacial dystosia, Weaver syndrome, cerebrocostomandibular syndrome, and Treacher-Collins syndrome, present with glossoptosis of the geniohyoid and genioglossus muscles. Glossoptosis results in hypopharyngeal obstruction due to the altered relationships between the mandible and the hyoid and appears to be worsened by cleft anomalies. Defects such as bifid epiglottis, laryngomalacia, webs and strictures, and cleft larynx also contribute to OSA.

Prevention

As in adults, obesity in children is associated with sleep-disordered breathing. In a study of nearly 400 children ages 2–18, obese children were 4–5 times more likely to have sleep-disordered breathing than nonobese children. Although obesity in children has been strongly associated with sleep-disordered breathing, it is important to remember that not all children with OSA are obese. Also, although blacks represented 27% of those studied, they represented 56% of children with an RDI > 10 events/h, indicating a disproportionate representation of children with sleep-disordered breathing. Black children are 3–4 times more likely to have sleep-disordered breathing than are white children. Factors such as age, gender, and exposure to cigarette smoke were not found to significantly correlate with presence of sleep-disordered breathing.

An increased prevalence of sleep-disordered breathing was also observed in children with chronic cough, occasional wheeze, persistent wheeze, asthma, and sinus-related problems. Chronic cough was the strongest predictor of sleep-disordered breathing (with an odds ratio of 8.83), and although both were significantly correlated with sleep-disordered breathing, *persistent* wheeze was found to be a stronger predictor of sleep-disordered breathing than *occasional* wheeze (odds ratio of 7.45 versus 3.29, respectively). Sinus-related disease was related to sleep-disordered breathing with a 5.10 odds ratio, and asthma was related to sleep-disordered breathing with an odds ratio of 3.83.

Clinical Findings

A. Signs and Symptoms

As in adults, children exhibit the stereotypical nighttime symptoms such as snoring (quiet or loud), choking or gasping, restless sleep, witnessed apneas, and enuresis. It is important to remember that the quality or volume of snoring does not correlate well with the severity of OSA in children. Children exhibit a number of nonspecific daytime symptoms, such as chronic mouth breathing, hyponasality, dysphagia, and halitosis, as well as other symptoms not typically expressed by adults, such as aggression, hyperactivity, and learning disabilities. The physician can obtain subjective information from parents by having them complete the Obstructive Sleep Disorders-6 (OSD-6) survey, which has been validated and addresses the patient's physical suffering, sleep disturbance, speech or swallowing disorder, emotional distress, activity limitation, and the caregiver's concerns. Corroboration with schoolteachers can be helpful in attesting to the level of participation in school, learning progress, and school performance at the level of peers. Daytime sleepiness in children is not a typical manifestation in contrast to the adult population.

B. Physical Exam

All children should be evaluated for appropriate height and weight gain according to the American Association of Pediatricians (AAP) recommendations because children with OSA are 4–5 times more likely to be overweight than children without OSA. Treatment to control weight may be necessary as part of the overall treatment plan.

A thorough head and neck exam, including cranial nerve examination, begins with identifying stigmata associated with genetic syndromes. Although all portions of the upper airway need to be evaluated, significant attention should be directed to the nasopharynx and the oropharynx. Inspection of the nasal cavity for masses or rhinitis, the posterior nasal cavity for choanal stenosis or atresia, and the nasopharynx for the adenoids with nasopharyngoscopy is performed when possible.

Thorough inspection of the oral cavity for macroglossia and the oropharynx for obstructing tonsils can be performed by direct observation. As in adults, tonsils are described as 1, 2, 3, or 4+ in size, respectively, indicating a 0–25%, 25–50%, 50–75%, or > 75% lateral narrowing of the oropharynx. Palpation of the hard and soft palate is essential to diagnose submucous clefts. The hypopharynx and larynx can be inspected with fiberoptic endoscopy and assessed for abnormalities as well.

C. Special Tests

1. Polysomnography—Although overnight PSG has been standardized and is used frequently in diagnosing OSA in adults, it is neither standardized nor practical at this moment for the routine diagnosing of children with OSA. However, the American Thoracic Society (ATS) recommends that PSG be performed in children according to specific criteria, some of which are summarized in Table 40–2. The ATS consensus statement

Table 40–2. Sample American Thoracic Society indications for performing polysomnography in children.

1. Differentiating primary snoring from OSA-related snoring.
2. Evaluate EDS, cor pulmonale, failure to thrive, or polycythemia in the snoring child.
3. Uncertainty about whether results of exam are sufficient to warrant surgery.
4. Children with laryngomalacia with worsening symptoms during sleep.
5. Obesity in children associated with unexplained hypercapnia, snoring, or disturbed sleep.
6. Child with sickle cell anemia and symptoms of OSA or sleep-related vasoocclusive crises.
7. If weight loss or CPAP is selected as primary therapy (in order to titrate).

CPAP, continuous positive airway pressure; EDS, excessive daytime sleepiness; OSA, obstructive sleep apnea.

on PSG reporting in children defines an obstructive apnea as the cessation of airflow during thoracoabdominal excursion; however, it does not establish a maximally acceptable time interval as in adults. Some authors have stated that a normal apnea index in children is 0.1 ± 0.5 events/h; thus, it would seem that *any* duration of airflow cessation is abnormal in children. The ATS consensus statement defines hypopnea as a 50% reduction in airflow; however, others have defined hypopneas as 50% reduction in respiratory effort, 50% decreases in airflow with decreases in blood oxygen saturation, or combinations of the above. Since determining the end points of hypopneas can be difficult, end-tidal $CO_2 > 45$ mm Hg for more than 60% of sleep time has also been used to score a hypopnea. By strict criteria, children with an RDI > 5 events/h are considered to have OSA, although, as noted above, some believe that any apnea at all is abnormal. Routine use of PSG in the diagnosis of OSA in children is not recommended. Furthermore, children with upper airway resistance and significant sleep fragmentation often have normal sleep study results.

2. Other tests—Other studies such as sleep questionnaires; abbreviated PSG, which has been shown to have a 97% positive predictive value and a 47% negative predictive value; nighttime video and audio recording; and sleep somnography have also been evaluated, but remain unproven for routine diagnosis.

Complications

Children with OSA incur the same health complications as do adults with OSA, and these include a host of cardiopulmonary complications as well as consequences that are unique to children, such as failure to thrive, poor growth, short stature, learning disabilities, mental retardation, behavioral problems, and attention deficit/hyperactivity disorder. Studies comparing pre- and post-adenotonsillectomy data for height and weight demonstrate significant gains in height and weight following adenotonsillectomy, and performance in school is also demonstrated to increase after adenotonsillectomy.

Treatment

A. Nonsurgical Measures

1. CPAP therapy—Because the cause of OSA is more clearly defined in children and because surgical treatment is significantly more successful in children than in adults, CPAP therapy is reserved for patients with specific contraindications to surgery, patients with persistent OSA despite surgical treatment, and patients refusing surgical therapy. CPAP is approximately 85% effective in eliminating OSA in children and improves nadir SaO_2 as well as REM sleep. Children older than 2 years of age are noted to be poorly compliant with CPAP therapy and frequently complain of the same side effects that adults experience. As with adults, there are no conclusive data that CPAP use in children is beneficial in eliminating the long-term sequelae of OSA.

2. Weight loss—General measures used to treat children with OSA include weight loss and treatment of preexisting medical conditions deemed to influence the development of sleep-disordered breathing. Overweight children should be encouraged to lose weight; however, for patients with Down syndrome or Prader-Willi syndrome, this may not be practical. The ATS recommends that those choosing weight loss as the primary therapy undergo PSG to evaluate the severity of apnea and its progress.

3. Other treatment measures—Respiratory tract maladies such as rhinitis, sinus disease, wheezing, and asthma have also been linked to OSA; attempts to treat these conditions should parallel treatment of OSA. In addition, children with gastroesophageal reflux disease should also be treated with age-appropriate measures in coordination with a gastroenterologist or pulmonologist.

B. Surgical Measures

1. Adenotonsillectomy—Adenotonsillectomy is highly successful in eliminating OSA in children and should be recommended as first-line therapies if the family is amenable and there are no specific contraindications. Adenotonsillectomy is indicated in children with obligate mouth breathing, snoring, and obstructive sleep apnea, and care must be taken in patients with secondary palate or submucous clefts, because adenoidectomy may increase the risk of velopharyngeal insuffi-

ciency. Additional caution is advisable for surgery in children younger than 3 years of age owing to increased frequency of complications. By objective measures, adenotonsillectomy improves quality of life and is approximately 85–95% effective in *eliminating* OSA in children. A more recent study using the OSD-6 survey to evaluate the quality of life of children pre- and post-adenotonsillectomy demonstrated an 87.7% improvement in short-term quality of life with 74.5% reporting a large improvement in quality of life. Only 5.1% reported a worsening in quality of life.

2. Other surgical measures—Although they are performed less commonly because of the high success of adenotonsillectomy, the procedures performed on adults (UPPP, osteotomies and advancements, and tracheostomy) are performed in children as well. Because these procedures are performed less commonly and more frequently in patients with craniofacial disorders, their use and evaluation must be made on an individualized basis.

PROGNOSIS

The prognosis of untreated OSA in children can be severe, with such long-term consequences as hypertension, myocardial ischemia, congestive heart failure, and stroke. Clinicians must also be aware that untreated OSA in children presents additional complications such as failure to thrive, short stature, mental retardation, and learning disabilities. In contrast to management of adult cases, the management of OSA in children is frequently gratifying. For children, studies comparing pre- and post-adenotonsillectomy data for height and weight demonstrate significant gains in height and weight following adenotonsillectomy, and performance in school is also demonstrated to increase after this procedure.

American Academy of Pediatrics, Section on Pediatric Pulmonology, Subcommittee on Obstructive Sleep Apnea Syndrome. Clinical practice guideline: diagnosis and management of childhood obstructive sleep apnea syndrome. *Pediatrics.* 2002;109:704. [PMID: 11927742] (Published guidelines regarding the AAP's position on the diagnosis and treatment of obstructive sleep apnea in children.)

American Thoracic Society. Standards and indications for cardiopulmonary sleep studies in children. *Am J Respir Crit Care Med.* 1996;153:866. [PMID: 8564147] (Reviews the evidence for PSG in children and establishes guidelines for its use in children.)

Arens R et al. Magnetic resonance imaging of the upper airway structure of children with obstructive sleep apnea syndrome. *Am J Respir Crit Care Med.* 2001;164:698. [PMID: 11520739] (Use of MRI as a tool to identify structural risk factors in children with obstructive sleep disorders.)

de Serres LM et al. Measuring quality of life in children with obstructive sleep disorders. *Arch Otolaryngol Head Neck Surg.* 2000;126:1423. [PMID: 11115276] (Article addressing quality of life in children with obstructive sleep disorders.)

de Serres LM et al. Impact of adenotonsillectomy on quality of life in children with obstructive sleep disorders. *Arch Otolaryngol Head Neck Surg.* 2002;128:589. [PMID: 12003578] (Unique study using the OSD-6 survey to assess quality of life in children undergoing tonsillectomy and adenoidectomy.)

Nieminen P et al. Snoring children: factors predicting sleep apnea. *Acta Otolaryngol.* 1997;529(Suppl):190. [PMID: 9288307] (Addresses risk factors for obstructive sleep apnea in a population of children.)

Redline S et al. Risk factors for sleep-disordered breathing in children. Associations with obesity, race, and respiratory problems. *Am J Respir Crit Care Med.* 1999;159:1527. [PMID: 10228121] (Details risk factors for obstructive sleep apnea and associated upper and lower respiratory conditions in children.)

Tasker C et al. Evidence for persistent UA narrowing during sleep, 12 years after adenotonsillectomy. *Arch Dis Child.* 2002;86:34. [PMID: 11806880] (Long-term follow-up of 12 children with snoring who underwent tonsillectomy and adenoidectomy.)

SECTION X
Thyroid & Parathyroid

Disorders of the Thyroid Gland | 41

Grace A. Lee, MD, & Umesh Masharani, MRCP(UK)

■ ANATOMY & HISTOLOGY

The normal thyroid gland is located anterior to the trachea and midway between the apex of the thyroid cartilage and the suprasternal notch (Figure 41–1). Important neighboring posterior structures include the four parathyroid glands situated behind the upper and middle thyroid lobes, and the recurrent laryngeal nerves coursing along the trachea. The thyroid consists of two pear-shaped lobes connected by an isthmus. The typical dimensions of the lobes are 2.5–4.0 cm in length, 1.5–2.0 cm in width, and 1.0–1.5 cm in thickness. Also, in about 50% of patients, a small pyramidal lobe is present at the isthmus or adjacent part of the lobes. Microscopically, the thyroid consists of varying-sized follicles consisting of a central collection of colloidal material surrounded by a single layer of epithelial cells.

A normal thyroid gland weighs approximately 10–20 g, depending on dietary iodine intake, age, and weight. The thyroid gland usually grows posteriorly and inferiorly, since it is limited from upward extension by the sternothyroid muscle. In large multinodular goiters, substernal extension is not uncommon.

The thyroid gland has a rich blood supply, derived from the superior, inferior, and the small inferior ima artery (Figure 41–2). Venous flow returns via multiple surface veins draining into the superior, lateral, and inferior thyroid veins.

■ THYROID HORMONES

THYROID HORMONE SYNTHESIS

The synthesis of T_4 (thyroxine) and T_3 (triiodothyronine) occurs both within the cell and at the cell-colloid junction. The key components of thyroid hormone synthesis include thyroglobulin, a large thyroid hormone precursor sequestered in the colloid and thyroid peroxidase that catalyzes the iodination of thyroglobulin and the coupling of thyroglobulin residues to form T_4 and T_3. The six essential steps to thyroid hormone synthesis are (1) active uptake of iodide, (2) oxidation of iodide and iodination of thyroglobulin, (3) coupling of iodotyrosine molecules within thyroglobulin to form T_3 and T_4, (4) proteolysis of thyroglobulin and the release of free iodothyronines and iodotyrosines, (5) deiodination of iodotyrosines within the thyroid and recycling of the liberated iodide, and (6) in certain situations, deiodination of T_4 to T_3 (Figure 41–3). Thyroid hormone synthesis is mostly controlled by the hypothalamic-pituitary-thyroid axis, as illustrated in Figure 41–4.

THYROID HORMONE TRANSPORT

Thyroid hormones are mostly bound to carrier proteins; 99.96% of T_4 and 99.60% of T_3 are bound in the serum (Figure 41–5). The small fraction of unbound

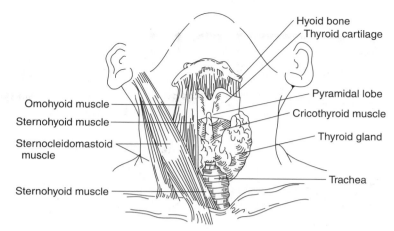

Figure 41–1. Gross anatomy of the thyroid gland. (Reproduced, with permission, from Greenspan FS: *Basic and Clinical Endocrinology.* Originally published by Appleton & Lange. New York: The McGraw-Hill Companies, 1983.)

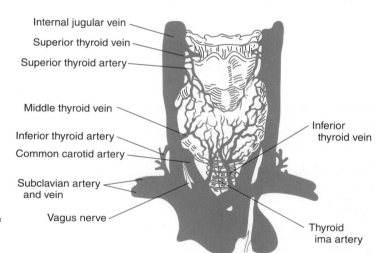

Figure 41–2. Arterial and venous blood supply of the thyroid gland. (Reproduced, with permission, from Lindner HH: *Clinical Anatomy.* Originally published by Appleton & Lange. New York: The McGraw-Hill Companies, 1989.)

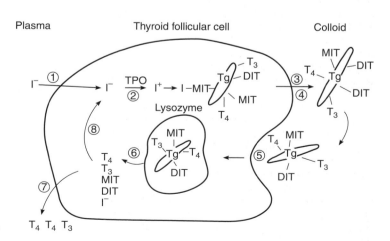

Figure 41–3. Thyroid hormone synthesis.

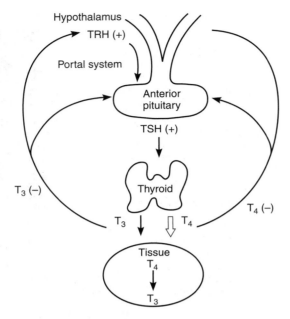

Figure 41–4. The hypothalamic-pituitary thyroid axis. The hypothalamus secretes thyroid-releasing hormone (TRH), which causes the pituitary to release thyroid stimulating hormone (TSH). In turn, TSH stimulates most of the thyroid hormone formation of T_4 and some of the formation of T_3. T_4 and T_3 negatively feed back on the hypothalamus and pituitary, completing the regulatory cycle.

T_4 and T_3 hormones are responsible for biologic activity. Thyroid hormones are transported throughout the body bound to three carrier proteins in the serum: (1) thyroxine-binding globulin (TBG); (2) thyroxine-binding prealbumin (TBPA), also known as transthyretin; and (3) albumin.

METABOLISM OF THYROID HORMONES

Biologic activity is dependent on the degree and location of iodination (see Figure 41–5). T_3 is 3–8 times more potent than T_4. T_4 is the predominant circulating thyroid hormone, whereas T_3 is the main peripherally active hormone. 5'-deiodinase converts T_4 into the active form T_3 in the peripheral tissues. Certain drugs can inhibit the conversion of T_4 to T_3: propylthiouracil, amiodarone, ipodate, glucocorticoids, and propranolol. T_4 has a half-life of approximately 7 days, whereas T_3 has a half-life of 1 day.

■ ASSESSMENT OF THYROID FUNCTION

THYROID FUNCTION TESTS

The most commonly used thyroid function tests in clinical practice are serum immunoassays for thyroid-stimulating hormone (TSH, or thyrotropin) and free thyroxine (or free T_4, also known as FT_4). TSH can be used alone in screening for overt thyroid disease, but both TSH and FT_4 are needed for the diagnosis, especially if pituitary or hypothalamic disease is suspected. With a normal hypothalamus and pituitary, TSH maintains an inverse relationship with FT_4. Figure 41–6 provides an algorithm for the evaluation of thyroid function tests. The common profiles of thyroid function tests in different disease states are outlined in Table 41–1. TSH is an extremely sensitive pituitary indicator of thyroid disease, but it requires

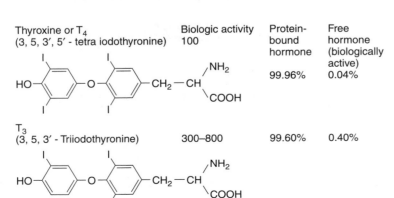

Thyroxine or T_4 (3, 5, 3', 5' - tetra iodothyronine)	Biologic activity 100	Protein-bound hormone	Free hormone (biologically active)
		99.96%	0.04%
T_3 (3, 5, 3' - Triiodothyronine)	300–800	99.60%	0.40%

Figure 41–5. Thyroid hormone structure and biologic activity.

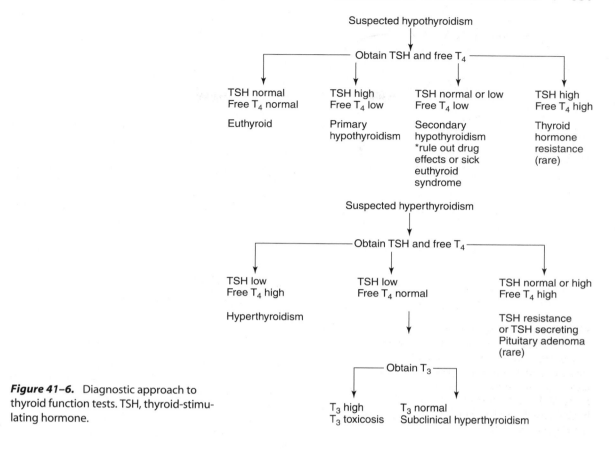

Figure 41–6. Diagnostic approach to thyroid function tests. TSH, thyroid-stimulating hormone.

Table 41–1. Patterns of thyroid function tests.

TSH	Free T$_4$	T$_3$	Diagnosis
Normal	Normal	Normal	Euthyroid
Normal	Low normal or low	Low or normal	Central hypothyroidism or sick euthyroid or drugs
High	Low	Normal or low	Primary hypothyroidism
High	Normal	Normal	Subclinical hypothyroidism
High	High	High	TSH resistance syndrome*
Low	High or normal	High	Hyperthyroidism
Low	Normal	Normal	Subclinical hyperthyroidism or drugs
Low	Normal	High	T$_3$ toxicosis*
Low	Low	Low	Central hypothyroidism or sick euthyroid or drugs

*Denotes rare conditions

4–6 weeks to reflect changes in thyroid hormone levels. FT_4 is a less sensitive indicator of thyroid hormone production, but it may be helpful in monitoring more acute changes in thyroid activity. In evaluating hyperthyroidism, it may also be helpful to obtain a total T_3 or FT_3 to rule out T_3 thyrotoxicosis.

Thyroid-Stimulating Hormone Immunoassay

The TSH assays currently used are immunoassays based on two monoclonal antibodies detecting different epitopes of the TSH. Most laboratories use either a second- or third-generation TSH assay, which detects levels as low as 0.10 and 0.01 mU/L respectively. TSH is a sensitive measure of the response of the pituitary gland to circulating FT_4 levels.

TSH levels are elevated mostly in primary hypothyroidism and are accompanied by a low level of FT_4. Table 41–2 lists situations in which the TSH is elevated (other than in hypothyroidism), including drugs, recovery from an acutely ill state, acute psychiatric admission, and the very rare TSH-secreting pituitary tumor.

A decreased TSH level should be interpreted in conjunction with the FT_4 level. A decreased TSH level with an elevated FT_4 level suggests primary hyperthyroidism. A low FT_4 level with a normal to decreased TSH level may indicate secondary or central hypothyroidism (< 5% of all cases of hypothyroidism), which are due to a pituitary or hypothalamic tumor. The diagnosis can be confirmed by performing a thyrotropin-releasing hormone (TRH) stimulation test, with elevation of the TSH 30 and 60 minutes postinjection, but this test is rarely necessary. A number of situations, including drugs and nonthyroidal illness, can also cause both low TSH and FT_4 levels (see Table 41–1).

Free Thyroxine Immunoassay (FT₄)

FT_4 is an assay measuring the serum concentration of T_4. It has largely replaced indirect measurements of FT_4 concentrations, such as the free T_4 index (FT_4I), which is the product of resin T_3 (or T_4) uptake and total T_4. Most laboratories use a chemiluminescent immunoassay to measure FT_4 levels. It is valid in most cases, except in patients with very high or low thyroid-binding proteins or severe illness. Under these circumstances, the measurement of FT_4 levels by equilibrium dialysis is more reliable. FT_4 is elevated in hyperthyroidism and decreased in hypothyroidism. Table 41–2 lists the conditions that affect FT_4 levels. Of note, the antiepileptic drugs phenytoin, carbamazepine, and rifampin can cause a significantly increased hepatic metabolism of T_4. Also, drugs and illness rarely suppress the TSH to undetectable levels. The measurement of FT_4 levels by dialysis is spuriously elevated by heparin, which activates lipoprotein lipase, which in turn generates fatty acids that displace T_4 from TBG.

Total Triiodothyronine (T₃)

Total T_3 measures both the free and bound T_3 in circulation. Total T_3 is helpful in diagnosing hyperthyroidism with elevated T_3 levels but normal T_4 levels (ie, T_3 toxicosis). The preferential secretion of T_3 can be seen in early Graves' disease or toxic multinodular goiter.

Free T₃

Free T_3 (FT_3) is a newer test that allows for the direct measurement of FT_3 levels via chemiluminescent assay or radioassay.

Antithyroid Peroxidase Antibody

Thyroid peroxidase (TPO) is the key enzyme that catalyzes the iodination of thyroglobulin and the coupling of iodinated tyrosyl residues to form T_3 and T_4. TPO is located on the microvilli at the thyroid-colloid interface. Almost all patients with Hashimoto's thyroiditis have antithyroid peroxidase (anti-TPO) antibodies present—these antibodies are usually measured to diagnose Hashimoto's thyroidi-

Table 41–2. Drugs and their effects on thyroid function tests.

True hyperthyroidism	Iodine and iodine-containing drugs (amiodarone, IV contrast), lithium, interferon alfa, interleukin 2
True hypothyroidism	Iodine and iodine-containing drugs (amiodarone, IV contrast), lithium, interferon alfa, interleukin 2
Suppressed TSH secretion	Glucocorticoids, dopamine, dobutamine, octreotide, amphetamines, opioids, nifedipine, and verapamil, dopamine antagonists, atypical antipsychotics, phenothiazines
Low T_4 by decreased absorption of T_4	Cholestyramine, soy-based foods, colestipol, aluminum hydroxide, calcium carbonate, iron sulfate, sucralfate
Low T_4 by increased T_4 clearance	Phenytoin, carbamazepine, phenobarbital, rifampin
High T_4 by inhibited T_4 to T_3 conversion	Amiodarone, iodine and iodine-containing substances, glucocorticoids, propylthiouracil, propranolol

tis. A large number of patients with Graves' disease also have anti-TPO antibodies. Both anti-TPO and thyroglobulin antibodies are positive in about 5–10% of normal subjects.

Thyroid Stimulating Immunoglobulin

Thyroid stimulating immunoglobulin (TSI) of the TSH receptor antibody is an indirect test that confirms the diagnosis of Graves' disease. TSI is positive in approximately 90% of patients with Graves' disease, and negative both in normal patients and patients with Hashimoto's thyroiditis. Patient serum is incubated with either human thyroid cell culture or hamster ovary cells that express recombinant human TSH receptor; cyclic adenosine monophosphate (AMP) activity is measured. TSI is also of diagnostic value in patients with normal thyroid function who have exophthalmos. The measurement of TSI is helpful during pregnancy—high titers increase the risk of neonatal thyrotoxicosis.

Serum Thyroglobulin

Serum thyroglobulin is the precursor protein required for the synthesis of T_4 and T_3. The normal measure is < 40 ng/mL in individuals with normal thyroid function, and < 5 ng/mL in patients after a thyroidectomy. Thyroglobulin is raised when the thyroid is overactive, such as with Graves' disease or multinodular goiter. In very large goiters, the elevated levels of thyroglobulin reflect the gland size. In subacute or chronic thyroiditis, thyroglobulin is released as a consequence of tissue damage.

Thyroglobulin is a very useful marker for thyroid cancer, both to assess treatment efficacy and to monitor for recurrence after total thyroidectomy and radioiodine ^{131}I therapy. Because thyroglobulin is made only by the thyroid gland, its level serves as an indicator of the presence of thyroid tissue, as in well-differentiated thyroid cancer. Under these circumstances, a thyroglobulin level of > 10 mg/dL indicates the presence of metastatic disease. It is necessary to measure for endogenous thyroglobulin antibodies as part of interpreting the measurement of the thyroglobulin level. These antibodies can interfere with the assay and give spuriously high or low levels, depending on the measurement method used.

Radioactive Iodine Uptake & Scan

Radionuclide imaging of the thyroid with ^{123}I or ^{99m}Tc is useful in evaluating the *functional activity* of the thyroid. The two tests that use radioactivity to assess the thyroid are the radioactive uptake and scan. Radioactive uptake evaluates thyroid function by reporting the percentage uptake of iodine, whereas the scan produces an image of the distribution of iodine in the thyroid. The radioactive scan gives information regarding the size and shape of the thyroid, as well as information about nodules that are either functioning ("hot" nodules) or nonfunctioning ("cold" nodules).

[123]I can be used to assess both radioactive uptake and scan, but ^{99m}Tc can only be used for scanning. A ^{99m}Tc study gives results within 30 minutes, whereas ^{123}I images are obtained at 4–6 hours and at 24 hours. [123]I delivers less radiation than ^{131}I because of its short half-life of 13 hours and the absence of beta radiation. Its gamma photo energy of 159 keV is ideally suited for thyroid scanning. Both ^{123}I and ^{99m}Tc are contraindicated in pregnancy.

[123]I allows assessment of the turnover of iodine by the thyroid gland. After 100–200 μCi of ^{123}I, radioactivity over the thyroid area is measured by scintigraphy at 4 or 6 hours and at 24 hours. The normal ranges of uptake vary with iodine intake. In areas of low iodine intake and endemic goiter, uptake may be as high as 60–90%. In the United States, with a relatively high intake, the normal uptake is 5–15% at 6 hours, and 8–30% at 24 hours.

Both ^{123}I uptake and scan are useful in delineating the cause of hyperthyroidism. Uptake is elevated in thyrotoxicosis due to Graves' disease and toxic multinodular goiter. Uptake is low in subacute thyroiditis, the active phase of Hashimoto's thyroiditis with the release of preformed hormone, exogenous thyroid hormone ingestion, excess iodine intake (from amiodarone, iodinate contrast dyes, or kelp pills), and hypopituitarism. More rare causes include ectopic thyroid hormone production from HCG (human chorionic gonadotropin), struma ovarii, and metastatic follicular thyroid carcinoma. [131]I uptake and scans are very useful in monitoring the recurrence of well-differentiated thyroid cancer. Typically, 2–3 mCi of ^{131}I is given to the patient, and images of the thyroid and the whole body are taken to look for recurrence or metastases. If the patient is treated with high-dose ^{131}I to ablate remnant thyroid cancer, a post-treatment thyroid and whole-body scan is often helpful to look for tumor tissue that weakly uptakes iodine.

Nonthyroidal Illness & Thyroid Function Tests

Severely ill patients exhibit altered thyroid function tests. Most hospitalized patients have lower serum T_3 concentrations due to inhibition of the peripheral conversion of T_4 to T_3 by 5' deiodinase. Severely ill patients (50% of patients in the ICU and 15–20% of hospitalized patients) can have a low serum T_4 level. This low level is mostly due to very low levels of thyroid-binding proteins, but the exact mechanism remains to be elucidated. The degree of T_4 depression has been directly correlated with overall patient outcome. Most hospitalized patients also have slightly depressed but detectable levels of TSH. It has been suggested that hospitalized patients may have a subtle form of central hypothyroidism as a protective mechanism against their ill health and an increased catabolism. Studies have shown that administering thyroxine to patients who are ill has no benefit and may, in fact, be harmful. In the recovery phase of nonthyroidal illness, the TSH level tends to transiently rise before it returns to normal levels.

The assessment of thyroid function in the setting of nonthyroidal illness is difficult and should be undertaken only when there is a strong suspicion of thyroid disease. A straightforward approach to thyroid function tests in a patient who is hospitalized is to measure both TSH and FT_4. An elevated TSH, especially > 20 μU/mL, is suggestive of primary hypothyroidism. In 75% of cases, patients with an undetectable TSH using a third-generation TSH assay are likely to have primary hyperthyroidism. A depressed but detectable TSH usually accompanied by a low T_4 level could indicate nonthyroidal illness, drug effect, subclinical hyperthyroidism, or central hypothyroidism. In these situations, other aspects of the patient history and examination may be helpful in making the diagnosis. The presence of a goiter, known pituitary disease, and thyroid test results obtained *before the illness* can direct the diagnosis and treatment. If nonthyroidal illness or a drug effect is highly suspected, the intermittent monitoring of thyroid function tests may be warranted.

Dayan CM. Interpretation of thyroid function tests. *Lancet.* 2001;357(9256):619. [PMID: 11558500] (A practical approach to thyroid function tests with a focus on common test pattern interpretation and the avoidance of pitfalls.)

Klee GG, Hay ID. Biochemical testing of thyroid function. *Endocrinol Metab Clin North Am.* 1997;26(4):763. [PMID: 9429859] (A more comprehensive analysis of thyroid function tests.)

PHYSICAL EXAMINATION

There are three basic maneuvers in examining the thyroid. The patient should be seated with only a slightly flexed neck to relax the sternocleidomastoid muscles. The thyroid should first be observed while the patient swallows a sip of water. An enlarged gland or nodules can be observed as the gland moves up and down. The thyroid gland should then be palpated from behind the patient, with the middle three fingers on each lobe of the gland. While the patient swallows, thyroid nodules or an enlargement can be noted as the gland passes beneath the examiner's fingers. A normal thyroid is usually found to be 2 cm in length and 1 cm in width. A generalized enlargement of the thyroid is called a **diffuse goiter** (from *gutta,* Latin for "throat"), whereas an irregular enlargement is termed a **nodular goiter.**

■ THYROID MASSES

THYROID NODULES

General Considerations

Thyroid nodules are common, with a 4% prevalence in the United States and a male-to-female ratio of 4:1. Although the incidence of thyroid cancer is only 0.004% per year, each nodule should be assessed to rule out the possibility of thyroid cancer.

Clinical Findings

The initial evaluation of a thyroid nodule involves a careful history taking and physical examination (Table 41–3). Age is an important risk factor, with adults younger than 30 or older than 60 years of age carrying a high risk for thyroid cancer. A patient family history of medullary thyroid carcinoma or personal radiation exposure, especially when young, should alert the physician to the possibility of thyroid cancer. Recent growth, or evidence of hoarseness, dysphagia, or obstruction, should also raise suspicion. An ultrasound study is particularly helpful in distinguishing a cyst from a solid nodule and also in identifying

Table 41–3. Clinical evaluation of thyroid nodules.

	Low Risk	High Risk
History	Family history of goiter	Family history of medullary cancer History of head and neck radiation Recent growth of nodule Hoarseness, dysphagia
Epidemiology	Older woman	Young adult, male, or child
Physical exam	Soft nodule Multinodular goiter	Solitary, firm nodule Vocal cord paralysis Firm lymph nodes
Serum factors	High titer of thyroid antibodies, hyper- or hypothyroidism	
^{123}I Thyroid scan	"Hot nodule"	"Cold nodule"
Ultrasound of thyroid	Pure cystic lesion	Solid or semicystic lesion
Thyroxine therapy	Regression	Increase in size of mass

other nonpalpable nodules. Ultrasound can also identify nodules that are more concerning for malignancy, that is, those that have microcalcifications, irregular borders, and increased blood flow.

After primary thyroid disease is ruled out with normal thyroid function tests, the diagnostic procedure of choice is a fine-needle aspiration (FNA) biopsy of the thyroid nodule. Indications for biopsy include solitary thyroid nodules, multiple nodules, or dominant or growing nodules that exist within a multinodular goiter. Although in the past, multinodular goiters and multiple nodules were thought to have a decreased incidence of thyroid cancer, recent data have suggested that the incidence of thyroid cancer may be higher. FNA biopsy is performed using a 23- to 25-gauge needle with or without local anesthesia, and usually with ultrasound guidance. Several passes are made into the thyroid nodule, and the aspirated material is used in thin smear slides that are both air dried and alcohol preserved.

Cytopathologic examinations are typically reported as benign; suspicious or indeterminate (eg, follicular neoplasms); malignant; or nondiagnostic. One review of thyroid biopsy reported that 70% of FNAs were benign, 10% were suspicious or were follicular neoplasms, 5% were malignant, and 15% were nondiagnostic. Cystic lesions yield serous fluid with immediate involution of the nodule. Although a malignant growth is less likely to occur in a purely cystic lesion, the fluid should still be sent for cytologic examination. If the cyst has tissue in the wall, then FNA of this region should be performed under ultrasound guidance. FNA is considered nondiagnostic if the specimens show a lack of follicular epithelium or the presence of excessive bloody dilution. A recent review of more than 5000 FNA procedures revealed an accuracy of over 95%, with a false-negative rate of 2.3% and a false-positive rate of 1.1%.

Treatment

An algorithm of thyroid nodule management can be found in Figure 41–7. The management of a malignant growth, as indicated by FNA, requires total thyroidectomy, with careful attention paid to local, palpable lymph nodes that may require neck dissection at the time of surgery. Follicular adenomas are often deemed "indeterminate" because they are difficult to distinguish from follicular carcinomas on FNA. Evidence of vascular or capsular invasion is required for the diagnosis of follicular carcinoma. Roughly 10–20% of all suspicious lesions actually prove to be follicular carcinoma on excision. A ^{123}I scan can be helpful in distinguishing between an adenoma or carcinoma—if the lesion is hyperfunctioning or "hot," then it is unlikely to be malignant and can be observed or radioablated if the patient is hyperthyroid. In contrast, if the lesion is hypofunctioning or "cold," then the patient is referred for partial thyroidectomy to rule out follicular carcinoma.

Benign thyroid nodules are usually followed up clinically; these growths may enlarge, stay the same size, or involute. Ultrasound is particularly helpful in follow-up measurements. Suppressive therapy of benign thyroid nodules is controversial. Most studies have not shown regression of solitary nodules with exogenous thyroxine, whereas some studies have shown a 20–30% reduction. Currently, most authorities do not recommend L-thyroxine therapy in the treatment of solitary nodules. Nodules that increase in size raise concern for a malignant growth and require reexamination with repeat FNA or surgical removal. Cystic lesions quickly involute on aspiration but are more prone to recur. In addition, FNA of cystic lesions can yield nondiagnostic cytology because of the difficulty of performing a biopsy of the thin cystic wall. Repeat FNAs are often required, and ultimately surgical removal may be needed. One small randomized trial showed that suppressive therapy for cystic nodules was not helpful.

An increasing number of incidental thyroid nodules are being identified as a result of the frequent use of ultrasonography by the primary care physicians in the evaluation of the thyroid gland. It is recommended that patients with nodules that are ≥ 1.0 cm or that have

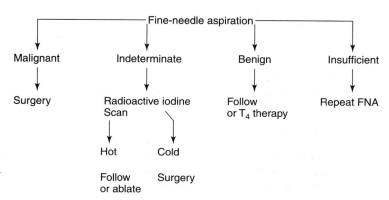

Figure 41–7. Algorithm for the management of thyroid nodules.

suspicious sonographic appearance proceed with FNA-guided ultrasound. Incidental thyroid nodules identified on positron emission tomography (PET) scans should undergo particularly careful evaluation because up to two thirds of these hypermetabolic lesions have been found to be cancers.

MULTINODULAR GOITER

General Considerations

With multinodular goiter, the thyroid gland is usually large, weighing from 60 to 1000 g. On pathologic examination, it contains nodules that vary in size, number, and appearance. Some nodules contain colloid and others are cystic, containing brown fluid that indicates previous hemorrhage. Some of the nodules have autonomous function. The spectrum of function of these goiters ranges from the euthyroid state, with some degree of autonomous function, to thyrotoxicosis (eg, toxic multinodular goiter).

Clinical Findings

The principal clinical features of a nontoxic goiter are the same as those of a thyroid enlargement. Large goiters can cause dysphagia, a choking sensation, and inspiratory stridor. Hemorrhage into a nodule can present with acute painful enlargement and may induce or enhance obstructive symptoms.

Treatment

The treatment for an enlarged asymptomatic multinodular goiter is suppressive therapy. Up to 60% of these goiters respond to such treatment. Long-term treatment is required because stopping the suppression results in regrowth of the gland. It is important to start with a low dose of L-thyroxine and carefully monitor the FT_4 and TSH levels, aiming for a level of FT_4 in the normal range and a level of TSH in the low–normal range. Careful follow-up is necessary to monitor both for the development of autonomous function within the gland and for thyrotoxicosis. Surgery should be considered in patients when either the gland grows on suppressive treatment or there are obstructive symptoms. Surgical complications, such as recurrent laryngeal nerve damage and hypoparathyroidism, can be as high as 7–10%. Radioactive iodine treatment can result in a reduction of the thyroid volume and is safe in the treatment of a nontoxic multinodular goiter. Hypothyroidism can occur in 22–40% of subjects within 5 years after ^{131}I treatment.

For a toxic multinodular goiter, control of the hyperthyroid state with antithyroid drugs followed by subtotal thyroidectomy is the treatment of choice. If the patient is a poor surgical candidate, then a ^{131}I treatment dose is a reasonable option. Patients who have some degree of autonomous function in their multinodular goiter can develop overt thyrotoxicosis when exposed to an iodine load (eg, amiodarone treatment or IV contrast). This iodide-induced thyrotoxicosis can be treated with methimazole and beta-adrenergic blockade. [131]I treatment may not be possible because of the large iodine pool. Total thyroidectomy is curative but is feasible only if the patient can withstand the stress of surgery.

Hermus AR, Huysmans DA. Treatment of benign nodular thyroid disease. *N Engl J Med.* 1998;338(20):1438. [PMID: 9580652] (Practical review of the management and treatment of nontoxic and toxic multinodular goiter.)

Meier CA. Thyroid nodules: pathogenesis, diagnosis and treatment. *Baillieres Best Pract Res Clin Endocrinol Metab.* 2000;14:559. [PMID: 11289735] (Review of currently recommended approach to thyroid nodules.)

Siegel RD, Lee SL. Toxic nodular goiter. Toxic adenoma and toxic multinodular goiter. *Endocrinol Metab Clin North Am.* 1998;27(1):151. [PMID: 9534034] (Practical review of current theories of the pathogenesis and treatment of solitary toxic adenoma and toxic multinodular goiter.)

■ THYROID CANCER

Thyroid cancer represents only 1% of all cancers, with an estimated incidence of 19,500 new cases in 2001. In the past three decades, the incidence of thyroid cancer has increased by almost 50%; however, mortality rates have declined by 20%. This may be due to earlier detection by FNA and subsequent treatment. There are four main pathologies encountered in thyroid cancer: papillary, follicular, medullary, and anaplastic carcinomas (Table 41–4).

Table 41–4. Frequency of thyroid cancer.

Cancer	Percentage
Papillary carcinoma	75%
Follicular carcinoma	16%
Medullary carcinoma	5%
Undifferentiated	3%
Other	1%
(Lymphoma, fibrosarcoma, squamous cell carcinoma, teratomas, hemangioendothelioma, and metastatic carcinomas)	

PAPILLARY CARCINOMA

General Considerations

Papillary carcinoma is the most common thyroid cancer, representing 75% of all thyroid cancers. It has the best prognosis, with a 5% mortality rate at 20 years for patients with no evidence of local invasion at diagnosis. In addition to a history of childhood exposure to radiation, risk factors for papillary carcinoma include familial papillary carcinoma, Cowden syndrome (eg, multiple hamartomas of the skin and mucous membranes), and familial adenomatous polyposis coli.

Clinical Findings

Microscopically, papillary carcinoma consists of single layers of thyroid cells arranged in avascular projections or papillae, which manifest as large pale nuclei, intranuclear inclusion bodies, and anaplastic features. "Psammoma bodies" are laminated calcified spheres and are usually diagnostic of papillary carcinoma. Papillary carcinoma can be either purely papillary or mixed with follicular carcinoma; both are treated with similar therapies. Certain histopathologic variants, such as tall cell, columnar cell, and diffuse sclerosing types, are associated with a higher risk of recurrence.

Papillary carcinoma typically has an indolent natural history. Usually unencapsulated, these lesions grow slowly, with intraglandular metastasis and local lymph node extension. In the late stages, it can spread to the lung. In older patients, chronic low-grade papillary carcinoma may rarely convert to an aggressive anaplastic carcinoma.

Treatment

Because papillary carcinoma retains the ability to synthesize thyroglobulin and to concentrate iodine in the early stages, radiation therapy is often effective. The initial treatment involves either partial thyroidectomy or total thyroidectomy with possible modified neck dissection (Figure 41–8).

A. Surgical Measures

Patients can be classified as having either a low or a high risk for thyroid cancer based on their age, the size of the lesion, and evidence of extrathyroidal spread. Patients younger than 45 years of age who have lesions < 1 cm with no evidence of intra- and extrathyroidal involvement are considered to have a low risk for thyroid cancer. All other patients should be considered at high risk. For both low-risk and high-risk patients, total thyroidectomy is generally recommended, although a partial thyroidectomy may be adequate for the former group. If lymphatic spread is present on the initial evaluation, the patient should undergo a modified neck dissection as well; however, neck dissection is not indicated in the absence of lymphatic

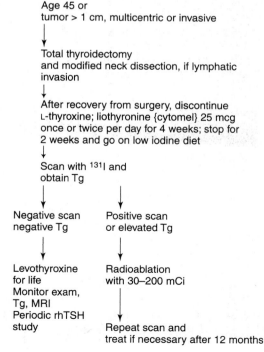
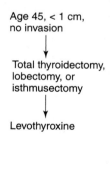

Figure 41–8. Algorithm for the management of papillary or follicular cancer. Tg, thyroglobulin; TSH, thyroid-stimulating hormone.

spread. In the hands of a skilled surgeon, thyroid surgery portends less than a 1% complication rate; the primary complications are hypoparathyroidism and recurrent laryngeal nerve damage. Immediately after surgery, the patient should be placed on suppressive T_4 therapy.

B. POSTSURGICAL MEASURES

After undergoing a total thyroidectomy, patients should receive radioiodine to ablate the remnant thyroid bed to decrease the likelihood of recurrent disease. Radioablation also allows the physician to subsequently follow thyroglobulin levels as a marker for thyroid cancer activity.

The usual protocol requires thyroxine therapy to be stopped for 6 weeks and L-triiodothyronine (25 to 50 mcg) to be initiated for 4 weeks. The patient is then taken off all thyroid hormone therapy and goes on a low iodine diet for 2 weeks. This dietary modification allows for a rise in the patient's TSH level, which stimulates iodide uptake by the residual tumor. At maximal TSH stimulation (usually a TSH of > 50 µU/mL), thyroglobulin is drawn and 2–5 mCi of ^{131}I is administered to the patient. The patient is scanned for residual radioactive iodine uptake 24–72 hours later. An undetectable thyroglobulin level at a time when the serum TSH is elevated is the most sensitive test to determine that all thyroid tissue has been eradicated. If thyroglobulin is increased or radioactive iodine uptake is evident, a treatment dose of ^{131}I is given (see Figure 41–8).

The amount of ^{131}I given for the treatment of thyroid cancer depends on the degree of disease, the response to previous treatments, and the amounts of ^{131}I administered in the past. Approximately 30–50 mCi of ^{131}I is used to ablate the thyroid remnant in a postsurgical patient who does not have metastatic disease; uptake is limited to the thyroid bed. For metastatic or recurrent disease, patients are generally treated with a 100–200 mCi dose of ^{131}I. Side effects from doses larger than 100 mCi include sialadenitis, xerostomia, and temporary oligospermia. With cumulative doses of up to 300 mCi, no permanent sterility has been reported in women and < 10% of men have permanent sterility. Cumulative doses larger than 500 mCi have been associated with infertility, pancytopenia (in < 4.0% of cases), and leukemia (in 0.3% of cases). However, cumulative doses over 800 mCi have been associated with permanent sterility in up to 60% of women and 90% of men. A week after the treatment dose of ^{131}I, a posttreatment scan is performed. This scan is very useful in locating any subtle residual thyroid cancer that was not identified by the low-dose, pretreatment ^{131}I scan.

With postradioactive iodine treatment, the patient is placed on suppressive L-thyroxine therapy, with the goal TSH level ranging from below normal (< 0.1 mU/L) to undetectable. The patient is monitored at regular intervals, with either careful neck examination for new masses or lymphadenopathy with measurements of serum thyroglobulin, FT_4, and TSH. Repeat radioactive iodine scans are performed at 12-month intervals with concomitant radioactive treatments as necessary. Once a negative scan and negative thyroglobulin are achieved at the time of elevated TSH, the patient may be followed up with a recombinant TSH radioactive scan instead of withdrawal from thyroid hormone therapy. Recombinant TSH allows the patient to avoid the discomfort of severe hypothyroidism and disrupting suppressive T_4 therapy. On the first 2 days, patients are injected intramuscularly with recombinant TSH. On the third day, a 3–5 mCi dose of ^{131}I is administered to the patient; on the fifth day, a whole-body scan is performed. TSH and thyroglobulin are measured on the third and fifth days. Because thyroglobulin is the most sensitive test for residual tumor, in some circumstances the uptake and scan can be deferred. The patient is likely to be free from disease if the serum thyroglobulin is < 1 ng/mL and the scan is negative. Thyroid cancer with a negative scan but a positive thyroglobulin positive thyroid level poses a diagnostic dilemma. As thyroid cancer dedifferentiates, it can potentially lose the ability to concentrate iodine and thus lose responsiveness to radioactive iodine treatment. Once excessive iodine intake is ruled out, patients generally undergo further imaging such as ultrasound, MRI, CT scanning, PET/CT scanning, or thallium or technetium-MIBI scanning to locate metastatic disease. If active thyroid disease is found, patients may undergo modified neck dissection to remove the metastatic disease.

Thyroglobulin antibodies in patient's serum can interfere with the thyroglobulin assay, and so the test is not reliable as a tumor marker. Under these circumstances, the patient may have to be followed with periodic imaging such as ultrasound or MRI.

C. NONSURGICAL MEASURES

External radiation therapy may be useful in a variety of situations. Nonfunctional bone metastases respond well to external-beam therapy. Solitary metastatic lesions that do not concentrate radioactive iodine may respond to local external beam therapy. Brain metastases usually do not respond to ^{131}I and are best treated by either resection or gamma knife radiation therapy.

Prognosis

The overall prognosis of well-differentiated thyroid cancer is assessed by the initial staging and the adequacy of treatment. Table 41–5 describes the TNM staging system as well as 5- and 10-year survival rates. In this system, the staging is related to the age of the patient, recognizing that for patients who are younger than 45 years of age at the time of diagnosis, papillary tumors are relatively indolent. Stage 1 patients have an excellent 5-year survival rate of 99% and a 10-year survival rate of 98%.

The treatment modality, including the type of surgery, the radioactive treatment, and adequate L-thyroxine

Table 41–5. TNM staging and survival rates for adults with appropriately treated differentiated thyroid carcinoma.

Stage	Description	5-year Survival Rate	10-year Survival Rate
1	Under 45: any T, any N, no M Over 45: T < 1 cm, no N, no M	99%	98%
2	Under 45: any T, any N, any M Over 45: T > 1 cm, no M, no M	99%	85%
3	Over 45: T beyond capsule, no N, no M Or: any T, regional N, no M	95%	70%
4	Over 45: any T, any N, any M	80%	61%

suppressive therapy, also affects the prognosis. Patients with tumors > 1 cm who receive partial thyroidectomies have a mortality rate that is 2.2 times greater than that of patients who undergo total thyroidectomies. Patients who have never undergone radioablation carry a two-fold increased mortality rate at 10 years compared with patients who receive radioablation. Adequate suppressive therapy decreases the mortality rate but must be weighed against the possible side effects of tachycardia, arrhythmias, angina, and osteoporosis.

FOLLICULAR CARCINOMA

General Considerations

Follicular carcinoma is the second most common thyroid cancer, accounting for 16% of all thyroid cancers.

Clinical Findings

Microscopically, follicular cancer forms small follicles that contain small, cuboidal cells with poor colloid formation. The distinction between carcinoma and adenoma requires the presence of capsular or vascular invasion. It is often difficult to distinguish a follicular carcinoma from a follicular adenoma on an FNA biopsy; therefore, a frozen section at the time of surgery is necessary. Like papillary carcinoma, follicular carcinoma retains the ability to synthesize thyroglobulin and concentrate iodine and is therefore responsive to radioactive iodine treatment. Rarely, follicular carcinoma synthesizes T_3 and T_4 and presents with hyperthyroidism and distant metastases. Follicular carcinoma tends to be slightly more aggressive than papillary carcinoma; it may spread to local lymph nodes or by the blood to bone or lung. Histologic variants, such as Hürthle cell and poorly differentiated carcinoma, rarely take up radioiodine and have a higher risk of metastases and recurrence.

Treatment & Prognosis

The treatment and prognosis of follicular carcinoma are the same as for papillary carcinoma (see previous section).

MEDULLARY CARCINOMA

General Considerations

Medullary carcinoma represents only 5% of thyroid cancers. Papillary and follicular carcinomas involve thyroid epithelial cells; medullary carcinoma is a disorder of the parafollicular or C cells.

Clinical Findings

The neuroendocrine cells of medullary carcinoma appear as sheets of cells with abundant, interspersed amyloid that stains Congo red. In addition to secreting calcitonin, medullary carcinoma can secrete histaminase, prostaglandins, serotonin, and other peptides. Local extension often occurs into the lymph nodes, surrounding muscle, and the trachea. In addition, medullary carcinoma can spread via the blood to the lungs and viscera. Treatment involves surgical resection, since radiation therapy has no effect.

Medullary carcinoma has a natural history that is more aggressive than papillary or follicular thyroid carcinoma. Patients with multiple endocrine neoplasia (MEN) type 2b have the most aggressive form, whereas the cancers found in patients with MEN 2a and familial medullary thyroid carcinoma (FMTC) are the least aggressive. This cancer also has a strong familial association; one third of cases are sporadic, a second third are associated with MEN type 2, and the other third of cases are familial without other associated endocrinopathies. MEN 2a is composed of medullary carcinoma, pheochromocytoma, and hyperparathyroidism, whereas MEN 2b consists of medullary carcinoma, pheochromocytoma, and multiple mucosal neuromas. A patient with a diagnosis of medullary carcinoma should be screened for other endocrinopathies found in MEN type 2, and the patient's family members should be screened for medullary carcinoma and MEN type 2. Genetic screening for the *RET* proto-oncogene has replaced measurements of serum calcitonin after a calcium gluconate bolus.

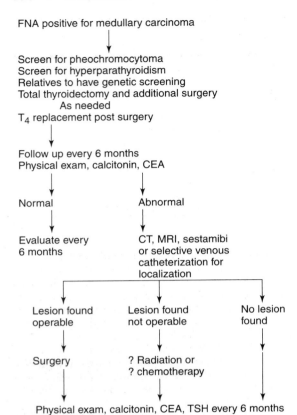

FNA positive for medullary carcinoma

Screen for pheochromocytoma
Screen for hyperparathyroidism
Relatives to have genetic screening
Total thyroidectomy and additional surgery
As needed
T_4 replacement post surgery

Follow up every 6 months
Physical exam, calcitonin, CEA

Normal | Abnormal

Evaluate every 6 months

CT, MRI, sestamibi or selective venous catheterization for localization

Lesion found operable | Lesion found not operable | No lesion found

Surgery | ? Radiation or ? chemotherapy

Physical exam, calcitonin, CEA, TSH every 6 months

Figure 41–9. Management of medullary carcinoma. CEA, carcinoembryonic antigen; TSH, thyroid-stimulating hormone.

Treatment

Patients with medullary carcinoma should undergo total thyroidectomy with regional lymph node dissection if indicated. Postoperatively, patients are placed on suppressive L-thyroxine therapy. There is no role of ^{131}I or chemotherapy in the treatment of medullary carcinoma. Patients should be monitored for the recurrence of disease with serum calcitonin or carcinoembryonic antigen (CEA) measurements (Figure 41–9). In addition, family members should be screened for familial medullary carcinoma and the *RET* proto-oncogene associated with MEN 2a and 2b. Imaging modalities include MRI of the neck and chest, PET scanning, indium-labeled somatostatin scanning, or sestamibi scanning.

ANAPLASTIC CARCINOMA

General Considerations

Undifferentiated (anaplastic) carcinoma represents 1% of all thyroid cancers. Histopathologic types include small cell, giant cell, and spindle cell carcinomas. Anaplastic carcinoma is the most aggressive form of thyroid cancer and rapidly expands by local extension into surrounding structures. It results in death in 6–36 months.

Clinical Findings

The typical presentation of anaplastic thyroid carcinoma is an older patient with a long history of goiter with sudden rapid expansion of the gland followed by compressive symptoms or vocal cord paralysis.

Treatment & Prognosis

Anaplastic thyroid carcinoma is resistant to all treatment modalities. Treatment is palliative and includes isthmectomy to prevent tracheal compression, and external-beam therapy plus suppressive L-thyroxine therapy. Although chemotherapy is generally not effective with anaplastic carcinoma, doxorubicin may be useful in patients who cannot undergo other forms of therapy. Anaplastic carcinoma carries a very poor prognosis because of the aggressiveness of the disease and a lack of responsiveness to treatment.

OTHER THYROID CANCERS

Other types of malignant thyroid disorders represent approximately 3% of all thyroid cancers. These include lymphomas, metastatic carcinomas, fibrosarcomas, squamous cell carcinomas, malignant hemangioendotheliomas, and teratomas. Lymphoma can present rapidly in patients with long-standing Hashimoto's thyroiditis, or it may develop in association with generalized lymphoma. The thyroid lymphoma associated with Hashimoto's thyroiditis can sometimes be difficult to distinguish from chronic thyroiditis. In the absence of systemic spread, thyroid lymphoma is responsive to radiation therapy. Common metastatic cancers of the thyroid include breast, renal cell, and bronchogenic cancers, as well as melanoma.

Brandi ML, Gagel RF, Angeli A et al. Guidelines for diagnosis and therapy of the MEN type 1 and type 2. *J Clin Endocrinol Metab.* 2001;86(12):5658. [PMID: 11739416] (International consensus statement regarding the diagnosis and management of MEN type 1 and type 2, including screening and genetic counseling.)

Cooper DS, Doherty GM, Haugen BR et al. Management guidelines for patients with thyroid nodules and differentiated thyroid cancer. *Thyroid.* 2006;16. [PMID: 16420177] (Recommendations of the American Thyroid Association Guidelines Taskforce on the Evaluation of Thyroid Nodules and Treatment of Thyroid Cancer.)

Hay ID. Papillary thyroid carcinoma. *Endocrinol Metab Clin North Am.* 1990:19:545. [PMID: 2261906]

Kebebew E, Clark OH. Medullary thyroid cancer. *Curr Treat Options Oncol.* 2000;1(4):359. [PMID: 12057161] (Review of the management of medullary thyroid cancer, with a focus on surgical treatment strategies.)

Ladenson PW, Braverman LE, Mazzaferri EL et al. Comparison of administration of recombinant human thyrotropin with withdrawal of thyroid hormone for radioactive iodine scanning in patients with thyroid carcinoma. *N Engl J Med.* 1997;337:888. [PMID: 9302303] (Landmark clinical trial comparing the efficacy of recombinant human thyrotropin to the withdrawal of thyroid hormone for radioactive iodine scanning in recurrent, well-differentiated thyroid cancer.)

Mazzaferri EL, Kloos RT. Clinical review 128: current approaches to primary therapy for papillary and follicular thyroid cancer. *J Clin Endocrinol Metab.* 2001;86(4):1447. [PMID: 11297567] (Comprehensive review of the management of well-differentiated thyroid cancer.)

Mazzaferri EL, Kloos RT. Using recombinant human TSH in the management of well-differentiated thyroid cancer: current strategies and future directions. *Thyroid.* 2000;10(9):767. [PMID: 11041042] (Review of the clinical trials to date on the use of recombinant human thyroid-stimulating hormone in well-differentiated thyroid cancer, as well as a review of the National Cancer Center Network's consensus practice guidelines.)

St. Louis JD, Leight GS, Tyler DS. Follicular neoplasms: the role for observation, fine-needle aspiration biopsy, thyroid suppression, and surgery. *Semin Surg Oncol.* 1999;16:5. [PMID: 9890733] (Practical review of the diagnosis, management, and treatment of follicular neoplasms.)

NONMALIGNANT THYROID DISORDERS

HYPERTHYROIDISM & THYROTOXICOSIS

Thyrotoxicosis is a clinical syndrome that results from excessive levels of circulating thyroid hormone. The most common causes of thyrotoxicosis are due to overproduction of thyroid hormone by the thyroid gland, but other sources of thyroid hormone may exist, including exogenous ingestion of thyroid hormone or ectopic secretion (Table 41–6).

Patients with thyrotoxicosis classically present with a large number of symptoms related to hypermetabolism; these symptoms, listed in Table 41–7, include anxiety, insomnia, a racing heartbeat, palpitations, hand tremors, increased stool frequency, weight loss, heat intolerance, and increased perspiration. Older patients may exhibit "apathetic hyperthyroidism," which is characterized by weight loss, severe depression, and the potential for slow atrial fibrillation.

On physical examination, patients may be hyperkinetic with an inability to sit still; they may also present with fine tremor and hyperreflexia. Lid retraction is responsible for the characteristic "stare" and lid lag may be evident whereby the sclera can be seen above the iris when the patient is asked to gaze downward slowly. Lid retraction and lid lag are due to the hyperadrenergic state

Table 41–6. Causes of hyperthyroidism (in order of frequency).

Graves' disease
Toxic multinodular goiter
Solitary hyperfunctioning adenoma
Subacute thyroiditis
Exogenous thyroid hormone
Iodine-induced hyperthyroidism
Rare forms of hyperthyroidism
Struma ovarii
Metastatic follicular thyroid carcinoma
Trophoblastic tumors
TSH-secreting pituitary adenoma
Pituitary resistance to thyroid hormone

and should not be confused with exophthalmos, which is unique to Graves' disease. The patient's skin may have a velvety, moist texture, and the hair is thin and fine. Cardiovascular signs include tachycardia, widening of the pulse pressure with an increase in systolic pressure and a decrease in diastolic pressure, and a hyperdynamic precordium. Atrial fibrillation occurs in approximately 10% of patients with thyrotoxicosis. Examination of the neck may reveal a diffusely enlarged or multinodular goiter, a single nodule, or a painful and tender thyroid. A bruit may be present and is most often heard over the gland in Graves' disease.

The diagnosis is confirmed by laboratory analysis. Overt thyrotoxicosis typically has a suppressed TSH and elevated FT_4 and FT_3 concentrations. A normal T_4 but an elevated T_3 is consistent with T_3 toxicosis, usually seen in the early phase of toxic multinodular goiter and Graves' disease. The diagnosis of the etiology of thyrotoxicosis can be aided by the physical examination—the presence of ophthalmopathy, diffuse goiter, and pretibial myxedema is suggestive of Graves disease. Additional laboratory tests,

Table 41–7. Signs and symptoms of hyperthyroidism.

Symptoms	Signs
Irritability	Tachycardia, atrial fibrillation
Insomnia	Systolic hypertension
Heat intolerance	Extremity tremor
Diaphoresis	Warm, moist skin
Heart racing and palpitations	Fine or thin hair
Weight loss with increased appetite	Lid lag or retraction
Diarrhea	Goiter with bruit
Oligomenorrhea, loss of libido	

such as TSI (thyroid-stimulating immunoglobulin), anti-TPO (thyroid peroxidase), and ESR (erythrocyte sedimentation rate) can be helpful in diagnosing Graves' disease, the hyperthyroid phase of Hashimoto's disease, and viral thyroiditis. Radioactive thyroid uptake and scan are occasionally needed to confirm the cause of thyrotoxicosis.

GRAVES' DISEASE

General Considerations

Graves' disease is an autoimmune disorder characterized by the production of immunoglobulins that bind and activate the TSH receptor, which stimulates thyroid growth and hormone secretion. It tends to occur in women between the ages of 20 and 40, with an incidence of 1.9% in women. Females are five times more likely to be affected than males. There is a strong family predisposition in that 15% of patients have a close relative with the disorder.

Clinical Findings

In addition to the signs and symptoms of hyperthyroidism, several signs and symptoms are unique to Graves' disease, including ophthalmopathy, dermopathy, and osteopathy. Infiltrative ophthalmopathy is by far the most common sign. For unclear reasons, increased inflammation and the accumulation of glycosaminoglycans cause swelling of extraocular and retroorbital muscles, as well as displacement of the eye forward (also known as proptosis or exophthalmos). Patients can experience eye irritation; excessive tearing worsened by cold air, bright lights, or wind; diplopia; blurred vision; and, rarely, loss of vision.

Other physical findings in Graves' disease include dermopathy and osteopathy. Glycosaminoglycans can accumulate in the dermis layer, causing thickening of the skin, especially over the anterior tibia (pretibial myxedema). Osteopathy may occur with subperiosteal bone formation and swelling. The extrathyroidal manifestations often have a course independent of the thyroid disease itself and can persist despite restoration of the euthyroid state.

Laboratory Tests

The diagnosis of Graves' disease can be made from evidence of ophthalmopathy on the physical exam, as well as a decreased TSH and an increased FT_4 or FT_3. If ophthalmopathy is absent, obtaining a measure of TSI can be helpful. TSI is specific for Graves' disease but the lack of a TSI elevation does not exclude the diagnosis. Anti-TPO and antithyroglobulin can also be elevated but are nonspecific. In the absence of eye signs or an elevated TSI, a radioactive scan and uptake constitutes the gold standard for diagnosing Graves' disease.

Treatment

There are three aspects in the treatment of Graves' disease: (1) the control of hyperadrenergic symptoms, (2) the short-term restoration of the euthyroid state, and (3) the long-term control of excess thyroid hormone production.

A. Control of Adrenergic Excess

To control the symptoms of adrenergic excess, beta-blockers—either propranolol or atenolol—are used. These agents should be instituted even before determining the cause of hyperthyroidism. Propranolol has the advantage of inhibiting peripheral T_4 to T_3 conversion, whereas atenolol is more convenient with once-daily dosing. A typical starting dose is 10–20 mg of propranolol—three to four times a day, or 25 mg of atenolol once daily. These drugs are then titrated up over a few days while the patient's pulse and blood pressure are monitored.

B. Restoration of Euthyroid State

Thionamides (methimazole or propylthiouracil) act by inhibiting thyroid peroxidase-mediated iodination of thyroglobulin to form T_4 and T_3 within the thyroid gland and are generally used to restore the patient to the euthyroid state before deciding on long-term management. Methimazole has the advantage of once-daily dosing with no risk of irreversible hepatitis, a rare side effect of propylthiouracil therapy. Also, in patients for whom ^{131}I treatment is planned, methimazole is preferable to propylthiouracil because propylthiouracil may inhibit radioactive iodine uptake for weeks or months after discontinuation. Typically, a patient is started on a daily 20–40 mg dose of methimazole for 1–2 months, and then titrated down to a maintenance dose of 5–10 mg. Titration of the drug dose is based on the measurement of TSH and FT_4, as well as on the signs and symptoms of hyper- or hypothyroidism.

Propylthiouracil (but not methimazole) blocks the peripheral conversion of T_4 to T_3 and is traditionally used in the treatment of thyrotoxic crisis (as noted in the following section on "Thyrotoxic Crisis"). It also is more protein bound and is therefore the preferred drug in pregnancy and during breastfeeding. The typical starting dose of propylthiouracil is 100–150 mg three times a day; after 1–2 months it is titrated down to 50–100 mg twice daily. In pregnancy, if the initial dose of propylthiouracil is 300 mg or less and the maintenance dose is 50–150 mg daily, the risk of fetal hypothyroidism is extremely low. Propylthiouracil is titrated to maintain FT_4 at the upper limit of normal.

Both methimazole and propylthiouracil cause a rash in approximately 5.0% of patients. Agranulocytosis, which occurs in about 0.5% of patients, is usually heralded by a severe sore throat and fever. Patients should be counseled to stop the drug if they get a sore throat or fever and to see their physician. If the white blood cell count is normal, then the antithyroid drug can be resumed. Other serious side effects requiring discontinuation of drug include arthritis with both drugs; cholestatic jaundice with methimazole; angioneurotic edema, hepatocellular toxicity, and vasculitis with propylthiouracil.

C. LONG-TERM THERAPY

The choice of long-term therapy is based on the age of the patient, the severity and duration of the hyperthyroidism, the size of the gland, and the potential for a future pregnancy. In the one randomized trial that assessed the efficacy of drug treatment, radioablation, and surgery, all three modalities were found to be equally effective. However, there are several guidelines for choosing a treatment modality.

1. Methimazole—Methimazole treatment is chosen for long-term therapy, particularly in adolescents and young patients with small glands and less severe disease. The drug is usually given for up to 18 months to allow the disease to remit spontaneously. This remission occurs in 30–40% of patients treated for 18 months.

2. Radioactive iodine—Radioactive iodine ablation is the treatment of choice in patients 21 years and older. From a survey performed by the American Thyroid Association, 69% of American thyroid specialists recommended radioablation as the therapy of choice. In contrast, only 22% and 11% of European and Japanese thyroid doctors recommended radioablation as a first-line therapy.

With this treatment modality, patients are dosed with radioactive iodine based on their uptake scan. Restoration of the euthyroid state can take from several months to a year. Patients with severe hyperthyroidism, serious thyroid enlargement, or a history of heart disease should be adequately returned to the euthyroid state with methimazole prior to radioablation, with methimazole discontinued about 5 days prior to radioablation. Most patients subsequently become hypothyroid and require thyroid hormone replacement. Approximately 10% of patients have unsuccessful radioablation and may require a second dose. Radioactive iodine treatment is contraindicated in pregnancy, and it is important to advise women who may become pregnant in the near future that they should wait at least 6 months after ^{131}I treatment to allow for the resolution of any transient effects of the radiation on the ovaries. Alternative options should be offered to a female patient who cannot wait that long.

3. Subtotal thyroidectomy—Subtotal thyroidectomy should be considered in patients with a very large gland (ie, > 150 g) or in the patient who wants to get pregnant soon. Pretreatment is important to reduce the vascularity of the hyperthyroid gland. Patients should be given thionamides until a euthyroid state is achieved (approximately 6 weeks), and a saturated solution of potassium iodide—5 drops twice daily for the 2 weeks before surgery. The degree of the thyroidectomy is variable among surgeons, but generally 2–3 g of thyroid tissue is left intact. Most patients require hormone replacement therapy postoperatively.

Complications

A. THYROID CRISIS (THYROID STORM)

Thyroid crisis is an acute exacerbation of all symptoms of thyrotoxicosis. It occurs in patients with inadequately controlled thyrotoxicosis who undergo surgery, radioactive iodine treatment, parturition, and severe stressful illnesses such as infections, uncontrolled diabetes, and myocardial infarction. This disorder results from hypermetabolism and excessive adrenergic response.

Systemic symptoms include fever (38–41 °C), flushing, and sweating. Cardiac symptoms and signs include tachycardia, atrial fibrillation, and congestive cardiac failure. Neurologic symptoms and signs include agitation, restlessness, delirium, and coma. Gastrointestinal symptoms include nausea, vomiting, diarrhea, and jaundice.

Thyroid crisis is a medical emergency and should be treated promptly. Propranolol, either in a dose of 1–2 mg given as a slow IV injection, or in a dose of 40–80 mg administered orally, is given to control tachyarrhythmias. Propylthiouracil (PTU) is traditionally favored because it partially blocks peripheral T_4 to T_3 conversion. It is given in a 250-mg dose every 6 hours. If the patient cannot take oral medications, then 400 mg of PTU every 6 hours or 60 mg of methimazole every 24 hours can be administered rectally. An hour *after* a dose of PTU or methimazole has been given, hormone release can be retarded by giving an oral, saturated solution of potassium iodide (10 drops twice daily). The oral cholecystographic agents (sodium ipodate or iopanoic acid) similarly retard hormone release and also potently block T_4 to T_3 conversion, but they are not currently available in the United States. Sodium iodide (1 g) can be given intravenously over 24 hours. In addition, 50 g of hydrocortisone is administered intravenously every 6 hours, then tapered as clinical improvement occurs. Supportive measures include intravenous fluids and the management of electrolytes and nutrition. Aspirin should be avoided because it can displace T_3 from TBG.

B. GRAVES OPHTHALMOPATHY

The American Thyroid Association has classified Graves ophthalmopathy into six classes: (1) Class 1, spasm of the upper eyelids; (2) Class 2, soft tissue involvement with periorbital edema and conjunctival chemosis; (3) Class 3, proptosis; (4) Class 4, muscle involvement that limits gaze; (5) Class 5, corneal involvement (eg, keratitis); and (6) Class 6, visual loss due to optic nerve involvement.

The treatment of Graves ophthalmopathy involves (1) reversal of the hyperthyroid state; (2) symptomatic treatment with eye lubrication, glucocorticoids, or both; and (3) with severe symptoms, the surgical decompression of the orbit. Most patients have mild disease; one study found that approximately 65% of patients treated with thionamide therapy alone had no progression of eye disease, and only 8% demonstrated deterioration.

Restoration of the euthyroid state can be achieved by thionamide therapy, radioablation, and surgery. Radioablation can aggravate the ophthalmopathy, especially in smokers. Treatment with a short course of prednisone (40–60 mg/d) tapered over 4–6 weeks at the same time as ^{131}I treatment can prevent this exacerbation.

In most patients, symptomatic treatment involves alleviating corneal irritation and wearing dark glasses. Glucocorticoid therapy is indicated for worsening chemosis, diplopia, or proptosis. Surgical decompression is warranted for progressive eye disease despite glucocorticoids, optic nerve changes, corneal ulceration or infection, and cosmetic reconstruction. A loss of vision, which is heralded by a loss of color vision, is considered a medical emergency; the patient should be treated with high-dose glucocorticoids and surgical decompression.

Bartalena L, Marcocci C, Bogazzi F et al. Relation between therapy for hyperthyroidism and the course of Graves' ophthalmopathy. *N Engl J Med.* 1998;338(2):73. [PMID: 9420337] (Landmark article correlating radioactive iodine treatment with more serious cases of Graves' ophthalmopathy, and providing evidence that prednisone can prevent the progression of eye disease after radioactive iodine treatment.)

Bartalena L, Pinchera A, Marcocci C. Management of Graves' ophthalmopathy: reality and perspectives. *Endocr Rev.* 2000;21(2):168. [PMID: 10782363] (Comprehensive review of the management of mild and severe cases of Graves' ophthalmopathy, including treatment strategies, prevention, and future therapeutics.)

Kaplan MM, Meier DA, Dworking HJ. Treatment of hyperthyroidism with radioactive iodine. *Endocrinol Metab Clin North Am.* 1998;27(1):205. [PMID: 9534037] (Review of the role of radioactive iodine in treating various hyperthyroid states.)

Weetman AP. Graves' disease. *N Engl J Med.* 2000;343(17):1236. [PMID: 11071676] (Comprehensive review of the pathogenesis, clinical signs and symptoms, diagnosis, and treatment of Graves' disease.)

OTHER FORMS OF THYROTOXICOSIS

1. Amiodarone-Induced Hyperthyroidism

General Considerations

The antiarrhythmic drug amiodarone contains 37.3% iodine and has a half-life of about 50 days. Although amiodarone-induced hypothyroidism is far more common than hyperthyroidism, 2% of patients on amiodarone will develop hyperthyroidism. The symptoms of amiodarone-induced hyperthyroidism may be blunted by the antiadrenergic effects of amiodarone itself, and hyperthyroidism often develops years after starting this medication.

Etiology & Clinical Findings

There are two etiologies responsible for hyperthyroidism that manifests in the setting of amiodarone: (1) excess iodine in an underlying abnormal gland causes excessive hormone production; and (2) thyroiditis caused by amiodarone itself. Thyroid ultrasound may be useful in differentiating between the two causes, with an increased Doppler flow in excess hormone production and a decreased Doppler flow in thyroiditis. However, most patients may have a mixed etiology, and it is often difficult to differentiate between the two forms.

Treatment

Patients may be treated with higher-dose thionamides, such as 40–60 mg of methimazole, and beta-adrenergic blockade. If there is inadequate control, a 40-mg daily dose of prednisone is often helpful, especially in cases of amiodarone-induced thyroiditis. Total thyroidectomy should be considered since it is curative, but patients often have a poor operative status.

Bogazzi F, Bartalena L, Gasperi M, Braverman LE, Martino E. The various effects of amiodarone on thyroid function. *Thyroid.* 2001;11(5):511. [PMID: 11396710] (Comprehensive review of amiodarone-induced hypothyroidism and hyperthyroidism.)

2. Subacute Thyroiditis

General Considerations

Subacute granulomatous thyroiditis is an acute inflammatory disorder of the thyroid gland presumed to be due to viral infection. Subacute granulomatous thyroiditis may also be referred to as de Quervain thyroiditis, subacute thyroiditis, and subacute nonsuppurative thyroiditis.

Clinical Findings

The classic signs and symptoms are fever, malaise, and soreness of the neck; the thyroid gland is extremely tender on examination. Patients need a changing pattern of thyroid function tests throughout the course of the disease. Initially, with thyroid follicle damage and the release of preformed thyroid hormones, TSH is decreased, with an increase in T_4 and T_3 and a low radioactive iodine uptake. After 2–6 weeks, patients enter a euthyroid phase as T_4, T_3, and TSH levels return to normal. A transient hypothyroid phase of 2–8 weeks ensues while thyroid hormone stores are exhausted and the thyroid follicles regenerate. Most patients return to the euthyroid state once the thyroiditis has resolved; however, a hypothyroid state may be permanent in 10% of patients.

Diagnosis

The diagnosis of subacute thyroiditis is made clinically. A markedly elevated ESR as high as 100 mm/h is strongly suggestive of the diagnosis. Additional helpful laboratory findings include negative thyroid autoantibodies.

Treatment

Patients are usually treated symptomatically with beta-blockers and nonsteroidal anti-inflammatories (NSAIDs); prednisone is usually reserved for more severe cases. Patients who become hypothyroid should be administered L-thyroxine.

3. Rare Forms of Thyrotoxicosis

A. THYROTOXICOSIS FACTITIA

Thyrotoxicosis factitia is a psychoneurotic disorder in which patients purposely take thyroid hormones, usually for weight control. In addition, patients may be given thyroid hormones by psychiatrists to facilitate the treatment of depression. Clinical findings include the absence of a goiter, a suppressed TSH level, mild elevation of T_4 and T_3, a negative radioactive iodine uptake level, and a low thyroglobulin level.

B. STRUMA OVARII

Teratoma of the ovaries may contain functioning thyroid tissue, which results in hyperthyroidism. Radioactive iodine uptake in the neck is absent, but a whole body scan shows an increased uptake in the pelvis. Curative treatment involves resection of the teratoma.

C. METASTATIC FOLLICULAR CARCINOMA

Follicular thyroid carcinoma usually does not retain the ability to produce active hormone, but in rare instances, as in the presence of metastatic disease, follicular carcinoma can produce a hyperthyroid state. A radioactive body scan usually shows an increased uptake in the lungs or bones.

D. HYDATIDIFORM MOLE

Hydatidiform moles do not produce thyroid hormone; rather, they produce chorionic gonadotropin, which displays TSH-like activity. Clinical evidence of hyperthyroidism is usually not present, but a laboratory workup can reveal a suppressed TSH and a mild elevation of serum T_4 and T_3. Resection of the mole is curative.

HYPOTHYROIDISM

General Considerations

The failure of thyroid hormone production results in a generalized hypometabolic state and seriously impairs normal growth and development if it occurs early in life. Hypothyroidism may be due to a primary disease of the thyroid gland, or it may be secondary to a pituitary deficiency. Hypothalamic dysfunction, resulting in a TSH deficiency or peripheral resistance to the action of thyroid hormone, is a rare cause (Table 41–8).

Clinical Findings

In adults, the onset of symptoms of hypothyroidism is often insidious. These symptoms include fatigue, weight gain, intolerance to cold, and a delayed relaxation phase to deep tendon reflexes (Table 41–9).

Hashimoto's thyroiditis is the most common cause of hypothyroidism. It is an autoimmune disease characterized by lymphocytic infiltration, destruction of thyroid follicles, and fibrosis. Several autoantibodies are present, including anti-TPO, antithyroglobulin antibody, and TSH-receptor blocking antibody. Thyroperoxidase antibodies remain positive for many years and are useful for diagnosis. There may or may not be a goiter. The goiter in Hashimoto's thyroiditis is usually moderate in size and firm in consistency. In older patients, the thyroid may be totally destroyed by the immune process, and the gland is found to be small on examination.

Table 41–8. Causes of hypothyroidism (in order of frequency).

Primary Hypothyroidism
1. Hashimoto's thyroiditis
2. Iatrogenic:
   a. Radioactive iodine therapy for Graves' disease
   b. Subtotal thyroidectomy for Graves' disease or nodular goiter
3. Excessive iodide intake (kelp, radiocontrast dyes)
4. Transient hypothyroidism
   a. Subacute lymphocytic thyroiditis
   b. Subacute granulomatous thyroiditis
   c. Postpartum thyroiditis
5. Lithium, antithyroid drugs (methimazole, propylthiouracil); (rare)
6. Iodide deficiency (rare)
7. Inborn errors of thyroid hormone synthesis (rare)
Secondary Hypothyroidism
1. Hypopituitarism due to a pituitary adenoma
2. Pituitary ablative therapy
Tertiary Hypothyroidism
1. Hypothalamic dysfunction (rare)

Table 41–9. Signs and symptoms
of hypothyroidism.

Symptoms	Signs
Fatigue, weakness	Bradycardia
Cold intolerance	Delayed tendon reflexes
Dyspnea on exertion	Slowed movement and speech
Weight gain	Dry, rough skin, loss of eyebrows
Constipation	Nonpitting edema, periorbital edema
Hoarseness	Muscle stiffness, proximal weakness
Menorrhagia	Carotenemia
Rare: Dementia	Rare: Pleural and pericardial effusions
	Depressed ventilatory drive
	Diastolic hypertension

Diagnosis

The diagnosis of suspected hypothyroidism is outlined
in an algorithm listed in Figure 41–6. In primary
hypothyroidism, the TSH is elevated with a low FT_4
level. In secondary hypothyroidism, the TSH level is
low or inappropriately normal with a low FT_4 level.
Secondary hypothyroidism may also present with other
signs of pituitary deficiency, including hypogonadism
and adrenal insufficiency.

Treatment

Treatment involves hormone replacement with L-thyroxine; the average replacement dosage in adults is 1.6
mcg/kg/d. In young, healthy adults, a starting dosage of
75–100 mcg can be used, followed by a dosing adjustment every 4–6 weeks. Elderly patients or patients with
coronary artery disease should be started on much
smaller doses of 12.5–25.0 mcg/d, and then increased
by 12.5–25.0 mcg every 4–6 weeks until the TSH level
normalizes between 0.5 and 2 mU/L. Once stabilized,
patients should be monitored once or twice a year
with TSH and FT_4. T_4 has a half-life of about 7 days
and therefore needs to be given only once daily.

Desiccated thyroid is unsatisfactory because of its
variable hormone content and should not be used. The
use of T_3 is controversial. The current preparation is rapidly absorbed, has a short half-life, and a rapid biological
effect. Patients who experience malabsorption or who
ingest drugs such as calcium and iron, which impair T_4
absorption, may require an increase in T_4 dosing. Since

the half-life of T_4 is long, it is not a problem omitting
the drug for a few days if the patient is unable to take oral
medications. Alternately, the patient can be given parenteral L-thyroxine at 75% of the usual oral dose.

MYXEDEMA COMA

General Considerations

Severe, untreated hypothyroidism can result in a hypo-
thermic coma. It tends to occur in elderly patients and
is frequently fatal (> 20% incidence).

Clinical Findings

Myxedema coma is characterized by hypothermia, bradycardia, alveolar hypoventilation with CO_2 retention,
hyponatremia, hypoglycemia, and either stupor or coma.
The diagnosis is often difficult because the coma and
hypothermia may be due to other causes, such as stroke.
Heart failure, pneumonia, excessive fluid administration,
and sedatives or narcotic use can precipitate myxedema
coma.

Treatment

Treatment consists of L-thyroxine administered intravenously, at an initial loading dose of 300–400 mcg, followed by 80% of the calculated full replacement dose
intravenously daily. Ventilatory support may be required
for hypoventilation and hypercarbia. Hyponatremia is
treated with fluid restriction. Active rewarming is contraindicated, because it may induce vasodilation and vascular collapse. The patient should be screened for concomitant adrenal insufficiency by a cosyntropin stimulation
test. Until the cortisol results are available, the patient
should be treated with hydrocortisone (100-mg IV bolus
followed by 50 mg intravenously every 6 hours).

Jordan RM. Myxedema coma: pathophysiology, therapy, and factors
affecting prognosis. *Med Clin North Am.* 1995;79(1):185.
[PMID: 7808091] (General review of the diagnosis and treatment of myxedema coma.)

Lindsay RS, Toft AD. Hypothyroidism. *Lancet.* 1997;349(9049):413.
[PMID: 9033482] (Practical, concise review of hypothyroidism,
including the causes of hyperthyroidism and its diagnosis and
treatment.)

Woeber KA. Subclinical thyroid dysfunction. *Arch Intern Med.*
1997;157(10):1065. [PMID: 9164371] (Review focusing on
the prevalence, natural history, and potential consequence of
subclinical hypothyroidism and subclinical thyrotoxicosis.)

Malignant Thyroid Neoplasms

42

Michael C. Scheuller, MD, & David W. Eisele, MD

ESSENTIALS OF DIAGNOSIS

- *Painless, firm thyroid nodule.*
- *Euthyroid.*
- *Fine-needle aspiration (FNA) biopsy is diagnostic.*

General Considerations

Thyroid cancer accounts for approximately 1.5% of all cancers in the United States. Thyroid cancer, moreover, makes up 92% of endocrine gland cancers and accounts for approximately 12,000 new cases in the United States annually. However, only 1200 people succumb to thyroid cancer each year in the United States, making it one of the more survivable cancers. The incidence of well-differentiated thyroid cancer is approximately 2–3 times greater in women than in men. Poorly differentiated thyroid cancers are seen in equal proportions in men and women.

The spectrum of malignant thyroid disorders ranges from very indolent tumors, such as most papillary carcinomas, to highly aggressive tumors, such as anaplastic or undifferentiated carcinoma. Papillary carcinoma typically is seen in young adults and often metastasizes regionally to the lymphatics of the neck. Even in the presence of regional metastasis, however, patients with papillary carcinoma have very low mortality rates. Conversely, patients are typically in their sixth or seventh decade when a diagnosis of anaplastic thyroid cancer is made. Only 10% of patients with anaplastic thyroid cancer will survive one year after the diagnosis, with a median survival of approximately 6 months.

Pathogenesis

The two types of cells found in thyroid gland tissue include the neuroendocrine calcitonin-producing C cell (the parafollicular cell) and the follicular cell, derived from the endoderm, which synthesizes thyroglobulin. Thyroid malignancies derive from these two types of cells. Papillary carcinoma, follicular carcinoma, Hürthle cell carcinoma, and anaplastic carcinoma are derived from the follicular cells. Medullary carcinoma is derived from the parafollicular cells.

The cause of most malignant thyroid growths is unknown; however, patients whose thyroid glands have been exposed to low-dose therapeutic radiation therapy are at an increased risk of developing thyroid cancer. In general, there is a long latency period (> 20 years) between the exposure to radiation and the onset of carcinoma. Children who receive ionizing radiation (as little as 10 cGy) are more likely to develop thyroid carcinoma later in life than adults who receive equal amounts of ionizing radiation. Also, medical personnel and others exposed to radiation have a significantly higher prevalence of thyroid carcinoma than do control groups.

Medullary thyroid carcinoma is familial approximately 25% of the time. The sporadic form of medullary thyroid cancer tends to be unilateral, and the familial form is almost always bilateral and multifocal. Papillary carcinoma can also be familial, by itself or in association with familial adenomatous polyposis, Gardner syndrome, and Cowden syndrome.

Clinical Findings

A. SYMPTOMS AND SIGNS

Usually, the only presenting symptom of a patient with thyroid cancer is the presence of a palpable thyroid mass or an enlarged cervical lymph node. It is unusual for these masses to be symptomatic. Occasionally, patients present with more problematic symptoms and signs, which alert the physician to the possibility of a malignant condition. These symptoms and signs include hoarseness, localized or referred pain, dysphagia, shortness of breath, hemoptysis, and a hard, fixed thyroid nodule or neck mass. Although these symptoms may also occur with benign disease, their presence increases the suspicion of a malignant growth.

The physical examination of patients with possible thyroid cancer should include a thorough examination of the head and neck. Laryngoscopy is essential to evaluate vocal cord function because invasive cancers can invade the recurrent laryngeal nerve and cause vocal cord paralysis. Also, it is important to document any preexisting functional abnormalities of the vocal cords prior to thyroidectomy.

B. LABORATORY FINDINGS

FNA biopsy is a very accurate diagnostic test and is the primary diagnostic test for the evaluation of a thyroid nodule. The most important factors that influence the accuracy of FNA for thyroid nodules are the experience of the cytopathologist and the adequacy of the cyto-pathologic specimen. The cytopathologic finding is reported as being malignant, benign, indeterminate (eg, for follicular or Hürthle cell neoplasm), or insufficient for the diagnosis. If an FNA biopsy is deemed insufficient, it should be repeated.

Patients with thyroid neoplasms are typically euthyroid. However, the serum thyroid-stimulating hormone (TSH) and serum calcium levels should be checked preoperatively in order to determine thyroid and parathyroid function.

C. IMAGING STUDIES

1. Radionuclide imaging—If an FNA biopsy is indeterminate or insufficient for the diagnosis, other imaging studies can be used to help determine the possibility of a thyroid nodule being malignant. Radionuclide imaging with radioiodine (^{131}I) demonstrates the ability of the thyroid nodule to concentrate iodine. Nodules that actively concentrate radiolabeled iodine are considered to be "hot" nodules. Almost all "hot" nodules (99.6%) are benign. "Cold" nodules, which do not take up radioiodine ^{131}I, are more likely to be malignant. However, most "cold" nodules (80%) are also benign.

2. Ultrasonography—Ultrasonography is another imaging modality that can be used to determine the nature of a thyroid nodule. One advantage of ultrasound is its ability to determine if a thyroid nodule has a cystic component. In addition, other nonpalpable nodules may be detected. Purely cystic masses are almost always benign. Mixed lesions and completely solid lesions are potentially malignant. Ultrasound can also help guide FNA when thyroid nodules are small and difficult to palpate. Ultrasound can also detect nonpalpable extrathyroidal lymphadenopathy.

3. Other imaging studies—When further evaluation of the neck is important to determine the extent of regional metastases in thyroid cancer, magnetic resonance imaging (MRI) can sometimes be useful. In general, computed tomography (CT) scanning with contrast is to be avoided because iodinated contrast material can interfere with subsequent ^{131}I scanning or therapy, if they become necessary.

D. DIAGNOSTIC SURGERY

A diagnostic thyroid lobectomy and isthmusectomy are indicated for nodules that exhibit suspicious cytology on FNA, follicular neoplasms, nodules that enlarge on thyroid suppression therapy, and clinically suspicious nodules. Intraoperative frozen sections are not helpful in differentiating follicular adenomas from follicular carcinomas.

■ BENIGN THYROID NEOPLASMS

Benign thyroid adenomas are derived from follicular cells and represent the most common neoplasm of the thyroid gland. Adenomas typically occur in women older than 30 years of age. Surgical excision of thyroid adenomas is appropriate (1) when there is a history of ionizing radiation to the thyroid; (2) if the mass is symptomatic or cosmetically displeasing; or (3) if it is autonomously functioning, resulting in hyperthyroidism.

■ THYROID CARCINOMAS

WELL-DIFFERENTIATED THYROID CARCINOMAS

Staging

The three most commonly used staging systems for well-differentiated thyroid carcinoma are the MAICS, TNM, and AMES systems.

The **MAICS staging system** evaluates **M**etastasis, **A**ge, **I**nvasion, **C**ompleteness (of surgical resection), and **S**ize (of the tumor). Each variable is mathematically scored to determine the predicted survival rate (Table 42–1).

Table 42–1. MAICS scoring system.

Prognostic Variables	Score
Presence of distant **M**etastasis	Yes = 3, No = 0
Age at the time of diagnosis	< 39 years = 3.1, > 40 = 0.08 × age
Invasion beyond the thyroid gland	Yes = 1, No = 0
in **C**omplete surgical resection	Yes = 1, No = 0
Size of the tumor	0.3 × size in centimeters

20-year survival rate according to MAICS score.				
MAICS Score	< 6.00	6.00–6.99	7.00–7.99	> 8.00
20-year survival	99%	89%	56%	24%

Table 42–2. TNM staging system for well-differentiated thyroid carcinoma.

Stage	Age < 45	Age > 45	Incidence of Local Recurrence	Incidence of Distant Recurrence	Mortality
I	Any T Any N M0	T1 N0 M0	5.5%	2.8%	1.8%
II	Any T Any N M1	T2 or T3 N0 M0	7%	7%	11.6%
III	n/a	T4 N0 M0 Any T Any N M1	27%	13.5%	37.8%
IV	n/a	Any T Any N M1	10%	100%	90%

In addition to patient age, the **TNM staging system** of the American Joint Committee on Cancer (AJCC) prognosticates the survival rate based on **T**umor size, **N**odal metastasis, and distant **M**etastasis (Table 42–2).

The **AMES staging system** uses **A**ge, **M**etastases, **E**xtent of the primary tumor, and **S**ize of the tumor to predict survivability (Table 42–3). In this system, patients are classified as either low-risk with a mortality rate of 1.8%, or high-risk with a mortality rate of 46%.

PAPILLARY CARCINOMA

The most common malignant neoplasm of the thyroid gland is papillary carcinoma, which represents approximately 80% of all thyroid cancers. Papillary carcinoma, a well-differentiated carcinoma, arises from thyroid follicular cells. Women are affected two to three times more frequently than men, and the incidence peaks between the third and fourth decades of life. Papillary carcinomas are often multicentric and are found in both lobes of the thyroid up to 80% of the time. A multifocal presentation is particularly common in patients with prior low-dose radiation therapy to the neck. This tumor spreads via the regional lymphatics to the central and lateral cervical lymph nodes. Up to 40% of patients present with cervical or mediastinal metastases at the time of the initial diagnosis. Despite the high incidence of cervical metastases, their presence

does not increase the overall mortality. However, patients with metastatic neck disease have a greater risk of regional recurrence. The 20-year survival rate of noninvasive papillary carcinoma is very high (95%).

Histologically, papillary carcinoma is characterized by finger-like projections of follicular cells interposed with calcifications, intranuclear vacuoles, and psammoma bodies. Intranuclear vacuoles are often referred to as "Orphan Annie eyes" because of their characteristic rounded appearance. Psammoma bodies are present in just over 50% of papillary carcinomas; when they are found in extrathyroidal tissue, they are strongly suggestive of metastatic papillary carcinoma. The follicular variant of papillary carcinoma has a similar behavior to classic papillary carcinoma.

Treatment of papillary carcinoma is thyroidectomy as well as the removal of regional neck nodes by selective neck dissection when lymph nodes are involved. Total thyroidectomy is recommended by most surgeons, although lobectomy and isthmusectomy is acceptable for microcarcinomas (ie, < 1.0 cm). The advantages of total thyroidectomy include a decreased recurrence rate and the ability to use thyroglobulin and radioactive iodine scans for the diagnosis of recurrent disease postoperatively. Patients with tumors > 1.5 cm and high-risk patients benefit from postoperative ^{131}I therapy. In addition, all patients with well-differentiated thyroid carcinomas should be treated indefinitely with suppressive doses of L-thyroxine (levothyroxine).

Table 42–3. AMES staging system.

Low Risk = 1.8% Mortality Rate	High Risk = 46% Mortality Rate
Men < 41 years old and women < 51 years old All patients without distant metastases	All patients with distant metastases
All men > 41 years old and women > 51 years old with: 1. Intrathyroidal papillary carcinoma OR 2. Follicular carcinoma with minor capsular involvement AND 3. Primary tumor < 5 cm in diameter AND 4. No distant metastases	All men > 41 years old and women > 51 years old with: 1. Extra-thyroidal papillary carcinoma OR 2. Follicular carcinoma with major capsular involvement AND/OR 3. Primary cancer ≥ 5 cm in diameter

FOLLICULAR CARCINOMA

Follicular carcinoma, like papillary carcinoma, is another well-differentiated thyroid carcinoma. Approximately 10–15% of all thyroid cancers have a follicular histology. It occurs two to three times more frequently in women than in men. It typically occurs later in life than papillary carcinoma and usually arises with a mean age at presentation in the fifth or sixth decade of life.

Even though papillary carcinoma is associated with a lower mortality rate than follicular carcinoma, follicular carcinoma is still considered a highly survivable cancer. The 10-year survival rate is approximately 85% and the 20-year survival rate is approximately 70%. Compared with papillary carcinoma, follicular carcinoma does not metastasize via the lymphatics as frequently, and few patients have regional metastases at the time of the initial diagnosis. Follicular carcinoma is more likely than papillary carcinoma to spread via hematogenous pathways and tends to spread to the lungs, liver, and bone.

Histologically, follicular carcinoma can be difficult to distinguish from normal thyroid tissue. The presence of capsular or vascular invasion differentiates follicular carcinoma from follicular adenoma. The treatment of follicular carcinoma is total thyroidectomy followed by ^{131}I ablation and L-thyroxine suppression therapy.

HÜRTHLE CELL CARCINOMA

Hürthle cell carcinoma is considered to be an aggressive variant of follicular carcinoma and accounts for approximately 2% of thyroid carcinomas. Hürthle cell carcinoma is composed of Hürthle (oxyphilic) cells, which are eosinophilic follicular cells that contain large amounts of mitochondria. Approximately 70% of patients with Hürthle cell carcinoma present with intrathyroid disease alone, 20% with regional cervical lymph node metastasis, and 10% with distant metastases. The treatment of Hürthle cell carcinoma is total thyroidectomy. Patients with regional metastases require selective neck dissection. Most Hürthle cell carcinomas exhibit low ^{131}I uptake.

INVASIVE WELL-DIFFERENTIATED CARCINOMA

Both papillary carcinoma and follicular cell carcinoma can invade adjacent structures, including the trachea, the larynx, the esophagus, the laryngeal nerves, and blood vessels. Invasive well-differentiated carcinomas are much more likely to metastasize (up to 80%) and are associated with higher mortality rates than noninvasive well-differentiated carcinoma (up to 20% at 10 years). Patients presenting with either hemoptysis or dyspnea and thyroid carcinoma are particularly likely to harbor an invasive form of carcinoma. These neoplasms are best treated with complete surgical resection, including total thyroidectomy with postoperative ^{131}I therapy. Select patients may also benefit from adjuvant external beam radiation therapy.

OTHER THYROID CARCINOMAS

MEDULLARY CARCINOMA

Medullary thyroid carcinoma originates from the parafollicular cells (C cells) of the thyroid. It accounts for approximately 5–10% of malignant thyroid neoplasms. The incidence is almost equal in men and women. Approximately 75% of medullary carcinomas occur sporadically, but 25% are familial in origin. Familial medullary carcinoma occurs in three forms: (1) MEN 2a (multiple endocrine neoplasia syndrome), (2) MEN 2b, and (3) non-MEN familial. Patients with MEN 2a and non-MEN familial medullary carcinoma have a better prognosis than patients with either MEN 2b or the sporadic type. The mean survival rate for all medullary thyroid cancers is approximately 50%. Regional lymph node involvement is common (50%). The diagnosis of medullary carcinoma is typically made by an FNA biopsy. An elevated serum calcitonin level is characteristic. Serum carcinoembryonic antigen (CEA) levels may also be elevated.

Mutation of the *RET* proto-oncogene is seen in most cases of familial medullary carcinoma. The family members of patients with familial medullary thyroid carcinoma should be considered for screening for this point mutation in *RET*. Individuals determined to have the mutation for MEN 2a should undergo prophylactic total thyroidectomy before 6 years of age. In patients with the more aggressive MEN 2b, prophylactic thyroidectomy is recommended before the age of 2.

Surgery is the only effective therapy for medullary carcinoma. Before surgery, it is important to rule out a concomitant pheochromocytoma. Total thyroidectomy and a central neck dissection are recommended for all patients with medullary carcinoma. An ipsilateral selective neck dissection is also recommended. Select patients may benefit from external-beam radiation therapy postoperatively.

Postoperatively, a serum calcitonin level should be obtained. Elevation of the serum calcitonin level indicates persistent disease. Localizing studies for residual carcinoma include ultrasound, MRI, and radionuclide scans, such as DMSA. Selective venous sampling of calcitonin can also be performed. Laparoscopy is the most sensitive study for distant metastases. Surgical resection is recommended for select patients with identifiable residual disease or palliation of locoregional recurrences despite distant metastases.

ANAPLASTIC CARCINOMA

Anaplastic (undifferentiated) carcinoma is a highly lethal cancer that is associated with a mortality rate of greater than 90% within 2 years of the initial diagnosis. Anaplastic carcinoma constitutes approximately 1% of all malignant thyroid disorders. Its incidence is equal in men and women and patients typically are older than 65 years of age. This disorder usually arises from a well-differentiated thyroid carcinoma.

Anaplastic carcinoma is frequently locally invasive into adjacent structures. It often metastasizes regionally as well as distally. Histologically, this tumor has large numbers of mitoses and is seen in three main forms: spindle cell, giant cell, and small cell.

Treatment is generally palliative with radiation therapy and chemotherapy. Infrequently, localized anaplastic carcinomas can be cured with surgery and postoperative radiation therapy. Tracheotomy and gastrostomy tube placement are often beneficial adjuncts for the palliative care of most patients with anaplastic carcinoma.

THYROID LYMPHOMA

Thyroid lymphoma represents 1–5% of malignant thyroid disorders, and its incidence is increasing. Patients with Hashimoto thyroiditis have a 70-fold increased risk of thyroid lymphoma compared with that of the general population. Thyroid lymphoma occurs approximately eight times more frequently in women than in men. The mean age of patients diagnosed with thyroid lymphoma is over 60 years. Patients typically present with a rapidly growing thyroid mass, neck swelling, hoarseness, neck pain, and dysphagia.

Non-Hodgkin lymphoma (NHL) accounts for the majority of thyroid lymphomas and is often classified as histiocytic lymphoma. NHL of the thyroid gland usually arises from the thyroid gland itself. Hodgkin lymphomas tend to occur in other locations and either invade or metastasize to the thyroid gland. Differentiating thyroid lymphoma from anaplastic carcinoma can be problematic and an open biopsy may be necessary.

Treatment for thyroid lymphoma is primarily radiation therapy for localized disease and chemotherapy for systemic disease. The 5-year survival rate with lymphoma confined to the thyroid gland is more than twice as high (85%) as with extrathyroidal cervical disease (35%).

THYROGLOSSAL DUCT CARCINOMA

Carcinoma of the thyroglossal duct is typically papillary carcinoma, although other malignant types, except medullary thyroid carcinoma, can occur. The diagnosis can be made by FNA or following the removal of a presumed thyroglossal duct cyst. Treatment is surgical resection by the Sistrunk procedure and L-thyroxine suppression therapy.

METASTATIC CARCINOMA TO THE THYROID

Melanoma, lung carcinoma, breast carcinoma, and renal cell carcinoma are the most common neoplasms to metastasize to the thyroid gland. FNA biopsy is usually helpful in the diagnosis of metastatic carcinoma of the thyroid gland. In particular, renal cell carcinoma may be difficult to differentiate from a primary thyroid neoplasm unless proper immunohistochemical staining is performed.

■ TREATMENT CONSIDERATIONS

COMPLICATIONS OF THYROIDECTOMY

The complications of thyroidectomy are unusual and include neck hematoma, recurrent laryngeal nerve injury, and hypoparathyroidism. Neck hematoma can cause airway compromise and must be evacuated immediately. Injury to the recurrent laryngeal nerve causes ipsilateral vocal cord paralysis and occurs in approximately 1% of cases. Bilateral recurrent laryngeal nerve injury can cause airway obstruction, which often requires a tracheotomy. Hypoparathyroidism occurs in less than 2% of patients who undergo total thyroidectomy or thyroid lobectomy following prior contralateral lobectomy. Treatment for hypoparathyroidism requires supplemental calcium replacement therapy, with or without calcitriol (ie, Rocaltrol). If the intraoperative removal of all parathyroid tissue is suspected, parathyroid tissue can be autotransplanted into a muscle and should, in most cases, regain function.

Blankenship DR, Chin E, Terris DJ. Contemporary management of thyroid carcinoma. *Am J Otolaryngol.* 2005;26(4):249. [PMID: 15991091] (Review article discussing approaches to thyroid malignancies.)

D'Avanzo A, Treseler P, Ituarte PH, et al. Follicular thyroid CA: histology and prognosis. *Cancer.* 2004;100(6):1123. [PMID: 15022277] (Retrospective study describing the behavior of follicular thyroid carcinoma.)

Sniezek JC, Holtel M. Rare tumors of the thyroid gland. *Otolaryngol Clin North Am.* 2003;36(1):107. [PMID: 12803012] (Review article on the diagnosis and treatment of rare thyroid malignancies.)

Wein RO, Weber RS. Contemporary management of differentiated thyroid carcinoma. *Otolaryngol Clin North Am.* 2005;38(1):161. [PMID: 15649506] (Review article on well-differentiated malignant thyroid disorders.)

Parathyroid Disorders

43

Karsten Munck, MD, & David W. Eisele, MD

■ EMBRYOLOGY & ANATOMY

The parathyroid glands are typically composed of four glands: two superior and two inferior. Although 85% of the population has four glands, 3–7% have more than four glands, and 3–6% have fewer. Both pairs of glands are formed during the fifth week of embryogenesis. The superior glands arise from the fourth branchial pouch, and the inferior glands are derived from the third branchial pouch. They subsequently detach from the pharynx and migrate caudally, coming to lie in their final positions during the seventh week of gestation.

The superior parathyroid glands are usually located in the fat posterior to the superior lobe of the thyroid, near the site where the recurrent laryngeal nerve enters the larynx. The inferior parathyroid glands tend to be found within or in close proximity to the thymic tissue that extends from the inferior pole of the thyroid gland.

The parathyroid glands tend to remain fairly constant in their anatomic location, with each gland exhibiting positional symmetry with the contralateral gland. Considerable anatomic variability, however, can occur. The superior parathyroid gland and the lateral lobe of the thyroid remain in close proximity as they migrate together during embryogenesis. Therefore, the superior parathyroid gland may be directly embedded within the lateral lobe of the thyroid gland. Occasionally, the superior parathyroid gland may be located in a retropharyngeal, retrolaryngeal, or retroesophageal position. The gland may also continue to migrate caudally along the esophagus, into the posterior mediastinum.

The inferior parathyroid gland descends with the thymus and can exhibit variability in its final location. The gland can be found anywhere from the level of the carotid bifurcation to the anterior mediastinum. Regardless of its location, it is generally associated with the thymus or thymic tissue (eg, the parathymus). Infrequently, the inferior parathyroid gland can be intrathyroidal.

The inferior thyroid artery usually supplies both the inferior and the superior parathyroid glands, but on occasion an anastomotic branch between the inferior and the superior thyroid artery supplies the superior parathyroid gland.

■ HYPERPARATHYROIDISM

Hypercalcemia has an incidence of approximately 0.5% in the general population. Although the differential diagnosis of hypercalcemia is extensive, hyperparathyroidism is the most common cause of hypercalcemia in nonhospitalized patients (Table 43–1). Primary hyperparathyroidism, due to a parathyroid adenoma, is the most common of the parathyroid disorders. Secondary and tertiary hyperparathyroid disease is mostly seen in patients with renal disease.

PRIMARY HYPERPARATHYROIDISM

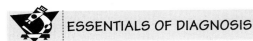 ESSENTIALS OF DIAGNOSIS

- *Elevated serum calcium.*
- *Elevated serum parathyroid hormone.*
- *Familial hypocalciuric hypercalcemia may be incorrectly diagnosed as primary hyperparathyroidism.*

General Considerations

Primary hyperparathyroidism is most common in postmenopausal women, with a peak incidence in the third to fifth decades. Primary hyperparathyroidism is characterized by the production and secretion of excess parathyroid hormone (PTH) and has been associated with low-dose radiation therapy. Primary hyperparathyroidism can be attributed to a single parathyroid adenoma (83%), double adenomas (2–3%), multigland hyperplasia (12%), or, rarely, carcinoma of the parathyroid gland (1%). The overproduction of PTH results in the mobilization of calcium from bone and inhibition of the renal absorption of phosphate.

Clinical Findings

Historically, renal disease and skeletal manifestations have been the presenting problems of patients with primary hyperparathyroidism. Currently, most patients are diag-

Table 43–1. Causes of hypercalcemia.

Hyperparathyroidism
Malignant neoplasms
    Breast, lung, kidney, prostate, and thyroid malignant
      growths, as well as multiple myeloma, leukemia, and
      PTH-secreting cancers
Endocrine disorders
    Hyperthyroidism, adrenal insufficiency, pheochromocy-
      toma, and VIPoma
Granulomatous diseases
    Sarcoidosis, tuberculosis, histoplasmosis, coccidiomycosis,
      and leprosy
Drugs and vitamins
    Thiazide diuretics, lithium, aluminum, and vitamins A and D
Immobilization
Milk alkali syndrome
Renal disease
Benign familial hypocalciuric hypercalcemia

nosed with the disease through routine laboratory tests. Many patients are asymptomatic or have nonspecific symptoms that resolve after successful surgical treatment.

A. Symptoms and Signs

The signs and symptoms of primary hyperparathyroidism include the following categories: neurologic, renal, gastrointestinal, and cardiovascular. They can be loosely described as "stones, bones, abdominal groans, psychic moans, and fatigue overtones."

1. Neurologic symptoms—The neurologic signs and symptoms include muscular weakness, fatigue, depression, anorexia, confusion, headache, and memory loss.

2. Renal symptoms—Polyuria, polydipsia, renal colic, and nephrocalcinosis are the most common renal symptoms.

3. Gastrointestinal symptoms—Patients may present with constipation, nausea, vomiting, pancreatitis, peptic ulcer disease, or abdominal pain.

4. Cardiovascular symptoms—Hypertension and cardiac arrhythmias are the most common cardiovascular symptoms.

5. Other symptoms—Other common presenting signs and symptoms include arthralgia, myalgia, and pruritus.

B. Laboratory Findings

1. Calcium—Hypercalcemia is the most important biochemical finding when evaluating patients for primary hyperparathyroidism. It is important to recognize that hypoalbuminemia can give the appearance of a normal total calcium level, despite an elevated level of ionized serum calcium.

2. Parathyroid hormone—An elevated serum PTH level in the setting of an elevated serum calcium level is virtually diagnostic for primary hyperparathyroidism. PTH is low for essentially all other causes of hypercalcemia.

3. Phosphate—PTH tends to increase the renal excretion of phosphate, causing the serum level of phosphate to be decreased in hyperparathyroidism.

4. Urine calcium—Patients with primary hyperparathyroidism should have a high or normal 24-hour urinary calcium level. If the patient is noted to have a low 24-hour urinary calcium level, the cause of the patient's hypercalcemia can be secondary to familial hypocalciuric hypercalcemia syndrome rather than primary hyperparathyroidism.

C. Imaging Studies

Preoperative localization imaging studies are indicated for patients who are candidates for minimally invasive parathyroidectomy, failed prior surgery, or recurrent primary hyperparathyroidism.

1. Ultrasound—High-resolution ultrasound has been used for the preoperative localization of parathyroid adenoma. The sensitivity of ultrasound in preoperatively detecting parathyroid adenoma has been reported to be in the range of 60–90%. This modality is highly dependent on the experience of the individual performing the imaging study and may help to explain the large variability in the sensitivities reported.

2. Sestamibi scans—One of the main advances in both the imaging of the parathyroid glands and the preoperative localization of parathyroid adenoma has come with the use of technetium-99m sestamibi scans. The sensitivity of sestamibi scans is in the range of 70–80% for the localization of parathyroid adenoma. Recently, the use of delayed technetium-99m sestamibi single-photon emission computed tomography (SPECT) has allowed for the localization of an adenoma in two-dimensional space. Sestamibi SPECT scans have been reported to have a sensitivity of 87%, an accuracy of 94%, and a positive predictive value of 86%. The sensitivity of sestamibi SPECT scans is similar in patients undergoing operative exploration and subsequent surgery.

3. Methylene blue—The preoperative injection of methylene blue (ie, methylthionine chloride) has been reported by some clinicians to facilitate the intraoperative identification of parathyroid adenoma. The sensitivity of this technique has been reported to be similar to sestamibi scans. When these two modalities have been used together, they have been reported to increase diagnostic sensitivity to 96%. Neurotoxicity has been reported with higher doses of methylene blue in patients on selective reuptake inhibitors. Similar side effects have been avoided with lower doses and without degradation in efficacy.

Treatment

Surgery is the only effective treatment for primary hyperparathyroidism. Nephrolithiasis, bone disease, and neuromuscular symptoms all respond very well to the surgical removal of diseased parathyroid tissue. Historically, only patients with symptomatic hyperparathyroidism or extremely high calcium levels were considered to be good surgical candidates. At present, it is generally accepted that all patients with either symptomatic or asymptomatic hyperparathyroidism will benefit from surgery. Early surgical intervention can not only alleviate symptoms, but it can also prevent the potential future complications of hyperparathyroidism and in most cases reverse some of the associated bone loss.

A. PRINCIPLES OF OPERATIVE INTERVENTION

Bilateral neck exploration has previously been considered the gold standard surgical approach for primary hyperparathyroidism. The operation is accomplished through a transverse incision in the lower neck. This incision is carried down through the platysma muscle. Subplatysmal flaps are elevated. The strap muscles are divided in the midline and retracted laterally. One thyroid lobe is exposed and retracted medially, and the parathyroid glands are identified.

If a bilateral neck exploration fails to reveal four parathyroid glands that are located relatively symmetrically, the thymic pedicle should be explored. In addition, the thyroid lobe on the side of the missing gland should be mobilized and palpated, which then allows for exploration of the retrolaryngeal area, the tracheoesophageal groove, and the great vessels of the neck (Table 43–2).

Once the parathyroid glands have been identified, an intraoperative decision has to be made regarding the extent of resection. Although a single adenoma is most likely, both double adenomas and multigland hyperplasia must be considered. If a single abnormal-appearing parathyroid gland is identified, it is removed and parathyroid tissue is confirmed by frozen section.

In the event that a four-gland hyperplasia is identified, there are two acceptable surgical options. The first option is a **total parathyroidectomy** with autotransplantation of

Table 43–2. Aberrant locations of parathyroid adenoma.

Anterior mediastinum
Posterior mediastinum
Retroesophageal area
Retrolaryngeal area
Tracheoesophageal groove
Intrathyroidal area
Carotid bifurcation

parathyroid tissue into either the sternocleidomastoid muscle or the brachioradialis muscle of the nondominant arm. This technique offers the advantage of easy access to the implanted tissue if the patient requires a reoperative procedure for recurrent or persistent hyperparathyroidism. The main disadvantage of total parathyroidectomy is the potential for permanent hypoparathyroidism if the transplanted gland tissue does not function. The second approach is a **subtotal parathyroidectomy** with removal of three and one half of the parathyroid glands, leaving a portion of a parathyroid gland in situ. The advantage of this approach is that the parathyroid tissue remains attached to its native blood supply.

B. INTRAOPERATIVE PARATHYROID HORMONE MONITORING

The intraoperative use of a rapid PTH assay has become an important adjunct in helping the surgeon determine the adequacy of the parathyroid gland resection. The normal half-life of PTH is approximately 3–5 minutes, making it easy to evaluate a decrease in serum PTH following the resection of adenomatous or hyperplastic parathyroid tissue. A decrease in the PTH level by 50% or more at 10 minutes after adenoma excision—compared with the preexcision baseline PTH—reliably predicts surgical success. Compared with frozen sections, intraoperative PTH has been shown to be indispensable in guiding the operative strategy during focused exploration parathyroid surgery.

C. AUTOTRANSPLANTATION OF PARATHYROID TISSUE

If parathyroid tissue is removed with the intent of autotransplantation, it should be promptly placed in iced saline. When the surgeon is ready to perform the autotransplantation, the specimen is removed from the saline and sectioned into 1–2 mm pieces. Individual muscle beds are created for each slice of parathyroid tissue in either the sternocleidomastoid or the brachioradialis muscle of the arm. Once the parathyroid tissue has been transplanted into the muscle, the site of implantation is marked with a surgical clip. In most cases, within 2–3 months from the time of autotransplantation, the graft is neovascularized and functioning. Parathyroid tissue can also be sent for cryopreservation for up to 18 months. If the initial autotransplantation of the graft fails and is nonfunctional after 2 months, the sample, which has been cryopreserved, can be autotransplanted with a 50% chance of eventual function.

Complications of Parathyroidectomy

Postoperative hypocalcemia can occur following parathyroidectomy. The chronic stimulation of the bone with PTH results in the skeletal depletion of calcium. The normalization of PTH causes the bone reuptake of calcium, with a resultant fall in serum calcium; this condition is clinically referred to as the "hungry bone syndrome." The preoperative elevation of serum alkaline phosphatase predicts this problem. Permanent hypoparathyroidism may complicate parathyroidectomy in < 2% of cases of adenoma and in 10–30% of cases of hyperplasia. Conversely, persistent hyperparathyroidism complicates 5% of the operative procedures of primary hyperparathyroidism; it may reoccur in up to 16% of patients with nonfamilial hyperplastic parathyroid disease and in 26–36% of patients with familial hyperplastic disease. Permanent recurrent laryngeal nerve injury occurs in < 1% of patients undergoing parathyroidectomy. Neck hematoma and infection are unusual complications after parathyroidectomy.

SECONDARY HYPERPARATHYROIDISM

Hyperparathyroidism can develop as a consequence of chronic renal failure, which results in increased serum phosphate levels and a decrease in 1-hydroxylase (ie, α-1-hydroxylase) activity in the kidney. These factors act in synergy to cause hypocalcemia, which causes the parathyroid glands to be chronically stimulated. Treatment of this disorder is focused on treating the underlying renal failure.

TERTIARY HYPERPARATHYROIDISM

Some patients with secondary hyperparathyroidism develop tertiary hyperparathyroidism. In this condition, the parathyroid glands autonomously secrete PTH, despite correction of the underlying cause of the hyperparathyroidism (eg, after kidney transplantation).

HYPERPARATHYROIDISM IN PREGNANCY

Hyperparathyroidism in pregnancy is a rare disorder that can have detrimental consequences for the fetus. Surgical exploration should be accomplished during the second trimester of pregnancy to minimize the potential complications of neonatal tetany, stillbirth, and spontaneous abortion. Total parathyroidectomy with autotransplantation is the treatment of choice for this disorder.

During pregnancy, the PTH of the mother does not cross the placenta, which results in chronic suppression of the fetal parathyroid glands. After birth, the neonate's serum calcium level quickly drops without the maternal calcium via the placenta. It takes approximately 7–10 days for the newborn's parathyroid glands to respond to the hypocalcemia by secreting adequate PTH. Thus, profound hypocalcemia can occur in the early perinatal period.

■ OTHER PARATHYROID DISORDERS

MULTIPLE ENDOCRINE NEOPLASIA

Multiple endocrine neoplasia (MEN) syndromes are characterized by an autosomal dominant hereditary pattern with a predilection to develop tumors of the endocrine organs, including the parathyroid glands. Parathyroid hyperplasia is seen in several of these disorders, which results in elevated PTH in patients with MEN 1 and MEN 2a. MEN 1 is characterized by concurrent parathyroid hyperplasia, pancreatic islet cell tumors, and pituitary adenomas. MEN 2a consists of medullary carcinoma of the thyroid, pheochromocytoma, and parathyroid hyperplasia.

PARATHYROID CARCINOMA

Carcinoma of the parathyroid gland is a rare entity, accounting for < 1% of all patients with hyperparathyroidism. The histologic criteria for the diagnosis of parathyroid carcinoma include one of the following: (1) metastases to lymph nodes or distant organs, (2) capsular or local invasion, or (3) local recurrence following resection. Distant metastases tend to occur in the liver, lung, and bone.

Patients with parathyroid carcinoma typically present with symptomatic hypercalcemia and markedly elevated PTH levels. They may have symptoms of local invasion. A firm mass may be palpable on examination of the neck.

During the operative resection for parathyroid carcinoma, invasion of the surrounding tissue is usually noted. It is important to obtain wide local resection of the involved gland, usually with resection of the ipsilateral thyroid lobe. In cases of clinically involved neck nodes, a neck dissection is indicated. Patients who are treated with this approach have a 50% cure rate. In cases of recurrence, patients should undergo surgical resection for control of locoregional disease. Symptomatic control from hypercalcemia has been achieved in some patients using bisphosphonates and a new class of drugs known as calcimimetics. Recurrence is common in patients with parathyroid carcinoma; therefore, these patients require close follow-up.

Akerstrom G, Malmaeus J, Bergstrom R. Surgical anatomy of human parathyroid glands. 1984;95:14. [PMID: 6691181] (Review of 503 autopsy cases involving the parathyroid glands.)

Chen H, Pruhs Z, Starling JR, Mack E. Intraoperative parathyroid hormone testing improves cure rates in patients undergoing minimally invasive parathyroidectomy. *Surgery.* 2005;138(4):583.

Clark O. Diagnosis of primary hyperparathyroidism. In: Clark O, Duh Q, eds. *Textbook of Endocrine Surgery.* Philadelphia: WB Saunders, 1997. (Textbook on endocrine surgery.)

Giordano A, Rubello D, Casara D. New trends in parathyroid scintigraphy. *Euro J Nucl Med.* 2001;28:1409. [PMID: 11585302] (Review of recent advances in parathyroid scintigraphy.)

Halsted WS, Evans HM. The parathyroid glandules: their blood supply and their preservation in operations upon the thyroid gland. *Ann Surg.* 1907;46:489. (Historical article on the anatomy of the parathyroid gland.)

Iacobone M, Scarpa M, Lumachi F, Favia G. Are frozen sections useful and cost-effective in the era of intraoperative qPTH assays? *Surgery.* 2005;138(6):1164. [PMID: 16360404] (Compares the cost of using frozen sections for intraoperative diagnosis of parathyroid adenoma versus rapid parathyroid hormone.)

Kacker A, Komisar A. Unilateral versus bilateral neck exploration in parathyroid surgery: an assessment of 55 cases. *Ear Nose Throat J.* 2001;80:530. [PMID: 11523470] (Retrospective review of 55 cases comparing unilateral with bilateral neck exploration in parathyroid surgery.)

Kearns AE, Thompson GB. Medical and surgical management of hyperparathyroidism. *Mayo Clin Proc.* 2002;77:87. [PMID: 11794462] (Review of the medical and surgical management of hyperparathyroidism.)

Kebebew E, Arici C, Duh Q, Clark O. Localization and reoperation results for persistent and recurrent parathyroid carcinoma. *Arch Surg.* 2001;136:878. [PMID: 11485522] (Retrospective review of the clinical experience in reoperative surgery for parathyroid carcinoma.)

Krauz Y, Bettman L, Guralnik L et al. Technetium-99m-MIBI SPECT/CT in primary hyperparathyroidism. *World J Surg.* 2006;30(1):76. [PMID: 16369710] (Describes the use of combined nuclear and CT imaging to provide three-dimensional localization.)

Majithia A, Stearns MP. Methylene blue toxicity following infusion to localize parathyroid adenoma. *J Laryngol Otol.* 2006;120(2):138. [PMID: 16359577] (Describes complications from the use of methylene blue for intraoperative identification.)

Mandell DH, Genden EM, Mechanick JI, Bergman DA, Diamond EJ, Urken ML. The influence of intraoperative parathyroid hormone monitoring on the surgical management of hyperparathyroidism. *Arch Otolaryngol Head Neck Surg.* 2001;127:821. [PMID: 11448357] (Retrospective review of the clinical use of intraoperative parathyroid hormone levels.)

Nobori M, Saiki S, Tanaka N et al. Blood supply of the parathyroid glands from the superior thyroid artery. *Surgery.* 1994;115:417. [PMID: 8165531] (Anatomic description of blood supply to the parathyroid glands.)

Orloff LA. Methylene blue and sestamibi: complementary tools for localizing parathyroids. *Laryngoscope.* 2001;111:1901. [PMID: 11801966] (Nonrandomized study evaluating the use of methylene blue in operative localization of the parathyroid glands.)

Poorten VL, Debruyene F, Delaere PR. Recent trends in the initial surgical treatment of primary hyperparathyroidism: a review. *Acta Otorhinolaryngol Belg.* 2001;55:159. [PMID: 11441475] (Review of the evaluation of parathyroid surgery.)

Silverberg SJ. Natural history of primary hyperparathyroidism. *Endocrinol Metab Clin North Am.* 2000;29:451. [PMID: 11033755] (Provides history of primary hyperparathyroidism.)

Udelsman R. Complications of parathyroid surgery. In: Eisele DW, ed. *Complications in Head and Neck Surgery.* St. Louis: Mosby, 1993. (Textbook on complications of head and neck surgery.)

Thompson N, Eckhauser F, Harness J. The anatomy of primary hyperparathyroidism. *Surgery.* 1982;92:814. [PMID: 7135202] (Retrospective review of the anatomic location of parathyroid adenomas.)

Ulanovski D, Feinmesser R, Cohen M, Sulkes J, Dudkiewicz M, Shpitzer T. Preoperative evaluation of patients with parathyroid adenoma: the role of high-resolution ultrasonography. *Head Neck Surg.* 2001;24:1. [PMID: 11774396] (Prospective evaluation of ultrasonography in the preoperative localization of parathyroid adenomas.)

SECTION XI
Otology

Anatomy & Physiology of the Ear · 44

John S. Oghalai, MD, & William E. Brownell, PhD

Sound (detected by the cochlea) and gravity and rotational acceleration (detected by the vestibular organs) are forms of mechanical energy. Sound is a mechanical vibration (eg, as produced by a vibrating piano string). This vibration sets up small oscillations of air molecules that, in turn, cause adjacent molecules to oscillate as the sound propagates away from its source. Sound is called a pressure wave because when the molecules of air come closer together, the pressure increases (**compression**)**;** as they move further apart, the pressure decreases (**rarefaction).**

A sound is characterized by its frequency and intensity. The **frequency** of a sound is its pitch. Middle C on a piano has a frequency of 256 cycles per second, whereas high C (7 white keys to the right) has a frequency of 512 cycles per second (Figure 44–1). People with normal hearing can tell the difference between two sounds that differ by less 0.5%. To appreciate how small a difference in frequency this is, one needs only to realize that middle C differs from C sharp (the black piano key immediately to the right of middle C) by more than 5%. Human hearing is limited to sound waves between 20 Hz and 20,000 Hz. Many other mammals can hear ultrasound (> 20,000 Hz), and some, such as whales, approach 100,000 Hz.

The **intensity** of a sound determines its loudness and reflects how tightly packed the molecules of air become during the compression phase of a sound wave. The ear can detect sounds in which the vibration of the air at the tympanic membrane is less than the diameter of a hydrogen molecule. The mammalian ear has the ability to discriminate a wide range of intensities—over a 100,000-fold difference in energy (120 dB).

To maximize the transfer of sound energy from the air-filled environment to the fluid-filled inner ear, land animals evolved external ears as sound collectors and middle ears as mechanical force amplifiers (Figure 44–2).

The task of the cochlea is to analyze environmental sounds and transmit the results of that analysis to the brain. The inner ear first determines how much energy is present at the different frequencies that make up a specific sound. The cochlea can do this because of its **tonotopic organization,** whereby different frequency tones stimulate different areas of the cochlea. This mapping of frequency information is just one of several strategies that the ear uses to code incoming information. The frequency analysis of environmental sounds begins in the external ear.

EXTERNAL EAR

1. Pinna

The external ear consists of the pinna and the external auditory canal. The pinna is a three-layered structure. The central framework consists of elastic cartilage surrounded on either side by a layer of skin. There is minimal subcutaneous tissue between the skin and the perichondrium (Figure 44–3).

Physiologically, the pinna acts to funnel sound waves from the outside environment into the ear canal. The intricate shape of the pinna affects the frequency response of incoming sounds differently, depending on the vertical position from which the sound originated. This information is used by the brain to localize the sound source in three-dimensional space. Overall, the shape of the external ear provides approximately 20 dB of gain to sounds in the middle frequency range (2–4 kHz).

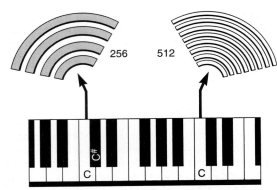

Figure 44–1. The pressure waves of sound are represented by the advancing concentric lines radiating away from the vibrating source. Middle C has a frequency of 256 cycles per second, while upper C (one octave higher) has a frequency of 512 cycles per second.

2. External Auditory Canal

The external auditory canal consists of a lateral cartilaginous portion and a medial bony portion. Each portion of the canal takes up approximately half of its length. The tragus forms the anterior cartilaginous canal. Directly in front of it lies the parotid gland. The facial nerve exits the stylomastoid foramen 1 cm deep to the tip of the tragus (the tragal pointer). Within the anterior and inferior portions of the cartilaginous ear canal, there are small fenestrations through the cartilage called the **fissures of Santorini.** Infection of the ear canal (otitis externa) can spread to the parotid gland through these fissures and may lead to skull base osteomyelitis. The tympanic portion of the temporal bone forms most of the bony ear canal. Anterior to the bony canal is the temporomandibular joint. The skin of the ear canal is thicker in the cartilaginous canal and contains glands that secrete cerumen (ear wax). The skin of the bony ear canal is very thin and fixed to the periosteum. No cerumen is secreted in the bony ear canal.

The great auricular nerve (from nerve roots C2 and C3) provides sensory innervation to the skin overlying the mastoid process as well as to most of the pinna. Cranial nerves V (the trigeminal nerve), VII (the facial nerve), and X (the vagus nerve) innervate the external auditory canal.

MIDDLE EAR

1. Tympanic Membrane

The tympanic membrane consists of three layers: outer, middle, and inner. The outer layer arises from the ectoderm, which consists of squamous epithelium. The inner layer originates from the endoderm and consists of cuboidal mucosal epithelium. The middle layer originates from the mesenchyme and is called the middle fibrous layer. The middle fibrous layer of the tympanic membrane consists of both radial and circumferential fibers. These fibers are important in maintaining the strength of the tympanic membrane as well as in aiding the proper vibration of the tympanic membrane with different frequency sounds.

The tympanic membrane has an oval shape and is approximately 8 mm wide and 10 mm high (Figure 44–4). The tympanic membrane is sloped so that the superior aspect is lateral to the inferior aspect. In addition, the tympanic membrane is tented medially by the long process of the malleus (manubrium). Around the circumference of the tympanic membrane is the fibrous annulus, which sits in the tympanic sulcus, a groove in the bone at the medial end of the external auditory canal. The annulus is incomplete superior to the anterior and the posterior malleal folds. This section of the

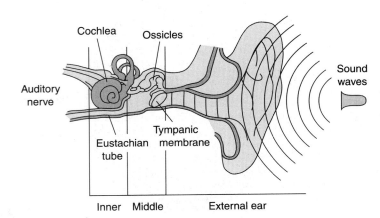

Figure 44–2. Anatomy of the ear. The external ear collects sound pressure waves and funnels them toward the tympanic membrane. The middle ear ossicles transmit the sound waves to the inner ear (cochlea). The middle ear acts to match the impedance difference between the air of the external environment to the fluid within the cochlea. This permits maximal sound transmission.

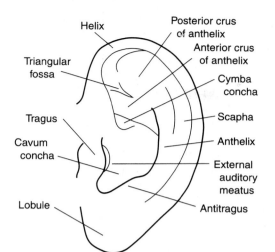

Figure 44–3. Anatomy of the pinna. The pinna consists of a cartilaginous framework covered by skin.

tympanic membrane above the anterior and posterior malleal folds is the pars flaccida, while the section inferior to the folds is the pars tensa. The pars flaccida is also known as the **Shrapnell membrane.** The middle fibrous layer of the pars flaccida is weaker than that of the pars tensa. Hence, this area of the tympanic membrane can easily retract inwardly when the middle ear pressure is less than the environmental air pressure. Moreover, this area is often the starting point of an attic

cholesteatoma. Blood vessels enter the tympanic membrane through the superior external auditory canal skin (the vascular strip) as well as circumferentially from around the fibrous annulus.

2. Middle Ear Cavity

The middle ear cavity (Figure 44–5) originates embryologically from the first branchial pouch. It is connected to the nasopharynx via the eustachian tube. Posterior to the middle ear cavity are the mastoid air cells, which connect with the attic portion of the middle ear cavity through the aditus ad antrum. The middle ear cavity and mastoid air cells are lined with ciliated mucosal epithelium. Anatomically, the middle ear space can be divided into five portions based on their relationship to the tympanic annulus: the mesotympanum, the hypotympanum, the attic, the protympanum, and the retrotympanum (see Figure 44–5). The retrotympanum includes the sinus tympani and facial recess.

The blood supply of the middle ear and mastoid originate from the internal and external carotid arteries. Vessels off the external carotid artery include the anterior tympanic artery and the deep auricular artery (branches of the internal maxillary artery), the superior petrosal and superior tympanic arteries (branches of the middle meningeal artery), and the stylomastoid artery (a branch of the occipital artery that runs up the stylomastoid foramen). In addition, the caroticotympanic artery, a branch of the internal carotid artery, forms a plexus over the promontory of the middle ear.

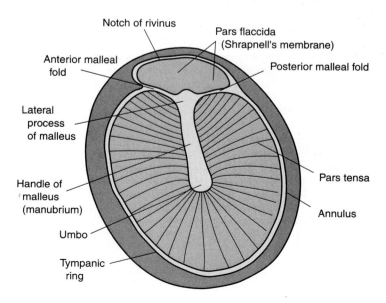

Figure 44–4. Anatomy of the tympanic membrane (a left ear).

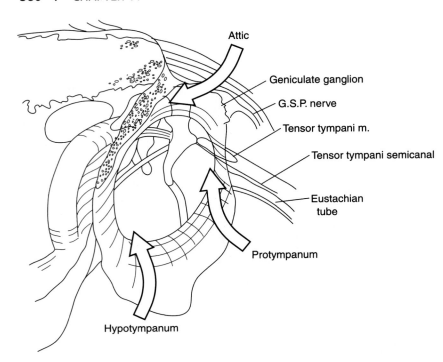

Attic

Geniculate ganglion

G.S.P. nerve

Tensor tympani m.

Tensor tympani semicanal

Eustachian tube

Protympanum

Hypotympanum

Figure 44–5. Spaces of the middle ear (a right ear). The mesotympanum is the portion of the middle ear directly behind the tympanic membrane. The attic, protympanum, and hypotympanum are superior, anterior, and inferior to the mesotympanum, respectively. The facial recess and sinus tympani are posterior to the mesotympanum (also see Figure 44–8). GSP, greater superficial petrosal.

3. Ossicular Chain

There are three ossicles (Figure 44–6): the malleus, the incus, and the stapes. The malleus has a long process, a short process, and a head. The malleus is bonded to the tympanic membrane from the tip of the long process (the umbo) to the short process. The head of the malleus articulates with the body of the incus in the attic.

The incus has a long process and a short process. The short process is tethered to the posterior wall of the middle ear cavity for structural support and the long process is connected to the stapes capitulum. The distal portion of the long process of the incus is known as the lenticular process. The blood supply to the ossicular chain is most tentative at the lenticular process. Hence, this is the first portion of the ossicular chain to be resorbed in patients with chronic otitis media, producing ossicular discontinuity.

The stapes consists of a footplate and a superstructure. The superstructure includes the anterior and posterior crus, which are attached at the capitulum. The footplate is the bony covering that sits within the oval window.

The stapedius muscle originates from the pyramidal eminence (Figure 44–7). The tensor tympani muscle is anchored by the cochleariform process where it turns 90° and becomes a tendon that connects to the malleus (Figure 44–8). The ponticulus is a ridge of bone between the round window and the oval window. The subiculum is a ridge of bone just anterior to the round window. The promontory is the medial wall of the middle ear cavity. Medial to the promontory is the cochlea.

The embryologic development of the ossicles is complex. The ossicular portions that are found in the attic are formed from the first branchial arch. This includes the head of the malleus and the body and short process of the incus. The ossicular portions that are found within the mesotympanum originate from the second branchial arch. This includes the long process of the malleus, the long process of the incus, and the stapes superstructure. The stapes footplate originates from the otic capsule (the primordial otocyst), rather than from a branchial arch. The ossicles are full-sized cartilage models by 15 weeks of gestation, and endochondral ossification is complete by 25 weeks.

4. Nervous Structures

The facial nerve is the major nerve traversing the middle ear cavity (Figure 44–7). After entering the temporal bone via the internal auditory canal, the labyrinthine segment courses to the geniculate ganglion, immediately superior to the cochlea. The facial nerve then turns (first genu) and runs horizontally through the middle ear space (the tympanic portion of the facial nerve). The nerve lies superior to the oval window and the bone is often missing (dehiscent facial nerve) at this point. The nerve then turns again (second genu) and runs vertically (the vertical portion of the facial nerve). The nerve exits the temporal

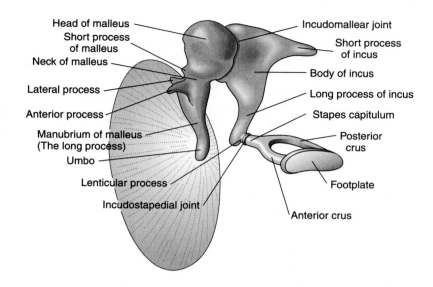

Figure 44–6. The middle ear ossicles.

bone through the stylomastoid foramen, which is medial to the digastric muscle but lateral to the styloid process.

There are three branches of the facial nerve within the temporal bone. The greater superficial petrosal nerve branches off at the geniculate ganglion and delivers parasympathetic nerves to the lacrimal gland and to the minor salivary glands of the nose. Another branch of the facial

nerve goes to the stapedius muscle. Finally, the chorda tympani nerve branches off from the vertical portion of the facial nerve and runs underneath the tympanic membrane, medial to the malleus, before exiting the middle ear space through the petrotympanic fissure. It joins up with cranial nerve V3 and supplies both taste to the anterior two thirds of the tongue as well as parasympathetic innervation to the

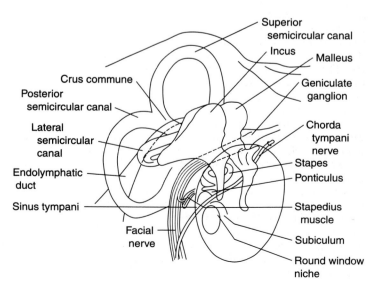

Figure 44–7. Relationship of the middle ear structures with the inner ear (a right ear).

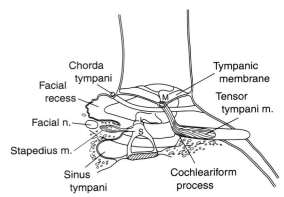

Figure 44–8. The facial recess and sinus tympani (a right ear viewed from below). malleus (m); staples (s).

sublingual and submandibular glands. The cell bodies of these nerves that supply special visceral afferent innervation (taste) to the anterior two thirds of the tongue and the palate are found in the geniculate ganglion.

Cranial nerve IX (the glossopharyngeal nerve) has a branch that runs across the tympanic promontory called the tympanic nerve or Jacobson's nerve. It innervates the mucosa of the middle ear space and Eustachian tube as well as provides parasympathetic innervation to the parotid gland. There is also a branch of the vagus nerve within the middle ear cavity called Arnold's nerve, which supplies innervation to the external auditory canal. Patients often cough when their ear canal is cleaned because of the referred sensation to the throat.

5. The Facial Recess & the Sinus Tympani

The area around the second genu of the facial nerve is critical to understand in order to perform proper middle ear surgery (Figure 44–8). The bony ear canal ends at the level of the annulus. The space medial to the end of the ear canal, but lateral to the facial nerve, is the facial recess. Medial to the facial nerve is another pocket of space called the sinus tympani. It is impossible to visualize the sinus tympani by looking either through the ear canal or through an opening made through the mastoid. Residual cholesteatoma is often found here because of remnants left behind (and not seen) during primary surgery.

Physiology of the Middle Ear

The middle ear provides an acoustic impedance match between the environmental air and the fluid-filled inner ear. The middle ear amplifies the airborne sound vibra-

tion in two ways. First, the large surface area of the tympanic membrane, compared with the small surface area of the stapes (14:1), imparts an increase in vibrational amplitude. Second, the lever arm effect of the malleus and incus imparts a further increase in vibrational amplitude (1.3:1.0). Thus, the total middle ear gain is between 20 and 35 dB. In addition, the mass and stiffness of the ossicular chain affect its frequency response. Overall, the middle ear acts as a band-pass filter, with a maximum energy transfer over the range of 1–10 kHz.

Changing the mass and stiffness of the middle ear modulates its frequency response, which can be observed clinically. For example, the stapedius and tensor tympani muscles contract through a neural reflex arc mediated by loud sounds (> 80 dB). They act to stiffen the ossicular chain and protect the inner ear from noise damage, particularly at low frequencies. In contrast, cholesteatoma formation in the middle ear can contact the ossicular chain, increasing the total mass, causing a predominantly high-frequency conductive hearing loss.

The middle ear is aerated through the eustachian tube to keep it at the same pressure as that of the ear canal. If the eustachian tube is blocked (eg, by edema of the nasopharynx secondary to allergy, adenoid hypertrophy, nasopharyngeal tumor, etc.), the middle ear pressure becomes lower than atmospheric pressure, pulling the tympanic membrane inward. As the tympanic membrane is richly innervated, this can be painful. The occasional opening of the eustachian tube, with a resultant change in middle ear pressure, can cause a patient to experience a popping sensation, pain, and a mild fluctuation in the sensation of hearing. If the tube becomes chronically blocked, a serous middle ear effusion with conductive hearing loss can develop.

INNER EAR

Development

The inner ear begins as a thickening of the ectoderm on the side of the embryo (the otic placode) and is first noted at 3 weeks of gestation. The otic placode invaginates to form the otic pit. It then pinches off and begins to enlarge, forming the otocyst. Beginning in weeks 5–6, the otocyst elongates and partitions itself into what will become six different sensory structures (three semicircular canals, two otolithic organs, and the cochlea) and the endolymphatic duct and sac. By 12 weeks, the formation of the membranous labyrinth is complete and the sensory cells have differentiated. By 16 weeks, cartilage has formed around the membranous labyrinth; by 23 weeks, this has undergone complete endochondral ossification to form the adult-size otic capsule (Figure 44–9). By 26 weeks, the human inner ear is sending auditory information to the brain.

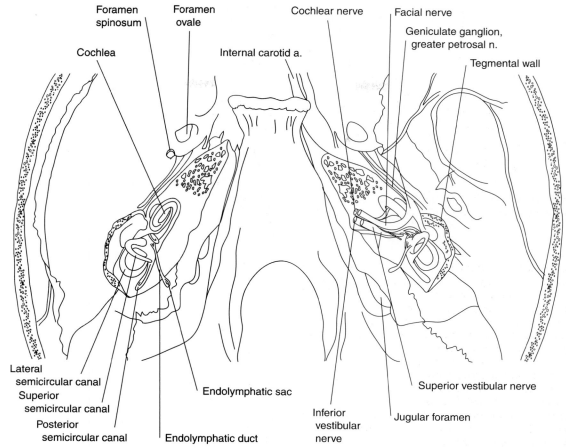

Foramen spinosum
Foramen ovale
Cochlear nerve
Facial nerve
Geniculate ganglion, greater petrosal n.
Cochlea
Internal carotid a.
Tegmental wall
Lateral semicircular canal
Superior semicircular canal
Posterior semicircular canal
Endolymphatic sac
Endolymphatic duct
Inferior vestibular nerve
Superior vestibular nerve
Jugular foramen

Figure 44–9. The location of the inner ears within the skull base.

1. Fluid Compartments

The inner ear is divided into two fluid-filled chambers, one inside the other (Figure 44–10). The fluid in the two chambers differs on the basis of the kind of salt that each contains. The fluid in the outer or bony chamber is filled with a sodium salt solution called **perilymph,** which resembles cerebrospinal fluid. The inner or membranous chamber is filled with a high potassium salt solution called **endolymph,** which resembles intracellular fluid. Marginal cells in the stria vascularis (see Figure 44–21) actively pump potassium into the membranous chamber to maintain the difference in the sodium and potassium concentrations. The difference in the chemical composition between perilymph and endolymph provides the electrochemical energy that powers the activities of the sensory cells. The inner ear is unique because the sensory cells rely on energy provided by other cells. In virtually all other systems, whether it is heart muscles, the brain, or the retina of the eye, the principal cells must combine nutrients and oxygen to produce the energy they use to perform their functions.

2. Hair Cell Function

Hair cells (Figure 44–11) are the sensory receptor cells of hearing and balance and are the most important cells in the inner ear. Their name derives from the fact that they have about 100 stereocilia at their apical end. Individual stereocilia are packed with a filamentous actin cytoskeleton. Hair cells are specialized mechanoreceptors that convert the mechanical stimuli associated with hearing and balance into neural information for transmission to the brain. The conversion of one type of energy to another is called **transduction.**

The stereocilia of each hair cell are arranged in a precise geometry. This arrangement is asymmetrical and polarized because the stereocilia are arranged in

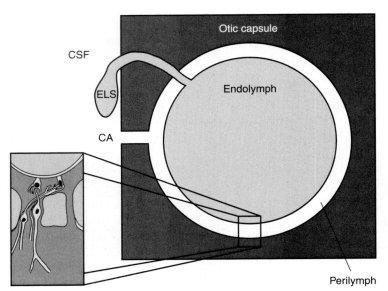

Figure 44–10. Schematic diagram showing the organization of the inner ear organs of hearing and balance. The inner ear contains two fluid chambers, a membranous and a bony chamber. The membranous chamber is filled with endolymph while the bony chamber is filled with perilymph. CA, cochlear aqua duct; CSF, cerebrospinal fluid; ELS, endolymphatic sac.

rows of short, intermediate, and tall stereocilia. A single kinocilium is located adjacent to the tallest row. It has a 9 by 2 microtubule organization similar to motile cilia found elsewhere in the body. The kinocilium is thought to establish the morphologic polarization of the stereocilia bundle and is not required for mechanoelectrical transduction. It is present in embryonic cochlear hair cells but is resorbed by the time cochlear hair cells mature.

There is a stepwise progression from the shortest row to the tallest row. The organization of the bundle from short to tall rows is related to the functional consequences of bending the bundle on the cell's membrane potential. The mechanoelectrical transduction channels that are in the wall of the stereocilia are tethered to adjacent stereocilia by "tip links" (see Figure 44–11). The deflection of the stereocilia toward the tallest row causes shearing between the stereocilia, which causes the tip links to pull on the transduction channels, opening them. Deflection in the other direction releases the tension of the tip link, causing the transduction channels to close. Bending the bundle in the direction of the tallest row leads to entry of K^+ and Ca^{2+} ions into the hair cell through channels that open at the tips of the stereocilia. This causes the hair cell to depolarize. Bending the bundle in the opposite direction promotes channel closure and results in hair cell hyperpolarization.

Within the stereociliary bundle, there is movement of the bundle back and forth parallel with the axis of symmetry through the kinocilium. Movement in this direction produces a maximal receptor potential (change in

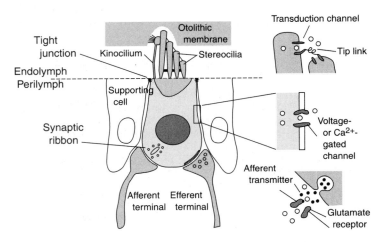

Figure 44–11. A stereotypical hair cell. The sensory cells are called hair cells because of their stereocilia. Each hair cell has a tuft of stereocilia arranged in rows that increase in length toward one side of the cell. A single kinocilium sits in front of the longest stereocilia. Neurotransmission from the hair cells to afferent neurons occurs at their basal pole. Some hair cells also receive efferent input that regulates their sensitivity. Voltage- and calcium-gated ion channels in the basolateral hair cell membrane shape the electrical response of the hair cell to mechanical stimuli.

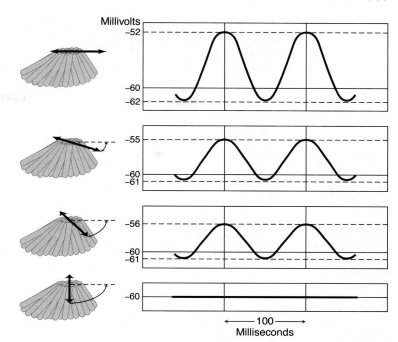

Figure 44–12. Mechanoelectrical transduction in the hair cell stereocilia. (Used, with permission, from Estate of Bonji Tagawa.)

intracellular voltage). As the bundle is moved at larger angles away from this axis, the receptor potential is reduced. In Figure 44–12, note that the receptor potential is asymmetric, with larger depolarizing swings compared with hyperpolarizing swings. This is because the current-voltage characteristics of the hair cell are nonlinear and are shaped by the various voltage- and calcium-dependent ion channels in its basolateral plasma membrane. The lowest tracing (see Figure 44–12) demonstrates that deflection of the stereociliary bundle perpendicular to the bundle's axis of symmetry produces no receptor potential.

Hair cells have synapses located at their basal pole. When a hair cell is mechanically stimulated, it releases a chemical that modulates the electric activity of the afferent neurons (Figure 44–13). This neurotransmitter release is regulated by changes in the membrane poten-

tial of the hair cell in response to bending its stereocilia bundle. Efferent synapses at the termination of the fibers originating deep in the brainstem are also present. The neural signals from the brain conveyed by these efferent fibers modulate the gain (amplification) of the hair cells they innervate.

3. The Organs of Hearing & Balance

The inner ear sensory epithelia are among the smallest organs in the body, containing less than 20,000 sensory cells. (By comparison, about 1 million photoreceptors are in the eye.) The inner ear organs must be small because any increase in their size would increase their mass. An increase in mass would increase the mechani-

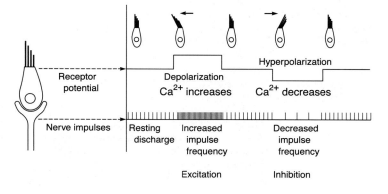

Figure 44–13. Modulation of afferent nerve fiber activity by stereociliary bundle deflection. The normal afferent eighth nerve has a resting spontaneous discharge rate. Depolarization of the hair cell leads to an increase in this rate and hyperpolarization leads to a decrease in this rate.

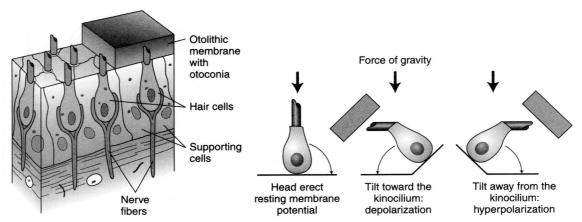

Figure 44–14. Organization and physiology of the maculae.

cal force that would be required to make them vibrate. Any increase in the driving force would represent a decrease in the sensitivity of the system (a hearing loss). The small number of cells in the hearing organ means that the loss of even a small number affects hearing.

Inner ear sensory organs differ in the way the stereocilia bundles of the hair cells are mechanically bent. The hair cells in each organ are grouped in one of three types of sensory epithelia. The maculae (Figures 44–14 and 44–15) and the cristae (Figure 44–16) are the sensory epithelium of the vestibular system (balance) and the organ of Corti (Figure 44–17) is the sensory epithelium of the cochlea. There are two maculae (the saccule and the utricle), three cristae, and one organ of Corti on each side of the head.

VESTIBULAR SYSTEM

Anatomy & Physiology of the Vestibular Organs

The maculae (see Figure 44–15) of the otolithic organs are responsible for sensing gravity (linear acceleration). The maculae are flat, ovoid structures that are covered with hair cells across their surface. The stereocilia of the hair cells protrude upward and are embedded in the gelatinous otolithic membrane, which contains calcium carbonate crystals called **otoconia.** Otoconia have a density greater than water, so when the head is tilted from side to side, gravity causes a shearing force between the otolithic membrane and the surface of the maculae. This results in a bending of the stereocilia. The deflection of the stereocilia in the direction of the longer stereocilia causes the transduction channels to open and hair cell depolarization to occur. The deflection of stereocilia toward the shorter stereocilia causes the transduction channels to close and the cell to hyperpolarize.

The utricle and saccule take advantage of this bidirectional coding because there are hair cells oriented in both directions across their surface. In this way, a single macule can produce both excitatory and inhibitory signals with a change in head position. The striola is defined as a thinning in the center of the otolithic membrane in the utricle and a thickening in that of the saccule (see Figure 44–15). This roughly defines the area on the sensory epithelium that divides hair cells oriented in one direction from those oriented in the opposite direction. Both the utricle and the saccule have a gentle curved orientation. Two-dimensional information is able to be detected by a single otolithic organ because of the distributed orientation of the hair cell stereociliary bundles in all directions.

Hair cells have a mechanism for adjusting their set point, which is particularly important to the otolithic organs. When a steady-state head tilt occurs, hair cell stereocilia are deflected and a receptor potential occurs within the cell. However, over the next few seconds, the intracellular potential partially returns to normal levels, which is termed *adaptation.* It permits the hair cell to respond to further changes in head position rather than resting unresponsively in a fully deflected position. Actin-myosin motors within the stereocilia are thought to be activated in a manner that keeps the tip links between adjacent stereocilia tight.

The ampullae (see Figure 44–16) of the semicircular canals are responsible for sensing head turning (angular acceleration). The semicircular canal ampulla contains the crista, which has a shape similar to a horse saddle. Hair cells sit on the surface of the crista. The stereocilia protrude upward off the surface of the crista and into a gelatinous material called a **cupula.** With a turn of the head, the inertia of the endolymph within the semicircular canal causes the cupula to move, deflecting the hair cell stereocilia and stimulating transduction. The

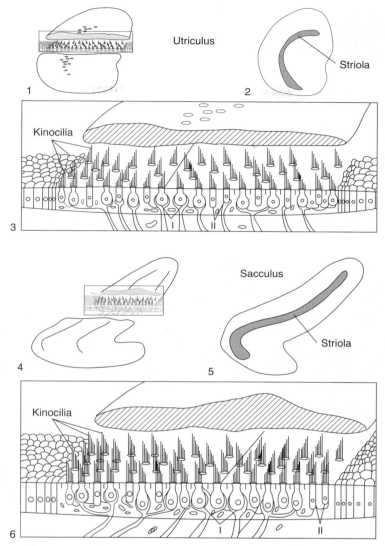

Figure 44–15. Organization of the utricle and saccule.

three semicircular canals (lateral, superior, and posterior) are perpendicular to one another and thereby provide sensory signals from any type of head rotation.

Each semicircular canal is paired with one in a parallel plane on the opposite side of the head (see Figure 44–9). For instance, both lateral canals are in the same plane, the left posterior canal is in the same plane as the right superior canal, and the right posterior canal is in the same plane as the left superior canal. One vestibular organ gives an excitatory response, and the other vestibular organ gives an inhibitory response for rotation in a given plane. This paired input is then integrated by the

brainstem to control balance. The kinocilia of the hair cells in the lateral semicircular canals are oriented toward the utricular side; therefore, the displacement of the cupula toward the vestibule provides an excitatory response **(ampullopetal endolymph flow).** In contrast, the kinocilia of the superior and posterior semicircular canals are oriented toward the canal side. Therefore, the displacement of the cupula toward the canal provides an excitatory response **(ampullofugal endolymph flow).**

Within the otolithic organs and the semicircular canals are two different types of hair cells, Type I and Type II (Figure 44–18). Physiologically, these cells act

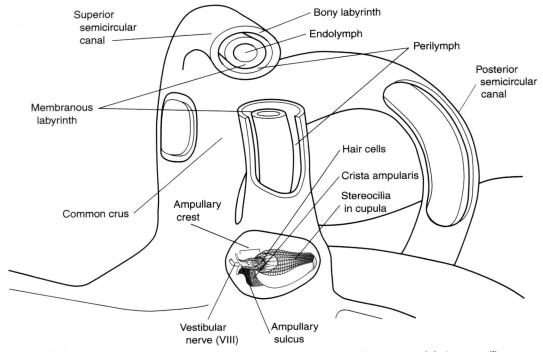

Figure 44–16. The semicircular canals and ampullae. The hair cells sit on the crista, and their stereocilia are embedded in the gelatinous cupula. Angular acceleration (head rotation) causes the endolymph within the semicircular canal to bend the cupula, resulting in stereociliary deflection. The three semicircular canals (lateral, superior, and posterior) are perpendicular to one another, permitting detection of head rotation in any direction.

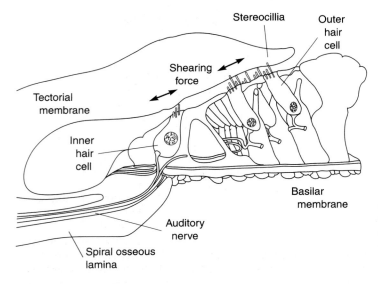

Figure 44–17. The organ of Corti. The central axis of the spiraling cochlea is to the left of the drawing. Eighth nerve fibers pass through a bony shelf (the spiral osseus lamina) on their way to the hair cells.

Type I hair cell   Type II hair cell

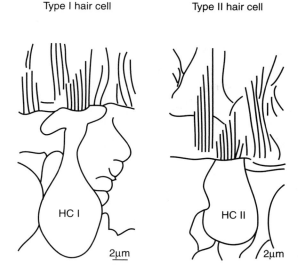

HC I   HC II

2μm   2μm

Figure 44–18. Vestibular hair cells. Two types of vestibular hair cells are found in both the otolithic organs and in the semicircular canals, Type I and Type II. Type I hair cells (left) have a flask shape with a narrow neck, whereas Type II hair cells (right) are more cylindrical.

differently, although both are mechanoreceptor cells that transduce the head position and send this information to the brain.

Neurophysiology

Eighth nerve (vestibulocochlear) fibers innervate ipsilateral vestibular nuclei. The neural signals coming from the semicircular canals start the vestibuloocular reflex (Figure 44–19). The **vestibuloocular reflex** is critical to the ability to visually fixate on an object while one's head is turning. In contrast, keeping one's head still while trying to follow a moving target with the eyes is predominantly under cortical and cerebellar control. This is a much slower, multisynaptic, response compared with the three-neuron reflex arc of the vestibuloocular reflex.

An excitatory response from one semicircular canal results in an excitatory signal that crosses the midline of the brainstem via a second neuron to the contralateral abducens nucleus. The abducens nucleus then sends inputs via the sixth cranial nerve (the abducens nerve) to the lateral rectus muscle in the contralateral eye, causing the eye to deviate away from the side of the vestibular excitation. In addition, the abducens nucleus sends an excitatory input via the medial longitudinal fasciculus to the ipsilateral ocular motor nucleus. This controls the

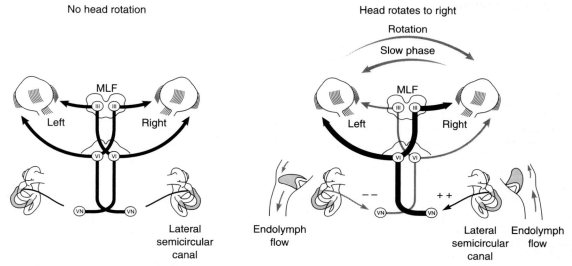

No head rotation

Head rotates to right

Rotation

Slow phase

MLF   MLF

III   III   III   III

Left   Right   Left   Right

VI   VI   VI   VI

VN   VN   − −   + +   VN   VN

Lateral   Endolymph   Lateral   Endolymph
semicircular   flow   semicircular   flow
canal   canal

Figure 44–19. The vestibuloocular reflex. Horizontal head rotation stimulates the ipsilateral lateral semicircular canal and inhibits the contralateral canal. A three-neuron reflex arc involving the abducens (VI) and oculomotor (III) brainstem nuclei leads to stimulation of the contralateral lateral rectus muscle and stimulation of the ipsilateral medial rectus muscle. The corresponding antagonistic muscles (the contralateral medial rectus and ipsilateral lateral rectus) are inhibited. MLF, medial longitudinal fasciculus; VN, vestibular nucleus.

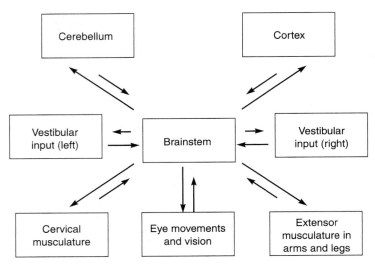

Figure 44–20. Balance control involves the vestibular system, the cervical musculature, the visual system, and the extensor musculature. The cerebellum and cortex provide control over the sensory integration and motor control process that occurs predominantly in the brainstem. Normal balance processes act to keep the head upright. When falling asleep (for example, during a lecture), the loss of cortical input reduces the tonic output of the vestibulospinal pathways, causing your head to fall forward.

ipsilateral medial rectus muscle, causing the ipsilateral eye to deviate away from the side of the vestibular excitation. Because this input is paired, inhibitory signals from the other ear cause precisely the opposite response.

Balance is a complex interplay among input from the inner ear, the eyes, and musculature in the body and cervical spine. These signals are integrated in the brainstem, the cerebellum, and the cortex (Figure 44–20). The utricle and saccule send information regarding head position to the brain and to the spinal cord, relaying changes in orientation to the antigravity musculature. These vestibulospinal reflexes are important for postural maintenance, equilibrium, and resting muscular tone. The cerebellum modulates these effects as well. The muscles responsible for postural control include the abdominal and paraspinal muscles around the hip, the hamstrings and quadriceps in the thigh, and the gastrocnemius and tibialis anterior in the calf. The vestibulospinal reflexes are carried by many distinct vestibulospinal tracts. The most important is the lateral vestibular spinal tract. Fibers within this tract cause a monosynaptic excitation of the ipsilateral extensors and disynaptic inhibition of contralateral extensors. Hence, a unilateral labyrinthine lesion causes increased contralateral extensor activation. For example, patients who have an acoustic neuroma and decreased vestibular input from one side tend to fall toward the side of the lesion because of the contralateral extensor activation.

AUDITORY SYSTEM

1. The Cochlea

The cochlea achieves a greater mechanical sensitivity than the vestibular organs. The energy required for this process is provided by the stria vascularis (Figure 44–21). This structure forms the outer wall of the scala media and sits within the spiral ligament. It is highly vascular and metabolically active in order to maintain the high potassium concentration within the scala media. The stria vascularis acts as a battery whose electrical current powers hearing. In addition to elevated potassium concentrations, it creates a positive potential within the endolymph relative to the perilymph. This increases the electrochemical gradient that drives a constant flow of K^+ ions from the endolymph into the hair cells. This "silent current" is modulated as hair cell stereocilia are deflected. Potassium ions are recycled back to the stria vascularis by diffusion

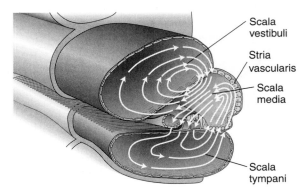

Scala vestibuli
Stria vascularis
Scala media
Scala tympani

Figure 44–21. Cross-section of the cochlea. There are three fluid-filled chambers: the scala vestibuli and scala tympani are connected at the apex of the cochlea and contain perilymph; the scala media contains endolymph. The stria vascularis maintains the endolymphatic potential and drives the silent current (arrows) that provides the energy for hearing.

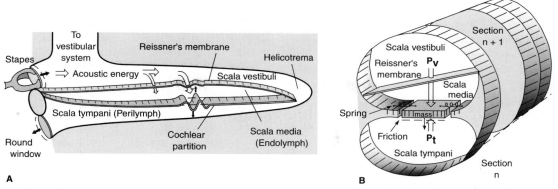

Figure 44–22. The traveling wave. The basilar membrane varies in mass and stiffness along the length of the cochlea (here shown unrolled). This creates a tonotopic organization in which different segments of the basilar membrane are most sensitive to different frequencies. The pressure wave introduced from movement of the stapes propagates up the cochlea and is dissipated at its characteristic frequency place. The cochlea can be modeled as having multiple sections, each with a distinct mass and stiffness of the basilar membrane. (Adapted from Geisler CD. *From Sound to Synapse: Physiology of the Mammalian Ear.* New York: Oxford University Press, 1998.)

through the perilymph and through supporting cells via gap junctions. The gap junction proteins are called connexins, and mutations of their genes result in sensorineural hearing loss. Connexin mutations are the most common mechanism of genetic hearing loss.

Passive Mechanics within the Cochlea

The hair cells in the organ of Corti vibrate in response to sound. Their stereocilia insert into the overlying tectorial membrane. Differential movements between the basilar membrane and the tectorial membrane bend the stereocilia bundle (see Figure 44–17). In this figure, the flexible basilar membrane is anchored to the bony shelf on the left and a ligament (not shown) on the right. A single flask-shaped inner hair cell is shown on the left, and three rows of cylindrically shaped outer hair cells are seen on the right. The tips of the outer hair cell stereocilia are embedded in a gelatinous mass called the **tectorial membrane,** which lies on top of the organ of Corti. When sound is transmitted to the inner ear, the organ of Corti vibrates up and down. Since the basilar membrane is attached to bone and ligament at its two ends, the area of maximal vibration is near the third (furthest right) row of outer hair cells. The basilar membrane is fixed at the osseous spiral lamina, whereas the tectorial membrane is fixed at a different position. Movement of the basilar membrane up and down, induced by sound waves within the cochlear fluids, causes a shearing force to deflect the hair cell stereocilia.

The cochlea acts as both a passive and an active filter. Passive filtering produces a traveling wave in response to sound vibrations (Figure 44–22). The location of the

peak of the traveling wave changes with the frequency of the sound played into the ear. The change in location results from the tonotopic organization of the organ of Corti. There are systematic differences in its mass and stiffness along its length that determine the frequency response at any specific location. At the base of the cochlea (the high-frequency region), it has a lower mass and a higher stiffness. In contrast, at the apex of the cochlea (the low-frequency region), the organ of Corti has a higher mass and a lower stiffness. Sound vibrations that enter the cochlea at the stapes footplate propagate along the length of the cochlear duct and are maximal when they match the characteristic frequency at a specific location.

Active Processes within the Cochlea

Analyses of the cochlea based only on passive mechanical properties such as mass and stiffness cannot explain the exquisite frequency selectivity of human hearing or the frequency selectivity that could be measured from individual auditory nerve fibers. However, the frequency selectivity of the cochlea can be enhanced if a source of mechanical energy is present in the cochlea. The concept that a source of mechanical energy exists in the cochlea appeared validated when in the late 1970s it was discovered that sound is produced by the inner ear. These sounds can be measured by placing a sensitive microphone in the ear canal. They were called otoacoustic emissions, and they are now routinely measured in the clinic to assess hearing. Within 5 years, it was discovered that the outer hair cell could be made to elongate and shorten by electrical stimulation. The function of the outer hair cell in hearing is now perceived as that of a cochlear amplifier that refines the sensitivity and frequency selectivity of the mechanical vibrations of the cochlea.

2. Outer Hair Cells

The organ of Corti is a highly organized sensory structure that sits on the **basilar membrane** (see Figure 44–17). There is a single row of inner hair cells, and there are three rows of outer hair cells. These rows of hair cells run the length of the cochlea and are positioned on top of the basilar membrane by various supporting cells. There are tight junctions between the apex of the hair cells and the surrounding supporting cells that form the barrier (the reticular lamina) between the endolymph and the perilymph.

Pressurization of the Outer Hair Cells

Most cells have a cytoskeleton to maintain cell shape. Because such an internal skeleton would impede electromotility, a central cytoskeleton is missing in the cylindrical portion of the outer hair

cell, thereby improving the cell's flexibility. The outer hair cell must be more than flexible; it must also be strong enough to transmit force to the rest of the organ of Corti. As a result, outer hair cells are pressurized.

Most cells do not tolerate internal pressure because their membrane is weak.

The outer hair cell has reinforced its membrane with a highly organized actin-spectrin cytoskeleton just underneath the plasma membrane (Figure 44–23). The shape of the outer hair cell is maintained by a pressurized fluid core that pushes against an elastic wall. The wall is reinforced by additional layers of cytoskeletal material and membranes. The lateral wall of the outer hair cell is about 100 nm thick and contains the plasma membrane, the cytoskeleton, and an intracellular organelle called the subsurface cisternae. Particles sit within the plasma membrane and may be related to electromotility. The cytoskeleton consists of actin filaments that are oriented circumferentially around the cell and that are cross-linked by spectrin molecules. Pillar molecules tether the actin-spectrin network to the plasma membrane. The plasma membrane may be rippled between adjacent pillar molecules.

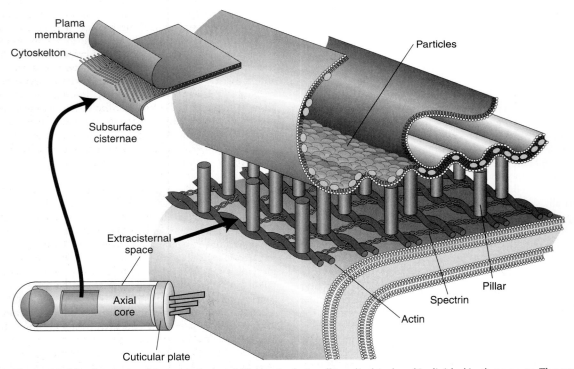

Figure 44–23. Anatomy of the outer hair cell. The outer hair cell is cylindrical and is divided in three parts. The top part is capped with a cuticular plate (CP) into which the stereocilia are inserted. The base of the cell is hemispheric. It contains the cell nucleus and synaptic structures (not shown). The central part of the cell is cylindrical.

Electromotility of Outer Hair Cells

Outer hair cells have a cylindrical shape (Figure 44–24). They vary in length from approximately 12 μm at the basal or high-frequency end of the cochlea to > 90 μm at the low-frequency end. Their diameter at all locations is approximately 9 μm, which is slightly larger than the diameter of a red blood cell. Their apical end is capped with a rigid flat plate into which the stereocilia are embedded, and their synaptic end is a hemisphere (compare with the typical hair cell shown in Figure 44–11).

Each of these three regions (flat apex, middle cylinder, and hemispheric base) has a specific function. The stereocilia at the apex of the cell are responsible for converting the mechanical energy of sound into electrical energy. Synaptic structures are found at the base of the hair cell and are responsible for converting electrical energy into chemical energy by modulating the release of neurotransmitters. The apex and the base of the

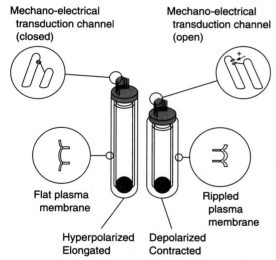

Figure 44–24. Outer hair cell electromotility. When the mechanoelectrical transduction channels are closed (cell on the left), the outer hair cell is hyperpolarized and elongated. When the channels are open (cell on the right), the outer hair cell is depolarized and shortened. The plasma membrane may flatten and ripple during this process, although this concept is hypothetical. These length changes occur at speeds of up to 100 kHz, and function to amplify the sound pressure waves (the cochlear amplifier). (Adapted from Synder KV, Sachs F, Brownell WE. The outer hair cell: a mechanoelectrical and electromechanical sensor/actuator. In: Barth FG, Humphrey JAC, Secomb TW, eds. *Sensors and Sensing in Biology and Engineering.* Wien: Springer-Verlag, 2003.)

outer hair cell perform functions that are common to all hair cells. The elongated cylindrical portion of the outer hair cell is where electrical energy is converted into mechanical energy. This function is unique to the outer hair cell. No other hair cell is able to change its length at acoustic frequencies in response to electrical stimulation. These length changes can be greater than 1% of the cell's original length if the electrical stimulation is large.

The electromotility of the outer hair cells is based on a novel membrane-based motor mechanism in the plasma membrane of the cells' lateral walls. The membrane protein *prestin* and intracellular chloride ions are required for the motor to work. The mechanical force generated by the membrane is communicated to the ends of the cell by means of an elegant cytoskeletal structure immediately adjacent to the plasma membrane (see Figure 44–23). This motor mechanism is a biological form of piezoelectricity similar to that used in sonar or ultrasound imaging. Both cochlear and vestibular hair cells from humans have similar properties to those of rodents, the animal models in which most research has been done.

Humans are able to discriminate between sounds that are very close in frequency because the outer hair cell acts as the cochlear amplifier. The role of the outer hair cell in hearing is both sensory and mechanical. When the organ of Corti begins to vibrate in response to the incoming sound, each hair cell senses the vibration through the bending of its stereocilia. The bending results in a change in the voltage within the outer hair cell, causing electromotility. If the resulting mechanical force is at the natural frequency of that portion of the cochlea, then the magnitude of the vibration increases. If the electromotile force is at a different frequency, the vibrations decrease. The system now has greater sensitivity and frequency selectivity than when the outer hair cells are missing or damaged.

One consequence of having an active system is that oscillations can occur even when no energy is coming into the system from the outside. This happens in the cochlea, and the resulting sound vibrations can be measured in the ear canal. These are called spontaneous otoacoustic emissions and are observed only in living ears. Other types of otoacoustic emissions can be measured as well, including distortion product otoacoustic emissions and transient evoked otoacoustic emissions. These can be triggered as needed by playing certain types of sound stimuli into the ear and are therefore more useful clinically than the measurement of spontaneous otoacoustic emissions. Measuring otoacoustic emissions has become an important diagnostic tool for determining if outer hair cells are working, particularly in newborn hearing screening (see Chapter 45, Audiologic Testing).

Sensorineural hearing loss is a common clinical problem and has many possible causes, including noise expo-

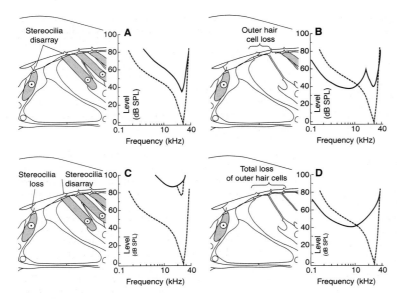

Figure 44–25. Various forms of hair cell damage found with noise trauma and their effect on eighth nerve tuning curves. The dotted lines represent normal turning curves and the solid lines are pathologic. (Adapted from Kiang NY, Liberman MC, Sewell WF, Guinan JJ. Single unit clues to cochlear mechanism. *Hear Res.* 1986;171.)

sure, ototoxicity, and age-related hearing loss (presbycusis). The common site of pathology for all of these conditions within the inner ear is the outer hair cell (see Figure 44–24). The attachments of outer hair cell stereocilia to the tectorial membrane can be broken, even with mild noise exposure. This reduces the ability of outer hair cell electromotility to provide positive feedback, leading to a temporary hearing loss. With further damage, the actin core of the outer hair cell stereocilia can fracture. With enough trauma, hair cell death occurs and a permanent hearing loss results because mammalian cochlear hair cells do not regenerate. After outer hair cells begin to degenerate, further structures within the cochlea die as well, including inner hair cells, supporting cells, and auditory nerve cells.

A low level of trauma that produces disarray of both inner and outer hair cell stereocilia proportionally elevates tuning curve thresholds (Figure 44–25A). When outer hair cells are lost, only the sharp peak of the tuning curve is lost (Figure 44–25B and D). Loss of inner hair cells produces a dramatic elevation in tuning curve thresholds (Figure 44–25C). Outer hair cell damage blocks the cochlear amplifier, but the passive tuning properties of the cochlea are retained. In contrast, inner hair cell damage reduces cochlear function overall. In summary, outer hair cells are responsible for the cochlear amplifier, whereas inner hair cells provide afferent input.

THE CENTRAL PATHWAYS: BRAINSTEM NUCLEI & THE AUDITORY CORTEX

Input from both cochleae are integrated, and the acoustic environment is reconstructed in the brainstem and auditory cortex. This begins with the conversion of mechanical vibrations of the organ of Corti into changes of inner hair cell membrane potentials. Synaptic transmission to the afferent eighth nerve fibers (the auditory nerve) modulates the ongoing action potential discharge of the fiber. As a result of the faithful link between basilar membrane mechanics and the afferent fiber, each auditory nerve fiber is tuned to a particular characteristic frequency (see Figure 44–25). In this way, the central nervous system knows that there is energy at that specific frequency entering the ear.

Auditory brainstem-evoked response (ABR) is a clinical test to verify that the pathway from the cochlea to the midbrain is intact. Electrodes placed on the scalp (similar to those used with an electroencephalogram) can measure the electrical signals being relayed from the cochlea to the auditory cortex. By playing a "click" into the ear, a large number of auditory nerve fibers are excited simultaneously. This is called the compound action potential, and is Wave 1 of the ABR (see Chapter 45, Audiologic Testing). ABR Waves 2, 3, 4, and 5 represent the sequential activation of neurons as the signal is passed up the brainstem (distal auditory nerve, cochlear nucleus, superior olivary complex, and lateral lemniscus). Each wave should occur within a certain timeframe after the previous wave. If delayed, a conduction block can be diagnosed, which may represent brainstem pathology. The most common conduction delays are measured between Waves 1 and 3 and Waves 1 and 5, which may suggest the presence of an acoustic neuroma that is slowing conduction along the eighth cranial nerve. Many other types of pathology, including other cerebellopontine angle tumors, multiple sclerosis, chronic meningitis, and brainstem malformation, need to be included in the differential diagnosis. In most instances, an abnormal ABR indicates the need to order an MRI with and without gadolinium contrast to evaluate for retrocochlear pathology.

In all sensory systems, an important part of the neural code is determined by what location of the sensory organ is stimulated. In the case of the eye, a spot of light falls on a few photoreceptors and they excite nerves that map a representation of the visual world in the brain. In the ear, the acoustic world is coded by a one-dimensional representation of frequency. This frequency map then projects to the brain, which reconstructs the three-dimensional acoustic "world." Parts of the auditory cortex contain a true three-dimensional representation of the outer world so that the sound of a twig snapping behind an individual excites nerve cells in one location while a twig snapping on the right of an individual excites nerve cells in another spatially precise location. The analysis of speech appears to take place in parts of the brain that are highly developed only in humans. The amazing machinery that accomplishes the reconstruction of the acoustic world relies on the delicate structures of the inner ear that deconstruct the original sounds.

Brownell WE, Spector AA, Raphael RM, Popel AS. Micro- and nanomechanics of the cochlear outer hair cell. *Annu Rev Biomed Engl.* 2001;3:169. [PMID: 11447061] (Review of the mechanical properties of the outer hair cell.)

Dallos P, Fakler B. Prestin, a new type of motor protein. *Nat Rev Mol Cell Biol.* 2002;3:104. [PMID: 11836512] (Review of the prestin protein found in outer hair cells, which is involved with electromotility force generation.)

Fettiplace R, Hackney CM. The sensory and motor roles of auditory hair cells. *Nat Rev Neurosci.* 2006;7:19. [PMID: 16371947] (Recent review.)

Geisler CD. *From Sound to Synapse: Physiology of the Mammalian Ear.* New York: Oxford University Press, 1998.

Kiang NY, Liberman MC, Sewell WF, Guinan JJ. Single unit clues to cochlear mechanism. *Hear Res.* 1986;171. (A classic in the field.)

Oghalai JS. The cochlear amplifier: augmentation of the traveling wave within the inner ear. *Curr Opin Otolaryngol.* 2004;12:431. [PMID: 15377957] (Review of the cochlear amplifier.)

Weitzel EK, Tasker R, Brownell WE. Outer hair cell piezoelectricity: frequency response enhancement and resonance behavior. *J Acoust Soc Am.* 2003;114:1462. [PMID: 14514199] (Describes how outer hair cell piezoelectric behavior benefits high-frequency mammalian hearing.)

Audiologic Testing

Robert W. Sweetow, PhD, & Jennifer Henderson Sabes, MS

Otolaryngologists often rely on audiologic test results to determine the course of treatment for a given patient. Many of the tests constituting the diagnostic audiologic battery of 20 years ago have now been replaced with newer procedures with greater specificity, sensitivity, and site of lesion accuracy. This is exemplified by the fact that the terms "sensory" or "neural" can now frequently replace the term "sensorineural." In addition, audiologic tests have gone beyond the realm of identifying anomalies in structure to identifying anomalies in function. The logical extension of this advancement is to provide the audiologist and otolaryngologist with information related to prognosis and rehabilitation.

Audiologic tests can be classified according to measures of hearing threshold, suprathreshold recognition of speech, assessment of middle ear function, assessment of cochlear function, determination of neural synchrony and vestibular function. The test correlates associated with these measures are pure-tone audiometry, speech recognition, immittance battery, otoacoustic emissions, electrophysiology (including auditory brainstem, middle latency responses, auditory steady state response, electrocochleography, and evoked cortical potentials), and electronystagmography (discussed in Chapter 46).

Audiologic test results should always be interpreted in the context of a battery of tests because no single test can provide a clear picture of a specific patient. In addition, the combination of objective and subjective (behavioral) tests provides a cross-check of the results. It is vital to remember that there are no age restrictions for audiologic testing; it is now possible to test newborns within hours of birth.

■ AUDIOMETRY

The **audiogram** is a graph that depicts threshold as a function of frequency (Figure 45–1). **Threshold** is defined as the softest intensity level that a pure tone (single frequency) can be detected 50% of the time. Intensity is designated on a normalized decibel hearing level (HL) scale that takes into account the differences in human sensitivity as a function of frequency. The typical range of frequencies tested does not cover the entire range of human hearing (20–20,000 Hz). Instead, the range includes the frequencies considered to be essential for understanding speech (250–8000 Hz). Most testing is administered at discrete octave frequencies. However, when threshold differences between adjacent octaves exceed 15 dB, inter-octave frequencies should be tested. This is particularly true at 3000 and 6000 Hz, where "notches" in audiometric configuration often typify noise-induced hearing loss. Thresholds are measured clinically in 5-dB steps. There is a test-retest variability of ±5 dB. Therefore, a change of 10 dB may not necessarily represent a true threshold shift.

Thresholds can be obtained using **air conduction** (AC) or **bone conduction** (BC). Because sound transmission via earphones, foam inserts, or loudspeakers requires the movement of air molecules, it is termed air conduction. This testing assesses the entire auditory system from the outer ear to the auditory cortex. Testing through loudspeakers does not isolate differences between ears. The advantages of insert earphones over over-the-ear (supraaural) earphones include the prevention of collapsing ear canals, greater attenuation from ambient noise (excessive noise above permissible standards), and greater interaural attenuation (the loss of sound energy that occurs as the signal travels from one ear to the other either around the head or through the bones of the skull). Interaural attenuation is also referred to as "crossover." The amount of interaural attenuation varies as a function of the transducer type and frequency; it is typically 0 dB for bone conduction, 40–60 dB for supra-aural earphones, and 55–70 dB for insert earphones. AC thresholds are marked on the audiogram with an "O" for the right ear and an "X" for the left ear. BC thresholds are obtained using a small vibrator placed on the forehead or on the mastoid bone. Thresholds are typically indicated on the audiogram with the symbols "<" ">" (unmasked) or "[" "]" (masked). Because the skull vibrates as a whole, BC thresholds primarily reflect the contribution of the inner ear, mostly bypassing the function of the outer and middle ear. The comparison of AC thresholds and BC thresholds provides an initial differentiation between conductive, mixed, and sensorineural involvement. Sensorineural hearing loss is characterized by equivalent air and bone conduction (ie, air-bone gaps of less than 10 dB). Conductive hearing loss is characterized by

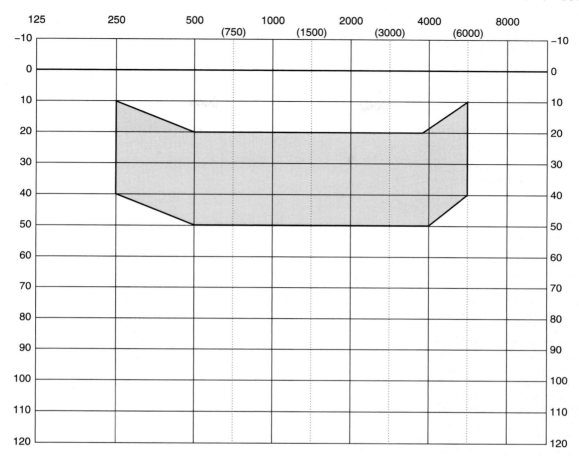

EARPHONES _____   **INSERTS** _____

AIR CONDUCTION		BONE CONDUCTION		SOUND FIELD
WITHOUT MASKING	WITH MASKING	WITHOUT MASKING	WITH MASKING	**S** Sound field (unaided)
◯ Right ear	△ Right ear	< Right ear	[Right ear	
X Left ear	□ Left ear	> Left ear	] Left ear	SSS filtered speech
↓ No response at maximum limits or audiometer		⊓ Better cochlea		**A** Sound field (aided)

Figure 45–1. An audiogram. The shaded area is called the "speech banana," which is the area where speech sounds are concentrated.

BC thresholds within normal limits, with a concurrent gap between the poorer AC and better BC thresholds of at least 10 dB. A mixed hearing loss contains air-bone gaps with the bone conduction thresholds outside of the normal range (Figure 45–2).

Both air and bone conduction thresholds may be obtained using an approach that ascends or descends in intensity but are typically determined using a bracketing technique. If tones are presented at high intensity levels, both air- and bone-conducted stimuli can evoke vibrotactile sensations. For AC, vibrotactile thresholds may occur at 90 dB HL at 250 Hz, and at 110 dB HL at both 500 and 1000 Hz. For BC, vibrotactile thresholds may occur at 30–35 dB HL at 250 Hz, 55 dB HL

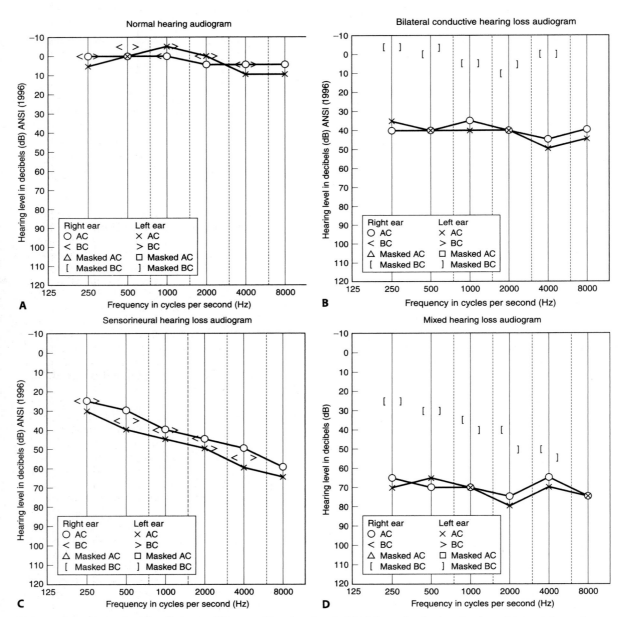

Figure 45–2. Examples of audiograms. **(A)** normal hearing thresholds, **(B)** conductive hearing loss, **(C)** sensorineural hearing loss, and **(D)** mixed hearing loss.

at 500 Hz, and 65–70 dB at 1000 Hz. Therefore, patients with severe hearing loss may appear to respond at lower (softer) levels than their true auditory thresholds. For that reason, the tester should ask the patient whether the stimulus was heard or felt when approaching the aforementioned intensity levels. Furthermore, BC greater than approximately 45–60 dB HL in the lower frequencies and 70–75 dB HL in the mid- and higher frequencies cannot be measured due to equipment output limits for bone-conducted stimuli. Thus, listeners with severe or profound losses may have real, but nonmeasurable, air-bone gaps, and one must not automatically assume that a profound hearing loss is exclusively sensorineural. This is one of several reasons why a battery of diagnostic test results should always be considered, as opposed to any single measure.

MASKING

One of the most important yet confusing aspects of hearing testing is to ensure that the auditory function of each ear is measured independently. In some situations, a noise is presented to the non-test ear to prevent it from responding to a signal presented to the test ear. This is referred to as masking. Masking is required for AC whenever the difference between the air conduction presentation level and the non-test ear BC thresholds exceed approximately 40 dB for the lower frequencies and 60 dB for the higher frequencies. For BC testing, masking should be used whenever there is any difference in the AC and BC thresholds, since there is essentially no interaural attenuation by bone conduction. When the masking presented to the non-test ear crosses over to the test ear, a masking dilemma results. Usually, this occurs when a patient has a large bilateral conductive hearing loss. The use of insert earphones greatly minimizes these occurrences because of the greater interaural attenuation they provide. Failure to mask or the inappropriate use of masking may have potentially serious medical and audiologic consequences.

CATEGORIES OF HEARING LOSS

Table 45–1 provides a very general guideline for interpreting degrees of hearing loss based on audiometric findings. Levels should be categorized somewhat more stringently for children.

■ SPEECH TESTING

One commonly used speech measure is the speech reception threshold (SRT). The SRT is the lowest intensity level at which a patient can correctly repeat 50% of common bisyllabic words like "hotdog" or "baseball." These

Table 45–1. Guidelines for interpreting hearing loss.

Hearing Threshold	Interpretation
0–25 dB	Hearing within normal limits.
26–50 dB—Mild hearing loss	Has difficulty with soft sounds, background noise, and when at a distance from the source of the sound
51–70 dB—Moderate hearing loss	Has significant difficulties with normal conversational level speech and will rely on visual cues
71–90 dB—Severe hearing loss	Cannot hear conversational speech and misses all speech sounds. Can hear environmental sounds, such as dogs barking and loud music
91+ dB—Profound hearing loss	Hears only loud environmental sounds, such as jackhammers, airplane engines, and firecrackers

results should correspond with pure-tone thresholds. However, caution must be exercised in using the SRT as the only indication of hearing sensitivity. An example of how the SRT can provide misleading information is shown in Figure 45–3. Note that for this patient, the SRT is 5 dB, well within the range of normal hearing. This value reflects the normal auditory sensitivity at 500 and 1000 Hz. Further inspection of the audiogram illustrates that this patient has a moderate hearing loss above 1000 Hz and will have considerable difficulty hearing in many acoustic environments. The only true purpose of the SRT is to validate the pure-tone findings.

A variation of the SRT is the **speech detection threshold (SDT)** or **speech awareness threshold (SAT),** which is the softest level at which a person detects (as opposed to understands) speech sounds. Pure-tone testing and SRT, SAT, or SDT yield information about hearing sensitivity. Most listening is actually done at suprathreshold levels. Therefore, to define a person's true auditory capacity, measures reflecting suprathreshold listening and clarity must be included. **Word recognition testing** (formerly referred to as *speech discrimination testing*) assesses a patient's ability to identify monosyllabic words. A list of words are presented to the patient at a suprathreshold level at approximately 40 dB above the SRT, or at a comfortable listening level if 40 dB is either too loud for the patient or incongruous with the audiometric configuration.

The type and degree of hearing loss can often affect word recognition scores. Given the relatively low face validity of monosyllabic word testing (because we do not typically listen to single-syllable words all day), the audiologist can further define hearing by assessing con-

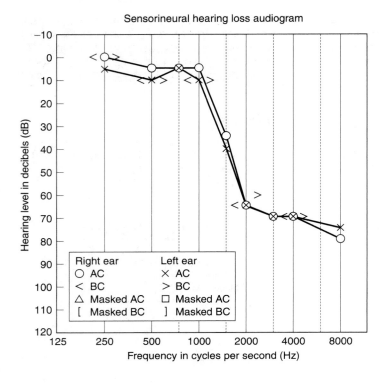

Figure 45–3. An example of an audiogram in which the SRT could give misleading information regarding a patient's hearing. Note that the patient has normal hearing to 1000 Hz, which then drops to a moderate hearing loss in the high frequencies.

versational speech or sentence recognition both in quiet and in noise.

NONORGANIC (FUNCTIONAL) HEARING LOSS

Pseudohypacusis is defined as functional hearing loss. Occasionally, patients willfully or subconsciously exaggerate their hearing loss. The signs in test behavior that suggest a functional component include (1) inconsistent responses, (2) significant differences between the thresholds obtained using ascending and descending administration of test stimuli, (3) a discrepancy of more than 8 dB between the SRT and the pure-tone average of 500–2000 Hz, and/or (4) a positive Stenger test. The **Stenger test** may be used to identify unilateral or asymmetrical functional hearing loss. It is based on the concept that when both ears are stimulated simultaneously by a tone equal in frequency and phase, the auditory percept is lateralized to the ear with better hearing. Systematic manipulation of the relative intensities delivered to each ear provides the audiologist with an estimate of the true threshold in the ear that has a more significant hearing loss. When speech stimuli are used, the test is called a **Speech Stenger test** or a **Modified Stenger test.** Other objective measures that may disclose functional involve-

ment include acoustic reflexes, auditory brainstem responses, and otoacoustic emissions. These tests are discussed later in this chapter.

Shoup AG, Roeser RJ. Audiologic evaluation of special populations. In: Roeser RJ, Valente M, Hosford-Dunn H, eds. *Audiology: Diagnosis.* New York: Thieme Medical Publishers, 2000. (Review of diagnostic procedures for possible functional hearing loss.)

ACOUSTIC IMMITTANCE TESTING

Acoustic immittance testing, an integral part of the test battery, consists of tympanometry, acoustic reflexes, and static compliance. These tests measure the function of the tympanic membrane, middle ear, and acoustic reflex arc pathway. They are not direct measures of hearing sensitivity.

TYMPANOMETRY

Tympanometry is based on the amount of sound reflected back from the tympanic membrane when an

85-B sound pressure level (SPL) low-frequency (226 Hz) probe tone is introduced into the sealed ear canal and pressure in the ear canal is varied. When the pressure in the ear canal corresponds with the pressure in the middle ear cavity, the tympanic membrane is at its most compliant point and thus absorbs, rather than reflects, the most sound. The **tympanometric peak,** or maximum flow of acoustic energy into the middle ear, occurs when the pressure in the ear canal and middle ear is equal. If eustachian tube function is normal, peak pressure occurs near 0 daPa. If the middle ear is not properly aerated, the middle ear pressure will be negative (> 100 daPa). Thus, the ear canal

pressure corresponding to the tympanometric peak provides an estimate of middle ear pressure. For infants and neonates, tympanograms obtained using a 226-Hz probe tone may appear normal erroneously; therefore, a higher-frequency probe tone (660 or 1000 Hz) must be used.

Classification

Traditionally, tympanograms have been classified as Type A, Type B, or Type C (Figure 45–4). Some clinicians prefer describing the tympanogram in a more specific narrative form.

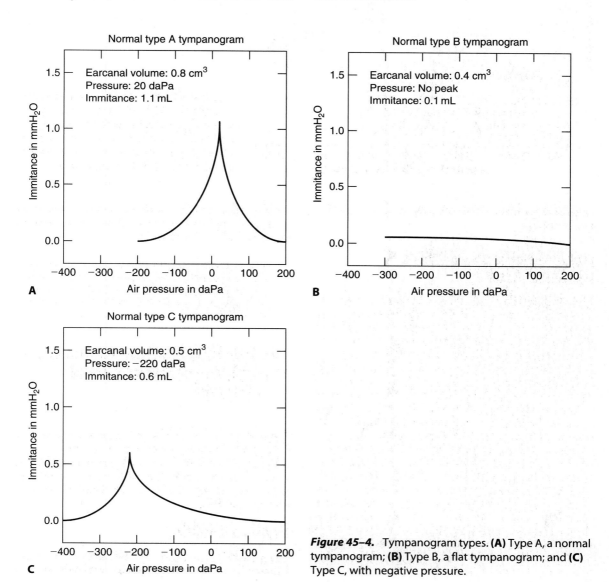

Figure 45–4. Tympanogram types. **(A)** Type A, a normal tympanogram; **(B)** Type B, a flat tympanogram; and **(C)** Type C, with negative pressure.

A. TYPE A

Type A tympanograms have normal peak height and pressure. Two variations of the Type A tympanogram also are normal in pressure, but may be shallow (A_S), reflecting otosclerosis or middle ear effusion, or peaked very high (A_D), reflecting ossicular discontinuity or a monomeric eardrum.

B. TYPE B

The Type B tympanogram is flat in appearance, indicating lack of compliance. The volume measurement that is simultaneously performed with tympanometry helps to differentiate between a flat tympanogram suggesting an intact eardrum with middle ear effusion and a perforated eardrum or patent ventilating tube.

C. TYPE C

The Type C tympanogram has negative peak pressure.

ACOUSTIC REFLEX

An acoustic reflex occurs when the stapedius muscle contracts in reaction to a loud sound. Acoustic reflex thresholds refer to the softest intensity levels that can trigger the response. They usually occur at 70–90 dB *above* the patient's threshold. When the muscle contracts, the stapes footplate rocks in the oval window and stiffens the ossicular chain and tympanic membrane, thus decreasing compliance. The change in compliance coincident with the presentation of an intense acoustic signal is measured with the same instrument as that used for tympanometry. Because monaural stimulation results in contraction of the stapedius muscles in both ears, the reflex can be measured either ipsilaterally or contralaterally. When the reflex is recorded in the stimulated ear, it is called an ipsilateral reflex; if it is recorded in the opposite ear, it is called a contralateral reflex. The following four stimulus-probe configurations can be measured: (1) right ipsilateral (stimulus to the right ear, probe to the right ear); (2) right contralateral (stimulus to the right ear, probe to the left ear); (3) left ipsilateral

(stimulus to the left ear, probe to the left ear); and (4) left contralateral (stimulus to the left ear, probe to the right ear). Figure 45–5 depicts the acoustic reflex arc. Knowledge of this pathway allows the clinician to compare the results of the various testing configurations to interpret the findings.

Patients with mild or moderate cochlear (sensory) hearing loss yield contralateral and ipsilateral acoustic reflex thresholds at approximately the same intensity levels as those with normal hearing. Acoustic reflexes are absent in the presence of a severe or profound hearing loss. A significant conductive hearing loss typically eliminates the response on either ear whenever the affected side is stimulated. This is because the stimulating sound is not loud enough to trigger the reflex when the affected ear is stimulated, and the middle ear abnormality (eg, otosclerosis or middle ear effusion) prevents the stapedius muscle from contracting even when the opposite (normal) ear is stimulated. Therefore, any disorder of the stapedius muscle can also cause absent acoustic reflexes. Thus, the only reflex that will occur for a unilateral conductive loss is the ipsilateral reflex to the normal ear. A bilateral conductive loss eliminates the reflex in all four conditions. A lesion of cranial nerve VIII can eliminate both the contralateral and ipsilateral acoustic reflexes whenever the affected side is stimulated. However, contralateral and ipsilateral reflexes are usually present when the normal ear is stimulated. For pathologies affecting the central crossed pathways, reflexes are present in both ipsilateral conditions, but may be absent in the two contralateral conditions. A lesion of the seventh nerve (eg, Bell palsy) can eliminate the acoustic reflex whenever the affected side is measured, regardless of which ear is stimulated. This pattern can be distinguished from the conductive pattern because in a conductive loss, both the measured and the stimulated ear typically show absent contralateral reflexes. In seventh nerve pathology, the acoustic reflex also can help to determine whether the lesion is proximal or distal to the branching of the stapedius muscle. If the lesion is proximal to the stapedius muscle, acoustic reflexes are absent; if the lesion is distal to the muscle, reflexes are present. Any central nervous system depressant, including alcohol, can depress the ampli-

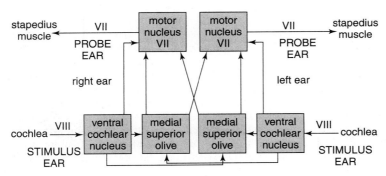

Figure 45–5. An acoustic reflex arc.

tude of the response. A functional hearing loss may be suspected if reflexes occur below the volunteered pure-tone thresholds or possibly (though not always) if less than 20 dB above threshold. When hearing loss exceeds 70 dB HL, it becomes difficult to determine whether absent reflexes are due to a cochlear or a retrocochlear hearing loss.

ACOUSTIC REFLEX DECAY

The measurement of acoustic reflex decay may be useful when a retrocochlear lesion is suspected. For this procedure, a 500- or 1000-Hz signal is presented to the ear contralateral to the probe ear, at 10 dB above the patient's acoustic reflex threshold for 10 seconds. If the response amplitude decreases more than 50%, it is considered abnormal (positive) and suggestive of a lesion on cranial nerve VIII. Usually, acoustic reflex decay is only measured contralaterally at 500 or 1000 Hz, because higher frequencies and ipsilateral stimulation may show decay even in normal subjects. The sensitivity and specificity of reflex decay are not as high as the auditory brainstem response (ABR) for identifying acoustic neuromas. Also, care must be taken in deciding whether or not to administer decay testing, especially in patients with tinnitus or hyperacusis, because of the intense stimulus levels that are often required.

Harris PK, Hutchison KM, Moravec J. The use of tympanometry and pneumatic otoscopy for predicting middle ear disease. *Am J Audiol.* 2005;14(1):3. [PMID: 16180966] (Describes tympanometry and multifrequency tympanometry and assesses the predictive potential of tympanometry for otitis media.)

■ ELECTROPHYSIOLOGY

AUDITORY BRAINSTEM RESPONSE

Auditory brainstem response (ABR) testing objectively assesses the neural synchrony of the auditory system from the level of the eighth nerve to the midbrain. The obtained results can be extrapolated to provide information regarding hearing sensitivity and also can be used for **neurodiagnostic** purposes. To administer the ABR test, electrodes are placed on the patient's head, and a series of sounds are presented. The patient must remain still and, with children, it may be necessary to sedate the patient to obtain valid results. The diagnostic (not screening) test procedure typically requires 45–90 minutes. The ABR consists of a series of 5–7 waves that occur within the first 10–15 ms following the stimulus. These potentials are shown in Figure 45–6. Waves I and II are thought to be generated in the eighth nerve

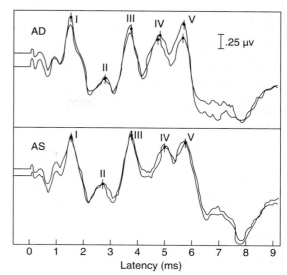

Figure 45–6. An example of a normal auditory brainstem response.

of the stimulus ear; Waves III–V are thought to be generated in the brainstem and midbrain. For neurologic purposes, the latencies (absolute, **interwave,** and **interaural**) and amplitudes (absolute and relative) of Waves I, III, and V are analyzed. Clicks are the most commonly used stimuli because their abrupt rise time and broad spectrum enhance **neural synchrony;** however, the results are dominated by the high-frequency region.

The other primary use of electrophysiologic measures is to estimate the auditory thresholds for AC and BC in patients who are unwilling or unable to provide accurate behavioral audiometric thresholds. For these patients, the lowest intensity level at which Wave V can be visualized and repeated is considered the threshold. Because interwave latencies are not measured, faster stimulation rates (25–50/s) may be used. ABR is frequently used for newborn hearing screening, because it provides accurate information in a fairly short amount of time. For better definition across the frequency range, **frequency-specific** stimuli, such as tone pips, are used. Because tonal signals have a slower rise-fall time than clicks, the wave morphology may be degraded, making threshold identification more difficult. Normative values from research centers for gender and age are available; however, to be accurate, each clinic should establish its own equipment-specific normative values. Recent additions to the electrophysiologic battery include **ASSR** (auditory steady-state response), which allows for a potentially more rapid means of establishing frequency-specific thresholds, stacked ABR (a more sensitive and specific method for the detection of small tumors), and **CHAMP** (cochlear hydrops analysis masking procedure) for detection of Meniere disease.

ABR Interpretation

Interpretation of the ABR depends on knowledge of the relevant recording and subject variables. Age and gender, as well as the type, degree, and configuration of the hearing loss, may substantially affect the latencies and amplitudes of the ABR. The following statements summarize the expected outcomes:

A. Normal Hearing

The latencies for Waves I, III, and V are within the normal range and the interaural (between ears) latencies are equal (within 0.2 to 0.3 ms).

B. Conductive Hearing Loss

The absolute latencies of all waves are prolonged, but the interwave latencies are not substantially affected. This pattern occurs regardless of the stimulus intensity. The configuration of the hearing loss may also contribute to variability in the latencies.

C. Cochlear Hearing Loss

The degree and configuration of the hearing loss may affect the latencies of Waves I, III, and V. A relatively flat hearing loss of less than 60 dB HL should not impact the ABR latencies, but high-frequency hearing loss may reduce the amplitudes and prolong the absolute latencies of the waves, without increasing the interwave I–V latency difference when stimuli are presented at high intensities.

D. Retrocochlear Hearing Loss

A variety of effects on the latencies and morphology of the ABR may occur. These may include the absence of waves, prolonged absolute or relative latencies (2 or 3 standard deviations beyond the mean), or prolonged interaural latencies. Wave I may be within normal limits, but the absolute latency for Wave V, and consequently the I–V interwave latency, is prolonged beyond the normal limits.

MIDDLE LATENCY RESPONSE

The middle latency response (MLR) occurs between 10 ms and 100 ms. The MLR is used primarily to estimate the hearing threshold. Because it requires less neural synchrony than the ABR, the MLR can be recorded in some cases in which the ABR cannot because of disruption of the neural synchrony by hearing loss or neural pathology. However, the use of the MLR for diagnostic purposes is limited by the fact that the origins are not well documented, the pathways are complex, and the response is variable.

ELECTROCOCHLEOGRAPHY

Electrocochleography (ECoG or ECochG) evaluates the electrical activity generated by the cochlea and the eighth cranial nerve, which usually occurs during the first 2–3 ms subsequent to a stimulus. The active electrode can be placed in the ear canal, on the tympanic membrane, or through the tympanic membrane; the reference electrode can be placed on the vertex or the contralateral earlobe or mastoid. The closer the active electrode is to the cochlea, the larger the response. The principal potentials that are evoked through ECoG are the cochlear microphonic, the summating potential, and the compound action potential. Most commonly, only the summating potential and the compound action potential are of interest. The main application of the ECoG is to help determine if a patient has Meniere disease. The amplitude of the summating potential (reflecting activity of the hair cells) is compared with that of the compound action potential (reflecting whole nerve activity). If the ratio is larger than normal (0.3–0.5), it is considered indicative of Meniere disease. The increased usage of CHAMP may render ECoG less applicable, especially since ECoG is somewhat variable unless the electrode is placed either on or through the tympanic membrane.

Don M, Kwong B, Tanaka C, Brackmann D, Nelson R. The stacked ABR: a sensitive and specific screening tool for detecting small acoustic tumors. *Audiol Neurootol.* 2005;10(5):274. [PMID: 15925862] (Introduction and basic explanation of the stacked auditory brainstem response test.)

Picton TW, John MS, Dimitrijevic A, Purcell D. Human auditory steady-state responses. *Int J Audiol.* 2003;42(4):177. [PMID: 12790346] (Review of the auditory steady-state response test protocol.)

■ OTOACOUSTIC EMISSIONS

Otoacoustic emissions (OAE) are objective, noninvasive, and rapid measures (typically less than 2 minutes) used to determine cochlear outer hair cell function. It is believed that OAE are a by-product of the **biomechanical motility** of the outer hair cells. Emissions are recorded from a small microphone placed in the ear canal via a soft probe. A good probe fit and low ambient and patient noise levels are essential to record OAE because the OAE response is very small (usually < 20 dB SPL).

OAE are usually detected in the presence of normal or near-normal hearing. Using current measurement protocols, emissions typically are not detected if there is a conductive or sensorineural hearing loss greater than

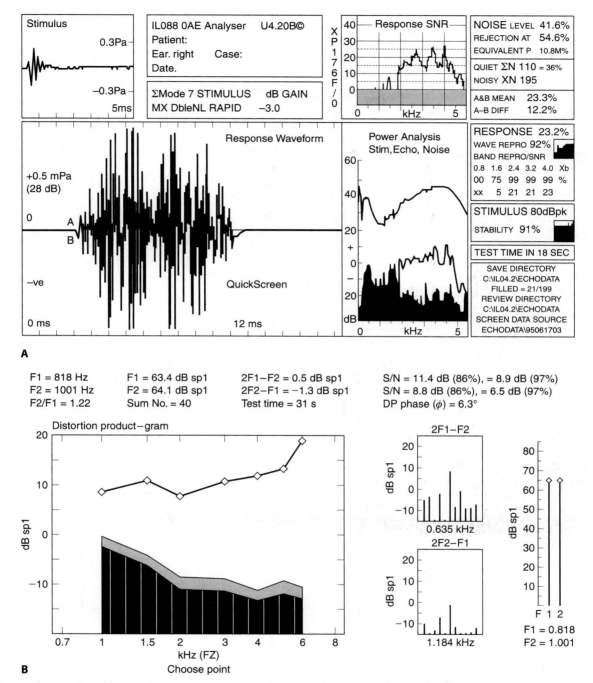

Figure 45–7. Examples of otoacoustic emissions. **(A)** In transient evoked otoacoustic emissions, the patient has normal hearing to 4000 Hz; and **(B)** in distortion product otoacoustic emissions, the patient has normal hearing.

25–30 dB HL. Although produced in the cochlea, a pathology in the outer or middle ear may obliterate OAE because of the reduction in stimulation signal intensity and also because the signal must travel distally through the middle and outer ear to be measured by the recording microphone.

The three main types of OAE are spontaneous, transient evoked, and distortion product.

SPONTANEOUS OTOACOUSTIC EMISSIONS

Spontaneous otoacoustic emissions (SOAE) occur even in the absence of a stimulus. SOAE are the product of a healthy cochlea; however, they are found in less than half of the normal hearing population and therefore cannot be used in hearing screening. They have limited clinical use at this time.

TRANSIENT EVOKED OTOACOUSTIC EMISSIONS

Transient evoked otoacoustic emissions (TEOAE) occur when the ear is stimulated by transient or brief signals, such as clicks. Even though the stimulus is a broadband signal, the TEOAE do provide frequency-specific results. As the traveling wave progresses through the cochlea, the basal (high frequency) turn of the cochlea is first to be stimulated by the click and responds earliest, followed by the more middle- and low-frequency (apical) portions, thus allowing the response to be analyzed in both the frequency and time domain.

DISTORTION PRODUCTION OTOACOUSTIC EMISSIONS

Distortion production otoacoustic emissions (DPOAE) are produced when two tones of different, but related, frequencies (F1 and F2) are presented to the cochlea simultaneously. F2 is usually 1.21 times the frequency of F1. In response to these two tones, a normal cochlea will generate tones, called distortion products, at frequencies that are related to F1 and F2. This is due to the **nonlinearity** of the healthy cochlea. The information obtained from DPOAE is frequency specific because tonal stimuli are used to generate the response. Although the results do show a relationship with the audiometric configuration, the relationship is not precise. More research is needed to determine the specific recording parameters and criteria for predicting peripheral hearing loss. Figure 45–7A and B show examples of TEOAE and DPOAE recorded from a patient with normal hearing.

The clinical applications of OAE are significant. Because OAE are specific to cochlear function, they can be very useful in differentiating between cochlear and retrocochlear lesions in sensorineural hearing loss. In fact, their use often renders the term "sensorineural" obsolete. Even though OAE assess cochlear outer hair cell function, the results are often used in predicting the likelihood of hearing impairment. As such, OAE testing is commonly used in newborn hearing screening because of its speed and noninvasive nature. It also is used in confirming pure-tone test results obtained from young children, in patients for whom a functional hearing loss is suspected, for audiometric configuration confirmation, for ototoxic drug monitoring, and in hearing aid candidacy. More recently, OAE, in conjunction with ABR, can be used in identifying individuals with **auditory neuropathy**, also termed auditory dyssynchrony.

Ellison JC, Keefe DH. Audiometric predictions using stimulus-frequency otoacoustic emissions and middle ear measurements. *Ear Hear.* 2005;26(5):487. [PMID: 16230898] (Estimating hearing loss from otoacoustic emission data.)

Lonsbury-Martin BL, Martin GK. Otoacoustic emissions. *Curr Opin Otolaryngol Head Neck Surg.* 2003;11(5):361. [PMID: 14502067] (Review of otoacoustic emissions.)

Vestibular Testing

46

Bulent Satar, MD

PATIENT HISTORY

Before performing any vestibular test, taking a thorough medical history and ascertaining the patient's symptoms constitute the first steps in caring for a patient with a vestibular disorder. Sometimes the patient history alone may suggest a diagnosis.

Symptoms

Taking a patient history should include determining the patient's symptoms, including balance, hearing, vision, somatosensation, and motor function. The first task for a neurotologist in evaluating a patient with a balance disorder is to allow the patient to describe what he or she senses, using his own descriptions. However, the clinician may help the patient in choosing the correct terms to describe his complaints.

A. VERTIGO

Vertigo can be described as an unreal sense of rotationary movement. It should be distinguished from dizziness, which describes any kind of altered sense of orientation. A history of vertigo is of great value in identifying the presence of vestibular pathology but not in localizing its origin. Vertigo results from impaired tonic symmetry in the inputs of the vestibular nuclei. Therefore, a vestibular lesion can occur anywhere within the vestibular endorgans, the vestibular nuclei, the cerebellum, the pathways connecting these structures in the brainstem, and, rarely, within the cortex.

The differentiation between peripheral and central nervous system (CNS) lesions may be based on detailed features of vertigo, even though these features may not apply to every patient. The clinician should determine whether the vertigo occurs in episodes or continuously. If it is episodic, it should be ascertained how often the episodes occur and how long they last. In peripheral causes, vertigo occurs in episodes with an abrupt onset. It disappears in varying time periods, from seconds to days, based on the underlying pathology. The origin of intensive, episodic vertigo that lasts up to a minute is more likely **benign paroxysmal positional vertigo** (BPPV) if it is provoked with particular positions. Other causes of brief but recurrent vertigo or dizziness, especially if pre-cipitated by body straining, is **perilymph fistula.** Vertigo that lasts 2–20 minutes is consistent with a **transient ischemic attack,** which affects the posterior circulation if it is associated with visual deficits, ataxia, and localized neurologic findings. **Meniere disease** causes recurrent vertigo attacks that can last between 20 minutes and 24 hours. An isolated attack of vertigo that lasts more than 24 hours is suggestive of **vestibular neuronitis.** Autonomic symptoms such as nausea, vomiting, and sweating are common presenting symptoms. Generally, the more intense symptoms a patient has, the more likely it is that the vertigo is caused by a peripheral lesion.

B. LIGHTHEADEDNESS

Lightheadedness describes the sensation of unsteadiness and falling or the symptoms similar to those preceding syncope, such as blurred vision and faded facial color. It should be distinguished from both vertigo and visual disorientation. Most often, lightheadedness occurs with nonvestibular causes such as cardiac or vasovagal reflex.

C. IMBALANCE

Imbalance is described as the inability to maintain the center of gravity. It causes the patient to feel unsteady or as if about to fall. The causes may be sensory or motor.

D. OTHER SYMPTOMS

The physician should also ascertain the presence of other associated symptoms such as hearing loss, tinnitus, and facial weakness. A positive history of precipitating factors (eg, rapid head movement) may lead the clinician to variants of BPPV. However, identifying the factors that induce vertigo may not be helpful in distinguishing peripheral lesions from CNS lesions because vertigo precipitated by rapid head movements may result from either decompensated peripheral vestibular lesions or CNS lesions. The physician should ascertain whether the patient has a history of falling with no loss of consciousness; this symptom may be associated with Meniere syndrome. Determining whether noise is a precipitating factor may be useful in identifying **Tullio phenomenon.** A history of brief episodes of vertigo induced by Valsalva-like maneuvers, which increase middle ear pressure, may be indicative of a perilymph

Gaze - Both Eyes

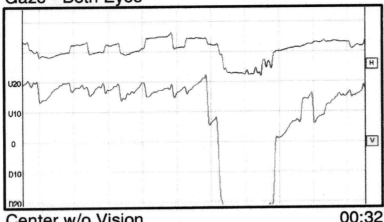

Center w/o Vision   00:32

Figure 46–1. Upbeating nystagmus in a patient with superior canal dehiscence syndrome as proven by coronal temporal bone CT. Upper trace (H) indicates horizontal eye movement and the bottom trace (V) vertical eye movement. There is no nystagmus in the horizontal record. However, the vertical trace shows upbeating nystagmus with gradually increasing slow-phase velocity (from 5°/s to 9.9°/s) as hyperventilation deepened.

fistula, Chiari malformation, or dehiscence of the superior semicircular canal (SCC). Figure 46–1 shows upbeating nystagmus induced by hyperventilation in a patient with superior canal dehiscence syndrome.

Drug Use

Determining the patient's drug history and current drug use (prescription or other) is crucial in evaluating dizziness. Vestibulotoxic drug intake may cause bilateral vestibular end-organ damage, which results in oscillopsia.

Psychological Factors

The clinician should also query patients about psychological factors. The specific site where dizziness occurs should be identified. Panic attacks or agoraphobia may be suspected if lightheadedness occurs in crowded areas or public places.

Family History

A positive family history of a balance disorder may contribute to the diagnosis, especially in Meniere syndrome, neurofibromatosis, migraine, and a narrow endolymphatic duct.

PATIENT EVALUATION

Physical Exam

The physical examination of a patient with a balance disorder should begin with a complete ear, nose, and throat exam. A detailed neurotologic examination should also be performed; it should include an evaluation for nystagmus and oculomotor function, as well as positional tests, postural control tests, and a cranial nerve examination.

Testing & Evaluation

A. OCULOMOTOR FUNCTION TESTS

Oculomotor function is tested by asking the patient to gaze at the tip of the clinician's index finger. The clinician should first hold her or his finger 25 cm away from the patient's eyes and then move it laterally and vertically, which is the tracking function. The clinician should assess whether the patient's eye movements are conjugate or disconjugate. In testing the horizontal tracking function, anything other than a smooth horizontal eye movement is assumed to be indicative of vestibulocerebellar pathology. During the vertical tracking test, a superimposed horizontal eye movement (ie, a saccadic intrusion) may occur in patients with a central oculomotor lesion. An imbalance in the tonic levels of activity that underlies the otolith-ocular reflexes leads to static ocular torsion, head tilt, and a skew deviation, which is a vertical misalignment of the eyes that is observed upon switching the cover from one eye to the other.

1. Nystagmus testing—In assessing for the presence of nystagmus, the clinician should be aware of possible changes in findings at the time of either the acute or chronic phase of the vertigo or dizziness.

    a. Spontaneous nystagmus—Spontaneous nystagmus is identified by having the patient wear Frenzel glasses. If nystagmus is found, the direction of its fast phase, frequency, and amplitude are noted. Determining the characteristics of the nystagmus would give the physician an overall indication, before electronystagmographic testing is performed, if there is an obvious asymmetry in the vestibular system. If primary positional nystagmus is purely vertical or purely torsional, a CNS disorder, usually in the vestibulocerebellum, the

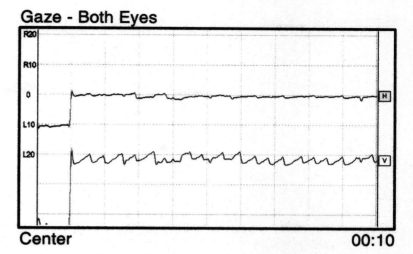

Figure 46–2. Downbeating nystagmus in a patient with diffuse cerebellar atrophy. Upper trace (H) indicates horizontal eye movement and the bottom trace (V) vertical eye movement. No nystagmus is noted in the horizontal record. Downbeating nystagmus (slow-phase velocity 7.8°/s) is clearly seen in the vertical trace.

vestibular nuclei, and their connections within the interstitial nucleus of Cajal in the midbrain, is likely. Figure 46–2 shows downbeating nystagmus in a patient with diffuse cerebellar atrophy. Spontaneous nystagmus that is peripheral in origin is characteristically diminished by visual fixation and increased only when fixation is canceled.

b. Gaze nystagmus—Gaze nystagmus is identified by holding the index finger at off-center positions. **Central origin nystagmus** may change its direction with different gaze positions. The direction of **peripheral origin nystagmus** is fixed in all gaze positions. A low-velocity, direction-fixed nystagmus (ie, 1–2°/s) or a direction-changing, gaze-evoked nystagmus, both of which present only in darkness, can occur as a nonspecific finding both in nonsymptomatic individuals and patients with organic peripheral or central vestibular lesions. While gazing at a distant object, the passive rotation of a patient's head at the frequency of 1 Hz over 20 seconds causes a patient with oscillopsia to make saccadic corrections and to view the object as no longer being stationary.

c. Head-shaking nystagmus—Head-shaking nystagmus is evaluated in the same way as gaze nystagmus; however, in head-shaking nystagmus, patients either wear Frenzel glasses or close their eyes. The frequency and speed of the patient's head shaking should be maintained at sufficiently high levels (at least 160°/s) to elicit the nonlinearity of the diseased vestibular labyrinth. The direction of head-shaking nystagmus may be toward either the side with the lesion or the side without it, and it may be monophasic, biphasic, or triphasic. If a head-shaking nystagmus beats toward the side without the lesion in a patient with no spontaneous nystagmus, the presence of a statically compensated peripheral lesion should be considered.

2. Nonlinearity testing—Dynamic nonlinearity in the SCCs can be tested at the bedside by observing the effect of head rotations on eye movements. With this test, the malfunction of individual canals is examined by applying high-acceleration head thrusts, with the eyes beginning about 15° away from the primary position in the orbit and the amplitude of the head movement such that the eyes end near the primary gaze position. The patient is asked to fix his or her gaze on the examiner's nose. Any corrective saccade shortly after the end of the thrusts is a sign of an inappropriate and compensatory slow-phase eye movement. Each canal can be tested in its plane.

3. Fistula testing—The presence of a fistula is suspected if nystagmus occurs or if the patient perceives movement of a visual target that is fixed after applying positive pressure to the outer ear canal. A positive test result (ie, **Hennebert sign**) suggests either a perilymph fistula or Meniere disease. Tullio phenomenon occurs in the same clinical entities when a loud noise is applied. Hyperventilation may induce symptoms in patients with anxiety and phobic disorders, but it seldom produces nystagmus.

B. POSITIONAL TESTS

Positional tests can be described as either dynamic or static. Static positional tests are discussed in the Electronystagmography section of this chapter.

The dynamic positional test is called the **Dix-Hallpike maneuver.** This test is performed to elicit typical nystagmus of BPPV of the vertical SCCs. The patient may be asked to wear Frenzel glasses. In the test, the patient sits on the examination table with his head rotated 45° from the sagittal plane to one side. The patient is then moved quickly into a position where his head hangs over the edge of the table. After a 20-second waiting period, if nystagmus is not observed, the patient is returned to his initial sitting position. The patient then rotates his head 45° from the sagittal plane to the alternate side. Then he is again brought quickly into a position where his head hangs over the edge of the table. Nystagmus is again sought. If rotational or torsional nystagmus is observed in any of the head-hanging positions, then typical nystagmus reversal is expected when the patient returns to the initial sitting position. The horizontal variant of BPPV is investigated in a different way; the patient is placed in the supine position with head raised 30° by the clinician. Horizontal geotropic or ageotropic nystagmus is identified when the clinician rotates the patient's head to both sides with nystagmus observation time-interval. The side of the lesion is determined based on the intensity of horizontal nystagmus produced by head movement toward each side. It is the side of lesion to which head movement creates more intense nystagmus.

C. Visual Acuity Testing

Visual acuity is the patient's ability to read an eye chart while his or her head is moving. The head is rotated passively at a frequency of 1–2 Hz/s. A drop in acuity of two lines or more from the baseline suggests an abnormal vestibuloocular reflex gain.

D. Postural Control Tests

The examination of postural control includes the following tests: (1) the Romberg test, (2) the pastpointing test, (3) the tandem gait test, and (4) the Fukuda stepping test. Postural control tests are considered to have mild sensitivity and specificity in identifying lesions. Depending on the nature and phase of the pathology, the side of the lesion cannot reliably be identified from these tests. Excessive swaying toward one side in the Romberg test, deviation to one side in the pastpointing test, or rotation to one side in the Fukuda stepping test may all indicate either a paretic lesion of the labyrinth in that side or an irritative lesion in the opposite side. The patient may show sway, rotation, or deviation toward the unaffected side if the peripheral lesion is at the compensated phase.

1. Romberg test—During the Romberg test, which is used to identify vestibular impairment, the patient is asked to stand still with eyes closed and feet together. An increased sway or fall toward either side is considered abnormal. The Romberg test can be made more sensitive by asking the patient to stand with the feet in a heel-to-toe position and with arms folded against the chest.

2. Pastpointing test—The patient and clinician both stand facing each other; they then stretch their arms forward with index fingers extended and in contact with one another. The patient is asked to raise his arms up and

bring his index fingers again into contact with the clinician's index fingers, which are fixed. The patient performs this movement 2–3 times with eyes open; later, the patient repeats the same maneuver with eyes closed. Deviation to one side is considered abnormal.

3. Tandem gait test—The patient is asked to take tandem steps with eyes closed. Healthy individuals can take at least 10 steps without deviation. Patients with vestibular disorders fail this test.

4. Fukuda stepping test—The patient is asked to march in place with eyes closed. After 50 steps, a rotation > 30° toward one side is considered abnormal.

E. Cranial Nerve Evaluation

An evaluation of cranial nerve function may reveal hypoesthesia of the outer ear canal and an absent corneal reflex, as found in acoustic neuromas. Facial nerve paralysis may be associated with herpes zoster oticus. Eye muscle restrictions may be elicited by evaluating the functioning of cranial nerves III (oculomotor nerve), IV (trochlear nerve), and VI (abducens nerve) before the electronystagmogram.

Fetter M. Assessing vestibular function: which tests, when? *J Neurol.* 2000;247:335. [PMID: 10896264] (Relevant points of examining and testing patients with balance disorders.)

Katsarkas A, Smith H, Galiana H. Head-shaking nystagmus (HSN): the theoretical explanation and the experimental proof. *Acta Otolaryngol.* 2000;120:177. [PMID: 11603767] (Investigating the consistency of the head-shaking nystagmus as a bedside examination with rotary chair testing.)

Rosenberg ML, Gizza M. Neuro-otologic history. *Otolaryngol Clin North Am.* 2000;33:471. [PMID: 10815031] (Definitions of the terms vertigo, visual disorientation, lightheadedness, and imbalance, as well as the precipitating factors and symptoms associated with vertigo and dizziness.)

Walker MF, Zee DS. Bedside vestibular examination. *Otolaryngol Clin North Am.* 2000;33:495. [PMID: 10815033] (Detailed neurotologic examination and findings.)

ELECTRONYSTAGMOGRAPHY

Electronystagmography (ENG) is the fundamental test and the first step in a vestibular testing battery to evaluate the vestibuloocular reflex in patients with a balance disorder. It is based on recording and measuring eye movements or eye positions in response to visual or vestibular stimuli.

A. Equipment

Standard ENG equipment consists of the following components: (1) an amplifier for amplification of the corneal-retinal potential that occurs following eye movement, (2) band-pass and notch filters, (3) a signal recorder, (4) a light array, and (5) water and air caloric stimulators. The techniques available to record eye movements are electrooculography (EOG), infrared recording, magnetic search coil, and video-recording systems.

An ENG analysis consists mainly of three tests: (1) oculomotor tests, (2) positional tests, and (3) caloric tests. Before each test, the system needs to be calibrated to maintain accuracy. The calibration is performed via a saccade test that is discussed in the section on Oculomotor Tests.

B. UTILITY OF ELECTRONYSTAGMOGRAPHY

ENG is very useful in diagnosing vestibular pathology. No other test provides information on the site of the lesion. The data obtained from an ENG test battery support the diagnoses of horizontal BPPV, vestibular neuronitis, Meniere disease, labyrinthitis, and ototoxicity. With acoustic neuromas, it may be helpful to predict the nerve from which the tumor originates; caloric weakness may be associated with a tumor that originates from the superior vestibular nerve. ENG may also predict whether the patient will experience vertigo after acoustic tumor removal. However, relying on ENG alone to identify lesions in the CNS would not be appropriate.

Abnormal findings in ENG testing do not necessarily indicate a definite CNS lesion. One study investigated the ratio of patients with abnormal results as reported by magnetic resonance imaging (MRI) to patients with abnormal ENG findings in different age groups and found a better correlation between MRI and ENG findings in a group of elderly patients. Overall, MRI confirmed a central lesion in 52% of patients with abnormal ENG findings. In contrast, ENG findings were abnormal in 15 of 21 patients (71%) with an abnormal MRI. In two recent studies, only 30–37% of the patients with abnormal ENG findings had abnormal MRI scans.

1. Oculomotor Tests

Oculomotor tests measure the accuracy, latency, and velocity of eye movements for a given stimulus. The standard oculomotor test battery includes saccade tests, smooth pursuit tests, optokinetic nystagmus testing, gaze tests, and fixation suppression testing. All oculomotor tests are performed with the patient seated upright, with the head stabilized. For oculomotor tests, the ENG device should have a light array on which LED (light-emitting diodes) are given as a stimulus. The light array may be rotated vertically for calibration purposes as well as for testing vertical saccades. The center of the light arrays should be at the same level as the patient's eyes.

Saccade Test

Saccades are rapid eye movements that bring objects in the periphery of the visual field onto the fovea. The latency of saccades is very brief. Because peak velocity can be as high as 700°/s, vision is not clear during saccadic movement. Saccades are controlled by the occipitoparietal cortex, the frontal lobe, the basal ganglia, the superior colliculus, the cerebellum, and the brainstem.

To test saccadic eye movement, the patient is asked to follow the LED with as much accuracy as possible. The LED flashes sequentially in two positions: at the center of the array, and then 15–20° to the right or left from the center. The interval between flashes is usually a few seconds. The test is repeated vertically.

Three parameters are of clinical significance in evaluating saccades: latency, peak eye velocity, and accuracy of the saccades.

Latency is the time difference between the presentation of a target and the beginning of a saccade. The mean latency is 192 ± 32 ms in normal subjects. Abnormalities in latency include prolonged latency, shortened latency, and differences in the latency between the right eye and the left eye. These abnormalities are observed in the presence of neurodegenerative disease.

The **peak velocity** is the maximum velocity that eyes reach during a saccadic movement. It ranges from 283 to 581°/s for 20° of amplitude in normal subjects. Abnormalities in the saccadic velocity are slow saccades, fast saccades, or a difference in the velocity between the right eye and the left eye. Reasons for saccadic slowing include the use of sedative drugs, drowsiness, cerebellar disorders, basal ganglia disorders, and brainstem lesions. Fast saccades can be observed in calibration errors and eye muscle restrictions. The asymmetry of velocity is observed in internuclear ophthalmoplegia, eye muscle restrictions, ocular muscle palsies, and palsy of cranial nerves III and VI (the oculomotor and abducens nerves, respectively).

Accuracy is the final parameter in the evaluation of saccades. Saccadic accuracy is determined by saccadic movement by comparing the patient's eye position relative to the target position. Figure 46–3 provides a record of normal saccadic movement with accurate square tracing. If the saccadic eye movement goes farther than the target position, it is referred to as a **hypermetric saccade** (or **overshoot dysmetria**). If the saccadic movement is shorter than the target position, it is referred to as **hypometric saccade** (or **undershoot dysmetria**). Undershooting by 10% of the amplitude of the saccade may be observed in healthy subjects, whereas hypermetric saccades rarely occur in healthy subjects. Inaccurate saccades suggest the presence of a pathologic condition in the cerebellum, brainstem, or basal ganglia.

Smooth Pursuit Test

Smooth pursuit is the term used to describe eye movement that is created when the eyes track moving objects. Similar central pathways to those of saccadic movement produce smooth pursuit movement. The

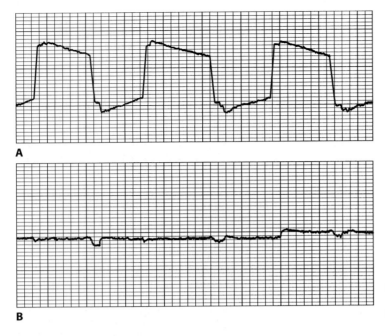

A

B

Figure 46–3. An EOG recording of normal saccadic eye movement. **(A)** A horizontal record. **(B)** A vertical record.

neural pathways serving the "pursuit system" are distributed in the cortical and subcortical areas of the brain. Smooth pursuit function also involves the fovea.

In a commonly used stimulus paradigm of the smooth pursuit test, the LED moves back and forth between two points on a light bar at a constant frequency and velocity. The patient is asked to follow this moving target. The frequency of the test stimulus should be between 0.2 and 0.8 Hz/s. A typical pursuit velocity is between 20 and 40°/s. Performance declines with higher velocities and increasing patient age.

The primary parameters for evaluation are gain, phase, and trace morphology. **Gain** is the ratio of peak eye velocity to the target velocity. For a stimulus of 0.5 Hz with a sweeping amplitude of 40° a gain > 0.8 is considered normal. A low gain is suggestive of a CNS disorder. **Phase** is the difference in time between eye movement and target movement. Under optimal conditions, healthy subjects can track a target with a phase angle of 0°. The level of attention and drugs affecting the CNS can destroy pursuit performance.

A morphologic assessment of the trace is also important. Figure 46–4 shows a record of normal tracking eye movement. A morphologic abnormality is referred to as a staircase of saccades, in which the trace shows staircase-like eye movement while the target is followed. Pursuit traces can be impaired symmetrically or asymmetrically. An asymmetrically impaired pursuit is more suggestive of a CNS lesion than is a symmetrically impaired pursuit. Acute peripheral vestibular lesions can also impair smooth pursuit contralateral to the affected side when the eyes are moving against the slow phase of a spontaneous nystagmus.

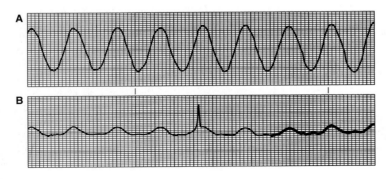

A

B

Figure 46–4. EOG recording of normal tracking eye movement. **(A)** and **(B)** are horizontal and vertical records of the tracking movement, respectively.

Testing of Optokinetic Nystagmus & Optokinetic Afternystagmus

Optokinetic nystagmus (OKN) is an involuntary oculo-motor response to a moving target that fills at least 90% of the visual field.

A. EQUIPMENT

The best optokinetic stimulator is a 360° turning cloth drum with black and white stripes. Because this drum can be unwieldy, it is preferable to use an optokinetic projector.

B. TEST ADMINISTRATION

The normal response to an optokinetic stimulator is a smooth eye movement that follows the direction of the visual stimulus both clockwise and counterclockwise. OKN aims to stabilize the visual field onto the retina. OKN is produced by cortical and brainstem structures, which is the same as the pursuit. Optokinetic afternys-tagmus (OKAN) is a form of nystagmus that is pro-duced by the brainstem after a 10-second, constant-velocity optokinetic stimulus. It lasts about 30 seconds.

OKN can be stimulated with a constant target speed between 20 and 60°/s or a sinusoidal target speed of up to 100°/s. Each target speed needs to be repeated in both clockwise and counterclockwise directions. The patient is asked to gaze straight ahead while the target is moved in front of his or her field of vision. The type of stimulus chosen is presented for 1 minute. When a con-stant-velocity optokinetic stimulus is used, the patient's eyes reach a constant velocity after 10 seconds of stimu-lation in one direction. Once this stimulus is discontin-ued, the room light is turned off and the recording is continued for OKAN until the OKAN is decayed. The same stimulus is then applied in the opposite direction. It should be noted that a sinusoidal stimulus cannot be used to test OKAN.

C. TESTING PARAMETERS OF OPTOKINETIC NYSTAGMUS

In testing of OKN, the most useful parameters are gain and phase.

1. Gain—The normal value of gain is ≥ 0.5, as well as symmetry on both sides (ie, in both eyes) for a stimulus of 60°/s. A gain in OKN may be reduced symmetrically or asymmetrically. A symmetrically reduced gain is observed in visual disorders, fast-phase disorders, and congenital nystagmus. Unilateral parietal-occipital lesions cause an asymmetrically reduced gain.

2. Phase—As a testing parameter, phase is applied only for the sinusoidal stimulus of OKN. The testing of OKN is less sensitive than a pursuit test. The sensitivity and specificity of OKN elicited by stimulation of the full visual field are 46% and 92%, respectively, which is superior to the sensitivity and specificity of OKN elic-ited by stimulation of the partial visual field.

D. TESTING PARAMETERS OF OPTOKINETIC AFTERNYSTAGMUS

The testing of OKAN is evaluated by three parameters: the initial velocity, the time constant, and the slow-cumu-lative eye position. The **initial velocity** is calculated from the OKAN at the 2nd second. This initial velocity is approximately 10°/s for a stimulus of 60°/s. The **time constant** is the length of time required for the slow-phase velocity to decline to 37% of the initial velocity. The **slow cumulative eye position** is a function of both the initial velocity and the time constant. Because it shows less inter-subject variability compared with the other two, it is the most useful parameter. The normative value of the slow cumulative eye position varies among the vestibular laboratories. Abnormalities in OKAN present as symmet-rically reduced OKAN, which is bilateral; asymmetrically reduced OKAN; and hyperactive OKAN. A complete bilateral loss of OKAN is observed in a bilateral vestibular loss, which may be either peripheral or central. Asymme-try in OKAN is indicative of a unilateral vestibular loss. Hyperactive OKAN may be seen in mal de debarquement syndrome.

Gaze Test

The gaze test is performed by recording eye movements while the patient fixes his vision on the center of a tar-get; the patient then fixes his gaze 30–40° to the right, to the left, and then above and below the center of the target. The patient's gaze, as well as a recording of that gaze, are sustained for at least 30 seconds. A gaze test may reveal peripheral or CNS lesions that are either vestibular or nonvestibular in origin. It may also reveal either congenital or spontaneous nystagmus. Patients with gaze nystagmus cannot maintain stable conjugate eye deviation away from the primary position; there-fore, the focus of the patient's vision is brought back to the center by resetting the corrective saccades. Vestibu-lar spontaneous nystagmus is seen during and after uni-lateral vestibular dysfunction and beats away from the afflicted side. It is seen as a horizontal nystagmus in an ENG recording, but it is actually both horizontal and torsional in nature. The intensity of vestibular sponta-neous nystagmus increases when the patient's gaze is directed toward the direction of the nystagmus.

A typical gaze-evoked nystagmus that is peripheral in origin is unidirectional on a horizontal plane; it is both horizontal and torsional. Its intensity increases when gaze is directed toward the direction of the nystagmus. A gaze-evoked nystagmus with a CNS origin may change direc-tion with the patient's gaze. A nystagmus that results from a vertical gaze is always suggestive of CNS lesions.

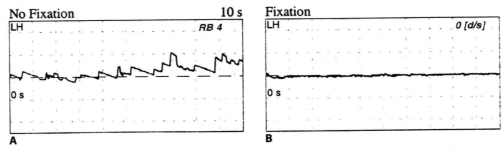

Figure 46–5. (A) A right-beating spontaneous nystagmus with a slow-phase velocity of 4°/s. **(B)** Note that the nystagmus disappears with fixation. (Reprinted, with permission of Hussam K. El-Kashlan, MD; University of Michigan, Ann Arbor, Department of Otolaryngology–Head & Neck Surgery.)

Gaze nystagmus may be classified as symmetric, asymmetric, rebound, or disassociated. In **symmetric gaze nystagmus,** the eyes move in equal amplitude in both directions. The ingestion of drugs that affect the CNS, as well as multiple sclerosis, myasthenia gravis, and cerebellar atrophy, may all cause symmetric gaze nystagmus. **Asymmetric gaze nystagmus** is indicative of a lesion within the brainstem or the cerebellum. **Rebound nystagmus** begins in lateral gaze positions and reverses its direction to the primary position, even though there is no evidence of nystagmus in the primary position at the beginning of testing. It is also a strong indicator of cerebellar or brainstem lesions. **Dissociated (disconjugate) nystagmus** is the difference in eye movements during the gaze. It results from lesions of the medial longitudinal fasciculus.

Fixation Suppression Testing

Spontaneous nystagmus is determined by placing the patient, with eyes closed, in a totally darkened room without any visual or positional stimuli. If spontaneous nystagmus is found, its slow-phase velocity is recorded. The patient is then asked to fixate on the center of a visual target (central gaze). The ratio of the slow-phase velocity with fixation to the slow-phase velocity without fixation is then calculated. This calculation provides a **fixation-suppression index.** This index should be < 50%. Nystagmus that results from a peripheral origin decays to more than 50% with fixation. Figure 46–5 shows the effect of fixation on a spontaneous nystagmus that is peripheral in origin.

2. Positional Tests

The purpose of positional testing is to determine the effect of different stationary head positions (and not head movements) on eye movements. The assumption of these tests is that the patient's nystagmus is generated as a result of the orientation of the patient's head to gravity. The patient is asked to wear Frenzel glasses (or the test can be performed while the patient's eyes are closed), and the patient is brought slowly into the following positions: the patient's head (1) is turned right and then left while sitting, (2) is turned right and then left in the supine position, (3) is turned right and then left in a decubitus position, and (4) hangs straight down. Each position is maintained for at least 20 seconds. Positional nystagmus may be intermittent or persistent, and the direction may be fixed or changing.

The identification of positional nystagmus is not a localizing finding since it may be observed in patients with both peripheral and CNS lesions. Two features may help to distinguish the positional nystagmus that results from a peripheral lesion from one that results from a central lesion: (1) positional nystagmus caused by a peripheral lesion is suppressed by fixation; (2) the direction changing nystagmus may be indicative of a CNS lesion. The clinician must be careful about the contamination of spontaneous nystagmus with positional changes. If persistent nystagmus is noted, it should be observed for at least 2 minutes. This observation is especially important with periodic alternating nystagmus, in which the nystagmus reverses direction every 2 minutes. It is found that this type of nystagmus is caused by CNS lesions.

3. Caloric Tests

Caloric tests are based on comparing magnitude of the induced nystagmus on the right and left sides. Since the outer ear canal is close to the horizontal SCC, most of the response origins come from the horizontal SCC. Therefore, the nystagmus is horizontal. The temperature gradient produced by a cold stimulus causes the cupula to move away from the utricle, thereby creating a nystagmus that beats toward the opposite side. A warm stimulus causes the endolymph to rise, resulting in a nystagmus that beats toward the stimulus side.

Caloric testing is an important tool in assessing the vestibular system. It allows for the separate stimulation of each ear. Therefore, it provides data about the site of the lesion. However, there are some disadvantages of this test. Heat transfer from the ear canal to the horizontal SCC may vary among individuals, depending on the differences in the temporal bone pneumatization among patients. Another disadvantage is the fact that a caloric stimulus can provide a means of evaluating the vestibular response, but at only one frequency. The last disadvantage is that the caloric test allows only for the evaluation of the horizontal SCC.

A. EQUIPMENT

The caloric test uses a caloric stimulator, either a water or air irrigator, in addition to the EOG recording equipment. Two types of water stimulators are available: open loop and closed loop. The difference between the two stimulators is where the water circulates. An **open-loop stimulator** delivers water directly into the outer ear canal. In **closed-loop systems,** the water circulates in an expandable rubber medium to preserve its temperature. Open-loop systems are thought to provide more reliable and reproducible results than closed-loop systems. Caloric testing with either air or a closed-loop water stimulus should be reserved for patients who have a tympanic membrane perforation.

B. TEST ADMINISTRATION

The patient should be in the supine position, with his head tilted 30° upward to bring the horizontal SCC into the earth vertical position—this position makes the horizontal SCC more sensitive. The test can be performed with either a bithermal or a monothermal caloric stimulus. The **bithermal caloric test** provides the most useful data on the vestibular system, which is stimulated by warm and cold water or air. To enhance the nystagmus response, mental tasks are given to the patient during the test. The recording can be performed with the patient's eyes opened in total darkness, with his eyes opened and wearing Frenzel glasses, or with his eyes closed.

In performing caloric testing, temperatures seven degrees below and above body temperature (30° and 44° C) are used as cold- and warm-water stimuli. A total volume of 250 mL of water is given to the outer ear canal over a period of 30 or 40 seconds. As an alternative to the water stimulus, two air stimuli that are 24° C and 50° C are used with a flow rate of 8 L/min for 60 seconds. Four caloric stimuli are given with an interval of no less than 5 minutes to prevent superimposition or conflicting responses. The following order of stimuli is preferred: (1) right–warm, (2) left–warm, (3) right–cold, and (4) left–cold. In response to the caloric stimulus, the nystagmus begins just before the end of the caloric stimulus and reaches a peak at approximately 60 seconds of stimulation; it then slowly decays over the

next minute. When it reaches its peak, patients are asked to fixate their eyes on a central point to check the fixation suppression index.

C. TESTING PARAMETERS

The most reliable and consistent parameter is the peak slow-phase velocity of the induced nystagmus. The peak slow-phase velocity is averaged over a 10-second period and is calculated for each side.

The values obtained for each caloric stimulus are placed into equations, with each used for specific conditions that define vestibular function. Unilateral weakness (ie, canal paresis) indicates a significantly weak response on one side relative to the other. It is formulated as follows:

$$(R\ 30°C + R\ 44°C) - (L\ 30°C + L\ 44°C) \times 100\% \div$$
$$(R\ 30°C + R\ 44°C + L\ 30°C + L\ 44°C)$$

The difference between the sides $\geq$ 20–25% indicates the presence of a **unilateral weakness.** However, normative data for this critical percentage should be determined for each laboratory. Unilateral weakness is not a localizing finding and may be caused by lesions from the labyrinth to the root entry zone of the eighth cranial nerve (ie, the vestibulocochlear nerve) in the brainstem, such as Meniere disease, labyrinthitis, vestibular neuronitis, acoustic neuromas (and other tumors pressing on the eighth nerve), and multiple sclerosis.

Directional preponderance (ie, unidirectional weakness) refers to a condition in which the mean-peak, slow-phase velocity of the nystagmus beating toward one side is significantly greater than the mean-peak, slow-phase velocity of the nystagmus beating toward the opposite side. It is determined by the following equation:

$$(R\ 30°C + L\ 44°C) - (R\ 44°C + L\ 30°C) \times 100\% \div$$
$$(R\ 30°C + R\ 44°C + L\ 30°C + L\ 44°C)$$

A difference > 20–30% assumes the existence of a directional preponderance. This critical percentage should be determined by a testing laboratory. The directional preponderance is often associated with a spontaneous nystagmus because a spontaneous nystagmus enhances the nystagmus beating toward its direction and eliminates the nystagmus beating toward the opposite direction. The directional preponderance simply shows the existence of bias in the tonic activity of the vestibular system. However, the directional preponderance is considered to reflect an asymmetry in the dynamic sensitivity between the left and the right medial vestibular neurons, as opposed to the reason behind the spontaneous nystagmus, which is reflected in asymmetry in the resting activity. The directional preponderance is a poor localizing finding. It may be observed in lesions from the labyrinth to the cortex. The directional preponderance is toward the lesion site for labyrinth and eighth nerve lesions, and toward the uninvolved site for lesions of the brainstem and cortex. It is controversial that a directional preponderance without a spontaneous nystagmus is suggestive of a CNS disorder. One retrospective study showed that 5% of patients with an isolated directional preponderance had a CNS lesion. Other patient groups had peripheral lesions or no definite diagnosis. Directional preponderance and unilateral weakness may be observed together, which is suggestive of acute unilateral peripheral lesions.

Caloric weakness may be found in both sides, which is referred to as **bilateral weakness.** The level of response that is considered a bilateral weakness varies based on the normative data. However, several physicians give their own normative measurements. For both sides, the total response to a warm stimulus (< 11°/s) and the total response to a cold stimulus (< 6°/s) is considered bilateral weakness. Patients with bilateral weakness often present with oscillopsia. A bilateral weakness is often associated with vestibulotoxic antibiotherapy or bilateral Meniere disease. However, it is also observed in patients with lesions of the vestibular nuclei, Lyme disease, Cogan syndrome, pseudotumor cerebri, and neurodegenerative diseases of the brainstem and cerebellum.

Hyperactive caloric responses may also be observed. The numeric criteria for these responses varies among laboratories from 40°/s to 80°/s. Hyperactive caloric responses are associated with a cerebellar lesion or atrophy due to removal of the cerebellar inhibitory effect on the vestibular nuclei.

Failure (ie, an abnormal finding) of the fixation suppression test may be found in the caloric test. The patient is asked to fixate on a central point during the peak caloric response. Vestibular nystagmus is normally suppressed by visual fixation. The fixation index expresses this attenuation quantitatively, which is the difference between the slow-phase velocity in the dark and in the light divided by the slow-phase velocity in the dark. The normal value for the visual suppression of the caloric response is > 50%. If it fails—that is < 50%—impaired fixation suppression results. Cerebellar lesions affecting the flocculus cause impaired fixation suppression.

The **inversion of caloric nystagmus** is observed in patients with a tympanic membrane perforation. It occurs because of the cooling effect of the evaporation of moisture in the middle ear mucosa when warm air is used as a caloric stimulus.

Premature caloric reversal is the finding that can be observed in patients with **Friedreich ataxia** and brainstem lesions. The normal caloric response starts to decay at 90 s of the stimulation and disappears after 200 s, with a nystagmus beating toward the opposite side. In premature caloric reversal, nystagmus reversal occurs earlier than 140–150 s. It is worth noting that one should not refer to a preexisting spontaneous nystagmus as a premature caloric response.

Bhansali SA, Honrubia V. Current status of electronystagmography testing. *Otolaryngol Head Neck Surg.* 1999;120:419. [PMID: 10064649] (Brief description including the methodology and interpretation of oculomotor tests, the positional test, and the caloric test.)

Henry DF. Test-retest reliability of open-loop bithermal caloric irrigation responses from healthy young adults. *Am J Otol.* 1999;20:220. [PMID: 1010026] (Presents normal caloric response with standard deviations and seeks correlation between measurements obtained from repeated open-loop caloric irrigations.)

Maire R, Duvoisin B. Localization of static positional nystagmus with the ocular fixation test. *Laryngoscope.* 1999;109:606. [PMID: 10201749] (Describes the features of positional nystagmus that result from peripheral and central origins.)

Steering Committee of the Balance Interest Group. Recommended procedure. *Br J Audiol.* 1998;33:179. [PMID: 10439144] (The article gives a recommended caloric test protocol.)

Stoddart RL, Baguley DM, Beynon GJ, Chang P, Moffat DA. Magnetic resonance imaging results in patients with central electronystagmography findings. *Clin Otolaryngol.* 2000;25:293. [PMID: 10971536] (Abnormal electronystagmographic findings and their reliability in diagnosing central lesions.)

van der Stappen A, Wuyts FL, van de Heyning PH. Computerized electronystagmography: normative data revisited. *Acta Otolaryngol.* 2000;120:724. [PMID: 11099148] (Presentation of methodology and normative values of computerized oculomotor tests, positional tests, and caloric tests.)

van der Torn M, van Dijk JE. Testing the central vestibular functions: a clinical survey. *Clin Otolaryngol.* 2000;25:298. [PMID: 10971537] (Assesses the reliability of abnormal findings in saccade, smooth pursuit, fixation suppression, and sinusoidal acceleration tests.)

ROTARY CHAIR TEST

The rotary chair test, which is also referred to as **rotational testing,** is used to evaluate the pathway between the horizontal SCC and the eye muscles. This pathway is known as the **horizontal vestibuloocular reflex** because the patient is positioned so that only the horizontal SCC is stimulated. Rotational testing has three main functions: (1) to confirm the bilateral impairment of horizontal functioning of the SCC, (2) to provide evidence of a central vestibular dysfunction, and (3) to quantify the progress of a known vestibulopathy.

A. EQUIPMENT

A typical rotary chair test consists of a stimulus device, a response recording and its analysis, a light-proof booth, a video camera, and a two-way communication system. The stimulus device is a chair whose rotational speed is precisely controlled by a computer within certain speed and frequency limits. The response recording is made with electrodes, which are placed to record horizontal eye movements.

B. STIMULUS TYPES

Rotary chair testing includes basically two types of stimuli. Different protocols for each type of stimulus are used in different laboratories. One type of stimulus is called a **sinusoidal harmonic acceleration;** a series of rotational stimuli is used at the octaves of frequencies from 0.01 Hz to 1.28 Hz, to the right and to the left. The velocity of the chair is set at 50–60°/s. The rotational stimulus at a given frequency is used for multiple cycles. The second type of stimulus is a **velocity step test,** which applies a series of velocities. The test is started with an acceleration impulse of 100°/s² until a fixed, desirable rotational stimulus of 60–180°/s is achieved. Once the fixed velocity has been reached and applied for 46–60 s, the chair is decelerated to 0°/s, with the same magnitude of the acceleration. The test is then repeated in the opposite direction.

After each stimulus protocol, the computer detects slow-component eye velocity, omitting the fast component of the induced nystagmus. During the tests, the eye position, eye velocity, and chair velocity (ie, head velocity) are monitored.

C. TEST ADMINISTRATION

The patient sits in the chair with his or her head secured in the head support. The seatbelt should be fastened. Eye movements are recorded with an infrared camera or electrodes placed lateral to both outer canthi. The patient should be informed of the stimulus type to be given and instructed not to move throughout the test unless told to do so. Throughout the test, the patient should be kept mentally alert with arithmetic tasks (eg, counting cities or states in alphabetical order). Before the rotational test, the system should be calibrated. The test is performed in total darkness, with the patient's eyes opened. Throughout the test, the patient's eyes should be monitored with a video camera. A two-way communication system is used to give instructions and arithmetic tasks to the patient.

D. TESTING PARAMETERS

In a sinusoidal harmonic acceleration test, there are three parameters to be evaluated: phase, gain, and symmetry data.

1. Phase—The phase demonstrates a timing relationship between the head velocity and the slow-component eye velocity through the frequencies tested. The difference between the two is defined as the phase angle and is expressed in a measure of degrees. The fact that the eye velocity is greater than the head velocity is known as the **phase lead.** The opposite is known as the **phase lag.** For maintaining the position of objects in the retina, the eye velocity needs to be equal to the head velocity. Under this circumstance, the phase angle would be 180°. An alternative measure of the phase angle is the time constant of the response, which is inversely correlated to it.

2. Gain—The gain is the ratio of slow-component eye velocity to the head velocity, which represents the response capability of the vestibular system through the frequencies tested. The values outside of the normal range, based on normative data, are considered abnormal as long as the system is calibrated and the patient is alert.

3. Symmetry data—Symmetry data demonstrates whether slow-component eye velocities are equal on both sides.

The main testing parameter in the velocity step test is the time constant, which is the time needed for slow-component eye velocity to decline to 37% of the initial value. The second parameter of the velocity step test is the gain, whose definition is the same as its counterpart in the sinusoidal harmonic acceleration test.

In a sinusoidal harmonic acceleration test, an increased phase angle may imply a peripheral system insult or, less commonly, vestibular nucleus involvement. A decreased phase angle may imply a lesion in the cerebellum. Low gain is consistent with bilateral peripheral insult; high gain may be seen in cerebellar lesions. Asymmetry can be suggestive of the involvement of a central or decompensated peripheral vestibular system. If the central system is intact, a paretic lesion where either asymmetry or an irritative lesion in the opposite side is present is likely. It is analogous with the directional preponderance in the caloric test. In the velocity step test, an acute peripheral insult results in low gain and a shortened time constant of the response to the rotational stimulus toward the side of the lesion. Figure 46–6 presents a comparative analysis of caloric and rotary chair testing.

The relationship between the horizontal vestibuloocular reflex generated by the rotational stimulus and the caloric stimulus is significant. There is no linear relationship between the gain and canal paresis because as the magnitude of canal paresis increases, the gain decreases somewhat and then remains stable. However, the time constant decreases proportionally with increasing canal paresis.

HIGH-FREQUENCY ROTATIONAL TESTS

High-frequency rotational tests are tools for testing horizontal and vertical vestibuloocular reflexes generated by the patient making active or passive head move-

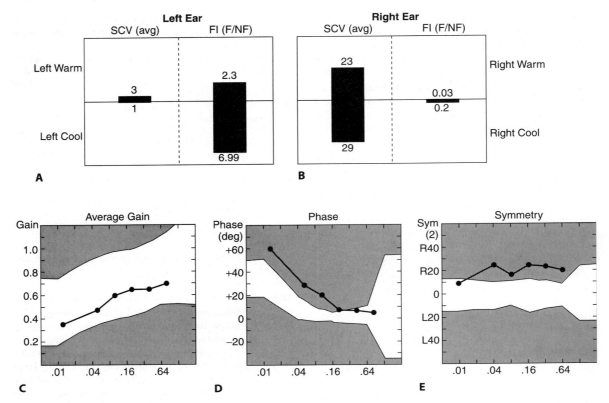

Figure 46–6. **(A)** This panel demonstrates left unilateral weakness (88%) in a patient with an acute peripheral vestibular insult. Left-sided irrigations produce very weak responses (3°/s and 1°/s) compared with **(B)** right-sided irrigations (23°/s and 29°/s). There is no directional preponderance (13%). Fixation indices (FI) in both sides are within the normal range. The patient had right-beating spontaneous nystagmus (6°/s). The sinusoidal harmonic acceleration test in the same patient displays **(C)** normal gain throughout the test frequencies, **(D)** an increased phase angle at lower frequencies, and **(E)** right asymmetry at frequencies higher than 0.01 Hz. Note that there is no asymmetry at 0.01 Hz, which corresponds to an absent directional preponderance on the caloric test. Stippled areas represent the 95th percentile values. (Reprinted, with permission, of Hussam K. El-Kashlan, MD; University of Michigan, Ann Arbor, Department of Otolaryngology–Head & Neck Surgery.)

ments like those encountered in everyday life. High-frequency and high-acceleration rotational stimuli are expected to unmask the inherent asymmetry in the vestibular system. The tests have some advantages over the rotary chair test. For example, the equipment is more affordable. Testing time is very short (almost 20 s). The equipment is not heavy machinery in contrast to the rotary chair. The tests investigates vestibuloocular reflex by means of active or passive rotationary head movements in both horizontal and vertical planes.

A. EQUIPMENT

The two types of high-frequency rotational tests **are** the head thrust test and the head (vestibular) autorotation test. The equipment is almost the same. The equipment

mainly consists of skin electrodes or one of the other eye-movement recording systems, a software calculating gain and phase data, a headband carrying a motion sensor for detecting head movements.

B. TEST ADMINISTRATION

Test room is dark in both types of high-frequency rotational tests. There is a target in front of the patient who is sitting upright. The patient keeps his or her eyes on the target during the test. The main difference between the two tests is the way of applying stimulus. Stimuli in the head thrust test are passive (applied by the examiner). Stimuli in the vestibular autorotation test are actively generated by the patient but based on computer-driven tonal stimuli. For the vestibular autorotation test, the patient shakes his or her head like "no" (a movement in horizontal plane) and then "yes" (a movement in vertical plane) while looking at the target. Frequency of the head movement is sinusoidally increased from 2 to 6 kHz in accordance with auditory stimulus. For the head thrust test, rotational stimuli are given manually at an unpredictable onset time and in a randomly varied direction; 20 to 40 head thrusts are analyzed.

C. Testing Parameters

There are two parameters for each test: (1) gain and phase for the vestibular autorotation test and (2) gain and response delay for the head thrust test. Description of the gain and phase is the same as in the sinusoidal harmonic acceleration test (rotary chair test). The response delay is the time between the onsets of head and eye movements.

For healthy subjects, the gain is almost 1 at low frequencies and declines somewhat at the higher frequencies. The phase is almost zero (ie, 180°) at the low frequencies and lags somewhat at the higher frequencies. In case of vestibular lesion, the most common pattern is decreased gain (below 0.7 when especially ipsilesional head movement is performed) and/or increased phase angle. The response delay does tend to be longer. It was shown that sensitivity to identify an abnormality in the vestibuloocular reflex is higher for the head thrust test than for the vestibular autorotation test because of the reflex augmentation in predictable stimulus paradigm used in the latter. A comparative study showed that the vestibular autorotation test provides additional information that could be missed by the caloric testing in diagnosing an abnormality in vestibuloocular reflex caused by a labyrinthine lesion and vestibular schwannoma.

Della Santina CC, Cremer PD, Carey JP, Minor LB. Comparison of head thrust test with head autorotation test reveals that the vestibulo-ocular reflex is enhanced during voluntary head movements. *Arch Otolaryngol Head Neck Surg.* 2002;128:1044. [PMID: 12220209] (Presents a comparison among the head autorotation test, active and passive head thrust tests in healthy subjects and patients with unilateral labyrinthectomy.)

Halmagyi GM, Yavor RA, McGarvie LA. Testing the vestibulo-ocular reflex. *Adv Otorhinolaryngol.* 1997;53:132. [PMID: 9226050] (Practical evaluation of nystagmus, including the methodology and the interpretation of caloric and rotational testing.)

Hirvonen TP, Aalto H, Pyykko I, Juhola M. Comparison of two head autorotation tests. *J Vestib Res.* 1999;9:119. [PMID: 10378183] (Compares and presents differences in normative data of gain and phase values of vestibuloocular reflex obtained by two equipments of high-frequency rotational test available in the market.)

Hirvonen TP, Aalto H, Pyykko I. Decreased vestibulo-ocular reflex gain of vestibular schwannoma patients. *Auris Nasus Larynx.* 2000;27:23. [PMID: 10648064] (Presents abnormally low gain of vestibuloocular reflex obtained with the head autorotation test in patients with vestibular schwannoma.)

Ng M, Davis LL, O'Leary DP. Autorotation test of the horizontal vestibulo-ocular reflex in Meniere's disease. *Otolaryngol Head*

Neck Surg. 1993;109(3 Pt 1):399. [PMID: 8414555] (Presents the most common abnormality pattern of vestibular autorotation test in Meniere patients.)

Ruckenstein MJ, Shepard NT. Balance function testing: a rational approach. *Otolaryngol Clin North Am.* 2000;33:507. [PMID: 10815034] (Pertinent descriptions and interpretations of the results of balance function tests.)

Saadat D, O'Leary DP, Pulec JL, Kitano H. Comparison of vestibular autorotation and caloric testing. *Otolaryngol Head Neck Surg.* 1995;113:215. [PMID: 767548] (Investigates the advantages of the high frequency of vestibular autorotation test over the caloric test in detecting abnormality of vestibuloocular reflex.)

Wade SW, Halmagyi GM, Black FO, McGarvie LA. Time constant of nystagmus slow-phase velocity to yaw-axis rotation as a function of the severity of unilateral caloric paresis. *Am J Otol.* 1999;20:471. [PMID: 10431889] (Comparison of the parameters of rotary chair testing with canal paresis of caloric testing.)

SUBJECTIVE VISUAL VERTICAL & HORIZONTAL TESTS

Subjective visual vertical and horizontal tests are measures of otoliths, and especially of utricular function. The bilateral gravitational input from the otoliths dominates the patients' perception of vertical and horizontal positions. To test for the subjective visual vertical or the subjective visual horizontal, the subject sits with head fixed in an upright position and looks at an illuminated line (either on a computer display or projected with a laser galvanometer system) in complete darkness. The subject is asked to adjust the line several times from starting positions at different angles to his subjective visual vertical or subjective visual horizontal. In acute peripheral vestibular lesions, including of the utricles, there is a typical deviation of the subjective visual vertical or subjective visual horizontal of about several degrees to the affected side. With central compensation, gradual improvement occurs in the patient's perception of tilt.

Tribukait A, Bergenius J, Brantberg K. Subjective visual horizontal during follow-up after unilateral vestibular deafferentation with gentamicin. *Acta Otolaryngol.* 1998;118:479. [PMID: 9726670] (Results of subjective visual horizontal test during the early and late stages of unilateral vestibular deafferentation with gentamicin and the effects of vestibular compensation on subjective visual horizontal.)

Vibert D, Hausler R, Safran AB. Subjective visual vertical in peripheral unilateral vestibular diseases. *J Vestib Res.* 1999;9:144. [PMID: 10378186] (Methodology of subjective visual vertical and the results in peripheral vestibular lesions.)

COMPUTERIZED DYNAMIC POSTUROGRAPHY

Computerized dynamic posturography is an established test of postural stability. It is an important tool to quantitatively assess individual and integral patterns of visual, proprioceptive, and vestibular signal processing, as well as overall balance function, in response to simulated tasks similar to those encountered in daily life.

A. EQUIPMENT

The computerized dynamic posturography test described here is the EquiTest platform (Neurocom International, Inc.).

Computerized dynamic posturography measures the force applied by the body to a platform equipped with strain gauges. The device, which is controlled by a computer, measures postural sway in several test conditions and allows for the manipulation of somatosensory and visual feedback. The information obtained with this test includes the vertical and horizontal shear forces generated by the patient during postural sway. Ground reaction forces are used to infer particular types of postural sway.

The test includes some requirements for testing personnel and patients. The patient should be able to stand still, unassisted and with eyes open, for at least 1 minute. The safety harness should be appropriately fastened so that the patient can move freely with no external support. The patient's feet and medial malleolus should be placed at designated points on the force plate.

Testing consists of three main protocols: (1) the sensory organization test, (2) the posture-evoked response, and (3) motor control tests. Of the three tests, the sensory organization test is the most useful in the assessment of patients with vestibular disorders.

Sensory Organization Test

The sensory organization test evaluates whether a patient with a balance disorder appropriately *does* utilize visual, vestibular, and somatosensory cues, and picks the appropriate cue under conflicting conditions to maintain balance.

A. SENSORY CONDITIONS

The sensory organization test includes six sensory conditions of gradually increasing difficulty that disrupt somatosensory cues, visual cues, or both. In **sensory condition 1,** the patient is asked to stand still with eyes open. The support surface and visual surround are fixed. **Sensory condition 2** is like sensory condition 1 except that the patient's eyes are closed. In **sensory condition 3,** the support surface is fixed. The visual surround leans forward, which is called sway referenced. The patient keeps eyes open. **Sensory condition 4** requires the patient to stand on the tilted support surface with eyes open and the visual surround fixed. **Sensory condition 5** is like condition 4 except that the patient's eyes are closed. In **sensory condition 6,** the support surface is tilted and the visual surround leans forward, which means that the visual and support conditions are sway referenced.

B. TEST ADMINISTRATION

This protocol consists of three repetitions of each sensory condition. Before each trial, the patient is asked to stand as still as possible and ignore the visual surround and the support surface motions. During each condition of the sensory organization test, force plates monitor the sway of the patient's center of gravity for periods of 20 seconds. Stability is quantified by an equilibrium score that is the percentage expression of the ratio of anteroposterior peak-to-peak sway amplitude during the trials to the theoretical anteroposterior limits of the stability. Equilibrium scores near 100% show little sway, whereas scores closer to zero are associated with a sway near the limits of the stability. Theoretical limits of stability are calculated on the basis of the maximum backward and forward center of gravity sway angles to which healthy subjects can move without losing balance.

C. TESTING PARAMETERS

The primary testing parameters are the composite equilibrium score and the sensory analysis.

1. Composite equilibrium score—The composite equilibrium score, which is a weighted average of all trials, provides an overall idea of the patient's balance performance. Abnormally low scores may be associated with either a malingering circumstance or vestibular, somatosensory, or visual dysfunction.

2. Sensory analysis—The sensory analysis quantifies the differences in the equilibrium scores between two conditions. The equilibrium score for sensory analysis is the average of each of the three trials of the conditions 1–6. Differences are sought in four ratios: (1) the somatosensory ratio, (2) the visual ratio, (3) the vestibular ratio, and (4) the vision preference ratio. The vestibular dysfunction pattern should also be considered in the sensory analysis.

a. **Somatosensory ratio**—In the somatosensory ratio, a comparison is made of the equilibrium scores of conditions 1 and 2. Abnormally low ratios are associated with dysfunction of the somatosensory system.

b. **Visual ratio**—The visual ratio is the ratio of the equilibrium scores of conditions 1 and 4. Low ratios are associated with a poor processing of visual cues.

c. **Vestibular ratio**—The vestibular ratio compares the equilibrium scores of conditions 1 and 5. Low scores are considered indicative of a dysfunction of the vestibular system (Figure 46–7B).

d. **Vision preference ratio**—The vision preference ratio compares the sum of the equilibrium scores of conditions 3 and 6 with the sum of the equilibrium scores of conditions 2 and 5. It tests whether the patient uses inappropriate and inaccurate visual cues. Low ratios are considered an abnormal preference of visual inputs. Normal sub-

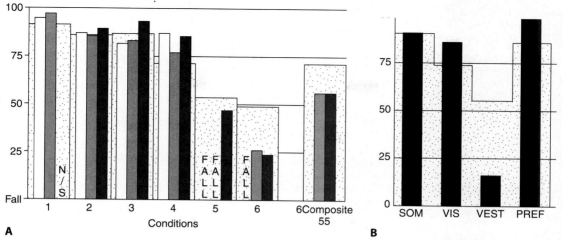

Figure 46–7. A vestibular pattern in the sensory organization test. **(A)** Normal or near-normal equilibrium scores are found in conditions 1 through 4, with falls and low scores demonstrated in conditions 5 and 6. The composite score is also low. **(B)** Sensory analysis reveals a low vestibular ratio. Stippled areas reflect the confidence level of the 95th percentile. SOM, somatosensory ratio; VIS, visual ratio; VEST, vestibular ratio; PREF, vision preference. (Reprinted, with permission of Hussam K. El-Kashlan, MD; University of Michigan, Ann Arbor, Department of Otolaryngology–Head & Neck Surgery.)

jects suppress inaccurate visual inputs, whereas a patient with a vision preference shows unsteadiness when many stimuli are moving simultaneously. A free-fall is usually enough to rule out an exaggeration or malingering circumstance because it is difficult for a patient to fall freely without a causative disorder.

The vestibular dysfunction pattern in sensory analysis is seen in bilateral vestibular loss or decompensated unilateral vestibular loss. In these cases, the equilibrium scores are expected to be within the normal range for conditions 1 through 4, but below the lower limit of the range for conditions 5 or 6 (or both) (Figure 46–7A). However, the vestibular dysfunction pattern alone is not enough to make a distinction between peripheral and central vestibular lesions. An abnormal vision preference usually occurs in patients following head trauma. It can be associated with a vestibular dysfunction pattern, depending on whether vestibular compensation develops. Multisensory dysfunction patterns, including combinations of vestibular and vision systems or vestibular and somatosensory systems, suggest CNS lesions.

Utility of Computerized Dynamic Posturography

The clinical usefulness of computerized dynamic posturography in neurotologic practice has been assessed in the literature. It is agreed that this test is quite useful in

the following conditions and situations: (1) chronic dysequilibrium; (2) persistent dizziness or vertigo despite treatment; (3) patients with normal results in other vestibular tests; (4) measuring the baseline postural control prior to treatment; (5) monitoring the results of vestibular ablative treatments; and (6) selecting the most useful rehabilitation strategy. The identification of malingering individuals is possible with this test. Strong indicators of a poor response are (1) a substandard performance on the sensory organization test in conditions 1 or 2 (or both), with great intertrial differences; (2) a relatively better performance in conditions 5 and 6 compared with that in conditions 1 and 2; (3) circular sway without falling; (4) exaggerated motor responses to small platform translations; and (5) inconsistent motor responses to small and large, forward and backward platform translations. However, computerized dynamic posturography alone does not localize and lateralize the site of the lesion and cannot aid in establishing a diagnosis. Moreover, the results of this test may be at odds with the results of the ENG and rotary chair test because computerized dynamic posturography assesses the vestibulospinal and postural control systems, whereas the other two rely on the vestibuloocular reflex.

Black FO, Paloski WH. Computerized dynamic posturography: what have we learned from space? *Otolaryngol Head Neck Surg.* 1998;118:S45. [PMID: 9525491] (Describes the method of sensory organization test, its results in astronauts and usefulness of computerized dynamic posturography.)

Furman JM. Role of the posturography in the management of vestibular patients. *Otolaryngol Head Neck Surg*. 1995;112:8. [PMID: 7816461] (Summarizes computerized dynamic posturography [CDP] protocols, and addresses the evaluation of patients with vestibular disorders, as well as the usefulness of CDP.)

Gianoli G, McWilliams S, Soileau J, Belafsky P. Posturographic performance in patients with the potential for secondary gain. *Otolaryngol Head Neck Surg*. 2000;122;11. [PMID: 10629476] (Describes the Sensory Organization Test analysis of malingering individuals as well as their clinical impression, audiometric and electronystagmographic evaluations.)

Monsell EM, Furman JM, Herdman SJ, Konrad HR, Shepard NT. Computerized dynamic platform posturography. *Otolaryngol Head Neck Surg*. 1997;117:394. [PMID: 9339802] (Addresses the technological aspects of posturography, and reviews the indications and clinical validity of the information.)

VESTIBULAR EVOKED MYOGENIC POTENTIALS

The vestibular evoked myogenic potentials (VEMP) are short latency electromyograms that are evoked by acoustic stimuli in high intensity and recorded from surface electrodes over the tonically contracted sternocleidomastoid muscle. The origin of VEMP has been shown to be the saccule. The response pathway consists of the saccule, inferior vestibular nerve, lateral vestibular nucleus, lateral vestibulospinal tract, and sternocleidomastoid muscle. The test provides diagnostic information about saccular and/or inferior vestibular nerve function. An intact middle ear is required for the response quality.

A. EQUIPMENT AND RECORDING

A commercially available evoked potential unit can be used for recording the VEMP. The patient is tested while seated upright with the head turned away from the tested ear to increase tension of the muscle. A non-inverting surface electrode is placed at the middle third of the sternocleidomastoid muscle. An inverting electrode is located at the sternoclavicular junction. A ground electrode is placed on the forehead. Rarefaction click (at 100 dB normalized hearing level [nHL]) or tone-burst stimuli (2-0–2 ms at 500 or 750 Hz and 120 dB peak sound pressure level [SPL]) are delivered monoaurally at the rate of 5/s. Electromyogenic activity of the muscle is amplified (× 5000) and bandpass filtered from 10 to 2000 Hz. Analysis window is adjusted to 100 ms. Responses are averaged over a series of 128 or more based on the response stability.

B. WAVEFORM OF THE RESPONSE

The VEMP waveform is characterized by a positive peak (P13 or wave I) at 13 (13–15) ms, and a negative peak (N23 or wave II) at 23 (21–24) ms. Peak-to-peak amplitude of P13–23 is measured.

Stimulus intensity, stimulus frequency, and tonic electromyogenic activity may affect response amplitude but not response latency. Click-evoked VEMP threshold ranges from 80 to 100 dB nHL in subjects with normal audiovestibular function. In tone burst-evoked VEMP recordings, robust responses are obtained with 500, 750, and 1000 Hz tone bursts, and thresholds ranges from 100 to 120 dB peak SPL across frequency.

C. PARAMETERS AND EVALUATION

For clinical purposes, the main interest is amplitude and threshold asymmetries between the right and left sides. However, controlling the tonic state of the sternocleidomastoid muscle is important for the accurate interpretation of interaural amplitude difference. Asymmetry ratio (AR) between the right and left ears is formulated as:

$$AR = 100 \, (A_L - A_R)/(A_L + A_R)$$

where A_L and A_R indicate peak-to-peak amplitude of P13 and 23, respectively. When the ratio exceeds 36%, it is interpreted as an indicator of saccular hydrops and called "augmented VEMP." The augmented VEMP has been reported in almost 33% of affected ears. This finding was found to correlate with flat and high-frequency hearing loss. VEMP may also be absent in up to 54% of Meniere patients. The absent VEMP correlates with low scores in sensory condition 5 of posturography and also low-frequency hearing loss, which is an indicator of apical hydrops. The test is also useful in detecting vestibular schwannoma originating from the inferior vestibular nerve. In this circumstance, elevated VEMP threshold or absent VEMP is expected. In vestibular neuronitis, VEMP may be absent. Superior canal dehiscence syndrome causes lowered VEMP thresholds or increased amplitudes. In otosclerosis, absent VEMP is expected. However, despite conductive hearing loss, if there is still normal VEMP, one should suspect the superior canal dehiscence syndrome rather than otosclerosis. Latency of the VEMP peak was focused on less than the parameters aforementioned. However, prolonged P13 latency was reported to correlate with retrolabyrinthine lesions such as large vestibular schwannoma and multiple sclerosis.

Akin FW, Murnane OD, Proffitt TM. The effects of click and tone-burst stimulus parameters on the vestibular evoked myogenic potential (VEMP). *J Am Acad Audiol*. 2003;14:500. [PMID: 14708838] (Examines the effects of click and tone-burst level and stimulus frequency on the latency, amplitude, and threshold of vestibular evoked myogenic potentials in healthy subjects.)

de Waele C, Huy PT, Diard JP, Freyss G, Vidal PP. Saccular dysfunction in Meniere's disease. *Am J Otol*. 1999;20:223. [PMID: 10100527] (Investigates VEMP characteristics in Meniere disease and correlation of these findings with degree and type of hearing loss, caloric test, and posturography results.)

Murofushi T, Shimizu K, Takegoshi H, Cheng PW. Diagnostic value of prolonged latencies in the vestibular evoked myogenic potential. *Arch Otolaryngol Head Neck Surg.* 2001;127:1069. [PMID: 11556854] (Describes conditions in p13 latency prolongation.)

Ochi K, Ohashi T, Nishino H. Variance of vestibular-evoked myogenic potentials. *Laryngoscope.* 2001;111:522. [PMID: 11224786] (Investigation of variations in VEMP and its diagnostic parameters and presentation of VEMP characteristics in vestibular schwannoma and neurolabyrinthitis.)

Ochi K, Ohashi T, Watanabe S. Vestibular-evoked myogenic potential in patients with unilateral vestibular neuritis: abnormal VEMP and its recovery. *J Laryngol Otol.* 2003;117:104. [PMID: 12625881] (Incidence of inferior vestibular nerve disorders in patients suffering from unilateral vestibular neuritis and the recovery of these disorders.)

Streubel SO, Cremer PD, Carey JP, Weg N, Minor LB. Vestibular-evoked myogenic potentials in the diagnosis of superior canal dehiscence syndrome. *Acta Otolaryngol Suppl.* 2001;545:41. [PMID: 11677740] (Presents VEMP characteristics in superior canal dehiscence syndrome.)

Welgampola MS, Colebatch JG. Characteristics and clinical applications of vestibular-evoked myogenic potentials. *Neurology.* 2005;64:1682. [PMID: 15911791] (Reviews VEMP evoked by clicks, tones, and alternative stimuli, and describes its usefulness in diagnosis of peripheral and central vestibular lesions.)

Young YH, Wu CC, Wu CH. Augmentation of vestibular evoked myogenic potentials: an indication for distended saccular hydrops. *Laryngoscope.* 2002;112:509. [PMID: 12148863] (Describes differentiating features of VEMP in Meniere disease and sudden deafness.)

SECTION XII
External & Middle Ear

Diseases of the External Ear | 47

Eli Grunstein, MD, Felipe Santos, MD, & Samuel H. Selesnick, MD

ANATOMY

Morphology

The pinnae of the external ear are bilaterally symmetric elastic cartilaginous frames that aid in focusing and localizing sound. Each pinna is anchored to the cranium by skin, cartilage, the auricular muscles, and extrinsic ligaments. The anatomy of the pinna is illustrated in Figure 47–1.

The external auditory canal (EAC) is typically 24 mm in length with a volume of 1–2 mL. The lateral third of the canal is made of fibrocartilage, whereas the medial two thirds are osseous. During early childhood, the canal is straight, but takes on an "S" shape by the age of 9. The EAC has an important relationship with the mastoid segment of the facial nerve, which lies posterior to the EAC as it descends toward the stylomastoid foramen. The temporomandibular joint is anterior to the EAC, and disease processes affecting this joint may lead to otalgia.

Skin

The EAC is lined by stratified squamous epithelium that is continuous with the skin of the pinna and the epithelial covering of the tympanic membrane. The subcutaneous layer of the cartilaginous portion of the canal contains hair follicles, sebaceous glands, and ceruminous glands, and is up to 1 mm thick. The skin of the osseous canal does not have subcutaneous elements and is only 0.2 mm thick (Figure 47–2). The epithelium of the EAC has the capacity to migrate laterally, allowing the canal to remain unobstructed by debris. The rate of epithelial migration is 0.07 mm/d and is thought to occur at the basal cell layer.

The ceruminous glands are modified apocrine sweat glands surrounded by myoepithelial cells; they are organized into apopilosebaceous units (Figure 47–3). Cerumen prevents canal maceration, has antibacterial properties, and has a normally acidic pH, all of which contribute to an inhospitable environment for pathogens.

Innervation

The pinna is innervated laterally, inferiorly, and posteriorly by the great auricular nerve (cervical plexus). Arnold's nerve (a branch of the vagus nerve) innervates the inferior bony canal, the posterosuperior cartilaginous canal, and corresponding segments of the tympanic membrane and the cymba concha. The posterosuperior bony EAC is innervated by branches of the facial nerve. The auriculotemporal branch of V3 supplies the anterior portion of the pinna. The glossopharyngeal nerve contribution to the external ear is not well delineated.

Lymphatic Drainage

The anterior and superior wall of the EAC and tragus are drained by the preauricular lymph nodes. The infra-auricular lymph nodes drain the helix and the inferior wall of the EAC, whereas the concha and antihelix are drained by the mastoid nodes.

Vascular Supply

The posterior auricular artery and the superficial temporal artery arise from the external carotid artery and supply the auricle and lateral EAC. The deep auricular branch of the maxillary artery supplies the more medial aspects of the

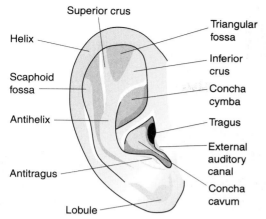

Figure 47–1. Anatomy of the pinna.

canal and the external surface of the tympanic membrane. The posterior auricular and superficial temporal veins drain the external ear.

PHYSIOLOGY

The external ear aids in the efficient transmission of sound to the tympanic membrane by serving as a functional resonator and, in particular, boosts transmission in the speech frequencies.

The hairs in the later canal, as well as the depth and tortuosity of the EAC, protect the tympanic membrane and structures of the middle ear.

EMBRYOLOGY

The mammalian ear is divided into external, middle, and inner ear components, which differ in their embryologic origin (Figure 47–4). The external ear consists of the pinna, the EAC, and the tympanic membrane, is embryologically derived from the first and second branchial arches, and includes both ectodermal and mesodermal components. The mesenchymal tissue of the arches is composed of paraxial mesoderm and neural crest cells. The pinna is formed by the gradual change in shape and fusion of components of the six auricular hillocks, which are derived from the first and second branchial arches (Figure 47–5). Formation of the external auditory meatus results from an ingrowth of a solid epithelial plate of ectodermal cells, the meatal plug, which eventually resorbs with only the lining of the canal remaining. The canal is lined by epithelial cells of ectodermal origin. The tympanic membrane begins to develop during the 28th week of gestation and arises from the most medial aspect of the meatal plug, which eventually becomes the external layer of the tympanic membrane.

■ CONGENITAL ANOMALIES OF THE EXTERNAL EAR

General Considerations

Congenital anomalies of the external ear include a spectrum of malformations of the pinna as well as varying degrees of atresia and stenosis of the EAC. The causes of these disorders may be genetic or secondary to environmental exposures. These disorders include variants of microtia, lop ear, cup ear, Stahl's ear, cryptotia, and prominent ear. Patient evaluation requires a thorough head and neck examination to exclude additional congenital anomalies. The list of associated syndromes is extensive and includes Goldenhar (hemifacial microsomia), branchio-otorenal, Treacher Collins, and Robinow syndrome.

Pathogenesis

Multiple genes may have redundant roles in outer ear formation, which can account for phenotypically similar malformations. The sequence of such dysregulation is only beginning to be understood with the help of murine knock-out and knock-in models. The auricular hillocks that give rise to the pinna arise during the sixth week of embryogenesis, whereas the inner two thirds of the EAC are not formed until the 26th week. Unto-

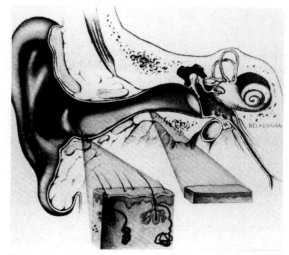

Figure 47–2. Coronal section of the ear canal. The skin of the cartilaginous and osseous canals are magnified. (Reproduced, with permission, from Lucente F, ed. *The External Ear.* Copyright Elsevier, 1995.)

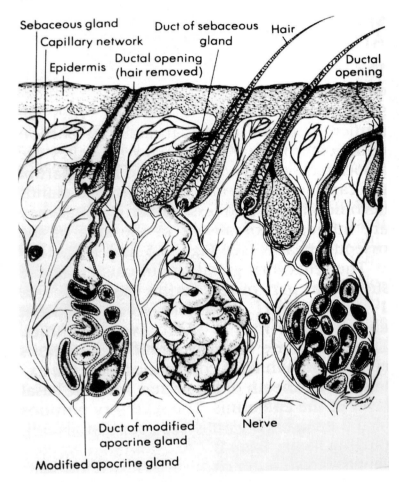

Sebaceous gland
Capillary network
Epidermis
Ductal opening (hair removed)
Duct of sebaceous gland
Hair
Ductal opening
Duct of modified apocrine gland
Nerve
Modified apocrine gland

Figure 47–3. Skin of the cartilaginous portion of the external auditory canal depicting apopilosebaceous units. (Reproduced, with permission, from Main T, Lim D: The human external auditory canal: an ultrastructural study. *Laryngoscope.* 1976;86:1164. Copyright LWW.)

ward events throughout this period could give rise to structural anomalies of the external ear.

Prevention

Genetic counseling should be made available to parents who are known carriers of genetic anomalies associated with external ear deformities. However, many anomalies of the external ear occur without known patterns of genetic transmission. In these cases, genetic counseling opportunities are limited. Isotretinoin, vincristine, colchicine, cadmium, and thalidomide are among the known teratogens associated with anomalous hypoplasia of the external ear and should be avoided during pregnancy.

MICROTIA

Clinical Findings

Patients typically present at birth with obvious auricular malformations. Several classification systems are used to

further subcategorize this entity, one of which is detailed below.

A. GRADE I

The ear exhibits mild deformity, typically with a slightly dysmorphic helix and antihelix. This group includes lowset ears, lop ears, cupped ears, and mildly constricted ears. All major structures of the external ear are present to some degree. The lop ear is characterized by inferiorly angled positioning of the auricular cartilage, whereas the cup ear protrudes with a deep conchal bowl.

B. GRADE II

All pinna structures are present, but tissue deficiency and significant deformity exist.

C. GRADE III

Also known as classic microtia or peanut ear, type III microtia has few or no recognizable landmarks of the auri-

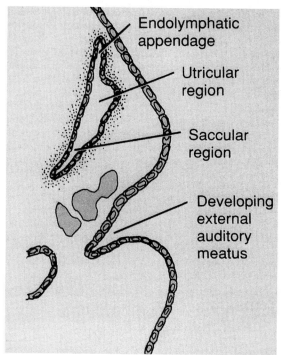

Figure 47–4. Development of the ear at 29 days' gestation. (Reproduced, with permission, from Larsen WJ, ed. *Human Embryology*, 2nd ed. Churchill Livingstone, 1997. Copyright Elsevier.)

cle. The ear lobule is usually present and anteriorly positioned. This subgroup includes anotia, which is complete absence of the external ear.

Treatment

Classically, microtia has been treated by a multistage auricular reconstruction. Patients undergo observation until the age of 5 to allow for growth of rib cartilage, which is harvested for reconstruction, and the development of the contralateral ear. This approach offers the benefit of reconstruction with autogenous material, which ultimately requires little or no maintenance. However, it is difficult to achieve a perfect cosmetic result. Typically, reconstruction occurs in four stages:

A. STAGE I: AURICULAR RECONSTRUCTION

The goals of this stage include symmetry in the position of the reconstructed cartilaginous ear framework with the normal ear. Postoperatively, the patient must be assessed for pneumothorax, which may arise with rib harvest.

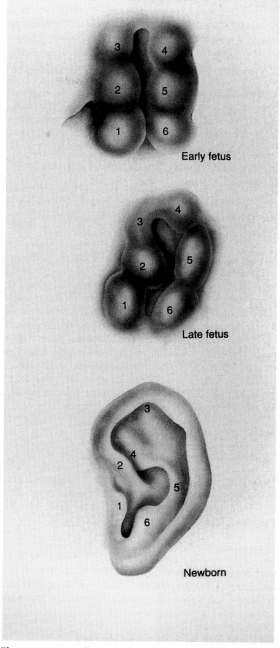

Figure 47–5. Differentiation of the six auricular hillocks. (Reproduced, with permission, from Larsen WJ, ed. *Human Embryology*, 2nd ed. Churchill Livingstone, 1997. Copyright Elsevier.)

B. STAGE II: LOBULE TRANSPOSITION

This procedure should be performed 2–3 months after Stage I reconstruction and aligns the lobule with the reconstructed cartilage framework.

C. STAGE III: POSTAURICULAR SKIN GRAFTING

A postauricular sulcus is created to allow the ear to project away from the mastoid. This step should be performed 3 months after Stage II reconstruction. Skin for the creation of the sulcus may be harvested from the groin, lower abdomen, buttocks, contralateral postauricular sulcus, or back.

D. STAGE IV: TRAGAL RECONSTRUCTION AND SOFT TISSUE DEBULKING

This should be performed several months after Stage III reconstruction.

E. OTHER TREATMENT OPTIONS

Another option for reconstruction includes the placement of a prosthesis. This can be either glued on or anchored to bone. If the patient selects a bone-anchored prosthesis rather than auricular reconstruction, he or she must be aware that daily maintenance is required and that the anchor may compromise the vascularity of non–hair-bearing skin, complicating future reconstructive surgery if the patient becomes dissatisfied with the prosthesis. However, the cosmetic result of a bone-anchored prosthesis is usually excellent. Complications of all types of auricular reconstructions include infection, hematoma formation, skin-flap necrosis, scar contracture, and poor contouring.

PROTRUDING EARS

Clinical Findings

An increase in distance from the helical rim to the mastoid is thought to be due to a lack of the antihelical fold and prominence of the conchal bowl. This entity is most frequently bilateral.

Treatment

Otoplasty is the mainstay of treatment for protruding ears. Often used techniques include recreating the antihelical fold, postaurical skin excision, and conchal-mastoid suture.

ATRESIA & STENOSIS OF THE EXTERNAL AUDITORY CANAL

Clinical Findings

Congenital anomalies of the EAC range from mild stenosis to complete atresia. These are often seen in association with malformations of the pinna and the structures of the middle ear. EAC cholesteatoma can develop

in the face of severe of EAC stenosis. Audiologic evaluation via behavioral or electrophysiologic measures should be performed to confirm normal hearing in the contralateral ear in unilateral disease, and to assess for ipsilateral sensorineural hearing loss. The typical pattern of hearing loss in affected ears is a conductive hearing loss of 50–70 dB. Axial and coronal computed tomography (CT) scans are essential in the evaluation of patients with canal atresia or stenosis. CT scanning assesses for ossicular, facial nerve, and otic capsule abnormalities as well as for the degree of temporal bone pneumatization. In addition, CT scanning can be used to identify a cholesteatoma medial to a canal stenosis.

Treatment

A discussion on reconstruction for aural atresia can be found in Chapter 48, Congenital Disorders of the Middle Ear.

◼ EXTERNAL EAR TRAUMA

The external ear is subject to a wide variety of injuries. All trauma patients require appropriate stabilization and triage of associated injuries based on their severity. Adherence to basic surgical principles and wound care prevents complications and improves the likelihood of a successful outcome.

AURICULAR HEMATOMA

 ESSENTIALS OF DIAGNOSIS

- *History of auricular trauma.*
- *Edematous, fluctuant, and ecchymotic pinna with loss of normal cartilaginous landmarks.*
- *Early diagnosis and treatment necessary to minimize cosmetic deformity.*

General Considerations

Auricular hematoma refers to the accumulation of blood in the subperichondrial space, usually secondary to blunt trauma.

Pathogenesis

Cartilage lacks its own blood supply; it relies on the vascularity of the surrounding perichondrium via diffusion. Shearing forces secondary to blunt trauma to the pinna lead to an accumulation of blood in the subperichondrial space. This creates a barrier for diffusion between the cartilage and the perichondrial vascularity, leading to necrosis of the cartilage and predisposing it to infection and further injury.

Clinical Findings

A patient with an auricular hematoma usually presents with an edematous, fluctuant, and ecchymotic pinna, with loss of the normal cartilaginous landmarks. Failure to evacuate the hematoma may lead to cartilage necrosis and permanent disfigurement known as "cauliflower ear."

Treatment

The evacuation of hematomas can be performed using a skin incision parallel with the natural auricular skin folds. The irrigation of evacuated hematomas with topical antibiotics reduces the likelihood of infection. Splinting after drainage prevents the reaccumulation of hematomas, and options include cotton bolsters, plaster molds, silicon putty, and water-resistant thermoplastic splints.

AURICULAR LACERATIONS

Sharp or severe blunt trauma may lead to laceration or avulsion of the auricle. The expeditious repair and prevention of infection are essential. Auricular lacerations should be cleansed and débrided prior to repair. Simple lacerations can be closed primarily, whereas extensive injuries with tissue loss may require undermining, flap reconstruction, or tissue grafts. In certain circumstances, even completely avulsed segments may be re-attached. Repairs should be covered with pressure dressings to prevent edema and hematoma formation, and cartilage-penetrating antibiotics should be prescribed. Excellent cosmetic results can be achieved, even with extensive lacerations.

Pham TV, Early SV, Park SS. Surgery of the auricle. *Facial Plast Surg.* 2003;19(1):53. [PMID: 12739182] (A thorough review of external ear anatomy and embryology, as well as the surgical management of auricular deformities and trauma.)

OTITIS EXTERNA

 ESSENTIALS OF DIAGNOSIS

- *Otalgia, otorrhea, pruritus, hearing loss, history of water exposure.*
- *Tender pinna and canal; canal erythema, edema, and purulent debris.*
- *Culture for refractory cases.*

General Considerations

Otitis externa is an inflammatory and infectious process of the EAC. *Pseudomonas aeruginosa* and *Staphylococcus aureus* are the most commonly isolated organisms. Less commonly isolated organisms include *Proteus* species, *Staphylococcus epidermidis*, diphtheroids, and *Escherichia coli*. Fungal otitis externa is discussed in the next section.

Pathogenesis

In the preinflammatory stage, the ear is exposed to predisposing factors, including heat, humidity, maceration, the absence of cerumen, and an alkaline PH. This can cause edema of the stratum corneum and occlusion of the apopilosebaceous units. In the inflammatory stage, bacterial overgrowth ensues, with progressive edema and intensified pain. Incomplete resolution or persistent inflammation for more than 3 months refers to the chronic inflammatory stage.

Clinical Findings

Symptoms of otitis externa may vary, depending on the stage and extent of disease. The clinical diagnosis is suggested by the presence of otalgia, otorrhea, aural fullness, pruritus, tenderness to palpation, and varying degrees of occlusion of the EAC. The patient may also present with hearing loss that results from occlusion of the EAC by edema and debris. Signs of otitis externa include pain on distraction of the pinna, EAC erythema, edema, otorrhea, crusting, and, in more advanced disease, lymphadenopathy of the periauricular and anterior cervical lymph nodes. Skin changes of cellulitis may be present as well. In the chronic stage, the skin of the EAC may be thickened. A culture may be helpful for infections that are refractory to treatment.

Treatment

Treatment for otitis externa involves meticulous atraumatic debridement of the EAC with the aid of a microscope. Analgesia can be achieved with nonsteroidal anti-inflammatory drugs (NSAIDs), opioids, or topical steroid preparations. After cleansing is complete, otic drop preparations that are antiseptic, acidifying, or antibiotic (or any combination of these) should be used. If the degree of stenosis of the canal is severe, a wick may be carefully placed in an effort to deliver the drops to the medial portion of the canal.

Available antiseptic preparations include acetic and boric acids, ichthammol, phenol, aluminum acetate, gentian violet, thymol, thimerosal (eg, Merthiolate), cresylate, and alcohol. Available antibiotic preparations include ofloxacin, ciprofloxacin, colistin, polymyxin B, neomycin, chloramphenicol, gentamicin, and tobramycin. Polymyxin B and neomycin preparations are often used in combination for the treatment of *S aureus* and *P aeruginosa* infec-

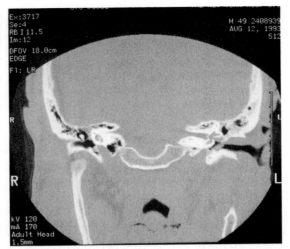

Figure 47–6. High-resolution coronal CT scan demonstrating soft tissue edema of the left external auditory canal consistent with otitis externa.

tions. Ofloxacin and ciprofloxacin are single-agent antibiotics with an excellent spectrum of coverage for pathogens encountered in otitis externa. Preparations with steroids help to reduce edema and otalgia. Systemic antibiotics are indicated for infections that spread beyond the EAC. For chronic otitis externa, a canalplasty may be indicated for thickened skin that has caused canal obstruction. Patients must be instructed to avoid EAC manipulation and water exposure if they have a history of recurrent otitis externa (Figure 47–6).

OTOMYCOSIS

 ESSENTIALS OF DIAGNOSIS

- *Pruritus, otalgia, otorrhea, fullness, hearing loss, no response to topical antibiotics.*
- *Fungal elements on physical examination.*
- *Positive KOH prep or fungal culture.*

General Considerations

Otomycosis is an inflammatory process of the external ear canal due to infection with fungi and is responsible for more than 9% of the diagnoses of otitis externa. In 80% of cases, the etiologic agent is *Aspergillus*, whereas *Candida* is the next most frequently isolated fungus. Other more rare fungal pathogens include *Phycomycetes*, *Rhizopus*, *Actinomyces*, and *Penicillium*.

Pathogenesis

Otomycosis has similar predisposing factors to bacterial otitis externa. Patients with diabetes mellitus or an immunocompromised state are particularly susceptible to otomycosis.

Clinical Findings

Patients with otomycosis most frequently present with pruritus, aural fullness, and otorrhea, and may also complain of otalgia and hearing loss. The hearing loss associated with otomycosis usually results from the accumulation of mycotic debris.

Otoscopy often reveals mycelia, establishing the diagnosis. The EAC may be erythematous and fungal debris may appear white, gray, or black. Patients have typically been tried on topical antibacterial agents with no significant response. The diagnosis can be confirmed by identifying fungal elements on a KOH preparation or by a positive fungal culture.

Treatment

The treatment of otomycosis includes cleansing and debriding the EAC, acidifying the canal, and administering antifungal agents. Nonspecific antifungal agents include thimerosal (eg, Merthiolate) and gentian violet. Commonly used specific antifungals include clotrimazole, Nystatin (otic drops or powder), and ketoconazole. Itraconazole is the only orally administered antifungal agent that is effective against *Aspergillus*.

SKULL BASE OSTEOMYELITIS

 ESSENTIALS OF DIAGNOSIS

- *Immunosuppressed patients with intense otalgia, otorrhea, hearing loss, fullness, and pruritus.*
- *Edema and erythema of the EAC, granulation tissue at the bony–cartilaginous junction, cranial neuropathies in advanced stages.*
- *Elevated erythrocyte sedimentation rate (ESR) or C-reactive protein (CRP). Culture of EAC. CT, MRI, and bone scan diagnostic; gallium scan to follow resolution.*

General Considerations

Skull base osteomyelitis, also known as malignant external otitis or necrotizing external otitis, is a bacterial infection of the EAC and skull base. This disease process is most frequently seen in elderly diabetics and immunocompromised patients. It most commonly begins as an external otitis that progresses to involve the temporal bone, and it may progress to fatal meningitis, sepsis, and death.

Pathogenesis

Skull base osteomyelitis commonly begins as an external otitis that progresses to cellulitis, chondritis, osteitis, and, ultimately, osteomyelitis. Unlike otitis media, which spreads through the pneumatized portion of the temporal bone, skull base osteomyelitis disseminates through the haversian canals and vascularized spaces of the skull base. As this progresses along the base of the skull, the facial nerve (stylomastoid foramen); hypoglossal nerve (hypoglossal canal); the abducens and trigeminal nerves (petrous apex); and the glossopharyngeal, vagus, and spinal accessory nerves (jugular foramen) may be involved. Cranial neuropathies portend a grave prognosis.

The most frequently isolated causative organism is *P aeruginosa*, which may exhibit high levels of antibiotic resistance. *Aspergillus* may also be an etiologic organism and is thought to originate from the middle ear or mastoid. Elderly diabetics are thought to be particularly susceptible because of the microangiopathic changes that blunt an already attenuated immune response.

In children, the clinical course of the disease progresses more rapidly, often manifesting with pseudomonal bacteremia. In contrast to that seen in adults, the tympanic membrane and middle ear are often involved.

Clinical Findings

A. Symptoms and Signs

Patients may present with intense otalgia, otorrhea, aural fullness, pruritus, and hearing loss. As the disease advances to involve the temporal bone, granulation tissue is seen on the floor of the EAC at the osteocartilaginous junction. Bony sequestra can also be found in the EAC. Edema, periaural lymphadenopathy, and trismus may be present. Cranial neuropathies occur in more advanced presentations of disease, and the facial nerve is the most frequently affected cranial nerve. Further progression may lead to sigmoid sinus thrombosis, meningitis, sepsis, and death.

B. Diagnostic Tests

Inflammatory markers such as ESR and CRP may be elevated. Cultures and sensitivity should be obtained to aid in selecting appropriate antibiotics.

CT and MRI are useful in the initial evaluation to determine the extent of disease. Bone scans are sensitive for assessing bony involvement but are not specific (Figures 47–7, 47–8, and 47–9). Gallium scans are used to track the resolution of the infection, since bone scans often remain positive long after the infection has resolved (Figure 47–10).

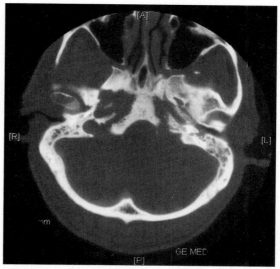

Figure 47–7. Axial high-resolution CT scan demonstrating skull base osteomyelitis with evidence of petroclival bone erosion.

Differential Diagnosis

Carcinomas of the EAC, chronic granulomatous disease, Paget disease, fibrous dysplasia, and nasopharyngeal carcinomas must be considered in the differential diagnosis.

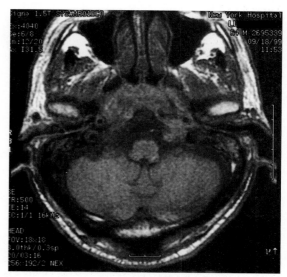

Figure 47–8. Axial T1-weighted MRI depicting the replacement of bone marrow in the clivus with inflammatory tissue.

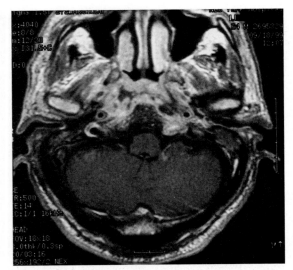

Figure 47–9. Axial T1-weighted MRI, with gadolinium enhancement, with evidence of petroclival bone erosion and enhancement of inflammatory tissue secondary to skull base osteomyelitis.

Treatment

Long-term parenteral antibiotics are the treatment of choice. Aminoglycosides (eg, tobramycin) and antipseudomonal β-lactam antibiotics, including piperacillin, ticarcillin, or ceftazidime, may be used. Some physicians recommend the use of outpatient fluoroquinolones such as ciprofloxacin or ofloxacin; however, this is appropriate

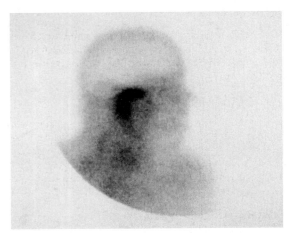

Figure 47–10. Sagittal image of a bone scan in a patient with skull base osteomyelitis revealing focal enhancement of the skull base.

only for patients with early presentations who can be followed up closely. Control of hyperglycemia and immunosuppression is necessary to maximize treatment. Surgical debridement may be necessary to remove necrotic tissue. The use of hyperbaric oxygen has been described in cases refractory to antibiotics, with variable results. In an effort to prevent skull base osteomyelitis, all diabetic and immunocompromised patients must be followed up closely and treated aggressively if they present with symptoms suggestive of external otitis.

Rubin Grandis J, Branstetter BF IV, Yu VL. The changing face of malignant (necrotizing) external otitis: clinical, radiological, and anatomic correlations. *Lancet Infect Dis.* 2004;4(1):34. [PMID: 14720566] (An overview of the diagnosis and management of skull base osteomyelitis.)

■ DERMATOLOGIC DISEASES OF THE EXTERNAL EAR

 ESSENTIALS OF DIAGNOSIS

- *Atopic dermatitis—pruritic erythematous patches or weeping plaques.*
- *Psoriasis—oval salmon-pink plaques with silvery scales on elbows, knees, scalp, and buttocks.*
- *Seborrheic dermatitis—pruritic greasy scales with erythematous bases on ears, scalp, forehead, eyebrows, glabella, or nasolabial folds.*
- *Contact dermatitis—pruritic, indurated, and erythematous lesions after exposure to allergen or irritant.*

ATOPIC DERMATITIS

General Considerations

Atopic dermatitis is a chronic skin disease of immune-mediated origin. It may remit spontaneously or endure as a chronic condition. Lesions presenting on the ear may be pruritic and erythematous. Patients often have a personal or family history of atopy and allergy.

Atopic dermatitis often manifests in infancy on extensor surfaces and the face. Children may present with skin lesions on flexural areas and on the hands.

Pathogenesis

Though not completely understood, the clinical presentation of atopic dermatitis is thought to be secondary to immune dysfunction. Atopic skin lesions have been shown to have higher levels of Th2 T-lymphocytes, which produce inflammatory mediators such as interleukin 4, 5, and 10.

Clinical Findings

The diagnosis of atopic dermatitis is a clinical one. There is variability in skin lesions ranging from erythematous patches to weeping plaques. Lesions presenting on the ear are often pruritic and erythematous. Lesions typically persist for more than 1 month. Secondary infections with *S aureus*, herpes simplex virus, vaccinia, and molluscum contagiosum may occur.

Atopic dermatitis is characterized by the absence of specific laboratory and histologic markers. Elevated IgE and eosinophilia may be present yet are not specific for the diagnosis.

Differential Diagnosis

The differential diagnosis includes seborrheic dermatitis and psoriatic dermatitis.

Treatment

Topical corticosteroids are the mainstay of treatment. Antihistamines and lubricants may be used for the treatment of accompanying pruritus. Moisturizers and mild soaps are preferred to minimize exposure to potential allergens found in many cosmetic products. Food elimination and desensitization are not recommended. Though often self-limited, the disease may recur spontaneously and can become chronic. Bacterial superinfection may require topical and systemic antibiotics.

PSORIASIS

General Considerations

Psoriasis is a chronic inflammatory disorder of the skin. Eighteen percent of patients with psoriasis have some involvement of the external ear, which may be secondary to extension from the scalp. Plaques may present on the concha and meatus of the EAC and are variably pruritic.

The incidence of psoriasis in the United States ranges from 2% to 5%. Males and females are equally affected, with the onset of disease typically occurring in adolescence.

Pathogenesis

The cause of psoriasis is unknown, yet there is a strong genetic component. Attacks of psoriasis may be triggered by certain drugs such as NSAIDs, beta blockers, lithium carbonate, and antimalarial agents, as well as by infection, trauma, and stress.

Clinical Findings

Psoriasis is characterized by erythematous papules that coalesce to form round or oval salmon-pink plaques with silvery white scales found on the elbows, knees, scalp, and buttocks. These lesions bleed in pinpoint areas when scratched (Auspitz sign). Opacification or "oil spots" of the nails, as well as pitting and subungual hyperkeratosis, are also suggestive of this disease. Psoriatic lesions may present over areas of trauma, an entity known as Koebner phenomenon. Psoriatic arthritis occurs in 5–10% of all psoriatic patients.

Treatment

Patients should avoid excessive drying of the skin. For the ears and face, treatment includes low-dose topical nonfluorinated corticosteroids such as alclometasone, mometasone, desonide, clocortolone, hydrocortisone valerate, and butyrate creams and topical calcipotriene. Warm-water soaks, 1–5% coal tar treatment, and topical anthralin C may also be helpful. Oral psoralens and UVA phototherapy for patients with widespread disease may be necessary. Antihistamines are used to treat the associated pruritus. Methotrexate may be required for severe cases and for psoriatic arthritis. The response to treatment is variable, and the condition may become chronic.

SEBORRHEIC DERMATITIS

General Considerations

Seborrheic dermatitis is a chronic inflammatory skin disease of unknown etiology with a predilection for areas of the skin rich with sebaceous glands. Seborrheic dermatitis affecting the ear is often distributed along the concha, scaphoid region, EAC, and postauricular crease.

Pathogenesis

The cause of seborrheic dermatitis remains unknown, but an association with *Pityrosporum ovale* and *Malassezia furfur* has led to the approval of ketoconazole shampoo for treatment.

Clinical Findings

Seborrheic dermatitis is characterized by greasy scales overlying erythematous and often pruritic plaques. The distribution is frequently not limited to the ears and often involves the scalp, forehead, eyebrows, glabella, and nasolabial folds. Scaling of the scalp or dandruff is common. Superimposed infection and edema may also occur.

Differential Diagnosis

Seborrheic dermatitis may be confused with atopic or psoriatic dermatitis, and scaling within the EAC may be confused with external otitis or otomycosis.

Treatment

Medicated shampoos with sulfur, tar, selenium sulfide, or zinc are helpful in the treatment of the associated dandruff. Intermediate- or high-dose glucocorticosteroids (eg, betamethasone or fluocinonide) are needed for more severe presentations and to alleviate pruritus. Fluorinated topical glucocorticoids may worsen lesions when used on the face or ear. Ketoconazole cream and shampoo are helpful in refractory cases. Seborrheic dermatitis can often become chronic with periods of exacerbation and remission. Super-infection should be treated with warm compresses, topical antibiotics, and selective use of oral antibiotics.

CONTACT DERMATITIS

General Considerations

Contact dermatitis can be an acute or chronic inflammatory disorder of the skin caused by contact with an allergen or irritant. This process may occur anywhere along the pinna or the EAC. Eruption may occur secondary to instrumentation, foreign objects—including jewelry, ear plugs, and hearing aids—and other objects used to scratch pruritic lesions. In addition, cosmetics and hair products are frequent culprits.

Pathogenesis

Allergic contact dermatitis is a Type IV hypersensitivity reaction, and cutaneous manifestations are often delayed by 1–3 days. This is in contrast to irritant-mediated contact dermatitis, which usually manifests earlier.

Clinical Findings

Allergic contact dermatitis is characterized by an indurated, erythematous, pruritic, and poorly demarcated process. This is in contrast to irritant dermatitis, which often presents with well-defined areas of exposure.

Skin testing to identify contact allergens may be of use.

Treatment

The avoidance of exposure to irritants and allergens and high-dose topical glucocorticoids are the mainstays of therapy.

FIRST BRANCHIAL CLEFT ANOMALIES

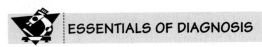 ESSENTIALS OF DIAGNOSIS

- Cyst or tract along anterior border of sterno-cleidomastoid muscle; corresponding tract at the bony-cartilaginous junction of the EAC.
- Recurrent neck or ear drainage and infection.
- CT scan may be helpful to identify tract.
- May be intertwined with the facial nerve.

Pathogenesis

First branchial cleft anomalies occur as a result of anomalous fusion of the first and second branchial arches, with incomplete obliteration of the first branchial cleft.

Clinical Findings

Patients may present with a cyst or tract along the anterior border of the sternocleidomastoid muscle. One may also see a corresponding tract at the junction of the bony and cartilaginous ear canal. The patient may have a history of recurrent infection and drainage from the ear or neck. A Work type 1 anomaly is a duplication anomaly of the EAC. A Work type 2 anomaly may be intertwined with the facial nerve.

Treatment

The treatment for first branchial cleft anomalies is complete excision. Incomplete excision predisposes the patient to recurrence and re-infection. The tract may be intimately involved with the facial nerve, which is at risk during excision.

AURICULAR FROSTBITE

 ESSENTIALS OF DIAGNOSIS

- Cold exposure.
- Auricle initially numb, then subsequently painful.
- Auricle initially pale, cyanotic, and hypesthetic, then subsequently erythematous with bullae.

Pathogenesis

Freezing temperatures lead to both direct cellular injury as well as vascular compromise. Prolonged exposure to cold temperatures can lead to vasoconstriction, cold-mediated dehydration, endothelial injury, thrombosis, and ischemia of auricular tissue. In the early stage, this process may be reversible, but over time, it leads to tissue necrosis.

Clinical Findings

Temperatures below 10° C may lead to hypesthesia, and the person is frequently unaware of impending frostbite. The ear is initially pale and then cyanotic. Ultimately, as the ear thaws, pain, erythema, and subcutaneous bullae secondary to extravasated extracellular fluid or blood may develop.

Treatment

The initial treatment for auricular frostbite consists of rapid rewarming of the ear to 40–42 °C. Nonhemorrhagic blisters may be débrided, and patients should be given pain medicine and antibiotics. Aloe vera has antithromboxane properties and, together with ibuprofen, may aid in reestablishing circulation. More aggressive débridement should be delayed for several weeks until demarcation is complete.

Petrone P, Kuncir EJ, Asensio JA. Surgical management and strategies in the treatment of hypothermia and cold injury. *Emerg Med Clin North Am.* 2003;21(4):1165. [PMID: 14708823] (An overview of the current recommendations for the management of frostbite, including frostbite of the external ear.)

AURICULAR BURNS

 ESSENTIALS OF DIAGNOSIS

- *Superficial burn—erythema and pain.*
- *Partial-thickness burn—painful blisters.*
- *Full-thickness and subdermal burns—painless, gray/black eschar.*

General Considerations

Thermal injury can be classified by the degree of the burn. Superficial burns involve the superficial layer of the epidermis. Partial-thickness burns extend into, but not through, the dermis. Full-thickness burns extend through the full thickness of the dermis. Subdermal burns extend into the subcutaneous tissue, including fat, muscle, tendon, cartilage, and bone.

Clinical Findings

Superficial auricular burns present with erythema secondary to dermal capillary dilation and vessel congestion. These burns are red and moderately painful. Patients with partial-thickness burns usually present with blisters that blanch on direct pressure and are very painful. Deep partial-thickness burns are associated with less pain, and there may be an eschar. Full-thickness and subdermal burns are painless because dermal nerve endings have been destroyed. The wound surface is of varying color, but may be gray or black and charred.

Treatment

Superficial burns do not scar and may be treated with moisturizing creams. The blisters of partial-thickness burns should be débrided, and bacitracin ointment applied. When not deep, these burns heal without scarring as well. Full-thickness, subdermal, and deep partial-thickness burns of the auricle heal with scarring and contracture and may be complicated by suppurative chondritis. These burns should be treated with both topical (usually silver based) and systemic cartilage penetrating antibiotics. Early débridement and closure with skin grafts should be considered. Secondary reconstruction is usually performed at approximately 1 year after injury.

DeSanti L. Pathophysiology and current management of burn injury. *Adv Skin Wound Care.* 2005;18(6):323. [PMID: 16096398] (An overview of the current recommendations for the management of burns, including those of the external ear.)

FOREIGN BODIES OF THE EXTERNAL EAR

General Considerations

Foreign bodies within the external ear may present in both children and adults. Common objects include erasers, pills, batteries, and insects.

Clinical Findings

Patients may present with pain, pruritus, conductive hearing loss, and bleeding. A persistent foreign body may lead to infection and the formation of granulation tissue. Batteries lodged within the EAC, when in contact with moisture, may cause liquefaction necrosis, low-voltage injury, or pressure necrosis of the EAC skin or tympanic membrane.

Treatment

The removal of foreign objects should be done in an atraumatic manner. Injury to the EAC is minimized with direct visualization using the operating microscope and proper instrumentation (eg, right angle pick, curet, forceps, and suction) as well as minimizing patient movement. In children, general anesthesia is often required. Irrigation may help dislodge cerumen or smaller objects. Cerumen impaction may require prior softening with an otic preparation. Two percent lidocaine may be used for the removal of insects both to achieve topical anesthesia and also to kill the insect. Complete occlusion of the EAC with cyanoacrylate adhesives (ie, "superglue") may require surgical removal with a postauricular approach.

NEOPLASMS OF THE EXTERNAL EAR

 ESSENTIALS OF DIAGNOSIS

- *History of chronic sun exposure; usually found on sun-exposed areas of body.*
- *Basal cell carcinoma—nodular, ulcerated, and/or bleeding lesion.*
- *Squamous cell carcinoma—plaque, nodule, or ulceration.*
- *Melanoma—lesion with increasing size, ulceration, or bleeding.*
- *Any suspicious skin lesion should be biopsied.*
- *CT/MRI if concern regarding local extension or regional disease.*

BASAL CELL CARCINOMA OF THE AURICLE

General Considerations

Basal cell carcinomas are the most common malignant neoplasm of the auricle, representing 45% of auricular carcinomas.

Pathogenesis

Chronic long-term sun exposure is the predominant cause of basal cell carcinoma. Specifically, UVB radiation has been identified as a major carcinogen. The incidence of cancer increases with age. Other risk factors include fair skin, outdoor occupations, and a history of skin carcinoma.

Classification

A. NODULAR BASAL CELL CARCINOMA

The most common and least aggressive subtype, nodular basal cell carcinoma appears as a telangiectatic, pearly papule.

B. ULCERATIVE BASAL CELL CARCINOMA

This subtype presents with a central ulceration and pearly border.

C. PIGMENTED BASAL CELL CARCINOMA

This carcinoma is similar in gross appearance to the nodular form, but with brown pigmentation.

D. SUPERFICIAL BASAL CELL CARCINOMA

This subtype occurs predominantly on the trunk, appearing as indurated, erythematous scaly patches. These lesions may be mistaken for other dermatologic conditions, including eczema and psoriasis.

E. MORPHEAFORM BASAL CELL CARCINOMA

Occurring predominantly on the face, morpheaform basal cell carcinoma presents as yellowish cicatricial plaque lesions.

F. DIFFERENTIATED BASAL CELL CARCINOMA

This subtype is characterized by slow-growing lesions with histologically differentiated glandular or ductal elements.

G. BASALOID BASAL CELL CARCINOMA

Composed of highly invasive keratinized lesions, this subtype represents 1% of basal cell carcinomas.

Clinical Findings

Patients may initially present with a skin lesion that is nodular, ulcerated, and/or bleeding. Basal cell carcinomas of the auricle typically occur on the posterior surface of the pinna and in the preauricular area. The diagnosis of any suspicious lesion should be confirmed with biopsy. CT scans and MRI may be used to evaluate advanced disease with tumor extension to the adjacent temporal bone and soft tissue structures of the head and neck. The overall rate of metastasis is 0.003–0.1%.

Staging

Carcinomas of the EAC can be staged using the American Joint Committee on Cancer (AJCC) general staging system for nonmelanoma cancer of the skin, which is a TNM (tumor, node, metastases) staging system. This staging system is limited by the fact that it does not account for histologic subtypes or the anatomic variability of the skin of the external ear compared with other skin sites.

Differential Diagnosis

Given the variability of subtypes, the differential diagnosis includes benign nevi, amelanotic melanomas, cutaneous squamous cell carcinomas, eczema, and scleroderma.

Treatment

A. NONSURGICAL MEASURES

1. Topical 5-fluorouracil

2. Radiation therapy—Indicated for poor surgical candidates or unresectable lesions.

B. Surgical Measures

1. Curettage with electrodissection—Operator dependent and typically used to excise nodular lesions and desiccate the base.

2. Cryosurgery—Indicated for small basal cell carcinomas (< 1 cm) with well-defined borders.

3. Local excision—Ninety-five percent of basal cell carcinomas < 2 cm in size can be successfully treated with local excision with a surgical margin of at least 4 mm. Auricular reconstruction may be required for large defects.

4. Mohs surgical technique—Refers to complete micrographic excision of the tumor using intraoperative histopathology to assess for positive margins. This technique is particularly useful for recurrent basal cell carcinomas, those larger than 2 cm, or those with an aggressive histology. Five-year cure rates using Mohs technique should approach 97.1%.

Prevention

Minimizing sun exposure between 10:00 AM and 3:00 PM, wearing protective clothing, and using UV-B-protective sunscreens are helpful measures for preventing basal cell carcinoma.

CUTANEOUS SQUAMOUS CELL CARCINOMA

General Considerations

Squamous cell carcinomas account for 20% of all cutaneous malignant neoplasms and commonly occur in elderly males.

Pathogenesis

Risk factors for squamous cell carcinoma include immunosuppression, advanced age, a nonhealing ulcer, and exposure to chemicals such as arsenic, soot, coal, tar, paraffin, and petroleum oil. The most important risk factor is exposure to UV radiation.

Classification

A. Adenoid Squamous Cell Carcinoma

This is a **classic nodular, ulcerative lesion.**

B. Bowenoid Squamous Cell Carcinoma

This type of carcinoma has the **histologic appearance of Bowen's disease, with invasive properties.**

C. Generic Squamous Cell Carcinoma

Generic squamous cell carcinoma is the **most common histologic group.**

D. Verrucous Squamous Cell Carcinoma

The carcinoma is composed of wartlike lesions that are locally invasive.

E. Spindle Cell Squamous Cell Carcinoma

This type of squamous cell carcinoma consists of aggressive and deeply penetrating tumors named for their elongated fusiform cells.

Clinical Findings

The appearance of these tumors is variable and includes plaques, nodules, and ulcerations. They may be friable and prone to bleeding. Auricular lesions frequently occur on the helix or pre-auricular region, but may occur on any sun-exposed areas.

CT scanning and MRI may be used to evaluate advanced disease with tumor metastasis to the adjacent temporal bone and soft tissue structures of the head and neck. The proper diagnosis should be made with biopsy. The overall risk of metastasis for cutaneous squamous cell carcinoma of the external ear is approximately 6–18%.

Staging

Carcinomas of the EAC can be staged using the AJCC general staging system for nonmelanoma cancer of the skin (ie, the TNM staging system). This staging system is limited by the fact that it does not account for histologic subtypes or the anatomic variability of the external ear skin compared with other skin sites.

Differential Diagnosis

The differential diagnosis includes basal cell carcinoma, actinic keratosis, seborrheic keratosis, keratoacanthomas, scars, psoriatic lesions, melanomas, and sarcomas.

Treatment

A. Nonsurgical Measures

Radiation therapy may be indicated for unresectable lesions or those that may lead to significant cosmetic disfigurement with surgery.

B. Surgical Measures

1. Local excision—Ninety-five percent of squamous cell carcinomas < 2 cm can be successfully treated with local excision with a surgical margin of at least 6 mm. Auricular reconstruction may be required for large defects.

2. Mohs surgical technique—This technique is particularly useful for recurrent lesions, those > 2 cm, or those with an aggressive histology.

Prevention

As with basal cell carcinoma, minimizing sun exposure between 10:00 AM and 3:00 PM, wearing protective clothing, using UVB-protective sunscreens, and avoiding the sun are paramount for risk reduction.

Prognosis

In addition to the patient's age and overall immune status, the prognosis for squamous cell carcinoma is dependent on the histologic subtype, size, and location of the tumor. A better prognosis is associated with a well-differentiated histology. The 5-year cure rate for squamous cell carcinomas ranges from 75% to 92%.

MELANOMA OF THE EXTERNAL EAR

General Considerations

The incidence of melanoma in the United States is 11.1 cases per 100,000 individuals. Auricular melanoma accounts for 1% of all melanomas.

Classification

A. LENTIGO MALIGNA MELANOMA

This subtype is characterized by hyperpigmented macules occurring on sun-exposed areas. The lesions expand laterally and may progress for years. This subtype carries the best prognosis.

B. SUPERFICIAL SPREADING MELANOMA

This subtype accounts for approximately 75% of melanomas and often occurs on the lower extremities or the back. The lesions are irregular and hyperpigmented and may develop central nodularity. The natural history of these lesions begins with a superficial spreading lesion (radial growth phase) and subsequently ulceration, bleeding, and dermal invasion (vertical growth phase). Lesions that have already begun the vertical growth phase portend a worse prognosis.

C. NODULAR MELANOMA

Blue-black nodules of nodular melanoma invade deeply into the dermis. They occur predominantly on the trunk, but may present on the head and neck. This subtype carries the worst prognosis.

Clinical Findings

Most melanomas involving the ear present on the helix. Though initially painless, these lesions may change in size, ulcerate, and bleed. A thorough head and neck examination requires attention to enlarged lymph nodes that may occur with regional spread of disease.

The diagnosis of melanoma is dependent on the histologic evaluation of a biopsy. At a minimum, metastatic evaluation should include a chest x-ray to rule out lung metastases and liver function tests to rule out liver metastases. CT scanning and MRI have added sensitivity in detecting metastatic disease. Radionuclide bone scans can be used to diagnose bony metastases.

Staging

At present, melanomas are staged using one of two systems: (1) the TNM staging system or (2) the staging system of the AJCC. Both systems incorporate the depth of invasion, measured in millimeters. Deeper lesions and lesions with ulceration are associated with higher stages and higher mortality rates.

Differential Diagnosis

The differential diagnosis is diverse and includes benign lesions as well as basal cell and squamous cell carcinomas.

Treatment

A. NONSURGICAL MEASURES

Adjunctive radiation therapy may have a role in palliation.

B. SURGICAL MEASURES

The extent of excision, including surgical margins, is dependent on the histologic type and stage of disease. Management of the regional lymphatics is controversial and may include elective regional lymph node dissection and parotidectomy. Recently, sentinel lymph node biopsy has become a well-accepted approach in the management of the N0 neck for lesions more than 1 mm deep.

Prevention

The avoidance of and protection from sun exposure are important in preventing disease, as is early detection. Early detection is also extremely important in improving prognosis.

GLANDULAR TUMORS OF THE EXTERNAL AUDITORY CANAL

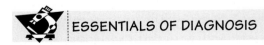

ESSENTIALS OF DIAGNOSIS

- *Otorrhea, fullness, otalgia, and conductive hearing loss.*

- Sensorineural hearing loss indicates inner ear extension.
- CT and MRI to define tumor and surrounding anatomy.
- Biopsy essential.

Classification

Glandular tumors of the EAC are rare and include four types: (1) adenoid cystic carcinomas; (2) ceruminous adenomas; (3) ceruminous adenocarcinomas; and (4) pleomorphic adenomas.

A. ADENOID CYSTIC CARCINOMA

These are capsular tumors most often found in salivary gland tissue. They have a predilection for perineural, perivascular, and fatty infiltration. Patients with perineural invasion often present with otalgia. Histologically, these tumors may show cribriform, tubular, or solid patterns of cellular arrangement. Lymph node metastases are rare, but late distant metastasis is not an uncommon feature of these tumors.

B. CERUMINOUS ADENOMA

Ceruminous adenoma consists of benign painless masses that may grow undetected for prolonged periods of time. Patients may present with a conductive hearing loss or otitis externa. They are histologically characterized by double-layered cuboidal or columnar cells, and the epithelium may show apical "snouts" of apocrine secretion.

C. CERUMINOUS ADENOCARCINOMA

These tumors share histologic features with ceruminous adenomas, but they have higher rates of mitoses and cellular atypia. Invasion into adjacent structures may be present, and lymph node metastases are rare.

D. PLEOMORPHIC ADENOMA

These tumors vary histologically but are characterized by epithelial and mesenchymal elements. These benign tumors do not display features of invasion.

Clinical Findings

Patients with glandular tumors of the EAC may present with otorrhea, aural fullness, otalgia, and conductive hearing loss. Sensorineural hearing loss signifies tumor extension into the inner ear. CT imaging is helpful in determining the amount of bony erosion and the size of the tumor. Generous tissue samples are important for histologic diagnosis.

Treatment

Benign glandular tumors are treated with wide local excision. Malignant tumors are treated with a variant of temporal bone resection, and consideration should also be given to adjuvant radiation.

Devaney KO, Boschman CR, Willard SC, Ferlito A, Rinaldo A. Tumours of the external ear and temporal bone. *Lancet On-col.* 2005;6(6):411. [PMID: 15925819] (Overview of the diagnosis and management of malignancies that affect the external and middle ear.)

OSTEOMAS & EXOSTOSES OF THE EXTERNAL AUDITORY CANAL

 ESSENTIALS OF DIAGNOSIS

- Usually asymptomatic; may present with cerumen impaction, otitis externa, or conductive hearing loss.
- Osteoma—pedunculated bony EAC lesion.
- Exostoses—multiple EAC lesions.

General Considerations

Osteomas are benign osseous neoplasms. Exostoses are firm, bony, broad-based lesions composed of lamellar bone (Figure 47–11). Exostoses are formed by reactive bone formation and have been associated with cold

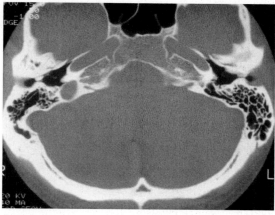

Figure 47–11. High-resolution axial CT scan revealing right anterior and posterior external auditory canal exostoses.

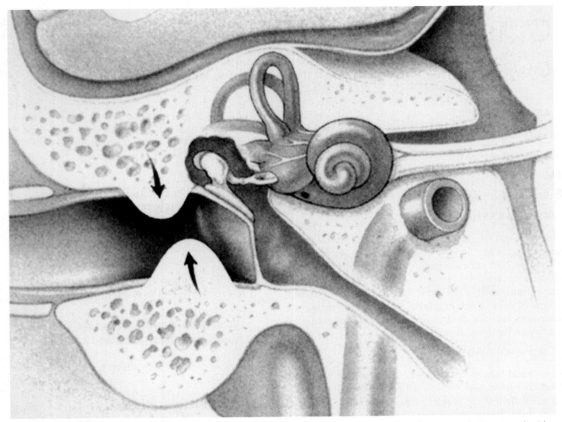

Figure 47–12. Coronal view of superior and inferior exostoses of the external auditory canal. (Reprinted with permission of Jackler RK.)

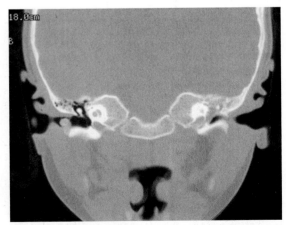

Figure 47–13. High-resolution coronal CT scan demonstrating an inferiorly based osteoma of the right external auditory canal.

water exposure. Both osteomas and exostoses arise from the bony portion of the EAC (Figure 47–12).

Clinical Findings

Osteomas are usually pedunculated and often have a vascular core (Figure 47–13). Exostoses commonly present as multiple lesions. Although most osteomas and exostoses are asymptomatic, occlusion of the EAC with an enlarged lesion may lead to cerumen impaction, external otitis, and a conductive hearing loss on audiogram.

Treatment

Most exostoses and osteomas require no intervention. If surgery is necessary, a transcanal or postauricular approach can be used, depending on the size of the lesions. The preservation of skin flaps speeds healing.

Congenital Disorders of the Middle Ear

48

Abtin Tabaee, MD, Vicki Owczarzak, MD, & Samuel H. Selesnick, MD

◼ EMBRYOLOGY & DEVELOPMENT

INITIAL STAGES OF DEVELOPMENT

Beginning at week 4, the tubotympanic sulcus develops as an extension of the endodermal epithelium of the first pharyngeal (branchial) pouch and eventually forms the middle ear canal and the eustachian tube. The tubotympanic recess has elongated and constricted to form the primordial tympanic cavity and eustachian tube by week 8. Simultaneously, the expanding end of the tubotympanic sulcus comes into proximity with the medial aspect of the ectodermal first pharyngeal cleft, the primordial external auditory canal. Although intimately related, the two linings remain separated by a layer of mesenchyme known as the pharyngeal membrane. This trilaminar relationship develops into the adult tympanic membrane, which comprises the outer cutaneous, middle fibrous, and inner mucosal layers. As the middle ear cavity expands, the tympanic sinus is created by the pneumatization of already ossified temporal bone. By 9 months, pneumatization of the tympanum and epitympanum is virtually complete. At the same time, the mastoid antrum is formed by the growth of the tympanic cavity into the mastoid portion of the temporal bone. The attachment of the sternocleidomastoid on the temporal bone promotes the formation of the mastoid process. Although the development of the mastoid air cells begins in fetal life, full maturation does not occur until age 2.

Early in development, the middle ear cavity is filled with loose mesenchyme that spans the gap between the primordial tympanic membrane and oval window. However, during the last 2 months of pregnancy, this mesenchyme is systematically reabsorbed, leaving the nearly mature ossicles suspended in the middle ear cavity. Beginning sometime between weeks 4 and 7, a condensation of neural crest ectoderm embedded within the mesenchyme begins to form the ossicles.

Meckel cartilage, which is derived from the first pharyngeal (branchial) arch, gives rise to the head of the malleus and the body of the incus. The remainder of Meckel cartilage develops into the mandible and sphenomandibular ligament (Meckel ligament). The first pharyngeal arch is also associated with the mandibular division of the trigeminal nerve, the muscles of mastication, the tensor tympani muscle, and the tensor veli palatini muscle. The second pharyngeal arch gives rise to Reichert cartilage, which eventually forms the manubrium of the malleus, the long process of the incus and the stapes suprastructure. The facial nerve, the muscles of facial expression, the stapedius muscle, the upper portion of the hyoid bone, and the stylohyoid ligament are also derived from the second pharyngeal arch mesoderm. It is important to note that although the pharyngeal arches are mesenchymal, the ossicles are derived from neuroectoderm that is embedded within the mesenchyme. This partly explains the association between ossicular malformations and disorders of neuroectoderm.

STAPES

The stapes requires the longest period of development and is therefore the most frequently malformed. The earliest stages of development begin at 4 weeks, and ossification does not occur until week 26. Development of the stapes footplate is induced by a depression on the otic capsule, the lamina stapedialis. This occurs between weeks 6 and 9. Ultimately, the lamina stapedialis becomes the annular ligament and the vestibular portion of the footplate. Failure of this precise association between the stapes footplate and the lamina stapedialis may result in a malformed or atretic oval window.

The primordial stapes is characterized as a chondral ring. Resorption, periosteal erosion, and ossification shape this cartilaginous precursor into an adult-like ossified stirrup. As a result of this developmental process, the adult stapes is fragile; a "plate" of endosteal bone overlying the original layer of cartilage forms the head and base, and thin periosteal bone makes up the crura. This contrasts with the relatively dense incus and malleus, which form from the repeated layering of endosteal bone on a cartilaginous framework. Furthermore, in contrast to the stapes, the malleus and incus do not undergo morphologic changes, which minimizes the complexity of the shaping process and the potential for error.

MALLEUS & INCUS

The developmental process of the malleus and incus is rapid. The chondral elements reach adult size by week 15 and are fully ossified skeletal structures by week 25. Before the full development of the ossicular ligaments, projections from the endodermal lining of the middle ear cavity help to support the position of the ossicles. Invaginations of the endodermal lining between the ossicles also serve to separate the developing ossicles from each other and from the walls of the tympanic cavity. Failure of this results in ossicular fusion. The articulations between the ossicles develop early, with the incudomalleolar joint forming at 7 weeks. Adult size and relationships are fully established by the ninth month. Full ossicular mobility, however, does not occur until 2 months after birth, when the mesenchyme of the middle ear cavity is fully reabsorbed.

STAPEDIAL ARTERY

The developing intracranial vasculature originates from six paired aortic arches and their associated arteries. During the fourth week of development, the stapedial artery arises from the hyoid artery (second aortic arch) near the origin of the proximal internal carotid artery (third aortic arch). It enters the anteroinferior quadrant of the middle ear and courses over the promontory and through the primordial stapes to form the obturator foramen. It then proceeds anteriorly to pierce the horizontal facial canal and enter the cranial cavity. The artery subsequently divides into an upper (supraorbital) division and lower (maxillomandibular) division. The supraorbital division provides the vasculature to the orbit and to the supraorbital areas early in fetal development. However, as the ophthalmic artery matures to assume these distributions, the supraorbital division largely involutes and persists as the middle meningeal artery. The maxillomandibular division exits the cranial cavity through the foramen spinosum and contributes to the fetal vasculature of the lower face, as well as to the inferior alveolar and infraorbital areas. By the third month, this division is largely replaced by branches of the external carotid artery. The proximal trunk of the stapedial artery normally atrophies, whereas the distal portion, the middle meningeal artery, persists and is supplied by the external carotid artery.

■ VASCULAR ANOMALIES

JUGULAR VEIN ANOMALIES

 ESSENTIALS OF DIAGNOSIS

- *Dehiscence of the jugular bulb may lead to aberrant position within the middle ear.*
- *This may be asymptomatic or may lead to tinnitus or conductive hearing loss.*
- *Visible on CT and MRI/MRA.*
- *Avoidance is most prudent management.*

Between the third and fourth weeks of development, paired cardinal veins first appear in the primordial neck. The cranial portion of the anterior cardinal vein ultimately gives rise to the internal jugular vein, whereas the cephalad portion forms the jugular bulb. The sigmoid sinus and the inferior petrosal sinus converge at the jugular bulb, which drains into the jugular vein in the neck. Normally surrounded by a layer of bone within the jugular fossa, the bulb is subject to congenital dehiscence and an aberrant position within the middle ear. A "high-riding" bulb may be defined anatomically as a bulb that rises above the inferior aspect of the bony annulus or the basal turn of the cochlea. It is present in 5% of temporal bone specimens and may be related to the poor pneumatization of the mastoid air cells and middle ear. The bony covering of the bulb may be thin or absent, resulting in dehiscence and protrusion into the middle ear cavity. Tinnitus, vestibular symptoms, and conductive hearing loss due to ossicular, tympanic membrane, or round window compression have been described. However, dehiscent jugular bulbs are often discovered incidentally on otoscopic examination. Typically, a blue mass is seen in the posteroinferior quadrant of the tympanic membrane.

Contrast-enhanced computed tomography (CT) scanning, magnetic resonance imaging (MRI), and magnetic resonance angiography (MRA) help delineate a vascular mass in the middle ear, whereas a high-definition temporal bone CT scan will reveal a bony defect in the floor of the hypotympanum. Venography may differentiate this lesion from other vascular masses in difficult cases. The lack of a fascial covering over the jugular bulb predisposes it to inadvertent laceration during myringotomy. Therefore, avoidance during middle ear surgery represents the most judicious management of these lesions.

INTERNAL CAROTID ARTERY ANOMALIES

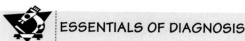 ESSENTIALS OF DIAGNOSIS

- *Agenesis, aneurysm, and aberrancy of the intratemporal carotid artery have been described.*
- *Symptoms include hearing loss, pulsatile tinnitus, aural fullness, otalgia, and vertigo.*
- *Pulsatile red mass is seen in the middle ear.*
- *Imaging studies differentiate this from other vascular lesions.*

General Considerations

Anomalies of the intratemporal internal carotid artery (ICA) are extremely rare. Typically, there is a female preponderance, and these anomalies first present in the third decade of life with conductive hearing loss, bloody otorrhea, headache, pulsatile tinnitus, or cranial nerve palsies. Conductive hearing loss is due to impingement by the aneurysm on the ossicles or tympanic membrane. Otoscopic exam may reveal a red and pulsatile mass in the middle ear or blood in the external auditory canal. However, it is presumed that most intratemporal aneurysms of the ICA are asymptomatic and go unrecognized.

Pathogenesis

The ICA normally enters the carotid canal in the petrous portion of the temporal bone medial to the styloid process. The initial vertical segment is anterior to the cochlea, separated from the internal jugular vein by the carotid ridge and from the tympanic cavity by a thin bony wall, 0.5 mm thick. When laterally displaced, this portion of the ICA is found in the hypotympanum with possible extension over the oval window. Displacement of the tympanic membrane and ossicles, as well as erosion of the cochlear promontory, may also be present. Although temporal bone studies have revealed an incidence of < 1% of an aberrant carotid artery, gross and micro-dehiscences of the carotid canal have a reported incidence of 7% and 15%, respectively.

Multiple etiologies for an aberrant ICA have been proposed, including (1) agenesis of the bony carotid canal; (2) lateral traction of the ICA by persistent embryonic vessels (eg, stapedial artery); and (3) agenesis of the vertical ICA with compensatory vascular communication from branches of the developing external carotid artery system. The latter theory also explains the association of aberrant ICAs with other vascular anomalies, such as persistent stapedial artery.

Clinical Findings

A. SYMPTOMS AND SIGNS

The presenting signs and symptoms of an aberrant ICA include pulsatile tinnitus, otalgia, aural fullness, vertigo, hearing loss (61% conductive, 6% sensorineural, and 33% normal) and a pulsating, red mass in the anteroinferior quadrant of the middle ear. There may be a right-sided predominance of this anomaly, and bilateral involvement has been described.

Although hypoplasia, agenesis, aneurysm, and aberrancy of the ICA have all been reported, the low incidence of these lesions demands a high clinical suspicion if disastrous complications are to be avoided. Agenesis and hypoplasia are most often found incidentally on radiographic imaging and may be unilateral or bilateral. These lesions may remain clinically silent since they may be well compensated by the vertebrobasilar, external carotid, or contralateral internal carotid systems. Alternatively, they may present with neurologic symptoms secondary to cerebral insufficiency or aneurysm formation. The latter occurs in 24–34% of cases.

B. IMAGING STUDIES

Radiographic imaging is essential and should include high-resolution CT scanning of the temporal bones (Figure 48–1), MRA, and angiography. CT and MRA are noninvasive and may delineate the vasculature and bony anatomy. A temporal bone CT scan in patients with carotid agenesis shows the complete absence of the petrous carotid canal. Angiographic findings include persistent fetal branches of the external carotid artery (ECA), such as the hyoid, caroticotympanic, inferior tympanic, and stapedial arteries, as well as other intracranial vascular anomalies. Findings suggestive of an aberrant ICA include the following: (1) a vascular mass in the hypotympanum, (2) an enlargement of the inferior tympanic canaliculus, and (3) a lack of bony canal wall over the vertical ICA. This last feature helps distinguish aberrancy from a glomus tumor.

Several clinicians advocate angiography as the gold standard in the diagnosis of vascular lesions of the middle ear. The classic angiographic finding of an aberrant ICA is identification lateral to a vertical line drawn through the lateral border of the vestibule. Angiography also allows for occlusion testing to define the adequacy of the contralateral carotid circulation if ligation is to be considered.

Differential Diagnosis

The rarity of ICA anomalies dictates that a broad differential diagnosis for vascular masses of the middle ear be

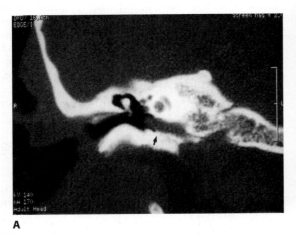
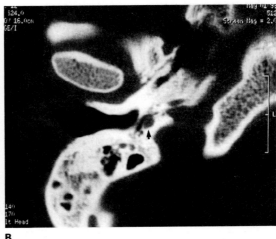

A
B

Figure 48–1. **(A)** Aberrant position of the internal carotid artery. **(B)** Coronal CT scanning demonstrates extension of the internal carotid artery into the hypotympanum (arrow).

considered. Also included in this list are glomus tympanicum, glomus jugulare, vascular tumors of the temporal bone, dehiscent jugular bulbs, arteriovenous malformations, and arterial fistulas.

Treatment

The treatment of aneurysms and aberrancy of the ICA should be determined on a case-specific basis. Most authors agree that if the patient's only symptom is pulsatile tinnitus or if the patient is asymptomatic, the lesions may be followed expectantly. Indications for definitive therapy include debilitating or progressive symptoms, the prevention of aneurysm formation, embolic phenomenon from an aneurysm, and the destruction of middle ear structures. Aneurysms may be embolized during angiography. Covering an aberrant vessel with fascia, a bone graft, or a Silastic (ie, polymeric silicone) sheet has been described but carries a significant risk of distal ischemia from compression. Inadvertent injury to an aberrant or aneurysmal ICA during myringotomy or middle ear surgery may result in severe hemorrhage. In these situations, the middle ear should be tightly packed. If this fails, surgical ligation of the internal or common carotid artery may be necessary to prevent exsanguination.

Botma M, Kell RA, Bhattacharya J, Crowther JA. Aberrant internal carotid artery in the middle ear space. *J Laryngol Otol.* 2000;114:784. [PMID: 11127152] (Highlights radiographic findings and clinical presentation of aberrant internal carotid artery.)

Windfuhr JP. Aberrant internal carotid artery in the middle ear. *Ann Otol Rhinol Laryngol Suppl.* 2004;192:1. [PMID: 15053213]
(Case series and literature review evaluating the incidence, signs and management of patients with an aberrant internal carotid artery.)

PERSISTENT STAPEDIAL ARTERY

ESSENTIALS OF DIAGNOSIS

- *Usually asymptomatic, but may cause pulsatile tinnitus and hearing loss.*
- *May be associated with other anomalies and may complicate middle ear surgery.*
- *Retraction or avoidance may be the most prudent management.*

A persistent stapedial artery (PSA) is a rare vascular anomaly of the middle ear. The reported prevalence of 0.48% in cadaveric studies of temporal bones is significantly less than the 0.02–0.05% found in surgical series.

Normally atrophied by 3 months of fetal development, the stapedial artery may persist as a 1.5- to 2.0-mm branch of the petrous internal carotid artery. As a result of this anomaly, the middle meningeal artery arises from the stapedial artery, and the foramen spinosum is absent. Although pulsatile tinnitus, conductive hearing loss, and sensorineural hearing loss have been described, most cases are clinically asymptomatic and found incidentally at the time of middle ear surgery. Case series have also noted multiple congenital anomalies associated with PSA, including aberrant internal carotid artery, Paget disease, anencephaly, anomalous stapes, anomalous facial nerve, thalidomide deformities, and trisomies 13 and 15.

Although the pathophysiology of these associations is poorly understood, an awareness of its possible existence at the time of surgery remains the most important aspect of treating PSA. Inadvertent transection during exploration of the middle ear may result in profuse hemorrhage. This has been described as a complicating factor for cholesteatoma surgery, stapes surgery, and cochlear implants. Some clinicians have described surgical ligation at the time of exploration, but this poses a theoretical risk of ischemic stroke. Generally, avoidance or retraction of a PSA is advocated.

Silbergleit R, Quint DJ, Mehta BA et al. The persistent stapedial artery. *Am J Neuroradiol.* 2000;21:572. [PMID: 10730654] (Case series and review of persistent stapedial artery, with a detailed discussion of embryology and developmental anatomy.)

CHOLESTEATOMAS

CONGENITAL CHOLESTEATOMA

 ESSENTIALS OF DIAGNOSIS

- *Commonly present as small pearl in the anterosuperior quadrant of the mesotympanum.*
- *May result from persistence of fetal epidermoid rests.*
- *Often asymptomatic and not associated with a history of otitis media, tympanic membrane perforation, or eustachian tube dysfunction.*
- *Timely surgical removal is indicated to avoid complications.*

General Considerations

Historically, congenital cholesteatoma has been defined as a middle ear cholesteatoma in the presence of an intact tympanic membrane without a history of perforation, otitis media, otorrhea, or otologic surgery. However, subsequent physicians have argued that these findings should not represent exclusionary criteria for congenital cholesteatoma given the high incidence of middle ear infections or effusions in the general population.

Several features help distinguish acquired from congenital cholesteatoma. Patients with acquired lesions present in the setting of frequent episodes of otitis media, structural pathology of the tympanic membrane, eustachian tube dysfunction, and diseased mastoid cavities. The developing mass is frequently symptomatic, causing otorrhea, otalgia, and hearing loss, and on examination it is found to expand in direct continuity with a tympanic membrane perforation or retraction pocket.

In contrast, congenital cholesteatomas are not associated with a history of recurrent otitis media and develop in the setting of a normal tympanic membrane, a functional eustachian tube, and a well-aerated mastoid cavity. Furthermore, they are often clinically silent and discovered on routine examination.

Pathogenesis

Multiple theories have been put forth to describe the pathophysiology of congenital cholesteatoma. The presence of the epidermoid formation in the anterior epitympanum of the developing fetal temporal bone between weeks 10 and 33 of gestation has been described. This implies that congenital cholesteatoma of the anterosuperior quadrant may result from the failure of the normal involution of this epidermoid tissue. This theory, however, does not account for posterior lesions. Proposed etiologies of posterior congenital cholesteatoma include the posterior migration of anterior epidermoid tissue, presence of amniotic cellular material in the middle ear, or ingrowth of external canal epithelium through a defect in the tympanic ring. To date, no single theory has been able to adequately account for the clinical spectrum of congenital cholesteatoma.

Clinical Findings

A. SYMPTOMS AND SIGNS

Lesions occurring "classically" in the anterosuperior quadrant of the mesotympanum account for anywhere from 27% to 67% of all cases. These typically present as small pearls adjacent to the long process of the malleus, with minimal ossicular involvement or hearing loss. Lesions in the posterosuperior mesotympanum, considered a minor variant in older series, develop near the incudostapedial joint and have recently been reported to account for 33–78% of all congenital cholesteatomas. These tend to be larger, with more frequent ossicular involvement and hearing loss. Bilateral congenital cholesteatoma (3% of cases), as well as extension into the epitympanum, sinus tympani, and facial recess, has been described.

Congenital cholesteatoma in any location is often clinically silent for years but may eventually present with a combination of tinnitus, vertigo, 30–40 dB conductive hearing loss, or sensorineural hearing loss. Although classically described as occurring in an ear free of structural pathology, a congenital cholesteatoma presenting at an advanced stage may perforate through the tympanic membrane or obstruct the eustachian tube and predispose to otitis media, making the distinction between a congenital and an acquired lesion difficult. No single symptom complex is diagnostic for congenital cholesteatoma, although the presence of a discrete, round white lesion seen in the anterosuperior quadrant of an otherwise normal tympanic membrane is suggestive. There is a male predilection, with a male-to-female ratio of approximately 2–3:1. The average age at presentation is 2–4 years for anterior lesions and 12 years for posterior lesions.

B. SPECIAL TESTS

The diagnosis of a congenital cholesteatoma is clinical and based initially on the history and otoscopic examination. Audiometry is performed to evaluate and document preoperative hearing, and temporal bone CT scans help determine the extent of disease. A common finding in these studies is a well-aerated mastoid cavity, in contradistinction to patients with acquired cholesteatoma.

Treatment

In general, the management of congenital cholesteatoma is timely surgical removal. Nonoperative intervention or observation may result in progressive growth of the lesion with progressive erosion of the ossicles. Although multiple surgical approaches have been advocated, the goal of complete extirpation remains universal. Simple myringotomy with or without the insertion of ventilation tubes should be avoided because this may lead to partial removal, middle ear adhesions, or seeding of the cholesteatoma, all of which make future surgical efforts more challenging.

Most lesions located in the anterior mesotympanum may be successfully removed via a traditional or an extended tympanotomy. A significant portion of posterior or extensive lesions may also be approached in this manner but may ultimately require an atticotomy or mastoidectomy. In contrast to acquired cholesteatoma, congenital lesions result in minimal inflammatory reactions or adhesions between the matrix and the middle ear mucosa. A clear plane can be easily developed between the cholesteatoma and the surrounding mucosa of the middle ear or ossicles, especially if prior surgeries have not been performed. Evidence of bony erosion in the mastoid on preoperative imaging studies are contraindications to attempted removal via an extended tympanotomy.

Lesions involving the attic, epitympanum, or the region of the aditus can initially be approached as a tympanotomy extended to an atticotomy. The mastoid air cells in patients with congenital cholesteatoma tend to be well pneumatized, and bony resection to the limits of the lesion in cases involving the mastoid cavity often spare the majority of the air cells. Most clinicians, therefore, recommend intact canal wall procedures in patients with congenital cholesteatoma in an effort to prevent creating a large open cavity with its associated lifelong burden of care. Congenital cholesteatoma is associated with ossicular erosion (most commonly the incus) in most cases. Ossicular reconstruction can be staged with a "second look" procedure and ossicular reconstruction 1 year later.

Prognosis

Congenital cholesteatomas recur in approximately 30–55% of cases after surgical removal. The incidence of recurrence is notably higher in patients with involvement of the posterior-superior quadrant, attic, or mastoid. The mean time to recurrence ranges from 8 to 14 months in patients with disease limited to the middle ear, and 30 months for patients with more extensive disease. The high rate of recurrence in patients with a history of surgery for congenital cholesteatoma requires that these patients be followed clinically for a significant period of time.

Nelson M, Roger G, Koltai PJ et al. Congenital cholesteatoma. *Arch Otolaryngol Head Neck Surg.* 2002;128:810. [PMID: 12117341] (Retrospective review to derive a classification system for congenital cholesteatoma and assess whether it is a reliable guide for surgical intervention, reexploration, and hearing outcome.)

Potsic WP, Korman SB, Samadi DS et al. Congenital cholesteatome: 20 years' experience at the Children's Hospital of Philadelphia. *Otolaryngol Head Neck Surg.* 2002;126:409. [PMID: 11997782]

Yeo SW, Sung-Won K, Ki-Hong C, Byung-Do S. The clinical evaluations of pathophysiology for congenital middle ear cholesteatoma. *Am J Otolaryngol.* 2001;22:184. [PMID: 11351288] (Case series with review of the literature and thorough discussion of congenital cholesteatoma.)

■ OSSICULAR ANOMALIES

 ESSENTIALS OF DIAGNOSIS

- *May occur in isolation or as part of a syndrome.*
- *Varying degrees of stable, conductive hearing loss may be present.*

- *Treatment is individualized based on the ossicular lesion, the patient's overall health, and the degree of hearing loss.*

General Considerations

Ossicular anomalies may be unilateral or bilateral and may be associated with anomalies of the external ear (atresia), the middle ear (facial nerve, stapedial muscle, tendon, or pyramidal eminence), or with a multiorgan syndrome (Treacher Collins or Goldenhar syndrome) (Table 48–1).

Classification

Historically, congenital malformations of the ear have been divided into major and minor types with the latter limited to the middle ear alone. Teunissen's classification system is based on the site of involvement and aids in determining the appropriateness for surgery (Table 48–2).

Surgical experience in patients with stapes ankylosis (Class I) and stapes ankylosis combined with ossicular anomaly (Class II) has been favorable, with a 73% rate of postoperative air-bone gap < 20 dB. In contrast, patients with mobile footplates, ossicular discontinuity, epitympanic fixation (Class III), or dysplasia of either the round or oval windows (Class IV) are poor surgical candidates. Finally, multiple ossicular anomalies with subtle but significant variations have been described (Figure 48–2 and Table 48–3).

Clinical Findings

A. Symptoms and Signs

Isolated ossicular anomalies are rare, as is evident from large retrospective reviews of otologic practices documenting only dozens of cases. Approximately 1–2% of patients with congenital conductive hearing loss have isolated middle ear anomalies. In addition to this low incidence, other factors make accurate preoperative diagnosis difficult. With the exception of malleus-incus fusion, hypoplasia of the malleus, and middle ear aplasia, the otoscopic examination is unremarkable. Furthermore, audiometric evaluation demonstrates a similarly moderate-to-severe conductive hearing loss that is fixed over time with most anomalies. These factors mandate a high index of suspicion to ensure both an accurate diagnosis and appropriate management.

A general examination of the patient is performed to evaluate the overall health and to search for any findings suggestive of a syndrome. Otoscopic examination of patients with anomalies of the malleus or combined ossicular anomalies may demonstrate loss of the tympanic membrane landmarks. Furthermore, the nonin-

volved ear should be evaluated for possible bilateral disease (25–40%).

B. Specials Tests and Imaging Studies

Audiometry demonstrates a stable moderate-to-severe conductive hearing loss, determines the severity of the air-bone gap, excludes bilateral or sensorineural disease, and can differentiate between ossicular discontinuity and fixation. A speech reception threshold worse than 30 dB has been defined as an indication for surgery. A high-resolution CT scan of the temporal bones may define the ossicular anomaly as well as the anatomy of the facial nerve and inner ear structures.

Treatment

Multiple factors are important in determining a patient's candidacy for operative intervention. Children with multisystem syndromes may be at a considerably higher anesthetic risk if there is involvement of the upper airway, heart, lungs, or kidneys. For children in overall good health, the indications, timing, and ideal method of surgical correction remain a source of controversy. The patient should be assessed for a delay in speech acquisition and the presence of cognitive and learning delays. Deferring surgery until at least the age of 5 is associated with a decreased incidence of otitis media, improved patient cooperation, and more sophisticated audiometric testing.

Surgery for unilateral disease in the setting of a normal contralateral ear either can be performed at the age of 5 or delayed until the patient is able to participate fully in the decision-making progress. Delaying surgery remains a source of controversy since the beneficial effects of binaural hearing on speech and development are continually being discovered. Finally, amplification with hearing aids, as a transition or an alternative to surgery, should be offered to the patient and family.

MALLEUS ANOMALIES

Although multiple anomalies of the malleus have been described, the incidence is lower than anomalies of the incus or stapes. Hypoplasia or aplasia of the malleus results from a failure of embryogenesis between weeks 7 and 25. Given the common pharyngeal arch origin, hypoplasia of the malleus is often associated with hypoplasia of the incus. An ossicular replacement prosthesis can be placed at the time of middle ear exploration in these cases. Fixation of the head of the malleus represents 80% of all isolated congenital anomalies of the malleus (Figure 48–3). Exploration of the temporal bone in these patients reveals bony bridges between the head of the malleus and the lateral epitympanum in 75–80% of cases. The term "malleus bar" has been used when this bridge connects to the posterior tympanic wall. Malleus fixation, in general, is presumed to result from failure of mesenchymal absorption and is correctable by either laser division of the connecting bridge or

Table 48–1. Syntromes with known middle ear anomalies.

Syndrome	Cardinal Features	Middle Ear Anomalies
Apert	Patent cochlear aqueduct, enlarged internal auditory canal, craniofacial dystosis, brachiocephaly, spina bifida, hypertelorism, syndactyly, cleft palate	Fixed stapes
Beckwith-Wiedemann	Exophthalmos, macroglossia, gigantism, auricular deformities, facial nevus flammeus, midface hypoplasia, organomegaly of viscera, genitourinary anomalies, advanced bone age, neonatal hypoglycemia	Fixed stapes
CHARGE	Coloboma, heart anomalies, choanal atresia, mental retardation, genital anomalies, external and internal ear anomalies	Aplasia or malformation of stapes and incus, aplasia of oval and round windows
Congenital heart disease, deafness and skeletal malformation	Fused carpal and tarsal bones, mitral valve insufficiency	Stenosis of EAC, fixed stapes
Congenital rubella	Inner ear anomalies, mental retardation, microcephaly, ocular abnormalities, thrombocytopenia, cardiovascular deformities, deformities of lower extremities	Fixed malleus head, hypoplasia of incudal ligament, malformation of stapes, fixed stapes, persistent mesenchyme
Congenital syphilis	Malformation of the temporal bone, inner ear anomalies, perforated nasal septum, interstitial keratitis, Hutchinson teeth	Fixed and hyperplastic malleus, spongy long process of incus, malformation of stapes
Crouzon	Premature craniosynostoses, midfacial hypoplasia, ocular and auricular deformities, underdevelopment of periosteal portion of labyrinth, reduced periosteal layer of petrous bone, hard cleft palate, cleft palate	Fixed malleus, malformed or fixed stapes, hypoplasia of middle ear
DiGeorge	Auricular deformities, hypoplastic thymus, aortic arch anomalies, patent ductus arteriosus, thyroid agenesis, acrania, microcephaly, micrognathia, short philtrum, cleft palate or bifid uvula	Atresia of EAC, aplasia of ossicles, aplasia of oval window, hypoplastic facial nerve, absent stapedius muscle, hypoplasia of tympanic cavity
Duane	Unilateral (left) aberrant innervation of lateral rectus muscle, ocular muscle anomalies, auricular deformities, facial asymmetry, skeletal deformities, congenital skin lesions, CNS disorders, seizures, genitourinary anomalies	Atresia of EAC, fused ossicles, malformation of stapes, thin membrane covering oval window, ossicular mass separated from stapes
Fanconi	Auricular deformities, aplastic anemia, hypoplasia of cochlea, short cochlear duct, skin pigmentation, skeletal and renal anomalies, mental retardation	Atresia of EAC, fixed stapes
Fetal hydantoin (anticonvulsant drug-induced malformations)	Cleft lip and palate, craniofacial and skeletal anomalies, auricular deformities, inner ear anomalies, mental retardation, cardiovascular, gastrointestinal, and genitourinary malformation	Malformation of ossicles, aplasia of oval and round window
Goldenhar	Unilateral facial hypoplasia, dermoids, lipodermoids, lipomas of eyes, vertebral anomalies, malformation of pinna, micrognathia, cleft lip and palate, laryngeal anomalies	EAC atresia, malformation or aplasia of ossicles, hypoplasia of oval window, chorda tympani, facial nerve
Hurler	Dwarfism, auricular deformities, hepatosplenomegaly, mental retardation, hypertelorism, facial deformities, skeletal deformities, broad stubby fingers, increased body hair, cardiac anomalies	Aplasia of incudomalleal joint, malformation of stapes, fibrous tissue replacement of otic capsule, persistent mesenchyme overlying oval and round window, underdevelopment of mastoid air cells, hypertrophied mucosa

648

Syndrome	Clinical features	Otologic findings
Klippel-Feil	Fused cervical vertebrae, pectoral girdle deformities, auricular deformities, inner ear anomalies, spina bifida, cleft palate	Atresia of EAC, aplasia of ossicles, malformation of malleoincudal joint, fused short process of incus, aplasia of lenticular process, fused long process of incus, fixed stapes, fistula of stapes footplate, aberrant course of facial nerve
Knuckle pads with leukonychia	Knuckle pad deformities	Aplasia of ossicles and facial nerve, high jugular bulb, absent facial canal
Larsen	Multiple joint dislocations, facial abnormalities	Bulbous lenticular process of incus, incudostapedial joint laxity, fixed stapes
Madelung deformity, Leri Weill syndrome	Short-limbed dwarfism, deformed radius, ulna and proximal carpal bones	Stenosis of EAC, aplasia of malleus, malformation of stapes and incus
Melnick needles (osteodysplasty)	Auricular deformities, cranial anomalies, small facial bone with prominent eyes, delay in paranasal sinus development, small mandible, skeletal deformities	Stenosis of EAC, aplasia of round window, mastoid sclerosis
Mixed hearing loss, low-set malformed ears, and mental retardation	Auricular deformities, mental retardation, high arched palate, small stature	Single posterior malleus-shaped ossicle, aplasia of incus and stapes, aplasia of round window
Möbius	Microtia, auricular deformities, inner ear anomalies, absent abductors of the eye, musculoskeletal deformities, cranial nerve palsies, expressionless face, short stature	Atresia of EAC, aplasia of stapes, ossicular mass, aplasia of oval window, round window and facial nerve
Mohr	Facial deformities, hypoplastic body of mandible, lobulated tongue, digital anomalies, brachydactyly	Malformation of long process of incus, aplasia of incudostapedial joint
Noonan (pseudo-Turner)	Normal karyotype, auricular deformities, short stature, short neck, micrognathia, hypertelorism, antimongoloid palpebral fissures, cardiovascular anomalies, skeletal anomalies	Aplasia of long process of incus and aberrant position of stapes
Osteogenesis imperfecta	Blue sclerae, multiple bone fractures, skeletal deformities, abnormal tooth dentin, weak joints, cardiovascular and platelet anomalies, macrocephaly	Malformation of stapes head and crura, fragile stapes, otosclerosis
Otopalatodigital	Frontal and occipital bossing, inner ear anomalies, hypertelorism, broad nasal root, small mandible, cleft palate, dwarfism, skeletal abnormalities, mental retardation	Fetal-shaped ossicles, fixed stapes, aplasia of round window
Pierre Robin	Auricular deformities, small internal auditory canal, cochlear malformations, mental retardation, hydrocephalus, microcephaly, ocular defects, cleft palate, mandibular hypoplasia, cardiac defects	Thickened stapes crura and footplate, hypoplastic facial nerve, dehiscent facial canal, aplasia of middle ear
Potter	Bilateral renal agenesis, auricular deformities, inner ear anomalies, facial deformities, pulmonary hypoplasia, GI malformations, genital deformities, anomalies of the lower extremities	Atresia of EAC, malformation of incus, fixed malleus and incus, aplasia of ossicles and oval window, persistent mesenchyme, dehiscent fallopian canal, aberrant course of facial nerve

(continued)

Table 48-1. Syndromes with known middle ear anomalies. *(Continued)*

Syndrome	Cardinal Features	Middle Ear Anomalies
Proximal symphalangia	Symphalangia of proximal interphalangeal joints	Stenosis of EAC, fixed stapes, elongated long process of incus
Thalidomide ototoxicity	Auricular deformities, inner ear anomalies, coloboma, short stature, absent long bones, hemangiomas, cardiovascular defects, renal hypoplasia, intestinal atresia	Atresia of WAC, malformation of the tympanic membrane, fixed malleus, malformation of long process of incus, aplasia of stapes, facial nerve, chorda tympani nerve and oval window, persistent stapedial artery, hypoplastic tympanic cavity
Treacher-Collins	Antimongoloid palpebral fissure, coloboma, micrognathia, hypoplasia of malar bones and infraorbital rim, short palate, cleft lip and palate, auricular deformities, clinodactyly and sternal deformities, mild mental retardation	Atresia or stenosis of EAC, aplasia of tensor tympani muscle, stapedial muscle and tendon, malformation of ossicles, aberrant course of facial nerve, hypoplasia of epitympanum and mesotympanum
Trisomy 13 (Patau syndrome)	Auricular deformities, microcephaly, arrhinencephaly, inner ear anomalies, ocular anomalies, hypertelorism, cleft lip and palate, VSD, simian crease	Stenosis of EAC, thick manubrium of malleus, malformation of incudostapedial joint and stapes, hypoplastic facial nerve, aplasia of stapedius muscle and tendon, persistent stapedial artery, dehiscent facial canal, hypoplasia of mastoid cavity
Trisomy 18 (Edward syndrome)	Auricular deformities, inner ear anomalies, ptosis of eyelids, micrognathia, flexion deformities, mental retardation	Atresia of EAC, malformation of malleus and incus, fetal form or columella-type stapes, absent stapedius tendon, hypoplasia of facial nerve, aberrant course of facial and chorda tympani nerves
Trisomy 21 (Down syndrome)	Auricular deformities, hypertelorism, epicanthal fold, protruding tongue, high arched palate, inner ear anomalies, cardiovascular defects, mental retardation	Stenosis of EAC, persistent mesenchyme, wide angle of facial genu, malformation of ossicles, high jugular bulb, poor mastoid pneumatization, eustachian tube stenosis
Trisomy 22	Auricular deformities, mental retardation, inner ear anomalies, hypertelorism, micrognathia, coloboma, cardiovascular defects, renal agenesis, anal atresia	Atresia of EAC, aplasia of stapes and oval window, poor pneumatization of middle ear, aplasia of round window
Turner	XO chromosome, auricular deformities, short stature, sexual gonadal dysplasia, short and thick neck, antimongoloid palpebral fissure, cardiovascular anomalies, renal malformations, mandibular hypoplasia	Underdevelopment of mastoid air cells, malformation of ossicles
VATER	Vertebral defects, anal atresia, tracheoesophageal fistula with esophageal atresia, renal defects, skeletal deformities, cardiac defects	Hypoplasia of facial nerve, chorda tympani, malformation of stapes
Wildervanck	Sensorineural deafness, auricular deformities, fused cervical vertebrae, ocular muscle anomalies, inner ear anomalies, facial asymmetry, torticollis, dermoids, cleft palate	Atresia of EAC, fused malleus and incus, malformation of ossicles, aplasia or fixation of stapes, aplasia of oval window, ossified stapedius tendon

EAC, external auditory canal.

Table 48–2. Teunissen's classification of ossicular anomalies.

Class	Anomaly
I	Congenital stapes ankylosis
II	Stapes ankylosis with ossicular anomaly
III	Ossicular anomaly with mobile footplate
	Ossicular discontinuity
	Epitympanic fixation
IV	Aplasia or dysplasia of round or oval window
	Aplasia or dysplasia with crossing facial nerve
	Aplasia or dysplasia with persistent stapedial artery

resection of the head and placement of a stapes to a manubrium ossiculoplasty prosthesis.

INCUS ANOMALIES

Hypoplasia or aplasia of the incus typically occurs in conjunction with hypoplasia of the malleus but may occur in isolation. Ossicular replacement techniques used for patients with acquired erosion of the incus secondary to chronic otitis media are, similarly, effective for patients with these congenital lesions. The incus is also susceptible to fixation to the epitympanum. Treatment involves sectioning of the bony bridge with a laser.

STAPES ANOMALIES

Isolated congenital anomalies of the stapes represent approximately 40% of all congenital ossicular lesions. The stapes requires the longest period of embryologic development and therefore has the greatest potential for malformation. In addition, the stapes is derived from both branchial arch and otic capsule precursors, adding to the complexity of the development of this ossicle.

Numerous anomalies with variable morphologies exist. Congenital stapes footplate fixation is the most common isolated ossicular anomaly and is thought to result from ossification of a portion of cartilage in the annulus of the oval window. Footplate fixation also frequently occurs in Fanconi anemia and Apert syndrome. Surgical therapy involves either stapedotomy or total stapedectomy. However, outcomes have been mixed, with postoperative cerebrospinal fluid otorrhea and decreased hearing (30%) reported as known complications.

Although aplasia of the stapes is rare, multiple forms of hypoplasia that include small or absent crura and small, blob-like stapes have been described. The surgical options include total stapedectomy in cases with a fixed footplate, or replacement with a stapes prosthesis in cases of a mobile footplate. In contrast, isolated hyperplasia of the stapes is often an incidental finding that does not require therapy.

This anomaly is thought to result from a failure of the resorption and remodeling that occurs during the final stages of stapes development and accounts for up to 20% of all ossicular anomalies.

Several crural anomalies have been described, including thin, absent, fused, and angled crura. The crura may also be replaced with a columella-like structure. Laser resection followed by stapes prosthesis replacement is effective in symptomatic crural lesions and columella stapes. The incomplete absorption of mesenchyme may result in bony bridges between the facial canal and either the head or crus of the stapes that result in a symptomatic conductive hearing loss. Laser division of these bony attachments is effective. Equally effective is laser removal of a bony bar that spans the pyramidal eminence and stapes neck in cases of ossified stapedius tendon.

MULTIPLE OSSICULAR ANOMALIES

Ossicular anomalies involving more than one ossicle occur as frequently as isolated anomalies. Complete agenesis of the ossicles occurs in conjunction with multisystem syndromes (eg, DiGeorge syndrome) and is not amenable to reconstruction. Fusion of the heads of the malleus and incus results from a failure of formation of the incudomalleolar joint at 7 weeks and is a common finding in aural atresia (Figure 48–4). Furthermore, the handle of the malleus is typically fixed to the atretic plate and posterior canal wall. This placement, in combination with the atresia of the external auditory canal, results in a maximal conductive loss.

Many management strategies have been proposed for appropriate surgical candidates. The incus-malleus complex may be removed and replaced with a partial ossicular replacement prosthesis. Alternatively, a combination of laser and a drill may be used to enlarge the canal and free the ossicular mass from the atretic plate and canal wall. Finally, the ossicular mass may be disarticulated from the stapes, remodeled, and used for reconstruction. All three ossicles may be fused either as a single mass or at specific articulation points (the malleus handle, the incus long process, or the stapes head). Although the treatment of complete ossicular fusion is limited secondary to fusion to the oval window, lesions involving fusion at single articulation points are amenable to reconstruction with a prosthesis.

One third of all anomalies of the stapes are associated with anomalies of the long process of the incus. The incudostapedial joint forms during week 8 of fetal development as the incus precursor migrates to articulate with the future stapedial ring. The fibrous union of this joint results in a conductive hearing loss of approximately 30 dB and may be transmitted in an autosomal dominant fashion. Treatment options include incus removal and prosthesis replacement, stapedectomy, or cartilage interposition. Other congenital lesions of the incus and stapes include bony fusion

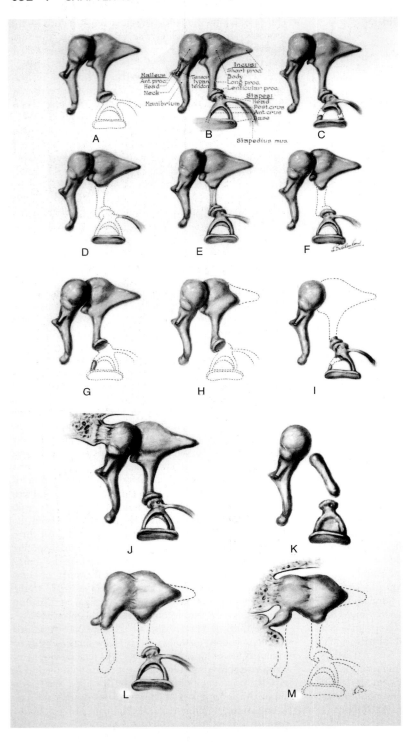

Figure 48–2. Congenital ossicular anomalies. **(A)** Absent stapes and stapedius muscle. **(B)** Anterior stapes fixation and hypoplasia of the oval window. **(C)** Stapes with incomplete anterior and posterior crus. **(D)** Absence of long crus of incus and crural arch of stapes. **(E)** Connective tissue strand replacing long crus of incus. **(F)** Absence of long crus of incus. **(G)** Absence of stapes and stapedius muscle except for small remnant of anterior crus. **(H)** Absence of stapes, stapedius muscle, and short process of incus. **(I)** Absence of anterior crus of stapes and absence of incus except for lenticular process. **(J)** Bony fixation of the lateral attic wall and head of malleus. **(K)** Solid stapes and hypoplasia of incus with only long crus present. **(L)** Conglomerate mass of incus and malleus. **(M)** Absent stapes and conglomerate mass of malleus and incus with fusion to the lateral attic wall. (Reproduced, with permission, from Paparella MM, Shumrick DA, Gluckman JL, Moeyerhoff WL. *Otolaryngology,* 3rd ed. Philadelphia: WB Saunders, 1991.)

Table 48–3. Congenital ossicular anomalies.

Location	Anomaly
Malleus	Hypoplasia or aplasia
	Head fixation
	Manubrium fixation
	Manubrium aplasia
	Manubrium separation from head
	Spindle handle
Incus	Hypoplasia or aplasia
	Long process hypoplasia
	Lenticular process hypoplasia
	Fixation
Stapes	Hypoplasia or aplasia
	Aplasia of the head or crus
	Hyperplasia
	Columellar stapes
	Superstructure fixation
	Head fixation
	Obturator foramen obliteration
	Stapedius tendon ossification
	Footplate fixation, absence, or doubling
	Juvenile otosclerosis
Combined	Ossicular agenesis
	Malleus-incus fusion
	Incudostapedial joint disarticulation, absence, or fixation
	Ossicular mass

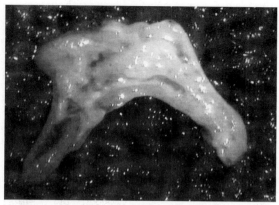

Figure 48–4. Fusion of the incus with the head of the malleus.

and aplasia of the articular joint. Both lesions are amenable to laser remodeling followed by interposition grafts.

Raveh E, Hu W, Papsin BC, et al. Congenital conductive hearing loss. *J Laryngol Otol.* 2002;116:92. [PMID: 11827579] (Results of 67 patients undergoing exploratory tympanotomy for nonserous congenital conductive hearing loss suggest exploring the ear, but in a more realistic, informed way.)

Teunissen EB, Cremers CWRJ. Classification of congenital middle ear anomalies. Report on 144 ears. *Ann Otol Rhinol Laryngol.* 1993;102:606. [PMID: 8352484] (Classic description of congenital ossicular anomalies, including their classification scheme and surgical interventions.)

◼ ANOMALIES OF THE OVAL & ROUND WINDOWS

ESSENTIALS OF DIAGNOSIS

- *Abnormal development of the oval window may be associated with failure of stapes insertion, a maximal conductive hearing loss and abnormal position of the facial nerve.*
- *Round window aplasia is commonly associated with stapes ankylosis and results in unsuccessful stapedectomy.*

OVAL WINDOW ANOMALIES

Hypoplasia or aplasia of the oval window is a rare anomaly and may occur in isolation or in conjunction with other

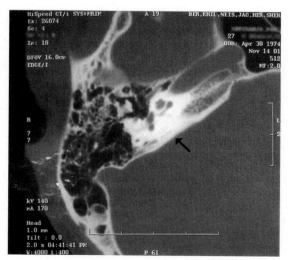

Figure 48–3. Coronal CT scan of a patient with external canal atresia and lateral fixation of the head of the malleus (arrow).

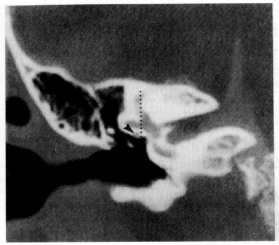 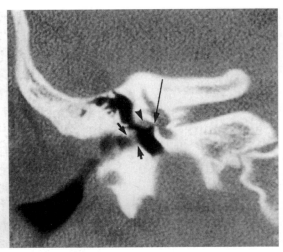

A　　　　　　　　　　　　　　　　　　　　**B**

Figure 48–5. Congenital oval window aplasia. **(A)** Coronal CT scan demonstrating obliteration of the oval window by a bony plate and a normal facial nerve canal (arrow) lying lateral to the anterior junction of the anterior and superior semicircular canals (vertical line). **(B)** Partial absence of the oval window (long arrow) in a patient with external canal stenosis (short arrows) and a large horizontal facial nerve (arrowhead). (Reproduced, with permission, from Zeifer B, Sabini P, Sonne J. Congenital absence of the oval window: radiologic diagnosis and associated anomalies. *Am J Neuroradiol.* 2000;21:322.)

anomalies. Failure of the normal association between the primordial oval window niche (the otic capsule) and the developing stapes footplate between the fifth and sixth weeks of development results in aplasia of the oval window and is most commonly associated with anterior displacement of the tympanic segment of the facial nerve. Additional anomalies of the stapes, round window, and inner ear may be present. A maximal conductive hearing loss (60 dB) is usually detected in early childhood, and an absent oval window may be visualized on high-resolution CT scanning (Figure 48–5). Radiographic imaging may also be used to confirm the presence of normal inner ear structures, determine the anatomy of the facial nerve, and detect any associated ossicular anomalies.

The management of oval window aplasia remains controversial. Options include hearing aids, vestibulotomy with prosthesis insertion, fenestration and piston insertion above the aberrant facial nerve, or fenestration of the horizontal semicircular canal. The success of all these different surgical approaches has been mixed. Furthermore, the facial nerve and the inner ear are at considerable risk for injury during these surgical approaches.

ROUND WINDOW ANOMALIES

Aplasia or hypoplasia of the round window may be associated with endemic cretinism and mandibulofacial dysostosis. Non-syndromic cases of round window anomalies are rare, with fewer than 10 reports described

in the literature. More commonly, the round window position and size may vary without functional consequence. The significance and management of round window aplasia remain unclear. During week 11 of fetal development, a condensation of connective tissue forms at the future site of the round window. This develops into a cartilage ring that prevents ossification of the round window niche. Failure of the development of this ring results in bony obliteration of the primordial niche.

Round window aplasia is often associated with stapes ankylosis and a 40-dB conductive hearing loss. When stapedectomy is unsuccessful in reversing this hearing loss, the absence of the round window may be diagnosed in retrospect. Although high-resolution CT scans may detect aplasia of the round window, most cases are diagnosed after unsuccessful stapedectomy. Attempts at surgical fenestration have met with poor results and carry a significant risk of sensorineural hearing loss. Therefore, amplification represents the most practical therapy.

Martin C, Tringali S, Bertholon P et al. Isolated congenital round window absence. *Ann Otol Rhinol Laryngol.* 2002;111:799. [PMID: 12296334] (Case report describing the diagnosis of congenital absence of the round window using a high-resolution computed tomography scan.)

Zeifer B, Sabini P, Sonne J. Congenital absence of the oval window: radiologic diagnosis and associated anomalies. *Am J Neuroradiol.* 2000;21:322. [PMID: 10696017] (Radiographic diagnosis and clinical evaluation of oval window aplasia.)

Otitis Media

Philip D. Yates, MB ChB, FRCS, & Shahram Anari, MD, MRCS

The term otitis media (OM) refers to an inflammatory process within the middle ear cleft. Otitis media can be either acute or chronic. There is no absolute time period, but, in general, disease that persists for more than 3 months should be considered as chronic.

A subclassification of acute and chronic OM is summarized in Table 49–1. Otitis media associated with cholesteatoma is considered separately in Chapter 50, Cholesteatoma. The eustachian tube appears to be central to the pathogenesis of all forms of OM (with the possible exception of cholesteatoma). The normal physiologic functions of the eustachian tube are to (1) maintain the gaseous pressure within the middle ear cleft at a level that approximates atmospheric pressure; (2) prevent reflux of the contents of the nasopharynx into the middle ear; and (3) clear secretions from the middle ear by both mucociliary transport and a "pump action" of the eustachian tube.

The failure of any or all of these normal functions of the eustachian tube can result in OM. Both anatomic and functional obstruction of the eustachian tube results in the failure of normal regulation of the middle ear pressure. **Anatomic obstruction** is most commonly caused by inflammation of the eustachian tube mucosa or extrinsic compression by tumor or large adenoids. **Functional obstruction** usually occurs as a result of either the failure of the normal muscular mechanism of eustachian tube opening, as seen in cleft palate, or insufficient stiffness of the cartilaginous portion of the eustachian tube, often seen in infants and young children. The more acute angle of the eustachian tube seen in children, compared with adults, may also result in the impaired function of the eustachian tube opening. If the eustachian tube is abnormally patent or short, its normal protective function against the reflux of nasopharyngeal contents is lost. These abnormalities are often seen in patients with Down syndrome, which may account for the high rate of OM in this particular patient population. Normal function of the eustachian tube is also dependent on ciliary function; therefore, any condition that affects mucociliary clearance, such as viral infection, bacterial toxins, or inherited abnormalities of ciliary structure, can predispose to OM.

Bluestone CD. Studies in otitis media: Children's Hospital of Pittsburgh-University of Pittsburgh progress report. *Laryngoscope.* 2004;114(11 Pt 3 Suppl 105):1. [PMID: 15514559] (Reviews epidemiology, risk factors, anatomy of eustachian tube, pathophysiology, and microbiology of otitis media.)

Lim DJ. Recent advances in otitis media. Report of the Eighth Research Conference. *Ann Otol Rhinol Laryngol.* 2005;114(1 Pt 2 Suppl 194):1. (Comprehensive report on the recent studies on different aspects of otitis media.)

ACUTE OTITIS MEDIA

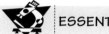 ESSENTIALS OF DIAGNOSIS

- *Otalgia.*
- *Pyrexia.*
- *Thickened, bulging, hyperemic tympanic membrane.*
- *Hearing loss.*
- *Otorrhea.*

General Considerations

Acute otitis media (AOM) is one of the most common infectious diseases seen in children, with its peak incidence in the first 2 years of life. Most of the population will suffer at least one episode of AOM at some point in their childhood. It can occur in suppurative, nonsuppurative, and recurrent forms. In nonsuppurative AOM, inflammation of the middle ear cleft mucosa occurs either without formation of an effusion or with a sterile effusion. This type of AOM is often seen prior to, or in the resolution stage of, the acute suppurative OM; however, resolution may occur before frank suppuration. Recurrent AOM is defined as ≥ 3 episodes of acute suppurative OM in a 6-month period, or ≥ 4 episodes in a 12-month period, with complete resolution of symptoms and signs between the episodes.

The epidemiology of AOM and otitis media with effusion (OME) overlaps to such an extent that the risk factors apply to both conditions. Both environmental and host factors play a role in the epidemiology of OM Table 49–2). Attendance at day-care facilities is one of the major risk factors for OM. Child care results in

Table 49–1. Classification of otitis media.

Acute Otitis Media
  Suppurative
  Nonsuppurative
  Recurrent
Chronic Otitis Media
  Suppurative
    Tubotympanic
    Cholesteatoma
  Nonsuppurative
    Otitis media with effusion

many children being in close contact, which increases the exposure to respiratory tract pathogens responsible for OM. The risks associated with child care attendance are variable and are related to the number of children in a facility, the hours spent in child care, the child's age at entry, and whether siblings are in child care. Breast-feeding appears to have a protective effect against OM, particularly when breast-feeding is used exclusively for at least the first 3–6 months of life. The protective mechanism of breast-feeding has not been clearly demonstrated, but is likely to be related to antibacterial and immunologic benefits conferred by breast milk.

Exposure to cigarette smoke has been implicated in the etiology of OM. Passive smoking results in inflammation of the mucosa of the middle ear cleft as well as impaired mucociliary clearance, which lead to an increased susceptibility to infection. There is a seasonal variation in the incidence of OM; it is more common in winter months, which mirrors the incidence of upper respiratory tract infections.

Genetics play an important role in the etiology of OM. Males have a higher incidence of OM than females, a fact that is true of most infections of infancy and childhood. The sibling, maternal, and paternal histories of OM are all independently related to a child's risk of developing OM.

Table 49–2. Factors relevant to the epidemiology of otitis media.

Environmental Factors
  Day-care attendance
  Not being breast-fed
  Exposure to tobacco smoke
  Seasonal variation in respiratory infections
Host Factors
  Genetics
  Immunodeficiency
  Birth defects
    Cleft palate
    Down syndrome

Although OM is largely a uniform worldwide condition, some racial variations in the rates of OM exist; this condition is more prevalent in Native Americans, Alaskan and Canadian Eskimos, and Australian Aboriginals. These genetic variations may be related to anatomic and physiologic variations in the eustachian tube.

Otitis media is seen almost universally in children with cleft palate. Because the tensor veli palatini muscle lacks its normal insertion into the soft palate, it is unable to open the eustachian tube properly on swallowing. A small number of patients suffering from OM have an abnormal host defense owing to various conditions such as immunoglobulin deficiency, malignant neoplasms, immunosuppressive therapy, and AIDS.

Pathogenesis

In most cases of AOM, an antecedent viral upper respiratory tract infection leads to disruption of eustachian tube function. Inflammation of the middle ear mucosa results in an effusion, which cannot be cleared via the obstructed eustachian tube. This effusion provides a favorable medium for proliferation of bacterial pathogens, which reach the middle ear via the eustachian tube, resulting in suppuration.

Although viral infection is important in the pathogenesis of AOM, the majority of patients develop subsequent bacterial colonization, and therefore AOM should be considered a predominantly bacterial infection. Many studies, using tympanocentesis, have identified *Streptococcus pneumoniae* (up to 40%), *Haemophilus influenzae* (25–30%), and *Moraxella catarrhalis* (10–20%) as the organisms most commonly responsible for AOM. Less frequently identified pathogens include group A streptococci, *Staphylococcus aureus,* and gram-negative organisms such as *Pseudomonas aeruginosa.* In all studies of the microbiology of AOM, a significant number of cultures prove negative. This finding may occur for a variety of reasons, including (1) antibiotic therapy before tympanocentesis; (2) nonbacterial pathogens (eg, viruses, chlamydia, and mycoplasma); and (3) pathogens that do not proliferate in classic culture conditions (eg, mycobacteria and anaerobic bacteria). Recent studies on bacteriology of AOM show that the polymerase chain reaction (PCR) methods produce positive results in patients in whom cultures have been negative by the conventional methods.

The role of the adenoids (ie, the pharyngeal tonsils) in the pathogenesis of AOM and OME remains unproven. There are two mechanisms by which the adenoids may influence OM: (1) physical obstruction of the eustachian tube when the adenoids are enlarged and (2) a reservoir of pathogenic bacteria harbored in the adenoid tissue, which predisposes the patient to repeated episodes of AOM.

Prevention

Strategies for the prevention of AOM include prophylactic antibiotics, vaccines, and surgery. The most commonly recommended regimen for antibiotic prophylaxis of recurrent AOM is once-daily oral amoxicillin at 20 mg/kg/d. Although antibiotic prophylaxis has been demonstrated to significantly reduce the number of episodes of AOM, this effect has to be considered along with the increased incidence of antibiotic-resistant organisms emerging as a direct result of the widespread prescription of antibiotics.

A pneumococcal vaccine has been introduced for use in infants and children younger than 2 years as well as in children older than 2 years who are at a high risk of recurrent AOM. However, until vaccines for other bacteria and viruses commonly responsible for AOM are available, the effect of vaccination will be limited. The prophylactic use of tympanostomy tubes (not myringotomy alone) has been demonstrated to reduce the number of episodes of AOM and hence the need for antibiotics. Adenoidectomy also has a demonstrable effect, though more modest than that seen with tympanostomy tubes.

Clinical Findings

A. SYMPTOMS AND SIGNS

Before the onset of symptoms of AOM, the patient frequently has symptoms of an upper respiratory tract infection. Older children usually complain of earache, whereas infants become irritable and pull at the affected ear. A high fever is often present and may be associated with systemic symptoms of infection, such as anorexia, vomiting, and diarrhea. Otoscopy classically shows a thickened hyperemic tympanic membrane, which is immobile on pneumatic otoscopy.

Further progression of the infective process may lead to the spontaneous rupture of the tympanic membrane, resulting in otorrhea. If this occurs, the otalgia and fever often subside. At this stage, it is often not possible to visualize the tympanic membrane because of the discharge in the ear canal.

B. SPECIAL TESTS

In most cases of AOM, no further investigations are necessary since the diagnosis is clinical. If symptoms are severe, a blood count often reveals a leukocytosis, and blood cultures may detect bacteremia during episodes of high fever. A culture of the ear discharge is helpful in guiding antibiotic therapy in patients in whom the first-line treatment is unsuccessful. If recurrent AOM occurs along with recurrent infections in other systems, then an underlying immune deficiency (commonly IgA and IgG deficiency) should be considered and appropriate investigations requested. Ciliary motility disorders need to be considered if recurrent AOM

is associated with recurrent/chronic respiratory or sinus infections. Radiologic investigation is not recommended unless complications are suspected.

Differential Diagnosis

In any patient who has otorrhea, particularly if it is recurrent, a diagnosis of chronic suppurative otitis media (CSOM), either tubotympanic or with cholesteatoma, should be considered. Otitis externa also presents with otalgia and otorrhea and may be the primary diagnosis, or it may be secondary to the infected discharge from the middle ear.

If otalgia is the primary complaint, then referred pain should be considered, particularly when otoscopy reveals a normal tympanic membrane. The common sites of origin of referred otalgia are the teeth and temporomandibular joints. In adults, malignant neoplasms of the pharynx and larynx may present with otalgia as the only symptom.

In neonates and infants with a high fever and systemic upset, the possibility of meningitis should be considered.

Treatment

A. NONSURGICAL MEASURES

1. Watchful waiting—The current practice guidelines advise on an initial watchful waiting without antibiotic therapy for healthy 2-year-olds or older children with nonsevere illness (mild otalgia and fever < 39 °C) because AOM symptoms improve in most within 1–3 days. However, guidelines should not replace clinical judgment. Watchful waiting is not recommended for children < 2 years old if AOM is certain.

2. Antibiotic therapy—If AOM does not settle after the watchful waiting period, then antibiotic therapy should begin. The use of antibiotics is probably beneficial, but there is a trade-off between benefits and side effects. There is no difference demonstrated in recurrence rates or the development of complications among different antibiotics. Amoxicillin (80 mg/kg/d given in three divided doses for 10 days) remains the first-line therapy for AOM, although with increasing numbers of resistant strains of bacteria, it may be necessary to use more broad-spectrum antibiotics in the future. In resistant cases, amoxicillin should be given in combination with clavulanate.

3. Adjunctive therapy—The adjunctive therapy for AOM should include analgesics and antipyretics. There is no role for oral decongestants or antihistamines in the treatment of AOM.

B. SURGICAL MEASURES

A minority of patients with AOM fail to respond to medical therapy or develop a complication. Myringotomy is then indicated to allow the drainage of pus from the middle ear space. Randomized trials have shown myringotomy to be ineffective in uncomplicated AOM.

Prognosis

The vast majority of uncomplicated episodes of AOM resolves without any adverse outcome. In some cases, suppuration resolves, but a sterile middle ear effusion persists. If this effusion persists for more than 3 months, then a diagnosis of OME should be made. Of patients who develop a perforation of the tympanic membrane with otorrhea, a small proportion go on to develop CSOM because of the failure of the tympanic membrane to heal.

American Academy of Pediatrics Subcommittee on Management of Acute Otitis Media. *Pediatrics.* 2004;113(5):1451. [PMID: 15121972] (Practice guidelines for the AOM. The online version and updated information can be accessed at http://www.pediatrics.org/cgi/content/full/113/5/1451.)

Flynn CA, Griffin G, Tudiver F. Decongestants and antihistamines for acute otitis media in children (Cochrane Review). *The Cochrane Library.* Issue 3, 2001. Oxford Update Software. [PMID: 11406002] (Meta-analysis of the use of decongestants and antihistamines for AOM.)

O'Neill P, Roberts T. Acute otitis media in children. *Clin Evid.* 2005;13:227. [PMID: 16135262] (Evidence-based review of trials for AOM treatment.)

OTITIS MEDIA WITH EFFUSION

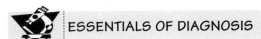

ESSENTIALS OF DIAGNOSIS

- *Persistent hearing loss.*
- *Dull, immobile tympanic membrane.*
- *"Flat" tympanogram.*

General Considerations

Otitis media with effusion is defined as the persistence of a serous or mucoid middle ear effusion for 3 months or more. Various terms, such as *chronic secretory otitis media, chronic serous otitis media,* and "glue ear," have been used to describe the same condition. It is the most common cause of hearing loss in children in the developed world and has peaks in incidence at 2 and 5 years of age. The risk factors for OME are closely interrelated with those associated with AOM and have already been described in the previous section. In fact, the formation of a middle ear effusion frequently occurs after an episode of AOM, and children with OME are far more likely to suffer from recurrent AOM.

Pathogenesis

Under normal conditions, the middle ear mucosa constantly secretes mucus, which is removed by mucociliary transport into the nasopharynx via the eustachian tube. As a consequence, factors resulting in an overproduction of mucus, an impaired clearance of mucus, or both can result in the formation of a middle ear effusion.

Both viral and bacterial infection can lead to the increased production and viscosity of secretions from the middle ear mucosa. Infection also leads to inflammatory edema of the mucosa, which may obstruct the eustachian tube. Temporary paralysis of cilia by bacterial exotoxins further impedes the clearance of an effusion. Bacteriologic studies have demonstrated that the bacteria commonly responsible for AOM are cultured from about half of chronic effusions. The fact that not all patients with OME have a history of infection suggests that other mechanisms are involved in the formation of a middle ear effusion. Experimental studies have confirmed that the failure of eustachian tube opening can result in a middle ear effusion. Because gas is constantly being absorbed into the microcirculation of the middle ear mucosa, a negative pressure develops in the middle ear cleft if the eustachian tube is blocked. This negative pressure results in the transudation of fluid into the middle ear cleft. The fact that a middle ear effusion can develop as a result of barotrauma (eg, scuba diving) supports this theory for the pathogenesis of middle ear effusions. Allergy has also been implicated in the pathogenesis of OME; however, evidence to support this theory is lacking.

Exposure to passive smoking is also likely to contribute to ciliary dysfunction and hence to OME. There is an optimum viscosity of mucus at which effective mucociliary transport occurs. If the mucus formed in a middle ear effusion is either too serous or too mucoid, then the cilia will be unable to clear it efficiently. Recently, the concept of biofilms in the pathogenesis of otitis media has been raised, but the evidence is not conclusive. Biofilms are the structured community of bacterial cells adherent to the mucosa and have antibacterial resistance property.

Prevention

Since OME often occurs as a direct result of AOM, the measures for preventing AOM previously described should also reduce the incidence of OME. Avoidance of risk factors (see Table 49–2) could also reduce the chance of a child developing OME, but its effectiveness remains unproven.

Clinical Findings

A. SYMPTOMS AND SIGNS

Otitis media with effusion may be completely asymptomatic and detected only on routine audiologic screening. The most common symptom of OME is hearing loss. Although older children may complain of reduced hearing, in many cases the hearing loss is noticed by

Table 49–3. Types of tympanogram.

Tympanogram Type	Middle Ear Pressure	Typical Appearance of Trace
A	−99 daPa to +200 daPa	
B	No compliance peak	
C	−400 daPa to −100 daPa	

daPa = deca Pascal.

parents, nursery nurses, or teachers. In younger children, the only symptom may be delayed speech development or behavioral problems. Another common symptom is a "blocked" feeling in the ear, which may cause infants and young children to pull at their ears. More rarely, symptoms of earache, tinnitus, or balance disorder may be present.

Otoscopy classically reveals a dull gray- or yellow-colored tympanic membrane that has reduced mobility on pneumatic otoscopy. If the tympanic membrane is translucent, an air-fluid level or small air bubbles within the middle ear effusion may be seen.

B. SPECIAL TESTS

1. Tympanometry—Tympanometry is a valuable tool for the investigation of OME. It is easy to use, provides reproducible results, is inexpensive, and is widely tolerated by patients—even young children. By measuring the compliance of the middle ear transformer mechanism, it provides an objective assessment of the status of the middle ear. Tympanometry produces a peak (ie, maximal compliance) when the pressure in the external ear canal equals that of the middle ear. By varying the pressure in the external ear, the tympanometer is able to provide information on the status of the middle ear (Table 49–3). If there is an effusion in the middle ear, then compliance does not vary with changes in canal pressure, and a flat (Type B) tympanogram is produced. If the air in the middle ear is at or near atmospheric pressure, then a normal (Type A) tympanogram is produced. Negative middle ear pressure results in a Type C tympanogram, with the compliance peak being at less than −99 daPa (deca Pascal).

2. Audiometry—Patients who have OME usually have a moderate conductive hearing loss. Audiometry provides an assessment of the severity of hearing loss and is therefore important in both monitoring the progress of the condition and providing information useful for management decisions. For example, in patients with hearing thresholds of 20 dB or better, it is unlikely that surgical intervention is indicated, despite the presence of OME.

Differential Diagnosis

There is considerable overlap between AOM and OME, and it may be difficult to distinguish between the two on first presentation unless otalgia and fever are prominent. Other causes of conductive hearing loss in childhood are much less common than OME, and congenital abnormalities of the ossicular chain are frequently associated with abnormalities of the external ear or present as part of a syndrome.

In adults presenting with a unilateral middle ear effusion, the possibility of a nasopharyngeal carcinoma should be considered.

Treatment

A. OBSERVATION

A large number of patients with OME require no treatment, particularly if the hearing impairment is mild. Spontaneous resolution occurs in a significant proportion of patients. A period of watchful waiting of 3 months from the onset (if known) or from the diagnosis (if onset unknown) before considering intervention is therefore advisable. Ideally, early treatment should be initiated in patients in whom spontaneous resolution is unlikely. A multicenter randomized controlled trial identified both the season of attendance (ie, July to December) and a bilateral hearing impairment of > 30 dB as factors that make spontaneous resolution less likely. Early intervention should be considered if there is a significant delay in speech and language development or if OME is present in an only hearing ear.

B. NONSURGICAL MEASURES

The medical treatment of OME is controversial and there is a wide geographic variability in practice. Autoinflation with purpose-built nasal balloon has been shown to be beneficial, although compliance is generally poor. Medical treatments include antibiotics, steroids, decongestants, and antihistamines. The use of antibiotics in OME has been shown to be effective in a small proportion of patients, but the effect is likely to be short-lived. The small chance of benefit from antibiotic therapy needs to be considered along with the fact that a number of patients treated with antibiotics develop significant side effects, such as gastroenteritis and atopic reaction. A meta-analysis of the use of topical and systemic steroids for the treatment of OME found a short-term improvement in hearing, but no lasting benefit. Steroids are therefore not recommended in the treatment of OME. There is no evidence to support the use of decongestants, antihistamines, or mucolytics for the treatment of OME.

C. SURGICAL MEASURES

The surgical options for OME are tympanostomy tubes and adenoidectomy. Myringotomy and aspiration of middle ear effusion without ventilation tube insertion has a short-lived benefit and is not recommended.

1. Insertion of tympanostomy tubes—The aim of tympanostomy tube insertion is to allow ventilation of the middle ear space—hence to improve hearing thresholds. The prolonged ventilation of the middle ear may also allow resolution of chronic inflammation of the middle ear mucosa. Complications include myringosclerosis, purulent otorrhea, and residual perforation after extrusion. There are two main types of tympanostomy tubes: **short-term tubes** (eg, **grommets**), which remain in the tympanic membrane for an average of 12 months, and **long-term tubes** (eg, **T-tubes**), which can remain for several years. The high incidence of residual perforation following the use of long-term ventilation tubes indicates that they should not be used in uncomplicated cases.

2. Adenoidectomy—Controversy still exists over the role of adenoidectomy in the treatment of OME. The rationale for adenoidectomy is that it relieves nasal obstruction, improves eustachian tube function, and eliminates a potential reservoir of bacteria. Evidence does suggest that adenoidectomy is effective in reducing the morbidity of OME. However, because of the potential risks associated with adenoidectomy (primarily hemorrhage and, rarely, velopharyngeal insufficiency), many surgeons use tympanostomy tubes alone as a first-line treatment and consider adenoidectomy when repeated tympanostomy tube insertion is required for recurrent OME.

Prognosis

There is a sharp decline in the prevalence of OME in children over 7 years of age, which reflects improved eustachian tube function and maturation of the immune system.

American Academy of Family Physicians. American Academy of Otolaryngology–Head and Neck Surgery. American Academy of Pediatrics Subcommittee on Otitis Media with Effusion. *Pediatrics.* 2004;113(5):1412. [PMID: 15121966] (Practice guidelines for otitis media with effusion. The online version and updated information can be accessed at http://www.pediatrics.org/cgi/content/full/113/5/1412.)

Haggard MP, Cannon MM, Birkin JA et al. Risk factors for persistence of bilateral otitis media with effusion. *Clin Otolaryngol Allied Sci.* 2001;26:147. [PMID: 1309057] (A multicenter randomized controlled trial assessing multiple risk factors for persistence of OM with effusion.)

Rosenfeld RM, Kay D. Natural history of untreated otitis media. *Laryngoscope.* 2003;113(10):1645. [PMID: 14520089] (A systematic review and meta-analysis to estimate the natural history of acute otitis media and otitis media with effusion.)

CHRONIC SUPPURATIVE OTITIS MEDIA (TUBOTYMPANIC)

 ESSENTIALS OF DIAGNOSIS

- Chronic or recurrent otorrhea or both.
- Hearing loss.
- Tympanic membrane perforation.

General Considerations

Chronic suppurative otitis media is defined as a persistent or intermittent infected discharge through a non-intact tympanic membrane (ie, perforation or tympanostomy tube). Chronic perforation of the tympanic membrane can occur without suppuration and is often referred to as "inactive" CSOM.

Chronic suppurative otitis media is particularly prevalent in developing countries and is more common in lower socioeconomic groups in the developed world. Many of the epidemiologic factors discussed in the section on AOM equally apply to the development of CSOM.

Pathogenesis

There are a number of mechanisms by which a persistent tympanic membrane perforation may develop. In most cases, CSOM occurs as a consequence of an episode of AOM with perforation, with subsequent failure of the perforation to heal. There is also an association between OME and chronic perforation. The continued presence of a middle ear effusion leads, in some cases, to degeneration of the fibrous layer of the tympanic membrane. This weakness of the tympanic membrane both predisposes to perforation and reduces the likelihood of spontaneous healing. Although most tympanic membranes heal spontaneously after the extrusion of ventilation tubes, a small percentage do not. Traumatic perforations, particularly if large, may fail to heal.

There are two main mechanisms by which a chronic perforation can lead to continuous or repeated middle ear infections: (1) Bacteria can contaminate the middle ear cleft directly from the external ear because the protective physical barrier of the tympanic membrane is lost. (2) The intact tympanic membrane normally results in a middle ear "gas cushion," which helps to prevent the reflux of nasopharyngeal secretions into the middle ear via the eustachian tube. The loss of this protective mechanism results in the increased exposure of the middle ear to pathogenic bacteria from the nasopharynx.

The most commonly isolated bacteria responsible for CSOM are *P aeruginosa, S aureus,* and the *Proteus* species.

Clinical Findings

A. SYMPTOMS AND SIGNS

Typically, a patient with CSOM presents with a history of otorrhea, which may be either intermittent or continuous, and hearing loss. The discharge is usually mucopurulent, although chronic infection of the middle ear may lead to polyp or granulation tissue formation, which can result in bloodstained otorrhea. Pain is not a usual feature of CSOM and its presence should alert the physician to the possibility of a more invasive pathology.

Inspection may reveal scars from previous surgery for chronic ear disease. To properly visualize the tympanic membrane, it is necessary to suction the discharge from the external auditory canal with an operating microscope. The middle ear mucosa, seen through the perforation, is edematous, sometimes to the point of polyp formation. If the perforation is of sufficient size, it may be possible to identify the presence of ossicular discontinuity due to necrosis of the long process of the incus.

B. SPECIAL TESTS

A swab of the discharge should be sent for culture and sensitivity, preferably before beginning antimicrobial therapy. An audiologic evaluation is necessary, because the majority of patients have an associated conductive hearing loss.

Since the diagnosis of CSOM can be made clinically, radiologic investigation is not usually indicated. Computed tomographic (CT) scans are useful in demonstrating bony anatomy and are essential if an intracranial extension of the infection is suspected. However, CT scanning is poor in differentiating between the soft tissue opacity caused by CSOM and cholesteatoma.

Differential Diagnosis

The primary differential diagnosis is the presence of a cholesteatoma. Both pathologies present with a very similar clinical course, and the presence of severe inflammation or granulation tissue can cause difficulty with the diagnosis. Reexamination after a course of medical treatment usually provides an accurate diagnosis.

If granulations are severe and unresponsive to antimicrobial therapy, then chronic granulomatous conditions such as Wegener granulomatosis, mycobacterial infection, histiocytosis X, and sarcoidosis should be considered. Biopsy of the granulation or polyp in these circumstances is recommended.

Pain is not usually a prominent feature of CSOM, and its presence should raise the possibility of necrotizing otitis externa (particularly in the immunocompromised, eg, AIDS patients or elderly diabetics) or a malignant neoplasm of the eternal canal or middle ear.

Treatment

The treatment goals of uncomplicated CSOM are to eliminate infection, prevent further infection, and restore normal functioning to the middle ear. Both medical and surgical interventions play a role in achieving these aims (Table 49–4).

A. NONSURGICAL MEASURES

1. Aural toilet—Aural toilet is important for the successful treatment of CSOM, particularly when topical medication is used. Clearing the discharge from the external auditory canal allows the topical agent to reach the middle ear in an adequate concentration.

2. Topical antibiotics—Although topical antibiotics are more effective than systemic antibiotics in the treatment of CSOM, many contain aminoglycosides, which are potentially ototoxic. Ototoxicity has been demonstrated in animal models, and the use of gentamicin for vestibular ablation in Meniere disease is well documented. However, sensorineural hearing loss as a result of the use of topical aminoglycosides in CSOM is rarely reported. This circumstance is probably due to a combination of the relatively low concentration of aminoglycoside reaching the middle ear and edema of the middle ear mucosa, which prevents the direct absorption of the drug through the round window. Despite the risk of ototoxicity, topical aminoglycosides are widely prescribed by otolaryngologists for the treatment of CSOM because the benefits of effective treatment outweigh the risks. The recent availability of topical ofloxacin preparations may prove to be as effective as topical aminoglycosides without the ototoxic potential.

Table 49–4. Treatment summary for otitis media.

	Acute Otitis Media (AOM)	Otitis Media with Effusion	Chronic Suppurative Otitis Media
Watchful waiting	Up to 72 hours with analgesia/antipyretics if nonsevere and patient > 2 years old	For 3 months from onset or diagnosis	NI
Medical therapy	Antibiotics (amoxicillin)	NI	Aural toilet and topical antibiotics (quinolones)
Surgical intervention	Myringotomy for refractory AOM Cortical mastoidectomy in nonresponding mastoiditis	VT insertion if unresolved after 3 months Adenoidectomy on second VT insertion	Tympanoplasty Tympanomastoid surgery if refractory to medical therapy

NI, not indicated; VT, ventilation tube.

3. Systemic antibiotics—Systemic antibiotics tend to have a poor penetration of the middle ear and are therefore less effective than topical antibiotics. Because *P aeruginosa* is the primary pathogen responsible for CSOM, the choice of oral systemic antibiotics is limited. Both ciprofloxacin and ofloxacin have good antipseudomonal activity. Unfortunately, these quinolone antibiotics are not recommended in children owing to the possibility of causing arthropathies. This circumstance limits the choice of systemic antibiotics in children to broad-spectrum penicillins, such as piperacillin and cephalosporins, which must be administered parenterally.

B. SURGICAL MEASURES

Some cases of CSOM resolve with medical treatment, and if the patient is asymptomatic, then no further intervention is required. However, if otorrhea recurs or persists despite medical treatment or if the patient feels handicapped by a residual conductive hearing loss, surgical therapy should be considered.

1. Tympanoplasty—Ideally, surgery should be carried out when the infection has been adequately treated and the middle ear mucosa is healthy, since the chance of a successful outcome is increased. In this situation, a tympanoplasty, with repair of the tympanic membrane and ossicular chain (if required), is recommended.

2. Tympanomastoid surgery—In cases that are refractory to medical treatment, it is necessary to perform tympanomastoid surgery (tympanoplasty combined with a cortical mastoidectomy). The aims of this procedure are to aerate the middle ear and mastoid, remove chronically inflamed tissue, repair the tympanic defect, and reconstruct the ossicular chain. The achievement of all of these goals often requires more than one procedure.

Acuin J. Chronic suppurative otitis media. *Clin Evid.* 2004;12:710. [PMID: 15865672] (Evidence-based review of the literature on treatment of chronic suppurative otitis media.)

Acuin J, Smith A, MacKenzie I. Interventions for chronic suppurative otitis media (Cochrane Review). *The Cochrane Library.* Issue 3, 2001. Oxford: Update Software. [PMID: 17096720] (Meta-analysis of randomized trials investigating the medical management of chronic suppurative otitis media.)

SEQUELAE & COMPLICATIONS OF OTITIS MEDIA

The sequelae and complications of otitis media can be found in Table 49–5.

1. Sequelae

Tympanosclerosis

Tympanosclerosis is characterized by hyalinization and the deposition of calcium in the tympanic membrane, middle ear, or both. It often occurs as a result of inflammation or trauma and is therefore commonly seen after recurrent episodes of AOM and OME and after ventilation tube insertion. The typical clinical appearance is of white plaques in the tympanic membrane. If the process is limited to the tympanic membrane (ie, myringosclerosis), then hearing is usually unaffected. However, if the middle ear is involved, then the ossicular chain can become immobilized, resulting in a conductive hearing loss. Attempts at surgical correction by tympanoplasty may initially be successful, but refixation of the ossicles is not uncommon.

Atelectasis

Atelectasis refers to the presence of a grossly retracted or collapsed tympanic membrane. It probably occurs as a result of prolonged negative middle ear pressure secondary to chronic eustachian tube dysfunction. The whole of the tympanic membrane can be affected, but if collapse is only partial, then a localized retraction pocket is formed. The presence of an atelectatic tympanic mem-

Table 49–5. Sequelae and complications of otitis media.

Sequelae
  Tympanosclerosis
  Atelectasis
Intratemporal Complications
  Mastoditis
    Acute
    Subacute ("masked")
  Petrositis
  Facial nerve paralysis
  Suppurative labyrinthitis
Intracranial Complications
  Meningitis
  Intracranial abscess
    Brain abscess
    Extradural
    Subdural
  Lateral sinus thrombosis
  Otic hydrocephalus

---

brane may not produce any symptoms, but more commonly results in a mild conductive hearing loss. Prolonged contact between the tympanic membrane and the ossicles can result in ossicular erosion, particularly of the long process of the incus; consequently, a more significant hearing loss results. Another consequence of persistent atelectasis is that the normal migration pattern of squamous epithelium from the tympanic membrane may be disrupted, leading to the accumulation of squamous debris and cholesteatoma formation. This situation is a particular risk if the retraction pocket is located in the pars flaccida or the posterosuperior pars tensa.

The management of atelectasis is controversial. If eustachian tube dysfunction is still considered to be present, the insertion of ventilation tubes could potentially reverse the changes in the tympanic membrane by normalizing the pressure in the middle ear space. If no improvement is observed and the location of the retraction raises the concern of subsequent cholesteatoma formation, then excision and grafting of the affected portion of the tympanic membrane are recommended. The recurrence of tympanic membrane retraction after this procedure is not uncommon; therefore, prolonged observation is advised.

2. Intratemporal Complications

Mastoiditis

The fact that the mastoid air cell system is part of the middle ear cleft means that some degree of mastoid inflammation occurs whenever there is infection in the middle ear. In most cases, this infection does not progress to clinically apparent acute mastoiditis. However, if pus collects in the mastoid air cells under pressure, necrosis of the bony trabeculae occurs, resulting in the formation of an abscess cavity. The infection may then progress to periostitis and subperiosteal abscess, or to a more serious intracranial infection.

A. ACUTE MASTOIDITIS

Typically, acute mastoiditis presents as a complication of AOM in a child. Pain and tenderness over the mastoid process are the initial indicators of mastoiditis. As the infection progresses, edema and erythema of the postauricular soft tissues with loss of the postauricular crease develop. These changes result in anteroinferior displacement of the pinna. Fullness of the posterior wall of the external auditory canal is frequently seen on otoscopy as a result of the underlying osteitis. If a subperiosteal abscess has developed, fluctuance may be elicited in the postauricular area. Rarely, a mastoid abscess can extend into the neck (Bezold's abscess) or the occipital bone (Citelli abscess). Once the diagnosis of acute mastoiditis is suspected, the radiologic investigation of choice is a CT scan, which provides information about the extent of the opacification of the mastoid air cells, the formation of subperiosteal abscess, and the presence of intracranial complications.

In some cases, acute mastoiditis can be successfully managed by antibiotic therapy alone, but some patients require surgical intervention. When there is no clinical or radiologic indication of a subperiosteal abscess or an intracranial extension of disease, then high-dose broad-spectrum intravenous antibiotics should be commenced. If, after 24 hours of treatment, there is no evidence of resolution or if symptoms progress, a cortical mastoidectomy should be performed, along with myringotomy if spontaneous perforation of the tympanic membrane has not occurred. If a subperiosteal abscess or an intracranial extension of disease is suspected, surgery in combination with high-dose intravenous antibiotics should be the first-line therapy.

B. SUBACUTE MASTOIDITIS

Subacute or "masked" mastoiditis may occur when inadequate treatment of AOM results in a low-grade infection of the mastoid air cells. The symptoms and signs are equivalent to those of acute mastoiditis, but are less severe and more persistent. Most cases resolve with ventilation of the middle ear combined with appropriate antibiotic therapy. If this treatment fails to resolve the infection, cortical mastoidectomy is indicated.

Petrositis

This rare complication of suppurative OM occurs in both acute and chronic forms. In the **acute form,** there is extension of acute mastoiditis into a pneumatized petrous apex. The **chronic form** of petrositis usually occurs as a result of mucosal or cholesteatomatous CSOM; pneumatization of the petrous apex is not a prerequisite as the infection spreads by thrombophlebitis, hematogenous dissemination, or direct extension. Because of the close relationship of the ophthalmic division of the trigeminal nerve and the abducens nerve to the petrous apex, the classic features of petrositis are otorrhea associated with retroorbital pain and lateral rectus palsy (Gradenigo syndrome).

Because of the high incidence of an intracranial extension of infection from petrositis, a combination of antibiotics and surgical drainage of the petrous apex is the management of choice.

Facial Nerve Paralysis

Facial nerve palsy can occur as a result of either acute or chronic OM. There are two mechanisms by which OM can result in facial nerve paralysis: (1) as a result of the locally produced bacterial toxins or (2) from direct pressure applied to the nerve by cholesteatoma or granulation tissue. If there is a congenital dehiscence of the bony canal of the facial nerve in the middle ear, then an episode of AOM can lead to inflammatory edema of the nerve and a subsequent paresis. This situation should be managed by myringotomy with aspiration of pus from the middle ear along with antibiotic therapy, which will mostly result in the rapid resolution of paralysis. Further surgical exploration of the facial nerve is not indicated unless the paralysis fails to resolve. If facial nerve paralysis occurs as a result CSOM, urgent surgical exploration, with decompression of the facial nerve, is indicated.

Suppurative Labyrinthitis

Infection of the middle ear can lead to direct bacterial invasion of the inner ear, usually via the round window, resulting in acute suppurative labyrinthitis. Erosion of the bony capsule of the inner ear by a cholesteatoma (most commonly the lateral semicircular canal) provides an alternative route of entry to the inner ear. Suppurative labyrinthitis presents with sudden sensorineural hearing loss, severe vertigo, nystagmus, and nausea and vomiting. The cochlear aqueduct provides a direct communication between the perilymph and the cerebrospinal fluid; therefore, there is a significant risk of developing meningitis.

The aim of treatment is to eradicate infection, thereby preventing meningitis. Surgical intervention is often required for underlying chronic middle ear disease, although the timing of surgery is controversial. Cochlear and vestibular functions are invariably permanently lost and, as healing occurs, obliterative osteitis of the inner ear commonly develops.

3. Intracranial Complications

The incidence of intracranial complications has been considerably reduced since the introduction of antibiotics. Despite this fact, once an intracranial complication develops, it carries a significant risk to life. Therefore, early recognition and treatment are vital to improve the prognosis. It is not uncommon for more than one intracranial complication to occur simultaneously. The most common early symptoms of intracranial extension of infection are persistent headache and fever. Other features include lethargy, irritability, and neck stiffness. A decreasing level of consciousness and seizures are late signs associated with a poor prognosis. Once suspicion of an intracranial infection is raised, an MRI of the brain is the investigation of choice, along with lumbar puncture if meningitis is suspected. The causative organism depends on whether the complication has developed as a consequence of acute or chronic OM; the initial antibiotic therapy should be prescribed accordingly until the results of bacterial cultures and sensitivity are available.

Meningitis

Acute otitis media is the most common cause of bacterial meningitis. It can occur as a result of hematogenous spread, of direct extension from the middle ear through a bony dehiscence, or through the cochlear aqueduct via the inner ear. The most common organisms responsible for otic meningitis are *S pneumoniae* and *H influenzae* type B. The classic presentation is with headaches, photophobia, neck stiffness, and fluctuating levels of consciousness. The evaluation should include an MRI of the brain to rule out other intracranial complications as well as a lumbar puncture. If meningitis is secondary to AOM, then a myringotomy should be performed once antibiotic therapy has been initiated. In the case of CSOM resulting in meningitis, the patient should be fully stabilized before considering surgical management of the chronic ear disease.

Intracranial Abscess

Brain, subdural, and extradural abscesses can all arise as a complication of middle ear infections (commonly associated with chronic disease). Intracranial abscesses are usually caused by multiple aerobic and anaerobic bacteria. Commonly cultured organisms include streptococci, *S aureus*, *S pneumoniae*, *H influenzae*, *P aeruginosa*, *Bacteroides fragilis*, and *Proteus* species.

A. Brain Abscess

Most otogenic brain abscesses develop within the temporal lobe or cerebellum. The progression of symptoms from a brain abscess can be gradual, occurring over days or even weeks. In addition to the generalized symptoms, focal neurologic signs can develop depending on the anatomic location of the abscess within the brain. As the abscess enlarges, features typical of raised intracranial pressure develop. Once a brain abscess has been diagnosed, urgent neurosurgical intervention is indicated to drain the abscess. Surgery for the associated ear disease is less urgent and should be planned when the patient's condition is more stable.

B. SUBDURAL ABSCESS

A subdural abscess forms between the dura mater and the arachnoid mater. Symptoms and signs tend to progress much more rapidly than those seen with a brain abscess. Drainage of the abscess is the mainstay of treatment.

C. EXTRADURAL ABSCESS

Extradural abscesses are typically formed in the middle fossa between the dura mater and the thin bony plate of the tegmen. They can also occur in the posterior fossa, where they are commonly associated with lateral sinus thrombosis. The clinical features are often nonspecific and may fluctuate if a dehiscence in the tegmen is present, allowing the abscess to partially drain into the mastoid cavity. As with other intracranial complications, headache and fever are the most common features. Because of its location, an extradural abscess can usually be drained through a mastoidectomy approach while treating the underlying middle ear disease.

Lateral Sinus Thrombosis

Because of its close proximity to the mastoid air cells, the lateral, or sigmoid, sinus is prone to involvement in middle ear infections, which may lead to thrombosis. Once an infected thrombus has formed in the lateral sinus, it may propagate both distally and proximally and may give rise to infected emboli. Typically, there are intermittent episodes of high pyrexia associated with rigors. If the thrombus propagates into the neck, there will be neck tenderness along the internal jugular vein and neck stiffness or torticollis. Proximal extension of the thrombus to the sagittal sinus can result in symptoms and signs of raised intracranial pressure. MRI most reliably makes the diagnosis of lateral sinus thrombosis. The management of lateral sinus thrombosis requires broad-spectrum antibiotics and surgery. A complete mastoidectomy should be performed, with exposure of the lateral sinus. Once the diagnosis has been confirmed by needle aspiration, the sinus is opened and the infected thrombus evacuated. If symptoms persist after this procedure, consideration should be given to ligation of the ipsilateral internal jugular vein, once the possibility of other intracranial complications has been excluded.

Otic Hydrocephalus

Otic hydrocephalus is a rare complication in which raised intracranial pressure develops as a result of a middle ear infection, but its pathophysiology is poorly understood. The usual features are headache, vomiting, disturbed mental state, visual disturbance, and papilledema associated with a middle ear infection. Imaging of the brain reveals the ventricular size to be normal, but lumbar puncture confirms raised cerebrospinal fluid pressure. Management is aimed at resolving the middle ear infection while normalizing intracranial pressure with the use of steroids, diuretics (eg, mannitol), and, if required, intermittent drainage of cerebrospinal fluid.

Agrawal S, Husein M, MacRae D. Complications of otitis media: an evolving state. *J Otolaryngol.* 2005;34(Suppl 1):S33. [PMID: 16089238] (Discussion of diagnosis, workup, and management of otitis media complications.)

Cholesteatoma

50

C.Y. Joseph Chang, MD

ESSENTIALS OF DIAGNOSIS

- *Squamous epithelium in the middle ear or mastoid.*
- *Otorrhea and conductive hearing loss.*
- *Retraction of the tympanic membrane with a squamous debris collection or a whitish mass behind an intact tympanic membrane.*
- *Testing includes computed tomography (CT) scanning, which can be useful in delineating disease extent but is not critical to making a diagnosis in most cases.*

General Considerations

A. ACQUIRED CHOLESTEATOMA

Cholesteatoma is the presence of squamous epithelium in the middle ear, mastoid, or epitympanum. The most common form of cholesteatoma is the acquired variety, which is classified as primary and secondary acquired cholesteatoma. **Primary acquired cholesteatoma** is the most common of these types and forms as a retraction of the tympanic membrane. In most cases, the retraction occurs in the pars flaccida, although pars tensa retractions can also occur (Figure 50–1). **Secondary acquired cholesteatoma** forms as a result of either squamous epithelial migration from the tympanic membrane or implantation of squamous epithelium into the middle ear during surgery, such as ventilation tube placement or tympanoplasty.

B. CONGENITAL CHOLESTEATOMA

Cholesteatomas that occur without tympanic membrane retraction or implantation of squamous epithelial material are considered to be congenital in origin. This type comprises a minority of cholesteatoma cases. It is classically defined as an embryonic rest of epithelial tissue in the ear without tympanic membrane perforation and without a history of ear infection. This definition has been modified in recent years, but essentially it is a condition typically seen in young children without evidence of the acquired type of cholesteatoma.

Derlacki EL, Clemis JD. Congenital cholesteatoma of the middle ear and mastoid. *Ann Otol Rhinol Laryngol.* 1965;74:706. [PMID: 5834665] (Classic definition of congenital cholesteatoma.)

Pathogenesis

The pathogenesis of primary acquired cholesteatoma remains unclear. Factors that appear to be associated with formation of cholesteatoma retractions of the tympanic membrane include poor eustachian tube function and chronic inflammation of the middle ear, as in chronic otitis media. In theory, chronic negative middle ear pressure leads to retractions of the structurally weakest area of the tympanic membrane, the pars flaccida. Once the retractions form, the normal migratory pattern of the squamous epithelium is disrupted, resulting in the accumulation of keratin debris in the cholesteatoma sac. Chronic infection and inflammation ensue, leading to biochemical changes in the local environment that foster the further growth and migration of the squamous epithelium and increased osteoclastic activity, resulting in bone resorption. The local inflammatory response further inhibits eustachian tube function, increases mucosal edema and mucous secretion, and disrupts the drainage pathways of the temporal bone. This environment also fosters the growth of bacteria, including *Pseudomonas aeruginosa, Streptococcus, Staphylococcus, Proteus, Enterobacter,* and anaerobes, which increase the host's inflammatory response and continue the cycle. It is not understood why only a small percentage of patients with poor eustachian tube function develop cholesteatoma and why some patients form pars tensa retractions rather than the more common pars flaccida retraction.

The pathogenesis of congenital cholesteatoma is unclear, but the most prevalent theory is the failure of involution of the epithelioid formation in the middle ear during fetal development. Other theories include metaplasia of the middle ear mucosa and, more recently, direct microretractions of the tympanic membrane near the malleus long process that are self-limited, but leave squamous epithelial rests in the middle ear.

Albino AP, Kimmelman CP, Parisier SC. Cholesteatoma: a molecular and cellular puzzle. *Am J Otol.* 1998;19:7. [PMID: 9455941] (Review of pathogenesis.)

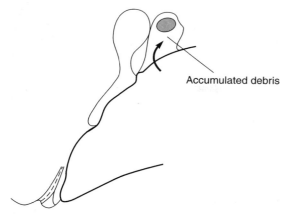

Figure 50–1. Formation of primary acquired cholesteatoma in the pars flaccida portion of the tympanic membrane.

Sudhoff H, Tos M. Pathogenesis of attic cholesteatoma: clinical and immunohistochemical support for combination of retraction theory and proliferation theory. *Am J Otol.* 2000;21:786. [PMID: 11078064] (Theory of cholesteatoma pathogenesis.)

Tos M. A new pathogenesis of mesotympanic (congenital) cholesteatoma. *Laryngoscope.* 2000;110:1890. [PMID: 11081605] (New theory on congenital cholesteatoma origin and review.)

Prevention

There are currently no known methods by which congenital cholesteatoma can be prevented. Secondary acquired cholesteatomas are often iatrogenic and therefore could theoretically be prevented if the surgeon takes all steps possible to prevent implantation of squamous epithelium into the middle ear.

Although the pathogenesis of primary acquired cholesteatoma is not clearly understood, if it is assumed that eustachian tube dysfunction is required for its formation, restoring eustachian tube function should help prevent the formation of this type of cholesteatoma. Unfortunately, there is no way to correct eustachian tube function directly. However, providing secondary ventilation to the middle ear space can reduce the complications related to poor eustachian tube function. This can be accomplished by inserting a ventilating tube. If early progressive tympanic membrane retractions are detected, this intervention could potentially prevent future progression of the disease to cholesteatoma. In addition, the successful control of infection and the inflammatory state of the middle ear, followed by regular débridement of the cholesteatoma sac in an office setting, can prevent future progression of the cholesteatoma in some cases.

Clinical Findings

A. SYMPTOMS AND SIGNS

Patients with acquired cholesteatomas typically present with recurrent or persistent purulent otorrhea and hearing loss. Tinnitus is also common. However, some patients with cholesteatoma may not develop otorrhea for a long period of time. In rare cases, vertigo or dysequilibrium can result from the inflammatory process in the middle ear or, in rare cases, from direct labyrinthine erosion by cholesteatoma. Facial nerve twitching, palsy, or paralysis can also result from the inflammatory process or from mechanical compression of the nerve.

Physical findings are usually diagnostic in cases of acquired cholesteatoma. In primary acquired cholesteatoma, there will be a retraction of the pars flaccida in most cases, and less commonly in the pars tensa (Figure 50–2). Both types of retractions contain a matrix of squamous epithelium, which may or may not be visible, and often keratin debris. Other typical findings include purulent otorrhea, polyps and granulation tissue, and ossicular erosion. In secondary acquired cholesteatoma, the findings depend on the cause. If the cholesteatoma developed from a tympanic membrane perforation, the squamous epithelial matrix, keratin debris, or both are usually visible through the perforation. If the cholesteatoma developed from either an implantation of squamous epithelium during surgery or a perforation that has closed, the tympanic membrane may in fact appear relatively normal. Once the middle ear cholesteatoma has enlarged to a sufficient size, it becomes visible behind the tympanic membrane. In patients whose tympanic

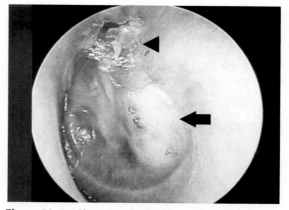

Figure 50–2. Photograph of primary acquired cholesteatoma in the pars flaccida portion of the left tympanic membrane. The arrowhead points to retraction. The arrow points to the cholesteatoma sac behind the tympanic membrane.

membrane is opaque, further studies, such as imaging, may be required.

Congenital cholesteatomas are usually asymptomatic until the mass grows to a sufficient size that the ossicular chain function becomes disrupted and hearing loss develops. In many cases, the cholesteatoma is noted on the routine ear examination of an asymptomatic child.

In all cases, cranial nerve function, especially that of the facial nerve (CN VII), should be examined. In addition, an office evaluation for nystagmus and balance function should be considered in patients who have any evidence of vestibular dysfunction. A fistula test can be performed, but it has a low sensitivity in detecting labyrinthine fistula.

B. IMAGING STUDIES AND SPECIAL TESTS

1. CT scanning—CT can be performed to delineate the extent of disease. Bone window axial and coronal cuts of 1.5-mm slices or less are ideal. It should be understood that a CT scan usually cannot make a definitive diagnosis regarding the nature of any existing temporal bone disease. CT findings that are suggestive of the presence of cholesteatoma include the erosion of bone, most commonly the scutum and ossicular chain (Figure 50–3). The presence of erosion of the labyrinth is highly suggestive of the presence of cholesteatoma, although neoplasms can also cause this finding. CT scanning cannot differentiate between fluid and tissue and, in particular, cannot distinguish between tissue types. The presence of fluid or soft tissue density in the middle ear and mastoid could indicate the presence of mucus, pus, inflammatory tissue such as granulations or polyps, thickened mucosa, cholesteatoma, neoplasm, encephalocele, or other conditions.

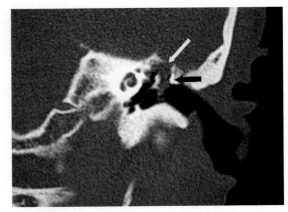

Figure 50–3. Coronal CT scan of the left temporal bone, showing pars flaccida cholesteatoma. The white arrow points to cholesteatoma. The black arrow points to eroded scutum.

CT scans are especially useful in patients with a history suggestive of secondary acquired cholesteatoma in which the middle ear cannot be visualized because the tympanic membrane is opaque. In these cases, the amount of inflammatory tissue may be minimal, and the soft tissue density of the cholesteatoma may be identifiable, thereby aiding in the diagnosis. CT scanning is also useful for delineating the extent of disease in congenital cholesteatoma. This imaging modality can assist the surgeon in determining whether a tympanoplasty alone is adequate for treatment or whether a mastoidectomy will also be needed.

Many surgeons find CT scanning useful in planning any surgical intervention. A CT scan can indicate the presence of low tegmen, anterior sigmoid sinus, labyrinthine erosion, ossicular erosion, and petrous apex involvement, all of which can affect the surgeon's approach to the disease. In some cases, facial nerve dehiscence and tegmen erosion can be detected, but these conditions are more accurately determined at the time of surgery. It should be noted that CT imaging is not a requirement prior to surgical intervention, because most of the relevant information that CT scanning provides becomes apparent at the time of surgery. In fact, many surgeons do not routinely obtain imaging unless there are specific indications, such as revision surgery, suspicion of labyrinthine fistula, or the possibility of petrous apex disease.

2. Magnetic resonance imaging (MRI)—Magnetic resonance imaging (MRI) can, in theory, differentiate between tissue types and may therefore aid in the diagnosis of cholesteatoma. In practice, the small confines of the ear and mastoid, and the frequent presence of inflammatory disease, make determination of tissue characteristics difficult using the current technology. However, MRI is useful if a neoplasm or an encephalocele is suspected.

3. Audiometry—An audiogram should be obtained in all cases. Patients with cholesteatoma usually exhibit various degrees of conductive hearing loss, depending on the status of the ear canal, the tympanic membrane, and the ossicular chain. The presence of an otherwise unexplained sensorineural hearing loss should alert the surgeon to the possibility of a labyrinthine fistula, although in most cases, this hearing loss results from a chronic or recurrent inflammatory process.

Differential Diagnosis

In most cases of primary acquired cholesteatoma, the diagnosis is quite clear after obtaining the history and performing a physical examination. However, diagnostic considerations in patients with recurrent or persistent otorrhea include chronic otitis media without cholesteatoma; otitis externa; malignant external otitis; neoplasms such as squamous cell carcinoma of the ear or other rare tumors, such as adenomas; adenocarcinoma; adenoid cystic carcinoma;

and cerebrospinal fluid otorrhea, such as from an encephalocele. If there is any doubt regarding the diagnosis, further workup, such as biopsy, laboratory studies, and imaging, should be considered.

The diagnostic considerations for cases in which the tympanic membrane appears intact or even normal, such as in cases of congenital and some cases of secondary acquired cholesteatoma, can be more problematic. In such children who present with conductive hearing loss, diagnostic considerations include congenital malformation of the ossicular chain, the most common of which is stapes fixation, or ossicular dysfunction resulting from either previous inflammatory disease of the ear or trauma. In adults presenting with normal tympanic membrane and conductive hearing loss, diagnostic considerations include otosclerosis and ossicular dysfunction resulting from previous inflammatory disease of the ear or trauma. A CT scan can be helpful in obtaining a diagnosis in these cases.

Complications

Cholesteatomas result in the continued slow growth of the keratin sac with chronic inflammation and infection in most cases. The major sequelae are bone erosion, which results in erosion of the ossicular chain, and otorrhea. In some cases, cholesteatomas can become complicated over time and result in sensorineural hearing loss, dizziness, facial nerve injury, and suppurative complications such as acute mastoiditis, subperiosteal abscess, sigmoid sinus thrombosis, meningitis, and brain abscess.

Treatment

A. Nonsurgical Measures

The initial goal of treatment for cholesteatomas is to reduce the level of the inflammatory and infectious activity in the involved ear. The mainstays of medical treatment are to remove infected debris from the ear canal, keep all water out of the ears to prevent further contamination, and apply ototopical agents that cover the usual bacterial organisms, which include *P aeruginosa,* streptococci, staphylococci, *Proteus, Enterobacter,* and anaerobes. Commercially available agents such as ofloxacin or neomycin-polymyxin B are usually adequate. If the middle ear is exposed, there is a theoretical danger of causing ototoxicity with the use of agents such as aminoglycosides. This risk has not been studied adequately but appears to be relatively low in cases of chronic inflammation; however, it may be in the patient's best interest to avoid ototoxic agents and instead use agents such as ofloxacin.

Some physicians favor the additional use of topical steroid agents to reduce both the level of inflammation and the volume of any inflammatory tissues that are present. The efficacy of this treatment modality has not been studied adequately, but in theory, the anti-inflammatory effects could be beneficial. However, it is also theoretically possible that steroids may inhibit the local immune responses, allowing progression of the infectious process.

In many cases, the infection fails to subside completely. This situation usually occurs in the presence of a cholesteatoma sac with infected keratin debris that is not effectively treated by any local or systemic agents. However, after surgical treatment, the otorrhea usually resolves.

B. Surgical Measures

1. Treatment goals—The definitive treatment of cholesteatoma should achieve several goals. The primary goal is to create a "dry and safe" ear. Essentially, this means that the processes that are causing bone erosion, chronic inflammation, and infection should be reversed permanently. To achieve this goal, all cholesteatoma matrices must be either removed or exteriorized. Failure to accomplish this usually results in persistent or recurrent disease. If a cholesteatoma matrix is exteriorized, as in cases of canal-wall-down tympanomastoidectomy or atticotomy, the cavity should be designed to be relatively self-cleaning so that it will not be prone to develop chronic otorrhea. A summary of surgical approaches is shown in Table 50–1.

2. Anatomic considerations—Cholesteatoma can involve any area of the middle ear, hypotympanum, protympanum, epitympanum, and mastoid. Since most cases of cholesteatoma arise from a retraction of the tympanic membrane, it follows that most cases involve the middle ear space in some form. Pars flaccida retractions are the most common. These cholesteatomas typically invade Prussack space, which is the area between the pars flaccida laterally and the malleus neck and the lower portion of the head medially. From here, the cholesteatoma can invade the middle ear inferiorly, the attic, and then the mastoid superiorly.

a. Middle ear—The most common location of cholesteatoma in the middle ear is in the area around the stapes superstructure and incus long process. This area is usually difficult to dissect because of the presence of the facial nerve and ossicular chain. The facial recess, sinus tympani, and posterior hypotympanum are also areas where the surgeon can easily leave behind cholesteatoma because surgical access to these locations is quite limited (Figure 50–4). The remainder of the mesotympanum is usually accessed without difficulty.

b. Epitympanum—After the mesotympanum, the epitympanum is the next most common location for cholesteatoma. The ossicular chain usually obstructs adequate visualization in this area, but removal of the incus and malleus head significantly improves the exposure. The area anterior to the malleus head can harbor cholesteatoma that can escape the surgeon's attention unless this area is adequately exposed. In some cases, the tegmen is so inferiorly

Table 50–1. Overview of surgical procedures for cholesteatoma.

Procedure	End Result	Advantages after Surgery	Disadvantages after Surgery
Tympanoplasty (canal wall up) with mastoidectomy	Ear canal with tympanic membrane	Low risk of otorrhea	Risk of recurrent pars flaccida cholesteatoma
Atticotomy	Ear canal with tympanic membrane and defect into epitympanum	Intermediate risk of otorrhea	Risk of recurrent pars flaccida cholesteatoma
Modified radical mastoidectomy (canal wall down)	Mastoid cavity with tympanic membrane	Low chance of recurrent pars flaccida cholesteatoma	Significant risk of otorrhea
Radical mastoidectomy (canal wall down)	Mastoid cavity without tympanic membrane	Low chance of recurrent pars flaccida and pars tensa cholesteatoma	Significant risk of otorrhea and poor hearing

positioned that access to the epitympanum is not adequate without removing the posterior and superior canal wall.

c. Mastoid—The mastoid can contain a large amount of cholesteatoma, but access to the mastoid is relatively straightforward using standard otologic techniques (Figure 50–5). In some cases, a very low tegmen and very anterior sigmoid sinus can make the surgical exposure inadequate, in which case the canal wall will need to be removed. Once the horizontal semicircular canal has been identified, the surgeon will become oriented to important structures such as the facial nerve and the remainder of the labyrinth.

d. Petrous apex—Occasionally, the cholesteatoma invades the petrous apex through various air cell tracts.

These include the subarcuate, retrolabyrinthine, supralabyrinthine, retrofacial, and infralabyrinthine tract. Petrous apex cholesteatomas usually cannot be accessed adequately using standard otologic techniques and may require neurotologic dissections, such as a middle fossa craniotomy.

3. Surgical techniques—The surgical exposure for cholesteatoma surgery usually requires either a postauricular or an endaural incision.

a. Facial nerve—Care must be taken during dissection of the posterior-superior mesotympanum to avoid injury to the horizontal course of the facial nerve and the stapes or stapes footplate. The facial nerve in the horizontal segment is at greatest risk for surgical injury

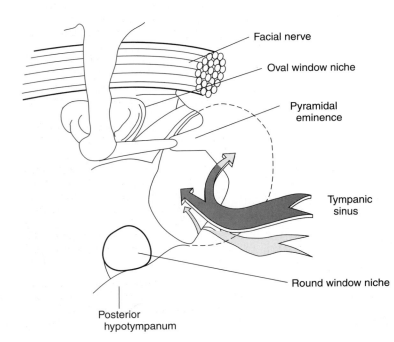

Facial nerve

Oval window niche

Pyramidal eminence

Tympanic sinus

Round window niche

Posterior hypotympanum

Figure 50–4. Diagram showing the anatomy of the posterior mesotympanum. Note the location of the facial nerve and ossicular chain.

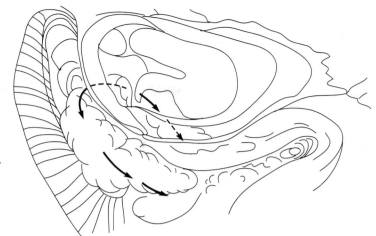

Figure 50–5. Diagram of the exposure obtained during a canal-wall-up mastoidectomy of the right ear. A cholesteatoma arising from the pars flaccida and extending into the mesotympanum, the epitympanum, and the mastoid is depicted.

since dehiscences of the fallopian canal are common here. In general, identification of the horizontal course of the facial nerve in a severely diseased middle ear is easiest from the antrum and attic, just anterior and inferior to the horizontal semicircular canal.

b. Facial recess and epitympanum—Adequate exposure of the posterior-superior mesotympanum usually requires dissection of the facial recess. This can be accomplished with either the canal-wall-up or canal-wall-down tympanomastoidectomy in most cases. The canal-wall-down technique provides reliable access to this area. If the canal wall is kept up, the facial recess exposure needs to be extended into the attic by removing the incus buttress and the incus itself to provide adequate exposure.

The epitympanum is usually best exposed using the canal-wall-down technique, but an adequate exposure is usually obtainable using the canal-wall-up technique as long as there is adequate space between the top of the external auditory canal and the tegmen.

c. Canal wall considerations—The issue of whether a canal-wall-up or a canal-wall-down surgery should be performed is based on various factors. The first consideration relates to the surgeon's training level and experience often influence the choice. The second consideration is the anatomy of the patient's temporal bone. In some cases, adequate exposure can be obtained with either approach, in which case the surgeon may choose the approach based on other factors. In other cases, the canal-wall-down approach is necessary because anatomic features such as a low tegmen or an anterior sigmoid sinus do not allow adequate exposure with any other technique.

The third consideration in surgical approach is the issue of recurrent disease and recidivistic (residual) disease. There are diverse opinions about whether the

canal-wall-up procedure leads to a higher incidence of recurrent or residual disease (or both). In general, the canal-wall-down procedure provides superior surgical exposure during chronic ear surgery, but in select cases, the canal-wall-up procedure with appropriate facial recess and epitympanum dissection provides an equivalent level of exposure. There are conflicting reports on whether the incidence of residual disease is higher in canal-wall-up cases, but the results are likely highly dependent on individual surgical techniques and the experience of the surgeon. However, there is compelling evidence that recurrence of cholesteatoma arising from the pars flaccida after the initial surgical treatment (new disease) is significantly higher in patients who have undergone the canal-wall-up procedure. Currently, this type of recurrence can be prevented only by performing canal-wall-down surgery, which essentially exteriorizes potential areas of recurrence such as the attic and the mastoid, or by obliterating these areas if the canal-wall-up or a canal–wall-reconstruction technique is used.

A cholesteatoma recurrence from the pars tensa is a less common problem, but this should be an important consideration, especially if the initial cholesteatoma was of this type. The preventive options include inserting a ventilation tube, placing cartilage grafts to stiffen the tympanic membrane, or obliterating the middle ear space by performing a radical mastoidectomy. The radical mastoidectomy is the most effective technique for preventing pars flaccida retractions, but this approach is not used routinely because patients' postoperative hearing results are uniformly poor.

d. Mastoid cavity—The canal-wall-down tympanomastoid surgery, whether it is a radical or modified radical mastoidectomy, results in a mastoid cavity. There is a substantial amount of data pointing to a relatively high incidence of otorrhea and debris collection in mastoid cavities, even without the presence of residual or recurrent cholesteatoma. There are many suggested causes for this, but the most common causes, excluding cholesteatoma, are anatomic problems such as a high facial ridge and the presence of mucosal tissue within the mastoid cavity. Anatomic problems occur as a result of technical failure by the surgeon in creating an appropriately shaped mastoid cavity. The mastoid cavity must not have any residual bony ledges, which could cause the retention of squamous debris. A meatoplasty that allows for the adequate inspection and cleaning of the cavity in the office setting is also critical. The formation of mucosal tissue within the mastoid cavity typically occurs when a canal-wall-down procedure is performed in a mastoid that is well pneumatized, and therefore, a canal-wall-up surgery should be considered in these cases.

If the canal wall must be taken down, options include reconstructing the canal wall, obliterating the mastoid cavity with local flaps, such as the temporalis muscle or mastoid periosteum, and covering all exposed areas of mucosa with fascia grafts. The key concept in preventing mucosal overgrowth within the mastoid cavity is to suppress the growth of mucosa by removal or coverage.

e. Staging—Another controversial area in the surgical treatment of cholesteatoma is whether treatment should be staged. The reasons for planning a second surgical procedure include removal of any residual cholesteatoma and the reconstruction of the ossicular chain. Although complete cholesteatoma removal is the goal during the primary procedure, the surgeon, in some cases, may suspect that small pieces of cholesteatoma that are not readily visible could have been left in the surgical field. The most common areas of recurrence include the mesotympanum, in the area of the ossicular chain, and secondarily in the epitympanum. Residual disease in the mastoid is much less common.

Second-look surgery, usually performed 8–12 months after the initial surgery, is often performed after canal-wall-up surgery and less commonly performed after canal-wall-down surgery. The mastoid and epitympanum are highly unlikely to harbor residual cholesteatoma if these areas have been adequately exteriorized during the initial surgery.

A reason for delaying the ossicular chain reconstruction is to prevent adhesion formation around the reconstruction, which may adversely affect the hearing results. If there has been significant mucosal damage in the area of the oval window niche, the surgeon may elect to place a sheet of polymeric silicone (ie, Silastic) or other material to allow the mucosa to heal and form an adequately aerated middle ear space. Once this has been achieved, the surgeon may elect to perform a secondary surgery to reconstruct the ossicular chain. The choice of primary versus delayed ossicular reconstruction is based on the surgeon's experience and the surgical findings.

f. Perilymph fistula—In general, cholesteatoma in the oval window niche is removed toward the end of the procedure so that management of any potential fistula into the vestibule can be instituted without the risk of compromising the repair during further dissection. The repair of an oval window or round window fistula usually consists of patching the defect with fascia or other soft tissue grafts.

Brown JS. A ten-year statistical follow-up of 1142 consecutive cases of cholesteatoma: the closed vs. the open technique. *Laryngoscope.* 1982;92:390. [PMID: 7070181] (Comparison of results of closed vs. open techniques, showing a difference in recurrence rates.)

Jackler RK. The surgical anatomy of cholesteatoma. *Otolaryngol Clin North Am.* 1989;22:883. [PMID: 2694067] (Review of surgical anatomy.)

Quaranta A, Cassano P, Carbonara G. Cholesteatoma surgery: open vs. closed tympanoplasty. *Am J Otol.* 1988;9:229. [PMID: 3177606] (Comparison of results of closed vs. open techniques, showing no difference in recurrence rates.)

Prognosis

There is a high rate of recurrent and residual cholesteatoma disease after primary surgical intervention. Over a time frame of 5 years or more, the combined rate of recurrent and residual disease has been reported to be as high as 40%. Many large series report a rate of 15–25% on follow-up of up to 10 years. The problem seems to be higher in the pediatric population.

The medical and surgical treatments that are available at this time cannot reverse all of the underlying physiologic elements in the ear that were responsible for the initial formation of the cholesteatoma. Chronic infection can usually be corrected, but if the underlying cause is significant eustachian tube dysfunction, this cannot be corrected primarily. The various surgical techniques discussed previously can help reduce the incidence of recurrent disease, but current techniques are not fully effective. Therefore, regular examinations over a course of 10 years or more after definitive treatment remain a critical part of the patient's care.

In most cases, patients are examined in the office setting once a year with the microscope. Symptoms suggestive of recurrent cholesteatoma are similar to those of an initial cholesteatoma, which were described previously. A recurrent cholesteatoma is relatively easy to detect based on the physical examination, at which point prompt treatment should be instituted to prevent both further damage to the temporal bone and other complications.

Parisier SC, Hanson MB, Han JC, Cohen AJ, Selkin BA. Pediatric cholesteatoma: an individualized, single-stage approach. *Otolaryngol Head Neck Surg.* 1996;115:107. [PMID: 8758639] (Rate of recurrence increases over 10-year follow-up.)

Vartiainen E. Factors associated with recurrence of cholesteatoma. *J Laryngol Otol.* 1995;109:590. [PMID: 7561462] (Pediatric recurrence rates are higher than those of adults.)

Otosclerosis

51

Derek Kofi O. Boahene, MD, & Colin L.W. Driscoll, MD

- *History of slowly progressive unilateral or bilateral hearing impairment.*
- *Onset fairly early in adult life, predominantly by the third and fourth decades.*
- *No clear preceding cause for hearing loss.*
- *History of paracusis.*
- *Worsening of hearing during pregnancy or estrogen therapy in females.*
- *Characteristically low-volume (soft) speech.*
- *Normal otoscopic examination or positive Schwartze sign.*
- *Present or previous audiogram demonstrating an air-bone gap.*
- *Family history of otosclerosis.*

General Considerations

Otosclerosis is a primary localized disease of the bony otic capsule. It is characterized by abnormal removal of mature bone of the otic capsule by osteoclasts, and replacement with woven bone of greater thickness, cellularity, and vascularity. Otosclerosis is distinct from other disorders of bone, such as Paget disease and osteogenesis imperfecta, in that it is restricted to the otic capsule and does not involve the generalized skeletal system. It has a predilection for the oval window, where involvement of the stapedial footplate may result in fixation and a resultant conductive hearing loss. Involvement of other parts of the otic capsule may result in sensorineural hearing loss and vestibular symptoms.

The true prevalence of otosclerosis is unknown. Estimates reported for clinical disease (ie, clinical otosclerosis) range from 0.5% to 1.0%. However, the incidence of non-clinical disease (ie, histologic otosclerosis) in unselected autopsy series has been reported as high as 13%; however, this rate needs to be confirmed with larger population-based studies. About 15 million people in the United States have otosclerosis, and it is considered among the most common causes of acquired hearing loss. The disease is more common among whites than black and Asian pop-

ulations, where it is rare. In practice, otosclerosis is seen more often in women than in men, by a ratio of approximately 2:1. It is possible that the incidence is the same in both sexes and that hormonal influences during pregnancy and menopause may cause a more rapid progression in women, bringing them to clinical attention sooner. Symptoms rarely become apparent before the late teens, with most patients presenting between the ages of 20 and 45.

Declau F, Van Spaendonck M, Timmermans JP. Prevalence of otosclerosis in an unselected series of temporal bones. *Otol Neurotol.* 2001;22(5):596. [PMID: 11568664] (The prevalence of otosclerosis correlated well with the rate of clinically significant disease.)

Lippy WH, Berenholz LP, Burkey JM. Otosclerosis in the 1960s, 1970s, 1980s, and 1990s. *Laryngoscope.* 1999;109(8):1307. [PMID: 10443838] (The audiometric patterns at presentation have changed over the past 37 years.)

Sakihara Y, Parving A. Clinical otosclerosis, prevalence estimates, and spontaneous progress. *Acta Otolaryngol.* 1999;119(4):468. [PMID: 10445163] (The prevalence of clinical otosclerosis increases with age and is twice as high in females.)

Pathogenesis

The otic capsule and stapes form from a cartilaginous anlage, which begins endochondral ossification by the 19th week of embryogenesis and is complete by the end of the first year of life. The vestibular surface of the footplate remains cartilaginous throughout life. Osteoblastic and osteoclastic activity that is typically seen in normal bone in other parts of the body is rarely evident in the adult otic capsule. However, in an area of otosclerosis, there is increased osteoblastic and osteoclastic activity and vascular proliferation. The otosclerotic focus is essentially an area of increased bony turnover and metabolic activity. The term "otospongiosis" is most descriptive of the histologic appearance at this stage of the disease. As the disease stabilizes or "burns out," the normal bone of the otic capsule is replaced with a focus of metabolically quiescent, dense mineralized bone. The most common location of the otosclerotic focus is the region of the otic capsule anterior to the stapes footplate (the region of the fissula ante fenestram). Fixation of the stapes begins as the lesion spreads to involve the annular ligament. Extension over the footplate may lead to total obliteration of the footplate. Some lesions extend into the inner ear, resulting in hyalinization of the spiral ligament and a sensorineural hearing loss. Rare cases of pure sensorineural hearing loss from isolated cochlear otosclerosis without ossicular involvement have been reported.

The inciting stimulus for the abnormal bone remodeling in otosclerosis is unknown and has been attributed to both genetic and environmental factors. Genetics play a role in the etiology of otosclerosis; the familial aggregation of individuals affected by otosclerosis has been well noted. Several studies have concluded that, in most cases, the disease is inherited as a simple autosomal dominant trait with incomplete penetrance. Recent findings suggest an association between the measles virus and otosclerosis. Whether the measles virus is a factor that can initiate the otospongiotic process remains to be determined. However, current efforts to immunize against this virus would be expected to drastically reduce the incidence of otosclerosis.

Chole RA, McKenna M. Pathophysiology of otosclerosis. *Otol Neurotol.* 2001;22(2):249. [PMID: 11300278] (Otosclerosis is a disease localized to the otic capsule of the temporal bone and does not occur outside of the temporal bone.)

Niedermeyer HP, Arnold W. Etiopathogenesis of otosclerosis. *ORL J Otorhinolaryngol Relat Spec.* 2002;64(2):114. [PMID: 12021502] (Various idiopathogenic factors may contribute to the genesis of otosclerosis.)

Niedermeyer HP, Arnold W, Schwub D, Busch R, Wiest I, Sedlmeier R. Shift of the distribution of age in patients with otosclerosis. *Acta Otolaryngol.* 2001;121(2):197. [PMID: 11349778] (The average age of patients with otosclerosis is increasing.)

Tomek MS, Brown MR, Mani SR et al. Localization of a gene for otosclerosis to chromosome 15q25-q26. *Hum Mol Genet.* 1998;7(2):285. [PMID: 9425236] (The study of a large family localized the gene for otosclerosis to chromosome 15 Q25-Q26.)

van Den Bogaert K, Govaerts PJ, Schatteman I et al. A second gene for otosclerosis, otsc2, maps to chromosome 7q34-36. *Am J Hum Genet.* 2001;68(2):495. [PMID: 11170898] (Genetic analysis in a Belgian family suggests otosclerosis may be related to an abnormality on chromosome 7Q.)

Prevention

Sodium fluoride, in moderate doses, may have a stabilizing effect on the otosclerotic focus and may also be beneficial in terms of both prevention and control of this disease. The role of fluorides and other bone-stabilizing agents that are used as preventive or stabilizing agents is discussed in the Treatment section.

Clinical Findings

A. SYMPTOMS AND SIGNS

The typical patient with otosclerosis presents with a history of slowly progressive hearing loss that is usually bilateral but asymmetric. Because of its insidious onset, the patient is often unaware of the hearing loss until it is brought to his or her attention by friends or family. Unilateral hearing loss may occur in 15% of patients. The disease may remain confined to one particular ear; the other ear may become involved later. Hearing loss typically becomes apparent when the loss reaches 25–30 dB and the patient has difficulty understanding speech. Patients characteristically have low-volume (soft) speech because they hear their own voices by bone conduction and consequently talk quietly. The ability to hear better in noisy surroundings (paracusis) during the early stages of hearing impairment is highly suggestive of otosclerosis. Tinnitus is a common complaint and may be an indication of sensorineural degeneration. Fluctuation is uncharacteristic but may occur during times of hormonal instability (eg, during pregnancy). Patients rarely have complaints of dizziness or vertigo.

B. PHYSICAL EXAM

A careful otoscopic examination is essential and is best performed with the operating microscope. The goal of the exam is to exclude other causes of conductive hearing loss, such as cholesteatoma, tympanosclerosis, and middle ear effusion or mass. In otosclerosis, the tympanic membrane is normal, the middle ear space is pneumatized, and the malleus should move with pneumatic otoscopy. In active disease, the experienced clinician may appreciate a reddish blush (Schwartze sign) over both the promontory and the oval window niche owing to the prominent vascularity associated with an otospongiotic focus.

C. IMAGING STUDIES

1. Computerized tomography (CT) scanning— Conventional radiography is of little use in the diagnosis of otosclerosis. However, high-resolution CT scanning provides an excellent visualization of the anatomy of the ossicles, the facial nerve (CN VII), the labyrinthine windows, and the otic capsule. It is valuable in assessing the pathology of the oval window and the footplate, and the extent of otic capsule involvement. CT scanning may show subtle areas of demineralization, which are typically located just anterior to the stapedial oval window, as well as thickening of the footplate. With cochlear involvement, there is a demineralization of the otic capsule, which yields the so-called "double ring sign" seen on CT as a low-density zone of demineralization outlining the cochlea (Figures 51–1 and 51–2).

In the sclerotic phase of the disease or after fluoride therapy, remineralization may occur and CT findings may be indistinguishable from the normal otic capsule. A CT scan is not necessary in most cases. CT scanning should be considered when the patient has vertigo, dizziness, tinnitus, or a sensorineural hearing loss. A CT

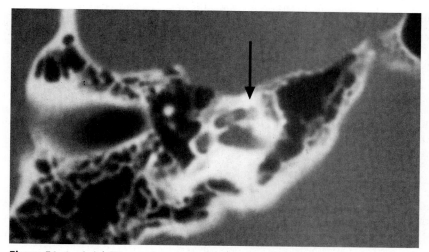

Figure 51–1. Axial CT scan demonstrating an area of radiolucent demineralization of the otic capsule.

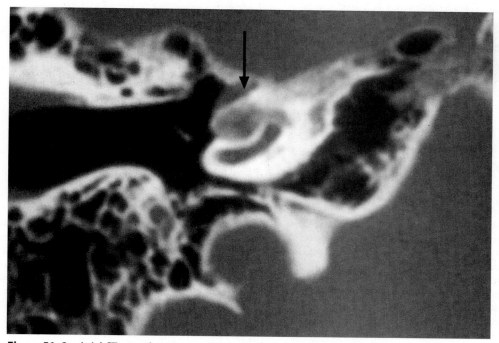

Figure 51–2. Axial CT scan showing extensive involvement of the apical portion of the cochlea and pericochlear otic capsule. The cochlea has a "smudged" appearance, with loss of the crisp demarcation between the endocochlear lumen and surrounding bone that is characteristic of a normal high-resolution CT scan of the temporal bone.

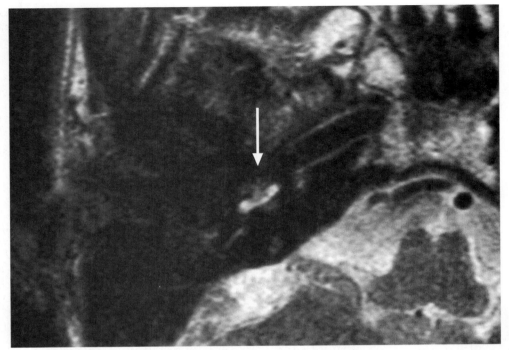

Figure 51–3. Axial T2-weighted scan demonstrating the lack of normal fluid signal from the cochlea due to inflammation or obliteration (or both) of the lumen. This scan correlates fairly closely anatomically to the axial CT scan of the same patient presented in Figure 51–2.

scan is always obtained in pediatric patients because of the higher risk of otic capsule and temporal bone malformations or abnormalities.

2. Magnetic resonance imaging (MRI)— MRI is not often obtained but can be useful, particularly in the active phase of the disease. It can detect congenital anomalies of the labyrinth (eg, enlarged vestibular aqueduct) and fibrosis within the cochlea. It can also exclude retrocochlear pathology, such as an acoustic neuroma. T1-weighted images show a loss of normal signal void from the otic capsule. Soft tissue or intermediate-signal density is noted in or around the otic capsule, and contrast-enhanced T1-weighted images show enhancement of the pericochlear otic capsule. T2-weighted images may demonstrate a loss of the normal fluid signal from the cochlea that results from inflammation or obliteration of the cochlea (Figure 51–3). MRI is reserved for patients with unusual features to their presentation—not classic otosclerosis.

D. SPECIAL TESTS

1. Rinne and Weber tuning fork tests—Tuning fork tests, including the Rinne and Weber tests, should be carefully performed at 256, 512, and 1024 Hz to confirm the findings of the audiogram. A negative Rinne test (bone conduction greater than air conduction) at 512 Hz usually indicates an air-bone gap of at least 25 dB. Typically, the tuning forks "reverse" in the higher frequencies, meaning that air conduction is greater than bone conduction (Table 51–1).

2. Tympanometry—Audiometric testing is one of the most important tools in evaluating a patient suspected of having otosclerosis. Testing patients who have a mixed hearing loss or far-advanced otosclerosis can be problematic because of masking dilemmas and audiometer limits. An experienced audiologist is invaluable in providing accurate and complete information on this type of testing.

Table 51–1. Classic audiometric findings.

Low-frequency conductive hearing loss
Carhart notch
Type A or A$_S$ (short/stiff) tympanogram
Diphasic or absent reflexes
Negative Rinne test

The gradual stiffening of the ossicular chain produced by progressive stapes fixation leads to specific and distinctive patterns of change on tympanometry. Because middle ear aeration is not affected by otosclerosis, patients with early- and mid-stage disease characteristically have a normal Type A tympanogram. Progressive stapes fixation often results in a Type A_S (A-short) tympanogram. The tympanogram pattern needs to be interpreted in conjunction with the otoscopic findings. An atrophic flaccid tympanic membrane results in both hypercompliance and an A_D (A-deep) tympanogram that may mask stapedial ankylosis. Alternately, an extensively tympanosclerotic membrane may reduce compliance, resulting in an A_S tympanogram, despite normal ossicular mobility.

3. Acoustic reflex—One of the earliest signs of otosclerosis is an abnormal acoustic reflex pattern. This pattern often precedes the development of an air-bone gap. In the normal hearing ear, the configuration of the acoustic reflex pattern is one of a sustained decrease in compliance owing to the contraction of the stapedial muscle that lasts the duration of the stimulus. In contrast, in early otosclerosis, a characteristic diphasic on-off pattern that is characterized by a brief increase in compliance at the onset and at the termination of the stimulus occurs, which is virtually pathognomonic for this condition. With disease progression, a reduction in the reflex amplitude is seen, followed by elevation of ipsilateral, then contralateral thresholds, and finally, the disappearance of the response. The most common finding at presentation is absent reflexes.

4. Pure-tone audiometry—On pure-tone audiometry, patients with early otosclerosis present with progressive low-frequency conductive loss, with a characteristic rising audiogram configuration. As otosclerosis spreads to involve the entire stapes, an increase in mass compounds the progressive increase in stiffness, resulting in (1) progression of loss in the high frequencies, (2) a gradual widening of the air-bone gap, and (3) a flat audiogram configuration. In the absence of a sensorineural component, the pure conductive hearing loss seen in a completely fixed stapes is limited to a 60- to 65-dB hearing level with a maximum air-bone gap across the frequency range. As the disease spreads to involve the cochlea, bone conduction thresholds increase, resulting in a mixed hearing loss in which most of the conductive component is confined to the low frequencies. A variant audiometric configuration with a "cookie bite" appearance is often seen with cochlear otosclerosis. Decreased bone conduction levels in the high frequencies usually represent a true sensorineural hearing loss.

The hallmark of bone conduction thresholds in otosclerosis is the Carhart notch. This is characterized by the elevation of bone conduction thresholds of approximately 5, 10, and 15 dB at 500, 1000, and 2000 Hz, respectively. The Carhart notch is thought to result from the disruption of normal ossicular resonance, which is approximately 2000 Hz. It is therefore a mechanical phenomenon and not a true reflection of cochlear reserve (see Table 51–1).

Goh JP, Chan LL, Tan TY. MRI of cochlear otosclerosis. *Br J Radiol.* 2002;75(894):502. [PMID: 12124236] (Cochlear otosclerosis can be diagnosed on MRI scans.)

Lopponen H, Laitakari K. Carhart notch effect in otosclerotic ears measured by electric bone conduction audiometry. *Scand Audiol Suppl.* 2001;(52):160. [PMID: 11318454] (Conventional and electric bone conduction testing both demonstrate the Carhart effect.)

Differential Diagnosis

The diagnosis of otosclerosis may be strongly suspected based on the history, physical exam, and audiometric findings. However, the diagnosis can only be confirmed at the time of surgery or upon histologic study of the temporal bone. Other lesions that may cause a conductive hearing loss are numerous (Table 51–2). Most of these can be excluded during the physical exam, but others, such as malleus fixation, are excluded at the time of surgery.

Treatment

Patients with otosclerosis have four treatment options: (1) observation, (2) nonsurgical measures, (3) amplification, and (4) surgery. Each option, and the advantages and disadvantages, should be discussed with the patient.

A. OBSERVATION

Observation is the least risky and least expensive option. It is often the strategy preferred for patients

Table 51–2. Lesions that may cause conductive hearing loss.

Tympanic Membrane Lesions
Tympanic membrane perforation
Tympanosclerosis
Middle Ear Lesions
Otitis media with effusion
Chronic adhesive otitis media
Cholesteatoma
Ossicular discontinuity
Malleus or incus fixation
Congenital footplate fixation
Middle ear tumor
Systemic Connective Tissue and Bone Diseases
Paget disease
Osteogenesis imperfecta (van der Hoeve syndrome)
Ankylosing rheumatoid arthritis

with unilateral disease and those with a mild conductive hearing loss (CHL). If the patient is not concerned about the hearing loss, then no intervention is indicated and audiograms are usually obtained on a yearly basis. The hearing loss typically progresses slowly, ultimately prompting further intervention.

B. Nonsurgical Measures

Therapeutic strategies to prevent the progression and control of otosclerosis have been directed at the suppression of bone remodeling with fluorides and bisphosphonates. However, the efficacy of these agents has not been definitively proved, and otologists vary widely in their recommendations regarding the use of these medications.

1. Sodium fluoride therapy—Fluoride reduces osteoclastic bone resorption and increases osteoblastic bone formation. Together, these actions may promote recalcification and reduce bone remodeling in actively expanding osteolytic lesions. Sodium fluoride is also thought to inhibit proteolytic enzymes that are cytotoxic to the cochlea and that may lead to a sensorineural hearing loss.

Fluoride therapy has been found to significantly arrest the progression of sensorineural hearing loss in the low and high frequencies. Sodium fluoride is typically dosed at 50 mg daily in a patient with evidence of active disease. With stabilization, as evidenced by hearing stabilization, reduced tinnitus, reduced dizziness, fading of an injected mucous membrane over an active focus (Schwartze sign), and radiologic signs of recalcification, a daily maintenance dose of 25 mg is administered.

Fluoride therapy is contraindicated in patients with chronic nephritis and chronic rheumatoid arthritis, as well as in pregnant and lactating women, children, and patients with a demonstrated allergy to fluoride. Gastrointestinal disturbances are the most common adverse effect of fluoride therapy. Taking enteric-coated capsules after meals largely prevents these adverse effects. Because there is also the rare possibility of skeletal fluorosis, a skeletal survey should be taken at intervals during the treatment.

Many otologists recommend the use of sodium fluoride in patients with new-onset otosclerosis, rapidly progressive disease, or inner ear symptoms such as sensorineural hearing loss and dizziness. The treatment is usually continued for 1–2 years. Patients with cochlear otosclerosis may be treated for longer periods of time or even indefinitely. Because the efficacy of this treatment is not clearly defined, each patient's response should be considered independently, with an assessment made of the risks versus the benefits.

2. Bisphosphonates—Bisphosphonates are potent antiresorptive agents that are useful for the prevention and treatment of osteoporosis and other conditions characterized by increased bone remodeling. They have been widely used in the treatment of osteoporosis and hold some promise in controlling otosclerosis. Following oral intake, bisphosphonates are incorporated into bone, where they inhibit osteoclastic activity. The most promising bisphosphonates in clinical use include alendronate, etidronate, risedronate, and zoledronate. These bisphosphonates potently inhibit bone resorption without significantly affecting bone deposition. The main side effects of oral bisphosphonates occur in the gastrointestinal tract. Nausea and diarrhea occur in 20–30% of patients treated with high doses of etidronate, but are rarely seen with the lower doses that are used for the treatment of otosclerosis.

3. Amplification—Most patients with otosclerosis have normal cochlear function with excellent speech discrimination and are therefore good hearing aid candidates. Before proceeding with surgery, patients should be encouraged to try a hearing aid (or aids). Some patients become successful hearing aid users and can therefore avoid surgery and its risks. However, although there is no risk to the patient with hearing aid use, there are some significant disadvantages when compared with the result of a successful surgery. The disadvantages include a poorer sound quality, cosmesis, cost, maintenance requirements, being able to hear only when the aid is in use, occlusion effect, and comfort. In practice, most patients under age 60 with good sensorineural reserve prefer to have surgery, but there are also many satisfied hearing aid users in this population.

C. Surgical Measures

1. Indications for surgery—Most patients with conductive hearing loss due to otosclerosis can be treated surgically (Table 51–3). The average patient with otosclerosis and a bone conduction level of 0–25 dB in the speech range and an air conduction level of 45–65 dB is a suitable candidate for surgery. An air-bone gap of at least 15 dB and discrimination scores of 60% or better are preferred. Clearly, the larger the existing air-bone gap,

Table 51–3. Contraindications to surgery.

1. A medically unfit patient.
2. Active otitis media.
3. Perforated tympanic membrane.
4. An only-hearing ear that does well with amplification.
5. Presence of vertigo and clinical evidence of labyrinthine hydrops.
6. Pregnancy.
7. Occupational considerations. Surgery may be inadvisable in individuals whose occupation or activities demand considerable physical strain or precise balance (eg, pilots, scuba divers, and construction workers).
8. Inner ear malformation.

the more there is to gain by surgical intervention. A subset of patients with a severe-to-profound mixed hearing loss have been referred to as having far-advanced otosclerosis. In far-advanced otosclerosis, the otosclerotic process has progressed to the point where there is no detectable air conduction threshold and bone conduction is difficult to interpret at high levels because of vibrotactile sensations. Some patients have been successfully treated with stapedectomy and amplification.

2. Preoperative counseling—Surgery for otosclerosis is an elective procedure and should be preceded by a thorough explanation of the treatment alternatives, including amplification. It is essential to explain the advantages and disadvantages of surgery and provide the patient with realistic expectations. The patient should also be prepared for potential failure in both the short and long terms, including the possible need for revision surgery. In the long term, patients with otosclerosis lose inner ear function at a more rapid rate than does the general population, and they are therefore more likely to eventually need a hearing aid, despite a successful surgery.

3. Preoperative considerations—Surgery can be performed under local or general anesthesia, depending on the preference of both the patient and the surgeon. There are several advantages to local anesthesia. (1) The patient's hearing can be tested after prosthesis placement by repositioning the tympanic membrane and either talking with the patient or performing tuning fork tests. (2) If the patient complains of vertigo during the procedure, the surgeon can alter his or her technique to reduce the vestibular irritation. (3) The patient can avoid the postoperative nausea that often accompanies general anesthesia; the newly reconstructed ear is therefore not subjected to the potentially extreme pressures associated with arousal from anesthesia and vomiting.

4. Surgical technique—Many subtle variations are used by various surgeons, but the basic concept and steps of the procedure are similar. After adequate cleaning of the ear and administration of both a local anesthetic and a vasoconstrictive agent, a tympanomeatal flap is elevated. If the stapes cannot be well visualized, the scutum is removed with a curet or drill. The ossicular chain is inspected and palpated to establish the diagnosis. Once the diagnosis is made, there is considerable variation in how a surgeon can handle the stapes superstructure and footplate. Ultimately, either a small fenestra stapedotomy or a total stapedectomy is performed, and the prosthesis is placed from the incus through the opening into the vestibule (Figure 51–4). The mobility of the prosthesis is assessed by gentle palpation of the malleus. Tissue or blood is used to seal the area around the prosthesis, and the tympanic membrane is repositioned. Most surgeons allow the patient to return home the day of the surgery. Prophylactic antibiotics are typi-

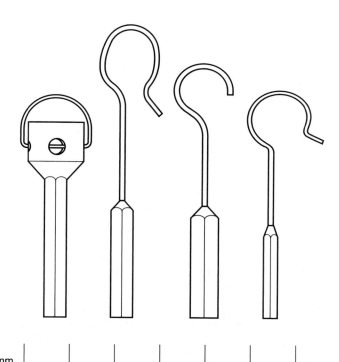

Figure 51–4. A wide variety of stapes prostheses are available, and only a few are shown here. On the left is a prosthesis that fits under the incus, with the lenticular process sitting in the bucket. The wire handle is then flipped over the long process of the incus for additional stabilization. The other prostheses are pistons of different configurations that are placed through the oval window and crimped over the long process of the incus. The materials used in virtually all prior and all current prostheses are MRI compatible (eg, stainless steel, platinum, and Teflon).

1mm

cally given in the operating room, and many surgeons send the patient home on a short course of antibiotic therapy; however, there is little evidence that the additional antibiotics are beneficial.

5. Laser use—Lasers are commonly used in otosclerosis surgery. The cited advantages of laser use are an improved ability to prepare a bloodless fenestra, a reduced risk of footplate subluxation, and precise cuts in the footplate without disturbing the otosclerotic focus. Various types of lasers have been used, including the CO_2, KTP, and argon lasers. Controversy exists surrounding the choice of laser type. The ideal laser should have the following properties: (1) precise optics for delivery, (2) a predictable laser-tissue interaction with both bone and collagen, and (3) no penetration or heating of perilymph. Some data suggest that the argon, KTP, and CO_2 lasers all could be used safely in primary cases; however, the CO_2 laser is recommended in revision cases in which there is a greater chance of exposure through an open vestibule.

6. Cochlear implantation—The pathophysiology of hearing loss in patients with otosclerosis differs from that seen in most cochlear implantation candidates. The otosclerotic process is usually focused on the lateral cochlear wall, resulting in degeneration of the spiral ligament and stria vascularis while mostly sparing the organ of Corti. The preservation of this neural element in otosclerosis may allow for greater electrical stimulation following implantation. One study reported that patients with profound hearing loss secondary to otosclerosis derived excellent benefits from cochlear implantation. In these patients, there is a reported higher incidence of facial nerve stimulation from current spread through the otosclerotic bone. Reprogramming the device and eliminating some of the offending channels can usually eliminate this undesirable side effect.

7. Revision surgery—Most patients should be encouraged to try a hearing aid before a revision procedure. However, a persistent or recurrent conductive hearing loss may benefit from revision surgery. The reasons for failure of the previous surgery can include incus erosion, a poorly positioned prosthesis (either too short or displaced), malleus or incus fixation, and reobliteration of the oval window. It is important to know the details of any prior surgeries and the experience level of the primary surgeon. A patient with a poor result after an operation by an experienced surgeon is not a good candidate for revision. In contrast, a patient who initially had a good result and lost function secondary to incus erosion can usually expect a successful outcome from revision surgery. Because the risk of hearing loss is higher in revision surgery, it is advisable to approach the surgery with the idea of exploring the ear and proceeding with the revision surgery if it appears favorable.

It is preferable to perform only an exploratory procedure than to attempt a difficult revision that results in a poor outcome.

In very rare cases, patients with a persistent perilymph fistula and subsequent dizziness may benefit from revision surgery.

8. Stapes surgery in children—Common indications for stapedial surgery in children include congenital footplate fixation and otosclerosis. The effectiveness of stapedial surgery in children has been less critically reviewed than in adults. However, some data noted a 91.7% success rate in achieving a 10-dB air-bone gap after 5 or more years of follow-up. Other studies reported an 82% success rate in primary otosclerosis cases but only a 44% success rate in cases of congenital footplate fixation.

The optimal time for surgery in children remains a point of controversy. With the higher incidence of otitis media during childhood, there is concern for the potential spread of infection through the oval window and the undesirable consequence of meningitis. Moreover, most children benefit from amplification, and delaying surgery until they are older is an acceptable option. However, delaying surgery may result in disease progression that may require more extensive drilling.

Brookler KH, Tanyeri H. Etidronate for the neurotologic symptoms of otosclerosis: preliminary study. *Ear Nose Throat J.* 1997;76(6):371. [PMID: 9210803] (Etidronate appears effective for the treatment of otosclerosis.)

de la Cruz A, Angeli S, Slattery WH. Stapedectomy in children. *Otolaryngol Head Neck Surg.* 1999;120(4):487. [PMID: 10187939]. (Stapedectomy can be safely performed in children.)

Derks W, de Groot JA, Raymakers JA, Veldman JE. Fluoride therapy for cochlear otosclerosis? An audiometric and computerized tomography evaluation. *Acta Otolaryngol.* 2001;121 (2):174. [PMID: 11349772] (Discusses fluoride therapy rest at the progression of sensorineural hearing loss in low and high frequencies.)

Lesinski SG, Palmer A. Lasers for otosclerosis: CO_2 versus argon and KTP-532. *Laryngoscope.* 1989;99:1. [PMID: 2498587] (The optical properties of the CO_2 laser are preferable to those of the argon and KTP-532 lasers.)

Ruckenstein MJ, Rafter KO, Montes M, Bigelow DC. Management of far-advanced otosclerosis in the era of cochlear implantation. *Otol Neurotol.* 2001;22(4):471. [PMID: 11449102]. (Patients with profound sensorineural hearing loss secondary to otosclerosis derive excellent benefit through cochlear implantation.)

Intraoperative Issues & Postoperative Complications of Otosclerosis Surgery

Table 51–4 details some of the potential complications that may result from stapedial surgery.

A. TYMPANIC MEMBRANE PERFORATION

If the tympanomeatal flap is either torn during elevation or too short after bone has been removed from the

Table 51–4. Potential postoperative complications of stapedial surgery.

Sensorineural loss
Tinnitus
Dysgeusia
Infection
Prosthesis displacement or loose wire
Incus necrosis
Tympanic membrane perforation
Dizziness
Fibrosis
Perilymph fistula
Postoperative granuloma
Phonophobia
Facial nerve paralysis

---

scutum, the defect should be repaired with fat, temporalis fascia, or tragal perichondrium.

B. DYSGEUSIA

All efforts should be made to preserve the chorda tympani nerve, especially in bilateral cases. Stretching this nerve may result in dysgeusia, with complaints of a salty or metallic taste. Typically, the taste disturbance gradually resolves over a few weeks or months, even if the nerve has been transected. Rarely, it persists indefinitely.

C. ABNORMALITIES OF THE FACIAL NERVE

Dehiscence of the facial nerve in the vicinity of the oval window is seen in about 0.5% of cases. It may bulge inferiorly—enough to obscure the footplate and make surgery difficult or inadvisable. Recognition of an aberrant or dehiscent facial nerve is critical to preventing injury, particularly if a laser is used. A facial nerve monitor may also be of benefit in preventing nerve injury. Periodically after surgery, a patient experiences an acute facial weakness due to the injection of local anesthetic. This weakness should abate over 2–4 hours as the medication effects dissipate. Occasionally, a patient develops a delayed paralysis 5–7 days after surgery. This paralysis is likely due to a viral reactivation within the nerve, analogous to Bell palsy, and is treated with prednisone and an antiviral medication. The prognosis is excellent for a full recovery.

D. MALLEUS AND INCUS FIXATION

After the middle ear has been exposed, it is important to palpate the long process of the malleus and assess the mobility of the malleus and the incus. The mobility of the stapes can be evaluated by light palpation by (1) pushing the superstructure side-to-side and (2) gently pushing toward the vestibule on the long process of the incus. With experience, it is possible to appreciate partial stapes fixation and subtle abnormalities in ossicular mobility. If the stapes is mobile and the malleus or incus is fixed, there are basically two options: (1) the ear can be closed and hearing aid use can be recommended to the patient, or (2) the incus and head of the malleus can be removed and a partial ossicular reconstruction prosthesis (PORP) or other graft or technique can be used to reconstruct the ossicular chain, as is commonly done in cholesteatoma or chronic ear surgery. Simple mobilization of the malleus or an attempt to remove a bony bridge between the malleus and surrounding bone usually fails to result in a good long-term hearing result due to refixation and fibrosis. Occasionally, a patient has both stapes and malleus fixation. In this situation, failure to make the correct diagnosis results in a substandard hearing result.

E. PERSISTENT STAPEDIAL ARTERY

A persistent stapedial artery can be mobilized or divided. Controlling bleeding can be a challenge.

F. PERILYMPH "GUSHER"

This complication is often discussed and, fortunately, is rare. When the footplate is opened, there is a brisk flow of perilymph. This flow is the result of either an abnormally patent cochlear aqueduct or malformation of the lateral end of the internal auditory canal, with a direct communication to the inner ear. It is more common in patients who have a congenitally fixed footplate; a preoperative CT scan is highly recommended in these cases. If these conditions are suspected preoperatively, surgery is contraindicated because of a high risk of causing a complete sensorineural hearing loss. If this complication occurs during surgery, fat or muscle grafts may be used to seal the leak. Postoperatively, the patient should be maintained in a head-elevated position. Severe leaks may require packing the middle ear and placing a temporary lumbar drain to reduce cerebrospinal fluid pressure postoperatively.

G. FLOATING OR SUBMERGED FOOTPLATE

A floating or submerged footplate presents a difficult technical challenge. The footplate may become mobile either while attempting to fracture the stapes superstructure or during manipulation of the footplate. If the footplate becomes mobile during an attempt to fracture the crura, it may be best to terminate the procedure; the result may be quite satisfactory. If refixation occurs, the ear can be reexplored at a later date. If the footplate is totally submerged, then no effort should be made to retrieve it, and a graft should be placed over the oval window. A mobile footplate in the normal anatomic location or a partially submerged footplate may be removed or retrieved using small hooks. Suction of the perilymph must be minimized, and any manipulation in the vestibule is very risky. If great care is not taken, there is a high likelihood of a sensorineural hearing loss, and abandoning the procedure should be considered.

H. Obliterative Otosclerosis

This condition presents the surgeon with a difficult intraoperative decision. Generally, the surgical results are less satisfying in these cases. The oval window tends to reobliterate, and the risk of an immediate sensorineural hearing loss is therefore higher. Strong consideration should be given to trying a hearing aid if the patient has not yet done so. If surgery is attempted, the obliterative bone is best removed with a drill rather than with a laser. In these cases, revision surgery is not recommended.

I. Vertigo

During stapedial surgery, vertigo may result from several causes, including diffusion of the anesthetic agent into the labyrinth, aspiration of perilymph, manipulations within the vestibule, a displaced footplate, and the introduction of a prosthesis that may be too long. One of the advantages of using local anesthesia is that, in a patient who is awake, vertigo is readily monitored during surgery. A delayed onset of vertigo may be the result of a perilymph fistula, an excessively long prosthesis, or labyrinthitis.

J. Sensorineural Hearing Loss

Severe sensorineural hearing loss occurs in about 1% of patients after primary surgery and in up to 10% of patients after revision surgery. Mild to moderate losses occur more commonly, particularly in the high frequencies, but the incidence is not known. The hearing loss may be either immediate or delayed. Possible causes of an immediate hearing loss include intraoperative trauma, postoperative infection, granuloma formation, and a perilymph fistula. The cause of a delayed loss is unknown. Many surgeons prefer to wait 1 year before considering surgery on the second ear because of this risk. In addition, some patients who find the hearing after surgery on one ear adequate or better may adapt and choose not to have surgery on the second ear.

K. Tinnitus

Most often, the tinnitus that is present preoperatively improves after surgery. If a sensorineural hearing loss has occurred, then any existing tinnitus may worsen. Preoperative preparation for this possible complication is exceedingly important; an inadequately informed patient who develops even a mild case of postoperative sensorineural hearing loss and tinnitus is frequently very dissatisfied.

L. Incus Dislocation, Fracture, and Necrosis

If the incus is moderately mobilized, it can simply be repositioned. If it is truly subluxated, it should be removed and a total ossicular reconstruction prosthesis (TORP) or malleus-to-footplate prosthesis used. If during crimping the long process is fractured, a number of options exist. A groove can be drilled proximally along the long process and the wire crimped in this location. A shape-memory (Nitinol) prosthesis may fit well without drilling a groove. Alternately, a prosthesis designed to fit under the long process of the incus can be used. If the incus is too short, a malleus-to-footplate wire can be used. Lastly, bone cements continue to improve and may be helpful in stabilizing a prosthesis in this situation. Incus necrosis is a common finding at revision surgery and is addressed in the same manner. It is important to have available a variety of prostheses for each surgery and to be facile with different reconstructive techniques.

Vincent R, Lopez A, Sperling NM. Malleus ankylosis: a clinical audiometric, histologic, and surgical study of 123 cases. *Am J Otol.* 1999;20(6):717. [PMID: 10565714] (Incudomallear ankylosis and stapes fixation can be addressed at the same surgery.)

Prognosis

The immediate success rate after stapedial surgery declines slowly over time owing to delayed conductive hearing loss and further sensorineural hearing loss. In one series that reported on primary stapedectomy cases, an air-bone gap closure of ≤ 10 dB was reported in 95.1% of cases after 1 year, in 94.7% after 2–5 years, and in 62.5% after 30 years. In revision cases, the reported rates of an air-bone gap closure measuring ≤ 10 dB was 71.1% after 1 year, 62.4% after 2–5 years, and 59.4% after 6–36 years. In a similar review, a residual air-bone gap of ≤ 10 dB was reported in 79% of primary cases, with a follow-up period ranging from 1 to 21 years, with a mean of 7 years. The decline in hearing after stapedotomy and stapedectomy has been estimated to occur at a rate of 3.2 dB and 9.5 dB per decade, respectively. Based on this predicted deterioration rate, it is estimated that a typical stapedectomy patient will reach the critical level of 40 dB, which will require amplification 13 years after surgery. In contrast, stapedotomy patients are not expected to reach this level for 21 years.

Causse JB, Causse JR, Parahy C. Stapedotomy technique and results. *Am J Otol.* 1985;6(1):68. [PMID: 3976862] (Review of stapedotomy technique and results of a large series from an experienced group.)

Kos MI, Montandon PB, Guyot JP. Short- and long-term results of stapedotomy and stapedectomy with a Teflon-wire piston prosthesis. *Ann Otol Rhinol Laryngol.* 2001;110(10):907. [PMID: 11642421] (Larger footplate perforations resulted in better correlation of air-bone gap at lower frequencies.)

Shea JJ Jr. Forty years of stapes surgery. *Am J Otol.* 1998;19(1):52. [PMID: 9455948] (Results of 14,449 stapedectomy operations performed by the author over a 40-year period.)

SECTION XIII
Inner Ear

Sensorineural Hearing Loss | 52

Anil K. Lalwani, MD

Anil K. Lalwani, MD

ESSENTIALS OF DIAGNOSIS

- *May affect patients of all ages.*
- *For patients who have unilateral hearing loss:*
- *Weber tuning fork test lateralizes to the unaffected side.*
- *Rinne tuning fork test demonstrates air conduction greater than bone conduction.*
- *Pure-tone thresholds result in equally diminished air and bone conduction.*
- *Speech discrimination testing less than 90% correct.*

General Considerations

Hearing loss is extremely common and has a wide spectrum ranging from a nearly undetectable degree of disability to a profound loss of ability to function in society. Nearly 10% of the adult population has some hearing loss. Often, this impairment presents early in life. One of every 1000 babies born in the United States is completely deaf, and more than 3 million children have hearing loss. However, hearing loss can present at any age. Between 30% and 35% of individuals over the age of 65 have a hearing loss sufficient to require a hearing aid. Forty percent of people over the age of 75 have hearing loss.

Hearing loss can result from disorders of the auricle, external auditory canal, middle ear, inner ear, or central auditory pathways. In general, lesions in the auricle, external auditory canal, or middle ear cause conductive hearing loss. The focus of this chapter is sensorineural

hearing loss that tends to result from lesions in the inner ear or eighth nerve. See Table 52–1 for a list of the common causes of hearing loss.

Classification

Sensorineural hearing loss may result from damage to the hair cells caused by intense noise, viral infections, fractures of the temporal bone, meningitis, cochlear otosclerosis, Meniere disease, and aging. The following drugs also can produce sensorineural hearing loss: ototoxic drugs (eg, salicylates, quinine, and the synthetic analogs of quinine), aminoglycoside antibiotics, loop diuretics (eg, furosemide and ethacrynic acid), and cancer chemotherapeutic agents (eg, cisplatin).

A. AGE-RELATED HEARING LOSS (PRESBYCUSIS)

Presbycusis, age-associated hearing loss, is the most common cause of hearing loss in adults. Initially, it is characterized by symmetric, high-frequency hearing loss that eventually progresses to involve all frequencies. More important, the hearing loss is associated with a significant loss in clarity.

B. CONGENITAL HEARING LOSS

Congenital malformations of the inner ear cause hearing loss in some adults. Genetic predisposition alone or in concert with environmental influences may also be responsible.

C. NEURAL HEARING LOSS

Neural hearing loss is due mainly to cerebellopontine angle tumors such as vestibular schwannomas (acoustic neuromas) or meningiomas; it also may result from any neoplastic, vascular, demyelinating (eg, multiple sclerosis), infectious, or degenerative

Table 52–1. Etiology of sensorineural hearing loss.

Category	Example
Developmental and hereditary	
Syndromic	Alport syndrome, Usher syndrome
Nonsyndromic	Large vestibular aqueduct syndrome
Infectious	Otitis media, viral, syphilis
Pharmacologic toxicity	Aminoglycosides, loop diuretics
Trauma	Head injury, noise-induced, barotrauma
Neurologic disorders	Multiple sclerosis
Vascular and hematologic disorders	Migraine, cryoglobinemia, sickle cell
Immune disorders	Polyarteritis nodosa, HIV
Bone disorders	Paget disease
Neoplasms	Vestibular schwannoma
Unknown etiology	Presbycusis, Meniere disease

disease or trauma affecting the central auditory pathways.

D. HIV-RELATED HEARING LOSS

Human immunodeficiency virus (HIV) infection leads to both peripheral and central auditory system pathology and is associated with sensorineural hearing impairment.

E. MIXED HEARING LOSS

A person can have both conductive and sensory hearing loss, which is termed mixed hearing loss. Mixed hearing losses are due to pathology that can affect the middle and inner ear simultaneously; causes include otosclerosis involving the ossicles and the cochlea, transverse and longitudinal temporal bone fractures, head trauma, chronic otitis media, cholesteatoma, and middle ear tumors. Some inner ear malformations also can be associated with mixed hearing loss. These include large vestibular aqueduct, lateral semicircular canal dysplasia, superior canal dehiscence, and a bulbous lateral end of the internal auditory canal (IAC); the latter is associated with the absence of the bony partition between the basal turn of the cochlea and the IAC (as seen in the stapes gusher syndrome).

Etiology

A. NONGENETIC CAUSES

The predominant etiology of hearing impairment in children has evolved with advances in medical knowledge and therapeutics. Historically, infectious disorders such as otitis media, maternal rubella infections, and bacterial men-

ingitis as well as environmental factors such as intrauterine teratogenic exposure or ototoxic insult were the dominant causes of congenital and acquired hearing losses. The introduction of antibiotics and vaccines, along with improved knowledge and enhanced awareness about teratogens, has led to a decline in hearing loss resulting from infections and environmental agents.

B. GENETIC CAUSES

Currently, more than half of childhood hearing impairment is thought to be hereditary; hereditary hearing impairment (HHI) can also manifest later in life. HHI may be classified as either **nonsyndromic hearing loss,** in which hearing loss is the only clinical abnormality, or **syndromic hearing loss,** in which hearing loss is associated with anomalies in other organ systems.

Pathogenesis

Hearing occurs by air conduction and bone conduction. In **air conduction,** sound waves reach the ear by propagating in the air, entering the external auditory canal, and setting the tympanic membrane in motion; the movement of the tympanic membrane, in turn, moves the malleus, incus, and stapes of the middle ear. The structures of the middle ear serve as an impedance-matching mechanism, improving the efficiency of energy transfer from the air to the fluid-filled inner ear. Hearing by **bone conduction** occurs when the sound source, in contact with the head, vibrates the bones of the skull; this vibration produces a traveling wave in the basilar membrane of the cochlea.

Cochlear neurons send fibers bilaterally to a network of auditory nuclei in the midbrain, and impulses are transmitted through the medial geniculate thalamic nuclei to the auditory cortex in the superior temporal gyri. At low frequencies, individual auditory nerve fibers can respond more or less synchronously with the stimulating tone. At higher frequencies, phase locking occurs so that neurons alternate in response to particular phases of the sound wave cycle. Three things encode the intensity of sound: (1) the amount of neural activity in individual neurons, (2) the number of neurons that are active, and (3) the specific neurons that are activated.

Nearly two thirds of hereditary hearing impairments are nonsyndromic and the remaining one third is syndromic. Between 70% and 80% of nonsyndromic HHI is inherited in an autosomal recessive manner; another 15–20% is autosomal dominant. Less than 5% is X-linked or maternally inherited via the mitochondria.

Extensive progress has been made in the identification of genes responsible for syndromic and nonsyndromic HHI. Nearly 100 loci harboring genes for nonsyndromic HHI have been mapped with an equal number of dominant and recessive modes of inheritance; 40 different genes have been cloned. In general, the hearing loss associated with dominant genes has its onset in adolescence or adulthood and varies in severity, whereas the hearing loss associated with recessive inheritance is congenital and profound. Among the genes associated with human deafness, *GJB2* encoding for connexin 26 is significant for being associated with nearly 20% childhood deafness. Furthermore, two frame-shift mutations, 35delG and 167delT, account for more than 50% of the cases making population screening feasible. The 167delT mutation is primarily prevalent in the Ashkenazi Jews where it is predicted that 1:1765 individuals will be homozygous and affected. The hearing loss associated with *GJB2* mutations can be variable but is generally severe to profound at birth. In addition, the hearing loss can be variable among the members of the same family, suggesting that other genes likely influence the auditory phenotype.

The contribution of genetics to presbycusis or age-associated hearing loss is also better understood. Several of the nonsyndromic genes are associated with hearing loss that progresses with age. Therefore, it is likely that presbycusis has both environmental and genetic components. Presbycusis is characterized by a loss of discrimination for phonemes, recruitment (abnormal growth of loudness), and particular difficulty in understanding speech in noisy environments. Between 30% and 35% of people over 65 years of age have a hearing loss that is sufficiently great to require a hearing aid.

More than 200 syndromes are associated with hearing loss. Common syndromic forms of hearing loss, among others, include the following: (1) **Usher syndrome** (retinitis pigmentosa and hearing loss), (2) **Waardenburg syndrome** (pigmentary abnormality and hearing loss), (3) **Pendred syndrome** (thyroid organification defect and hearing loss), (4) **Alport syndrome** (renal disease and hearing loss), and (5) **Jervell** and **Lange-Nielsen syndromes** (prolonged QT interval and hearing loss). As a direct result of the rapid advances in the fields of molecular biology and molecular genetics, the responsible genes for the aforementioned syndromes have all been identified. In addition, rapid progress in understanding the basis of these and related disorders has revealed a number of complexities. For example, identification of myosin 7A as the responsible gene for both syndromic and nonsyndromic deafness has led to the abandonment of the "one gene, one disease" dogma. Also, a single gene may cause syndromic or nonsyndromic forms of deafness or may be associated with autosomal dominant or autosomal recessive mode of inheritance.

Prevention

A. VACCINATION

The vaccination of infants against *Haemophilus influenzae* type B meningitis prevents a major cause of acquired deafness, as have immunizations for measles, mumps, and rubella. A vaccine against *Streptococcus pneumoniae,* the most common organism associated with otitis media, is also available and is having a positive impact on the reduction in the incidence of ear infections. In addition, careful monitoring of serum peak-and-trough levels can largely prevent the loss of vestibular function and deafness due to aminoglycoside antibiotics.

B. NOISE AVOIDANCE

Ten million Americans have noise-induced hearing loss and 20 million are exposed to hazardous noise in their employment. Noise-induced hearing loss can be prevented by avoiding exposure to loud noise or by the regular use of earplugs or fluid-filled muffs to attenuate intense sound. Noise-induced hearing loss results from recreational as well as occupational activities and often begins in adolescence.

1. High-risk activities—High-risk activities for noise-induced hearing loss include wood- and metalworking with electrical equipment as well as target practice and hunting with small firearms. All internal-combustion and electric engines, including snowblowers and leaf blowers, snowmobiles, outboard motors, and chain saws, require that the user wear hearing protectors.

2. Education—Almost all noise-induced hearing loss is preventable through education, which should begin before adolescence. Industrial programs of hearing conservation are required when the exposure over an 8-hour period averages 85 dB on the A scale. Workers in such noisy environments can be protected with preemployment audiologic assessment, the mandatory use of hearing protectors, and annual audiologic assessments.

Clinical Findings

A. EVALUATION GOALS

In a patient with auditory complaints, the goals in the evaluation are to determine: (1) the nature of the hearing impairment (conductive or sensorineural); (2) the severity of the impairment (mild, moderate, severe, profound); (3) the anatomy of the impairment (external ear, middle ear, inner ear, or central auditory pathway pathology); and (4) the etiology.

B. SYMPTOMS AND SIGNS

Initially, the history and the physical examination are critical in identifying the underlying pathology leading to the auditory deficit. The history should elicit hearing loss characteristics, including the duration of deafness, the nature of the onset (sudden or insidious), the rate of progression (rapid or slow), and the involvement of the ear (unilateral or bilateral). In addition, the presence or absence of the following conditions should also be ascertained: tinnitus, vertigo, imbalance, aural fullness, otorrhea, headache, facial nerve dysfunction, and head and neck paresthesia. Information regarding head trauma, ototoxic exposure, occupational or recreational noise exposure, and a family history of hearing impairment also may be critical in the differential diagnosis.

1. Sudden onset—A sudden onset of unilateral hearing loss, with or without tinnitus, may represent an inner ear viral infection or a vascular accident. Patients with unilateral hearing loss (sensory or conductive) usually complain of reduced hearing, poor sound localization, and difficulty hearing clearly with background noise.

2. Gradual progression—Gradual progression in a hearing deficit is common with otosclerosis, noise-induced hearing loss, vestibular schwannoma, or Meniere disease. People with small vestibular schwannomas typically present with any or all of the following conditions: asymmetric hearing impairment, tinnitus, and imbalance (although rarely vertigo). Cranial neuropathy, especially of the trigeminal or facial nerve, may accompany larger tumors. In addition to hearing loss, Meniere disease or endolymphatic hydrops may be associated with episodic vertigo, tinnitus, and aural fullness. Hearing loss with otorrhea is most likely due to chronic otitis media or cholesteatoma.

3. Family history—In families with multiple affected members across multiple generations, the family history may be crucial in delineating the genetic basis of hearing impairment. The history may also help identify environmental risk factors that lead to hearing impairment within a family. Sensitivity to aminoglycoside maternally transmitted through a mitochondrial mutation can be discerned through a careful family history. Susceptibility to noise-induced hearing loss or age-related hearing loss (presbycusis) may also be genetically determined.

C. Physical Examination

1. Examination of the ear—The physical examination should evaluate the auricle, external ear canal, and tympanic membrane. In examining the eardrum, the topography of the tympanic membrane is more critical than the presence or absence of the often-cited light reflex. The pars tensa (the lower two thirds of the eardrum) and the pars flaccida (the short process of the malleus) should be examined for retraction pockets that may be evidence of chronic eustachian tube dysfunction or cholesteatomas. Insufflation in the ear canal is necessary to assess tympanic membrane mobility and compliance.

2. Examination of other structures—A careful inspection of the nose, nasopharynx, and upper respiratory tract is indicated. Unilateral serous effusion in the adult should prompt a fiberoptic examination of the nasopharynx to exclude neoplasms. Cranial nerves should be carefully evaluated with special attention to trigeminal and facial nerve function as the dysfunction of these two nerves is most commonly associated with tumors involving a cerebellopontine angle.

3. Evaluation with a tuning fork—Evaluating hearing with a tuning fork can be a useful clinical screening tool to differentiate between conductive and sensorineural hearing loss. By comparing the threshold of hearing by air conduction with that elicited by bone conduction with a 256- or 512-Hz tuning fork, one can infer the site of the lesion responsible for hearing loss. The Rinne and Weber tuning fork tests are used widely both to differentiate conductive from sensorineural hearing losses and to confirm the audiologic evaluation results.

  a. Rinne tuning fork test—The Rinne tuning fork test is very sensitive in detecting mild conductive hearing losses if a 256-Hz fork is used. A Rinne test compares the ability to hear by air conduction with the ability to hear by bone conduction. The tines of a vibrating tuning fork are held near the opening of the external auditory canal, and then the stem is placed on the mastoid process; for direct contact, it may be placed on either teeth or dentures. The patient is asked to indicate whether the tone is louder by air conduction or bone conduction. Normally and in the presence of sensorineural hearing loss, a tone is heard louder by air conduction than by bone conduction. However, with a 30-dB or greater conductive hearing loss, the bone-conduction stimulus is perceived as louder than the air-conduction stimulus.

  b. Weber tuning fork test—The Weber tuning fork test may be performed with a 256- or 512-Hz fork. The stem of a vibrating tuning fork is placed on the head in the midline, and the patient is asked whether the tone is heard in both ears or in one ear better than in the other. With a unilateral conductive hearing loss, the tone is perceived in the affected ear. With a unilateral sensorineural hearing loss, the tone is perceived in the unaffected ear. As a general rule, a 5-dB difference in hearing between the two ears is required for lateralization.

The combined information from the Weber and Rinne tests permits a tentative conclusion as to whether a conductive or sensorineural hearing loss is present. However, these tests are associated with significant false-positive and -negative responses and therefore should be used only as screening tools and not as a definitive evaluation of auditory function.

D. Audiologic Assessment

The minimum audiologic assessment for hearing loss should include the following measurements: (1) pure-tone air-conduction and bone-conduction thresholds, (2) speech reception threshold, (3) discrimination score, (4) tympanometry, (5) acoustic reflexes, and (6) acoustic-reflex decay. This test battery provides a comprehensive screening evaluation of the whole auditory system. It allows the clinician to determine whether further differentiation of a sensory (cochlear) from a neural (retrocochlear) hearing loss is indicated. Refer to Chapter 45, Audiologic Testing, for additional details on audiologic assessment.

E. Imaging Studies

Appropriate radiologic studies may be needed to evaluate both the temporal bone and the auditory pathway. The radiologic evaluation of the ear is largely determined by what structures are being evaluated: the bony anatomy of the external, middle, and inner ear; or the auditory nerve and brain. Plain x-ray films of the ear have been supplanted by computed tomography (CT) and magnetic resonance imaging (MRI). Both CT scans and MRI are capable of identifying inner ear malformations; they are equally able to determine the cochlear patency in the preoperative evaluation of patients for cochlear implantation.

1. CT scans—Axial and coronal CT of the temporal bone with fine 1.00-mm cuts is ideal for determining the caliber of the external auditory canal, the integrity of the ossicular chain, and the presence or absence of middle ear or mastoid disease, and for detecting inner ear malformations. To reliably identify inner ear malformations, measurement of the cochlear height, lateral semicircular canal bony island width, and the vestibular aqueduct should be routinely performed on all temporal bone studies. CT scanning is also ideal for the detection of bone erosion often seen in the presence of chronic otitis media and cholesteatoma.

2. MRI—MRI is superior for imaging retrocochlear pathology such as vestibular schwannomas, meningiomas, other lesions of the cerebellopontine angle that may present with hearing loss, demyelinating lesions of the central nervous system, and brain tumors.

Differential Diagnosis

Synthesis of the findings on clinical history, otologic and physical examination, and audiologic testing is usually sufficient to establish both the nature and the probable cause of a hearing impairment. The different causes of sensorineural hearing loss generally fall into the following categories: (1) developmental and hereditary causes (eg, syndromic and nonsyndromic); (2) infectious disorders (eg, labyrinthitis, otitis media, and viral infection); (3) pharmacologic toxicity (eg, aminoglycosides, loop diuretics, antimalarials, and salicylates); (4) trauma (eg, head injury, acoustic trauma, barotrauma, and irradiation); (5) neurologic disorders (eg, multiple sclerosis); (6) vascular and hematologic disorders (eg, migraine and blood dyscrasias); (7) immune disorders (eg, primary and systemic); (8) bone disorders (eg, otosclerosis and Paget disease); (9) neoplasms (eg, vestibular schwannomas and meningiomas); and (10) disorders of

unknown etiology (eg, presbycusis and Meniere disease). See Table 52–1 for additional information.

Most patients with conductive hearing losses should have axial and direct coronal CT scans of the temporal bones to evaluate the external and middle ear. Patients with unilateral or asymmetric sensorineural hearing losses should have an MRI of the head with gadolinium enhancement to exclude tumors of the cerebellopontine angle. In the presence of vestibular symptoms, patients may require electronystagmography and caloric testing.

Treatment

A. Creating a Favorable Environment for Hearing

A variety of simple interventions can significantly enhance the ability to understand speech in people who are hard of hearing. A critical first step is to eliminate or reduce unnecessary noise (eg, radio or television) to enhance the signal-to-noise ratio. Speech comprehension is aided by lip reading; therefore, the impaired listener should be seated so that the face of the speaker can be seen at all times. Speaking directly into the ear is occasionally helpful; however, more is usually lost than gained in communication when the speaker's face cannot be seen. In addition, the lighting of the speaker's face should be considered. A person who is hard of hearing should sit with his or her back to the window so that the light is on the speaker's face. Speech should be slow enough to make each word distinct, but overly slow speech is distracting and loses contextual and speech-reading benefits. Although speech should be in a loud, clear voice, in sensorineural hearing losses in general and in elderly hearing-impaired individuals in particular, recruitment (the ability to hear loud sounds normally loud) may be difficult. Above all, optimal communication cannot take place unless both parties give it their full and undivided attention.

B. Amplification

Patients with mild, moderate, and severe sensorineural hearing losses are rehabilitated regularly with hearing aids that vary in configuration and strength. Hearing aids have been improved to provide greater fidelity. They also have been miniaturized; the current generation of hearing aids can be placed entirely within the ear canal, thus reducing the stigma associated with their use.

In general, the more severe the hearing impairment, the larger the hearing aid required for auditory rehabilitation. Digital hearing aids lend themselves to programming for the individual; in addition, multiple and directional microphones at the ear level help some individuals with the difficulty of using a hearing aid in noisy surroundings. Since all hearing aids amplify noise as well as speech, the only absolute solution to the problem is to place the microphone closer to the speaker than to the noise source. This arrangement is not possible with a self-contained, cosmetically acceptable device; it is cumbersome and requires a user-friendly environment.

In many situations, including at lectures and at the theater, hearing-impaired persons benefit from assistive devices that are based on the principle of having the speaker closer to the microphone than to any source of noise. Assistive devices include infrared and FM transmission; they also include an electromagnetic loop placed around the room for transmission to the individual's hearing aid. Hearing aids with telecoils also can be used with properly equipped telephones in the same way.

C. Cochlear Implants

In the event that a hearing aid provides inadequate rehabilitation, cochlear implants are appropriate. The criteria for implantation are undergoing constant revisions; an adult candidate has severe to profound hearing loss with a word recognition score of less than 40% under the best-aided conditions. Children with congenital and acquired profound hearing impairment are also appropriate candidates for cochlear implantation; many are being implanted as early as 6 to 9 months.

Cochlear implants are neural prostheses that convert sound energy to electrical signals and can be used to stimulate the auditory division of the eighth nerve directly. In most cases of profound hearing impairment, the auditory hair cells are lost, but the spiral ganglion cells of the auditory division of the eighth nerve are preserved. Cochlear implants are a specialized hearing prosthesis for the rehabilitation of profound deafness that convert mechanical sound energy into electrical signals that are delivered to the neurons of the cochlear nerve. The basic operation of the implant is as follows: A microphone is used to pick up acoustic information that is sent to an external speech processor (located on the body or at ear level). This processor converts the mechanical acoustic wave into an electric signal that is transmitted via the surgically implanted electrode array in the cochlea to the auditory nerve. A patient with cochlear implants experiences sound that helps with speech reading, allows open-set word recognition, and helps in modulating the individual's own voice. Usually within 3 months of implantation, adult patients can understand speech without visual cues. With the current generation of multichannel cochlear implants, almost 75% of the patients with these implants are able to converse on the telephone. Bilateral cochlear implants hold the promise of enhanced sound localization and improvement in understanding speech in the presence of background noise.

D. Brainstem Auditory Implant

For individuals who have had both eighth nerves destroyed by trauma or bilateral vestibular schwannomas (eg, patients with neurofibromatosis II), a brain-stem auditory implant placed near the cochlear nucleus may provide auditory rehabilitation. With additional advances in brainstem auditory implant technology, patients may eventually obtain benefits similar to individuals who have cochlear implants.

E. Therapy for Tinnitus

Tinnitus, a perception of abnormal sounds such as ringing or roaring noises, can often accompany hearing loss. The treatment of tinnitus is particularly problematic; the treatment does not cure it, and therapy is usually directed toward minimizing the appreciation of tinnitus.

The relief of tinnitus may be obtained by masking it with background music. Hearing aids also are helpful in tinnitus suppression, as are tinnitus maskers, devices that present a sound to the affected ear that is more pleasant to listen to than the tinnitus. The use of a tinnitus masker is often followed by several hours of inhibition of the tinnitus. Antidepressants are also beneficial in helping patients deal with tinnitus, although the exact mechanism by which they work is unknown.

Prognosis

A. Temporary Hearing Loss

Hearing loss due to an incident of noise exposure generally produces a temporary loss that recovers within 24 to 48 hours. However, if the noise is of high enough intensity or is repeated often enough, permanent hearing loss results.

B. Irreversible Hearing Loss

Sensorineural hearing loss is a condition that is generally irreversible. Presbycusis is a type of sensorineural hearing loss that is both progressive and irreversible.

Acoustic trauma consists of a single exposure to a hazardous level of noise resulting in a permanent loss without an intervening temporary loss. Given the poor prognosis for most causes of sensorineural hearing loss, the primary goals in management are the prevention of further losses and functional improvement with amplification and auditory rehabilitation.

Gates GA, Mills JH. Presbycusis. *Lancet.* 2005;366(9491):1111. [PMID: 16182900] (An excellent review of presbycusis.)

Kricos PB. Audiologic management of older adults with hearing loss and compromised cognitive/psychoacoustic auditory processing capabilities. *Trends Amplif.* 2006;10(1):1. [PMID: 16528428] (Overview of clinical management of older individuals who often have limitations in cognitive and psychoacoustic auditory processing capabilities.)

Purcell DD, Fischbein NJ, Patel A, Johnson J, Lalwani AK. Two temporal bone CT measurements increase recognition of malformations and predict SNHL. *Laryngoscope.* 2006;116(8):1439. [PMID: 16885750] (Inner ear measurements combined with visual inspection improves detection of temporal bone abnormalities.)

The Aging Inner Ear

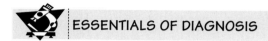

53

Anil K. Lalwani, MD

Presbycusis

- *High-frequency hearing loss.*
- *Reduced clarity of hearing.*
- *Absence of retrocochlear pathology.*

Presbystasis

- *Generalized imbalance.*
- *Absence of vertigo.*

General Considerations

Genetically determined and environmentally affected, the inner ear, like other organ systems, undergoes degenerative changes with aging. These changes result in a variable functional disability. In the United States, hearing difficulty is reported by 25% to 30% of people in the age group of 65 to 70 years and by nearly 50% of those over 75 years of age. It has been estimated that between 1.5% and 3.0% of the total population would benefit from hearing aids. Vestibular dysfunction is also common in the elderly, with reported prevalence of vertigo, dysequilibrium, or imbalance to be as high as 47% in men and 61% in women over the age of 70. The incidence of falling in individuals over the age of 65 is between 20% and 40% in those living at home and is twice as frequent for the institutionalized elderly. These falls are associated with significant morbidity and mortality and constitute one of the leading causes of death among the elderly.

The specialized neural cells of the auditory and vestibular systems are nonmitotic and thus cannot undergo replication and renewal. During the course of a lifetime, DNA transcription errors and insoluble pigments accumulate, and protein synthesis becomes increasingly inefficient. In addition, environmental and external factors such as noise trauma, physical trauma, ototoxic substances, and medications contribute to senescence. More recently, the contribution of genetics to age-related hearing loss is being appreciated.

Pathogenesis

A. AGE-RELATED HEARING LOSS

Hearing loss in the elderly is multifactorial and is due to the convergence of various risk factors. **Presbycusis** is the otherwise unexplained, slowly progressive, predominantly high-frequency symmetric hearing loss due to the aging process (Figure 53–1). Progressive high-frequency hearing loss has been clearly documented by numerous studies in populations over the age of 40 (Figure 53–2A). Older patients with presbycusis also have more diminished speech discrimination than younger patients with the same level of pure-tone averages (Figure 53–2B). This suggests that neural processing is affected in addition to end-organ dysfunction.

Central pathology includes increased synaptic time in the auditory pathway, increased information processing time, and decreased neural cell population in the auditory cortex. Thus, the older patient is handicapped by decreased hearing as well as the decreased ability to discriminate between similar words. The ability to discriminate between words further deteriorates in a noisy background. In addition, the ability to identify very small interaural time differences deteriorates. Consequently, there is a decrease in directional hearing, further limiting the understanding of speech.

The hearing loss that occurs with aging is not inevitable. Some individuals reach advanced age and maintain perfectly normal hearing. For example, the Mabaans, a Sudanese tribe who live in an almost silent environment, exercise daily, and abstain from smoking and eating animal fats, have significantly better hearing than age-matched control groups from industrialized areas in the United States. Similarly, other studies have shown that hearing loss is associated not only with noise exposure, but with hyperlipidemia, hypertension, and vascular disease. This has led some clinicians to consider presbycusis as "socio-acusis" and to suggest that preventive measures such as limiting exposure to noise may substantially reduce the hearing loss that accompanies aging. Through military, industrial, and recreational (eg, hunting or target practice) activities, men typically receive significantly greater noise exposure than women. Thus, the higher incidence and

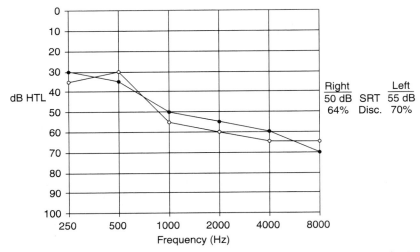

Figure 53–1. Presbycusis. The audiogram shows a moderate to severe downsloping sensorineural hearing loss, with a decreased speech discrimination score.

greater severity of presbycusis in men also argues in favor of the role of environmental causes.

Morphologic studies of human temporal bones have demonstrated an age-related loss of inner and outer hair cells and supporting cells, with the greatest loss being in the basal turn of the cochlea. There is greater loss of outer hair cells compared with inner hair cells; however, these changes have not been directly correlated with auditory function. Age-related loss in spiral ganglion cells, eighth nerve fibers, and neurons in cochlear nuclei have been demonstrated (Figure 53–2C). Some studies have reported changes in the brainstem-evoked response with aging, suggesting alteration at the level of the superior olivary complex, the lateral lemniscus, or the inferior colliculus. Thus, age-related auditory dysfunction results from aggregate deterioration of the entire auditory pathway.

The exact cause of presbycusis remains speculative, in part because of the difficulty in separating the contribution of various etiologic factors such as diet, nutrition, metabolism, arteriosclerosis, ototoxic exposure, and noise trauma. Many believe that genetic predisposition alone makes age-related biologic degeneration of the auditory system inevitable. Lifelong acoustic trauma and genetically programmed senescence are the most likely causes of age-related hearing loss.

B. AGE-RELATED BALANCE DISTURBANCE

Degenerative changes and atrophy have been noted throughout the vestibular apparatus, including the otoconia, vestibular epithelium, vestibular nerve, Scarpa ganglion, and cerebellum. In the otolithic organs (the utricle and saccule), statoconia progressively demineralize and

fragment, resulting in a decreased responsiveness to gravity and linear acceleration. The migration of degenerated otoconial debris into the dependant ampulla of the posterior semicircular canal may result in positional balance disturbances (cupulolithiasis or benign paroxysmal positional vertigo). After age 70, there is also a 20% decrease in the number of hair cells in the maculae of otolith organs and a 40% decrease in cristae of the semicircular canals. Type I hair cells are affected more than Type II hair cells.

In the sensory epithelium, there is accumulation of inclusion bodies, lipofuscin, and vacuoles. Atrophy and scar formation are also present in the sensory epithelia. A reduction in the number of ganglion cells in the Scarpa ganglion occurs earlier, by age 60. Beginning at age 50, there is a loss of nerve fibers between the vestibule and the Scarpa ganglion. The greatest loss occurs among the thick myelinated fibers of the cristae. Lipofuscin accumulation in the vestibular nuclei has also been observed. In the cerebellum, there is loss of Purkinje cells beginning in the fifth decade. **Presbyastasis** is a dysequilibrium that occurs with aging and should be used only as a diagnosis of exclusion.

Clinical Findings

A. PRESBYCUSIS

Classically, four types of presbycusis have been defined: sensory, neural, metabolic or strial, and conductive (Table 53–1). These types may occur in isolation or in combination.

1. Sensory presbycusis—Sensory presbycusis is audiometrically characterized as bilateral, symmetric high-tone hearing loss with an abruptly sloping threshold pattern

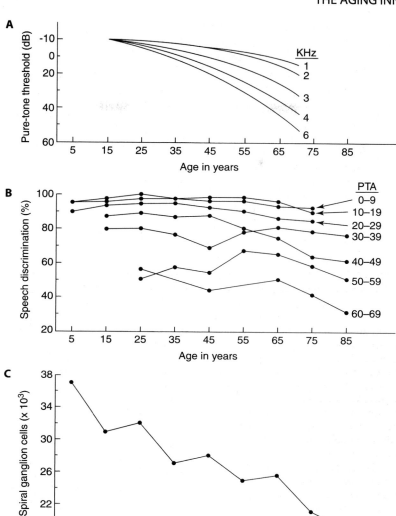

Figure 53–2. **(A)** Hearing level as a function of age. Pure-tone hearing level increases with age, and higher frequencies are affected more than the lower frequencies. **(B)** Speech discrimination as a function of age. For a given pure-tone hearing loss, the speech discrimination decreases with aging. **(C)** Total ganglion cell population versus age. There is progressive loss of cochlear neurons as a function of aging. (A, adapted from Glorig A, Davis H. Age, noise and hearing loss. *Ann Otol Rhinol Laryngol.* 1961;70:5571; B, adapted from Jerger J. Audiologic findings in aging. *Adv Otorhinolaryngol.* 1973;20:115; C, adapted from Otte J, Schuknecht HF, Kerr AG. Ganglion cell populations in normal and pathological human cochleae. Implication for cochlear implantation. *Laryngoscope.* 1978;88:1234.)

Table 53-1. Characteristics of hearing loss in presbycusis.

Type	Pure Tones	Speech Discrimination
Sensory	High tones, abrupt slope	Related to frequencies lost
Neural	All frequencies	Severe loss
Strial	All frequencies	Minimal loss
Cochlear conductive	High tones, gradual slope	Related to steepness of high-tone loss

that begins in middle age. Speech discrimination is directly correlated with the preservation of high-frequency hearing. Histologically, there is loss of a both hair cells and supporting sustentacular cells isolated to the basal turn of the cochlea. The initial flattening of the organ of Corti is followed by secondary neural degeneration. The middle and apical turns of the cochlea containing the speech frequencies are usually spared. These pathologic changes are similar to those seen with noise trauma.

2. Neural presbycusis—Neural presbycusis is characterized by a loss of cochlear neurons involving the whole cochlea and is associated with a significant loss of speech discrimination. The loss of speech discrimination is more profound than would be predicted on the basis of a pure-tone threshold level alone. Although it may occur at any age, hearing difficulty is not noted until the neuronal population falls below a critical number. A downward-sloping audiogram with a variable slope is characteristic. It has been shown that the magnitude of speech discrimination loss directly correlates with the extent of cochlear neuronal loss in the region corresponding to the speech frequencies in the cochlea.

3. Strial presbycusis—Strial presbycusis is characterized by a flat pure-tone audiogram with excellent speech discrimination. The stria vascularis is a metabolically active region of the cochlea that is responsible for the secretion of endolymph and the maintenance of ionic gradients across the organ of Corti. In strial presbycusis, a slowly progressive hearing loss begins in middle age. Pathologically, there is a patchy atrophy of the stria vascularis in the middle and apical turn of the cochlea, without loss of cochlear neurons. Strial atrophy may also involve the entire cochlea. The magnitude of atrophic changes correlates directly with the level of the hearing loss. The quality of endolymph is thought to be affected by strial degeneration, resulting in a loss of energy available to the end organ.

4. Conductive presbycusis—Changes in the mechanical characteristics of the basilar membrane have been suggested as causative of the gradually sloping high-frequency hearing loss of middle age. Cochlear conductive presbycusis lacks discernible pathologic changes within the inner ear. Without confirmation from direct micromechanical measurements, cochlear conductive presbycusis remains a theoretical category of presbycusis. The speech discrimina-tion is said to be diminished in relation to the magnitude of pure-tone loss.

B. NOISE TRAUMA

Noise trauma, in addition to presbycusis, is an important cause of sensorineural hearing loss in the elderly. Exposure to sounds greater than 85 dB for prolonged periods of time is potentially injurious to the cochlea and may result in a high-frequency biased hearing loss that is typically maximal at 4000 Hz (Figure 53–3). With continued acoustic trauma, the hearing loss progresses to involve the primary speech frequencies and therefore further affects speech communication. Because of the similarities between noise-induced hearing loss and presbycusis, assessing the relative contribution of each to auditory dysfunction in the elderly is often difficult. Preventive measures, including monitoring noise levels in the workplace, wearing earplugs and earmuffs, and avoiding loud noise exposure, should aid in diminishing noise-induced hearing loss.

C. PRESBYSTASIS

Vertigo is the cardinal symptom of vestibular disease. Although it is usually described as a rotatory sensation, it may take the form of any illusion of movement such as rocking, ground rolling, or a sense of falling forward or backward.

Dysequilibrium is a sense of poor coordination with erect posture or during a purposeful movement. Vertigo is usually episodic; dysequilibrium is typically continuous. The term **imbalance** implies an orthopedic (eg, hip disease) or neurologic (eg, hemiparesis) problem. **Dizziness** is an all-encompassing term used by the patient and may include vertigo, dysequilibrium, or imbalance. It may also be used to denote a light-headed feeling, as in postural hypotension or hypoglycemia, or to indicate an inability to concentrate.

Equilibrium problems are common in the elderly. Like the auditory system, the vestibular and balance systems also undergo degenerative changes, resulting in significant clinical disability. An estimated 50–60% of elderly patients living at home and 81–91% of patients in an outpatient geriatric clinic complain of dizziness. By age 80, one in three people will have suffered a fall associated with significant morbidity. Vestibular symptoms precede these falls in

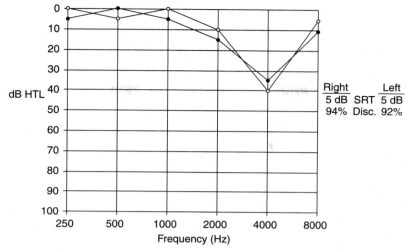

Figure 53–3. Noise-induced hearing loss. The audiogram shows a typical bilateral high-frequency sensorineural hearing loss, most severe at 4000 Hz, with a normal speech discrimination score.

more than half of the patients. The diagnostic evaluation of elderly patients complaining of dizziness yields a specific diagnosis in less than a third of the patients.

D. PATIENT EVALUATION

A thorough vestibular evaluation begins with a complete history, a general physical exam, and a specialized neurotologic examination.

E. IMAGING STUDIES

In the presence of asymmetric or sudden hearing loss or vestibular symptoms with associated neurologic findings, a magnetic resonance imaging (MRI) scan with contrast enhancement is indicated to rule out retrocochlear pathology. When inner ear malformations or superior canal dehiscence is suspected, computed tomography (CT) of the temporal bone may be revealing.

F. SPECIAL TESTS

Further evaluation may include electronystagmography, CT scanning, and MRI. **Electronystagmography** is a graduated series of evaluations of the vestibular and vestibuloocular systems that includes caloric responses. It may be useful in establishing the degree of vestibular function in an ear, determining the side of the pathology, and differentiating central from peripheral diseases. **Posturography** is a relatively new method for studying the ability of the subject to maintain balance with changing visual and somatosensory input.

   Rotational testing is available to evaluate the vestibuloocular reflex. After age 70, the elderly exhibit a decline in

caloric response. The relative energy required to maintain balance on the posturography test increases linearly with age until age 70. Studies of the vestibuloocular reflex in the elderly have shown a decreased sensitivity and shorter time constants over a wide range of frequencies of rotational stimuli. Overall, aging affects the vestibular, visual, and proprioceptive information available for central processing, as well as the ability of the central nervous system to process the sensory information and effect motor response.

Differential Diagnosis

A. HEARING LOSS

1. Ototoxicity—Not all hearing loss in the elderly is presbycusis. Ototoxic drugs such as aminoglycoside antibiotics, loop diuretics, and antineoplastic agents (especially cisplatin) may contribute to hearing loss in the elderly. Patients especially at high risk for injury to the auditory system from ototoxic drugs include those with a preexisting hearing loss, those undergoing simultaneous treatment with multiple ototoxic drugs, and those with renal insufficiency. The risk of ototoxic injury can be significantly reduced by monitoring ototoxic exposure with **serial audiometry.** Of course, serum peak-and-trough levels should be measured to establish the lowest possible dose compatible with therapeutic efficacy. Substitution with nontoxic therapy, whenever feasible, is paramount for prevention.

2. Sudden sensory hearing loss—Sudden loss of hearing in one ear is a relatively common occurrence in the elderly. Most cases are the result of thrombotic or embolic obstruction of the internal auditory artery. Although complete losses seldom recover, most partial losses experience some degree of spontaneous improvement within a few weeks to months. Empirical therapy with oral prednisone appears to be of some benefit. Although most sudden losses are idiopathic and presumably vascular, other etiologies, such as acute endolymphatic hydrops, perilymphatic fistula, tertiary syphilis, brainstem ischemia or infarction, demyelinating disease, and vestibular schwannoma, should be considered.

3. Asymmetric hearing loss—Most hearing losses in the elderly are bilateral and symmetric. Unilateral or asymmetric sensorineural hearing loss is atypical and demands further investigation to exclude disease of the central auditory system, such as **vestibular schwannoma.** The most common symptoms of vestibular schwannoma are sensorineural hearing loss, tinnitus, and dysequilibrium.

The initial screening test for the evaluation of asymmetric hearing loss is the **auditory brainstem response** (ABR), which records the changes in the electroencephalogram evoked by sound stimulation. Five waves may be observed in the first 10 ms, corresponding to the activation of the eighth cranial nerve (Wave I), the cochlear nucleus (Wave II), the superior olive (Wave III), the lateral lemniscus (Wave IV), and the inferior colliculus (Wave V). Absent ABR response or interaural latency differences in Wave V > 0.3 ms are suggestive of retrocochlear pathology and warrant further radiologic evaluation. Gadolinium-DTPA–enhanced MRI scanning is the gold standard for evaluating diseases involving the cerebellopontine angle and the internal auditory canal. MRI scanning may also detect brainstem pathology, such as multiple sclerosis or infarction, which can mimic the clinical presentation of vestibular schwannoma.

4. Other types of hearing losses—Less common causes of sensorineural hearing loss in the aged are numerous and include metabolic derangements (eg, diabetes, hypothyroidism, hyperlipidemia, and renal failure); infections (eg, measles, mumps, and syphilis); autoimmune disorders (eg, polyarteritis and lupus erythematosus); physical factors (eg, radiation therapy); and hereditary syndromes (eg, Usher syndrome). The identification of metabolic, infectious, or autoimmune sensory hearing loss is especially important because these hearing losses are occasionally reversible with medical therapy.

B. BALANCE DISTURBANCE

1. Vertebrobasilar insufficiency—In the elderly, vertebrobasilar insufficiency is an important cause of vertigo and dysequilibrium. It usually results from arteriosclerosis with insufficient collateral circulation, but may also be due to compression of vertebral arteries by cervical spondylosis, postural hypotension, or the subclavian steal syndrome. The full-blown clinical presentation of vertebrobasilar ischemia includes vertigo with head motion (especially looking up), dysarthria, numbness of the face, hemiparesis, headache, and diplopia. Less frequently, visual disturbances occur including oscillopsia, field defects, transient blindness, cerebellar ataxia, and dysphagia; drop attacks may also occur, reflecting ischemia of the brainstem and cerebellum. Vertigo or dysequilibrium may occur without other neurologic signs or symptoms. A definitive diagnosis may be established by **four-vessel cerebral angiography,** but is seldom indicated. Presently, there is no effective medical or surgical treatment for vertebrobasilar insufficiency, although rehabilitative measures may be beneficial.

2. Systemic disorders—A plethora of systemic disorders may affect equilibrium and balance in the elderly, including cardiovascular disease, cerebrovascular disease, peripheral vascular disease, neurologic disorders, visual impairment, metabolic disease, and musculoskeletal problems. Therapeutic drugs are frequently responsible for dysequilibrium and postural instability, especially the antihypertensive, antidepressant, and sedative-hypnotic classes.

3. Peripheral vestibular disorders—A host of peripheral vestibular disorders may cause vertigo, including benign paroxysmal positional vertigo (BPPV) or cupulolithiasis, labyrinthitis, vestibular neuronitis, Meniere syndrome, labyrinthine concussion due to trauma, superior canal dehiscence and perilymph fistulas, among others. In younger patients, BPPV is usually secondary to trauma, whereas in the elderly it is usually a result of degenerative processes. Patients complain of intermittent, irregular episodes of vertigo precipitated by rapid head motion. Vestibular suppressant medications are of limited usefulness except during periods of exacerbation. The severity of symptoms may diminish with repetition because of habituation. Patients usually respond to vestibular exercises, and spontaneous resolution occurs within 1 year in most cases.

4. Meniere syndrome—Meniere syndrome is characterized by episodic severe vertigo, fluctuating sensorineural hearing loss, tinnitus, and ear "fullness." Pathologically, there is distention of the endolymphatic system throughout the inner ear, presumably due to dysfunction of the endolymphatic sac. The clinical course is highly variable, with clusters of severe episodes interspersed with periods of remission of variable duration. Management may include a sodium-restricted diet, diuretics, vasodilators, vestibular suppressants, and, occasionally, surgery to decompress the endolymphatic system.

5. Acute labyrinthitis—Probably a viral infection of the inner ear, acute labyrinthitis causes both severe vertigo and hearing loss. Typically, it runs its course over a period of 1–2 weeks, although residual hearing loss and the periodic recurrence of vertigo are common sequelae. Vestibular neuronitis also presents with vertigo similar to labyrinthitis, but is unaccompanied by auditory symptoms.

Treatment

A. REHABILITATION OF HEARING LOSS

1. Hearing aids—Nearly 30 million people, or 10% of the US population, have hearing problems in one or both ears. In the elderly, the reduced ability to discriminate sounds and to understand speech in a noisy background can be minimized with auditory rehabilitation, usually through amplification. Contemporary hearing aids are comparatively free of distortion and have been miniaturized to the point where they often may be contained entirely within the ear canal. To optimize the benefit, a hearing aid must be carefully selected to conform to the nature of the hearing loss. Digitally programmable hearing aids have recently become available and promise substantial improvements in speech intelligibility, especially under difficult listening circumstances.

2. Assistive devices—Aside from hearing aids, many assistive devices are available to improve comprehension in individual and group settings to help with hearing television and radio programs and to assist in telephone communication.

a. Television devices—Television devices include headphones that plug into the listening jack of the television, listening loops for use with the telecoil on a hearing aid, and wireless infrared devices that send the television signal directly to the listener via a receiver.

b. Telephone amplifiers and devices—Portable and nonportable telephone amplifiers are available to increase the loudness of the telephone audio signal. Handset amplifiers built directly into the telephone base or earphones are widely available. Telephone devices for the deaf using message screens or paper printouts are available for severe or profoundly hearing-impaired individuals.

c. Cochlear implants—The cochlear implant, an electronic device that is surgically implanted to stimulate the auditory nerve, is playing an increasingly important role in the audiologic rehabilitation of the elderly with severe or profound sensorineural hearing loss.

B. REHABILITATION OF VESTIBULAR DYSFUNCTION

1. Nonsurgical measures

a. Pharmacologic agents—Many drugs have been used for the symptomatic relief of vertigo. The most commonly used drugs are antihistamines, sedative-hypnotics, and anticholinergics. Therapy with a combination of pharmacologic agents may be efficacious when single-drug therapy has been ineffective.

(1) Vestibular suppressants—Vestibular suppressants should be used to lessen the unpleasant sensation and alleviate vegetative symptoms such as nausea and vomiting. However, they should be used only for a short duration of 1–2 weeks because they adversely affect the process of central compensation following acute vestibular disease. In acute, severe vertigo, diazepam, 2.5–5.0 mg administered intravenously, may abate an attack.

(2) Antiemetics—Relief from nausea and vomiting usually requires an antiemetic delivered intramuscularly or by rectal suppository (eg, prochlorperazine, 10 mg intramuscularly, or 25 mg rectally, every 6 hours).

(3) Antihistamines—Antihistamines may be used for less severe vertigo. Examples include meclizine or dimenhydrinate, 25–50 mg administered orally every 6 hours.

(4) Anticholinergic medications—Transdermal scopolamine, which is in widespread use for the suppression of motion sickness, is also useful in the management of vertigo. In the elderly, however, anticholinergic therapy is frequently complicated by mental confusion and urinary obstruction; the latter is found especially in males. The use of transdermal scopolamine may also be limited owing to the side effects of dry mouth and blurred vision and is contraindicated in glaucoma patients. A therapeutic effect with fewer side effects may be achieved by cutting the patch in half or even to one quarter of its size. Careful hand washing after handling the patches is necessary to prevent inadvertent eye contact, which could result in prolonged pupillary dilatation and possible acute narrow-angle glaucoma.

b. Exercise and physical therapy—After nausea and vomiting have resolved, exercise should be encouraged to enhance central compensation following peripheral labyrinthine dysfunction. Physical activity is the single most important element in functional recovery after acute labyrinthine dysfunction. Patients should be instructed to repeatedly perform maneuvers that provoke "vertigo-up" to the point of nausea or fatigue in an effort to habituate them. Many patients find vestibular exercise programs (eg, Cawthorne exercises) helpful. A formal physical therapy program designed to identify and correct maladaptive compensation strategies may also prove beneficial.

2. Surgical measures—Surgical intervention may be helpful in selected patients who continue to have disabling symptoms despite a prolonged and varied course of medical therapy. Surgical therapy may include sectioning of the vestibular nerve in a hearing ear or a labyrinthectomy in a deaf ear.

Prognosis

Hearing loss associated with aging is progressive. However, the rate of progression is variable. Age-related hearing loss usually progresses at a rate of 1 dB/y. Rehabilitation of the older deaf individual is often less than satisfactory. Amplification, though helpful in making sound audible, usually does not adequately address the reduction in clarity. Cochlear implantation offers the hope of restoring audition and clarity to profoundly deaf individuals.

Imbalance can often be stabilized, but normal balance cannot be restored. Physical activity can play a critical role in the functional recovery of patients, allowing them to tend to routine daily activities with greater assurance.

Ekvall Hansson E, Mansson NO, Hakansson A. Benign paroxysmal positional vertigo among elderly patients in primary health care. *Gerontology.* 2005;51(6):386. [PMID: 16299419] (Benign paroxysmal positional vertigo may be very common in the elderly.)

Gates GA, Mills JH. Presbycusis. *Lancet.* 2005;366(9491):1111. [PMID: 16182900] (Excellent review of presbycusis.)

Hereditary Hearing Impairment

Nicolas Gürtler, MD

ESSENTIALS OF DIAGNOSIS

- *In most cases, sensorineural hearing loss of unknown origin.*
- *Positive family history often present.*
- *Vestibular symptoms possible, but rare.*
- *In syndromic cases, associated with other clinical abnormalities.*

General Considerations

Hearing loss is the most common sensory deficit in humans. The prevalence of congenital hearing loss in newborns is approximately 1–3 cases per 1000. More than 60% of these prelingual cases (ie, hearing loss before the acquisition of speech) are attributed to congenital causes. A further 1 in 1000 children becomes deaf before adulthood. In patients over 60 years of age, approximately half show a hearing loss > 25 dB. A large percentage of these populations is estimated to be likely affected by genetic influences, although age-related epidemiologic studies of the genetic contribution to hearing loss are not available. Finally, more than 100 deafness genes are believed to exist. These figures illustrate the impact of hearing loss on the public health system and the importance of genetic factors.

Classification

The most common and useful distinction in hereditary hearing impairment is syndromic versus nonsyndromic hearing impairment. Seventy percent of hereditary hearing impairments are nonsyndromic, whereas a minority of 15–30% are syndromic (Figure 54–1).

A. NONSYNDROMIC HEREDITARY HEARING IMPAIRMENT

Nonsyndromic hereditary hearing impairment is classified by the mode of inheritance. Autosomal recessive transmission (designated by prefix DFNB) is implicated in approximately 80% of cases, autosomal dominant transmission (DFNA) is present in approximately 20%

of cases, and X-linked (DFN) and mitochondrial transmission are responsible for < 2% of cases (see Figure 54–1). One single gene, *GJB2* (Gap-Junction Beta 2 or connexin 26), has emerged to be the most common cause of recessive deafness, and up to 40% of the onset of sporadic prelingual hearing impairment can be attributed to defects in this gene both in Europe and the United States. The prevalence is higher in southern Europe than in northern Europe, probably owing to one single gene mutation, 35delG. In a stretch of six guanines extending from position 30 to 35, one base pair is deleted. The high incidence of this mutation seems to be due to a common ancestor. Other common mutations include 167delT in Ashkenazi Jews and 235delC in the Japanese population. Recently, a common digenic pattern of inheritance involving *GJB2* and *GJB6* has been detected. Patients with a monoallelic mutation in *GJB2* harbor in addition a deletion of *GJB6*.

Mitochondrial genes constitute a small and unique group. Inheritance is entirely through the mother, because the maternal oocyte is the sole contributor of mitochondria. Although hearing loss occurs frequently in mitochondrial diseases, it is much more seldom the only symptom. The A1555G mutation in the *12srRNA* gene is the most important one among inherited hearing impairment with mitochondrial transmission.

B. SYNDROMIC HEREDITARY HEARING IMPAIRMENT

Syndromic hearing impairment means that hearing loss is accompanied by other clinical abnormalities. More than 400 syndromes that include hearing loss have been described in detail. Currently, syndromic hearing loss is categorized as follows: (1) syndromes due to cytogenetic or chromosomal anomalies; (2) syndromes transmitted in a classic monogenic or mendelian inheritance; or (3) syndromes due to multifactorial influences, in which the phenotype results from a combination of genetic and environmental factors. The breakdown of the genetic code of the various syndromes will most certainly lead to a classification based on molecular-genetic findings.

Cryns K, Van Camp G. Deafness genes and their diagnostic applications. *Audiol Neurootol.* 2004;9:2. [PMID: 14676470] (Detailed description of today's understanding of the molecular findings in hereditary hearing loss and clinical application.)

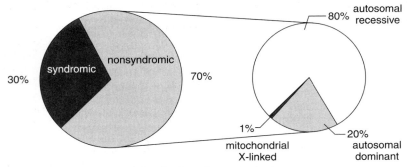

Figure 54–1. Causes and distribution of genetic deafness.

Del Castillo I, Villamar M, Moreno-Pelayo M et al. A deletion involving the connexin 30 gene in nonsyndromic hearing impairment. *N Engl J Med.* 2002;346(4):243. [PMID: 11807148] (First evidence for a digenic pattern of inheritance in hereditary hearing impairment.)

Pathogenesis

Several distinctions are typical of hereditary hearing impairment. Usually, the disease is genetically highly heterogeneous, with many different genes responsible for auditory dysfunction. To complicate things further, different mutations in one gene can cause variable phenotypes (eg, connexin genes in the skin or the ears) or even syndromic and nonsyndromic hearing loss as seen in genes *PDS* (Pendred syndrome and DFNB4), *MYH9* (May-Hegglin/Fechtner syndrome and DFNA17), and *WFS1* (Wolfram syndrome and DFNA6/DFNA14). Finally, a mutated gene can cause dominant and recessive forms of hearing loss. Typical examples include *GJB2* and *TECTA*.

A. NONSYNDROMIC HEREDITARY HEARING IMPAIRMENT

Most of the nonsyndromic genes that cause deafness are not restricted to the cochlea; the inner ear seems to be more sensitive to disruption of some cellular functions than are other organs. In most cases, the function of these genes is only slightly understood. Several genes involved in ion homeostasis and cytoskeleton (ie, hair-cell) structures that lead to deafness have been identified. Other genes include cell-to-cell interaction, transcription factors, extracellular matrix, and a few genes with unknown functions. Nonsyndromic genes discovered by the end of 2005 are listed in Table 54–1, which includes their function and mode of inheritance.

1. Homeostasis—In the homeostasis group, the connexins are the most well known. Three types of connexin genes have been discovered; *GJB2* is the most prevalent. The protein encoded by *GJB2* (connexin 26) belongs to a family of gap-junction proteins responsible for the intercellular transport of ions, metabolites, and second messengers. Based on its expression in the human cochlea in the stria vascularis, the basement membrane, the limbus, and the spiral prominence, as well as in animal studies, the role of *GJB2* seems to lie in recycling potassium ions back to the endolymph of the cochlear duct after stimulation of the sensory hair cells.

2. Hair-cell structure—Unconventional and conventional myosins represent the largest group of genes involved in hair-cell structure and motility. Myosins are actin-dependent molecular motors. Unconventional myosins are found in different locations in the inner ear, including the hair cells. Their various functions include endocytosis, the regulation of ion channels, the movement of vesicles in the cytoplasm, and anchoring stereocilia.

3. Transcription factors—Transcription factors are important for regulating the expression of other genes. The EYA4 protein, for example, regulates the early development of the organ of Corti and maintains its continued function postdevelopmentally.

4. Unknown functioning—The *Wolfram syndrome gene I* (*WFS1*) belongs in the group of genes with an unknown function and seems to cause a unique monogenous disorder. Interestingly, heterozygous missense mutations located at the end of the protein transcript cause hearing loss in the low frequencies only. Most families with low-frequency hearing loss demonstrate a mutation in *WFS1*. The disease-causing mechanism in mitochondrial genes is also mainly speculative. The pathophysiology of the mitochondrial *12srRNA* gene in aminoglycoside-induced ototoxicity is believed to lie in the structural similarity of the mutated gene to bacterial ribosomal RNA, which is the target of aminoglycosides.

Mburu M, Mustapha M, Varela A et al. Defects in whirlin, a PDZ domain molecule involved in stereocilia elongation, cause deafness in the whirler mouse and families with DFNB31. *Nat Gen.* 2003;34(4):421. [PMID: 12833159] (Good example of a deafness gene studied in mice and men.)

Table 54–1. Nonsyndromic hereditary hearing impairment: Genes (as identified by the end of 2001) according to their function and type of inheritance.

Gene	Function	Transmission
KCNQ4	Homeostasis	Autosomal dominant
PRES	Homeostasis	Autosomal recessive
CLDN14	Homeostasis	Autosomal recessive
OTOF	Homeostasis	Autosomal recessive
SLC26A4	Homeostasis	Autosomal recessive
GJB2 (Connexin 26)	Homeostasis	Both
GJB3 (Connexin 31)	Homeostasis	Both
GJB6 (Connexin 30)	Homeostasis	Both
MYOH9	Cytoskeletal system	Autosomal dominant
ACTG	Cytoskeletal system	Autosomal dominant
DIAPH1	Cytoskeletal system	Autosomal dominant
MYO6	Cytoskeletal system	Autosomal dominant
STRC	Cytoskeletal system	Autosomal recessive
ESPN	Cytoskeletal system	Autosomal recessive
MYO15	Cytoskeletal system	Autosomal recessive
WHRN	Cytoskeletal system	Autosomal recessive
CDH23	Cytoskeletal system	Autosomal recessive
MYO7A	Cytoskeletal system	Both
TMC1	Cytoskeletal system	Both
EYA4	Transcription factors	Autosomal dominant
TFCP2L3	Transcription factors	Autosomal dominant
POU4F3	Transcription factors	Autosomal dominant
POU3F4	Transcription factors	X-linked
COLL11A2	Extracellular matrix	Autosomal dominant
COCH	Extracellular matrix	Autosomal dominant
OTOA	Extracellular matrix	Autosomal recessive
TECTA	Extracellular matrix	Both
WFS1	Unknown	
MYO1A	Unknown	Autosomal dominant
DFNA5	Unknown	Autosomal dominant
TMPRRSS3	Unknown	
USH1C	Unknown	Autosomal recessive
TMIE	Unknown	Autosomal recessive

B. Syndromic Hereditary Hearing Impairment

The list of genes responsible for syndromic hearing impairment encompasses diverse molecules, such as enzymes, transcription factors, and cytoskeletal and extracellular matrix components. Although syndromic deafness is mostly inherited in an autosomal dominant fashion, in some cases, the transmission from parents to children does not occur. A classic example is neurofibromatosis, in which approximately 50% of genetic mutations are spontaneous. A summary of genetic findings is listed in Table 54–2.

1. Pendred syndrome—The gene for Pendred syndrome is named *PDS*. Findings based on the expression analysis suggest a putative role as an anion transporter involved in endolymphatic fluid resorption.

2. Waardenburg syndrome—Of the six genes identified in Waardenburg syndrome, four belong to the family of transcription factors that bind DNA and regulate its transcription. The other two genes are members of the group of endothelins and are involved in the development of neural crest–derived cells, which evolve into neurogenic or nonneurogenic sublineages, such as melanocyte precursors.

3. Usher syndrome—Among the 11 mapped loci connected to Usher syndrome, 8 genes are identified. The best studied gene is *MYO7A*, which is implicated in development and functioning of stereocilia.

4. Alport syndrome—Mutated collagen genes are responsible for the phenotype in Alport syndrome. Abnormalities in the basement membrane due to defective collagen Type IV have been demonstrated.

5. Branchio-oto-renal syndrome—Another transcription factor, *EYA1*, plays a predominant role in the pathologic mechanisms of branchio-oto-renal syndrome. Sixty percent of sporadic cases are accounted for by mutations in this gene.

6. Neurofibromatosis Type II—Merlin, the neurofibromatosis Type II gene product, acts as a tumor suppressor. Merlin exact mechanism of action is still under investigation.

7. Jervell-Lange-Nielsen syndrome—Disturbances in the hemostasis of endolymph through the defunct subunits of potassium channels (eg, *KCNE1* and *KVLQT1*) cause Jervell-Lange-Nielsen syndrome.

8. Treacher Collins syndrome—Most mutations in Treacher Collins syndrome result in the introduction of a stop codon with premature termination of the protein product, which plays an unspecified role in nucleolar-cytoplasmic transport.

9. Stickler syndrome—Mutated collagen genes are also responsible for the phenotype in Stickler syndrome. Some evidence points to the organ of Corti as the target organ, at least in Type III.

Table 54–2. Syndromic hereditary hearing impairment: Clinical findings besides hearing loss and associated genes. Most of the molecular analysis with regard to function and localization of the gene is based on the mouse model.

Syndrome	Clinical Findings	Gene		
		Name	Function	Localization
Pendred syndrome	Goiter	PDS	Anion transporter?	Endolymphatic duct and sac, utricle, saccule, cochlea
Waardenburg syndrome	Dystopia canthorum; pigmentary abnormalities of hair, iris and skin	MITF, PAX3, SOX10, SLUG	Transcription factors	Neural-crest-derived cells
		EDN3, EDNRB	Cell development	Melanoblast, neuroblast precursors
Usher syndrome	Retinitis pigmentosa	MYO7A	Cell maintenance?	Hair cells
		USH1C	Protein-protein interaction?	Organ of Corti, saccule, utricle
		CDH23	Cell organizer?	Inner, outer hair cell
		PCDH15	Development of hair cells?	Sensory epithelium, inner ear
		SANS	Development of hair cells?	Hair cells
		USH2A	Development/homeostasis?	Basement membrane
		VLGR1	?	?
		USH3	Cell synapsis?	hair cells, spiral ganglion
Alport syndrome	Renal dysfunction (hematuria with progressive renal failure); ocular abnormalities (lenticonus and retinal flecks)	COL4A3, COL4A4, COL4A5	Collagen formation	Outer sulcus, inner sulcus, basilar membrane, spiral ligament of cochlea
Branchio-oto-renal syndrome	Branchial-derived anomalies (cleft, cysts or fistulas); renal malformations	EYA1 SIX1	Role in development of inner ear	Vestibular organ, inner ear, sensory epithelium inner ear
Neurofibromatosis type II	Bilateral vestibular schwannomas, meningiomas, schwannoma, glioma, neurofibroma in the scalp; juvenile subcapsular cataract	NF2	Tumor suppressor gene	Schwannoma cells
Jervell-lange-nielsen syndrome	Prolonged QT interval with syncopal attacks	KVLQT1, KCNE1	Potassium channel	Stria vascularis
Treacher collins syndrome	Hearing loss due to malformations in the middle and inner ear; craniofacial abnormalities (mandibulofacial dysostosis)	TCOF1	Nucleolar cytoplasmic transport?	Neural folds, branchial arches
Stickler syndrome	Conductive hearing loss possible; eye findings (high myopia, cataract); arthropathy (spondyloepiphyseal dysplasia); cleft palate	COL2A1, COL11A1, COL11A2	Collagen protein	Tectorial membrane

Keats B, Savas S. Genetic heterogeneity in Usher syndrome. *Hum Genet.* 2004;130A:13. [PMID: 15578223] (Good short summary of the seven known genes in Usher syndrome.)

Neff B, Welling B, Akhmametyeva E, Chang LM. The molecular biology of vestibular schwannomas: dissecting the pathogenic process at the molecular level. *Otol Neurotol.* 2006;27:197. [PMID: 16540902] (Description of Merlin's role in schwannomas and genetic implications.)

Prevention

It is most important to detect infants born with nonsyndromic hearing loss early in order to support normal language development. The appropriate management of auditory function is greatly facilitated by early diagnosis. Children in whom intervention begins before 6 months of age can acquire normal language development, in contrast to late intervention, with developmental language quotients of only 50–60%. Even in using risk factors for the proper identification of these children, 50% of infants born with hearing loss will not be identified. Therefore, universal hearing screening programs have been established. They are based on the measurement of otoacoustic emissions and auditory brainstem responses. These methods have been proved to be objective and highly sensitive in identifying infants with greater than mild hearing loss. Only about 15% of hearing-impaired children will be missed by newborn hearing screening because their hearing loss will manifest postnatally, sometimes as late as school age.

Clinical Findings

A. Symptoms and Signs

A thorough history should be taken because it easily allows the physician to separate hereditary hearing impairment from other causes. Questions should cover embryopathies such as rubella, toxoplasmosis, or cytomegalovirus, as well as any ototoxic drug use. An audiologic assessment is mandatory and should include both parents and siblings. A pure-tone audiogram is usually sufficient. In children, testing of the auditory brainstem response and otoacoustic emissions can be performed. All forms of hearing loss can be seen in hereditary hearing impairment. Furthermore, a clear correlation between a characteristic form of hearing loss and a specific gene defect could not be demonstrated, with few exceptions such as *WFS1*. Likewise, a reliable prediction of the development of hearing loss cannot be made except in some syndromic cases. Guidelines on how to approach patients with hereditary hearing impairment are outlined in Figure 54–2.

A thorough physical examination is recommended, especially to detect syndromic hearing loss. The patient's ears should be examined for abnormalities such as auricles and preauricular pits; the patient should also be examined for pigmentary changes in the skin and hair and for a possible neck goiter. To complete a thorough assessment, an ophthalmologic examination and urinalysis/renal ultrasound have to be taken into account. In addition, other specialists, such as pediatricians, ophthalmologists, cardiologists, and others, should be consulted as part of the proper evaluation of these children.

1. Nonsyndromic hereditary hearing impairment— Most cases of profound prelingual hearing loss are associated with DFNB and are almost exclusively due to cochlear defects. In postlingual cases, an autosomal dominant inheritance is predominant; the hearing loss is less severe and besides sensorineural defects, conductive impairments are found. In X-linked disease, hearing impairment in males is earlier in onset and more severe than in females since the disease is transmitted

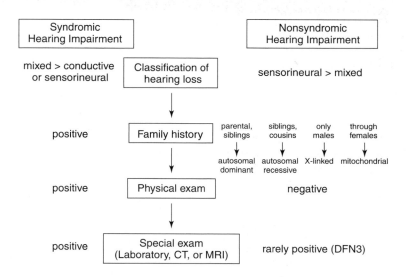

Figure 54–2. Guidelines for evaluating patients with hereditary hearing impairment.

Table 54–3. Clinical classification of Waardenburg syndrome and corresponding genes.

	Sensorineural hearing deficit Iris pigmentary abnormality Hair hypopigmentation ▼		
Type I	**Type II**	**Type III**	**Type IV**
+ dystopia canthorum	+ dystopia canthorum + upper limb abnormalities	– dystopia canthorum	– dystopia canthorum + Hirschsprung disease
PAX3	*MITF, SNAI2*	*PAX3*	*EDNRB, EDN3, SOX10*

only through female family members. Either all of the frequencies or the high frequencies are affected.

Patients with nonsyndromic hereditary hearing impairment demonstrate a few common features. Usually, the hearing loss is symmetric. The U-shaped or "cookie-bite" form is classically indicative for hereditary hearing impairment. In most cases, the hearing threshold is sloping in the middle and high frequencies; rarely, only the low frequencies are affected. The hearing loss can vary from moderate to profound and can be either stable or progressive. One of the best-studied genes, *GJB2*, which accounts for the majority of inherited deafness, has only been associated with a prelingual onset. The role of this gene in postlingual forms still is unclear, since only putative heterozygous mutations have been reported. Functional analysis of most mutations is incomplete or absent. The phenotype of patients with *GJB2* mutations varies enormously, even among siblings, from mild to profound, with audiometric curves that are either flat or sloping.

2. Syndromic hereditary hearing impairment— Syndromic hearing loss may be conductive, sensorineural, or mixed; other clinical features must be considered to allow for the recognition of a distinct entity. More than 400 syndromes that include hearing loss have been described. Most of these syndromes are characterized only clinically, with their underlying molecular mechanisms still unknown. At present, auditory-pigmentary diseases are the largest and best-characterized group and include more than 55 syndromes.

The clinical features of the syndromes that follow are summarized in Table 54–2.

a. Pendred syndrome—Pendred syndrome is the most common syndromic form of deafness, accounting for approximately 10% of cases. It presents with goiter and sensorineural hearing loss. Usually, the goiter is evident before puberty, but an adult onset has also been noted. Thyroid function is evenly divided, with 50% euthyroid patients and 50% hypothyroid patients. In most cases, the hearing loss is congenital, bilateral, moderate to profound, and sloping in the higher frequencies. An enlarged vestibular aqueduct is a consistent finding, and Mondini-type malformations have also been associated. In various studies, caloric testing showed diverging results, with both normal and depressed vestibular function.

b. Waardenburg syndrome—This syndrome is seen in at least 2–5% of patients with congenital hearing loss and includes the following clinical signs: dystopia canthorum; pigmentary abnormalities of the hair, iris, and skin; and sensorineural deafness in 20–50% of patients, depending on the classification type. Four clinical subtypes exist (Table 54–3). Abnormal functioning of the peripheral vestibular system can be found more often than hearing loss.

c. Usher syndrome—Three different types of Usher syndrome, the most common eye/ear syndrome, can be distinguished clinically by the type of hearing impairment, the absence or presence of vestibular responses, and the onset of retinitis pigmentosa (Table 54–4). The

Table 54–4. Classification of Usher syndrome by clinical type and corresponding genes.

Type	IA-F	IIA-C	III
Hearing impairment	Profound, congenital	Sloping, congenital	Progressive
Vestibular response	Absent	Normal	Variable
Onset of retinitis pigmentosa	First decade	First or second decade	Variable
Genes	*MYO7A, USH1C, CDH23, PCDH15, SANS*, 2 unknown	*USH2A, VLGR1*, 1 unknown	*USH3*

genetic classification is incomplete and includes 11 genes. The prevalence of this disorder among deaf children may be as high as 8%. The advancing failure of vision has the greatest impact on the quality of life in patients with this syndrome.

d. Alport syndrome—Alport syndrome is distinguished by hematuria with progressive renal failure, initial high-tone sensorineural hearing loss, and ocular abnormalities such as lenticonus and retinal flecks. The syndrome is seen in at least 1% of patients with congenital hearing impairment.

e. Branchio-oto-renal syndrome—The symptoms of this syndrome can be derived from its name: (1) branchial anomalies (clefts, cysts, or fistulas); (2) otologic anomalies (malformed pinna, preauricular pits, and hearing loss); and (3) renal malformations (hypoplastic kidneys and vesicoureteric reflux). Its prevalence is 2% in profoundly affected children. Sensorineural, conductive, or, most often, mixed hearing loss is seen. Hearing is affected with approximately 80% penetrance.

f. Neurofibromatosis Type II—Neurofibromatosis Type II is characterized by bilateral tumors of the eighth cranial nerve (the vestibulocochlear nerve) and any of the following: meningiomas, schwannomas, gliomas, or juvenile subcapsular cataracts. The symptoms mostly begin in late childhood to early adulthood. Hearing loss, predominantly unilateral, presents in approximately 50% of patients. A molecular diagnosis in sporadic patients is difficult because a high percentage of mosaicism for mutations is seen. Genetic screening should be considered in an asymptomatic, undiagnosed child, who is at risk for NF2 disease.

g. Jervell-Lange-Nielsen syndrome—The frequency of Jervell-Lange-Nielsen syndrome among those patients with a profound congenital hearing loss is approximately 0.25%. Sensorineural hearing loss is accompanied by syncopal attacks due to a prolonged QT interval. Death occurs in childhood if not treated.

h. Treacher Collins syndrome—In Treacher Collins syndrome, the clinical diagnosis is facilitated as distinct craniofacial abnormalities are found. The hearing loss can be related to radiographic findings of malformed cochlear and vestibular apparatus, including the ossicles and external ear canal.

i. Stickler syndrome—Three phenotypes corresponding to three defective genes have been described in Stickler syndrome. The clinical signs include eye symptoms (eg, myopia, astigmatisms, and cataracts), arthropathy, cleft palate, and sensorineural high-tone hearing loss, which has been noted in 80% of cases.

Mitchem KL, Hibbard E, Beyer LA, Bosom K, Dootz GA, Dolan DF, Johnson KR, Raphael Y, Kohrman DC. Mutation of the novel gene *Tmie* results in sensory cell defects in the inner ear of spinner, a mouse model of human hearing loss DFNB6. *Hum Mol Genet.* 2002;11(16):1887. [PMID: 12140191]

B. LABORATORY FINDINGS

Laboratory tests are helpful in distinguishing nonsyndromic from syndromic hereditary hearing impairment. However, full laboratory and radiographic evaluations are expensive, and the rate for obtaining a definite diagnosis is reported to be approximately 40–70%, although a thorough analysis has not been done. Therefore, laboratory tests should be undertaken after careful deliberation. Urinalysis is easy to perform and assesses the presence of proteinuria or hematuria (Alport syndrome). If Pendred syndrome is suspected, thyroid function tests should be requested.

C. IMAGING STUDIES

CT or MRI (fast-spin echo technique or gadolinium-enhanced) are the imaging studies of choice. Abnormalities in the bony structures of the inner ear are detectable on a CT scan. A CT scan is generally recommended in the evaluation of childhood sensorineural hearing loss to detect inner ear malformations that are associated with the higher risk of cerebrospinal fluid leak, meningitis, or traumatic hearing loss. However, most defects are located in the inner ear on a microscopic or molecular-genetic level and therefore are not detectable. The most common abnormality is a large vestibular aqueduct.

D. SPECIAL TESTS

1. Mutation screening—Various mutation detection methods exist and are in use. The methods are based on either conformation-based techniques such as single-stranded conformational polymorphism (SSCP) or on base-mismatch recognition such as denaturing gradient gel electrophoresis (DGGE). The former is more common. Both methods—SSCP, because of its simplicity, and DGGE, because of its high sensitivity—are the favored techniques. Recently, a relatively new technology for rapid automated mutation screening, denaturing high-performance liquid chromatography (DHPLC), has been assessed and found to be highly sensitive and specific for detecting *GJB2* mutations. However, each of these methods for detecting mutations has significant shortcomings, including expense, time, and limited sensitivity. Direct sequencing of the gene is the only method available to identify any number and type of mutation. Although its use is becoming increasingly automatic, the screening of a large population is expensive.

2. Perchlorate challenge test—The perchlorate challenge test can be performed with Pendred syndrome, although it is not specific and its sensitivity is unknown. The perchlorate ion is a competitor of radioactive iodine. In Pendred syndrome with an intrinsic organification defect, perchlorate will displace more iodine than in the normal thyroid gland, which results in a decrease in thyroid radioactivity over time compared with normal uptake.

E. SPECIAL EXAMINATIONS

An ophthalmologic examination (vision acuity, funduscopy, and electroretinogram to detect retinitis pigmentosa) is recommended to detect syndromic features (especially Alport, Stickler, and Usher syndromes) and to distinguish syndromic from nonsyndromic hereditary hearing impairments. Vestibular symptoms are not a typical feature of hereditary hearing impairment. However, if a patient reports dizziness or balance problems, functional testing of the peripheral vestibular system should be performed. For instance, absent vestibular responses can be seen in Usher syndrome Type I and in some forms of autosomal recessive deafness (DFNB4, etc.). Renal ultrasound scan may reveal dysplasia in branchio-oto-renal syndrome. In suspected Jervell-Lange-Nielsen syndrome, an electrocardiogram should be performed.

Gorlin RJ, Toriello HV, Cohen MM Jr. *Hereditary Hearing Loss and Its Syndromes.* New York, NY: Oxford University Press, 1995. (Very comprehensive and detailed description of all syndromes known to be associated with hearing loss.)

Grundfast KM, Siparsky N, Chuong D et al. Genetics and molecular biology of deafness. *Otolaryngol Clin North Am.* 2000;33:1367. [PMID: 11449793] (Very thoughtful proposal for a clinical approach to hereditary hearing disorders.)

Differential Diagnosis

In syndromic cases, the challenge lies more in correctly identifying the syndrome than in missing the inherited forms. In isolated cases of sensorineural hearing loss, all forms of cochleopathies—not just those that are due to hereditary causes—must be included in the differential diagnosis. In chronic noise-induced hearing loss, a history of noise exposure is pathbreaking. A dip in the hearing threshold between 3 and 6 kHz is typical for this condition. Tinnitus may be present and is much more common than in inherited hearing loss. Trauma of the labyrinth can be suggested by the patient history and often results in an asymmetric hearing loss. Metabolic disorders such as hyperlipidemia or uremia are still disputed to be causative for sensorineural hearing loss.

Cochlear otosclerosis is rare as a single entity and is usually accompanied by conductive hearing impairment. Blood and vascular disorders have been associated with hearing impairment. The use of ototoxic drugs and agents should be ascertained by taking the patient history, which should include the patient's profession and any history of pregnancy.

Treatment

Depending on the degree and onset of the patient's hearing loss, various hearing aids, including cochlear implants, have to be evaluated in patients with hereditary hearing impairment. Gene therapy for hearing disorders has potential future applications. Currently, most studies focus on gene delivery. The problems to be overcome are the targeted correction of gene function without systemic side effects, and sustainable changes in the inner ear.

Probst FJ. Correction of deafness in shaker-2 mice by an unconventional myosin in a BAC-gene. *Science.* 1998;280:1444. [PMID: 9603735] (The first time that hearing impairment was corrected by molecular-genetic methods.)

Prognosis

Generally, too little is known to make an accurate prediction in almost all cases of hereditary hearing impairment. Nonetheless, in some syndromic cases, patients can be counseled. In Waardenburg syndrome Type II and Usher syndrome Type III, the hearing loss may be progressive; in Alport syndrome, the hearing loss usually occurs during childhood only.

WEB SITES

[Centrum Medische Genetica]
  http://www.uia.ac.be/cmg/
(This website is a very comprehensive list of nonsyndromic loci and many syndromic loci, including genes, mouse models, and references.)
[The Connexin-Deafness Homepage]
  http://crg.es/deafness/
(This website is dedicated solely to connexin genes and deafness.)

Aural Rehabilitation & Hearing Aids　55

Robert W. Sweetow, PhD, & Troy Cascia, AuD

There has been much cynicism regarding the value of hearing aids. However, a study published in *JAMA* confirmed what audiologists have recognized for decades: Hearing aids do indeed provide substantial benefit and reduce communication problems. The National Council on Aging released the results of a study on the impact of untreated hearing loss in over 2000 hearing-impaired adults and their significant others. Data indicated that individuals with untreated hearing loss were more likely to report depression, anxiety, and paranoia, and less likely to participate in organized social activities compared to those who wear hearing aids. Other studies have indicated that hearing aid use is associated with significant improvements in the social, psychological, emotional, and physical aspects of the lives of hearing-impaired persons with all degrees of hearing loss.

Despite these findings and data indicating significant improvements in satisfaction related to the use of hearing aids featuring high technology (eg, multiple microphones), the percentage of hearing-impaired individuals who own hearing aids has remained steady or declined since 1984 and continues to hover around 20–22%. Many individuals continue to reject hearing aid use for a combination of reasons, including denial of need, stigma, cost, and lack of adequate benefit in the environments in which help is most needed (eg, noisy environments). In addition, patients are not likely to attempt to resolve problems that they are not highly motivated to address without the expressed recommendation of their physician.

Kochkin S. MarkeTrak VII: Hearing loss population tops 31 million people. *Hear Rev.* 2005;12(7)16. (A large survey of demographics and satisfaction among hearing aid users.)

National Council on Aging. The consequences of untreated hearing loss in older persons. *ORL Head Neck Nurs.* 2000;18(1):12. [PMID: 11147549] (Untreated hearing-impaired patients showed a wide range of significant hearing and emotional problems relative to those receiving amplification.)

Strom KE. Twenty trends influencing the hearing health care field. *Hear Rev.* 2005;12(13):16. (A detailed description of the demographics of hearing aid use in the United States.)

PATIENT CANDIDACY

Types of Hearing Loss

Decades ago, it was believed that the use of hearing aids was limited to individuals with conductive hearing impairment and would not be helpful for individuals with a sensorineural hearing loss. Patients were informed that hearing aids could make sounds louder, but would not make them clearer. Currently, technologic improvements and improved fitting strategies allow for the successful fitting of hearing aids in most individuals with a sensorineural hearing impairment.

Degree of Hearing Loss

Hearing loss is too complex to be characterized by a single measure. Indeed, an audiogram provides information only about one aspect of hearing: threshold sensitivity. The reality is that individuals rarely listen at their hearing threshold. Instead, speech occurs at suprathreshold levels, and the intensity levels that an impaired cochlea is exposed to are considerably higher than normal because of amplification. For some patients, stimulation at high intensity levels enhances auditory function, but for others, it may not. Thus, the prognostic value of amplification and determination of candidacy for hearing aids on the basis of the degree of hearing loss is, at best, a questionable practice. If necessary, however, the following broad guidelines may be used (for a motivated individual).

A. MILD HEARING LOSS (20–40 DB)

Hearing aid use may be helpful depending on the patient's communicative needs. Some may prefer to use amplification only on a part-time basis.

B. MODERATE HEARING LOSS (45–65 DB)

Amplification is needed and is usually successful if proper fitting strategies are used.

C. SEVERE HEARING LOSS (70–85 DB)

Amplification is necessary if the patient wishes to use the auditory channel as the primary receptive mode. Cochlear implants may be considered if hearing aids are unsuccessful.

D. PROFOUND HEARING LOSS (> 85 DB)

At a minimum, amplification is useful as a warning device; at a maximum, it allows the patient auditory use and likely enhances speech reading capabilities. Its effectiveness may depend on the age at which amplification is first used. Individuals with a profound hearing loss may be strong candidates for cochlear implantation.

Audiometric Configuration

With the versatility available in digital hearing aids, audiometric configuration is much less of an issue in determining candidacy.

Word Recognition (Speech Discrimination)

In general, patients with good word recognition scores are more likely to do better with hearing aids. However, it would be a mistake to conclude that either success or failure would depend on this single factor. Word recognition assessed in a sound-treated test booth is not reflective of the variety of difficult listening environments that many hearing-impaired users encounter. Word recognition ability becomes diminished because of four main factors: (1) reduced audibility, (2) cochlear distortions producing reduced frequency and temporal selectivity and resolution, (3) abnormal central auditory processing, and (4) diminished cognitive function. Modern hearing aid technology allows the audiologist the ability to correct reduced audibility. The other three factors, however, may not be subject to correction by amplification; they can, in fact, render a poor prognosis for success with amplification. Furthermore, word recognition testing is typically performed in a quiet environment. It is well known that individuals with a sensorineural hearing loss have considerably more difficulty understanding speech in a noisy environment. This difficulty is often a function of both peripheral and central disorders and may be particularly emphasized in elderly populations.

Patients presenting bilaterally asymmetrical word recognition scores often prefer monaural amplification for the better-hearing ear. There are many exceptions, however, so unless there are other contraindications (eg, extremely poor speech discrimination ability, an extremely limited dynamic range, or medical contraindications), low discrimination scores should not, by themselves, preclude a *trial* with amplification.

Other Factors

It is not unusual to find that the most important factors determining the success or failure of hearing aids are those unrelated to audiometric findings. Specifically, one must take into consideration *all* of the following: (1) the age and general physical and mental health of the patient; (2) the patient's, as opposed to only the family's, motivation; (3) finances; (4) cosmetic considerations; and (5) communication needs.

Unfortunately, despite need, many patients resist trying hearing aids. There is an unfortunate, yet undeniable social stigma attached to wearing hearing aids. The issue of cosmetic vanity is being addressed, in part, by the continuing trend toward miniaturization of hearing devices and the increased use of open coupler devices described later in this chapter. However, not all hearing-impaired listeners are candidates for these hearing aids. It is regrettable that hearing aids are often dispensed to patients who lack motivation for amplification. A poorly motivated patient is a poor candidate for amplification regardless of the degree of hearing loss and should not be forced into trying hearing aids. It is difficult to undo the damage that may be done if a candidate prematurely tries and fails with amplification. For these patients, it may be advisable to wait a year so that they may clearly perceive the need. However, encouraging patients to put forth the effort toward a trial period, with the understanding that it is possible they may be pleasantly surprised, is certainly worthwhile.

Occupational and social demands vary greatly among individuals. A judge who has a mild hearing loss may desperately need amplification, whereas a retired elderly patient with the same degree of hearing loss living alone may not. Patients must ask themselves if the ability to hear, albeit not understand, is acceptable and adequate for their needs. They must unselfishly examine whether they are becoming a burden to others, even if they do not personally recognize difficulty hearing. The critical variable is whether the patient experiences difficulty hearing or increased stress and fatigue in daily function. Amplification may simply relieve the strain of hearing, as opposed to improving word recognition or making sounds louder. This alone, however, can be a significant benefit. Thus, candidacy for amplification should be based on the patient's subjective needs rather than strictly on the basis of the audiogram.

Cox RM, Alexander GC, Gray GA. Who wants a hearing aid? Personality profiles of hearing aid seekers. *Ear Hear.* 2005;26(1):12. [PMID: 15692301] (Candidacy issues.)

NUMBER OF DEVICES REQUIRED

Over 80% of hearing aid fittings in the United States are binaural. A number of factors likely contribute to binaural superiority. Eliminating or minimizing the **head shadow** (the reduction in signal intensity from the side of the head opposite the signal) is important for listeners with a high-frequency hearing loss. Improved **localization** and the better balance of sounds result from hearing sounds from both sides. A central release from masking (**binaural squelch**) may result in better hearing in noise. With **binaural loudness summation**, absolute binaural thresholds are 2–3 dB better than monaural thresholds. This summation effect occurs near threshold but not for high intensities near uncomfortable levels. Thus, the dynamic range of listening is greater for binaural listening than for monaural listening.

Other factors to consider in choosing binaural versus monaural amplification include the possibility of tinnitus reduction regardless of a perceived dominant side because of increased stimulation to more cortical neural substrate, and the legal implications of the potential deprivation of an unaided ear.

The general rule should be that unless there is a significant asymmetry in sensitivity, tolerance to loudness, or word recognition ability, or unless a medical condition exists contraindicating the insertion of anything into the external auditory meatus, the standard should be at least to try binaural amplification. For these patients, a wired or wireless contralateral routing of signal (CROS) aid or transcranial CROS (placing a hearing aid in the "dead" ear, producing bone conduction stimulation of the "good" ear) may be tried. It should be noted that CROS devices should be applied only if the better ear has normal or near-normal hearing, and the transcranial CROS should be used only if the poorer ear has no residual hearing that might produce recruitment or other distortion factors. If the "good" ear is in need of amplification, a BICROS (bilateral contralateral routing of signal), in which microphones are located on both ears but the signal is routed only to the "good" ear, can be tried. In cases of unilateral impairment, candidacy should be based on the individual's communicative needs. It is also possible to try a bone-anchored hearing aid (BAHA) if the impaired ear is unaidable.

Niparko JK, Cox KM, Lustig LR. Comparison of the bone anchored hearing aid implantable hearing device with contralateral routing of offside signal amplification in the rehabilitation of unilateral deafness. *Otol Neurotol.* 2003;24(1):73. [PMID: 12544032] (Bone-anchored hearing aid versus contralateral routing of signal performance for unilateral loss.)

Wazen JJ, Spitzer JB, Ghossaini SN et al. Transcranial contralateral cochlear stimulation in unilateral deafness. *Otolaryngol Head Neck Surg.* 2003;129(3):248. [PMID: 12958575] (Candidacy for transcranial CROS amplification.)

HEARING AID STYLES

Hearing aids are available in a variety of styles, as shown in Figure 55–1. The general categories of hearing aids are (1) completely in the canal (CIC), (2) custom in the canal (ITC), (3) custom in the ear (ITE), (4) behind the ear (BTE), and (5) open-fit mini BTE. Unfortunately, many patients choose a style of hearing aid based strictly on cosmetic factors. Although cosmetic considerations cannot be ignored, decisions regarding which style aid is most appropriate for a specific patient should be based on physical factors such as shape of the pinna, depth of the concha, contour and diameter of the meatus; physical conditions such as drainage and exostoses, excessive production of cerumen, and manual dexterity; and audiologic factors such as degree of loss (patients with profound hearing loss are not candidates for CIC hearing aids), audiometric configuration (patients with regions of normal hearing, particularly in the low frequencies, are best served by systems that do not occlude the ear canal); need for special features (as discussed below); age of the patient; and cost of the devices (Table 55–1).

Probably the most common inquiry from patients today relates to whether they can use one of the small, "invisible" hearing aids. Hearing aids keep getting smaller, but smaller does not necessarily mean better. A canal-style hearing aid implies that no part of the hearing aid extends into the concha area. There are two types of canal-style hearing aids: the CIC and the ITC. The CIC is the smallest hearing aid and ideally is inserted several millimeters into the canal extending into the osseous portion of the meatus, and terminating within 5 mm of the tympanic membrane. The hearing aid is removed by a monofilament that lies near the tragal notch. The ITC is slightly larger, filling the cartilaginous portion (outer half) of the ear canal and is more visible than the CIC. Although CIC devices are the most cosmetically appealing for most ears, they are more difficult to keep clean because a small amount of wax can block the receiver. However, newer wax guard designs are significantly minimizing this problem. They are also the most expensive style of hearing aid and are more susceptible to acoustic feedback because of the close proximity of the microphone to the receiver, although digital feedback suppression decreases this concern. In addition, placement inside the meatus may produce a feeling of fullness and an occlusion effect that adversely impacts the perception of the user's own voice, giving the impression that one is talking inside a barrel. This occurs because low-frequency laryngeal vibrations are trapped inside the closed ear canal. To avoid this effect, it is often necessary to open the ear canal by venting the shell, although this may be problematic for small devices.

Although less cosmetically appealing than smaller instruments, larger devices may solve many of these above-mentioned problems. The ITE fills the entire concha, whereas the BTE consists of two parts: a hearing aid that hooks onto and rests behind the pinna and a custom earmold attached by a tube that secures the aid and directs sound into the ear canal. Because the microphones are further from the receiver, these devices are less prone to acoustic feedback, thus allowing for larger venting and more amplification for severe to profound losses. Also the larger batteries tend to last longer and are more easily handled by dexterity-challenged patients.

The newest style available, the open-fit mini BTE, combines many of the acoustic benefits of the larger styles with the cosmetic benefits of the smaller styles. Open-fit instruments consist of a small BTE device, a narrow tube that hooks over and closely follows the contour anterior to the crus of the helix, and a soft, nonoccluding coupler that directs sound into the ear canal. The open fit greatly reduces the occlusion effect and allows natural sound to enter the ear canal for patients with good low-frequency hearing. The instrument is very discreet and appealing to people with cosmetic concerns, and because it does not

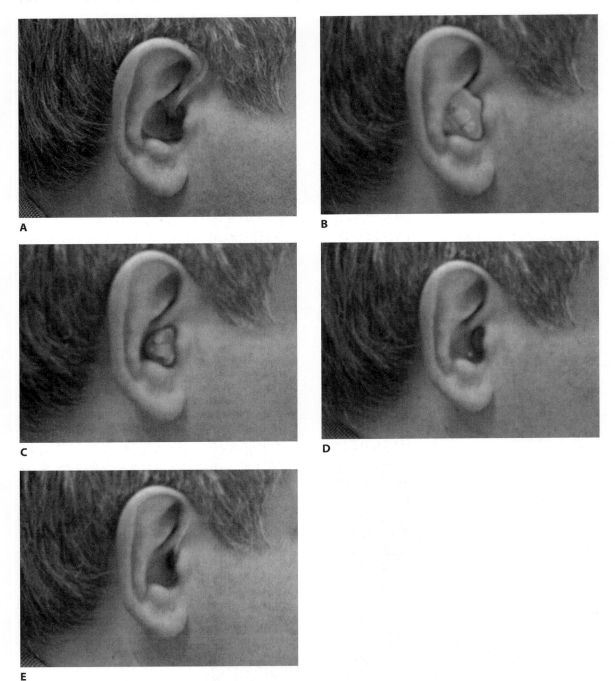

Figure 55–1. Five styles of hearing aids. **(A)** Behind the ear (BTE), **(B)** full shell in the ear (ITE), **(C)** in the canal (ITC), **(D)** completely in the canal (CIC), **(E)** open-fit mini BTE.

Table 55–1. Factors in determining appropriate hearing aid choice.

Shape of the pinna
Depth of the concha
Contour and diameter of the meatus
Manual dexterity
Physical condition (ie, drainage)
Excessive production of cerumen
Degree of loss
　Patients with profound hearing loss are not candidates for CIC (completely in canal) hearing aids
Audiometric configuration
　Patients with regions of normal hearing, particularly in the low frequencies, are best served by systems that do not occlude the ear canal
Special features, such as multiple microphones or the inclusion of a teleoil (ie, magnetic induction loops that allow the hearing aid to bypass the microphone and amplify signals presented either through the telephone or through assistive listening devices)

---

require custom molding, it can be programmed and fit in a single visit.

FEATURE ASSESSMENT

The last decade has brought a number of dramatic technologic advances in hearing aids. Earlier hearing aids contained variable screw potentiometers that allowed audiologists to alter the frequency response or output levels, but the majority of modern hearing aids are controlled via computerized programming. Because of the great flexibility in current hearing aids, the choice of which instruments are appropriate for a given individual is largely based on the features available. The most important features to be considered are (1) the type of processing, (2) compression, (3) multiple microphones, (4) multiple programs, and (5) the need for telecoils.

Processing Types

A. CONVENTIONAL HEARING AIDS

Less than 20% of hearing aids dispensed today fall into the conventional category. These devices are analog instruments that amplify, filter, and limit the maximum power via on-instrument screw-set controls, switches, or rotary wheels. They do not have the flexibility found in programmable or digital hearing aids. They typically use linear processing or contain relatively simple compression strategies. Many, though not all, have variable screw potentiometers that can be used to obtain a balance between low-frequency and high-frequency gain. In addition, most utilize user-operated volume controls.

B. PROGRAMMABLE HEARING AIDS

Digitally programmable hearing aids are hybrid instruments that process sound signals with analog components, but are programmed using a computer. Digitally programmable instruments are being phased out as fully digital instruments gain in popularity and are reduced in cost.

C. DIGITAL HEARING AIDS

Digital hearing aids are computer-controlled devices that use digital technology. Digitization means that incoming sounds are converted to numbers, which are then analyzed and manipulated via a set of rules (algorithms) programmed into the chip controlling the hearing aid. Digital signal processing (DSP) allows instruments to attempt a differentiation of noise from speech, not only on the basis of spectral composition, but also on the basis of temporal characteristics. Noise and speech have quite distinct temporal patterns. DSP hearing instruments assess the modulation pattern (rate and depth) of the input signal to predict whether or not that signal is primarily speech. If it is, full amplification is provided. If not, gain is attenuated within that frequency band. Studies have consistently shown subjective preferences for digital hearing aids, but, similar to binaural amplification, this perceived benefit may not always be reflected by word recognition scores, particularly in quiet.

One of the most demonstrable advantages of DSP is digital feedback reduction. This active approach is very different from traditional feedback management approaches in that, rather than simply reducing gain in certain frequency regions (generally, the high frequencies), digital feedback control seeks out and minimizes feedback by means of phase-shifting technology. Clinical measurements have shown that these systems provide feedback margins of at least 10 dB. This can be extremely important for patients because many users require significant high-frequency gain, but prefer ear molds that do not occlude their canals.

Sweetow RW (guest editor). Selection considerations for digital signal processing hearing aids. *Hear J.* 1998;51(11):35. (Article discusses a wide range of topics pertinent to the benefits and limitations of digital versus analog hearing aids and the selection of appropriate features.)

Compression

Because most hearing aid users have sensorineural hearing loss and because cochlear hearing loss is characterized by a loss of the linear processing provided by outer hair cells, most hearing aids now utilize compression (nonlinear amplification). Compression circuits both provide increased amplification for soft intensities (to compensate for the loss of the nonlinear outer hair cells) and prevent the amplified signal from reaching the loudness discomfort level of the wearer. Linear amplification provides constant **gain** (the difference in decibels between sound entering the microphone of the hearing aid and sound exiting the receiver) regardless of the input level until the output reaches a certain predetermined ceiling (saturation level). Thus, although it is useful in making soft sounds audible, louder sounds are frequently uncomfortable. Compression circuits automatically reduce gain once a predetermined level, referred to as the **kneepoint,** is reached.

A potential shortcoming of early compression circuits was that an input signal of any frequency reaching the kneepoint triggered a gain reduction across the frequency range, often reducing the gain of the high frequencies so much that the consonant sounds were not in the audible range of the listener. To combat this problem, many hearing aids contain **multiband compression** (ranging from 2 to as many as 20 bands). With multiband compression, if the offending signal is primarily low-frequency-based (as is common for noise stimuli), only the low-frequency gain would be reduced, without reducing the high-frequency gain. This can preserve audibility of the important high-frequency consonant sounds. This feature also allows for greater flexibility in shaping the frequency response (gain as a function of frequency) and compensation for recruitment (the abnormally rapid loudness growth characteristic of sensorineural impairment). The pattern of recruitment in any given individual cannot be predicted simply on the basis of a pure-tone audiogram. Therefore, it is beneficial to have adjustable characteristics for the various compression parameters such as the kneepoint (the activation level), the **compression ratio** (how severely the gain is reduced), and the **release time** (how soon the aid returns to a linear mode once the activating signal ceases).

Directional & Dual Microphones

Hearing-impaired patients frequently report that their primary communication difficulty is understanding speech in noisy environments. For these individuals to perform adequately, the signal-to-noise ratio (SNR) must be significantly higher than is necessary for individuals with normal hearing. Although the only true method of improving the SNR is to place the microphone in close proximity to the speaker's mouth using assistive listening devices like FM or infrared systems, an additional strategy is the use of directional or multiple microphones. Hearing aids with a directional microphone (one microphone with two entry ports) or dual microphones (two separate microphones) function by recognizing the difference in arrival time when sound reaches the front compared with the rear microphone (or port). Through sophisticated processing, this time delay directs the hearing aid to minimize the gain of sounds entering from the rear relative to the front, where, presumably, the person speaking would be located. Although single, omnidirectional microphones are often preferred for quiet listening, a significant improvement in noise is consistently shown in multiple microphone modes. However, it should be noted that the benefits from multiple and directional microphones can be minimized by highly reverberant environments. In addition, there is a minimal space requirement of at least 3 mm for dual microphones. Therefore, CIC hearing aids are too small for inclusion of this useful feature.

Bentler RA. Effectiveness of directional microphones and noise reduction schemes in hearing aids: a systematic review of the evidence. *J Am Acad Audiol.* 2005;16(7):473. Review. [PMID: 16295234] (Evidence-based review of the literature on directional microphones and noise reduction.)

Ricketts TA, Hornsby BW. Sound quality measures for speech in noise through a commercial hearing aid implementing digital noise reduction. *J Am Acad Audiol.* 2005;16(5):270. [PMID: 16119254] (Controlled study of subjective impact of noise reduction.)

Ricketts TA, Hornsby BW. Distance and reverberation effects on directional benefit. *Ear Hear.* 2003;24(6):472. [PMID: 14663347] (How multiple microphone performance changes as a function of distance and reverberation.)

Multiple Programs

Many hearing aids offer multiple programs so that at the touch of a button on the aid or in a remote control, the electroacoustic characteristics of the aid can be instantly changed to better compensate for the particular acoustic environment. Some audiologists also use the multiple program feature as a means of gradually introducing variations in amplified sound to the new user. For example, patients with a loss of high-frequency hearing initially may find that a sharply sloping high-frequency response sounds too "tinny." The optimal number of multiple programs to meet listening needs is unknown. Current multiple-program devices contain from two to four choices. If the device has no volume control yet the patient desires controllable changes in volume, devices having more programs might be beneficial so that program selection acts as a pseudo-volume control. In the past few years, many hearing aids have incorporated an automatic switching function dependent on internal sensors measuring the sound environment. Another use is for individuals with a fluctuating hearing loss, such as patients with Meniere disease. Rather than having to return to the audiologist each time hearing thresholds change, various memories can be programmed in anticipation of the expected amount of shift.

Telecoils

Many patients complain that they cannot hear well on the telephone with their hearing aids. Often, there is feedback that results from the physical proximity of the telephone receiver to the hearing aid microphone. To combat this problem, BTE and ITE hearing aids can contain a telecoil, a small inductance loop that picks up and amplifies electromagnetic leakage purposely produced from telephones. When the telecoil is activated, the microphone can be, but does not have to be, shut off, thus eliminating feedback. Telecoils also are used to interface with various assistive listening devices. The ability to program the telecoil separately from the microphone can be of great benefit. Certain cellular phones may be incompatible with telecoil usage; however, new FCC regulations are being phased in requiring increased compatibility compliance.

VALIDATION & VERIFICATION PROCEDURES

The verification and validation of a successful hearing aid fitting for patients should include the following: (1) the assessment of word and sentence recognition in quiet and noise; (2) the assessment of sound quality; (3) either functional gain or probe microphone measures, which verify the amount of amplified sound reaching the eardrum; and (4) subjective scaling.

Assessment of Word Recognition & Sound Quality

The primary goal of amplification is to enhance communication. For some hearing aid users, this corresponds with an improvement in word recognition. For others, the goal may be to ease listening effort. Word and sentence recognition scores (or both) and an assessment of sound quality should be obtained in both quiet and noisy environments. The use of adaptive speech measures (ie, maintaining a certain subjective intelligibility level, such as 50% of connected discourse in various SNRs) may be helpful in avoiding ceiling effects (eg, word recognition scores that are too high to show improvement).

Probe Tube Measures

Probe tube measurements allow for a noninvasive, rapid measurement of the sound received within approximately 5 mm of the tympanic membrane; they therefore take into account the effects of the ear canal. The goal of all hearing aid fittings is to package the amplified speech within the listener's **dynamic range** (defined as the range of the threshold to the loudness discomfort level). In other words, the amplified signal must be audible across the frequency range, but must not be uncomfortably loud for the listener at any frequency. Refined computer software packages are available that prescribe the amount of desired gain and output to

allow conversational speech to fall within these limits. If probe microphone measures are not available, one can use functional gain, the difference between aided and unaided thresholds, for verification.

Subjective Scaling

The quality and comfort of listening might be the most important factors determining the success of amplification for certain listeners. Therefore, it is important to validate the aided benefit with self-assessment scales. Several scales have been developed for this purpose. Some ask standardized questions, whereas others allow the individual patient to identify the situations most relevant to him or her.

Cox RM, Alexander GC, Gray GA. Audiometric correlates of the unaided APHAB. *J Am Acad Audiol.* 2003;14(7):361. [PMID: 14620610] (Discussion of subjective outcome measures.)

ASSISTIVE LISTENING DEVICES

Despite technologic advances, a basic problem remains for which wearable amplification falls short; that problem relates to the physical distance between the hearing aid microphone and the sound source. Intensity decreases by 6 dB for every doubling of the distance according to the inverse square law. Unfortunately, background noise often surrounds the listener, so although the intensity of the speech decreases with distance, the intensity of the noise may not. This is why hearing aids transmit sound well if the speaker talks directly into the microphone, but at longer, more realistic distances, reception diminishes. Ideally, sound produced at the source would transfer directly to the listener without losing any intensity. It is obviously impractical, however, to ask the speaker to move closer to the listener's ear.

Direct Audio Input

One way of achieving this effect is with direct audio input, in which the speaker holds a microphone that is hard-wired to the hearing aid itself. Many hearing aid wearers are reluctant to ask the speaker to do this, however. Fortunately, modern technology allows for a variety of wireless solutions.

Infrared, FM, & Inductance Loop Transmission

These systems are currently available in many theatres, concert halls, houses of worship, and households. Many of these systems are compatible with telecoils. One of the best uses is for television listening. A portable transmitter, typically smaller than most cable boxes, and microphone are located near the television loudspeaker. The sound picked up by the microphone is then transmitted to a receiver worn by the listener without any decrease in intensity. Other nonwearable devices that assist the hearing-impaired listener include telephone amplifiers, vibrating alarm clocks, closed-caption decoders for television, inexpensive personal handheld or body-borne amplifiers, visual alarm systems, and TDDs (telecommunication devices for the deaf).

Lesner S. Candidacy and management of assistive listening devices: special needs of the elderly. *Int J Audiol.* 2003;42(Suppl 2):2S68. Review. [PMID: 12918632] (Review of assistive listening devices.)

AURAL REHABILITATION

As professionals, our objective is to provide patients with better tools for hearing and listening. Although hearing aids are typically the vehicle for such an objective, other forms of aural rehabilitation, either in lieu of or in association with hearing aids, may be necessary. Just as physical therapy is provided to patients receiving artificial limbs, aural rehabilitation is important for hearing-impaired patients for whom central processing abilities have been compromised as a result of neural plasticity, cognitive changes, and aging processes. Adapting to hearing aid use takes time and should not be expected to occur automatically without instructions on how to manipulate the acoustic environment, supplement an impaired auditory system with visual cues, and enhance listening skills with compensatory strategies. These abilities can be abetted via individual or group aural rehabilitation sessions. In addition, patients should expect to receive written materials from their audiologist that address these issues. Because it may be difficult for some patients to return for frequent aural rehabilitation sessions, recent programs, such as Listening and Communication Enhancement, (LACE) have been introduced to allow patients to rehabilitate in their own home. For example, LACE is a computerized, adaptive training program designed to assist patients' listening skills in degraded speech environments, as well as to strengthen cognitive skills (speed of processing and auditory memory), and to teach communication strategies.

Sweetow R, Palmer C. Efficacy of individual auditory training in adults: a systematic review of the evidence. *J Am Acad Audiol.* 2005;16(7):494. [PMID: 16295236] (Review of literature on evidence-based studies of auditory training.)

Vestibular Disorders

56

Jacob Johnson, MD, & Anil K. Lalwani, MD

The value and function of the vestibular system may often be underestimated when considering the various special senses that we possess. However, of all the special senses, unilateral loss of the vestibular system may cause the most significant determent for our daily function and survival. Millions of people present annually to their physician with the complaint of dizziness. The goal of this chapter is to discuss the common disorders that affect the vestibular system and provide a framework for the evaluation, diagnosis, and treatment of patients with vestibular disorders.

Injury to the peripheral or central vestibular system causes asymmetry in the baseline input into the vestibular centers and this causes vertigo, nystagmus, vomiting, and a sense of falling toward the side of the injury. **Vertigo** is defined as the illusion of movement. However, the chief complaint of patients with injury to the vestibular system is usually not vertigo but dizziness. If the complaint is clarified to be vertigo, the duration, periodicity, and circumstance of the vertigo and the presence of other neurologic signs or symptoms allow for categorization of the vertigo.

The proximity of the vestibular system to the auditory system often causes vertigo to be coupled with hearing loss. The role of the otolaryngologist includes clarifying the subset of patients who have vertigo due to injury to the vestibular system and differentiating central from peripheral vestibular disorders. The evaluation includes a complete head and neck and vestibular exam (Table 56–1). The diagnostic evaluation includes audiology, vestibular testing, and imaging. Knowing the duration of the vertigo or disequilibrium and the presence or absence of hearing loss allows for a narrowing of the differential diagnosis (Table 56–2). The vertigo may be due to injury of the peripheral or central vestibular system. Often, the presence of other neurologic abnormalities leads to an investigation for a central cause of the vertigo. However, central vestibular injury due to a lesion or stroke may mimic a peripheral vestibular disorder.

Most patients with peripheral vestibular disorders have benign paroxysmal positional vertigo, Meniere disease, or vestibular neuronitis. These patients generally improve with supportive or conservative care (medical or physical therapy). The small percentage of medically recalcitrant patients can then be helped with surgical intervention. The surgical interventions, in general, ablate the vestibular system and rely on central compensation and vestibular rehabilitation to improve the patient's condition.

The central compensation for vestibular injury occurs via the cerebellum. The cerebellum provides a "clamping" response to the injured vestibular system to reduce the effects of the abnormal vestibular signal. In an acute injury such as vestibular neuronitis, the vertiginous response lasts 3–5 days, and then the central compensation is able to modulate the signal from the injured vestibular system. In episodic injuries, such as Meniere disease, the central compensation is not able to be as effective; therefore, with each new episode, there are acute vertiginous symptoms. In a slowly evolving process such as a vestibular schwannoma, the central compensation occurs in step with the vestibular dysfunction, and the patient may have minimal to no vestibular symptoms. The central compensation is enhanced by vestibular activity and delayed by the prolonged use of medical vestibular suppression. This observation has led to the development of vestibular rehabilitation programs.

Vestibular rehabilitation programs use three strategies: (1) habituation exercises, which facilitate central compensation by extinguishing pathologic responses to head motion; (2) postural control exercises; and (3) general conditioning exercises. Vestibular rehabilitation is critically important in the elderly because their ability to have optimal central compensation is diminished.

BENIGN PAROXYSMAL POSITIONAL VERTIGO

 ESSENTIALS OF DIAGNOSIS

- *Sudden vertigo lasting seconds with certain head positions.*
- *No associated hearing loss.*
- *Characteristic nystagmus (latent, geotropic, fatigable) with Dix-Hallpike test.*

Table 56–1. Steps in a vestibular evaluation.

1. Head and neck exam, including cranial nerves
2. Spontaneous and gaze-evoked nystagmus with Frenzel glasses
Direction: fixed-peripheral, changing-central Form: jerk-peripheral, pendular-central Fixation: suppression-peripheral, enchanced-central
3. Smooth pursuit—"Follow my fingers."
4. Saccades—"Look to my left or right finger when I say to."
Dysmetric: cerebellar Slow: brainstem Late: frontal lobe Disconjugate: multiple sclerosis
5. Head thrust
Normal: no refixation saccade Abnormal: refixation saccade (peripheral)
6. Headshake—"10 degrees, 2 cycles/second, 20 seconds."
Normal: no nystagmus Abnormal: horizontal, nystagmus-peripheral; vertical, nystagmus-central (brainstem)
7. Dynamic visual activity—"Look at Schnell chart with head shake."
Normal: < 3 line drop Abnormal: 3 or more line drop-bilateral vestibular loss
8. Fixation suppression—"Look at your thumb during rotation."
Normal: no nystagmus Abnormal: nystagmus-central (flocculus)
9. Positional testing—Dix-Hallpike
Normal: no nystagmus Abnormal: downbeating, fatigable, rotatory nystagmus
10. Cerebellum—finger to nose, rapid alternating movements, heel to shin
11. Posture—Romberg

Table 56–2. Differential diagnosis of vertigo based on the timeframe of vertigo and the presence or absence of hearing loss.

Time	No Associated Hearing Loss	Hearing Loss Present
Seconds	Benign positional paroxysmal vertigo	Perilymphatic fistula Cholesteatoma
Minutes	Vertebral basilar insufficiency Migraines	
Hours	Vestibulopathy	Meniere disease
Days	Vestibular neuronitis	Labyrinthitis
Weeks	Central nervous system disorders Lyme disease Multiple sclerosis	Acoustic neuroma Autoimmune processes Psychogenic

General Considerations

Benign paroxysmal positional vertigo (BPPV) is one of the most common types of peripheral vertigo, arising as a result of debris in the posterior semicircular canal. Patients complain of vertigo lasting seconds, with no associated hearing loss when in certain positions. The average age of presentation is in the fifth decade and there is no gender bias. The incidence may range from 10 to 100 cases per 100,000 individuals per year. Nearly 20% of patients seen at vertigo clinics are given the diagnosis of BPPV. Ten to fifteen percent of patients have an antecedent history of vestibular neuronitis and another 20% have a history of head trauma.

Pathogenesis

BPPV occurs because a semicircular canal has debris either attached to the cupula or free floating in the endolymph. The semicircular canal becomes stimulated by the movement of these particles in response to gravity. The study of temporal bones from patients with BPPV showed basophilic deposits adherent to the cupula; this finding was termed **cupulolithiasis.** Intraoperative findings during posterior canal occlusion in patients with resistant BPPV have shown free-floating debris in the endolymph. Electron microscopy of these particles shows that they are likely otoconia originating from the macula of the gravity-sensitive utricle. This process has been termed **canalolithiasis.**

The cupula of the semicircular canal has the same specific gravity as the endolymph and so is not sensitive to gravity. However, the debris in the semicircular canal moves in response to gravity and when the patient places the semicircular canal in a dependent position, the particles move and entrain endolymph with them and cause deflection of the cupula. The unexpected gravity-sensitive response from the semicircular canal causes vertigo. The majority of BPPV is due to debris in the posterior canal, but debris may also enter the horizontal and superior semicircular canals.

Clinical Findings

A. SYMPTOMS AND SIGNS

Patients usually complain of a sudden onset of vertigo that lasts 10–20 seconds with certain head positions.

The triggering positions include rolling over in bed into a lateral position, getting out of bed, looking up and back, and bending over. The vertigo may be associated with nausea. Patients have normal hearing (no new loss), no spontaneous nystagmus, and a normal neurologic evaluation.

B. Imaging Studies

Imaging is reserved for patients who do not have the characteristic nystagmus, have associated neurologic findings, or do not respond to treatment. The imaging choice is a magnetic resonance imaging (MRI) scan with gadolinium contrast to evaluate the brainstem, the cerebellopontine angle (CPA), and the internal carotid artery (IAC). The MRI is the most sensitive and specific test to identify posterior fossa tumors.

C. Special Tests

Patients should have no new hearing loss. The audiogram should show symmetric hearing with appropriate speech discrimination scores. The tympanogram should be normal. An asymmetric hearing loss calls into question the diagnosis of BPPV and further evaluation is required.

D. Special Examinations

BPPV is diagnosed by observing a characteristic nystagmus when performing the Dix-Hallpike test (Figure 56–1). There is a latency of 1–2 seconds before the onset of the nystagmus and vertigo. The nystagmus is mixed with a torsional and vertical component and is **geotropic** (downbeating, rotatory nystagmus). The nystagmus follows the Ewald law for excitation of the dependent posterior semicircular canal. The nystagmus is in the plane of the canal, and the fast phase is toward the stimulated canal. The vertigo and nystagmus increase and then decrease within 20 seconds; they are reduced with repeated Dix-Hallpike tests and so the nystagmus is fatigable. All these criteria need to be present to diagnose a patient with BPPV due to debris in the posterior semicircular canal.

Treatment

A. Nonsurgical Measures

The primary management for BPPV includes maneuvers to reposition the debris into the utricle. The most widely used set of repositioning maneuvers is depicted in Figure 56–2. The maneuver may be repeated if the patient is still symptomatic. A bone vibrator may also be placed on the mastoid bone during the maneuvers to loosen the debris. Eighty percent of patients are cured by a single repositioning maneuver. If the symptoms persist after a single maneuver or if patients have recurrent symptoms, the repositioning maneuver may be repeated. Other maneuvers and exercises are available for patients with symptoms resistant to medical management.

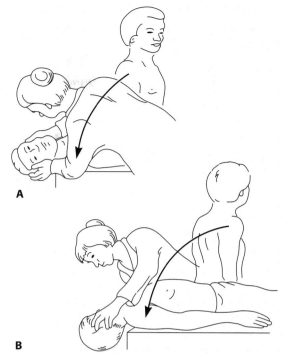

A

B

Figure 56–1. Dix-Hallpike test. **(A)** For testing the right posterior semicircular canal, the patient sits on the exam table and turns his or her head to the right 45 degrees. This places the posterior semicircular canal in the sagittal plane. The examiner stands facing the patient on the patient's right side or behind the patient. **(B)** The patient is then moved by the examiner from the seated to the supine position with the head slightly hanging over the edge of the table. The right ear is down and the chin is pointing slightly up. The eyes are observed for the characteristic nystagmus.

B. Surgical Measures

Surgical treatment is available for a very small number of patients with intractable BPPV. These patients have failed repositioning maneuvers and have no intracranial pathology on imaging studies. The primary surgical option is posterior semicircular canal occlusion. A standard mastoidectomy is performed and the posterior semicircular canal is fenestrated. The membranous canal is occluded with muscle, fascia, or bone pate, or collapsed with a laser. The occlusion prevents debris and subsequent endolymph movement to deflect the cupula. There may be a temporary mixed hearing loss that usually recovers. The success rate for an occlusion of the posterior semicircular canal is high. A more technically challenging surgical option with an increased risk to hearing involves ablating the nerve supply of the posterior semicircular canal via a singular neurectomy.

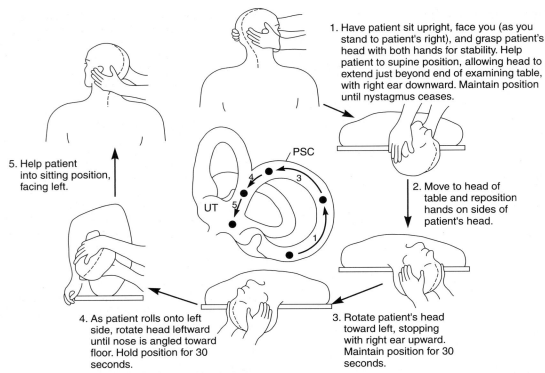

1. Have patient sit upright, face you (as you stand to patient's right), and grasp patient's head with both hands for stability. Help patient to supine position, allowing head to extend just beyond end of examining table, with right ear downward. Maintain position until nystagmus ceases.

2. Move to head of table and reposition hands on sides of patient's head.

3. Rotate patient's head toward left, stopping with right ear upward. Maintain position for 30 seconds.

4. As patient rolls onto left side, rotate head leftward until nose is angled toward floor. Hold position for 30 seconds.

5. Help patient into sitting position, facing left.

Figure 56–2. Epley maneuver. The patient is taken through four moves, starting in the sitting position with the head turned at a 45-degree angle toward the affected side. **(1)** The patient is placed into the Dix-Hallpike position (supine with the affected ear down) until the vertigo and nystagmus subside. **(3)** The patient's head is then turned to the opposite side, causing the affected ear to be up and the unaffected ear to be down. **(4)** The whole body and head are then turned away from the affected side to a lateral decubitus position, with the head in a face-down position. **(5)** The last step is to bring the patient back to a sitting position with the head turned toward the unaffected shoulder.

Prognosis

The natural history of BPPV includes an acute onset and remission over a few months. However, up to 30% of patients may have symptoms for longer than one year. Most patients improve with a repositioning maneuver. Patients may have unpredictable recurrences and remissions, and the rate of recurrence may be 10–15% per year. These patients may be retreated with a repositioning maneuver. A subset of patients who have adapted by not using certain positions in order to avoid the vertigo or who have other balance disorders can benefit from balance rehabilitation therapy.

Korres S, Balatsouras DG, Ferekidis E. Prognosis of patients with benign paroxysmal positional vertigo treated with repositioning manoeuvres. *J Laryngol Otol.* 2006;120:528. [PMID: 16556351] (Repositioning maneuvers are highly successful in treating BPPV.)

Shaia WT, Zappia JJ, Bojrab DI, LaRouere ML, Sargent EW, Diaz RC. Success of posterior semicircular canal occlusion and application of the dizziness handicap inventory. *Otolaryngol Head Neck Surg.* 2006;134(3):424. [PMID: 16500439] (Posterior semicircular canal occlusion is efficacious in the treatment of intractable BPPV.)

MENIERE DISEASE

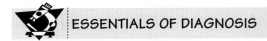

ESSENTIALS OF DIAGNOSIS

- *Episodic vertigo lasting hours.*
- *Fluctuating hearing loss.*
- *Tinnitus.*
- *Aural pressure.*

General Considerations

Meniere disease or endolymphatic hydrops is an idiopathic inner ear disorder characterized by attacks of vertigo, fluctuating hearing loss, tinnitus, and aural fullness. The incidence of Meniere disease ranges from 10 to 150 cases per 100,000 persons each year. There is no gender bias and patients typically present in the fifth decade of life. A new diagnosis of Meniere disease in someone younger than age 20 or older than age 70 is unusual. There is no right or left ear predilection for the disease.

Pathogenesis

The cause of Meniere disease remains elusive and has been attributed to anatomic, infectious, immunologic, and allergic factors. The focus of most studies has been the endolymphatic duct and sac based on the basic premise that there is increased endolymphatic fluid owing to impaired reabsorption of endolymphatic fluid in the endolymphatic duct and sac. Histopathologic studies have shown blockage in the longitudinal flow of endolymph in the endolymphatic duct, the endolymphatic sinuses, the utricular ducts, the saccular ducts, and the ductus reuniens. Studies have reported that the endolymphatic sacs in patients with Meniere disease are smaller, have less absorptive tubular epithelium, and have increased perisaccular fibrosis. Results of a blinded control study, however, did not show any difference in the connective tissue or fibrosis surrounding the endolymphatic sac in patients with Meniere disease. The vestibular duct has also been shown to be smaller in patients with Meniere disease. Recent studies have shown a decrease in Type II vestibular hair cells in cases of Meniere disease. The role and significance of the decrease of these Type II hair cells are currently not known. The endolymphatic sac has been shown to be important in inner ear metabolic homeostasis. The endolymphatic sac secretes glycoprotein conjugates in response to osmotic challenges, and preliminary studies have shown an alteration in glycoprotein metabolism in Meniere disease. There has been no conclusive proof of an infectious agent related to this disease.

The roles of allergy and immunology in Meniere disease are under active investigation. The "seat" of immunity in the inner ear may be the endolymphatic sac, which is able to process antigens and mount a local antibody response. The endolymphatic sac may be vulnerable to immunologic injury because of the hyperosmolarity of its contents and the fenestrations in its vasculature. These two properties increase the risk of immune complex deposition and injury. IgG deposition is seen in the endolymphatic sacs of patients undergoing shunt procedures of the endolymphatic sac. Patients with Meniere disease also have elevated IgM complexes and C1q component of complement, and low levels of IgA complexes in their serum. These patients have also shown vulnerability to autoimmune (cytotoxic) reactions. Thirty percent of patients with Meniere disease had autoantibodies to an inner ear antigen by Western blot analysis. The response of some patients to steroid therapy and the increased rate of expression of certain HLA antigens (eg, A3, Cw7, B7, and DR2) in patients with Meniere disease support the presence of an underlying immune mechanism.

A similar argument may be made regarding Meniere disease and allergy. A significant percentage (50%) of affected patients have concomitant inhalant or food allergies (or both), and treating these allergies with immunotherapy and diet modification has improved the manifestations of their allergies and Meniere disease. The fenestrated blood vessels of the endolymphatic sac may be vulnerable to vasoactive mediators, such as histamine, which are released during an IgE-mediated allergic reaction. Some physicians have suggested a synergistic role of allergy or viral infection in potentiating the immunologic abnormalities in Meniere disease.

The role of genetic influences in the pathogenesis in Meniere disease is also being elucidated. Mutation in the *COCH* gene is associated with Meniere disease. The family of water channels (AQPs) and ion channels have also been implicated.

Clinical Findings

A. SYMPTOMS AND SIGNS

Meniere disease occurs as episodic attacks lasting for hours. The four symptoms and signs include (1) a unilateral, fluctuating sensorineural hearing loss (often involving low frequencies); (2) vertigo that lasts minutes to hours; (3) a constant or intermittent tinnitus typically increasing in intensity before or during the vertiginous attack; and (4) aural fullness. The acute attack is also associated with nausea and vomiting and, following the acute attack, patients feel exhausted for a few days. Table 56–3 shows the diagnostic scale for Meniere disease created by the Committee on Hearing and Equilibrium of the American Academy of Otolaryngology—Head and Neck Surgery. As emphasized in the diagnostic scale, the diagnosis of Meniere disease is based on the longitudinal course of the disease rather than on a single attack.

B. LABORATORY FINDINGS

Meniere disease is a clinical diagnosis. The diagnostic evaluation primarily includes audiometry and a fluorescent treponemal antibody absorption (FTA-ABS) test to rule out syphilis. FTA-ABS testing is mandatory in any patient given the diagnosis of an idiopathic disease, because syphilis may perfectly imitate Meniere disease. Electrophysiologic studies, other serologic studies, and imaging are obtained as needed. The role of allergy testing continues to be defined. Initially, autoimmune ear disease may be clinically indistinguishable from Meniere disease.

Table 56–3. Diagnostic scale for Meniere disease of the AAO-HNS*

Certain Meniere Disease
Definitive Meniere's disease, plus histopathologic confirmation
Definitive Meniere Disease
Two or more episodes of vertigo of at least 20 minutes
Audiometrically documented hearing loss on at least one occasion
Tinnitus and aural fullness
Probable Meniere Disease
One definite episode of vertigo
Audiometrically documented hearing loss on at least one occasion
Tinnitus and aural fullness
Possible Meniere Disease
Episodic vertigo without documented hearing loss
Sensorineural hearing loss, fluctuating or fixed, with disequilibrium, but without definitive episodes

*In all scales, other causes must be excluded using any technical methods (eg, imaging, laboratory, etc.)

The distinguishing characteristics of an autoimmune ear disease include a more aggressive course and early bilateral involvement. Autoimmune serologic tests may also be helpful. There is no diagnostic test for Meniere disease.

C. IMAGING STUDIES

MRI with gadolinium contrast allows the exclusion of retrocochlear pathology, such as a vestibular neuroma. An imaging scan is not mandatory, with a classical course of Meniere disease leading to a clinical diagnosis. Imaging should be used if the initial presentation or course is unusual and nonmedical management is planned.

D. SPECIAL TESTS

1. Audiology—Audiologic assessment initially shows a low-frequency or a low- and high-frequency (inverted V) sensorineural hearing loss. As the disease progresses, there is a flat sensorineural hearing loss. A glycerol dehydration test involves measuring serial pure-tone thresholds and discrimination scores during diuresis. The diagnosis of Meniere disease is supported if there is improvement in the patient's hearing. The test is positive in only 50% of patients suspected to have the disease.

2. Electrocochleography—Electrocochleography (ECOG) measures the sound-evoked electrical potentials from the inner ear. The three phenomena measured from the external canal (tympanic membrane) or on the promontory in response to clicks include (1) the cochlear microphonic, (2) the summating potential, and (3) the action potential. The endolymphatic hydrops of Meniere disease causes a larger summating potential and so the ratio of the summating potential to the action potential (SP/AP) is elevated. ECOG lacks the specificity or sensitivity to reliably use the SP/AP ratio to consistently diagnose Meniere disease or predict the clinical course.

3. Electronystagmography (ENG)—ENG with caloric testing shows peripheral vestibular dysfunction. The caloric response decreases during the first decade of the disease and usually stabilizes at 50% of normal function.

4. Vestibular-evoked myogenic potential (VEMP) testing—VEMP is a vestibulo-collic reflex whose afferent limb arises from acoustically sensitive cells in the saccule, with signals conducted via the inferior vestibular nerve. VEMP is a biphasic, short-latency response recorded from the tonically contracted sternocleidomastoid muscle in response to loud auditory clicks or tones. VEMPs may be diminished or absent in patients with early and late Meniere disease, vestibular neuritis, BPPV, and vestibular schwannoma. On the other hand, the threshold for VEMPs may be lower in cases of superior canal dehiscence and perilymphatic fistula.

Differential Diagnosis

In addition to the vestibular system, dizziness may be caused by poor vision, decreased proprioception (diabetes mellitus), cardiovascular insufficiency, cerebellar or brainstem strokes, neurologic conditions (eg, migraines, multiple sclerosis), metabolic disorders, and the side effects of medications (see Table 56–2).

Treatment

A. NONSURGICAL MEASURES

Since the introduction of aminoglycoside therapy in 1948, no significant conceptual advances have been made in the treatment of Meniere disease. The current treatments focus on relieving vertigo without further injuring the patient's hearing. Hearing may be temporarily improved or stabilized by the current treatments, but the hearing does not have long-term stability.

1. Dietary modifications and vestibular suppressants—The primary management of Meniere disease involves a sodium-restricted diet ($\leq$ 1500 mg/d) and diuretics (eg, Diazide). In a crossover placebo study of Diazide, it was shown that diuretics seem to improve vestibular complaints but have no effect on hearing or tinnitus. Some patients benefit from dietary restrictions on caffeine, nicotine, alcohol, and foods containing theophylline (eg, chocolate). Acute attacks are managed with vestibular suppressants (eg, meclizine and diazepam [Valium]) and antiemetic medications (eg, prochlorperazine [Compazine] suppository). Most patients are controlled with conservative management.

2. Aminoglycoside therapy—Medically refractory patients with or without serviceable hearing may benefit from intratympanic gentamicin therapy. Intratympanic gentamicin is absorbed into the inner ear primarily via the round window and selectively damages the vestibular hair cells relative to the cochlear hair cells. Gentamicin may also decrease endolymph production by affecting dark cells in the stria vascularis. Intratympanic gentamicin has nearly a 90% vertigo control rate with a follow-up of at least 2 years; the extent of hearing loss depends on the protocol for gentamicin delivery. A variety of treatment protocols (daily, biweekly, weekly, or monthly injections) using fixed-dose or titration end-point regimens exist but a few trends are present. Treatments are stopped if there is persistent hearing loss. Vertigo control is nearly always obtained if vestibular function is ablated. However, the risk of hearing loss increases as the total dose and frequency of gentamicin injections are increased. Current protocols are reducing the dose and frequency of injections to decrease hearing loss and still obtain vertigo control. Vertigo control may be obtained with some residual vestibular function, and this residual function may be useful if patients develop bilateral Meniere disease. Recent studies with monthly injections have shown a nearly 90% vertigo control with a 17% (< 10 dB) hearing loss.

3. Steroid therapy—Acute exacerbation of Meniere disease may respond to a short burst of oral steroids. Intratympanic steroids have also been used to treat active disease and avoid the systemic complications associated with oral steroids.

B. SURGICAL MEASURES

Patients who have failed medical and gentamicin treatment may require surgical intervention. Endolymphatic sac surgery and vestibular nerve sections preserve hearing while labyrinthectomy ablates hearing.

1. Endolymphatic sac surgery—The role of endolymphatic sac surgery in the management of Meniere disease remains controversial. One double-blinded, placebo-controlled comparison of the endolymphatic mastoid shunt versus a simple cortical mastoidectomy showed no benefit of the sac surgery. A 9-year follow-up showed a 70% control of vertigo in both surgical groups. Re-analysis of the study suggested a greater benefit in the group who had endolymphatic sac surgery, and a recent study with a 5-year follow-up showed an 88% functional level 1 or 2 response after an endolymphatic mastoid shunt operation. Endolymphatic sac surgery involves a mastoidectomy and locating the endolymphatic sac on the posterior fossa dura (Figure 56–3A). The sac is medial to the sigmoid sinus and inferior to the posterior semicircular canal. The endolymphatic sac is also located along an imaginary line (**Donaldson line**) in the plane of the horizontal semicircular canal. The endolymphatic sac may be decompressed or have a shunt placed that communicates into the subarachnoid space or mastoid cavity. Endolymphatic shunt surgery provides a nondestructive option for patients who fail medical or aminoglycoside therapy and have good hearing. The role of endolymphatic surgery is currently in decline, with renewed interest in intratympanic aminoglycoside therapy.

2. Vestibular nerve section—A vestibular nerve section provides a definitive treatment of unilateral Meniere disease in patients with serviceable hearing. Ninety-five percent of patients achieve vertigo control, and hearing is preserved in more than 95% of patients. The vestibular neurectomy may be approached via a retrosigmoidal or middle fossa approach (Figure 56–3B). The risk to the facial nerve is < 1% in the retrosigmoidal approach and < 5% in the middle fossa approach. The patients are acutely vertiginous and have nystagmus (fast phase away from the operated ear) for a few days until central compensation takes effect. The hearing appears to degenerate in the postoperative patient in accordance with the natural history of Meniere disease.

3. Labyrinthectomy—A transmastoid labyrinthectomy with fenestration of the bony semicircular canals and vestibule and removal of the membranous neuroepithelium provides control of vertigo in nearly all patients with unilateral Meniere disease and poor hearing. The rate of control may decline in 10 years owing to the development of vertebral-basilar insufficiency (aging), poorer vision, and the development of Meniere disease in the contralateral ear. The complete loss of unilateral vestibular function due to the labyrinthectomy leads to unsteadiness in up to 30% of patients.

Prognosis

Meniere disease is characterized by remissions and exacerbations, making it difficult to predict the future behavior of the disease in any individual patient based on the patient's own history, diagnostic evaluations, or epidemiologic profiles. The initial manifestation may be vertigo or hearing loss, but within 1 year of onset, the typical syndrome—attacks of vertigo, tinnitus, fluctuating hearing loss, and aural fullness—is present. Longitudinal studies have shown that after 10–20 years, the vertigo attacks subside in most patients and the hearing loss stabilizes to a moderate to severe level (50 dB). Meniere disease is usually a unilateral disease, and the risk of developing this disease in the contralateral ear appears to be linear with time. Twenty-five to forty-five percent of patients may develop disease in the contralateral ear.

Banerjee AS, Johnson IJ. Intratympanic gentamicin for Meniere's disease: effect on quality of life as assessed by Glasgow benefit

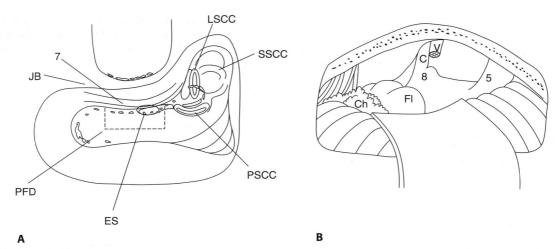

A   **B**

Figure 56–3. **(A)** Endolymphatic sac surgery. The sac surgery involves a mastoidectomy and identifying it within the posterior fossa dura. **(B)** Vestibular nerve section. Illustration shows a vestibular neurectomy via the posterior fossa craniotomy. LSCC, lateral semicircular canal; PSCC, posterior semicircular canal; SSCC, superior semicircular canal; ES, endolymphatic sac; PFD, posterior fossa dura; JB, jugular bulb; 7, facial nerve or cranial nerve 7; Fl, flocculus; 8, audiovestibular nerve or cranial nerve 8; C, cochlear division of the audiovestibular nerve; V, vestibular division of the audiovestibular nerve; 5, trigeminal nerve or cranial nerve 5; Ch, choroid plexus.

inventory. *J Laryngol Otol.* 2006;120:827. [PMID: 16707038] (Intratympanic gentamicin improves the quality of life in patients with Meniere disease.)

Lin MY, Timmer FC, Oriel BS et al. Vestibular evoked myogenic potentials (VEMP) can detect asymptomatic saccular hydrops. *Laryngoscope.* 2006;116(6):987. [PMID: 1673591] (VEMP may be useful in detecting saccular hydrops.)

VESTIBULAR NEURONITIS

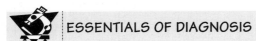

ESSENTIALS OF DIAGNOSIS

- *Vertigo lasting days after an upper respiratory infection.*
- *No hearing loss.*
- *No other neurologic signs or symptoms.*

General Consideration

Vestibular neuronitis is the third most common cause of peripheral vestibular vertigo after BPPV and Meniere disease. Vestibular neuronitis has no gender bias and typically affects middle-aged people. Less than half the patients have an antecedent or concurrent viral illness. The presentation includes acute vertigo. Like Meniere disease, the pathogenesis is not known but most patients recover with no seque-

lae. The primary role of the physician is to rule out a central cause of the acute vertigo. The treatment is primarily supportive care.

Pathogenesis

The proposed etiologies for vestibular neuronitis include viral infection, vascular occlusion, and immunologic mechanisms. The evidence to support a viral cause is limited by a lack of pathologic tissue for study. Furthermore, the evidence based on seroconversion remains unconvincing. The study of the available temporal bones of patients with vestibular neuronitis shows a spectrum of injury: from normal to significant degenerative changes in the vestibular nerve, Scarpa ganglion, and vestibular neuroepithelium. The injury is often seen in the superior vestibular nerve. There was no evidence of vascular occlusion affecting the vestibular system in any of these temporal bones.

Clinical Findings

A. SYMPTOMS AND SIGNS

The presentation of vestibular neuronitis includes the sudden onset of vertigo with nausea and vomiting. The patient has normal hearing and a normal neurologic exam. The patient may have postural instability toward the injured ear but is still able to walk without falling. He or she usually does not have a headache and has spontaneous nystagmus characteristic of an acute peripheral vestibular injury. The nystagmus is usually horizontal with a torsional component and is suppressed by visual fixation. The reduction in the vestibular signal in the injured ear leads to relative vestibular excitation in the opposite ear. The result is that the slow phase of nystagmus is toward the injured ear and the fast phase is away from the injured ear. The nystagmus is intensified by looking toward the fast phase and decreased by looking toward the slow phase or toward the injured ear. This principle is Alexander's law. The direction of the nystagmus does not change with changes in the direction of gaze.

B. IMAGING STUDIES

MRI, with emphasis on the identification of both infarction and hemorrhage in the brainstem and cerebellum, is obtained in patients with risk factors for stroke, with additional neurologic abnormalities, and who do not show improvement within 48 hours. Alternately, computed tomography (CT) scanning with thin cuts to evaluate the brainstem, cerebellum, and fourth ventricle may be obtained.

C. SPECIAL TESTS

In most patients, vestibular testing shows a complete or reduced caloric response in the injured ear. The caloric response eventually normalizes in 42% of patients. VEMP responses are attenuated or absent.

Differential Diagnosis

The diagnosis of vestibular neuronitis is based on the constellation of symptoms and signs described above; however, they may be mimicked by other disorders as well (see Table 56–2). The need for further evaluation is necessary only if there is a concern for a central cause of the acute vertigo or if the acute vertigo does not substantially improve in 48 hours. The primary central cause for acute vertigo lasting days is a brainstem or cerebellar stroke. In most cases, there are other neurologic findings: diplopia, dysmetria, dysarthria, motor and sensory deficits, abnormal reflexes, the inability to walk without falling, and a central nystagmus. Central nystagmus is not affected by visual fixation and may change directions with changes in gaze. A purely vertical or purely torsional nystagmus is highly suggestive of a central disorder. In the event of an isolated inferior cerebellar stroke, the presentation may be indistinguishable with vestibular neuronitis. Also, 25% of patients with risk factors for stroke who present with vertigo, nystagmus, and postural instability have had an inferior cerebellar stroke. Therefore, patients with significant risk factors for stroke should have an imaging study if they present with these symptoms.

Treatment

The primary management includes symptomatic and supportive care during the acute phase of the illness. The

patients are given vestibular suppressants and antiemetics to control the vertigo, nausea, and vomiting. These medications are withdrawn as soon as possible to avoid interfering with the central vestibular compensation.

Prognosis

The natural history of vestibular neuronitis includes an acute attack of vertigo that lasts a few days with complete or at least partial recovery within a few weeks to months. Some patients (15% in one study) may have significant vestibular symptoms even after 1 year. Recurrent attacks in the same or contralateral ear have been reported but are unusual. Some patients may later develop BPPV. Vestibular rehabilitation is of benefit in patients with residual symptoms.

Bartual-Pastor J. Vestibular neuritis: etiopathogenesis. *Rev Laryngol Otol Rhinol (Bord).* 2005;126(4):279. [PMID: 16496559] (There is substantial evidence for viral infection as the etiology of vestibular neuronitis.)

SUPERIOR SEMICIRCULAR CANAL DEHISCENCE

 ESSENTIALS OF DIAGNOSIS

- Vertigo or oscillopsia induced by loud sounds or pressure changes in the middle ear.
- Conductive or mixed hearing loss with presence of acoustic reflexes.
- Nystagmus align with the plane of the dehiscent superior semicircular canal.

General Considerations

In 1998, Lloyd Minor and colleagues described sound-and/or pressure-induced vertigo associated with the bony dehiscence of the superior semicircular canal. Patients complain of vertigo when exposed to loud noises (Tullio phenomenon), with Valsalva maneuvers, with pressure changes in the ear (Hennebert sign), or with factors that raise intracranial pressures. Auditory symptoms include sensitivity to bone-conducted sounds and autophony. Similar symptoms have also been noted with dehiscence of other semicircular canals.

Pathogenesis

The auditory and vestibular symptoms are due to exposure to external pressure along the dehiscent superior canal that is transmitted to the inner ear. Histologic and radiologic studies suggest that superior semicircular canal dehiscence is either congenital or developmental. Approximately 1% of temporal bone CT scans demonstrate significant thinning (≤ 0.1 mm) or dehiscence of the superior canal in the floor of the middle cranial fossa; this finding is usually bilateral. Over time, this thin bone may be further eroded by pressure transmitted by dura-encased temporal lobe.

Clinical Findings

A. SYMPTOMS AND SIGNS

Although dehiscence of the superior canal may be congenital, symptoms and signs usually do not present early in life; the youngest patients have been in their teens. Patients may complain of vestibular symptoms only, auditory and vestibular symptoms, or, less commonly, isolated auditory symptoms. Typically, loud noises, pressure on the external auditory canal, and factors that change intracranial pressure (Valsalva maneuver, jogging, jugular venous compression) lead to vertigo or oscillopsia. Many patients complain of chronic disequilibrium.

Patients report increased sensitivity to bone-conducted sounds, hearing their pulse sound, hearing their eye movements, and autophony. "Inner ear conductive hearing loss" is also common. The hearing loss is artefactual and mimics otosclerosis (low-frequency conductive hearing loss); in contrast to otosclerosis, the stapedius reflexes are present. The dehiscent portion of the superior canal acts as a third mobile window allowing acoustic energy to be dissipated there. The presence of stapedius reflex with low-frequency conductive hearing loss should prompt radiologic imaging of the inner ear to exclude the possibility of dehiscence of the inner ear.

B. IMAGING STUDIES

The presence of vestibular symptoms with loud noises or pressure changes, abnormally enhanced bone conduction hearing, or conductive hearing loss with normal stapedius reflexes should prompt radiologic imaging with high-resolution CT of the temporal bone. Superior semicircular canal dehiscence is best seen with 0.5-mm collimated helical CT scans with reformation of the images in the plane of the superior canal (instead of the tradition 1.0-mm collimated images in the axial and coronal plane) (Figure 56–4).

C. AUDIOLOGIC TESTING

Audiologic testing demonstrates low-frequency conductive hearing loss with the presence of stapedius reflex. In otosclerosis, with fixation of the stapes footplate, the reflexes are absent. Presentation of loud auditory signal may elicit typical symptoms of vertigo and eye movements.

D. SPECIAL EXAMINATIONS

Eye movements, examined with the use of Frenzel glasses (to prevent visual fixation and abolition of the nystagmus) typically align with the affected superior canal and follow Ewald law. The nystagmus is in the plane of the canal, and the fast phase is toward the stimulated canal. Loud noises, positive pressure in the ear canal, and the Valsalva maneuver against pinched nostril lead to excitation of the superior canal. The eye movements associated with the ampullifugal deflection of the cupula has the slow phase that is directed upward and torsion of the superior pole of the eye away from the affected ear. With inhibition of the superior canal due to negative pressure

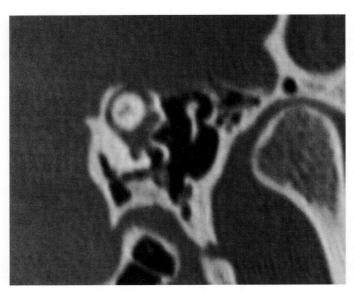

Figure 56–4. Superior semicircular canal dehiscence. CT scan of the temporal bone with reformation of the images in the plane of the superior canal demonstrating dehiscence of the superior semicircular canal.

in the ear canal, Valsalva against closed glottis, and jugular vein compression, the eye moves downward and torsions toward the affected ear.

VEMP testing is also useful in the evaluation of patients with SSCCD. Patients with superior semicircular canal dehiscence have lower than normal threshold for eliciting the VEMP response (81 dB NHL vs 99 dB NHL).

Treatment

A. NONSURGICAL MEASURES

Avoidance of symptom-provoking stimuli such as loud noises, jogging, or singing may be sufficient therapy for patients with mild symptoms. Correct diagnosis of superior semicircular canal dehiscence as the cause of low-frequency conductive hearing loss prevents unnecessary otosclerosis surgery.

B. SURGICAL MEASURES

Patients in whom the symptoms are associated with pressure in the ear canal can be treated with a tympa-nostomy tube. Patients with debilitating symptoms may require surgical repair of the dehiscence of the superior canal either through the middle cranial fossa approach or the transmastoid approach. The dehiscent area of the canal may be repaired with canal plugging or resurfacing procedure. Hearing loss following surgical repair is more common in revision surgery. The symptoms can recur following surgical repair.

Prognosis

Correct diagnosis of superior semicircular canal dehiscence is a critical first step in the management of patients with this clinical syndrome. Most patients can be helped by avoiding provoking stimuli. Surgery is reserved for the debilitated patient and is often curative.

Minor LB. Clinical manifestation of superior semicircular canal dehiscence. *Laryngoscope.* 2005;115:1717. [PMID: 16222184] (A comprehensive review of clinical manifestations of SSCD syndrome and therapeutic outcome.)

Diving Medicine

Allen M. Dekelboum, MD

Constantly increasing in number, the recreational and commercial diving community frequently presents with problems poorly understood by the average physician and otolaryngologist unless they have had some training in diving medicine. The consequences of breathing compressed gas mixtures under increasing barometric pressure and subsequent decreasing barometric pressure are confusing unless one understands the physics and physiology of the pressure environment. A well-trained otolaryngologist can be better prepared to treat the conditions that divers encounter by understanding the cause of these conditions.

DIVING PHYSICS

Living at sea level, our bodies are surrounded by one atmosphere of pressure (eg, 14.7 psi, 760 mm Hg, and 1 bar). The entire earth's atmosphere exerts this pressure, and it is exerted uniformly against our bodies. Pascal's principle states that any change in pressure in an enclosed fluid is transmitted equally throughout that fluid. The human body, being to a large extent fluid, is pushing out against the ambient pressure with the same force as the surrounding media. For this reason, divers can descend in the water to extreme depths with ease. It is only the air-filled spaces in our bodies that are affected by the changes in pressure. For each 33 feet of seawater (ie, 34 feet of fresh water, or 10 meters) through which we descend, we add an additional atmosphere of pressure. The pressure is doubled going from sea level to 33 feet of seawater, but is not doubled again until 99 feet of seawater is reached (Figure 57–1).

Conversely, as one ascends from depth, the pressure is decreased at the same rate. Boyle's law states that if the absolute temperature remains constant, the volume of a gas varies inversely as the absolute pressure. Because water temperature remains within a small absolute range, as a diver descends in the water, the air-filled spaces decrease in volume proportionately. As the diver ascends, the air-filled spaces increase in volume proportionately. Since we double the pressure from the surface to 33 feet of seawater and not again until 99 feet of seawater, the greatest pressure and volume changes occur closest to the surface. With the exception of decompression sickness, most divers' problems occur in the shallow depths, even as shallow as 4 feet of seawater.

Dalton's law of partial pressure states that in a mixture of gases (eg, air), the total pressure exerted by that mixture is equal to the sum of the partial pressures of each gas in the mixture. Both nitrogen and oxygen, composing most of the air we breathe, increase in partial pressure as the ambient pressure increases. Henry's law of solubility of gases states that as the partial pressure of a gas increases, more of that gas is dissolved in the surrounding liquid until saturation occurs. Since oxygen is utilized in metabolism, nitrogen, which is metabolically inert, is driven into solution in the circulating fluids of the body (eg, blood and lymph) in increasing amounts with increasing ambient pressure. Conversely, as ambient pressure is decreased, the dissolved gas becomes supersaturated and is released as gas bubbles. These latter two laws account for the indirect effects of pressure and are responsible for decompression sickness, or the bends, to be discussed later.

EXTERNAL EAR DISORDERS

Because divers spend much of their time in the water, they are subject to the same cutaneous problems of the external ear as are swimmers.

1. External Otitis

External otitis is very common and needs to be treated in the same fashion as external otitis that does not result as a complication of diving. In mild cases of pruritus, which are indicative of atopic external otitis, treatment can be limited to steroid drops both prophylactically and therapeutically. This is more of a chronic problem and treatment can be administered as needed. The more severe forms may require steroid-antibiotic drops with a wick being placed if the ear canal is completely closed. For severe infections, broad-spectrum antibiotics may be added. The prognosis is excellent and prophylaxis may prevent further infections. The use of acid-alcohol drops before diving and after leaving the water may prevent infection. One should wait until all the symptoms have resolved, the ear canal has returned to normal diameter, and hearing is restored. Prophylactic antibiotic drops may be needed for several weeks after the infection has cleared.

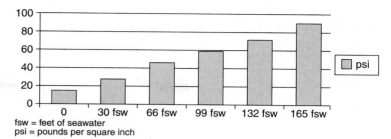

Figure 57–1. Ambient pressure relative to depth.

fsw = feet of seawater
psi = pounds per square inch

2. Foreign Bodies

Foreign bodies in the external ear canal, including cerumen, can be driven into the ear canal by the increasing water pressure and can either be lodged at the narrow portion of the canal or driven against the tympanic membrane. If they are lodged at the narrow portion of the ear canal and there is an air-filled space between the foreign body and the tympanic membrane, this air space is subject to Boyle's law, as stated above. The volume of the air space decreases with increasing ambient pressure, producing pain and hearing loss. There may be hemorrhage in the canal and on the outer surface of the tympanic membrane, and blebs and edema may be found after the foreign body is removed. Earplugs should never be used while diving unless they have a small vent hole. Treatment is removal of the foreign body and topical antibiotic eardrops.

Although exostoses can occur in divers who are also surfers, those who dive in cold water usually wear a thermal protective hood, which can prevent the formation of exostoses. If they are obstructive, they can be removed surgically.

Bove AA. *Bove & Davis' Diving Medicine,* 4th ed. Philadelphia: Saunders, 2004. (This text includes a very complete discourse on all aspects of diving medicine. The reader can consult it for much greater detail on the subjects included in this chapter.)

Edmonds C, Lowry C, Pennefather J, Walker R. *Diving and Subaquatic Medicine,* 4th ed. London: Arnold/Hodder Headline Group, 2002. (The fourth edition of one of the primary references in diving medicine, it includes detailed coverage of every subject and additional references at the end of each chapter.)

MIDDLE EAR DISORDERS

Etiology

As the diver descends in the water column, the air-filled space of the middle ear is subject to the effects of Boyle's law. With increasing pressure, the volume of the gas in the middle ear reduces proportionately and must be equalized by some technique (see Equalizing Techniques later in the chapter.). Frequent equalization is required near the surface as one descends and less so as the diver achieves greater depth. If equalization is not performed, the volume of the middle ear gas is reduced to the point that the tympanic membrane is retracted severely and fluid or blood (or both) is secreted into the middle ear, reducing the volume and equalizing the pressure. Alternately, the tympanic membrane may rupture.

Because of the unique etiology of diving disorders, the treating physician will see the entire spectrum of middle ear disease from eustachian tube obstruction, occurring rapidly, rather than over an extended period. Because this spectrum is caused by pressure changes, and usually on descent, it is referred to as barotrauma.

Occasionally, middle ear barotrauma can occur with ascent. In this case, the middle ear is equalized at depth, or partially so, and the diver ascends with an obstructed eustachian tube due to rebound rhinitis. The air in the middle ear space increases in volume with a decrease in ambient pressure, and if the middle ear is not vented via the eustachian tube, there will be pain and possible rupture of the tympanic membrane into the external ear canal. Descending to a deeper depth can relieve these symptoms; however, the diver is usually ascending because his breathing gas supply is low. Swallowing continually and ascending very slowly may partially relieve the symptoms, but if the gas supply is low, returning to the surface is mandatory. The symptoms, findings, and treatment are the same as for barotrauma of descent.

Prevention

Middle ear barotrauma can be prevented by not diving when there is any condition that might lead to eustachian tube obstruction (including upper respiratory infection or allergy). The diver should be able to easily equalize the middle ear. Prophylactic oral decongestants, short courses of nasal decongestants (no longer than 3 days because of possible rebound rhinitis), and steroid nasal sprays can assist in preventing obstruction.

Clinical Findings

Symptoms of middle ear barotrauma range from a dull feeling in the ear to pain and hearing loss. If a perforation of the tympanic membrane occurs, there will be vertigo with nausea and vomiting caused by the passage of water that is colder than body temperature into the middle ear; this water stimulates the lateral semicircular canal (a caloric stimulation).

Physical findings can be as simple as retraction, erythema and injection, or hemorrhage in the tympanic membrane. More severe findings include serous otitis, hemotympanum, and perforation of the tympanic membrane. Tuning fork tests and audiograms reveal a conductive hearing loss.

Treatment

Treatment of middle ear barotraumas consists of oral decongestants, short-term decongestant nasal sprays, and appropriate antibiotics if secondary infection is present. The diver should stay out of the water until the middle ear is healed and the diver can easily equalize the middle ear. If a perforation occurs, one must wait until the perforation heals and the tympanic membrane is intact again. If surgery is required for a nonhealing perforation, the above requirements must be met, usually requiring 3–4 months after surgery.

Divers should not return to diving until all the symptoms and findings have cleared. There should be ease of equalization of both middle ears confirmed by physical examination, tympanometry with a Valsalva maneuver, or both.

There remains controversy among otologists as to if or when divers who have had middle ear surgery can return to diving. The conditions that usually require myringoplasty or tympanoplasty are caused by eustachian tube obstruction. The surgical site and procedure should be completely healed with no evidence of difficulty in equalizing the middle ear. If ancillary conditions (eg, allergy or sinus disease) contributed to the need for middle ear surgery, they should be completely cleared, and if they recur, diving should be avoided.

Bove AA. *Bove & Davis' Diving Medicine,* 4th ed. Philadelphia: Saunders, 2004. (This text includes a very complete discourse on all aspects of diving medicine. The reader can consult it for much greater detail on the subjects included in this chapter.)

Edmonds C, Lowry C, Pennefather J, Walker R. *Diving and Subaquatic Medicine,* 4th ed. London: Arnold/Hodder Headline Group, 2002. (The fourth edition of one of the primary references in diving medicine, it includes detailed coverage of every subject and additional references at the end of each chapter.)

INNER EAR DISORDERS

1. Inner Ear Barotrauma

Etiology

Two mechanisms have been postulated as causing inner ear barotrauma. As the diver descends with difficulty in equalizing the middle ear space and continues to descend, attempting to forcefully equalize the middle ear, there can be a sudden opening of an obstructed eustachian tube with a rush of air into the middle ear space. This can rupture one of the windows between the middle ear and the inner ear—either the fenestra rotundum (ie, round window) or the fenestra ovalis (ie, oval window)—into the inner ear.

Conversely, if the diver descends with difficulty in equalizing the middle ear space and continues to descend, attempting to forcefully equalize the middle ear, and the eustachian tube does not open, the force is transmitted (as in a Valsalva maneuver) via the spinal fluid, through the cochlear aqueduct to the perilymphatic space of the inner ear. The round or oval windows can rupture into the middle ear.

Prevention

Prevention consists of avoiding situations that require forceful autoinflation of the middle ear, straining, or both.

Clinical Findings

Both mechanisms that cause inner ear barotrauma produce a perilymphatic fistula. The round window is more commonly affected than the oval window, but occasionally both windows rupture.

Symptoms include tinnitus, vertigo with nausea and vomiting, and hearing loss, which occur usually while descending. There may be pain due to a concomitant middle ear barotrauma. There is usually evidence of middle ear barotrauma, but the tympanic membrane may look perfectly normal. The hearing loss is sensorineural, accompanied by nystagmus and a positive fistula test.

Treatment

Treatment includes bed rest with the head of the bed elevated, anti-vertiginous medication, steroids (60–80 mg of prednisone or similar drugs initially, reducing the dosage over several days), and avoiding coughing, sneezing, and straining. Audiograms should be performed daily, and if there is improvement, continuation of nonsurgical treatment. Most patients recover spontaneously, but if the hearing loss and vertigo persist or worsen after 4–5 days, surgical exploration with repair of the fistula is recommended.

Many otologists trained in diving medicine recommend that the patient not return to diving, and many divers do return to diving in spite of the physician's recommendation. In addition, there have been no, or limited, recurrences. The diver should have no significant residual hearing loss (especially in speech frequencies), no significant defects in vestibular function, and no abnormalities of eustachian tube function with ease of equalization; however, she or he should not dive for at least 2 months after complete recovery. Divers should abort any dive in which there is difficulty in equalizing the middle ear. They should be advised that they might be at risk for further damage to the ear if they continue to dive.

Bove AA. *Bove & Davis' Diving Medicine,* 4th ed. Philadelphia: Saunders, 2004.

Edmonds C, Lowry C, Pennefather J, Walker R. *Diving and Subaquatic Medicine,* 4th ed. London: Arnold/Hodder Headline Group, 2002.

Pullen FW II, Rosenberg GJ, Cabeza CH. Sudden hearing loss in divers and fliers. *Laryngoscope.* 1979;89(9):1373. [PMID: 481042] (One of the original articles defining inner ear barotrauma and its treatment, a less conservative approach to management.)

Roydhouse N. Round window rupture. *South Pacific Underwater Med Soc J.* 1995;23(1):34. (This article supports the recommendations that divers may return to diving after suffering inner ear barotrauma. The late Dr. Roydhouse reported on a large series of divers with this problem.)

2. Inner Ear Decompression Sickness

Etiology

Decompression sickness follows Dalton's and Henry's laws. As one descends beneath the surface, the metabolically inert gas in the breathing mixture is dissolved in the fluids of the body with increasing pressure until that gas is saturated in solution. As one ascends, the dissolved gas comes out of solution as bubbles and is usually evacuated via the lungs. All divers ascend in a much shorter time than they spend under water; consequently, there is dissolved gas that now becomes supersaturated with decreasing pressure and is released as bubbles. Dive protocols have been created to allow the diver to ascend without the critical amounts of bubbles that produce symptoms of decompression sickness (or the bends).

Clinical Findings

If the diver violates protocols for ascending, or even when they are not violated, the bubbles can produce symptoms. The symptoms vary depending on the location of the bubbles. They can include cutaneous eruptions, pain, neurologic symptoms (including paralysis), and, rarely, death. If the bubbles lodge in the inner ear fluids, symptoms similar to inner ear barotrauma can occur and must be differentiated from that condition.

Inner ear decompression sickness is not a common problem with recreational divers who breathe gas mixtures principally containing nitrogen and oxygen (air and some mixtures with a higher content of oxygen and less nitrogen). It occurs more frequently in technical, commercial, and military divers who breathe gases that contain helium as one of the inert components. It is caused by gas bubbles being lodged in the fluids of the inner ear; these bubbles occur and enlarge on ascent.

Symptoms of tinnitus, hearing loss, severe vertigo with nausea and vomiting, ataxia, and syncope usually occur 10 minutes or longer after ascent from the dive. There is absence of tympanic membrane and middle ear barotrauma; however, the hearing loss is sensorineural and nystagmus is present.

Differential Diagnosis

Differentiating inner ear barotrauma and inner ear decompression sickness can usually be made by the history of the dive (Table 57–1). If there is doubt as to the differential diagnosis, patients should be treated for inner ear decompression sickness because it is the more severe condition and patients can be left with persistent vertigo and ataxia if this condition remains untreated.

Treatment

Treatment is recompression in a chamber, breathing 100% oxygen. Careful adherence to decompression schedules and ascent rates is the only prevention, but, as stated above, this condition can occur even if proper adherence to decompression schedules is followed.

Bove AA. *Bove & Davis' Diving Medicine,* 4th ed. Philadelphia: Saunders, 2004.

Table 57–1. Signs and symptoms of inner ear barotrauma and inner ear decompression sickness. These symptoms and signs can aid in the differential diagnosis of these two conditions.

Inner Ear Barotrauma	Inner Ear Decompression Sickness
Can occur on any dive	The dive usually exceeds the recommended depth and time
Usually presents with evidence of middle ear barotrauma	Normal tympanic membrane and middle ear
Sensorineural hearing loss	Sensorineural hearing loss
Usually occurs on descent, but can occur on ascent	Usually occurs shortly after ascending
Can result from any gas mixture	Usually occurs with gas mixes containing helium

Edmonds C, Lowry C, Pennefather J, Walker R. *Diving and Subaquatic Medicine,* 4th ed. London: Arnold/Hodder Headline Group, 2002.

Farmer JC. Diving injuries to the inner ear. *Ann Otol.* 1977;36:86. [PMID: 402882] (This letter to the editor offers the writer's lengthy experience to support divers returning to diving after suffering inner ear barotrauma. The late Dr. Roydhouse previously reported on a large series of divers with this problem.)

Nachum Z, Shupak A, Spitzer O, Sharoni Z, Doweck I, Gordon CR. Inner ear decompression sickness in sport compressed air divers. *Laryngoscope.* 2001;111(5):851. [PMID: 11359165] (One of the original reports of inner ear decompression sickness in sport divers.)

Parrell GJ, Becker GD. Inner ear barotrauma in scuba diving: a long-term follow-up after continuing diving. *Arch Otol.* 1993;119:455. [PMID: 8457309] (The first retrospective report of divers having no further problems returning to diving after suffering inner ear barotrauma.)

CAUSES OF VERTIGO WITH DIVING

Vertigo is a common symptom of diving injuries and has many causes common to the diving environment, including unequal vestibular stimulation (Table 57–2),

Table 57–2. Vertigo due to unequal vestibular stimulation.

Caloric
Unilateral external auditory canal obstruction
Cerumen
External otitis
Exostoses
Foreign body
Tympanic membrane perforation
Middle ear barotrauma
Shock wave
Middle ear barotrauma
Reverse block on ascent
Middle ear barotrauma of descent
Alternobaric vertigo—a condition in which one eustachian tube only opens on ascent. Usually self-limited, but can persist for several days
Inner ear barotrauma
Inner ear decompression sickness
Tulio phenomenon—caused by loud sounds
Seasickness
Temporomandibular joint syndrome

Table 57–3. Vertigo due to unequal vestibular responses.

Barotrauma
Gas toxicity
Inert gas narcosis—caused by increasing partial pressure of nitrogen with descent. Equivalent to one martini for every 30–50 feet dived. Immediately reversed on ascending to shallower depths
High-pressure nervous syndrome—caused by very deep diving using helium and oxygen mixtures. Can be prevented by slow ascent and by adding small amounts of nitrogen to the breathing mix
CNS oxygen toxicity
Carbon dioxide toxicity
Hypoxia, hypocarbia, carbon monoxide intoxication
Sensory deprivation—diving in low-visibility situations with significant water movement

unequal vestibular responses (Table 57–3), and central causes (Table 57–4).

Edmonds C, Lowry C, Pennefather J, Walker R. *Diving and Subaquatic Medicine,* 4th ed. London: Arnold/Hodder Headline Group, 2002.

OTHER CAUSES OF BAROTRAUMA

1. Barodontalgia

Barodontalgia is a condition producing dental pain on descent or ascent. It is caused by poor fillings, air pockets beneath the fillings, dental abscesses, or pressure-induced fluid leakage around the dentin of the tooth. It may be implosive on descent or explosive on ascent, occasionally forcing a filling, inlay, or crown to be extruded. This condition is rare and if dental pain in the upper teeth is a presenting symptom, one must first consider maxillary sinus barotrauma.

Table 57–4. Vertigo due to central causes.

CNS decompression sickness—bubbles produced in the central nervous system
Arterial gas embolus—bubbles in the arterial system produced by lung overpressure syndromes
Drug intoxication

2. Facial Nerve Baroparesis

Facial nerve baroparesis can occur. The facial nerve can be dehiscent of bone as it passes through the middle ear space. If there is extreme pressure due to inadequate equalization of the middle ear, temporary ischemia of the exposed portion my lead to palsy. It is usually self-limited, but can be repetitive.

TMJ Symptoms

Although not a true barotrauma condition, temporomandibular joint (TMJ) symptoms may occur. Novice divers have a tendency to bite down hard on their scuba mouthpieces, occasionally biting through the mouthpiece. The pain produced can mimic otologic conditions unless recognized. The ear examination is usually normal, and there is tenderness in the TMJ just in front of the tragus of the external ear. There may be teeth marks on the scuba mouthpiece.

Becker GD. Recurrent alternobaric facial paralysis resulting from scuba diving. *Laryngoscope.* 1983;93:596. [PMID: 684351] (The first description of recurrent facial palsy after scuba diving.)

Bove AA. *Bove & Davis' Diving Medicine,* 4th ed. Philadelphia: Saunders, 2004.

Edmonds C, Lowry C, Pennefather J, Walker R. *Diving and Subaquatic Medicine,* 4th ed. London: Arnold/Hodder Headline Group, 2002.

PARANASAL SINUS DISORDERS

The ostia of the paranasal sinuses are normally open unless obstructed by disease or anatomic deformities. Air freely exchanges between the nose and the sinus cavities. As long as this occurs, barotrauma of the paranasal sinuses does not occur. However, sinus barotrauma is very common, as are acute and chronic diseases of the sinuses. Preexisting allergy, acute infections, obstruction by polyps, or a deviated nasal septum can contribute to the inability of the sinuses to adequately aerate. The frontal sinuses are the most commonly involved, followed by the maxillary sinuses, the ethmoid sinuses, and, rarely, the sphenoid sinuses.

The symptoms, findings, and treatment are the same as for sinusitis. Pain, increasing with depth while descending, is the most significant symptom. Barodontalgia is a very rare condition. Maxillary sinus pain can mimic dental pain, and one must consider maxillary sinus barotrauma if the diver complains of upper dental pain.

The diagnosis is confirmed by radiographic examination, and diving should be withheld until there is complete clearing of the sinuses. The treatment of chronic nasal conditions is essential and the correction of anatomic abnormalities is sometimes necessary.

Bartley J. Functional endoscopic sinus surgery in divers with recurrent sinus barotrauma. *South Pacific Underwater Med Soc J.* 1995;25(2):64. (A review of endoscopic sinus surgery and criteria for returning to diving after this surgery.)

Edmonds C, Lowry C, Pennefather J, Walker R. *Diving and Subaquatic Medicine,* 4th ed. London: Arnold/Hodder Headline Group, 2002

CAUSES OF HEARING LOSS IN DIVING

Hearing loss is a common symptom in diving. At the scene of the diving accident, the examiner can frequently determine, with the use of tuning forks, whether the hearing loss was due to some interference with the conductive mechanism or to some damage to the sensory or neural pathway. Table 57–5 lists some of the causes of hearing loss that might occur in divers.

CONTRAINDICATIONS TO DIVING

Any condition that either prevents a diver from adequately equalizing the middle ear spaces and sinuses or puts the diver at risk if the condition was to occur under water must be recognized. Some conditions are controversial, and new evidence is helping to resolve the controversies. Several otolaryngologic conditions should preclude returning to diving. These include (1) a tympanic membrane perforation, (2) the presence of pressure-equalizing tubes in the tympanic membrane, (3) a radical or modified radi-

Table 57–5. Conditions that produce hearing loss in divers.

Conductive Hearing Loss
Negative pressure in the middle ear
Cerumen
Foreign body
External otitis
Exostoses
Tympanic membrane hemorrhage
Serous otitis media
Hemotympanum
Tympanic membrane perforation
Increased gas density—at extreme depths
Sensorineural Hearing Loss
Inner ear barotrauma
Inner ear decompression sickness
Noise-induced
Presbycusis

cal mastoidectomy (the lateral semicircular canal is exposed to water in the mastoid cavity, producing a caloric response), (4) any vertiginous condition that might occur under water, (5) the inability to inflate the middle ear, (6) chronic refractory sinusitis, (7) tracheotomy or tracheostoma, and (8) any condition that makes it impossible to hold a scuba regulator in the mouth. As noted previously, there is controversy with regard to inner ear barotrauma. Patients who have undergone stapes surgery have been advised not to return to diving. However, there is an increasing body of evidence that allows these individuals to dive safely (see references).

Temporary contraindications include (1) any acute or chronic otolaryngologic infection until resolved, (2) healed tympanic membrane perforations until they meet the criteria noted previously, (3) external otitis until cleared, (4) impacted cerumen, (5) middle ear barotrauma until resolved, (6) chronic nasal obstruction, (7) any acute sinus trauma until healed with no dehiscence of bone, (8) orthodontic appliances, and (9) current major dental therapy until completed.

Antonelli PJ, Adamcyzk M, Appleton CM, Parell GJ. Inner ear barotrauma after stapedectomy in the guinea pig. *Laryngoscope.* 1999;109(12):1991. [PMID: 10591361] (A basic research article supporting returning to diving after stapedectomy.)

Bove AA. *Bove & Davis' Diving Medicine,* 4th ed. Philadelphia: Saunders, 2004.

Edmonds C, Lowry C, Pennefather J, Walker R. *Diving and Subaquatic Medicine,* 4th ed. London: Arnold/Hodder Headline Group, 2002.

House JW, Toh EH, Perez A. Diving after stapedectomy: clinical experience and recommendations. *Otolaryngol Head Neck Surg.* 2001;1254:356. [PMID: 1159317] (A large clinical experience justifies allowing divers to return to diving after stapedectomy.)

EQUALIZING TECHNIQUES

Middle ear and sinus barotrauma are the most common injuries associated with exposure to increasing and decreasing pressure. Descent in the water adds approximately one-half pound of pressure for each foot of descent and diminishes a similar amount on ascent. According to Boyle's law, as the pressure increases on descent, the volume of a gas in an enclosed space decreases proportionately. As the pressure decreases on ascent, the volume of the gas increases proportionately. On descent, it is imperative that all enclosed air-filled spaces be equalized actively or passively. On ascent, the increasing gas volume usually vents itself naturally. As noted previously, the greatest pressure and volume changes occur closest to the surface.

For equalization to be effective, the diver should be free of nasal or sinus infections or allergic reactions. The lining of the nose, throat, and eustachian tubes should be as normal as possible. If this is the case, the following techniques are effective in reducing middle ear and sinus squeeze.

(1) Before descent and neutrally buoyant, with no air in the buoyancy compensator, the diver's ears should be gently inflated with one of the methods listed below. This gives the diver a little extra air in the middle ear and sinuses as he or she descends.

(2) The diver's descent should be feet first, if possible. This allows air to travel upward into the eustachian tube and middle ear, a more natural direction. A descent or anchor line should be used.

(3) The diver should inflate gently every 2 feet for the first 10–15 feet and less frequently as he or she descends more deeply.

(4) Pain is not acceptable. If there is pain, the diver has descended without adequately equalizing.

(5) If the diver does not feel the ears opening, he or she should stop, try again, and perhaps ascend a few feet to diminish the surrounding pressure. The diver should not bounce up and down, but should try to tilt the ear that is not opening upward.

(6) If the diver is unable to equalize, the dive should be aborted. The consequences of descending without equalizing could ruin an entire dive trip and, more important, produce permanent damage and hearing loss.

(7) If the diver's physician agrees, decongestants and nasal sprays may be used before diving to reduce swelling in the nasal and sinus passages, as well as in the eustachian tube.

Decongestants should be taken 1–2 hours before descent; they generally last from 8 to 12 hours. Nasal sprays should be taken 30 minutes before descent and usually last about 12 hours. Caution should be taken when using over-the-counter nasal sprays, since repeated use can cause a rebound reaction with a worsening of congestion and a possible reverse block on ascent.

(8) If at any time during the dive the diver feels pain, has vertigo (the "whirlies"), or notes sudden hearing loss, the dive should be aborted. If these symptoms persist, the diver should not dive again until consulting a physician.

(9) Equalizing techniques may be used.

The following techniques can be used by the diver to equalize the volume of gas in the middle ear.

(a) Passive. *This technique requires no effort.*

(b) Valsalva. *The diver can increase nasopharynx pressure by holding the nose and breathing against a closed glottis (throat).*

(c) Toynbee. *The diver swallows with mouth and nose closed. This technique is especially good for ascent.*

(d) Frenzel. *This technique involves the diver's using the Valsalva technique while contracting the throat muscles with a closed glottis.*

(e) Lowry (Valsalva plus Toynbee). *The diver holds the nose closed, gently trying to blow air out of the nose while swallowing. This technique is the easiest and best method to use after it is practiced.*

(f) Edmonds. *The diver juts the jaw forward and then performs the Valsalva technique, the Frenzel technique, or both. This method is very effective.*

(g) Miscellaneous. *Miscellaneous techniques include swallowing and wiggling the jaw. These techniques are especially good for ascent.*

Antonelli PJ, Adamcyzk M, Appleton CM, Parell GJ. Inner ear barotrauma after stapedectomy in the guinea pig. *Laryngoscope.* 1999;109(12):1991. [PMID: 10591361] (A basic research article supporting returning to diving after stapedectomy.)

Bartley J. Functional endoscopic sinus surgery in divers with recurrent sinus barotrauma. *South Pacific Underwater Med Soc J.* 1995;25(2):64. (A review of endoscopic sinus surgery and criteria for returning to diving after this surgery.)

Becker GD. Recurrent alternobaric facial paralysis resulting from scuba diving. *Laryngoscope.* 1983;93:596. [PMID: 684351] (The first description of recurrent facial palsy after scuba diving.)

Bove AA. *Bove & Davis' Diving Medicine,* 4th ed. Philadelphia: Saunders, 2004.

Edmonds C, Lowry C, Pennefather J, Walker R. *Diving and Subaquatic Medicine,* 4th ed. London: Arnold/Hodder Headline Group, 2002.

Farmer JC. Diving injuries to the inner ear. *Ann Otol.* 1977;36:86. [PMID: 402882] (This letter to the editor offers the writer's lengthy experience to support divers returning to diving after suffering inner ear barotrauma. The late Dr. Roydhouse previously reported on a large series of divers with this problem.)

House JW, Toh EH, Perez A. Diving after stapedectomy: clinical experience and recommendations. *Otolaryngol Head Neck Surg.* 2001;1254:356. [PMID: 1159317] (A large clinical experience justifies allowing divers to return to diving after stapedectomy.)

Nachum Z, Shupak A, Spitzer O, Sharoni Z, Doweck I, Gordon CR. Inner ear decompression sickness in sport compressed air divers. *Laryngoscope.* 2001;111(5):851. [PMID: 11359165] (One of the original reports of inner ear decompression sickness in sport divers.)

Parrell GJ, Becker GD. Inner ear barotrauma in scuba diving: a long-term follow-up after continuing diving. *Arch Otol.* 1993;119:455. [PMID: 8457309] (The first retrospective report of divers having no further problems returning to diving after suffering inner ear barotrauma.)

Pullen FW II, Rosenberg GJ, Cabeza CH. Sudden hearing loss in divers and fliers. *Laryngoscope.* 1979;89(9):1373. [PMID: 481042] (One of the original articles defining inner ear barotrauma and its treatment, with a less conservative approach to management.)

Roydhouse N. Round window rupture. *South Pacific Underwater Med Soc J.* 1995;23(1):34. (This article supports the recommendations that divers may return to diving after suffering inner ear barotrauma. The late Dr. Roydhouse reported on a large series of divers with this problem.)

WEB SITES

[Diving Medicine Online]
http://www.scuba-doc.com/

ADDITIONAL RESOURCES

The Divers Alert Network, maintained at Duke University, has a 24-hour number with trained medical personnel available to deal with diving accident problems: (800) 446-2671. They can refer you to the nearest recompression chamber and to the nearest physician trained in diving medicine who can handle your questions.

Occupational Hearing Loss

58

Sumit K. Agrawal, MD, David N. Schindler, MD, Robert K. Jackler, MD, & Scott Robinson, MPH, CIH, CSP

Noise-induced hearing loss (NIHL) ranks among the 10 most common occupational illnesses. NIHL is generally bilateral but not infrequently is an asymmetric, high-frequency sensory hearing loss. Sensory hearing loss results from deterioration of the structures within the cochlea, usually owing to the loss of hair cells from the organ of Corti. Among the many common causes of sensory hearing loss is the prolonged exposure to noise > 85 dB.

In an occupational setting, a high-frequency sensory hearing loss can be associated with head trauma or concussion. A mixed or conductive hearing loss can also be observed and is usually the result of direct head trauma (eg, tympanic membrane perforation due to a slag burn or ossicular discontinuity from a temporal bone fracture), indirect head trauma (ie, explosion or implosion), or barotrauma.

Although rarely seen in the occupational setting, ototoxicity may play a role in neurosensory hearing loss.

DIAGNOSIS

The most commonly encountered types of occupational hearing loss are NIHL, hearing loss due to physical trauma, and ototoxic hearing loss.

In evaluating a patient with occupational hearing loss, the following differential diagnosis must be considered: (1) presbycusis (ie, age-related hearing loss), (2) hereditary hearing impairment, (3) metabolic disorders (eg, diabetes mellitus, thyroid dysfunction, renal failure, autoimmune disease, hyperlipidemia, and hypercholesterolemia), (4) sudden sensorineural hearing loss, (5) hearing loss resulting from infectious origins (ie, bacterial or viral infections, including meningitis and encephalitis), (6) hearing loss resulting from central nervous system (CNS) disease (eg, cerebellopontine angle tumors, especially acoustic neuromas), (7) Meniere disease, (8) nonorganic hearing loss (ie, functional hearing loss).

EVALUATION OF HEARING

In all cases of occupational hearing loss, a complete pure-tone audiogram with speech reception thresholds (SRT) and word recognition scores (WRS) must be included. The audiometric equipment should be calibrated within 1 year to American National Standards Institute (ANSI) standards.

Functional hearing loss should always be considered, and the following tests can be used to help differentiate this from a genuine occupational hearing loss:

1. If SRT scores diverge more than 10 dB from the pure-tone average (PTA) for speech frequency, additional testing may be indicated to exclude the possibility of nonorganic or intentionally exaggerated hearing loss.
2. Audiometric evoked brainstem response (ABR)—normal in functional hearing loss.
3. Otoacoustic emissions (OAE)—normal in functional hearing loss.
4. Stenger test—based on the principle that if tones of the *same frequency* are presented to both ears, the patient will perceive only the loudest tone. A tone 5 dB above threshold is presented to the good ear and 5 dB below threshold is presented to the "bad" ear. A patient should state that he or she hears the tone in the good ear. A patient with functional hearing loss hears the tone in the "bad" ear and fails to respond.

NIHL

Definitions

Noise refers to unwanted, undesirable, or excessively loud sound experienced by an individual. The effects of noise depend on various characteristics of the sound: (1) intensity (more intense sounds > less intense sounds); (2) spectrum (higher frequencies > lower frequencies secondary to the protective effect of the acoustic reflex at lower frequencies); (3) cumulative lifetime exposure (longer exposures > shorter exposures); and (4) pattern (continuous exposures > interrupted exposures for the same overall duration and intensity).

Temporary threshold shifts (TTS) are changes in hearing after noise exposure which completely recover within 24 hours. **Permanent threshold shifts** (PTS) are hearing losses that are not recoverable with time. The noise exposure causes permanent loss of hair cell stereocilia with apparent fracture of the rootlet structures and destruction of the sensory cells, which are replaced by nonfunctioning scar tissue. Because TTS may mimic PTS, individuals should be given audiometric tests only after a recovery period of 24 hours following exposure to hazardous levels of noise.

Acoustic trauma occurs when high-intensity impulse noises (eg, explosions) penetrate the cochlea before the acoustic reflex has been activated. Impulse noises refer to either single or multiple noise events lasting 1 second or less, and high-intensity impulse noises of > 140 dB may cause immediate and irreversible hearing loss. The acoustic reflex is a reflex contraction of the stapedius muscle in response to noise > 90 dB. This reflex dampens sound transmission and is particularly protective against low-frequency noise. The delay from noise exposure to onset of the reflex is 25–150 ms, rendering it less effective against impulse noise compared with continuous noise.

Pathogenesis

NIHL results from trauma to the sensory epithelium of the cochlea. The sensory epithelium of the cochlea comprises one inner and three outer rows of stereociliated hair cells within the organ of Corti. In TTS, several potentially reversible effects include:

1. Regional decrease in the stiffness of stereocilia secondary to the contraction of rootlet structures which are anchored to the cuticular plate of hair cells

2. Intracellular changes within the hair cells including metabolic exhaustion and microvascular changes

3. Edema of the auditory nerve endings

4. Degeneration of synapses within the cochlear nucleus

In PTS, the changes become irreversible and include breaks in the rootlet structures, disruption of the cochlear duct and organ of Corti causing mixing of endolymph and perilymph, loss of hair cells, and degeneration of cochlear nerve fibers.

Acoustic trauma causes severe, irreversible hearing loss. High-intensity impulse noises can directly damage tympanic membrane, ossicles, inner ear membranes, and the organ of Corti.

Clinical Findings

Patients with NIHL frequently complain of a gradual, insidious deterioration in hearing. The most common complaint is difficulty in comprehending speech, especially in the presence of competing background noise. Background noise, which is usually low frequency in bias, masks the better-preserved portion of the hearing spectrum and further exacerbates problems with speech comprehension. Because patients with NIHL have a high-frequency bias to their hearing loss, they experience a distortion of speech sounds when listening to people with particularly high-pitched voices (eg, women and children) (Figure 58–1).

NIHL is frequently accompanied by tinnitus. Most often patients describe a high-frequency tonal sound (eg, ringing), but the sound is sometimes lower in tone (eg, buzzing, blowing, or hissing) or even nontonal (eg, popping or clicking). Often, the tinnitus frequency matches the frequency of the hearing loss seen on the audiogram and is approximately 5 dB above that threshold in loudness. Tinnitus in the absence of hearing loss is likely not related to noise exposure.

The diagnosis of occupational NIHL has been summarized in an evidence-based policy statement by the American College of Occupational and Environmental Medicine (2002).

The typical "4000 Hz notch" is thought to occur due to the (1) resonance frequency of the ear canal, (2) the acoustic reflex protecting the ear at lower frequencies, (3) intermittency protecting the ear at lower frequencies, and (4) outer hair cells being most susceptible at the base of the cochlea. Lower and higher frequencies become affected after many years of noise exposure, and a significant decrease in word recognition scores does not begin until frequencies < 3000 Hz are affected (Figure 58–2). Asymmetry can exist in the audiogram, particularly when the source of the noise is lateralized (eg, a rifle or shotgun firing).

Evoked otoacoustic emissions (OAE) may be useful in detecting early NIHL in persons with normal audiograms. Outer hair cells are affected early in NIHL, and both transient-evoked OAE and distortion-product OAE have been shown to detect subtle changes in outer hair cell function.

Predisposing Factors

A. SUSCEPTIBILITY

It has been observed that some individuals are able to tolerate high noise levels for prolonged periods of time, whereas others who are subjected to the same environment lose hearing more rapidly. The genetic basis of this variability has been studied in detail using a mouse model, and several strains have been found to be either susceptible or resistant to noise-induced damage. The risk is likely an interaction between genetic susceptibility and the duration and intensity of the noise exposure (Figure 58–3).

B. PRESBYCUSIS

NIHL and presbycusis often coexist in our aging population. Large studies have shown that the combined effect is additive over time, and attempts have been made to quantify this interaction.

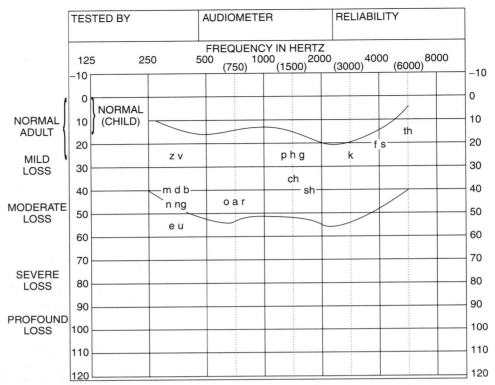

Figure 58–1. Relative consonant and vowel sounds on an audiogram are a function of frequency.

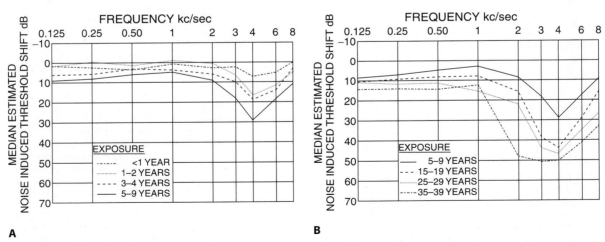

Figure 58–2. Estimated noise-induced threshold shift as a function of frequency, for various durations of exposure.

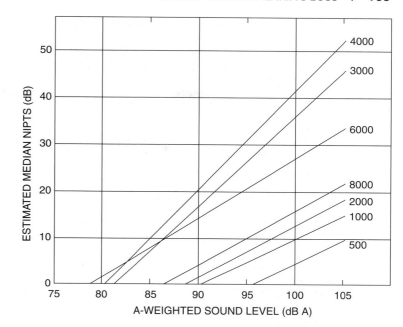

Figure 58–3. Estimated permanent threshold shifts at various frequencies produced by noise exposure of more than 10 years' duration.

C. Ototoxicity

Concurrent exposure to noise and ototoxic medications may potentiate hearing loss. These effects have been shown for both cisplatin and aminoglycosides. Loop diuretics and salicylates, however, have not been definitively shown to potentiate NIHL.

D. Vibration

There is recent evidence that vibration can interact with noise to cause both TTS and PTS. The mechanism of this interaction is not well understood.

ACOEM Noise and Hearing Conservation Committee Evidence-Based Statement. *Noise Induced Hearing Loss.* American College of Occupational and Environmental Medicine, 2002. (Update of the previous 1989 position statement by the ACOEM outlining diagnostic criteria of noise-induced hearing loss and worker evaluation.)

Borg E et al. Effect of the acoustic reflex on inner ear damage induced by industrial noise. *Acta Otolaryngol.* 1983;96:361. [PMID: 6637452] (Animal study investigating the stapedial reflex and its protective effect against temporary and permanent threshold shifts in noise exposure.)

Dobie RA. Noise-induced hearing loss. In: Baily BJ et al, eds. *Head and Neck Surgery—Otolaryngology.* Philadelphia: Lippincott Williams & Wilkins, 2001. (General chapter covering noise-induced hearing loss.)

Grati MM et al. Rapid turnover of stereocilia membrane proteins: evidence from the trafficking and mobility of plasma membrane Ca(2+)-ATPase 2. *J Neurosci.* 2006;26:6386. [PMID: 16763047]

Kim JJ et al. Fine structure of long-term changes in the cochlear nucleus after acoustic overstimulation: chronic degeneration and new growth of synaptic endings. *J Neurosci Res.* 2004;77:817. [PMID: 15334600] (Animal studying demonstrating synaptic degeneration in the cochlear nucleus following noise exposure.)

Lonsbury-Martin BL, Martin GK. Noise-induced hearing loss. In: Cummings CW et al, eds. *Cummings Otolaryngology—Head & Neck Surgery.* Philadelphia: Elsevier Mosby, 2005. (Chapter covering noise-induced hearing loss with a good review of basic science research.)

Oghalai JS. Cochlear hearing loss. In: Jackler RK, Brackmann DE, eds. *Neurotology.* Philadelphia: Elsevier Mosby, 2005. (Chapter on cochlear hearing loss and a sub-section on noise-induced hearing loss.)

Palmer KT et al. Raynaud's phenomenon, vibration induced white finger, and difficulties in hearing. *Occup Environ Med.* 2002;59:640. [PMID: 12205240] (Study examining the association between vibration and hearing loss.)

Sha SH et al. Differential vulnerability of basal and apical hair cells is based on intrinsic susceptibility to free radicals. *Hear Res.* 2001;155:1. [PMID: 11335071] (Study examining the viability of outer hair cells from the base and apex of guinea pig cochleas. It suggests that basal outer hair cells may be more susceptible to free-radical damage.)

Tan CT et al. Potentiation of noise-induced hearing loss by amikacin in guinea pigs. *Hear Res.* 2001;161:72. [PMID: 11744283] (Study suggesting that subtoxic doses of amikacin are sufficient to impair recovery from noise-induced threshold shifts in guinea pigs.)

Treatment

No medical or surgical treatments are available to reverse the effects of NIHL; therefore, prevention is the foremost priority. This often requires a team consisting of otolaryngology, audiology, and audiologic engineers. After the diagnosis has been established by otologic examination and by the administration of an audiometric test battery, the physician should counsel the patient on the likely consequences of continued exposure to excessive noise, including recommending techniques for avoiding further noise-induced damage.

Hearing amplification is reserved for patients whose hearing impairment is severe in social situations. Hearing aids must be carefully fitted to optimally meet the needs of the individual with regard to frequency bias and gain. In bilateral hearing losses, bilateral amplification usually provides more satisfactory rehabilitation. Although the decision to try hearing amplification is the patient's, a reasonable criterion for referral to a professional for hearing aid evaluation is a speech reception thresholds > 25 dB or a word recognition score < 80% when words are presented at a normal conversational level of 50 dB above threshold. There are some instances in which hearing aids may be recommended to assist the patient to hear in special circumstances, such as lectures or group situations. In patients with high-frequency hearing loss and relatively normal low-frequency hearing, hearing aids are generally the most helpful to those who have a significant hearing loss at 2000 Hz on a pure-tone audiogram. A borderline candidate may be a person with normal hearing through 1500 Hz, a mild hearing loss at 2000 Hz, and a moderate or greater hearing loss at 3000 Hz and above.

The two basic hearing aids that are available are the analog hearing aid and the newer, more expensive digitally programmable hearing aids. Before purchasing hearing aids, the patient should have a hearing aid evaluation and a trial period, with the patient wearing the aids in various circumstances. Numerous assistive listening devices are available (FM and infrared) to enhance comprehension in specific situations. Aural rehabilitation classes designed to enhance the patient's ability to comprehend speech may also be helpful and are usually available in urban areas.

There is no cure for tinnitus resulting from NIHL, although numerous amelioration measures are available. With no further inner ear injury, tinnitus gradually diminishes, usually over a course of weeks to months. A subtle degree of tinnitus often persists and is especially obvious when the patient is in a quiet room. For the few patients who find this to be extremely troublesome, masking the tinnitus with music or some other form of pleasant sound is often helpful. In those with significant hearing loss, the most successful treatment may be appropriate hearing amplification. Modified hearing aids (tinnitus maskers) designed to produce masking noises have generally been of limited success. The use of biofeedback has helped some patients suppress their tinnitus.

Patients should be informed of various support groups available and psychiatric referral may be necessary to medically manage associated depression and anxiety.

Prognosis

In patients with NIHL, hearing generally stabilizes if the patient is removed from the noxious stimulus. *NIHL does not progress after the worker is removed from the source of the hazardous noise.* If there has been further progression of hearing loss after a person has been removed from the source of noise, the progression of further hearing loss is the result of some other degenerative, congenital, or metabolic process (eg, presbycusis). Although adequate noise protection is essential and should always be recommended, even with adequate hearing protection, other factors may play a role in the patient's prognosis. Presbycusis can add to NIHL as the patient grows older, and coexisting NIHL may cause the patient to be more susceptible to the adverse effects of ototoxic substances such as aminoglycoside antibiotics, loop diuretics, and antineoplastic agents used in the treatment of other disorders (see Ototoxic Hearing Loss, which follows).

Prevention

A. OCCUPATIONAL SAFETY AND HEALTH ADMINISTRATION (OSHA) REGULATIONS

Noise has been measured by a number of governmental agencies, private corporate entities, and academic institutions. A list of common noise examples is included (Table 58–1).

The maximum permissible OSHA dB standard for nonimpulse noise is a time-weighted average of 90 dBA for 8 hours, with every increase of 5 dB halving the exposure time to a maximum of 115 dBA for 15 minutes (Table 58–2). OSHA has allowed for a maximum of 140-dB peak sound pressure for impulse noise. To protect against these maximal allowable exposures, workers exposed to 85 dBA or more require hearing protection and trigger the need to implement a hearing conservation program.

In 1998, the National Institute for Occupational Safety and Health (NIOSH) recommended limiting occupational noise exposure to a time-weighted average of 85 dBA for 8 hours, with a 3-dB exchange rate, although this has yet to become the enforced standard. Even with a time-weighted average of 85 dBA, the risk of impairment may be 10–15%. Each country uses its own standards and many have adopted programs similar to the revised criteria of the NIOSH.

B. HEARING CONSERVATION PROGRAM

The hearing conservation program is the recognized method of preventing NIHL in the occupational environment. Although there is a tendency to think of "hearing conservation" as the provision of audiometric tests

Table 58–1. Examples of noise in industry and noise in the environment.

Jet Engines-Flight Line	
FA-18E engine at 80% (rear) < 50 ft	130 dBA
FA-18E engine at idle (rear) < 50 ft	105 dBA
FA-18 after burner test (rear) < 50 ft	139 dBA
F104 engine at idle from 200 ft	91 dBA
Diesel hydraulic Jenny	107 dBA
Heavy Mobile Equipment	
Scrapers-loaders	117 dBA
Road graders	95 dBA
Tool Operations (Metal)	
Pneumatic grinders on aluminum	100–102 dBA
Chipping weld on large aluminum structure	120 dBA
Cut-off grinder cutting aluminum pipe	100 dBA
Cut-off grinder cutting galvanized pipe	96–98 dBA
Needle gun on 1/4-in. steel plate	108 dBA
Punch press 3/8-in. flat bar steel	118 dBA
Tool Operations (Woodworking)	
Cut-off saw	112 dBA
Radial arm saw	98 dBA
Router	93 dBA
Planer	106 dBA
Socioacusis	
Normal conversation	50–60 dBA
Motorboats	74–114 dBA
Motorcycles	up to 110 dBA
Snowmobiles	85–109 dBA
Lawnmowers	up to 96 dBA
Hunting weapons	143–173 dBA

Table 58–2. Permissible noise exposure in the workplace.

Hours Per Day	Sound Levels dBA (Slow Response)
16	85
8	90
6	92
4	95
2	100
1	105
0.5	110
0.25	115

and hearing protection, much more effort is required. An effective hearing conservation program integrates the following program elements: (1) noise monitoring, (2) engineering controls, (3) administrative controls, (4) worker education, (5) selection and use of hearing protection devices, and (6) periodic audiometric evaluations. Record keeping is important, and record-keeping requirements are described in the OSHA standard. Records should show a notation of NIHL on the OSHA log of injuries and illnesses.

1. Noise monitoring—If there is reason to believe that worker noise exposure equals or exceed a time-weighted average of 85 dBA, then noise monitoring is required. A sampling strategy must be designed to identify all workers who need to be included in the hearing conservation program. Using the appropriate noise-monitoring instrumentation, noise must be characterized in terms of the following: (1) frequency (predominantly high, predominantly low, or mixed); (2) intensity (how loud the sound is); and (3) type (continuous, intermittent, or impulse). Any time there is a change in production, the process, equipment, or controls, noise monitoring must be repeated.

2. Engineering controls—The information collected during noise monitoring—particularly octave band analysis, which indicates the sound level at selected frequencies—may be used to design engineering controls. Designers conceptualize possible engineering solutions in terms of (1) the source (what is generating the noise), (2) the path (the route or routes the generated noise may travel), and (3) the receivers (the noise-exposed workers).

To reduce noise exposure to workers, such controls may involve (1) enclosures (to isolate sources or receivers), (2) barriers (to reduce acoustic energy along the path), and (3) distance (to increase the path and ultimately reduce the acoustic energy at the receiver). In general, engineering controls are preferred but are not always feasible because of both their costs and the limits of technology.

3. Administrative controls—Administrative controls include (1) reducing the amount of time a given worker might be exposed to a noise source to prevent a time-weighted average of noise exposure from reaching 85 dBA, and (2) establishing purchasing guidelines to prevent the introduction of equipment that would increase the dose of noise to which workers are subjected. Though simple in principle, the implementation of administrative control requires management commitment and constant supervision, particularly in the absence of engineering or personal protection controls. In general, administrative controls are used as an adjunct to existing noise control strategies within a hearing conservation program rather than as an exclusive approach for controlling noise exposure.

4. Worker education—Workers and management must understand the potentially harmful effects of noise in order to satisfy OSHA requirements and—most important—to ensure that the hearing conservation program is successful in preventing NIHL. A good worker education program describes (1) program objectives, (2) existing noise hazards, (3) how hearing loss occurs, (4) the purpose of audiometric testing, and (5) how workers can protect themselves. In addition, the roles and responsibilities of the employer and the workers should be clearly stated. Training is required to be provided annually to all workers included in the hearing conservation program. Opportunities for maintaining awareness occur during periodic safety meetings, as well as during audiometric testing appointments, when testing results are explained.

5. Hearing protection devices—Hearing protection devices are available in a variety of types from a number of manufacturers. There are three basic types of hearing protection devices: (1) ear plugs or "aurals" (eg, premolded, formable, and custom molded); (2) canal caps or "semiaurals" (with a band that compresses each end against the entrance of the ear canal); and (3) earmuffs or "circumaurals" (which surround the ear). Each type of device has advantages and disadvantages that vary according to worker activity, noise characteristics, and the work environment. The selection of appropriate hearing protection devices should include input from the industrial hygienist, the audiologist, the physician of occupational medicine, and the workers who will use the device(s).

Although hearing conservation programs are triggered by the presence of noise levels $\geq$ an 8-hour, time-weighted average of 85 dBA, hearing protection devices must attenuate worker exposure to an 8-hour, time-weighted average of 90 dBA, which is the 8-hour level of permissible noise exposure mandated by OSHA.

An OSHA standard threshold shift occurs if the hearing level has changed by 10 dB or more in either ear in the average hearing thresholds of 2000, 3000, and 4000 Hz. If an employee has not had a baseline audiogram or is exposed to noise with a time-weighted average of 85 dBA and has a demonstrated standard threshold shift, then hearing protection devices must be provided and must attenuate noise levels to below an 8-hour time-weighted average of 85 dBA.

6. Audiometric evaluations—Audiometric testing provides the only quantitative means of assessing the overall effectiveness of a hearing conservation program. A properly managed audiometric testing program supervised by either a certified audiologist or a physician trained and experienced in occupational hearing conservation can detect changes in the response to environmental noise that might otherwise be overlooked. The results of audiometric testing must be shared with employees to ensure effectiveness. The overall results or trends noted in an audiometric testing program can be used to fine-tune the hearing conservation program,

including determining what types of hearing protection devices to offer to employees and the location where additional employee training is needed.

If a standard threshold shift occurs, the individual employee is notified and further action is required that may necessitate both modifying the hearing conservation program and notifying the appropriate authorities (eg, the employer or the appropriate government agency). In some cases, a referral to an otologist is indicated to determine the change in the hearing level from the previous audiogram or baseline audiogram.

Noise Reduction Ratings & Selection of Hearing Protection Devices

All hearing protection devices sold in the United States are assigned a standardized value known as the **noise reduction rating**. The manufacturers of hearing protection devices are required by the Environmental Protection Agency to have their products tested to obtain a noise reduction rate before placing these products on the market. Though useful in making preliminary purchasing decisions, assigned noise reduction ratings must be viewed and applied cautiously. Noise reduction ratings (measured in decibels) are based on laboratory attenuation data and achieved under ideal conditions. Actual noise reduction achieved under field conditions using any hearing protection device is much lower than the assigned rating.

The adjustment of an assigned noise reduction rating may be required before a device is prescribed for field use.

A. WEIGHTING SCALE ADJUSTMENT

Depending on the monitoring method used to determine the noise exposure, an initial adjustment to the noise reduction rating of a selected device may be required. Noise levels can be measured using either the "A" scale (dBA) or "C" scale (dBC). The A scale approximates the response of the human ear to speech frequencies and discounts much of acoustic energy from the low and high frequencies that are present in the work environment. Therefore, the A scale is often an underestimation of the total acoustic energy present. In contrast, the C scale is essentially flat across the frequency spectrum, and all of the acoustic energy present is integrated into the measurement.

If workplace noise levels are determined using the C scale (dBC) on the monitoring instrumentation, the assigned noise reduction rating may be subtracted *directly* from the actual measured time-weighted average noise levels to determine the legal "adequacy" of the device selected relative to the regulatory criterion of a time-weighted average of 90 dBA. If workplace noise levels are determined using the A scale (dBA) on the monitoring instrumentation, the assigned noise reduction rating must be reduced by 7 dB *before* being subtracted from the actual measured time-weighted average noise levels in order to determine the legal "adequacy" of the device selected relative to the regulatory criterion of 90 dBA. For employees who have either a demonstrated standard threshold shift or have not yet had a baseline audiogram, the criterion of a time-weighted average of 85 dBA is enforced regardless of which scale is used.

B. FIFTY PERCENT DE-RATING LEVELS

Although the effectiveness of hearing protection devices depends on whether they are properly used, noise reduction ratings are obtained in the laboratory under ideal conditions and reflect "best-case" attenuation. To predict more accurately (and conservatively) the noise reduction rating of hearing protection devices during *actual* use, the noise reduction rating of a product should be de-rated. In calculating the noise exposure to an individual using a hearing protection device in the work environment, OSHA de-rates the assigned noise reduction rating (after scale adjustment) by one half (50%) for all hearing protection devices. This is done to determine the "relative performance" of the device.

As a typical example, if a device has a noise reduction rating of 21 and workplace noise measurements were made using the A scale, then the predicted field attenuation (or relative performance) of the device would be 7 dB [(21 − 7) ÷ 2]. Such a device would be expected to provide protection (per the legal OSHA permissible exposure level of 90 dBA) when an 8-hour, time-weighted average noise level of up to 97 dBA [90 + 7] was present. As a worst-case example, the failure to make an adjustment for A scale noise measurements along with the failure to apply a 50% de-rating level could lead an uninformed evaluator to falsely believe that the hearing protection device would provide protection in environments with 8-hour, time-weighted average noise levels up to and including 111 dBA [90 + 21]. Workers in this situation would have an increased risk of sustaining an NIHL.

NIOSH has recommended a variable scheme for de-rating noise reduction ratings. For example, earmuffs are de-rated 25%; formable earplugs are de-rated 50%; all other earplugs are de-rated 70%. This scheme more accurately reflects the attenuation in actual work environments. It is important to remember that the de-rating level of hearing protection devices is not required; however, it does provide a conservative estimate of the attenuation in the working environment.

C. COMBINED HEARING PROTECTION DEVICES

Hearing protection devices may be combined (eg, earplugs and earmuffs used together) to provide more protection in high-noise environments. However, the noise reduction ratings of combined devices are not added together to determine the total noise reduction. Under such circumstances, OSHA advises its inspectors that 5 dB are to be added *after* the weighting scale adjustment is applied to the device with the *higher* noise reduction rating (OSHA does not require 50% de-rating levels in this circumstance). This is a conservative approach to determining the combined attenuation and actual field attenuation (and protection) is probably higher. As a practical matter, double protection is inadequate for noise levels over 105–110 dBA.

D. HEARING PROTECTION DEVICE ENFORCEMENT

For 8-hour, time-weighted average noise levels ≥ 85 dBA (a 50% noise dose) but < 90 dBA (a 100% noise dose), it is only requested that hearing protection devices be made available to the workers. However, for 8-hour, time-weighted average noise levels ≥ 90 dBA, hearing protection devices *must* be provided to workers. A suitable variety of hearing protection devices must be provided, and the employer is responsible for enforcing their proper use. The weighting scale adjustment of the noise reduction rating must be performed, and it is suggested that a 50% de-rating of the adjusted noise reduction rating be applied to ensure adequate protection of workers.

Very few randomized controlled trials have been performed to assess interventions to promote the wearing of hearing protection. A large review by Daniell revealed that current prevention and enforcement strategies in the United States may be inadequate. On average, 38% of employees did not routinely wear hearing protection when exposed to noise, and most companies relied primarily on hearing protection rather than noise control to prevent hearing loss.

Axelsson A. *Scientific Basis of NIHL.* New York: Thieme Medical Publishing, 1996. (Book covering the proceedings of the 5th International Symposium on the effects of noise on hearing.)

Berger EH et al. *The Noise Manual,* 5th ed. Fairfax, VA: American Industrial Hygiene Association Press, 1999. (Comprehensive textbook covering noise effects on hearing and hearing conservation.)

Berger EH et al. The naked truth about NRRs in *Earlog.* In: Berger EH et al, eds. *The Noise Manual.* Revised 5th ed. Fairfax, VA: American Industrial Hygiene Association Press, 2000. (Article examining noise reduction ratings and OSHA's 50% de-rating guidelines.)

Daniell WE et al. Noise exposure and hearing loss prevention programmes after 20 years of regulations in the United States. *Occup Environ Med.* 2006;63:643. [PMID: 166551755] (A study in Washington that reveals poor hearing protection by employees and inadequate enforcement and noise control by companies.)

El Dib RP et al. Interventions to promote the wearing of hearing protection. *Cochrane Database Syst Rev.* 2006;2:CD005234.

[PMID: 16625628] (Cochrane review finding that tailored interventions were not more effective than general interventions; however, school-based hearing loss prevention programs may be effective.)

Mansdorf SZ. *Complete Manual of Industrial Safety.* Fort Lee, NJ: Prentice Hall, 1993. (Book covering various aspects of industrial safety including hearing conservation strategies.)

National Institute of Health Consensus Development Conference: Noise and Hearing Loss. Consensus Statement 1990; 8:1. [PMID: 2202895] (Examines various aspects of noise-induced hearing loss, prevention strategies, and directions for future research.)

Royster JD, Royster LH. *Hearing Conservation Programs: Practical Guidelines for Success.* Albany, GA: Lewis Publishers, 1990. (Covers various aspects of designing and implementing cost-effective hearing conservation programs in the workplace.)

Sataloff RT, Sataloff J. *Occupational Hearing Loss.* New York: Marcel Dekker, 1987. (Comprehensive textbook covering all aspects of occupational hearing loss including etiology, diagnosis, and testing.)

US Department of Health and Human Services. *Occupational Noise Exposure—Revised Criteria 1998.* National Institute for Occupational Safety and Health, 1998. (Criteria proposed by the NIOSH for permissible noise levels. Proposed criteria include reducing the maximum permissible noise exposure to 85-dB time-weighted average and reducing the exchange rate to 3%.)

US Department of Labor, Occupational Safety, and Health Administration. *Occupational Noise Exposure: Hearing Conservation Amendment Final Rule.* Fed Reg. 1983;48:9738. (29CFR1910.95). (Federal regulations regarding noise exposure, hearing conservation programs, and reporting.)

HEARING LOSS DUE TO PHYSICAL TRAUMA

Etiology & Pathogenesis

Blunt head injury is by far the most common cause of traumatic hearing loss, and motor vehicle accidents account for approximately 50% of temporal bone injuries. The cochlear injury observed after blunt head trauma closely resembles, both histologically and from an audiologic perspective, the trauma induced by high-intensity acoustic trauma.

Penetrating injuries of the temporal bone are relatively rare, accounting for < 10% of cases. Other occupational causes of ear injury include falls, explosions, burns from caustic chemicals, open flames, and welder's slag injuries.

Examination & Treatment

In the conscious patient, hearing should be assessed immediately with a 512-Hz tuning fork. Even in an ear severely traumatized and filled with blood, sound lateralizes toward a conductive hearing loss and away from a sensorineural one. Complete audiometric examinations can be performed after the patient has been stabilized. Patients should also be checked for signs of vestibular injury (eg, nystagmus) and facial nerve trauma (eg, paralysis).

A. INJURIES CAUSING CONDUCTIVE HEARING LOSS

Blunt head trauma with or without temporal bone fracture may cause hematotympanum, a collection of blood in the middle ear. If this is the sole injury, hearing usually recovers over several weeks. Burns sustained when a piece of welder's slag penetrates the eardrum often heal poorly, and chronic infection often results. A loud explosion with sound pressure levels exceeding 180 dB may cause rupture of the tympanic membrane. Traumatic membrane perforations usually heal spontaneously if secondary infection does not develop, although hearing loss may persist; patients should be instructed not to get the ear wet during the healing period.

A conductive hearing loss that persists for more than 3 months after injury is usually due to a tympanic membrane perforation or disruption of the ossicular chain. These lesions are centrally suitable for surgical repair, usually on a delayed basis. Repair is accomplished by grafting the tympanic membrane or by reconstructing the ossicular chain with autograft or prosthetic materials.

B. INJURIES CAUSING SENSORINEURAL OR MIXED HEARING LOSS

Trauma to the inner ear most commonly results from blunt head injury. Labyrinthine concussion frequently occurs with transient vertigo, potentially with permanent hearing loss and tinnitus. These patients are generally treated with vestibular suppressants such as meclizine for symptomatic relief of vertigo. One should refer to the chapter on temporal bone trauma for a more detailed discussion.

OTOTOXIC HEARING LOSS

Etiology & Pathogenesis

Chemicals in the workplace can be absorbed through the skin or inhaled, and secondarily reach inner ear fluids via the bloodstream. Industrial chemicals are thought to damage both the cochlea and the central auditory structures via free-radical production.

According to Morata, the Human Field Studies Working Group has identified the following chemicals as having the highest priority for intervention in the workplace:

Solvents—toluene, styrene, xylene, *n*-hexane, ethyl benzene, white spirits/Stoddard, carbon disulfide, fuels, perchloroethylene

Asphyxiants—carbon monoxide, hydrogen cyanide

Metals—lead, mercury

Pesticides/herbicides—paraquat, organophosphates

Outside of the occupational setting, however, most ototoxic hearing loss is secondary to medications including aminoglycosides, loop diuretics, antineoplastic agents, and salicylates.

Prevention

Workplace controls must be in place to limit exposure to chemical ototoxins. High-risk workers should be identified based on ototoxic exposure, preexisting sensory hearing loss, and compromised renal or hepatic function. Audiometric evaluation is appropriate to identify and monitor ototoxic exposure, and the addition of otoacoustic emissions, evoked auditory brainstem potentials, and behavioral audiometry have been proposed to examine central effects of industrial chemicals.

Workers taking potentially ototoxic medications are at an increased risk for hearing loss when placed in noisy environments, since the combination of some ototoxic drug treatments and noise trauma can lead to a greater degree of hearing loss than either of these would produce by itself. Conversely, patients with any type of preexisting sensorineural hearing loss, including NIHL, may be more susceptible to the ototoxic effects of medications. Aspirin, however, though known to cause reversible sensorineural hearing loss, is probably not associated with an increased likelihood of NIHL.

Medicinal ototoxins should be administered in the lowest dose compatible with therapeutic efficacy. Serum peak and trough levels should be monitored to reduce the risk of excessive dosages. The simultaneous administration of multiple ototoxic drugs (eg, furosemide and an aminoglycoside antibiotic) should also be avoided, when possible, to minimize synergistic effects.

Morata TC. Chemical exposure as a risk factor for hearing loss. *J Occup Environ Med.* 2003;45:676. [PMID: 12855908] (Summary of the 2002 workshop "Combined Effects of Chemicals and Noise on Hearing" sponsored by the National Institute for Occupational Safety and Health and the National Hearing Conservation Association.)

MEDICAL-LEGAL ISSUES

1. Workers' Compensation

All states within the United States have workers' compensation programs to compensate the injured worker for injuries that arise from employment. Each state has developed its own method for handling the injured worker, and state statutes are not uniform across the country. Before assessing a worker compensation case, it behooves the medical examiner to understand the appropriate statutes of the state in which the claim is being filed.

To make matters more complicated, cases that fall under the purview of the federal government, such as

civilian federal employees under the Federal Employee Compensation Act (FECA), are handled differently from cases involving longshoremen under the Longshore and Harbor Workers Compensation Act (LHWCA), despite the fact that both acts are adjudicated by the US Department of Labor.

Cases involving maritime workers fall under the purview of the Jones Act, which covers workers such as merchant marines (seamen and ship crewmen), some divers, and pile drivers. Although Jones Act cases are under the auspices of the federal government, they are adjudicated differently from the Department of Labor cases.

Cases involving railroad workers involved in interstate commerce are handled by the Federal Employers Liability Act (FELA). Although the Jones Act and FELA are different from a practical point of view for the physician performing the evaluation, they are similar and are handled by medical examination and possible testimony in court rather than through a scheduled award (by a guideline that determines the percentage of hearing loss).

2. Calculation of Percentage of Hearing Loss

Several methods of calculating the percentage of hearing loss are in widespread use. The most current and frequently used method recommended by the American Academy of Otolaryngology (AAO, 1979) is as follows (Table 58–3):

1. **Thresholds.** The average hearing threshold level at 500, 1000, 2000, and 3000 Hz should be calculated for each ear.

2. **Monaural impairment.** The percentage of the impairment for each ear is calculated by taking the pure-tone average (500–3000 Hz), subtracting 25 dB, and multiplying the result by 1.5. The maximum 100% monaural loss is reached at 92 dB (high fence). This is based on the assumption that hearing loss only becomes a handicap beyond 25 dB and that the handicap increases at a rate of 1.5% per decibel after this point.

3. **Hearing handicap.** This is calculated by multiplying the smaller percentage (better hearing ear) by 5, adding this figure to the larger percentage (worse hearing ear), and dividing the total by 6. Because unilateral deafness is only considered a mild handicap, a 5 to 1 weighting is used for the better ear.

The AAO method of calculating the percentage of hearing loss described above is identical with the hearing impairment guidelines developed by the American Medical Association (AMA Guidelines on Evaluation of Permanent Impairment). The AAO method is now used by the majority of states in local worker compen-

Table 58–3. Calculation of hearing handicap.

Thresholds (dB)	Left Ear	Right Ear
500 Hz	dB	dB
1000 Hz	dB	dB
2000 Hz	dB	dB
3000 Hz	dB	dB
Pure-tone average (PTA)	$= \dfrac{\Sigma Thresholds(Left)}{4}$	$= \dfrac{\Sigma Thresholds(Right)}{4}$
Monaural impairment (MI)	$= 1.5(PTA_L - 25)$	$= 1.5(PTA_R - 25)$
Hearing handicap (HH)	$= \dfrac{5(MIb) + MIw}{6}$	

MIb, monaural impairment of better ear; MIw, monaural impairment of worse ear; PTA_L, pure-tone average of left ear; PTA_R, pure-tone average of right ear.

sation programs and by the US Department of Labor (eg, FECA and LHWCA).

Some states use the American Academy of Ophthalmology and Otolaryngology rule (AAOO, 1959). This method of calculating the percentage of hearing loss is similar to the AAO method, except that the 3000-Hz threshold is not included in the pure-tone average.

Generally, a statute of limitations determines when an employee is eligible to apply for compensation. This statute varies from state to state and with the federal government. In taking a history, the medical examiner should include a statement as to when the hearing loss occurred and when the employee may have realized that the hearing loss was related to noise.

Most states apportion a preexisting hearing loss; the US Department of Labor does not deduct for preemployment hearing loss. The US Department of Labor, FECA, and LHWCA ask only if the hearing loss was precipitated, accelerated, aggravated, or proximately caused by the accepted conditions of employment.

3. Assessment of Impairment

The normal range of speech reception thresholds is between 0 and 20 dB, with hearing losses designated according to the following measures: (1) mild (20–40 dB), (2) moderate (40–55 dB), (3) moderately severe (55–70 dB), (4) severe (70–90 dB), and (5) profound (> 90 dB). Of course, the extent of the disability suffered by the patient depends on many psychological, social, and work-related factors. *Disability* is a relative term. The assessment of an individual's ability to do his or her job requires knowledge about the various duties performed by that individual. Some typical work-related issues for consideration include the amount of communication with coworkers and others that is required on the job, the type of com-

munication (eg, in person or via the telephone), and the need to hear alerting signals or emergency warning alarms.

Police, firefighters, and other emergency and law enforcement personnel generally have to meet certain hearing requirements for employment. Guidelines for these occupations differ regionally; however, the guidelines for entry-level police officers and firefighters generally require a pure-tone average at 500, 1000, 2000, and 3000 Hz of 25–30 dB. Postemployment requirements vary greatly. There is an effort in some states to quantify hearing in a noisy environment; California now conducts "hearing in noise" tests (HINT).

To meet the Social Security Administration guidelines for total disability due to hearing impairment, an individual must have either (1) an average hearing threshold of ≥ 90 dB for the better-hearing ear based on both air and bone conduction at 500, 1000, and 2000 Hz, or (2) a speech discrimination score of 40% or less in the better-hearing ear. In both cases, hearing must not be restorable by hearing amplification devices.

In assessing cases of tinnitus, the otologist and audiologist may attempt to match the tinnitus with the intensity of the tinnitus in decibels and the frequency of the ringing in hertz. Tinnitus is a very subjective finding and may be described as minimal, slight or mild, moderate, or severe. Some states allow an award for tinnitus whereas other states do not. The examining physician should include a statement regarding the claimant's ability to perform his or her usual and customary occupation.

4. Compensation for Occupational Hearing Loss

An example of how occupational hearing loss is compensated is provided by the statistics of the US Department of Labor (FECA). In the fiscal year 1999–2000, there were 6745 claims. The cost to the federal government was $8,982,139 in medical costs and $30,925,247 in compensation for a total cost of $39,907,386. The average cost per claim was $5917. The general rise in costs per claim over the years reflects the rising costs of hearing aids. Many claimants are requesting newer digital hearing aids that cost between $2500 and $3100 each.

The relationship between NIHL and presbycusis is debatable at this time. Many studies have tried to address the issue of workers exposed to hazardous noise for a long period of time and their "presumed" hearing losses based on their age (ie, presbycusis). The International Organization Standards (ISO) published a report that attempts to quantify that relationship. As with all large series, attempts to estimate hearing for individuals at certain ages are also based on determining the median or averages of large populations at a given age. There is much debate whether epidemiologic hearing loss data can be applied to individuals.

Dobie RA. *Medical-Legal Evaluation of Hearing Loss,* 2nd ed. Singular/Thomson Learning, 2001. (Comprehensive book covering the medical-legal aspects of occupational hearing loss.)

International Organization for Standardization. *ISO-1999. Acoustics—Determination of Occupational Noise Exposure and Estimation of Noise Induced Hearing Impairment.* International Organization for Standardization, 1990. (ISO standard on estimating hearing impairment in occupational noise-induced hearing loss.)

Temporal Bone Trauma 59

John S. Oghalai, MD

EXTERNAL & MIDDLE EAR TRAUMA

 ESSENTIALS OF DIAGNOSIS

- *History of trauma to ear or foreign body insertion into the ear.*
- *Symptoms of pain and hearing loss.*
- *Bloody otorrhea.*

General Considerations

Injuries localized to the external or middle ear include auricular hematoma, external auditory canal abrasion or laceration, tympanic membrane perforation, and ossicular chain dislocation. Local trauma to the tympanic membrane and ossicles can occur by a penetrating injury with objects such as a cotton-tipped applicator, a bobby pin, a pencil, or a hot metal slag during welding. In addition, barotrauma, such as a slap to the ear or a blast injury, can cause a tympanic membrane perforation or ossicular chain dislocation.

1. Auricular Hematoma

An auricular hematoma may present after a forceful blow to the external ear. It can be recognized as a tender swelling of the pinna that is fluctuant on palpation. The hematoma arises after the perichondrium is sheared off the cartilage of the auricle. This fluid accumulation needs to be drained to prevent chondronecrosis and lead to a misshapen pinna, commonly known as a "cauliflower ear" or "wrestler's ear." After incision and drainage, a compression dressing is sutured through the pinna to bolster the skin and perichondrium against the auricular cartilage, preventing reaccumulation of the fluid.

2. External Auditory Canal Abrasion

Injuries to the external auditory canal most commonly occur when a patient is trying to remove his or her own earwax with a cotton-tipped applicator or bobby pin. The injury is usually a simple abrasion or laceration.

Treatment consists of using an antimicrobial otic drop to prevent bacterial or fungal superinfection of the area. Alternately, there may be a localized area of blood collection underneath the skin of the external auditory canal, called a *bulla*. Perforating the tense bulla with a sharp pick often helps to reduce the patient's discomfort. Patients with diabetes have a high risk of developing external otitis from this type of injury because of their poor microcirculation. These patients need to be followed up closely to verify wound healing.

3. Tympanic Membrane Perforation

A tympanic membrane perforation can occur after the use of a cotton-tipped applicator, a bobby pin, a pencil, or the entry of a hot metal slag into the ear canal during welding. Finally, barotrauma, such as a slap to the ear or a blast injury, can cause a perforation. In all cases, patients usually complain of pain and hearing loss, and the perforation can be diagnosed by otoscopy. It is important to note how much of the tympanic membrane has been perforated. A central perforation does not involve the annulus of the eardrum, whereas a marginal perforation does. In addition, the Weber tuning fork test should be performed to verify that it radiates to the affected ear, and the eyes should be checked for nystagmus. If the Weber test does not radiate to the affected ear and the patient has nystagmus, it is likely that stapes subluxation with sensorineural hearing loss has occurred. This is termed a perilymphatic fistula and requires urgent treatment (see Perilymphatic Fistula, Treatment).

If no evidence of sensorineural hearing loss is found, no specific treatment is required because traumatic tympanic membrane perforations, especially central perforations, typically heal spontaneously. However, strict dry ear precautions should be followed to prevent water from getting into the ear. Instructions to the patient include no swimming and the use of a cotton ball thoroughly coated with petrolatum (eg, Vaseline) in the affected ear during bathing. An audiogram should be performed after about 3 months to verify that hearing has returned to normal and that there is no ossicular chain discontinuity. If the perforation has not healed by 3 months, a tympanoplasty will likely need to be performed.

4. Ossicular Chain Dislocation

Penetrating trauma with objects such as a cotton-tipped applicator, a bobby pin, or a pencil can injure the ossicular chain (after perforating the tympanic membrane). Barotrauma, such as a slap to the ear, a blast injury, or rapid decent in an aircraft, can cause ossicular chain dislocation without tympanic membrane perforation. Ossicular chain dislocation with an intact eardrum manifests as a maximal (60 dB) conductive hearing loss. Ossicular chain dislocation with a perforated eardrum results in lesser degrees of hearing loss. The most common form of ossicular discontinuity is incudostapedial joint dislocation. The second most common is incudomalleolar joint dislocation. Also, fracture of the stapes crura may occur. Treatment in any case is middle ear exploration and ossicular chain reconstruction, with tympanoplasty if needed.

TEMPORAL BONE FRACTURES

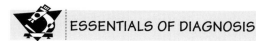

ESSENTIALS OF DIAGNOSIS

- *History of blunt head trauma.*
- *Symptoms of hearing loss and possibly vertigo and facial nerve palsy.*
- *Signs include Battle sign, hemotympanum, and bloody otorrhea.*

General Considerations

The skull base includes the frontal bone, the sphenoid bone, the temporal bone, and the occipital bone. A fracture of the skull base (otherwise known as a basilar skull fracture) must involve at least one of these bones and may involve all of them. Temporal bone fractures represent roughly 20% of all skull fractures. Risk factors include being male and under 21. The most common causes include motor vehicle accidents, falls, bicycle accidents, seizures, and aggravated assaults. Blunt trauma to the lateral surface of the skull (the squamous portion of the temporal bone) often results in a longitudinal fracture. A blow to the occipital skull may go through the foramen magnum and result in a transverse fracture of the temporal bone (Figure 59–1).

Pathogenesis

Longitudinal fractures involve the squamous portion of the temporal bone, follow the axis of the external auditory canal to the middle ear space, and then course anteriorly along the geniculate ganglion and eustachian tube, ending near the foramen lacerum. In a longitudinal temporal bone fracture, the otic capsule is spared. In contrast, transverse fractures course directly across the petrous pyramid, fracturing the otic capsule, and then extend anteriorly along the eustachian tube and geniculate ganglion. Longitudinal temporal bone fractures and transverse temporal bone fractures represent 80% and 20%, respectively, of temporal bone fractures.

Clinical Findings

A. SYMPTOMS AND SIGNS

Symptoms include hearing loss, nausea and vomiting, and vertigo. Clinical signs include Battle sign, which is a postauricular ecchymosis resulting from extravasated blood from the postauricular artery or mastoid emissary vein. The "raccoon" sign (periorbital ecchymosis) is associated with basilar skull fractures that involve the middle or anterior cranial fossa. Physical examination may demonstrate an external auditory canal laceration with bony debris within the canal. A hemotympanum is almost always identified. Cerebrospinal fluid (CSF) otorrhea or rhinorrhea may be seen. Tuning fork tests should always be performed on patients with a temporal bone fracture. The Weber tuning fork test radiates to the fractured ear if conductive hearing loss is present and radiates to the contralateral ear if sensorineural hearing loss is present. The presence or absence of facial nerve paralysis should be documented in all patients with temporal bone fractures.

B. IMAGING STUDIES

After initial resuscitation in the emergency room, computed tomography (CT) scanning of the head is usually the first study performed on patients with head trauma. It is critical to rule out an intracranial hemorrhage, which may require urgent neurosurgical treatment. It is at this point that a temporal bone fracture is usually identified. High-resolution CT scanning of the temporal bone is valuable in delineating the extent of the fracture, but it is not required unless a complication is suspected (eg, otic capsule fracture, facial nerve injury, or CSF leak). Patients with a longitudinal fracture associated with hemotympanum, without nystagmus, without evidence of CSF leak, with a Weber tuning fork test that radiates to the affected ear, and with normal facial nerve function typically do not need a CT scan of the temporal bone. Angiography may be performed if there is significant hemorrhage from the skull base to rule out vascular injury, but this is uncommon.

C. SPECIAL TESTS

1. Audiometry—Audiometry should be performed on all patients with a temporal bone fracture. However, this

Longitudinal fracture

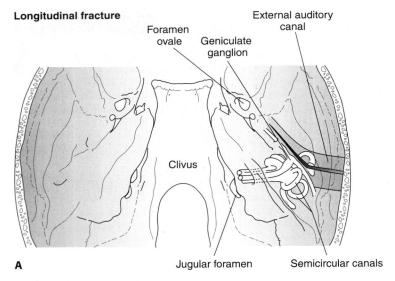

Foramen ovale
Geniculate ganglion
External auditory canal
Clivus
Jugular foramen
Semicircular canals

A

Transverse fracture

Foramen spinosum
Foramen lacerum

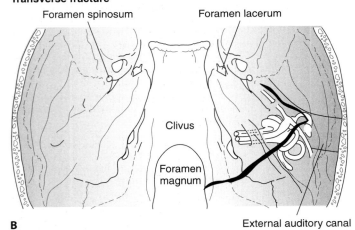

Clivus
Foramen magnum
External auditory canal

B

Figure 59–1. Types of temporal bone fractures. **(A)** Longitudinal fractures begin at the squamous portion of the temporal bone, run through the external auditory canal, and then turn anteriorly toward the foramen lacerum. **(B)** Transverse fractures begin from the foramen magnum, run through the otic capsule bone that surrounds the inner ear, and then turn anteriorly toward the foramen lacerum.

does not need to be done acutely unless the patient has signs or symptoms of inner ear dysfunction. If clinical examination is consistent with conductive hearing loss and there is no evidence of otic capsule fracture, audiometric assessment can be performed several weeks after the injury, permitting time for the hemotympanum to resolve.

2. Facial nerve testing—Facial nerve testing should be performed if a delayed, complete facial palsy occurs. The rationale is to identify patients with > 90% degeneration of the facial nerve, because these patients have poorer recovery of function and may benefit from surgical decompression. The **nerve excitability test (NET)** is performed by placing the two probes of a Hilger nerve stimulator across the stylomastoid foramen and slowly turning up the current until a facial twitch is just barely visible. This is the stimulation threshold of the facial nerve. A 3.5-mA difference between the injured and uninjured sides correlates with a > 90% loss of neural integrity.

Alternately, **electroneuronography (ENoG)** can be performed by a neurophysiologist. This involves stimulating both facial nerves with equal currents while simultaneously measuring the evoked myogenic potential in the muscles of facial expression. If the amplitude of the ipsilateral evoked potential is < 10% of that from the contralateral side, > 90% loss of neural integrity has occurred. Neither of these tests is accurate within 3 days of the injury because it takes about 72 hours for nerve fibers distal to the site of the injury to degenerate. Nonetheless, surgical decompression of delayed facial paralysis remains controversial.

Figure 59–2. Axial computed tomography scan of a patient who sustained a longitudinal temporal bone fracture several months previously. This patient had a 60-dB conductive hearing loss with a normal tympanic membrane on physical exam. **(A)** The inferior cut demonstrates the line of the fracture. **(B)** The superior cut shows dislocation of the malleus-incus joint. Note that the fracture runs directly along the geniculate ganglion, but the patient did not have facial nerve dysfunction.

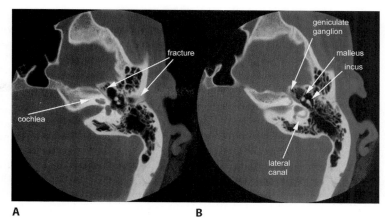

Complications

A. CONDUCTIVE HEARING LOSS

Conductive hearing loss is most commonly due to hemotympanum, but may also represent a tympanic membrane perforation or ossicular discontinuity. The most common form of ossicular discontinuity after temporal bone trauma is incudostapedial joint dislocation. The second most common is incudomalleolar joint dislocation (Figure 59–2). In addition, ossicular fixation may occur several months after the trauma if new bone formation at the line of the fracture fuses to the ossicular chain.

B. SENSORINEURAL HEARING LOSS AND VERTIGO

These complications are found in patients who sustain a transverse temporal bone fracture with otic capsule involvement (Figure 59–3). An audiogram usually demonstrates a complete sensorineural hearing loss in the affected ear. Acutely, clinical examination also reveals nystagmus, which is consistent with a unilateral vestibular deficit. Sensorineural hearing loss can also be sustained without otic capsule fracture if a labyrinthine concussion occurs. This is thought to involve shearing of the cochlear membranes or hair cell stereocilia due to the rapid acceleration and deceleration forces within the inner ear. Labyrinthine concussion manifests as a high-frequency hearing loss. Finally, patients exposed to traumatic noise exposure or blast injury may sustain a temporary threshold shift in their hearing. This is also felt to be representative of damage to the delicate structures within the inner ear, but this temporary sensorineural hearing loss resolves as these structures recover.

C. FACIAL NERVE INJURY

Facial nerve palsy occurs in 20% of longitudinal temporal bone fractures and 50% of transverse temporal bone fractures. The most important clinical feature to identify is whether the facial nerve palsy was of delayed or immediate onset. Patients with delayed-onset palsy present to the emergency room with normal facial nerve function that slowly worsens over the next several hours to days. This is thought to represent edema within the

Figure 59–3. Axial computed tomography scan of an 8-year-old child who sustained a transverse temporal bone fracture. This patient had nystagmus and a complete sensorineural hearing loss. His facial nerve function was normal. **(A)** The inferior cut demonstrates the line of the fracture that extends through the dense, white bone of the otic capsule. **(B)** The superior cut shows that the fracture extends to the facial nerve canal.

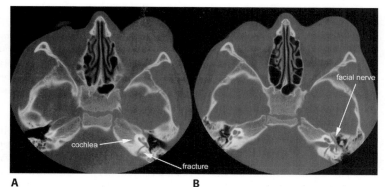

facial nerve without disruption of neural integrity. In contrast, immediate facial nerve injury is highly suggestive of facial nerve transection. Unfortunately, it is common to have an undetermined onset time of facial nerve palsy because patients with temporal bone fractures and facial nerve palsy typically have many other life-threatening issues that are being dealt with at the time of the initial evaluation. These patients are often comatose and therefore difficult to examine.

D. Cerebrospinal Fluid Leak

There is a 2% incidence of CSF leak in all skull fractures and a 20% incidence in temporal bone fractures. CSF leaks usually start within the first 48 hours of the trauma and are noted as clear fluid emanating from the ear or nose. Straining, standing up, or bending over worsens the CSF leak. Eighty percent of post-traumatic CSF leaks close spontaneously after 7 days, and the risk of meningitis is quite low (3%) within this time period. If the leak persists longer than 7–10 days, the risk of meningitis increases dramatically (23–55%). If clear fluid emanating from the nose or ear is suggestive of a CSF leak, the fluid is collected and sent for β_2 transferrin testing. β_2 transferrin is a protein found only in CSF; it is not found in other fluids of the body. The site of a CSF leak from the temporal bone is usually from a fracture in the otic capsule without new callous formation, which can be noted by a CT scan of the temporal bone. If it is not found on the scan, the injection of an intrathecal contrast during CT scanning often delineates the specific site of the leak.

E. Post-Traumatic Encephalocele

Post-traumatic encephalocele can result if a large defect in the floor of the middle cranial fossa occurs. Dura and temporal lobe brain can herniate down into the middle ear and mastoid. This can sometimes be visible on otoscopic examination of the ear as a white mass with blood vessels behind the tympanic membrane. A CSF leak can occur in combination with an encephalocele.

F. Perilymphatic Fistula

A perilymphatic fistula can occur after a fracture of the otic capsule or stapes subluxation of the oval window. It manifests as fluctuating vertigo and sensorineural hearing loss. This entity is fully described later in this chapter under Perilymphatic Fistula).

Treatment

A. Conductive Hearing Loss

A hemotympanum resolves spontaneously within 3–4 weeks of the injury with no sequelae. Traumatic tympanic membrane perforations have an excellent

chance of healing spontaneously. Within 1 month, 68% are healed; within 3 months, 94% are healed. If the perforation has not healed by 3 months, a paper-patch myringoplasty can be attempted in the office. This should be performed only if the perforation is quite small (< 25%) and does not involve the margins of the eardrum and if the middle ear mucosa appears uninfected and dry. The edges of the perforation are freshened with a Rosen needle and a paper patch (cigarette paper or a Steri-strip) is placed over the perforation.

If the perforation is large or has failed an attempt at paper-patch myringoplasty, the patient should be taken to the operating room for a standard tympanoplasty. The ossicular chain should also be explored to verify that it is intact during this procedure. A patient with a normal tympanic membrane and persistent conductive hearing loss probably has ossicular chain discontinuity. A middle ear exploration should be done through the canal by raising a tympanomeatal flap and carefully inspecting and palpating the ossicles. Ossicular chain reconstruction is based on the site of the injury.

B. Facial Nerve Paralysis

The treatment of delayed-onset palsy is based on conservative, nonsurgical management. It is expected that 94% to 100% of these patients will have complete and full recovery of their facial nerve function. However, patients with > 90% degeneration of neural integrity have been shown to have poor recovery. Presumably, the nerve is swollen within the bony fallopian canal, compressing itself within this confined space and therefore causing permanent injury to the nerve fibers.

The management of patients with > 90% degeneration is controversial. Although some neurotologists recommend facial nerve exploration and decompression, others recommend watchful waiting. In contrast, there is no controversy about patients with immediate-onset facial palsy. These patients should undergo facial nerve exploration as soon as the patient is medically stabilized. Human studies have not proved that early surgery improves the long-term facial nerve outcome, but animal studies suggest that intervention within 21 days of facial nerve transection is beneficial.

The exploration of post-traumatic facial nerve palsy is based on two routes. If the patient has normal hearing, a combined middle fossa-transmastoid facial nerve exploration is performed (Figure 59–4). This includes a subtemporal craniotomy with delineation of the facial nerve within the internal auditory canal from the *porus acousticus internus* to the geniculate ganglion. A mastoidectomy is also performed to explore the facial nerve from the middle ear to the stylomastoid foramen. If the patient has a complete sensorineural hearing loss, a

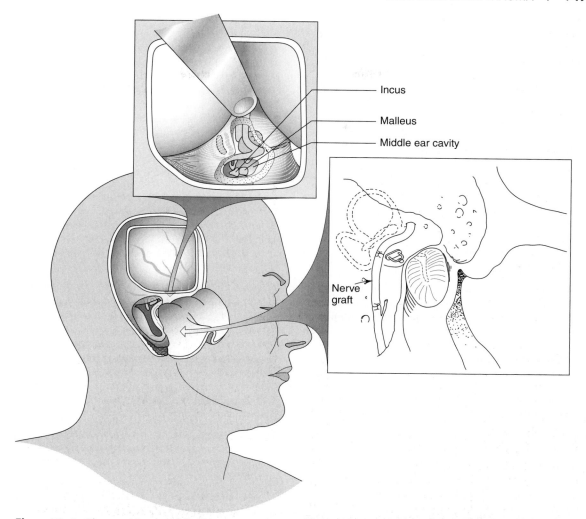

Incus

Malleus

Middle ear cavity

Nerve graft

Figure 59–4. The combined middle fossa-transmastoid approach. This approach is used for facial nerve exploration in patients with normal hearing. The middle fossa exposure permits visualization of the nerve from the brainstem to the geniculate ganglion, whereas the transmastoid route exposes the nerve from the geniculate ganglion to the stylomastoid foramen. In this example, an interpositional facial nerve graft has been placed within the vertical segment of the facial nerve.

translabyrinthine facial nerve exploration and repair can be undertaken (Figure 59–5). This approach allows for complete exposure of the facial nerve from the porous acousticus to the stylomastoid foramen completely through the mastoid.

Injuries are most commonly located in the area of the geniculate ganglion. If an intraneural hematoma is identified, the epineurium should be carefully opened and the hematoma evacuated. If bony fragments are impinging upon the nerve, these can be carefully removed as well. If there is an obvious fracture of the facial nerve, the two ends of the facial nerve should be freshened and anastomosed. If the segment of missing nerve is too long to be easily anastomosed without tension, an interposition nerve graft should be used from the greater auricular or sural nerve. If no pathology is visualized, the act of opening the bony canal of the facial nerve should allow adequate decompression and permit swelling of the nerve without impingement. The epineurium does not need to be incised.

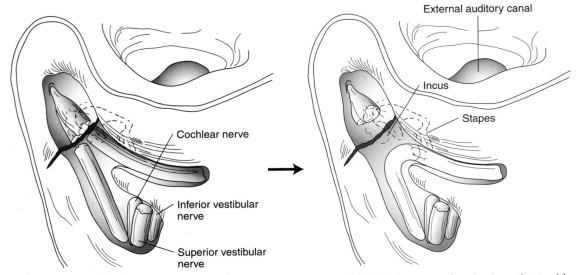

Figure 59–5. The translabyrinthine approach. This approach is used for facial nerve exploration in patients with complete sensorineural hearing loss and allows complete exposure of the nerve through one opening. In this example, a primary facial nerve anastomosis has been performed.

C. Cerebrospinal Fluid Leak and Encephalocele

Medical treatment is attempted initially. This includes head elevation, stool softeners, acetazolamide (to decrease CSF production), and the placement of a lumbar drain. Patients with intracranial hemorrhage who have undergone craniotomy often already have an intraventricular drain in place, in which case a lumbar drain is not needed. Short-term antibiotics have been shown to be useful in preventing meningitis. The most common organisms that cause meningitis in this situation are *Pneumococcus, Staphylococcus, Streptococcus,* and *Haemophilus influenzae.* If the CSF leak persists for more than 7–10 days, the risk of meningitis increases dramatically (> 20%) and surgical repair of the CSF leak should be performed. This situation is most common in patients who sustain a transverse temporal bone fracture with CSF leaking through the otic capsule. Otic capsule bone does not heal with new bone formation but by fibrous union, and this is often not strong enough to contain CSF.

An encephalocele should always be surgically repaired. If the patient has normal hearing, the repair of either a persistent CSF leak or an encephalocele is via a combined middle fossa craniotomy-transmastoid approach with suture repair of the dura. In a patient with no useful hearing, obliteration of the ear with an abdominal fat graft, plugging of the eustachian tube, and closure of the ear canal can be performed through the mastoid alone.

Darrouzet V, Duclos JY, Liguoro D, Truilhe Y, De Bonfils C, Bebear JP. Management of facial paralysis resulting from temporal bone fractures: our experience in 115 cases. *Otolaryngol Head Neck Surg.* 2001;125:77. [PMID: 11458219] (Management of facial paralysis after temporal bone fracture.)

Kahn JB, Stewart MG, Diaz-Marchan PJ. Acute temporal bone trauma: utility of high-resolution computed tomography. *Am J Otol.* 2000;21:743. [PMID: 10993469] (Role of CT scanning of the temporal bone for temporal bone fractures.)

McMurphy AB, Oghalai JS. Repair of iatrogenic temporal lobe encephalocele after canal wall down mastoidectomy in the presence of active cholesteatoma. *Otol Neurotol.* 2005;26:587. [PMID: 16015151] (How to repair a tegmen defect in a canal wall down cavity.)

PENETRATING TRAUMA TO THE TEMPORAL BONE

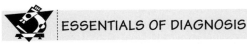 ESSENTIALS OF DIAGNOSIS

- *Usually caused by a gunshot wound.*
- *Significant soft-tissue deficit.*
- *High likelihood of facial nerve palsy and vascular injury.*

General Considerations

Penetrating trauma, predominantly from gunshot wounds, is much more damaging to the temporal bone than is blunt trauma. There is often significant injury to the external auditory canal, which requires local debridement of bone fragments and soft tissue, as well as stenting with Merocel wicks (a type of expandable, nonabsorbable sponge) to prevent stenosis. If stenosis does occur after several months, a canaloplasty may be required. Soft tissue loss may require regional or free-flap reconstruction. Tympanic membrane perforation, ossicular discontinuity, and labyrinthine fracture are also common entities with a gunshot wound to the temporal bone. Epithelial elements can be introduced into the mastoid or middle ear cavities and not be detected as a cholesteatoma until years later.

1. Vascular Injury

The most important aspect of penetrating trauma to the temporal bone is the potential for injury to the internal carotid artery, internal jugular vein, or dural sinuses. Vascular injury is found in 32% of patients with penetrating trauma to the temporal bone; therefore, these injuries should be considered as penetrating trauma to Zone III of the neck and treated accordingly. Angiography should be performed on all patients, with embolization or balloon occlusion used to control bleeding from the skull base. If the hemorrhage continues or there is evidence of major vessel injury on an angiogram, surgical exploration may be required. In the event that internal carotid artery laceration is found, Fogarty catheters can be used temporarily to control bleeding.

2. Facial Nerve Injury

The rate of facial nerve paralysis with penetrating trauma to the temporal bone is 36%. Facial nerve injury most commonly occurs in the tympanic and mastoid segments. Essentially all of these injuries are of immediate onset and occur because of nerve transection. Facial nerve electrophysiologic testing with a Hilger stimulator can be used to identify facial nerve trauma in a comatose patient. Facial nerve repair needs to be undertaken as soon as the patient is medically stable.

PERILYMPHATIC FISTULA

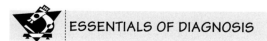

ESSENTIALS OF DIAGNOSIS

- *History of head trauma or previous stapedectomy.*

- *Fluctuating hearing loss and episodic vertigo worse with straining.*

General Considerations

There are many causes of perilymphatic fistula. The most common is head trauma. This may be either following a temporal bone fracture involving the otic capsule or with stapes subluxation into the oval window. Barotrauma during scuba diving, a rapid descent in an airplane, an explosion, or straining during a difficult childbirth may cause a perilymphatic fistula. A postsurgical perilymphatic fistula is also a well-recognized entity. It can occur after stapedectomy if the oval window fails to seal appropriately. Poor surgical technique while performing a mastoidectomy can lead to an iatrogenic lateral canal fistula. In addition, an expanding cholesteatoma can erode into the lateral semicircular canal or cochlea, causing a fistula. Finally, patients may present with a congenital perilymphatic fistula. These patients typically have stapes footplate anomalies or other temporal bone anomalies that are identified on CT scan. The superior semicircular canal dehiscence syndrome may be identified by CT scan, with a fistula from the superior canal into the intracranial space.

Clinical Findings

A. Symptoms and Signs

Patients with perilymphatic fistula present with disequilibrium and vertigo, which may be episodic in nature. They may have tinnitus and hearing loss, headache, and, occasionally, aural fullness. Most important, symptoms become much worse with any type of Valsalva maneuver, such as coughing, sneezing, or straining. Occasionally, an altitude change, such as going up and down in an airplane or in an elevator, can precipitate symptoms. Patients often complain of Tullio phenomenon, whereby loud noises precipitate a vertiginous attack. Clinically, the fistula test can be performed by insufflating air into the external auditory canal and observing the patient for evidence of nystagmus. This test is very insensitive and is positive in only about 50% of patients with a fistula. Also, it is nonspecific because many patients without a fistula experience disequilibrium during the test.

B. Laboratory Findings

The only definitive way to make the diagnosis of a perilymphatic fistula is surgical exploration with visualization of the leak. Even this evaluation is not necessarily definitive since it is difficult to verify that small amounts of clear fluid within the middle ear cavity represent a perilymphatic leak and not serous transudate from the middle ear mucosa. Fluid suggestive of perilymph can be sampled on an absorbable gelatin sponge (eg, Gelfoam pledget) and sent for β_2 transferrin testing. β_2 transferrin is a protein found only in CSF and perilymph; it is not found in other fluids of the body. Although the test result is not immediately available, it may be useful when following up these patients postoperatively.

C. IMAGING STUDIES

Computed tomography has a sensitivity estimated at 20%; however, if a fistula is identified on CT scan, this is obviously highly specific.

D. SPECIAL TESTS

Serial audiometry demonstrates a fluctuating sensorineural hearing loss. Vestibular testing may demonstrate a unilateral deficit. Nystagmus elicited by straining can be documented using electronystagmography monitoring and then evaluated.

Differential Diagnosis

The differential diagnosis includes all causes of dysequilibrium, most notably Meniere disease, cervical vertigo, psychogenic vertigo, disequilibrium related to aging (presbyastasis), vestibular neuritis, and labyrinthitis.

Complications

Fluctuating, but progressive, sensorineural or mixed hearing loss can occur. Also, these patients have progressive disequilibrium. Since there is a fistula from the middle ear space to the inner ear, an episode of acute otitis media is worrisome because bacteria in the middle ear can easily enter the inner ear and CSF. This may lead to permanent sensorineural hearing loss, meningitis, or both.

Treatment

Treatment is based on conservative therapy. The patient should be at bed rest with head elevated. Patients are placed on stool softeners and serial audiograms should be obtained to follow up for evidence of disease progression. If symptoms persist or the sensorineural hearing loss worsens, surgical treatment may be considered. One option is to simply draw blood from the patient's arm and inject it through the eardrum into the middle ear space. This blood seal may help allow a fistula to heal.

Alternately, a middle ear exploration can be performed. This is done by a transcanal approach with elevation of the tympanomeatal flap and careful examination of the oval and round windows. If a defect is noted, a graft of fascia or muscle should be laid over the defect. Many surgeons place fascia around both the oval and the round windows, even if a fistula is not definitively seen, since defects are considered to be difficult to detect.

Megerian CA, Hadlock TA. Case records of the Massachusetts General Hospital: weekly clinicopathological exercises. Case 40-2001: an eight-year-old boy with fever, headache, and vertigo two days after aural trauma. *N Engl J Med.* 2001;345:1901. [PMID: 11756582] (Good discussion of perilymphatic fistula.)

Michel O, Petereit H, Klemm E, Walther LE, Bachmann-Harildstad G. First clinical experience with beta-trace protein (prostaglandin D synthase) as a marker for perilymphatic fistula. *J Laryngol Otol.* 2005;119:765. [PMID: 16259651] (Beta-trace protein might be a promising marker in the diagnosis of perilymphatic fluid fistulas.)

Weber PC, Bluestone CD, Perez B. Outcome of hearing and vertigo after surgery for congenital perilymphatic fistula in children. *Am J Otolaryngol.* 2003;24:138. [PMID: 12761698] (Surgical repair may prevent further deterioration of hearing loss.)

SECTION XIV
Skull Base

Lesions of the Anterior Skull Base | 60

Michael J. Kaplan, MD

Although it remains a formidable problem, the anterior skull base is no longer an absolute barrier to the effective management of tumors that encroach on it. The otolaryngologist–head and neck surgeon involved in the multidisciplinary team that approaches this area will necessarily have an in-depth knowledge of surgical anatomy and tumor pathology, familiarity with radiologic assessment and the roles of interventional radiology, and experience with the various surgical approaches that have been used to access this area.

Most of the problems the surgical team encounters in anterior skull base surgery are either malignant tumors of the paranasal sinuses that extend superiorly to involve the anterior skull base, or benign or malignant processes such as meningiomas, which extend inferiorly from above. In addition, benign lesions of the paranasal sinuses, such as extensive inverted papillomas, extensive mucoceles, and selected benign fibro-osseous lesions, occasionally require these approaches to skull base surgery.

ANATOMY

The anterior skull base is the skull base superior to the orbit and the ethmoid and sphenoid sinuses. It includes the posterior wall of the frontal sinus, the ethmoid roof and cribriform plate, and the orbital roof. More posteriorly, it includes parts of the sphenoid bone, including the lesser wing of the sphenoid, the planum sphenoidale, and the roof of the sphenoid sinus.

Orbit

A thin fascial layer surrounds the orbital fat that lies just within the orbital periosteum. Preserving this layer allows for the resection of the orbital periosteum, when needed, while maintaining the integrity of the orbital contents. The significance of this layer is that the orbit is generally able to be preserved if the extraocular muscles, which are inside this fascial plane, are uninvolved. This is generally true when the patient has full extraocular motility preoperatively, and it may be true at times even when there is some diplopia secondary to mass effect. The actual invasion of orbit fat deep to this fascial plane usually suggests the need for orbital exenteration.

The optic canal transmits the optic nerve and the ophthalmic artery. The ophthalmic artery originates superiorly to superomedially from the internal carotid artery (ICA), but then courses laterally such that it is found lateral to the optic nerve at the anterior optic canal. The significance of this anatomy is that dissection of the *medial* surface of the optic nerves to the optic chiasm is generally safe with respect to its blood supply. The optic nerve, contained within a thin sheath of bone, is usually seen within the sphenoid sinus just superior to the ICA, which also is generally separated from the sphenoid sinus by bone. The optic nerve (and ophthalmic artery) borders the posterior ethmoidal air cells in about 10–15% of cases.

Imola MJ, Schramm VL Jr. Orbital preservation in surgical management of sinonasal malignancy. *Laryngoscope.* 2002;112:1357. [PMID: 12172245] (Orbital preservation is sound in selected cases. Although 30% of the 66 reviewed cases recurred locally, this was at the site of the initial orbit involvement in only 8% of these cases.)

Rhoton AL Jr. The anterior and middle cranial base. *Neurosurgery.* 2002;51:273. [PMID: 12234451] (Overview of the anterior and middle cranial base.)

Tiwari R, van der Wal J, van der Waal I, Snow G. Studies of the anatomy and pathology of the orbit in carcinoma of the maxillary sinus and their impact on preservation of the eye in maxillectomy. *Head Neck.* 1998;20(3):193. [PMID: 9570623] (Periocular fat is surrounded by a thin distinct fascial layer and is not in direct contact with the periorbita.)

Paranasal Sinuses

The variability in individual anatomy is such that a preoperative evaluation using magnetic resonance imaging (MRI) is essential in planning operative approaches. Sometimes, for example, tumor has eroded bone such that a particular approach becomes ideal.

Although the sphenoid sinus septum is usually midline anteriorly at the sphenoid rostrum, it almost always deviates laterally as it courses posteriorly. In addition, additional septa within the sphenoid sinus are common and can confuse an unwary surgeon. Intraoperative navigation can be useful so that the surgeon can be sure that the lateral limit of the sphenoid sinus has been accessed.

Traditionally, access to the sphenoid sinus is via the ethmoid sinuses from the front. However, if access to the skull base from above is needed for an individual, superb access to the sphenoid sinus, as well as the ethmoids and maxillary sinus, is possible from above.

Brain, Dura, Olfactory Nerves, & Frontal Bone

The cribriform plate is medial to the ethmoid roof and is separated from it by the superior attachment of the middle turbinate. Anatomically, the cribriform plate is usually 1–3 mm more inferior than the ethmoid roof and is perforated by the olfactory system. Dura at the cribriform plate is closely adherent to bone, unlike at the ethmoid roof where it can be separated more easily. The crista galli lies in the midline, directly above the superior extent of the nasal septum. The crista galli and nasal septum separate the left and right cribriform plates. Occasionally, the physician can consider saving the contralateral olfactory system when resecting a tumor that penetrates the skull base unilaterally in this area.

The involvement of the dura and the brain by malignant neoplasms of the paranasal sinuses is prognostically unfavorable. Dura is often resected in this area. The effective repair and subsequent segregation of brain and frontal bone plate from underlying sinuses is critical in preventing both cerebrospinal fluid (CSF) leaks and osteomyelitis of the bone flap.

LIMITS OF RESECTION

The limits of modern resection have changed in the past 25 years. A generation ago, it was generally felt that the skull base was unresectable, as was the pterygomaxillary space, the nasopharynx, and the ICA. Tumors that extend to the pterygomaxillary space, involve the orbital periosteum, or infiltrate the dura have a worse prognosis than those that do not. However, all three of these anatomic areas are technically resectable. A unilateral ICA can be resected with some degree of safety. A unilateral ICA can be resected with about a 5% risk of a cerebrovascular accident when a patient has successfully passed a balloon test occlusion. In this test, a transarterial balloon is placed by an interventional neuroradiologist into the ICA and inflated to occlude proximal blood flow to the brain. A patient is considered to have "passed" when he remains symptom-free and maintains adequate back pressures in the ICA distal to the balloon—even when, pharmacologically, the systemic blood pressure has been reduced 20 mm Hg.

Most surgeons feel that the optic chiasm is not resectable. Most surgeons also agree that patients with a malignant tumor that extends to involve the cavernous sinus are rarely helped by surgery. Similarly, surgery is unlikely to improve the prognosis when a malignant neoplasm extends from paranasal sinuses to beyond the mucosa and cartilage in the nasopharynx. The limits of resection today are posterior and superolateral: the osseous components of the nasopharynx, the cavernous sinus, and the optic chiasm.

MALIGNANT NEOPLASMS

Malignant tumors of the paranasal sinuses are fortunately rare, accounting for about 1:1,000,000 cases overall and representing < 2–3% of head and neck cancers. Most of these malignant tumors do not extend to the skull base, but skull base resection should be considered for the minority of tumors that do. In addition, benign processes that may also require anterior skull base resections include some angiofibromas, some fibro-osseous benign tumors, occasional inverted papillomas, and occasional sequelae of chronic sinusitis (eg, mucoceles).

1. Squamous Cell Carcinoma

The most common malignant tumor of the paranasal sinuses is squamous cell carcinoma (SCC). The antrum, the largest sinus, is the most common site of SCC, but extension posteriorly and superiorly may lead to the necessity of including a skull base resection in the overall management. About 10% of tumors present with neck nodes, and about 20% of patients develop cervical nodes if no elective neck irradiation is included in the treatment plan.

The radiologic assessment of the course of V2 is important to exclude perineural spread before surgery and as a baseline for future evaluation. For tumors that extend to the skull base, combining skull base surgery with postoperative irradiation has improved the overall local control and cure rates from < 50% to about 60%.

Le QT, Fu KK, Kaplan MJ, Terris DJ, Fee WE, Goffinet DR. Lymph node metastasis in maxillary sinus carcinoma. *Int J Radiat Oncol Biol Phys.* 20001;46(3):541. [PMID: 10701732] (The overall risk of developing cervical metastases from squamous cell carcinoma of the maxillary sinus was 28%; no patients who received elective neck irradiation subsequently developed nodal metastases.)

Paulino AC, Fisher SG, Marks JE. Is prophylactic neck irradiation indicated in patients with squamous cell carcinoma of the maxillary sinus? *Int J Radiat Oncol Biol Phys.* 1997;39(2):283. [PMID: 9308929] (Four of 42 patients presented with nodal metastases. Eleven [29%] of 42 patients with nodal metastases subsequently developed neck metastases, and because of this, the authors recommended prophylactic neck irradiation.)

2. Adenocarcinoma

Adenocarcinoma represents approximately 10–15% of paranasal sinus tumors. Involvement in the woodworking and leather industries is a causative factor in the development of adenocarcinoma, especially in Europe. Since distant spread is uncommon, local control is the goal. Results of surgery and postoperative irradiation suggest cure rates between 45% and 85%, with a meta-analysis suggesting that about two thirds of patients are cured.

3. Adenoid Cystic Carcinoma

Adenoid cystic carcinoma (ACC) represents about 10–15% of paranasal sinus tumors and tends to recur locally, despite surgery and irradiation. Approximately 15–20% of patients with ACC develop hematogenous metastases, especially to the lungs; therefore, an initial metastatic evaluation is important. Because it is advisable to resect isolated lung metastases, periodic metastatic evaluations remain an important part of post-treatment tumor follow-up. A baseline computed tomography (CT) scan of the chest followed by a chest scan repeated at least annually is recommended. When the initial tumor is bright on positron emission tomography (PET) scanning, it is logical to use PET as a total body screen; however, the use of periodic PET scans has not been established for this histology. Recent reviews suggest that the 5-year local control rate is as high as 60%, with a sizable number of patients—perhaps 15–20%—experiencing local recurrences but living with tumor. Like SCC, perineural spread should be specifically investigated by MRI, both initially and in follow-ups because there is evidence that gamma knife radiosurgery for perineural spread along the fifth cranial nerve is effective in both reducing pain and in controlling disease progression.

Pitman KT, Prokopakis EP, Aydogan B et al. The role of skull base surgery for the treatment of adenoid cystic carcinoma of the sinonasal tract. *Head Neck.* 1999;21(5):402. [PMID: 10402519] (Following surgery and radiation therapy, 36% recurred lo-

cally, 14% regionally, and 21% developed distant metastases. Skull base surgery facilitated gross total resection of lesions once deemed inoperable, but has not resulted in an overall improvement in the disease-free survival rate of 46%.)

4. Esthesioneuroblastoma (Olfactory Neuroblastoma)

A tumor of neuroendocrine origin, esthesioneuroblastomas are tumors of the olfactory nerve and are seen above and below the cribriform plate. An MRI evaluation is essential to determine the extent of intracranial involvement. At times, no involvement appears to exist superior to the cribriform plate, suggesting that resection of the dura around the olfactory groove would fully encompass the superior extent of the tumor. Occasionally, there is extensive involvement of dura and even brain. Nodal or distant metastases are rare at presentation. Eventually, about 10% of patients develop neck metastases.

Several staging classifications have been suggested based on the anatomic extent of tumor or based on the assessment of histologic parameters. Tumors that appear histologically aggressive and those with extension to the orbit or dura appear to do somewhat worse to the extent that the analysis of few cases can generalize.

The rarity of this tumor makes the comparison of different treatment regimens difficult. In most centers, surgery and radiation therapy are the mainstays of treatment, with 5-year cure rates frequently reported in the range of 74% to 86%. The role of chemotherapy remains unclear: some centers routinely include cisplatin-based treatment whenever there is bone erosion superiorly through the cribriform plate, whereas others reserve this for only the most advanced tumors. In addition, there are reports of chemotherapy and radiation therapy alone being used with initially good results, although the follow-up has been relatively brief.

Lund VJ, Howard D, Wei W, Spittle M. Olfactory neuroblastoma: past, present, and future? *Laryngoscope.* 2003;113(3):502. [PMID: 12616204] (A combination of skull base resection and irradiation, which was superior to surgery alone, is the standard to which other approaches must be judged. The 5- and 10-year disease-free actuarial survival was 77% and 53%, respectively, among the 24 patients so treated.)

5. Melanoma

Melanomas of the nose and paranasal sinuses portend a poor prognosis, with high rates of both local recurrence and distant metastases. When there are already metastases, participation in chemotherapy protocols is available. If disease appears to be locally confined, then surgical resection and irradiation are often plausible, despite the prognosis, as long as the morbidity is minimal. Whether radiation fractionation should be standard—1.8–2.0 Gy daily for 5 d/wk to a dose of 60–66 Gy—or provided as 6 Gy twice weekly to a total dose of 30 Gy is not definitively known. The 5-year survival rate of melanoma of the nose and paranasal sinuses has been reported to be in the range of 14% to 47%, with most reports citing 20–25%. When recurrences can be surgically resected with a minimum of morbidity, then a nasal airway may be maintained and epistaxis reduced.

Medina JE, Ferlito A, Pellitteri PK et al. Current management of mucosal melanoma of the head and neck. *J Surg Oncol.* 2003;83(2):116. [PMID: 12772206] (Reviews current management of this rare tumor that portends a poor prognosis.)

Patel SG, Prasad ML, Escrig M et al. Primary mucosal malignant melanoma of the head and neck. *Head Neck.* 2002;24(3):247. [PMID: 11891956] (Significant prognostic factors include advanced clinical stage, tumor thickness > 5 mm, the presence of vascular invasion, and the development of distant metastases.)

Thompson LD, Wieneke JA, Miettinen M. Sinonasal tract and nasopharyngeal melanomas: a clinicopathologic study of 115 cases with a proposed staging system. *Am J Surg Pathol.* 2003;27(5):594. [PMID: 12717245] (Reviews histologic and immunohistochemical parameters of sinonasal tract and nasopharyngeal melanomas.)

6. Sinonasal Undifferentiated Carcinoma

Sinonasal undifferentiated carcinoma is a rare and highly aggressive malignant tumor that is distinct from other apparently poorly differentiated small, round-cell tumors. At presentation, the tumor is invariably extensive, commonly involving the orbit and extending to or through the skull base. Neck metastases are seen in 20% of patients. The prognosis is very poor. An optimal treatment modality has not evolved; multimodality therapy is generally used. The goal of treatment should be the control of local disease, including the preservation of vision as long as possible and the prevention or at least delay of intracranial extension and its sequelae.

Mills SE. Neuroectodermal neoplasms of the head and neck with emphasis on neuroendocrine carcinomas. *Mod Pathol.* 2002; 15(3):264. [PMID: 11904342] (Clarifies the confusion in the literature regarding neuroendocrine carcinomas in the head and neck; suggests that sinonasal undifferentiated carcinoma is likely of neuroectodermal origin.)

Miyamoto RC, Gleich LL, Biddinger PW, Gluckman JL. Esthesioneuroblastoma and sinonasal undifferentiated carcinoma: impact of histological grading and clinical staging on survival and prognosis. *Laryngoscope.* 2000;110(8):1262. [PMID: 10942123] (Reviews Kadish clinical and Hyams histopathologic grading systems for sinonasal undifferentiated carcinoma [and esthesioneuroblastomas]. Although the prognosis for sinonasal undifferentiated carcinomas is poor, 2 of 14 patients had long-term survival, even with advanced disease.)

Musy PY, Reibel JF, Levine PA. Sinonasal undifferentiated carcinoma: the search for a better outcome. *Laryngoscope.* 2002;112:1450. [PMID: 12172261] (Reviews experience with chemotherapy, followed by skull base resection in 10 patients, with a 2-year survival rate of 64%.)

7. Chordoma

Chordomas are rare tumors of notochord origin that may be seen at the craniocervical junction. About 35% of these tumors are found in this sphenoclival area, with about 15% occurring in vertebrae and the rest in the region of the sacrum and coccyx. Although chordomas have been seen in infants and the elderly, the usual age at presentation is 35–50 years. These tumors are usually large at presentation but without evidence of metastases, and they may abut or encase the ICA in the cavernous sinus or the basilar artery. The typical symptoms are headache and diplopia secondary to paresis of cranial nerve VI (the abducens nerve). At times there may be numbness of the face via involvement of sensory branches of the trigeminal nerve.

Evaluation by MRI is critical in evaluating the extent of tumor involvement. Chordomas are usually bright on T2-weighted images and enhance heterogeneously with gadolinium. The goal of treatment is as complete a resection as possible by an appropriate approach, followed by irradiation. Although the appearance on MRI of a heterogeneously gadolinium-enhancing lesion that is also bright on T2-weighted images at the craniocervical junction is highly suggestive of a chordoma, this appearance is not pathognomonic. Other entities, such as nasopharyngeal carcinoma, meningioma, metastases, plasmacytoma, and pituitary adenoma, are included in the differential diagnosis. Frozen-section confirmation at the beginning of a resection is therefore recommended. A classic pathologic finding shows physaliphorous cells with abundant mucus or glycogen-rich vacuoles, mucoid microcysts, fibrovascular strands, and cords of eosinophilic syncytial cells. The results of surgery plus charged particle irradiation have demonstrated a 5-year survival rate of 76–80% for smaller tumors that had not been previously treated (see Radiation Therapy later in this chapter). At the skull base, about 90% of tumors fall into this favorable category. Larger tumors (> 75 cm³) and recurrent tumors did noticeably worse, with a 5-year cure rate of approximately 33%.

8. Lymphoma

Lymphomas represent about 10% of nonepithelial malignant tumors of the paranasal sinuses. The most common lymphoma is diffuse large cell B-cell lymphoma, with patients most often presenting in Stage 1E. Approximately 67% of these patients survive with modern multimodality therapy. CD56+ NK/T-cell lymphomas, especially with a positive finding of the Epstein-Barr virus, represent about 30% of lymphomas when only nasal involvement is seen. Although some Asian studies suggest a poorer prognosis compared with apparently similar patients in the United States, most patients survive. The role of surgery is generally limited to obtaining tissue for diagnosis if a fine-needle aspiration (FNA) of a lymph node is either not available or is insufficient for a definitive diagnosis.

BENIGN NEOPLASMS

Juvenile Angiofibroma

Juvenile angiofibromas are rare, benign but locally invasive, and highly vascular tumors that occur in male adolescents. They invariably originate at the level of the sphenopalatine foramen on the posterolateral nasal wall at the junction with the nasopharynx and may extend laterally into the pterygopalatine fossa, posteriorly to the sphenoid sinus, or superiorly to and through the skull base. As they extend anteriorly, they lead to nasal obstruction. Because of their high vascularity, recurrent epistaxis is typical. Their appearance on MRI is so typical that the diagnosis can be presumed. Angiography is indicated for preoperative embolization of the tumor and the ipsilateral internal maxillary artery. Treatment is interventional radiologic embolization followed by surgical excision. The approach used should be appropriate for the individual. Usually, a trans-sphenoethmoidal approach is sufficient to remove an angiofibroma completely. Some surgeons prefer a transpalatal approach (or a maxillotomy approach), which offers the advantage of avoiding even a small, well-camouflaged facial incision; however, this approach may either affect palate function or provide suboptimal exposure for larger tumors. If the tumor extends to the greater wing of the sphenoid, then a preauricular orbitozygomatic approach (sometimes combined with a middle cranial fossa approach) is necessary.

PATIENT EVALUATION

Because of the often poor prognosis and the possibility of significant surgical complications, it is important for the physician managing skull base problems to obtain a complete knowledge of the patient's comorbidities and to weigh different options based on the individual. This begins with a thorough history and physical examination. Although the symptoms of lesions of the anterior skull base often mimic those of chronic sinusitis, which is far more common, certain signs and symptoms suggest that the presenting disorder may be far more serious. These include unilateral, persistent lesions (especially if the onset occurs after the age of 50); bleeding; pain; diplopia, epiphora, and numbness (eg, V2).

The signs that suggest a possible malignant neoplasm include a visible mass that is either palpable subcutaneously or visible via an endoscopic exam, abnormal extraocular motility, facial dysesthesia or numbness (ie, V1–3), and a neck mass.

If the patient has a history of a malignant tumor, then metastasis should be considered in the differential diagnosis. If there is a history of tobacco use, SCC is a more likely finding; SCC is the most common malignant tumor of the paranasal sinuses, accounting for more than 50% of cases.

When the patient history and physical exam are suggestive of a malignant neoplasm, a radiologic evaluation is indicated before obtaining a biopsy. A high-quality MRI is always the examination of choice. T1-weighted images with and without gadolinium, T1-weighted images with fat suppression, and T2-weighted images are indicated. In addition to axial images, invasion through the cribriform area is best evaluated with coronal images, which are sometimes supplemented with sagittal images. Multiplanar images greatly assist the surgeon in visualizing a three-dimensional image of the tumor extent. MRI assesses the vascularity of the tumor and may, at times, strongly suggest a particular diagnosis, such as angiofibroma or lymphoma. Assessing the neck is usually indicated because a number of histologies have the potential to metastasize to the neck. Radiologic assessment is reviewed in more detail in Chapter 3, Radiology.

How extensive a metastatic evaluation should be completed before obtaining tissue for pathologic review depends on a number of factors. For example, if lymphoma is suspected, it might be more reasonable at times to pursue the noninvasive aspect of the evaluation as the physician may find an easily accessible node to biopsy. FNA of a neck node, when present, may yield a diagnosis of SCC, thus precluding the need for a nasal biopsy. However, the paranasal sinuses are frequently the sole site of involvement, however extensive, and establishing the diagnosis requires a biopsy. Depending on the individual circumstances, the biopsy may be done in advance of further planning; at times it may be performed at the beginning of a major resection, with the surgeon intending to proceed only if the frozen section diagnosis is definitive.

Both a thorough, detailed discussion with the patient and coordination with the primary care and referring physicians are imperative in planning the optimum treatment plan. The primary care physician may have considerable insight about how the patient reacts to bad news as well as how to best establish rapport with the patient and create a treatment plan. Where metastatic evaluations and medical evaluations will be done and how post-treatment follow-up is to be coordinated should all be discussed at this time. The patient must fully comprehend the treatment alternatives, the realistic goals and likelihood of the success of these alternatives, and the potential side effects and complications of each aspect of intervention. The surgeon, who is likely to lead the treatment team both for surgery and for long-term follow-up, must also understand how intervention is likely to affect the particular patient's daily life. He must respect the patient's own goals for treatment and recognize that what he thinks he might choose for himself may be different from what his patient chooses.

Plans for follow-up begin preoperatively. If PET scans are to be used in long-term follow-up, it may be helpful to obtain one preoperatively so that any areas that unexpectedly enhance can be evaluated. This approach occasionally also reveals unexpected metastases, which would make a curative surgical approach futile. The need for long-term radiologic and clinical follow-up should be discussed with the patient, the primary care physician and referring physician, and at times the patient's insurance carrier. A high-quality MRI obtained 2–3 months after the completion of all treatment is valuable as a baseline and is strongly recommended. This is the most sensitive way to detect subtle perineural spread, changes that suggest a possible recurrence, or possible radionecrosis.

RADIOLOGY, INTERVENTIONAL RADIOLOGY, & INTRAOPERATIVE NAVIGATION

Improved radiologic imaging, both preoperatively and for intraoperative guidance, has significantly enhanced accurate surgical planning; this allows the physicians to consider combining several low-morbidity approaches, resulting in adequate resection and reduced functional loss. High-quality MRI is imperative. Occasionally, CT scanning is complementary in assessing bone at the cribriform plate, the anterior clinoid process, or the posterior wall of the sphenoid bone. Imaging is reviewed in Chapter 3, Radiology.

For highly vascular tumors, the preoperative embolization of both the tumor and the distal internal maxillary artery is helpful in reducing blood loss. A common example of this is the treatment of juvenile angiofibromas. The anterior and posterior ethmoid arteries are branches of the ophthalmic artery. As such, they cannot be safely embolized; therefore, when indicated, they are controlled surgically, usually by a metallic clip.

Intraoperative navigation is frequently unnecessary because there are numerous adequate bony landmarks available to the surgeon. However, if important landmarks have been eroded by tumor or removed in a prior surgery or if a structure has been displaced by tumor, then intraoperative navigation may be invaluable. This is especially so if a critical structure within soft tissue cannot be easily found, despite adjacent landmarks. Dissection near the ICA and optic chiasm may often be aided in this manner.

TREATMENT

Preoperative Considerations

Before planning surgery, a metastatic evaluation, as indicated by the histology, is completed. The treatment goals, alternatives, risks, and expected postoperative course are thoroughly discussed with the patient. Follow-up strategies are also discussed with the patient and the referring physician. It is essential for the patient to clearly understand the limitations of surgery, the prognosis, and the alternatives, including palliative measures, even when a reasonably high possibility of a cure is anticipated. The poorer the prognosis, the more the physician should consider a PET scan to screen for metastatic disease; doing so may allow the physician to avoid surgery in patients for whom such an approach would prove futile. If a PET scan is to be considered as part of subsequent tumor surveillance, the physician should consider obtaining it initially to be sure the tumor is detected by the PET scan and to evaluate, in advance of the proposed surgery, any areas that are highlighted by the scan.

Surgical Measures

The surgical measures discussed here concentrate on the approaches appropriate for paranasal sinus tumors that extend superiorly to the anterior skull base. Such approaches can be expanded to the anterolateral skull base to access the middle cranial fossa floor and cavernous sinus. Similarly, an orbitozygomatic approach can be added if access to the superior infratemporal fossa is required. Access to the central skull base and the craniocervical junction for petroclival chordomas, chondrosarcomas, and meningiomas is also excluded.

The four major goals of the multidisciplinary surgical team that approaches a tumor of any part of the skull base are (1) safety; (2) adequate access for three-dimensional tumor resection, with negative surgical margins; (3) minimal brain retraction; and (4) reconstruction that preserves function and aesthetics. How best to accomplish these goals, as well as to succinctly coordinate the overlapping approaches required to do so, has led to the development of several classification schemes.

Approaches to the anterior skull base have evolved since their introduction 40–50 years ago. Initial approaches to the anterior skull base usually combined a bifrontal craniotomy with modifications of common otolaryngologic approaches, including lateral rhinotomy and external sphenoethmoidectomy. Current skull base surgery uses many complementary approaches to expose the tumor for resection while minimizing morbidity. Frontal brain retraction and edema are reduced by using lumbar subarachnoid drains and by adjusting the angle of approach, such as resecting and later replating the orbital rim when a tumor extends posteriorly to the planum sphenoidale. Facial skin incisions can often be eliminated by accessing the paranasal sinuses either via a bicoronal incision behind the hairline or by adding transoral, transmucosal incisions. For example, a combined glabellar and extended subcranial approach that provides adequate access to the sphenoethmoid and medial maxillary areas may eliminate an external ethmoidectomy incision. Often, all of the paranasal tumor resection can be done through a standard low bifrontal craniotomy, supplemented with a supraorbital rim approach, if needed, without a complete extended subcranial approach. Degloving approaches may be used to supplement the tumor resection. Endoscopic guidance for the paranasal sinus component of the resection may also be used.

Many surgeons favor minimizing central facial incisions for anterior skull base lesions. A low bifrontal craniotomy, supplemented as needed by a supraorbital rim approach, provides sufficient access to resect most paranasal sinus tumors that extend through the skull base. The supraorbital rim approach is added, when necessary, either to expose an orbital tumor or to reduce brain retraction when a far posterior exposure is required. When tumor involves bone in the glabellar area, requiring the resection of bone in this area, the extended subfrontal approach, in which the dural component is initially explored from below, provides excellent anterior dural exposure. Postoperative MRI has confirmed the clinical impression of excellent resections and shown only a modest incidence of encephalomalacia, with very few patients experiencing clinical symptoms. When needed, a limited facial incision (ie, a slightly extended external ethmoidectomy) results in good cosmesis.

A. BICORONAL CRANIOTOMY

If it is anticipated that the tumor can be resected without a facial incision, then the bifrontal craniotomy with or without a supraorbital rim approach is planned initially. A lumbar subarachnoid drain is usually placed. In contrast, when it is anticipated that resection can be accomplished extradurally or with the resection and repair of dura without a craniotomy, the transfacial approach is initially performed.

If intraoperative navigation is to be used, the patient is placed in fixation and the navigation system calibrated. Appropriate perioperative antibiotics are begun. The anesthesiologist monitors end-tidal CO_2.

The bicoronal skin incision from the top of one ear to the top of the other is placed approximately 1 cm posterior to the hairline. The hairline should be marked before shaving, with the patient choosing either a complete or anterior shave. If more skin reflection is needed, the incision can be extended inferiorly to just anterior to the root of the helix, toward the incision usually used for a parotidectomy. This incision incorporates the superficial temporal arteries into the skin flap. A pericranial-galeal flap is separated from the skin flap for later use. Its blood supply is from vessels coursing to it in the superomedial brow. At the end of the procedure, this flap is used to reinforce the dural closure and segregate the dura from the paranasal sinus

cavity below it. No bone graft or skin graft is necessary or indicated for a skull base repair, except perhaps in an infant. If the pericranial flap is unavailable because of either tumor involvement or prior surgery, then a microvascular free flap is often used instead, with superficial temporal vessels as the most convenient, correct-caliber vascular access to which to connect the vasculature of the flap.

1. Olfactory bulb preservation—If the tumor extends across the anterior midline, both olfactory bulbs are sacrificed. Invariably, this is necessary except in the smallest of tumors, such as a very small esthesioneuroblastoma.

2. Orbit preservation—If the extraocular motion is clinically normal, the orbit rarely needs to be sacrificed. Although MRI is the most effective evaluative tool to delineate tumor extent preoperatively, the radiologist and surgeon can misinterpret a film that suggests that orbital fat is medially invaded when, in fact, it is the periosteum and fat that are medially displaced; however, the fat is not involved per se. If the eye is functioning, the decision to preserve the eye or to do an orbit exenteration is likely to be an operative decision by the surgeon, based on whether the surgeon can remove the periosteum with negative margins while noting the fat is uninvolved.

If this decision appears to be a close one, it is often wise to leave it until the end of the case. If equally close margins are necessary elsewhere, as in the pterygomaxillary space or at the lateral sphenoid sinus, then it is unlikely that doing an orbit exenteration would substantially (if at all) improve the likelihood of local tumor control. The same holds true if the closest margin is the far posterior orbit where orbit exenteration would not materially improve the likelihood of overall tumor control.

Preservation of the orbit but partial resection of the orbit periosteum may make planning subsequent radiation fields difficult, requiring close cooperation of the radiation oncologist, neuroradiologist, and surgeon. Intensity-modulated radiation therapy (IMRT) would likely play an important role in planning radiation in this situation.

3. Optic nerve and chiasm—Tumors of the anterior skull base may extend to the optic nerves from an inferior and inferomedial direction. Occasionally, the optic nerve may be surrounded by tumor, in which case the overlying ICA may also be involved. Since the blood supply to the optic nerve does not run along its medial surface, the physician can generally dissect gently along the nerve without affecting the patient's vision. This is also true along the chiasm anteriorly. If the optic nerve or chiasm has been dissected, it is important that the placement of the pericranial-galeal flap at the conclusion of the procedure does not lead to pressure against the nerve. Occasionally, the optic nerve is nearly surrounded by tumor. If that is true, then particular attention must first be directed to the ICA, lying just above the optic nerve, to determine to what extent the tumor can be resected. Although the adjacent ICA will have been carefully examined on the preoperative MRI, the surgeon, intraoperatively, will need to closely inspect and confirm to what extent the tumor is resectable. For a tumor to be resectable there must be approximately 1 cm of uninvolved optic nerve anterior to the chiasm, as well as an uninvolved ICA.

4. Dural repair and pericranial-galeal flap—After tumor resection, the dura is repaired. This can be done using preserved bovine pericardium, fascia lata, or other materials. This repair is buttressed by the pericranial flap, or, if that is unavailable or in extensive skull base defects, by a microvascular free flap (rectus muscle or radial forearm myofascial flap). After hemostasis is achieved, pieces of absorbable gelatin sponge (ie, Gelfoam) are placed against the orbit periosteum and raw bone. Merocel sponges 8–10 cm in length are placed through the nostrils along the floor of the nasal cavity. A layer of small pieces of absorbable gelatin are then placed superior to the Merocel sponges, up to the axial plane of the skull base, to help support the pericranial flap. This layer also serves to segregate the Merocel sponges from the pericranial flap so that removal of these sponges 10 days later is unlikely to disturb the pericranial flap. The pericranial flap is then reflected over the central orbital rims and glabellas into the skull base defect and posteriorly rests on a shelf of remaining planum sphenoidale anterior to the chiasm. Care must be taken to ensure that there is sufficient redundancy (ie, the flap should not be stretched) so that the flap does not subsequently retract anteriorly. It may be helpful to tack the flap to the dura to prevent anterior displacement. Suctioning the air from beneath the flap while the flap is set may help the surgeon ensure an adequate length of flap on the bony defect. Any redundant flap may be reflected anterosuperiorly over the frontal dura. The Merocel sponge is left in place for approximately 10 days, and antibiotics are administered until the pack is removed.

In tumors that invade the sphenoid roof, there may be no remaining planum sphenoidale posteriorly (anterior to the chiasm) and therefore no bony shelf for the pericranial-galeal flap to rest on. In such cases, the skull base can be successfully sealed by placing the pericranial flap over the skull base defect where the ethmoidal roof, cribriform plates, and planum sphenoidale have been resected, and then turning it inferiorly to rest against sella and the posterior wall of the sphenoid sinus, which has been completely stripped of its mucosa. Gelfoam pledgets are placed in the sphenoid sinus first so that the Gelfoam is against the flap. The Merocel sponge is then placed through the nostril into the front of the sphenoid sinus and as the sponge expands, it presses the flap against bone. The pack is kept in place for 10 days.

5. Craniotomy closure and frontal sinus management—Subsequent closure of the craniotomy is routine; however, care should be taken at the end of the procedure to ensure there is no remaining mucosa in any frontal sinus that may have been part of the bone flap and is now superior to the pericranial-galeal flap. If there is any portion of frontal sinus within the bone flap, a diamond bur should be used to bur down the frontal sinus 1–2 mm in the same manner as the frontal sinus is prepared before obliteration of sinus by fat in an osteoplastic frontal sinus procedure. Some surgeons also prefer an active drain beneath the skin closure, depending in part on concern for some postoperative bleeding or oozing.

B. TRANSFACIAL APPROACHES

When necessary, a trans-sphenoethmoidal incision is planned. As mentioned earlier, this may supplement the craniotomy incision, or it may be performed as the sole approach. An example of its being performed as the sole approach is to access the craniocervical junction from the sphenoid sinus through the clivus to the foramen magnum and the arch of C1, the first cervical vertebrae. This incision is the same as for an external ethmoidectomy, but extends more inferiorly. It extends toward the medial ala but stops at the axial plane of the inferior limit of the nasal bone. A lateral rhinotomy at the ala and Weber-Ferguson incision is rarely needed. This extended external sphenoethmoidectomy provides access from the inferior clivus upward through the sphenoid sinus, the sella, the medial cavernous sinus, the ethmoid sinuses, and the frontal sinus. In the sphenoid sinus, the physician can access the area posterolateral to the carotid artery and, if needed, the area as far lateral as the abducens nerve. In addition, lateral access to the pterygomaxillary space, the lateral antrum, and the orbit is provided when the medial maxilla is removed. The preservation of the inferior turbinate reduces postoperative nasal crusting and discomfort and is possible unless tumor extirpation requires its removal.

C. TRANSORAL-TRANSPHARYNGEAL APPROACH

Additional routes to the skull base are available as needed, depending on the extent of tumor. A common approach for chordomas and for decompression of the cervical spinal cord at the craniocervical junction secondary to degenerative or inflammatory processes is a transoral-transpharyngeal approach. Whether this approach, a trans-sphenoethmoidal approach, or, occasionally, a combination of both approaches is best is determined on an individual basis by evaluating the sagittal images on MRI and determining the superior and inferior access afforded by each approach. If the patient has a small mouth or trismus, the exposure afforded by a transoral approach may be reduced.

Perioperative antibiotics are begun, an intraoral endotracheal tube, as small as is tolerable, is positioned and taped to the lower midline, and lidocaine with epinephrine (1:200,000) is infiltrated into both the midline soft palate and the posterior pharyngeal wall laterally.

The soft palate is divided in the midline (heading to one side or the other of the uvula posteriorly) and retracted laterally. Specialized intraoral retractors are available that keep the mouth open, retract the tongue inferiorly, and retract the soft palate laterally and also anteriorly, if needed. One way to access the inferior clivus, the dens (the body of the second cervical vertebra), and the arch of C1 is by creating an inferiorly based myomucosal flap that incorporates the longus colli muscle and superior constrictor muscles. The superior transverse part of the mucosal incision is placed as superiorly as needed, keeping in mind the following: (1) the surgeon can see more superiorly as he or she removes the posterosuperior odontoid and clival bone, and (2) closure of this superior incision can be difficult, even with specialized needles with a large radius of curvature (eg, C-type needles and absorbable suture materials).

The advantage of an inferiorly based flap is that it preserves maximal soft tissue, thus minimizing the risk of velopharyngeal insufficiency inherent in removing bone in this area, which posteriorly displaces the Passavant ridge. Depending on the individual, the physician can usually reach superiorly to the lower to mid-clivus and inferiorly to the junction of C2–C3. The exposure can be made greater or lesser, depending on the specific need of each case.

The arch of C1 is preserved or not, as needed. Laterally, this approach is limited by the vertebral arteries. Evaluation of the preoperative MRI demonstrates the distance from the midline of the left and right vertebral arteries. Usually, this distance is 12–15 mm, which provides an adequate 2.5- to 3.0-cm wide access to the central skull base. The odontoid and clivus can be removed as needed with long-handled narrow drills, with intraoperative spinal cord monitoring (in the case of serious spinal cord compression) or intraoperative anatomic monitoring (in the case of tumor resection), as indicated. Additional soft tissue at the posterior longitudinal ligament can also be removed as needed.

With this approach, entry into the dura is highly unusual. If it occurs, the direct repair of the CSF leak should be supplemented with the interposition of nearby muscle, along with the placement of a lumbar subarachnoid drain for 4–5 days. If there is no tongue edema, patients should be extubated at the end of the procedure, keeping a 32F (ie, 10 mm in diameter) nasal trumpet in place for 48 hours. If there is concern about the development of tongue edema from the retractor, then the patient may be intubated in the ICU for 2–3 days while the edema is monitored. In selected patients, a temporary tracheotomy may be performed at the beginning of the procedure, and decannulation may be planned before discharge. After repairing the posterior pharyngeal wall in one layer using absorbable sutures, a small-diameter nasogastric feeding tube is placed, taking care not to disrupt the pharyngeal suture line. The soft palate is then repaired in three layers, also using absorbable sutures.

D. ORBITOZYGOMATIC APPROACH

Access to the superior parapharyngeal space and access along the floor of the middle cranial fossa can be gained by a temporary removal, en bloc, of the zygomatic arch, the lateral orbit, and the part of the maxilla where they intersect. Care should be taken to avoid injury to the temporal branch of the facial nerve. The temporalis muscle can be separated from the temporal bone squama and reflected inferiorly, with some of the fibrous attachment left for resuturing at the conclusion of the procedure. Using this approach, the foramen ovale, posterolateral antrum, pterygomaxillary space, and lateral orbit are all in view, and the dura can be retracted as necessary. In addition, the floor of the middle cranial fossa can be resected.

Lalwani AK, Kaplan MJ, Gutin PH. The trans-sphenoethmoid approach to the sphenoid sinus and clivus. *Neurosurgery.* 1992;31:1008. [PMID: 1470312] (Reviews transfacial approach to sphenoid sinus and clivus, with diagrams showing the extent of exposure and discussing limitations.)

Van Buren JM, Ommaya AK, Ketcham AS. Ten years' experience with radical combined craniofacial resection of malignant tumors of the paranasal sinuses. *J Neurosurg.* 1968;28:341. [PMID: 5643926] (Reviews the early pioneering experience with this approach.)

Surgery-Related Complications

With a surgeon's increased surgical experience, complications have become less common. In the past decade, operative mortality has, in most US institutions, been reduced from about 2% to nearly 0%. The incidence of CSF leaks has similarly decreased from 10–15% to less than 2%. Serious central nervous system deficits (including cerebrovascular accidents, unanticipated blindness, and autonomic dysfunction) have remained constant at approximately 3%. Complications of intracranial infections, such as meningitis or brain abscess, have also remained at approximately 2%. The loss of the anterior bone flap secondary to osteomyelitis has been reduced from 8–13% to 0%. Pericranial-galeal flaps and, for larger defects and patients who have undergone prior irradiation, microvascular free flaps have reduced the incidence of postoperative CSF leaks as well as wound or bone infection. The incidence of intracranial hematoma has decreased from 2% to 0% as a result of tailoring approaches to minimize the need for brain retraction, thus reducing encephalomalacia as well as the risk of hematoma. Finally, nonlethal medical complications such as pneumonia, arrhythmias, and occasional myocardial infarction have been steady at 10%, sometimes extending the length of hospitalization.

Clayman GL, DeMonte F, Jaffe DM et al. Outcome and complications of extended cranial-base resection requiring microvascular free-tissue transfer. *Arch Otolaryngol Head Neck Surg.* 1995;121(11):1253. [PMID: 7576471] (Review of MD Anderson's outcomes and complications when microvascular flaps are needed in extensive skull base resections.)

Nonsurgical Measures

A. RADIATION THERAPY

In the past 25 years, numerous series have demonstrated that radiation therapy alone results in a survival rate no better than 50%, and, in most series, 25–35% for the more common malignant epithelial neoplasms of the paranasal sinuses. This poor prognosis has been the major impetus for developing anterior skull base surgery. However, most physicians agree that a multimodality approach for most malignant tumors in this area is superior to either surgery or radiation alone. Most centers plan surgery with postoperative radiation for resectable tumors.

The dilemma in planning radiation ports lies in the need to give a tumoricidal dose to the tumor volume while limiting the dose to adjacent critical structures such as the brain, optic nerve and chiasm, and the lens. The tolerance of the lens is about 50 Gy; above this dose, cataracts may develop. The optic nerve well tolerates doses below 50 Gy. There is approximately a 10% incidence of optic neuritis when the dose is 50–55 Gy, and above 65 Gy, this incidence is > 20%. Fortunately, a patient can often tolerate minimal radionecrosis of the inferior portions of the frontal lobe with a minimum of long-term symptoms. Although there is variation in the literature as to how much radiation should be given as the target volume, most centers aim for a minimum of 60 Gy, with many centers advocating a minimum of 65 Gy.

Before the development of intensity-modulated radiation therapy (IMRT), charged particles were often used when irradiating the anterior skull base. The rapid falloff in dose afforded by protons permitted, for example, a dose of 60–80 Gy to be administered to chordomas of the sphenoclival area without undue risk to the optic nerves and chiasm. At Harvard a 160-MEV proton beam was generated from their cyclotron. At the Lawrence Berkeley Laboratory, in conjunction with UCSF, a helium-neon beam was used until about 1991. Protons are also currently available at Loma Linda University in southern California.

In the last 5 years, IMRT has been applied to the anterior skull base. With IMRT, the radiation oncologist conceptually plots the target volume using CT scanning, often with additional diagnostic information provided by an MRI, and inputs this information into a computer. The computer then generates a plan for mul-

tifield conformal radiation, using as many ports as needed and with the ability to use as many as 55 fields. Machines are now increasingly available to implement this strategy. It is likely that with IMRT, there will be better uniformity of the dose to the target volume and therefore a reduction in damage to adjacent tissue.

B. CHEMOTHERAPY

As in SCC encountered elsewhere in the head and neck, the role of chemotherapy in the treatment of malignant neoplasms of the paranasal sinuses continues to be investigated. During the 1980s and early 1990s, neoadjuvant chemotherapy for SCC, usually using cisplatin and 5-fluorouracil, was widely studied. Except for nasopharyngeal carcinoma, no improvement in the overall survival rate was found, despite good response rates. These disappointing results led to a more intense investigation of concomitant chemotherapy-radiation strategies in which the chemotherapy agent was predominantly used as a radiosensitizer. The results of concomitant radiation therapy plus cisplatin in the initial treatment of SCC at a number of head and neck sites, including the paranasal sinuses, have been encouraging, with a meta-analysis suggesting a 5–8% improvement compared with radiation alone. Postoperatively, although the rationale remains sound, there is much less data comparing radiation alone with concomitant radiation therapy plus chemotherapy.

The role of chemotherapy for specific histologies, such as esthesioneuroblastoma and lymphoma, was discussed earlier in this chapter (see "Pathology"). Chemotherapy for metastases is also usually appropriate; the specific regimen chosen depends on the histology and the health and tolerance of the patient.

Adams EJ, Nutting CM, Convery DJ et al. Potential role of intensity-modulated radiotherapy in the treatment of tumors of the maxillary sinus. *Int J Radiat Oncol Biol Phys.* 2001;51(3):579. [PMID: 11597796] (Reviews intensity-modulated radiation therapy with respect to paranasal sinus tumors.)

Diaz EM Jr, Kies MS. Chemotherapy for skull base cancers. *Otolaryngol Clin North Am.* 2001;34(6):1079. [PMID: 11728933] (Review of the indications and results of chemotherapy for malignant tumors that affect the skull base.)

Rasch C, Eisbruch A, Remeijer P et al. Irradiation of paranasal sinus tumors, a delineation and dose comparison study. *Int J Radiat Oncol Biol Phys.* 2002;52(1):120. [PMID: 11777629] (Reviews details of radiation planning.)

Remouchamps V, Van Duyse B, Vakaet L, Lemmerling M, Vermeersch H, De Neve W. An implementation strategy for IMRT of ethmoid sinus cancer with bilateral sparing of the optic pathways. *Int J Radiat Oncol Biol Phys.* 2001;51(2):318. [PMID: 11567805] (Intensity-modulated radiation therapy is used to minimize the radiation dose to critical structures while retaining the adequacy and homogeneity of dose-to-tumor volume.)

Waldron JN, O'Sullivan B, Gullane P et al. Carcinoma of the maxillary antrum: a retrospective analysis of 110 cases. *Radiother Oncol.* 2000;57(2):167. [PMID: 11054520]. (Reviews the extensive experience of a single institution.)

Combined Surgery & Irradiation

Many series have documented that a combination of anterior skull base surgery and postoperative irradiation has improved the rates of local control for a number of malignant histologies, including esthesioneuroblastoma, adenoid cystic carcinoma, and adenocarcinoma. A review of the 5-year survival rate is summarized in Table 60–1. The survival rate is highest for esthesioneuroblastomas and adenocarcinomas. A number of tumors are associated with a fair prognosis, with 5-year survival rates that are approximately 50%. Melanoma and sinonasal undifferentiated tumors portend a poor prognosis, and treatment strategies for patients with these two histologies should stress the preservation of function; how best to incorporate chemotherapy protocols into the management of these tumors continues to be discussed.

Boyle JO, Shah KC, Shah JP. Craniofacial resection for malignant neoplasms of the skull base: an overview. *J Surg Oncol.* 1998;69:275. [PMID: 9881946] (Reviews the improvements in cure and the reduction in morbidity of Memorial Sloan-Kettering.)

Dulguerov P, Jacobsen MS, Allal AS, Lehmann W, Calcaterra T. Nasal and paranasal sinus carcinoma: are we making progress? A series of 220 patients and a systematic review. *Cancer.* 2001;92(12):3012. [PMID: 11753979] (Review of the UCLA experience; includes a good systemic literature review.)

Harbo G, Grau C, Bundgaard T et al. Cancer of the nasal cavity and paranasal sinuses. A clinico-pathological study of 277 patients. *Acta Oncol.* 1997;36(1):45. [PMID: 9090965] (Reviews the 28-year experience from the Aarhus University Hospital in Denmark.)

Table 60–1. Five-year survival rate with a combination of surgery and radiation therapy for malignant disorders of the anterior skull base.

Histology	5-year Survival Rate	Comment
Esthesioneuroblastoma	62–95%	Most: 80–95%
Adenocarcinoma	45–85%	Meta-analysis 78%
Adenoid cystic carcinoma	40–60%	AWD: + 15–20
Sarcomas	50–60%	AWD: + 20
Squamous cell carcinoma	30–65%	Meta-analysis 60%
Melanoma	<15–45%	Meta-analysis 23%
Sinonasal undifferentiated carcinoma and undifferentiated carcinoma	<10–15%	

AWD, alive with disease (ie, disease has recurred, but patient is alive).

Irish JC, Gullane PJ, Gentili F et al. Tumors of the skull base: outcome and survival analysis of 77 cases. *Head Neck.* 1994;16(1):3. [PMID: 8125786] (Reviews the outcomes from an experienced center in Toronto.)

Janecka IP, Sen C, Sekhar LN et al. Cranial base surgery: results in 183 patients. *Otolaryngol Head Neck Surg.* 1994;110(6):539. [PMID: 8208569] (Review of outcomes by a premier team.)

Janecka IP, Sen C, Sekhar L, Curtin H. Treatment of paranasal sinus cancer with cranial base surgery: results. *Laryngoscope.* 1994;104(5 Pt 1):553. [PMID: 8189985] (Review of outcomes by the same premier team as noted in the previous reference.)

Kraus DH, Shah JP, Arbit E, Galicich JH, Strong EW. Complications of craniofacial resection for tumors involving the anterior skull base. *Head Neck.* 1994;16(4):307. [PMID: 8056574] (Reviews and updates.)

Lund VJ, Howard DJ, Wei WI, Cheesman AD. Craniofacial resection for tumors of the nasal cavity and paranasal sinuses—a 17-year experience. *Head Neck.* 1998;20(2):97. [PMID: 9484939] (Reviews the outcomes and complications of a highly experienced team in England.)

McCaffrey TV, Olsen KD, Yohanan JM, Lewis JE, Ebersold MJ, Piepgras DG. Factors affecting survival of patients with tumors of the anterior skull base. *Laryngoscope.* 1994;104:940. [PMID: 8052078] (From the Mayo Clinic, a review of the prognostic factors in 54 patients, 24 of whom had esthesioneuroblastoma.)

O'Malley BW Jr, Janecka IP. Evolution of outcomes in cranial base surgery. *Semin Surg Oncol.* 1995;11(3):221. [PMID: 7638509] (Discusses methods used to decrease complications and improve overall results.)

Treatment of Recurrent Disease

A. PERINEURAL SPREAD

Perineural spread along V2 and less commonly along V1 is especially common in squamous cell and adenoid cystic carcinomas. It is suspected when there is a new onset of dysesthesias or when the patient experiences pain above the eye (V1) or along the lateral nasal area and the maxillary alveolar ridge (V2). MRI with gadolinium enhancement is diagnostic, especially if there have been serial MRIs indicating changes that correspond to patient symptoms. Gamma-knife radiosurgery has been used in such instances, with the control of pain usually achieved in approximately 6 months, and a 40% rate of disease control, with no progression radiologically or clinically, in 5 years.

B. NECK METASTASES

Neck metastases occur in approximately 20% of cases of SCC and in about 10% of cases of esthesioneuroblastoma. In both disorders, if the primary site is disease-free, it is likely that a neck dissection is indicated. If there has been no prior neck irradiation, then postoperative neck irradiation is also indicated. When there has been prior neck irradiation, then there may be a role for intraoperative radiation therapy.

C. LOCAL RECURRENCES

The local recurrence of malignant tumors of the paranasal sinuses portends a worse prognosis than the initial disease. There are usually limitations in the treatment of local recurrences owing to the prior use of irradiation and the scarring associated with prior surgery, which make subsequent surgery more difficult, if such surgery is even possible. In addition, a tumor that has recurred after prior postoperative irradiation is likely to have grown from a clonal population that is resistant to radiation. Because of some cross-resistance, it may also be resistant to chemotherapy. If a metastatic evaluation demonstrates no regional or distant disease, then the next step should be a thorough discussion with the patient of all the available modalities. Depending on the histology, chemotherapy protocols may be of some value. Protocols for subsequent treatment are useful for some patients. Depending on the patient's current symptoms and the extent of the recurrence, there may be a role for surgery that is palliative or, occasionally, even curative, although this latter is unlikely.

SPECIAL CONSIDERATIONS

In the past 30 years, surgery at the anterior skull base has evolved from a desperate attempt to improve dismal control rates fraught with daunting perioperative complications to a developed multidisciplinary subspecialty with proven results. Clearly, local control is now likely to be improved for the more common malignant tumors that occur in this area. Approaches have evolved that select an angle of approach that minimizes brain retraction while optimizing accessibility to structures requiring resection, and that simultaneously limit esthetic and functional side effects.

Initially, the approach that was routinely used was a transcutaneous transfacial approach via an extended external ethmoidectomy incision in association with a low bifrontal craniotomy, with or without a supraorbital rim approach. This allowed the exposure of an area from the frontal sinuses superiorly to the mid-clivus inferiorly, reaching laterally to the cavernous sinus and the carotid artery, orbit, and lateral antrum. This is an extension of an approach highly familiar to all otolaryngologists and requires no central facial plating. Its disadvantage is a facial incision, although one that heals with a generally well-camouflaged scar. With subsequent surgical experience, it was found that the transfacial incision could often be avoided, instead providing access solely from above. A subfrontal approach without brain retraction at all was occasionally possible when frontal bone and nasal bone necessarily needed to be removed because of tumor involvement.

At each institution where skull base surgery is performed, a multidisciplinary team has grown that involves, among others, otolaryngologist–head and neck surgeons, neurosurgeons, plastic surgeons, neuroradiologists, medical oncologists, radiation oncologists, and prosthodontists. Each team determines what classification schemes they find useful as an organizing and teaching tool, and with which sets of approaches, with variations, they are the most comfortable. This judgment may also be based on prior irradiation or surgical intervention as well as the patient's evaluation of the risks and alternatives.

Vestibular Schwannoma (Acoustic Neuroma)

61

Jacob Johnson, MD, & Anil K. Lalwani, MD

ESSENTIALS OF DIAGNOSIS

- *Asymmetric (unilateral) sensorineural hearing loss, tinnitus, and disequilibrium.*
- *Disproportionate speech discrimination score relative to pure-tone average.*
- *Facial and trigeminal nerve symptoms with larger tumors.*

General Considerations

Vestibular schwannomas (acoustic neuromas) are nerve sheath tumors of the superior and inferior vestibular nerves (cranial nerve VIII). They arise in the medial internal auditory canal (IAC) or lateral cerebellopontine angle (CPA) and cause clinical symptoms by displacing, distorting, or compressing adjacent structures in the CPA.

Vestibular schwannomas (VS) are by far the most common tumors involving the CPA. VS make up 80% of CPA tumors and 8% of all intracranial tumors. Various epidemiology studies have shown an incidence of 10 per 1 million individuals each year. This figure correlates with the 2000–3000 individuals diagnosed with VS each year in the United States. There is no gender bias and the age of presentation is between 40 and 60 years of age. Ninety-five percent of VS occur in a sporadic fashion. The remaining 5% of patients have neurofibromatosis type 2 (NF2) or familial VS. The age of presentation is earlier in nonsporadic VS and patients usually present in the second or third decades of life.

Anatomy

The CPA consists of a potential cerebrospinal fluid-filled space in the posterior cranial fossa bounded by the temporal bone, cerebellum, and brainstem. The CPA is a roughly triangular-shaped structure in the axial plane and is filled with cerebrospinal fluid (CSF) (Figure 61–1). The superior boundary is the tentorium and the inferior boundary is the cerebellar tonsil and medullary olives. The anterior border is the posterior dural surface of petrous bone and clivus, and the posterior border is the ventral surface of the pons and cerebellum. The medial border is the cisterns of the pons and medulla and the apex is the region of the lateral recess of the fourth ventricle. The lateral opening of the fourth ventricle, the foramen of Luschka, opens into the CPA. Cranial nerves V–XI traverse the cephalic and caudal extent of the CPA. The central structures crossing the CPA to and from the IAC are the facial (CN VII) and vestibulocochlear nerves (CN VIII), respectively.

Cranial nerves VII and VIII are covered with central myelin provided by neuroglial cells as they cross the CPA and carry a sleeve of posterior fossa dura into the IAC. The transition to peripheral myelin made by the Schwann cells occurs at the medial opening of the IAC. The vestibulocochlear nerve divides into three nerves: (1) the cochlear nerve and (2 and 3) the superior and inferior vestibular nerves in the lateral extent of the CPA or medial IAC. The IAC is divided into four quadrants by a vertical crest, called Bill's bar, and a transverse crest. CN VII comes to lie in the anterosuperior quadrant and is anterior to the superior vestibular nerve and superior to the cochlear nerve, while the inferior vestibular nerve lies in the posteroinferior quadrant and is inferior to the superior vestibular nerve and posterior to the cochlear nerve (see Figure 61–1). The anteroinferior cerebellar artery (AICA) is the main artery in the CPA and is the source of the labyrinthine artery. The labyrinthine artery via the IAC is an end artery for the hearing and balance organs. The AICA has a variable relationship to cranial nerves VII and VIII and to the IAC.

Pathogenesis

Vestibular schwannomas originate in the Schwann cells of the superior or inferior vestibular nerves at the transition zone (Obersteiner-Redlich zone) of the peripheral and central myelin. This transition zone occurs in the lateral CPA or medial IAC. Therefore, VS most often

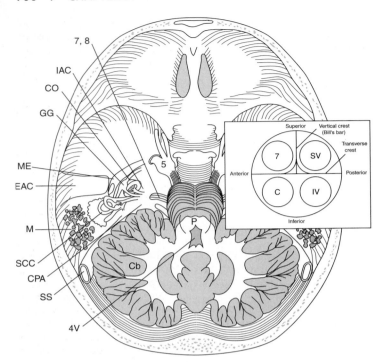

Figure 61–1. The anatomy of the cerebellopontine angle and its relationship to the temporal bone within the skull is shown. Inset shows the location of the cranial nerves within the internal auditory canal (IAC): the facial nerve (7) and the cochlear nerve (C) are in the anterior compartment whereas the superior and inferior vestibular nerves (SV and IV, respectively) are in the posterior half of the IAC. 5, trigeminal nerve; 7, facial nerve; 8, cochlear nerve; IAC, internal auditory canal; CO, cochlea; GG, geniculate ganglion; ME, middle ear; EAC, external auditory canal; M, mastoid; SCC, semicircular canal; CPA, cerebellopontine angle; SS, sigmoid sinus; 4V, 4th ventricle; Cb, cerebellum; P, pons.

arise in the IAC and occasionally in the CPA. These schwannomas rarely arise from the cochlear nerve and are rarely malignant. The propensity to develop from the vestibular nerves may be due to the vestibular ganglion in the IAC having the highest concentration of Schwann cells.

Recent studies have improved our molecular understanding of VS. VS occurs as a result of mutations in a tumor suppressor protein, merlin, located on chromosome 22q12. Merlin is a cytoskeletal protein and may control cell proliferation by regulating the abundance, localization, and turnover of cell-surface receptors. The formation of VS requires mutations of both copies of the merlin gene. One functioning merlin gene prevents the formation of VS. Somatic mutations in both copies of the merlin gene result in sporadic VS. The probabilities of two spontaneous, independent mutations at one locus predict a unilateral VS presenting in the fourth to sixth decades of life.

In contrast, familial VS occurring in NF2 only requires one occurrence of somatic mutation. People with NF2 inherit one mutated merlin gene and one normal merlin gene. A mutation in the normal allele leads to bilateral VS by age 20. Therefore, NF2 is an autosomal recessive mutation at the gene level since disease expression requires mutations in both alleles of the gene, but the inheritance is autosomal dominant (pseudodominant) since inheritance of one mutated allele often leads to a dis-

ease state. NF2 is a central form of neurofibromatosis, with affected patients having central nervous system tumors, including schwannomas, meningiomas, and gliomas. Most of these patients develop bilateral VS. In comparison, patients with NF type 1 (von Recklinghausen disease) have intra- and extracranial tumors, and < 5% of these patients develop unilateral VS. Genetic screens for the NF2 mutation have been developed and offer genetic counseling for family members of patients with NF2. The severity of mutation involving the merlin gene in NF2 can predict the severity of disease manifestation.

Clinical Findings

A. Symptoms and Signs

1. Hearing loss—Hearing loss is present in 95% of patients with VS. Conversely, 5% of patients have normal hearing; therefore, unilateral vestibular or facial complaints without hearing loss do not rule out retrocochlear disease. Of patients with hearing loss, most have slowly progressive hearing loss with noise distortion. Twenty percent have an episode of sudden hearing loss. The improvement of hearing loss with or without treatment does not rule out retrocochlear disease. The level of hearing loss is not a clear predictor of tumor size.

2. Tinnitus and disequilibrium—Tinnitus is present in 65% of patients. The tinnitus is most often constant with a high buzzing pitch. This symptom is often not reported by patients because of the focus on the accompanying hearing loss. Similarly, owing to the central compensation for the slowly evolving vestibular injury, patients tolerate and adapt well to the disequilibrium they experience. The majority of patients have self-limiting episodes of vertigo. The disequilibrium is initially mild and constant and often does not prompt a medical visit. Disequilibrium is present in 60% of patients.

3. Facial and trigeminal nerve dysfunction—Facial and trigeminal nerve dysfunction occurs after the auditory and vestibular impairments. The patients usually have midface (V2) numbness and also often have an absent corneal reflex. The motor supply of the trigeminal nerve of the muscles of mastication is rarely affected. The sensory component of the facial nerve is first affected and causes numbness of the posterior external auditory canal and is referred to as Hitselberger sign. Facial weakness or spasm occurs in 17% of patients and usually leads to a diagnosis of VS within 6 months.

4. Other symptoms—Patients with large VS tumors or tumors that have undergone rapid expansion have visual complaints of decreased visual acuity and diplopia due to compromise of CN II, IV, or VI. Hydrocephalus leads to complaints of headache, altered mental status, nausea, and vomiting and, on exam, increased intracranial pressure and papilledema. Compression of the lower cranial nerves IX and X causes dysphagia, aspiration, and hoarseness, and examination reveals a poor gag reflex and vocal cord paralysis.

B. IMAGING STUDIES

1. Magnetic resonance imaging—Magnetic resonance imaging (MRI) with gadolinium contrast is the gold standard for the diagnosis or exclusion of VS. An MRI scan also allows for surgical planning. The various lesions within the CPA may be differentiated based on their varying imaging and enhancing characteristics. The MRI characteristics of a VS include a hypointense globular mass centered over the IAC on a T1-weighted image with enhancement when gadolinium is added. VS are iso- to hypointense on T2-weighted images (Figure 61–2). High-resolution fast-spin echo T2-weighted sequence (FSE-T2), using CSF as the contrast agent, may obviate the need for contrast administration. FSE-T2 scans can be performed in 15–20 minutes and cost less compared with a standard MRI with intravenous contrast administration. More recently, however, lower sensitivity in identifying very small tumors has led to reduction in enthusiasm for FSE-T2 screening for VS.

2. Computed tomography scanning—In situations in which MRI scans cannot be used or are not accessible, a computed tomography (CT) scan with iodine contrast or an auditory brainstem response offers a reasonable alternate screening modality. CT scanning with contrast provides consistent identification of CPA tumors that are larger than 1.5 cm or that have at least a 5-mm CPA component. VS appear as ovoid masses centered over the IAC with nonhomogeneous enhancement. CT scans with contrast can miss intracanalicular tumors unless there is bony expansion of the IAC.

C. SPECIAL TESTS

1. Audiology—The average patient requires 4 years from the onset of symptoms to the diagnosis of VS. The diagnostic dilemma lies in choosing the appropriate patient to undergo audiometric and imaging studies. Although only a small percentage of patients with VS may present in an atypical fashion, most patients present with complaints of unilateral hearing loss or

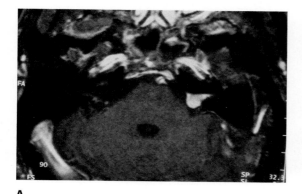

A

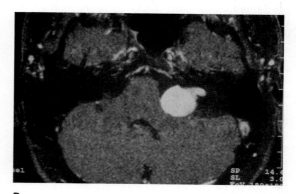

B

Figure 61–2. MRI with gadolinium enhancement demonstrating **(A)** a small and **(B)** a large vestibular schwannoma. While the smaller tumor fills the cerebellopontine angle, the large tumor is displacing the brainstem and cerebellum and compressing the fourth ventricle.

hearing distortion, unilateral tinnitus, vertigo or disequilibrium, or facial numbness, weakness, or spasm. Patients with unilateral auditory, vestibular, and facial complaints are not a diagnostic dilemma and need to undergo careful evaluation to rule out retrocochlear disease. The initial step in the evaluation includes an audiology exam. If the audiology exam suggests a retrocochlear lesion, then imaging of the CPA is performed to rule out a retrocochlear lesion. Vestibular testing lacks specificity in diagnosing VS.

The standard auditory evaluation should include pure-tone audiometry, a speech discrimination score (SDS), acoustic reflex thresholds, and acoustic reflex decay. Pure-tone audiometry of patients with VS shows asymmetric, down-sloping, high-frequency sensorineural hearing loss in almost 70% of patients. The hearing may also be normal, may involve only the low frequency, or may be a flat hearing loss or a trough or peak hearing loss. A retrocochlear-based hearing loss causes speech discrimination scores to be lower than predicted by the pure-tone thresholds. This out-of-proportion depression of speech discrimination scores is further accentuated when retested at a higher speech intensity. This phenomenon is called **rollover.** A poor SDS is present in about 50% of patients with VS. An abnormal SDS should trigger an imaging evaluation, but a normal SDS does not rule out a VS. A loss of acoustic reflexes or the presence of acoustic reflex decay is present in most cases of VS, but normal acoustic reflexes do not preclude VS.

2. Vestibular testing—Vestibular testing does not provide a sensitive or specific means of diagnosing VS. The most common test ordered to evaluate vestibular complaints includes an electronystagmogram (ENG). An ENG in a patient with VS will show a reduced caloric response in the problematic ear. The extent of the vestibular function predicts the amount of postoperative vertigo. The location of the VS on the inferior or superior vestibular nerve may also be predicted by the ENG because the ENG primarily evaluates the lateral semicircular canal. The lateral semicircular canal is innervated by the superior vestibular nerve.

3. Auditory brainstem response—An auditory brainstem response (ABR) is the measured electrical response of the cochlea and its brainstem pathway to short-duration, broad-band clicks. The evoked response is a characteristic waveform with five identifiable peaks (I–V). The absolute latency or timing of each wave is recorded. In patients with VS, the ABR is fully or partially absent, or there is a delay in the latency of Wave V in the affected ear. The delay may be an absolute delay based on normative data or a delay compared with the latency of Wave V in the opposite ear. An interaural delay of Wave V latency > 0.2 ms is considered abnormal. Overall, ABR has a sensitivity > 90% and a specificity of 90% in detecting VS. However, when considering only small intracanalicular tumors, 18–33% of tumors are missed. A stacked ABR may have greater sensitivity and specificity for smaller tumors when compared with standard ABR. As the detection limits and costs of imaging studies have improved, the role of ABR in diagnosis of VS has dramatically declined.

Differential Diagnosis

The three most common tumors of the CPA include schwannomas, meningiomas, and epidermoids (Table 61–1). Each of these tumors has a similar clinical presentation and each is primarily differentiated by its imaging characteristics. Other CPA lesions include congenital rest lesions (epidermoids, arachnoid cyst, lipoma), schwannomas of other cranial nerves, intra-axial tumors, metastasis, vascular lesions (paraganglioma, hemangioma) and

Table 61–1. Lesions of the cerebellopontine angle (CPA).

Common CPA Lesions
Schwannomas (especially involving cranial nerves V, VII, and VIII)
Meningiomas
Epidermoids
Congenital Rest Lesions
Epidermoids
Arachnoid cysts
Lipomas
Vascular Lesions
Hemangiomas
Paragangliomas (glomus jugulare)
Aneurysms
Hemangioblastoma
Intra-Axial Tumors
Medulloblastomas
Astrocytomas
Gliomas
Fourth ventricle tumors
Hemangioblastomas
Lesions Extending from the Skull Base
Cholesterol granulomas
Glomus tumors
Chordomas
Chondrosarcomas
Other Malignant Disorders
Metastasis

lesions extending from the skull base (cholesterol granulomas, chordoma).

Complications

The natural history of VS includes a slow rate of growth in the IAC and then into the cistern of the CPA. Studies show that periods of growth are intermixed with periods of quiescence. The average growth rate is 1.8 mm per year. This slow growth causes progressive and often insidious symptoms and signs since there is displacement, distortion, and compression of the structures first in the IAC and then in the CPA. This slow growth via cellular proliferation provides a predictable progression of symptoms and signs. Occasionally, the tumor may undergo rapid expansion due to cystic degeneration or hemorrhage into the tumor. A rapid expansion causes rapid movement along the subsequent phases of VS symptoms and may cause rapid neurologic deterioration.

The initial intracanalicular growth affects the vestibulocochlear nerve in the rigid IAC and causes unilateral hearing loss, tinnitus, and vertigo or disequilibrium. These three symptoms are the typical presenting complaint of not only patients with VS, but also of patients with other lesions of the CPA. It is interesting that the motor component of the facial nerve is resistant to injury during this phase of growth and patients have normal facial function. The tumor then grows into the CPA cistern and grows freely without causing significant new symptoms because structures in the CPA are initially displaced without injury (see Figure 61–2A). As the tumor approaches 3 cm, it abuts on the boundaries of the CPA and results in a new set of symptoms and signs. Compression of the CN V causes corneal and midface numbness or pain. Further distortion of CN VIII and now CN VII causes further hearing loss and disequilibrium and also facial weakness or spasms. Brainstem distortion leads to narrowing of the fourth ventricle (see Figure 61–2B).

Further growth leads to the final clinical spectrum of CPA syndrome. The patient develops cerebellar signs due to compression of the flocculus and cerebellar peduncle. The patient also develops obstructive hydrocephalus due to closure of the fourth ventricle. The increasing intracranial pressure manifests in ocular changes, headache, mental status changes, nausea, and vomiting. If the VS continues to grow without intervention, death occurs from respiratory compromise.

Treatment

The treatment of patients with CPA tumors includes surgical removal, observation, and irradiation. The primary management for vestibular schwannomas is surgical removal. Observation and radiation therapy are currently for patients who cannot tolerate a surgical procedure or who have a limited life expectancy. The role of radiation therapy is expanding. Most patients undergo surgical excision because the natural history of VS is to grow and eventually cause significant compression of the structures surrounding the CPA, as described previously. In addition, the ability to accomplish total tumor removal with the least morbidity is generally related to the size of the tumor, and so significant surgical delay is not recommended.

A. SURGICAL MEASURES

The surgical approaches to the CPA include translabyrinthine, retrosigmoidal, and middle fossa craniotomies (Figure 61–3A). The appropriate approach for a particular patient is based on the hearing status, the size of the tumor, the extent of IAC involvement, and the experience of the surgeon (Table 61–2). The approaches are either hearing preserving or hearing ablating. The retrosigmoidal and middle fossa approaches are hearing preserving. However, they have limitations of exposure to all aspects of the CPA and IAC. The middle fossa approach is well suited for patients with good hearing and a tumor that is < 1.5 cm in the CPA. The retrosigmoidal approach is well suited for patients with good hearing and a tumor < 4 cm and not involving the lateral IAC. The lateral IAC is usually only directly accessible via a retrosigmoidal approach by removing the posterior semicircular canal. The violation of the posterior semicircular canal leads to hearing loss. The translabyrinthine approach causes total hearing loss and so is well suited for patients with poor hearing (pure-tone average, or PTA, > 30) or patients with good hearing and tumors not accessible by the hearing-preserving approaches.

Three critical issues inherent in all three techniques are the extent of exposure of the IAC and CPA, the identification and preservation of the facial nerve, and the extent of brain retraction. These operations use electrophysiologic monitoring of CN VII and an ABR in hearing preservation approaches. The use of high-speed drills, craniotomies, and operating microscopes has brought VS removal into the modern age.

1. Translabyrinthine approach—The primary approach for removal of VS is the translabyrinthine approach. The boundaries of the approach include the mastoid facial nerve and cochlear aqueduct anteriorly, middle fossa dura superiorly, posterior fossa dura posteriorly, and jugular foramen inferiorly (see Figure 61–3A). These boundaries are approached via the familiar postauricular incision. A complete canal mastoidectomy is accomplished with identification of the incus, tegmen, sigmoid sinus, and facial nerve. A compete labyrinthectomy is then performed with medial skeletonization of the middle and posterior fossa dura and decompression of the sigmoid sinus to the jugular foramen. After bony skeletonization of the IAC, the dura of the IAC is opened, and the facial nerve is identified

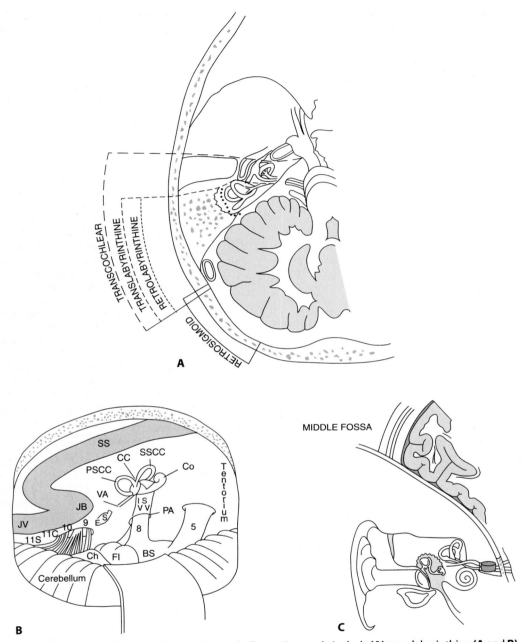

Figure 61–3. Surgical approaches to the cerebellopontine angle include **(A)** translabyrinthine **(A** and **B)**, retrosigmoidal, and **(C)** middle fossa craniotomies. The retrosigmoidal and middle fossa approaches can preserve hearing, whereas the translabyrinthine approach necessarily deafens the patient because it involves drilling the balance portion of the inner ear.

Table 61–2. Surgical approaches to the cerebellopontine angle (CPA) and indications.

Hearing Preservation
Retrosigmoidal approach: Patient has good hearing and tumor not involving the lateral internal auditory canal (IAC)
Middle fossa approach: Patient has good hearing and tumor ≤ 1.5 cm in the CPA or IAC
Hearing Ablation
Translabyrinthine approach: Patient has poor hearing or larger tumors not accessible by other approaches

medial to the transverse crest (Bill's bar). Once the facial nerve is identified in the fundus or lateral aspect of the IAC, tumor removal occurs from a lateral to medial direction along the IAC. In large tumors, the tumor is debulked internally and then the tumor capsule is removed from the surrounding structures, including the facial nerve. After tumor removal, abdominal fat is placed into the defect.

The three advantages of the translabyrinthine approach are the ability to remove tumors of all sizes, minimal retraction of the brain, and the ability to directly visualize and preserve the facial nerve. The rate of facial nerve preservation is 97%. The rate of CSF leakage presenting under the incision or draining through the nose via the eustachian tube is 5%. The majority of these CSF leaks resolve with conservative management, which includes mastoid dressing and fluid restriction. A minimal risk of meningitis is associated with a CSF leak.

2. Retrosigmoidal approach—The retrosigmoidal approach is a modification of the traditional suboccipital approach used by neurosurgeons to address most posterior fossa lesions. The retrosigmoidal approach is a versatile approach with a panoramic view of the CPA from the foramen magnum inferiorly to the tentorium superiorly (Figure 61–3B). The medial two thirds of the IAC is also accessible without violating the inner ear, therefore preserving hearing.

The surgical technique starts with a curvilinear skin incision 6 cm behind the ear over the retromastoid region. The soft tissue and posterior nuchal musculature are elevated to expose the mastoid and retromastoid bone. A 5 × 5 cm craniotomy is performed with the sigmoid as the anterior boundary and the transverse sinus the superior boundary. An elevation of a bone plate is technically difficult and so the bone may be removed by drilling. The bone fragments are collected and are replaced during closure. The bone fragments will reform a bone plate and prevent adherence of the musculature to the dura. If decompression of the sigmoid sinus is needed for exposure, a mastoidectomy

may also be performed. The dura is then opened along the sigmoid sinus and the cerebellum is seen. The CSF from the cisterna magnum needs to be released prior to retracting the cerebellum. Medial retraction of the cerebellum allows visualization of the CPA. To address the IAC component of the tumor, the posterior IAC bone needs to be removed. The bone dust created is carefully confined and removed to prevent meningeal irritation. The extent of IAC skeletonization is limited by the proximity to the inner ear. The endolymphatic duct and sac serve as landmarks to the proximity of the posterior semicircular canal and allow preservation of the inner ear and hearing. The facial nerve is normally anterior to the tumor or its position is ascertained with facial nerve monitoring. The tumor removal is as previously described. After tumor removal and hemostasis, air cells along the IAC and mastoid are closed with bone wax or bone cement to eliminate paths for CSF leak. A fat or muscle graft may also be placed into the petrosal defect to prevent CSF leak. The dura is closed and the bone plate or bone pate is replaced. The musculature and soft tissue are meticulously closed.

The primary advantage of the retrosigmoidal approach relative to the translabyrinthine approach is the ability for hearing preservation in properly selected tumors. If hearing preservation is not an issue, the retrosigmoidal approach allows a versatile approach to the CPA and IAC. The relative disadvantages compared with the translabyrinthine approach include persistent postoperative headache, increased difficulty in resolving CSF leaks, the need for cerebellar retraction, and the inability to have direct access to the facial nerve. The combination of intradural drilling leading to meningeal irritation by bone dust and dissection of suboccipital musculature causes nearly 10% of patients to have a persistent, severe, postoperative headache. In the case of extensive pneumatization of the IAC and mastoid, the air cells may be difficult to completely seal, and the inability to address the aditus-ad-antrum or the eustachian tube causes CSF leaks to be persistent, despite conservative treatment. The extent of cerebellar retraction is minimal in small tumors, but the amount of retraction increases with larger tumors. The surgical control of the facial nerve is adequate in the retrosigmoidal approach, but the exposure of the facial nerve is superior in the translabyrinthine approach.

3. Middle fossa approach—The middle fossa approach provides a hearing-preserving approach to intracanalicular tumors with a < 1.5 cm cisternal component. The surgical technique involves an inverted U-shaped incision centered over the ear. The temporal muscle is reflected inferiorly to expose the squamous portion of the temporal bone. A 5 × 5 cm temporal craniotomy is performed and is centered over the zygomatic root. Extradural elevation of the temporal lobe is accomplished to reveal the floor of the temporal bone. The greater superficial petrosal nerve leading to the geniculate ganglion reveals the anterior, lateral boundary of the IAC, and the arcuate eminence reveals the posterior boundary of the IAC (Figure 61–3C). These landmarks may be difficult to identify, and the IAC dura may have to be identified medially by drilling toward the porus acousticus. Once the IAC is identified and well skeletonized medially, the bone removal continues laterally. However, the extent of IAC skeletonization laterally is limited by the basal turn of the cochlea anteriorly and the superior semicircular canal posteriorly. The IAC dura is opened posteriorly to avoid injury to the facial nerve. The tumor is dissected free of the facial nerve and removed in a medial to lateral direction. Any air cells are sealed and the dural defect is covered with a fat or muscle plug. The craniotomy bone flap is replaced and the incision is closed.

The middle fossa approach is unique compared with the posterior fossa craniotomies because the entire IAC is accessible without violating the inner ear. This exposure allows for the removal of intracanalicular tumors while maintaining hearing preservation. The limitations of the middle fossa approach include tumors with a > 1.5 cm cisternal component. In situations of hearing preservation, an extended middle fossa approach with further removal of bone around the IAC, as well as the elevation or division of the superior petrosal sinus and tentorium allows improved exposure into the CPA. The relative merits of the procedure with increased temporal lobe retraction and limited access to the posterior fossa in the event of bleeding relative to a retrosigmoidal approach continues to be defined. The disadvantages of the middle fossa approach include temporal lobe retraction and a possible poor surgical position of the facial nerve relative to the tumor. Temporal lobe retraction may cause transient speech and memory disturbances and auditory hallucinations. The facial nerve, especially if the tumor originates from the inferior vestibular nerve, will be between the surgeon and the tumor. The increased manipulation of the facial nerve during tumor removal increases the risk of transient facial paresis.

B. Nonsurgical Measures

1. Observation—The predictable correlation between VS size and significant neurologic symptoms, and the relative slow growth of VS allows observation to be a management option for VS. Patients may be observed if their life expectancy is shorter than the growth time required for the VS to cause significant neurologic symptoms. The growth pattern of the VS should be assessed in these patients with a second radiologic evaluation in 6 months and then yearly radiologic evaluations. Studies have shown that 15–24% of patients undergoing conservative management require surgery or stereotactic radiation. If the growth rate in the first year exceeds 2–3 mm, then the patient is likely to need treatment of the VS. The patient should understand that initial conservative management, rather than immediate surgical intervention, may necessitate a resection of a larger tumor that is less amenable to hearing preservation or stereotactic radiation (or both) if intervention becomes necessary in the future.

2. Stereotactic radiation—The goal of stereotactic radiation is to prevent further growth of VS while preserving hearing and facial nerve function. This goal directly differs from the goal of complete tumor removal in microsurgical therapy. The mechanism of stereotactic radiation relies on delivering radiation to a specific intracranial target by using several precisely collimated beams of ionizing radiation. The beams take various pathways to the target tissue, therefore creating a sharp dose gradient between the target tissue and the surrounding tissue. The ionizing radiation causes necrosis and vascular fibrosis, and the time course of the effect is over 1–2 years. There is an expected transient swelling of the tumor for 1–2 years. The ionizing radiation is most commonly delivered using a 201-source cobalt-60 gamma knife system. The standard linear accelerator can also be adapted to deliver stereotactic radiation. The practical aspects include the patients wearing a stereotactic head frame, computer-assisted radiation planning using an MRI scan, and a single treatment for delivery of the radiation.

The success of stereotactic radiation in arresting tumor growth depends on the dose of radiation delivered. However, the rate of cranial nerve neuropathies, including hearing loss, is decreased by lowering the radiation dose. The current trend has been to lower the marginal radiation dose, and the long-term tumor control with these current dosing plans is under investigation. Since VS have a slow growth rate, these studies require 5- to 10-year follow-ups to provide reliable data about tumor control. Studies have shown control rates from 85% to more than 95%. The hearing preservation rate decreases each year after radiation and stabilizes after 3 years in 50% of patients. The rate of facial nerve dysfunction varies from 3% to 50% based on the radiation dose at the margin of the tumor and the length of the facial nerve in the radiation field. Approximately 20% of patients have trigeminal nerve neuropathy. The persistence and extent of these neuropathies with the lower dosing protocols continue to be studied. Hydrocephalus is also a complication of radiation.

As the long-term effectiveness and sequelae of stereotactic radiation are further defined, the indications for radiation therapy will become further refined. Radiation therapy is useful in patients in whom the arrest of tumor growth is acceptable. These patients have either short life expectancies or a high surgical risk. Compared with microsurgery, stereotactic radiation may allow improved hearing preservation in patients with 2–3 cm VS. Radiation therapy in large tumors (> 3 cm) or tumors causing brain compression will exacerbate symptoms because of initial tumor swelling.

Prognosis & Surgery-Related Complications

A. OPERATIVE COMPLICATIONS

The intraoperative complications for all three approaches include vascular injury, air embolisms, parenchymal brain injury, and cranial nerve injury. The anteroinferior cerebellar artery originates from the basilar artery and supplies the labyrinthine artery as well as the lower portion of the cerebellum and the vein of Labbé, which can be the only venous drainage of the temporal lobe. The anteroinferior cerebellar artery and vein of Labbé are vulnerable to injury during VS surgery. In the event of an air embolism via an open vein, the patient should be placed into a left lateral and Trendelenburg position to trap the air in the right ventricle; the air can then be aspirated via a central venous catheter. The cerebellum during a retrosigmoidal craniotomy and the temporal lobe during a middle fossa craniotomy are at risk from retraction injury.

B. POSTOPERATIVE COMPLICATIONS

Postoperative complications include hemorrhage, stroke, venous thromboembolism, the syndrome of inappropriate antidiuretic hormone (SIADH), CSF leak, and meningitis. Postoperative hemorrhage manifests as neurologic and cardiovascular deterioration and requires evacuation. Studies have shown that, postoperatively, low-molecular-weight heparin in addition to compression stockings and intermittent pneumatic compression devices may further reduce the risk of thromboembolism in high-risk patients (eg, elderly and obese patients) without increasing the risk of intracranial bleeding. The most common complication is CSF leak. CSF leak occurs in 5–10% of cases either via the wound or via a pneumatic pathway to the eustachian tube. Most of these leaks resolve with conservative care, which includes placing wound sutures at the leak site, replacing the mastoid dressing, decreasing intracranial pressure with acetazolamide (Diamox), fluid restriction, and bed rest. Some patients also require a lumbar subarachnoid drain (LSAD), and a very few patients need surgical reexploration. A related complication is meningitis.

Meningitis occurs in 2–10% of patients and may be aseptic, bacterial, or due to CSF leak and arachnoid irritation from the fat graft (lipoid). The distinction between aseptic and bacterial meningitis is necessary because the treatment for aseptic meningitis is a steroid taper and antibiotics for bacterial meningitis. Delayed meningitis should be considered bacterial and likely due to a CSF leak.

C. OPERATIVE PROGNOSIS AND REHABILITATION

The most concerning issues to patients are deafness, imbalance, and facial nerve weakness. The most important factors for hearing preservation are the tumor size and the preoperative hearing level. Hearing preservation ranges from 20% to 70%. Patients with contralateral hearing tolerate the unilateral loss but may benefit from bone-anchored hearing aids (BAHA). Patients with poor contralateral hearing may be rehabilitated with a CROS (contralateral routing of signal) hearing aid or a cochlear implant if the cochlear nerve fibers are preserved. Almost half the patients will have vertigo or imbalance beyond the postoperative period, but these symptoms have a minimal impact on daily activities.

The rapidity of vestibular compensation after unilateral vestibular loss is determined by the patient's efforts to exercise and challenge the vestibular system. Patients who continue to have disequilibrium in the extended postoperative period are referred for vestibular rehabilitation therapy. Facial nerve function is also best predicted by tumor size. In smaller tumors, more than 90% of patients are found to have House-Brackmann Grade 1 or 2 function (Grade 1 is normal and Grade 6 is complete paralysis). If all tumor sizes are considered, then approximately 80% of patients have Grade 1 or 2 function.

The rehabilitation of facial nerve injury is based on the general principles of nerve injury, recovery, and rehabilitation. If the nerve is transected intraoperatively, the nerve should be repaired primarily, if possible, or with a greater auricular interposition graft. The postoperative function may be predicted in an anatomically intact nerve by the intraoperative stimulability of the nerve. If the nerve stimulates at < 0.2 V, then there is a > 85% chance of Grade 1 or 2 function at 1 year. The lack of facial function (Grade 6) at 1 year and no reinnervation potentials on electromyograph (EMG) should lead to a hypoglossal-facial transposition, an interposition nerve graft, or a cross-facial graft. If facial rehabilitation has been delayed and there is electrical "silence" of the facial muscle on EMG, muscle transpositions with the temporalis or masseter muscle to the lip give improved tone and symmetry to the lower face. The upper face can be rehabilitated with a brow lift and gold weight for the eye. The eye must be protected with lubrication, ointment, and an eye bubble if there is either incomplete eye closure or a lack of sensation to the cornea due to trigeminal nerve involvement. The lack of eye care leads to corneal injury and blindness.

Arts HA, Telian SA, El-Kashlan H, Thompson BG. Hearing preservation and facial nerve outcomes in vestibular schwannoma surgery: results using the middle cranial fossa approach. *Otol Neurotol.* 2006;27(2):234. [PMID: 1643699] (Middle cranial fossa approach for the resection of small tumors is associated with excellent hearing preservation and facial nerve outcome.)

Beenstock M. Predicting the stability and growth of acoustic neuromas. *Otol Neurotol.* 2002;23(4):542. [PMID: 12170159] (One of many studies suggesting that VS growth follows a predictable pattern.)

Combs SE, Thilmann C, Debus J, Schulz-Ertner D. Long-term outcome of stereotactic radiosurgery (SRS) in patients with acoustic neuromas. *Int J Radiat Oncol Biol Phys.* 2006; 64(5):1341. [PMID: 16464537] (Stereotactic radiosurgery is associated with acceptable cranial nerve toxicities.)

Meyer TA, Canty PA, Wilkinson EP, Hansen MR, Rubinstein JT, Gantz BJ. Small acoustic neuromas: surgical outcomes versus observation or radiation. *Otol Neurotol.* 2006;27(3):380. [PMID: 16639278] (Small tumors are best treated by surgery for hearing and facial nerve preservation.)

Tufarelli D, Meli A, Alesii A et al. Quality of life after acoustic neuroma surgery. *Otol Neurotol.* 2006;27(3):403. [PMID: 16639281] (Treatment of vestibular schwannoma leads to patient perception of worsening of the quality of life.)

Nonacoustic Lesions of the Cerebellopontine Angle

Jacob Johnson, MD, & Anil K. Lalwani, MD

Vestibular schwannomas (acoustic neuromas) account for 80% of all lesions of the cerebellopontine angle (CPA). This chapter discusses some of the other common neoplasms (meningiomas and epidermoid cysts) as well as uncommon tumors of the CPA that commonly present with injury to the cochlear-vestibular system. Each of these tumors has a similar clinical presentation; they are primarily differentiated by their imaging characteristics.

The CPA consists of a potential space filled with cerebrospinal fluid (CSF) space in the posterior cranial fossa bounded by the temporal bone, the cerebellum, and the brainstem. The CPA is traversed by cranial nerves V–XI and most prominently the facial (CN VII) and vestibulocochlear (CN VIII) nerves. CPA tumors account for 10% of all intracranial tumors (Table 62–1). Nearly 90% of all CPA tumors include vestibular schwannomas (acoustic neuromas) and meningiomas. Other CPA lesions include congenital rest lesions (eg, epidermoid cysts, arachnoid cysts, and lipomas), schwannomas of other cranial nerves, intra-axial tumors, metastases, vascular lesions (eg, paragangliomas and hemangiomas), and lesions extending from the skull base (cholesterol granulomas and chordomas). CPA lesions become clinically symptomatic by causing compression of the neurovascular structures in and around the CPA. The classic description of these symptoms initially includes unilateral hearing loss, vertigo, altered facial sensation, facial pain that later progresses to nystagmus, facial palsy, vocal cord palsy, dysphagia, diplopia, respiratory compromise, and death (Table 62–2).

Lalwani AK. Meningiomas, epidermoids, and other nonacoustic tumors of the cerebellopontine angle. *Otolaryngol Clin North Am.* 1992;25(3):707. [PMID: 1625871] (A thorough review of nonacoustic lesions of the cerebellopontine angle.)

MENINGIOMAS

 ESSENTIALS OF DIAGNOSIS

- *Asymmetric (unilateral) sensorineural hearing loss, tinnitus, or both.*
- *More likely than vestibular schwannomas to have facial or trigeminal nerve findings, or both.*
- *Dural tail and calcification are distinctive on imaging.*

General Considerations

Meningiomas are the second most common CPA tumors and account for 3–10% of neoplasms at this location. Compared with schwannomas, meningiomas are a more heterogeneous group of tumors with regard to pathology, anatomic location, and treatment outcome. Most of these tumors are benign and slow growing; 1% will become symptomatic. Meningiomas differ in pathogenesis, anatomic location, and imaging characteristics from vestibular schwannomas but are nearly indistinguishable in terms of clinical presentation and audiovestibular testing. Meningiomas are primarily managed by surgical excision.

Pathogenesis

Meningiomas arise from arachnoid villi cap cells and are located along dura, venous sinuses, and neurovascular foramina. Meningiomas are most commonly sporadic but may occur in familial syndromes such as NF2, Werner syndrome, and Gorlin syndrome. More than one third of patients with NF2 have meningiomas. Molecular studies have shown deletions in chromosome 22 in nearly 75% of meningiomas. Specifically, mutations in the NF2 gene, merlin, have been shown in 30–35% of meningiomas. Although most meningiomas are benign, 5% are malignant. Chromosomal abnormalities in 1p, 6q, 9p, 10q, and 14q are seen in more aggressive or malignant meningiomas.

Clinical Findings

A. SYMPTOMS AND SIGNS

From the onset of symptoms, meningiomas take an average of 5 years to be diagnosed. The typical patient is a woman in her fourth or fifth decade of life. Unlike vestib-

Table 62–1. Lesions of cerebellopontine angle (CPA).

Common CPA Lesions
Schwannomas (cranial nerves V, VII, and VIII)
Meningiomas
Epidermoids
Congenital Rest Lesions
Epidermoid cysts
Arachnoid cysts
Lipomas
Vascular Lesions
Hemangiomas
Paragangliomas (glomus jugulare)
Aneurysms
Hemangioblastomas
Intra-Axial Tumors
Medulloblastomas
Astrocytomas
Gliomas
Fourth ventricle tumors
Hemangioblastomas
Lesions Extending from the Skull Base
Cholesterol granulomas
Glomus tumors
Chordomas
Chondrosarcomas
Metastasis
Breast cancer
Lung cancer
Melanoma
Prostate cancer

Table 62–2. CPA syndrome.

Unilateral hearing loss
Tinnitus
Vertigo
Hypesthesia and neuralgia
Nystagmus
Facial palsy
Vocal cord palsy
Dysphagia
Diplopia
Respiratory compromise
Death

1. Computed tomography (CT) scanning—CT scanning without contrast shows an iso- or hyperdense mass with areas of calcification in 10–26% of cases and provides information regarding hyperostosis or bony invasion. Meningiomas enhance homogeneously with CT contrast, and 90% of these neoplasms can be detected by contrast-enhanced CT.

2. Magnetic resonance imaging (MRI)—MRI is the study of choice for the diagnosis of meningiomas. Meningiomas are hypo- to isointense on MRI T1-weighted images and have a variable intensity on T2-weighted images. Areas of calcification appear dark on both T1- and T2-weighted images (Figure 62–1). Unlike vestibular schwannomas, meningiomas are broad based (sessile) and usually not centered over the porous acoustics. The broad-base attachment to the petrous wall leads to an obtuse bone–tumor angle. There is no widening of the internal auditory canal. Also unlike vestibular schwannomas, meningiomas more commonly herniate into the middle fossa. T1-weighted enhanced images can show an enhancing dural tail (meningeal sign) adjacent to the bulk of the tumor in 50–70% of meningiomas.

ular schwannomas, there is a 2:1 female bias. Meningiomas presenting in younger patients or multiple meningiomas in the same patient should prompt an evaluation for NF2. The most common complaints are the same as vestibular schwannoma and include unilateral hearing loss (80%), vertigo or imbalance (75%), and tinnitus (60%). The symptoms and signs more common to meningiomas relative to vestibular schwannomas include trigeminal neuralgia (7–22%), facial paresis (11–36%), lower cranial nerve deficits (5–10%), and visual disturbances (8%).

B. IMAGING STUDIES

Imaging provides the diagnosis of meningioma and allows the differentiation between meningioma and vestibular schwannoma (Table 62–3).

Table 62–3. Differential diagnoses of meningioma and vestibular schwannoma.

	Meningioma	Vestibular Schwannoma
Shape	Sessile	Globular
Internal auditory canal	Eccentric, extrinsic, and not eroded	Centered, penetrating, and eroded
Calcification	Present	Absent
Hyperostosis	Present	Absent
Tumor-bone angle	Obtuse	Acute
Meningeal sign	Present	Absent

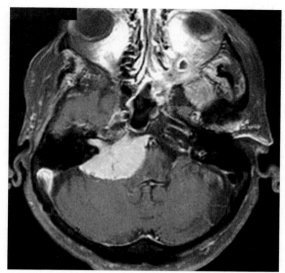

Figure 62–1. Meningioma of the cerebellopontine angle. A T1-weighted, gadolinium-enhanced MRI scan demonstrates a meningioma of the right cerebellopontine angle. The enhancing lesion has a broad dural base and does not expand the internal auditory canal.

C. Special Tests

The hearing loss on an audiogram has no characteristic pattern. The speech discrimination scores suggest a retrocochlear pathology in 50% of cases. The auditory brainstem response may be normal in 25% of cases.

Treatment

The two primary management options include surgery and observation. Observation is indicated in patients with limited life expectancy or in whom the expected morbidity of surgical excision is not justified.

A. Surgical Measures

Surgical treatment ideally consists of total meningioma removal, excision of a cuff of surrounding dura, and drilling of the underlying bone. The surgical approach is based on the tumor location and the patient's hearing status.

In contrast to vestibular schwannomas, the anatomic location of posterior fossa meningiomas is varied. The site of the meningioma is a major determinant of types of morbidity from the tumor and the success of treatment. A simple classification differentiates whether the tumor is medial or lateral to the internal auditory canal (IAC). Meningiomas medial to the IAC are more common. These meningiomas commonly arise along the inferior petrosal sinus and may involve the petrous

apex, the lateral clivus, and Meckel cave. Meningiomas lateral to the IAC involve the sigmoid sinus, the jugular bulb, and the superior petrosal sinus. In an uncommon pattern, meningiomas may be centered on the IAC and most closely mimic a vestibular schwannoma. IAC meningiomas may invade the inner or middle ear. Meningiomas may also be superior to the IAC and considered a midpetrosal meningioma.

Meningiomas lateral to the IAC are approached via a **retrosigmoidal approach.** The facial nerve in lateral meningiomas is most often displaced anteriorly and so does not lie between the surgeon and the tumor. Therefore, the facial nerve is less traumatized during tumor removal. The retrosigmoidal approach also allows for hearing preservation. Limited intracanalicular meningiomas may be managed by the **middle cranial fossa approach,** especially if hearing preservation is possible. Meningiomas involving the IAC in patients with poor hearing are approached via the **translabyrinthine approach.** If the tumor invades the cochlea and has an anteromedial extension to the clivus or Meckel cave, then a **transcochlear approach** should be considered. The transcochlear approach sacrifices hearing and requires rerouting of the facial nerve. Sixty percent of CPA meningiomas involve the middle fossa and may require a **craniotomy of the combined middle and posterior fossae.** The type of posterior fossa craniotomy in the combined approach depends on the need for hearing preservation and the extent of the surgical exposure required.

B. Adjunctive Therapies

Adjunctive therapies include external-beam radiation and stereotactic radiation therapy. Radiation therapy should be considered in cases of inoperable tumors, subtotal resection, recurrent tumors, and malignant tumors. The role of stereotactic radiation therapy in meningiomas continues to be defined.

Prognosis

Total tumor removal is accomplished in 70–85% of meningioma cases. Incomplete tumor removal is often associated with either adherence of the meningioma to the brainstem or cavernous sinus involvement. The long-term recurrence after total tumor removal is between 10% and 30%, whereas that of subtotal removal is more than 50%. In contrast to vestibular schwannoma, hearing preservation is more likely and approaches 70%. The facial nerve function has a 17% rate of deterioration from preoperative levels. Less frequently, gait disturbance and CSF leak may occur (8%). The mortality rate is between 1% and 9%.

Lalwani AK, Jackler RK. Preoperative differentiation between meningioma of the cerebellopontine angle and acoustic neuroma using MRI. *Otolaryngol Head Neck Surg.* 1993;109(1):88. [PMID: 8336973] (This paper defines the radiologic features that can be used to preoperatively differentiate a vestibular schwannoma from a meningioma.)

Nakamura M, Roser F, Dormiani M, Matthies C, Vorkapic P, Samii M. Facial and cochlear nerve function after surgery of cerebellopontine angle meningiomas. *Neurosurgery.* 2005;57(1):77. [PMID: 15987543] (Excellent postoperative facial nerve and cochlear nerve function is common; therefore, every attempt should be made to preserve the cochlear nerve.)

EPIDERMOID CYSTS

 ESSENTIALS OF DIAGNOSIS

- *Asymmetric (unilateral) sensorineural hearing loss, tinnitus, or both.*
- *More likely than vestibular schwannomas to have facial or trigeminal nerve findings, or both.*
- *A distinguishing characteristic relative to vestibular schwannomas and meningiomas is that epidermoid cysts show no enhancement with intravenous contrast.*

General Considerations

Epidermoid cysts are much less common than vestibular schwannomas or meningiomas. They account for approximately 5% of CPA lesions. Epidermoid lesions are slow growing and often grow to a significant size before causing CPA symptoms because they initially grow around structures via pathways of least resistance rather than cause compression. Epidermoid cysts are treated by surgical excision, but total removal is more difficult than vestibular schwannomas because they become adherent to normal structures.

Pathogenesis

Epidermoid cysts likely develop from ectodermal inclusions that become trapped during embryogenesis. These ectodermal inclusions lead to a keratinizing squamous epithelium in the CPA. The squamous epithelium produces a cyst filled with sloughed keratinaceous debris. The gross appearance is of a nodular cyst. The cyst is lined with squamous epithelium and filled with lamella of desquamated keratinaceous debris. Most epidermoid cysts are benign, with rare reports of squamous cell carcinoma arising in epidermoid lesions.

Clinical Findings

A. SYMPTOMS AND SIGNS

The presentation of epidermoid cysts is similar to other CPA lesions, with hearing loss being the most common symptom. Epidermoid cysts have a higher rate of preoperative facial and trigeminal nerve involvement—40% and 50%, respectively—compared with vestibular schwannomas. Patients may present with hemifacial spasm, facial hypesthesia, neuralgia, or wasting of the muscles of mastication.

B. IMAGING STUDIES

On CT scanning, epidermoid cysts are hypodense compared with the brain. A distinguishing characteristic relative to vestibular schwannomas and meningiomas is that epidermoid lesions show no enhancement with intravenous contrast. Epidermoid cysts have irregular borders, are not centered on the IAC, and do not usually widen the IAC (Figure 62–2). Epidermoid cysts have imaging characteristics similar to CSF on MRI imaging (hypointense on T1-weighted imaging and hyperintense on T2-weighted imaging) and do not enhance with gadolinium contrast.

C. SPECIAL TESTS

Audiovestibular testing does not show any patterns distinguishing for epidermoid cysts.

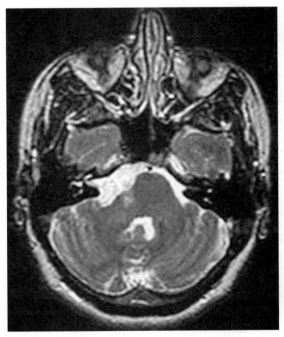

Figure 62–2. Epidermoid cyst of the cerebellopontine angle. A T2-weighted MRI scan demonstrates a bright lesion in the cerebellopontine angle with the same signal as CSF. The epidermoid cyst has the characteristic irregular borders and is not centered on the internal auditory canal.

Treatment

The primary treatment of epidermoid cysts is surgical. The approaches include a **retrosigmoidal approach** for hearing preservation and a **translabyrinthine approach** in patients with significant hearing loss. Any extension into the middle fossa can usually be removed via a **posterior fossa craniotomy.** The ability to completely remove the tumor is limited by the propensity of epidermoid cysts to adhere to neurovascular structures. Attempts at complete tumor removal may increase the rate of postoperative transient or permanent cranial nerve palsies.

Prognosis

Total tumor removal is accomplished in less than 50% of cases, and the recurrence rate may be as high as 50%. Regardless, most patients have excellent or good postoperative function.

Kountakis SE, Chang CY, Gormley WB, Cabral FR. Migration of intradural epidermoid matrix: embryologic implications. *Otolaryngol Head Neck Surg.* 2000;123(3):170. [PMID: 10964285] (Migratory properties of intradural epidermoid tumors of the cerebellopontine angle were indistinguishable from those of acquired cholesteatomas, suggesting that intradural epidermoid cysts are also derived from cells of the first branchial groove.)

Liu P, Saida Y, Yoshioka H, Itai Y. MR imaging of epidermoids at the cerebellopontine angle. *Magn Reson Med Sci.* 2003;2(3):109. [PMID: 16222102] (Hyperintense lesion on diffusion-weighted imaging is specific for cerebellopontine angle epidermoid cyst.)

NONVESTIBULAR SCHWANNOMAS

Nonvestibular schwannomas represent more than 95% of all CPA schwannomas. In addition to CN VIII (the vestibulocochlear nerve, schwannomas of cranial nerves V (the trigeminal nerve), VII (the facial nerve), IX (the glossopharyngeal nerve), X (the vagus nerve), XI (the accessory nerve), and XII (the hypoglossal nerve) can involve the CPA. CPA schwannomas share clinical, pathologic, and imaging characteristics. The primary treatment, similar to that for vestibular schwannoma, is surgical resection. The surgical approach is based on the location of the schwannoma and the patient's hearing status. Resection of cranial nerve schwannomas may lead to significant cranial nerve dysfunction; therefore, preoperative cranial nerve function and postoperative rehabilitation are important issues to consider.

1. Facial Nerve Schwannomas

Facial nerve schwannomas most commonly occur at the geniculate ganglion, but can involve any portion of the facial nerve. Similar to a vestibular schwannoma, a facial nerve schwannoma presents with hearing loss, tinnitus, and imbalance (CPA symptoms). Facial nerve symptoms such as facial spasm or weakness usually present with larger tumors. Audiovestibular testing shows an abnormality in acoustic reflex testing because of impairment of the CN VII motor supply to the stapedius muscle. Facial nerve schwannomas are associated with the reduction of electroneuronography (ENOG) potentials on the ipsilateral side, even when there is no clinically evident palsy. Imaging often does not allow for differentiation between a vestibular and a facial nerve schwannoma.

Distinguishing features on imaging of facial nerve schwannomas include expansion of the fallopian canal, extension from the geniculate ganglion into the middle fossa, and location of the schwannoma in the anterior superior portion of the IAC (a position eccentric to the axis of the IAC). These schwannomas may be observed until facial nerve function has deteriorated or a neurologic complication becomes imminent since resection usually requires division and grafting of the facial nerve. Mimetic function following interposition grafting is poor and is limited to House-Brackmann Grade 3 functioning at best.

2. Trigeminal Nerve Schwannomas

Trigeminal nerve schwannomas initially present with ipsilateral facial hypesthesia, paresthesias, neuralgia, and difficulties with chewing. Trigeminal schwannomas arise from the gasserian ganglion in the middle fossa and grow posteriorly to involve the CPA or arise from the root of the nerve and directly involve the anterior CPA and Meckel cave. These tumors frequently involve both the middle and posterior fossa and a combined approach may be necessary for resection.

3. Lower Cranial Nerve Schwannomas

Schwannomas of CN IX, X, and XI cause smooth enlargement of the jugular foramen and may grow superiorly into the CPA or inferiorly into the parapharyngeal space. Schwannomas of these cranial nerves produce symptoms based on their cranial nerve functions, thereby causing hypesthesia and weakness of the palate, vocal cords, and shoulders, respectively. Patients present with dysphagia, hoarseness, and shoulder weakness. CPA involvement also leads to CPA symptoms. Schwannomas of cranial nerve XII cause hemiatrophy of the tongue and expansion of the hypoglossal canal. The treatment is surgical removal and rehabilitation of the patient's functional deficit.

Friedman O, Neff BA, Willcox TO, Kenyon LC, Sataloff RT. Temporal bone hemangiomas involving the facial nerve. *Otol Neurotol.* 2002;23(5):760. [PMID: 12218631] (The authors recommend complete surgical excision of facial nerve hemangiomas with primary facial repair as the treatment of choice.)

Wiggins RH 3rd, Harnsberger HR, Salzman KL, Shelton C, Kertesz TR, Glastonbury CM. The many faces of facial nerve schwannoma. *AJNR Am J Neuroradiol.* 2006;27(3):694.

[PMID: 16552018] (MR imaging appearance of facial nerve schwannoma depends on the segment that is involved.)

CONGENITAL REST LESIONS

Congenital rest lesions involving the CPA include epidermoid cysts, arachnoid cysts, and lipomas. These lesions occur because of errors in embryogenesis that allow vestigial structures to remain and grow during adult life. These lesions are not aggressive but rather slow growing and have a tendency to envelop the neurovascular structures in the CPA. The presenting symptoms are very similar to, if not indistinguishable from, those of vestibular schwannoma, and only imaging allows their differentiation. The imaging characteristics on CT scan are very similar and include a well-encapsulated, hypodense mass that does not enhance with contrast. MRI allows differentiation based on the signal characteristics of desquamated epithelium, CSF, or fat. The treatment is surgical, but total removal is more difficult than in vestibular schwannoma and is not always necessary.

1. Arachnoid Cysts

Arachnoid cysts are CSF-filled cysts surrounded by an epithelial lining. This epithelial lining originates from a duplication of the arachnoid membrane and has secretory capabilities. The rate of growth is unpredictable and patients may present with arachnoid cysts in the CPA or IAC at any age. The key imaging point is that these cysts match the signal intensity of CSF on every MRI imaging sequence and do not enhance with gadolinium. The treatment involves diuretics, shunting procedures, and marsupialization of the cyst into the subarachnoid space.

2. Lipomas

Lipomas are rare lesions of the CPA and IAC. They are due to congenital malformations that lead to proliferation of adipocytes in subarachnoid cisterns or ventricles. MRI imaging parallels the intensities of fat, and so lipomas are hyperintense on T1-weighted imaging, show no enhancement with gadolinium, are hypointense on T2-weighted imaging, and become hypointense on T1-weighted imaging with fat suppression. The neurovascular structures of the CPA travel through the lipoma. Therefore, the surgical treatment of these lesions, if they become symptomatic, is conservative debulking.

Alaani A, Hogg R, Siddiq MA, Chavda SV, Irving RM. Cerebellopontine angle arachnoid cysts in adult patients: what is the appropriate management? *J Laryngol Otol.* 2005;119(5):337. [PMID: 15949094] (A small series suggesting that observation alone is often sufficient as management of arachnoid cyst.)

VASCULAR LESIONS

A variety of vascular lesions may directly or via extension involve the CPA. These include paragangliomas (glomus jugulare neoplasms), hemangiomas, and aneurysms.

1. Paragangliomas (Glomus Jugulare Neoplasms)

Glomus jugulare tumors arise from paraganglionic tissues (chief cells) and have intracranial extension in 15% of cases. These neoplasms are slow growing and present initially with pulsatile tinnitus and conductive hearing loss. Further growth at the jugular foramen causes lower cranial nerve neuropathies, and then intracranial extension into the posterior fossa may lead to sensorineural hearing loss and dizziness. Paragangliomas have a variable appearance on CT scans, but bone algorithms show the extent of temporal bone involvement. Paragangliomas cause irregular expansion of the jugular foramen, whereas lower cranial nerve schwannomas cause smooth enlargement of the jugular foramen. Paragangliomas have a "salt and pepper" appearance on T2-weighted MRI images, and MRI shows the extent of intracranial involvement. There is presence of flow voids and pronounced enhancement with gadolinium. Magnetic resonance angiography (MRA) and angiography provide information on the involvement of the great vessels and allow for preoperative embolization of larger neoplasms. The treatment requires surgical excision. Jugular bulb involvement may be addressed by a transmastoid-neck approach. Extension to the carotid artery or intracranial extension requires an infratemporal fossa approach.

2. Hemangiomas

Hemangiomas of the temporal bone often involve the geniculate ganglion and the internal auditory meatus. Hemangiomas are benign, slow-growing vascular hamartomas. The hemangiomas involving the geniculate ganglion cause progressive facial paresis. Patients also complain of facial twitches, tinnitus, and facial pain. Hearing loss, if present, is conductive because of middle ear involvement. The facial paresis occurs sooner with hemangiomas than with facial nerve schwannomas.

CT imaging shows a small, soft tissue mass at the geniculate ganglion, with surrounding smooth or irregular bony enlargement of the fallopian canal. The small size of the soft tissue mass, irregular bony erosion, and presence of calcium in the tumor are all suggestive of a geniculate ganglion hemangioma versus a facial nerve schwannoma. MRI shows isointense T1-weighted images, intense enhancement, and hyperintense T2-weighted images.

Hemangiomas in the IAC present similarly to vestibular schwannomas, and a preoperative differentiation may be very difficult. The treatment involves surgical removal when there is significant facial nerve dysfunction. Because hearing is often intact, the middle fossa approach provides good surgical exposure and allows for hearing preservation. The chance of an intact facial nerve after removal of a hemangioma is higher than with a facial nerve schwannoma. Regardless, facial nerve anastomosis or grafting is often still required.

3. Aneurysms

Aneurysms and vascular anomalies of the posterior circulation (anterior and posterior cerebellar artery, carotid artery, vertebral artery, and basilar artery) are rare but produce CPA symptoms by causing compression on neurovascular structures. Aneurysms are seen as enhancing lesions on CT scanning. In addition to MRI, MRA and angiography allow characterization of these vascular lesions.

Poznanovic SA, Cass SP, Kavanagh BD. Short-term tumor control and acute toxicity after stereotactic radiosurgery for glomus jugulare tumors. *Otolaryngol Head Neck Surg.* 2006;134(3):437. [PMID: 16500441] (A small series suggesting that stereotactic radiosurgery is effective in controlling symptoms and stabilizing tumor growth.)

INTRA-AXIAL NEOPLASMS

Intra-axial tumors of the brainstem (gliomas), cerebellum (medulloblastomas, astrocytomas, and hemangioblastomas), and fourth ventricle (ependymomas and choroid plexus papillomas) may extend into the CPA and present with CPA symptoms. The CPA extension occurs as a result of exophytic growth, growth into the CPA via the foramen of Luschka, and, rarely, extra-axial origin directly in the CPA from an embryonic rest.

To appropriately counsel and treat patients, intra-axial tumors involving the CPA must be differentiated from extra-axial CPA masses. The differentiation is based primarily on imaging characteristics. Imaging characteristics suggestive of an extra-axial neoplasm include bony changes, widening of the subarachnoid cistern, displacement of brain and blood vessels away from the skull or dura, and sharp definition of the tumor margin. Characteristics suggestive of intra-axial tumors include irregular and poorly defined brain tumor margins, widening of the foramen of Luschka, brain edema out of proportion to the CPA component of the tumor, and hydrocephalus. The management of intra-axial lesions includes angiography, conservative surgical resection, and adjunctive therapy.

Bonneville F, Sarrazin JL, Marsot-Dupuch K et al. Unusual lesions of the cerebellopontine angle: a segmental approach. *Radiographics.* 2001;21(2):419. [PMID: 11259705] (Reviews the critical role of CT and MRI findings in establishing the preoperative diagnosis for unusual lesions of the cerebellopontine angle.)

LESIONS EXTENDING FROM THE SKULL BASE

Lesions involving the skull base—specifically, the petrous apex (cholesterol granulomas), the clivus (chordomas), and the petrooccipital fissure (chondrosarcomas)—may grow posteriorly and laterally to involve the CPA. Each of these lesions has characteristic presentations and imaging criteria but at times may present solely with CPA symptoms. The treatment is primarily surgical.

1. Cholesterol Granulomas

The petrous apex of the temporal bone lies anterior and medial to the inner ear and posterior and lateral to the clivus and contains pneumatized air cells in one third of temporal bones. The obstruction of these air cells leads to inflammation and hemorrhage into the air cells. The phagocytosis of red cells leads to deposition of cholesterol crystals and a foreign body reaction in the petrous apex. This process leads to a cholesterol granuloma that may extend beyond the petrous apex to involve the CPA. Patients may have CPA symptoms in addition to symptoms of headache and sixth cranial nerve (the abducens nerve) dysfunction.

The key differential diagnosis in the petrous apex and CPA of a cholesterol granuloma is an epidermoid cyst. The distinguishing factor is that cholesterol granulomas are hyperintense on T1- and T2-weighted MRI images, whereas epidermoid cysts are hypointense on T1-weighted images. When symptomatic, the treatment is surgical drainage rather than complete excision. The petrous apex may be accessed via a transmastoid or transcanal approach.

2. Chordomas

Chordomas arise from remnants of the notochord, and skull base chordomas occur at the clivus (sphenooccipital synchondrosis). Patients usually present with headache and diplopia, but posterolateral extension to the CPA may lead to CPA symptoms. CT scans show an isodense mass with bone destruction, intratumor calcifications, and marked enhancement with contrast. MRI shows hypointense T1-weighted images, marked gadolinium enhancement, and hyperintense T2-weighted images. The midline location and bony destruction without sclerosis are characteristic of chordomas. The treatment is complete surgical excision and radiation for subtotal removal or recurrence.

3. Chondrosarcomas

The main differential diagnosis of chordomas is chondrosarcomas. These tumors arise along the sphenooccipital synchondrosis and are laterally located relative to chordomas. Chondrosarcomas may arise from embryonal cartilage rests located at the skull base synchondrosis. Tumor growth laterally causes involvement of the IAC and CPA. Hearing loss may very well be the presenting complaint. The differential diagnosis from chordoma may require immunohistochemistry stains since chondrosarcomas, unlike chordomas, do not stain positively with epithelial tissue markers.

Hoch BL, Nielsen GP, Liebsch NJ, Rosenberg AE. Base of skull chordomas in children and adolescents: a clinicopathologic study of 73 cases. *Am J Surg Pathol.* 2006;30(7):811. [PMID: 16819322] (Base of skull chordomas in children and adolescents treated with proton-beam radiation have better survival than chordomas in adults.)

METASTASES

Metastatic disease from the lungs, breasts, skin, prostate, nasopharynx, and kidney are the most common extraaxial malignant neoplasms of the CPA. In contrast to benign lesions of the CPA, malignant lesions of the CPA cause rapid progression of CPA symptoms. On imaging, the lesions are small, isointense to brain on T1- and T2-weighted images, and enhanced with gadolinium. There is high likelihood of parenchymal brain metastases and bilateral CPA lesions. The extent of treatment is based on the extent of the metastatic and primary disease and includes multimodality treatment with surgical biopsy or resection, radiation, and chemotherapy. The other aspect of treatment includes relieving symptoms of hydrocephalus or brainstem compression. The primary extra-axial malignant neoplasms of the CPA are exceedingly rare and include lymphomas, squamous cell carcinomas, malignant acoustic neuromas, and malignant meningiomas.

Eisen MD, Smith PG, Judy KD, Bigelow DC. Cerebrospinal fluid cytology to aid the diagnosis of cerebellopontine angle tumors. *Otol Neurotol.* 2006;27(4):553. [PMID: 16791049] (Patients with cerebellopontine angle tumors and progressive facial palsy should undergo cytologic examination of the cerebrospinal fluid before undergoing surgical intervention to evaluate for a malignant process.)

Neurofibromatosis Type 2

63

Anil K. Lalwani, MD

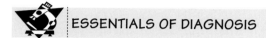

ESSENTIALS OF DIAGNOSIS

- Bilateral vestibular schwannomas.
- Posterior subcapsular lenticular opacities.
- Spinal tumors.
- Skin tumors or lesions.

General Considerations

Neurofibromatosis type 2 (NF2) is the official name for the syndrome whose hallmark is bilateral vestibular schwannomas (VS) (Figure 63–1). NF2 replaces a variety of synonyms that have been associated with this entity: central neurofibromatosis, bilateral acoustic neurofibromatosis, cranial neuromatosis, central schwannomatosis, neurofibromatosis universalis, familial bilateral acoustic neuroma syndrome, familial bilateral acoustic neurofibromas, Wishart-Gardner-Eldridge syndrome, neurinomatosis, and neurofibrosarcomatosis. The first known description of the clinical course and postmortem findings of NF2, almost two centuries ago, was of a patient who developed bilateral deafness, had intractable headaches and vomiting, and died at age 21.

NF2 has long been confused with classic von Recklinghausen syndrome and has only recently been recognized as a distinct diagnostic entity. In 1987, a consensus panel of the National Institutes of Health officially differentiated the clinical manifestations associated with classic von Recklinghausen syndrome or peripheral neurofibromatosis from those of a predominantly intracranial subtype or central neurofibromatosis. The two syndromes were designated neurofibromatosis type 1 (NF1) and NF2, respectively. Molecular genetic investigations confirmed this clinical differentiation: the gene responsible for NF1 was located near the proximal long arm of chromosome 17, whereas the gene responsible for NF2 was located on chromosome 22.

NF2 is much rarer than NF1, with an incidence estimated between 1:33,000 and 1:50,000. Inheritance of NF2 is autosomal dominant and gene penetrance is over 95%. NF2 most frequently presents in the second and third decades of life. VS represent approximately 8% of intracranial tumors and account for approximately 80% of the tumors found in the cerebellopontine angle. Most cases of VS occur sporadically, are unilateral, and present in the fifth decade. Patients with NF2 who also have bilateral VS represent 2–4% of patients with VS.

The recent identification of the gene responsible for NF2 has significantly advanced our understanding of the molecular pathology, as well as the factors responsible for the clinical heterogeneity among patients with NF2. The NF2 gene, merlin or schwannomin, has been shown to have homology to the ezrin-radixin-moesin (ERM) family of genes, which functions as membrane-organizing proteins. These proteins have a basic function indigent to all cells, which are postulated to link cytoskeletal proteins to the plasma membrane. It has been proposed to represent a recessive tumor suppressor, whose deletion or inactivation alters the abundance, localization, and turnover of cell-surface receptors, thus initiating tumorigenesis. Understanding the function of merlin in tumor formation will lead to the development of novel therapies that may eventually alleviate the suffering associated with NF2.

Pathogenesis

NF2 results from the inheritance of a mutation in the merlin (or schwannomin) gene on chromosome 22. The NF2 gene is spread over approximately 100 kb on chromosome 22q12.2 and contains 17 exons. The coding sequence of the messenger RNA is 1785 bp in length and encodes a protein of 595 amino acids. The gene product is similar in sequence to a family of proteins the include moesin, ezrin, radixin, talin, and members of the protein 4.1 superfamily. These proteins are involved in linking cytoskeletal components with the plasma membrane and are located in actin-rich surface projections such as microvilli. The N-terminal region of the merlin protein is thought to interact with components of the plasma membrane and the C-terminal with the cytoskeleton. Although the exact function of the NF2 protein is as yet unknown, the evidence available so far suggests that it is involved in cell-cell or cell-matrix interactions and that it is important for cell movement, cell shape, and commu-

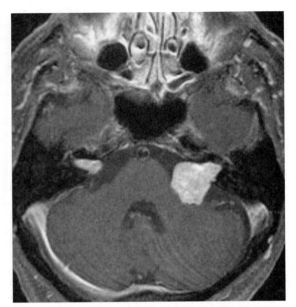

Figure 63–1. MRI scan with gadolinium, demonstrating bilateral vestibular schwannomas.

nication. The loss of function of the merlin protein therefore could result in a loss of contact inhibition and consequently lead to tumorigenesis. NF2 gene defects have been detected in other malignant disorders, including meningiomas, malignant mesotheliomas, melanomas, and breast carcinomas.

Approximately 50% of affected patients have no family history of NF2. Therefore, these patients represent new germ line mutations in the NF2 gene. To date, more than 200 mutations of the NF2 gene have been identified, including single-base substitutions, insertions, and deletions. Genotype-phenotype correlation studies suggest that mutations in the NF2 gene, which result in protein truncation, are associated with a more severe clinical presentation of NF2 (Wishart type), whereas missense and splice site mutations are associated with a milder (Gardner type) form of the disease. Retinal abnormalities were associated with the more disruptive protein truncation mutations of the NF2 gene. Although mutations in the NF2 gene play a dominant role in the biology of VS, it is also possible that other genetic loci contribute to the development of VS.

Maitra S, Kulikauskas RM, Gavilan H, Fehon RG. The tumor suppressors merlin and expanded function cooperatively to modulate receptor endocytosis and signaling. *Curr Biol.* 2006;16(7): 702. [PMID: 16581517] (Merlin protein may control cellular proliferation by regulating cell-surface receptors; in its absence, tumorigenesis occurs.)

Rouleau GA, Merel P, Lutchman M et al. Alteration in a new gene encoding a putative membrane-organizing protein causes neurofibromatosis type 2. *Nature.* 1993;363:515. [PMID: 8379998]. (Neurofibromatosis 2 is due to mutations in the merlin gene.)

Trofatter JA, MacCollin MM, Rutter JL et al. A novel moesin-, ezrin-, radixin-like gene is a candidate for the neurofibromatosis 2 tumor suppressor. *Cell.* 1993;72:791. [PMID: 8242753]. (Neurofibromatosis 2 is due to mutations in the merlin gene.)

Clinical Findings

A. SYMPTOMS AND SIGNS

Patients with NF2 usually present in the second and third decades of life, rarely after age 60. Patients' symptoms are attributable to VS, cranial meningiomas, and spinal tumors. The presentation of NF2 can vary considerably, but has been broadly divided into two subtypes based on the severity of disease: Gardner and Wishart NF2 subtypes (Table 63–1). The more severe Wishart type of NF2 is characterized by an early onset of tumors, a more rapid course of disease progression, and the presence of multiple other tumors in addition to bilateral VS. In contrast, the milder Gardner subtype is characterized by a later onset of symptoms, a more benign course of disease, and a tumor burden usually limited to bilateral VS. Many patients with NF2, however, cannot easily be categorized into these subtypes and have many overlapping features.

Hearing impairment is the presenting symptom in nearly 50% of patients. The hearing loss is usually progressive and is associated with poor speech discrimination. Auditory dysfunction is accompanied with tinnitus in 10% of patients. Although the tumors arise from the vestibular nerve, acute vertigo is uncommon since the slow growth pattern of the tumors allows the central nervous system to compensate. The tumor size at presentation is variable. Generally, younger patients have smaller tumors and older patients harbor larger tumors. VS are larger in patients with the more severe type of NF2 associated with spinal tumors or meningiomas.

Table 63–1. Characteristics of Gardner and Wishart NF2 subtypes.

Gardner	Wishart
Early onset	Later onset
Smaller tumors	Larger tumors
Few tumors	Multiple tumors
Slower-growing tumors	Faster-growing tumors
Hearing loss related to tumor size	Hearing loss not related to tumor size
Missense mutations	Truncation mutations

Skin tumors are present in nearly two thirds of patients with NF2. Café-au-lait spots, which are the hallmark of NF1, are also frequently found in patients with NF2. In contrast to patients with NF1, patients with NF2 invariably have fewer than six of these hyperpigmented lesions. Juvenile posterior subcapsular lenticular opacities are common and have been reported in up to 51% of patients with NF2. A proportion of these opacities are thought to be congenital and can be useful in the early diagnosis of NF2 in related family members. Retinal abnormalities are usually associated with the more disruptive protein truncation mutations of the NF2 gene. Muscular weakness or wasting is the initial presenting feature in up to 12% of patients with NF2. Distal, symmetric, sensorimotor neuropathy, though uncommon, may complicate NF2. Because of the heightened awareness of familial risks in individuals diagnosed with NF2, nearly 10–15% of patients diagnosed with NF2 are asymptomatic and are diagnosed as a result of screening.

B. Imaging Studies

Magnetic resonance imaging (MRI) with gadolinium-diethylenetriamine penta-acetic acid (DTPA) enhancement is the current gold standard for the radiologic investigation of VS and spinal tumors. VS are typically isointense or mildly hypointense to brain on T1-weighted images, but they enhance markedly with gadolinium. As a group, VS enhance far more than any other intracranial tumors, but there is sufficient overlap among tumors of different types that the degree of enhancement alone is not pathognomonic. The enhancement may or may not be homogeneous owing to cystic components in the schwannomas. Intratumoral hemorrhage may cause focal areas of hypointensity or hyperintensity, largely dependent on the age of the hemorrhage. With T2-weighted images, VS have an intensity between that of brain and cerebrospinal fluid (CSF).

The resolution of thin-sectioned gadolinium-enhanced MRI scans centered on the internal auditory meatus is such that lesions as small as 1 mm can be picked up. False-negative images are thought to be very rare, but the exact incidence is hard to establish because more sensitive study techniques currently are unavailable. Occasional false-positive gadolinium-enhanced MRI scans have been reported, most commonly as a result of viral mononeuronitis of the seventh or eighth cranial nerves. MRI imaging has an important role in the postoperative evaluation of patients with NF2. It also plays an important role in monitoring tumor growth rates when a nonsurgical approach is undertaken and in screening family members at risk of having NF2. MRI of the cervical spine should be performed on every patient with NF2 to exclude asymptomatic spinal cord lesions, assess therapeutic options in symptomatic patients, and assist in surgical planning.

C. Special Tests

1. Audiologic testing—Patients with NF2, as well as their family members, should undergo complete audiologic testing to assess the level of hearing. Although audiologic evaluation alone is not sufficient to screen patients or family members for NF2, it can play a valuable role in management. Pure-tone audiometry is useful as a means of monitoring the function in patients diagnosed with NF2, in deciding when function is deteriorating significantly, and in determining the better hearing ear.

It is a commonly held belief that sporadic VS have a more predictable audiologic profile when compared with that of NF2-associated vestibular tumors. This is incorrect. The auditory phenotype of a large number of patients with NF2 who were enrolled in an ongoing clinical and genetic study at the National Institutes of Health was studied. A significant association between increasing tumor size and a deterioration in pure-tone thresholds, speech reception threshold (SRT), word recognition scores, and loss of acoustic reflexes was demonstrated. The tumor dimension in the lateral to medial plane was the most useful dimension for audiologic prediction because it directly correlated with deterioration in the mid- and high-frequency averages for the total population. In fact, patients with NF2 demonstrated a more predictable audiologic profile for a given size tumor than has been previously described with sporadic VS. However, this association between tumor size and auditory findings did not hold true for the subgroup of patients with spinal tumors, meningiomas, or both.

Auditory brainstem response (ABR) testing has limited usefulness in reliably diagnosing VS in NF2. Interaural latency measurements are not useful in this population because of their bilateral tumors. ABR also is not reliable in detecting small tumors. The bilateral presentation of VS in NF2 means that there is potential for symmetric abnormalities in audiologic investigations; therefore, audiometry alone cannot be used to exclude NF2. Pure-tone audiometry, speech audiometry, acoustic reflexes, and brainstem-evoked response audiometry are poor screening modalities for patients with NF2.

2. Genetic testing—Genetic testing for the detection of mutations in the NF2 gene is available at some medical centers and private genetic testing centers. However, it is expensive and its exact role in the management of a patient with NF2 and the identification of family members at risk has not been clearly delineated.

Lalwani AK, Abaza MM, Makariow EV, Armstrong, M. Audiologic presentation of vestibular schwannomas in neurofibromatosis type 2. *Am J Otol.* 1998;19:352. [PMID: 9596188]. (This paper describes the relationship between the audiologic findings, the clinical severity of neurofibromatosis 2, and tumor size.)

Differential Diagnosis

The criteria for confirmed or definite NF2 are listed in Table 63–2. Some patients who do not meet the diagnostic criteria for NF2 should still be considered at risk for this disorder. These include people with a family history of NF2, those younger than 30 years of age with unilateral VS or meningioma, and those with multiple spinal tumors (Figure 63–2). In addition, it would be prudent to evaluate the following people for NF2: (1) patients with a unilateral VS plus any one of the following: meningioma, glioma, schwannoma, or juvenile posterior subcapsular lenticular opacity; (2) patients with two or more meningiomas and unilateral VS; and (3) patients with two or more meningiomas and one or more of the following: glioma, schwannoma, or a juvenile posterior subcapsular lenticular opacity.

NF2 should be differentiated from NF1. The diagnostic criteria for NF1 are met by an individual if two or more of the following are found: (1) six or more café-au-lait macules > 5 mm in greatest diameter in prepubertal individuals, and café-au-lait macules > 15 mm in diameter in postpubertal individuals; (2) two or more neurofibromas of any type or one plexiform neurofibroma; (3) freckling in the axillary or inguinal regions; (4) optic glioma; (5) two or more Lisch nodules (iris hamartomas); (6) a distinct osseous lesion (eg, sphenoid dysplasia or thinning of the long bone cortex) with or without pseudoarthrosis; or (7) a first-degree relative with NF1 by the above criteria.

The differential diagnosis of cerebellopontine angle lesions includes meningiomas, epidermoid tumors, lipomas, and arachnoid cysts. In cases of unilateral VS, consideration of NF2 should clearly arise when unilateral VS is encountered in a patient under the age of 30. NF2 is implicated in half of all cases of VS

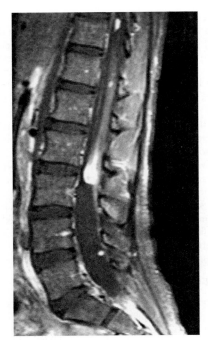

Figure 63–2. MRI scan with gadolinium demonstrating multiple spinal tumors.

presenting before the age of 20. In these young patients with unilateral VS, it behooves the clinician to obtain ophthalmologic consultation to look for posterior subcapsular cataracts associated with NF2. A spinal MRI scan should be performed to detect spinal tumors.

Treatment

The management of VS in patients with NF2 is a clinically challenging problem in contemporary neurotology. The bilaterality of vestibular tumors makes the common complications associated with surgical intervention more significant. Hearing loss following surgical removal in a patient with NF2 with a large contralateral VS or in what may be an only-hearing ear represents a significant morbidity. In patients with NF2 who are followed up medically, the complications associated with natural growth, including eventual hearing loss, cranial nerve palsies, and brainstem compression, are also important management considerations. The population of patients with NF2 often presents a difficult therapeutic dilemma because neither operative nor nonoperative management offers an acceptable risk-benefit ratio. Characteristics identifying the more aggressive or faster-growing tumors would be useful in planning treatment, such as choosing between expectant observation and the surgical extirpation of disease.

Table 63–2. Diagnostic criteria for NF2.

Bilateral Vestibular Schwannomas
or
Family History of NF2 and

1. Unilateral vestibular schwannoma or
2. Any two of:
   Meningioma
   Glioma
   Neurofibroma
   Schwannoma
   Posterior subcapsular lenticular opacity

A. Surgical Management

The decisions concerning the management of patients with NF2 are significantly different from those of sporadic unilateral VS, and are guided by the fact that patients with NF2 eventually develop bilateral profound deafness. It is advisable for these patients to learn lip reading at an early stage after the initial diagnosis. Patients with NF2 have a lifelong tendency to form intracranial tumors and are never cured of their underlying disease. The management priority should therefore be to maintain function even at the expense of incomplete tumor removal, if that is required. Once an ear has become deaf, total tumor resection should be performed. However, when both ears hear well, some divergence in opinion exists. Some surgeons advocate a resection of the larger tumor via a hearing-sparing approach, whereas others favor removal of the smaller tumor with the rationale that this provides a better chance of hearing preservation. The tumor associated with brainstem compression or central nervous system dysfunction should always be resected first, regardless of the hearing status. If the initial operation is successful in preserving hearing, the surgical excision of the second tumor could be undertaken. If the hearing is not preserved, the second tumor is followed expectantly until the hearing is lost, brainstem encroachment requires removal, or the tumor appears to be enlarging rapidly. Incomplete removal in an only-hearing ear has been recommended to preserve hearing. Unfortunately, even incomplete removal may impair or eliminate residual hearing.

The surgical treatment of spinal tumors, meningiomas, as well as VS, requires a team approach with a neurotologist, a neurosurgeon, a neuroanesthesiologist, and a neurophysiologist for cranial nerve monitoring. Spinal tumors and meningiomas are generally observed; signs of growth, neurologic compromise, or clinical deterioration usually lead to surgical intervention. Occasionally, a meningioma can be resected at the same time as another intracranial tumor, such as a VS, is being addressed.

B. Stereotactic Radiation Therapy

Stereotactic radiosurgery is a method of using ionizing radiation to destroy a precisely defined area of intracranial tissue. The technique combines a stereotactic delivery device with ionizing radiation. The radiation dose in stereotactic radiosurgery is delivered by several precisely collimated beams of ionizing radiation. The radiation dose gradient is extremely sharp at the target tissue, resulting in a sharply circumscribed area of high-dose radiation. As a result, the delivery of radiation to adjacent tissues and, hence, associated adjacent tissue damage is minimized.

Stereotactic radiosurgery as a treatment option is usually not recommended in patients with NF2. It is important to appreciate that VS are not especially radiosensitive and that stereotactic radiosurgery, at best, either will cause a reduction in the size of a VS due to necrosis or may arrest tumor progression. Stereotactic radiosurgery also has associated morbidity: progressive hearing deterioration, a transient facial paralysis, facial hypesthesia, hydrocephalus, and progressive tumor growth.

C. Hearing Restoration

The preservation of hearing, if technically possible, is far preferable to hearing restoration. Because of the short life expectancy of patients with NF2, partial tumor removal in an attempt to preserve hearing is more acceptable as a strategy in these patients. An increased awareness of NF2 and an earlier presentation and diagnosis mean that the likelihood that hearing will be preserved is increased. However, sooner or later, in all cases, hearing is lost owing to either tumor progression or the surgical intervention designed to remove the tumor.

1. Cochlear implants—A cochlear implant may be an option in patients in whom the cochlear nerve has been preserved. Of concern, however, is the impact of a cochlear implant on the ability of the patient to obtain MRI scans for diagnostic or follow-up purposes. This problem may be overcome by either removing the magnet from the receiver or by developing newer-generation implants without magnets.

2. Auditory brainstem implant—An auditory brainstem implant is a method of restoring hearing when hearing loss is due to the destruction of the auditory nerve. It is an alternate treatment option for the profoundly deaf because cochlear implants cannot be used in this patient population. The Nucleus 22-channel auditory brainstem implant design was first presented at the Second International Symposium on Cochlear Implants in Iowa in 1989. This is a multichannel brainstem prosthesis with transcutaneous signal transmission. The original design was slightly modified in 1993 and is now approved by the Food and Drug Administration. The implantation of an auditory brainstem implant can be carried out at the same time as tumor removal. During surgery, the visualization of the cochlear nucleus complex is necessary, with a recommendation for intraoperative monitoring of the facial and glossopharyngeal nerves. The measurement of electrically evoked auditory brainstem potentials is important in determining the optimum placement of the auditory brainstem implant on the cochlear nucleus complex.

Colletti V, Shannon RV. Open set speech perception with auditory brainstem implant? *Laryngoscope.* 2005;115(11):1974. [PMID: 16319608] (Tumor resection may negatively impact speech recognition outcome in patients with neurofibromatosis 2.)

Prognosis

The severity of the clinical phenotype determines the prognosis for patients with NF2. In turn, the severity of the clinical phenotype is determined by the underlying genotype or type of genetic mutation. Patients with nonsense and frameshift mutations in the NF2 gene have a clinically more severe disease with an earlier onset than those with missense mutations. The onset of hearing loss was earlier (20.2 years versus 28.4 years) and more prevalent (85% versus 81.3%) in patients with the more significant mutations. Therefore, the type of mutation of the NF2 gene is likely to have a large effect on the severity of the disease and the aggressiveness of the VS. Furthermore, because some sporadic VS are also associated with mutations in the NF2 gene, the variety of clinical presentations in these tumors could be related to the location and type of the mutation.

Ruttledge MH, Andermann AA, Phelan CM et al. Type of mutation in the neurofibromatosis type 2 gene (NF2) frequently determines severity of disease. *Am J Hum Genet.* 1996;59:331. [PMID: 8755919]. (Missense mutations in the NF2 gene are associated with a less severe clinical phenotype than nonsense mutations.)

Osseous Dysplasias of the Temporal Bone

Karsten Munck, MD, & Steven W. Cheung, MD

Patients with osseous dysplasias of the temporal bone, notably, fibrous dysplasia, Paget disease, osteopetroses, and osteogenesis imperfecta, present with hearing loss and external auditory canal obstruction that result in infection, lower cranial neuropathies, and temporal bone deformation. Differentiation among these entities is greatly helped by using coronal and axial high-resolution computed tomography (CT) imaging of the temporal bone and skull base. Outer, middle, and inner ear structures are detailed and foraminal stenoses are identified. Bone mineralization density appearance is the single most important imaging feature to secure a diagnosis.

FIBROUS DYSPLASIA

 ESSENTIALS OF DIAGNOSIS

- *External auditory canal stenosis.*
- *Progressive conductive hearing loss.*
- *Enlargement of the temporal bone.*
- *Abnormal skin pigmentation.*
- *Radiographic "ground glass" appearance.*

General Considerations

Fibrous dysplasia is perhaps the most common benign fibro-osseous disorder of the temporal bone. This poorly understood entity has three major classifications: (1) monostotic, (2) polyostotic, and (3) the McCune-Albright syndrome.

The **monostotic variant** is the most common variety, accounting for approximately 70% of all cases, and is seen late in childhood. The disease may enter a dormant phase in puberty. **Polyostotic disease** manifests as multiple bony lesions and often has long bone involvement. The active phase of the disease extends into the third and fourth decades. **McCune-Albright syndrome** affects mostly females and is characterized by

polyostotic fibrous dysplasia with endocrinopathy, cutaneous hyperpigmentation, and precocious puberty.

Pathogenesis

The radiographic appearance of fibrous dysplasia reflects the erosion of cortical bone by fibro-osseous tissue in the medullary cavity. Cortical bone is thinned by medullary fibrous tissue that is vascular, compressible, and weak. Histologically, there are interspersed regions of predominantly soft tissue or bone. Soft areas are abundant in collagen, and occasionally contain cysts. Areas of intermediate consistency are populated by fibroblasts.

Clinical Findings

A. SYMPTOMS AND SIGNS

Common clinical manifestations of fibrous dysplasia of the temporal bone include external auditory canal stenosis, progressive hearing loss, and increased temporal bone size presenting as postauricular swelling. The dysplastic process may entrap skin within the external auditory canal, resulting in conductive hearing loss. Uncommonly, facial nerve paralysis may result from infected or erosive cholesteatoma.

B. IMAGING STUDIES

The CT appearance of fibrous dysplasia may have several radiographic patterns: pagetoid, sclerotic, and cystic. **Pagetoid** is characterized by a mixture of dense and radiolucent areas of fibrosis with bone expansion. **Sclerotic** is homogeneously dense with bone expansion. **Cystic** has either spheric or ovale lucent regions with dense boundaries.

Treatment & Prognosis

The treatment for fibrous dysplasia is aimed at maintaining the patency of the external auditory canal and cranial nerve conduits. For ear canal stenosis, wide meatoplasty is performed to restore patency and exteriorize entrapped skin. Although sarcomatous degeneration is rare for those with fibrous dysplasia, the estimated incidences are 0.4% in monostotic and polyostotic disease, and 4% in McCune-

Albright syndrome. Clinical features that suggest sarcomatous degeneration include pain, swelling, and radiographic evidence of bony destruction. The prognosis for malignant transformation is poor.

OSTEOPETROSES

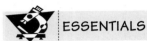

ESSENTIALS OF DIAGNOSIS

- *Conductive or sensorineural hearing loss.*
- *Cranial neuropathies.*
- *Facial dysfunction.*

General Considerations

The osteopetroses are a group of inheritable metabolic bone disorders. They result in diffuse, dense sclerosis and faulty bony remodeling. There are two forms: congenital and tarda. The **congenital** or **lethal form** is autosomal recessive, and manifests during infancy with pancytopenia secondary to obliteration of marrow spaces. Death due to hemorrhage, anemia, or overwhelming infection is common in infancy or childhood. The **tarda** or **adult form** is also known as Albers-Schönberg disease and is most commonly autosomal dominant. The adult form is benign and has a variable clinical course. Symptomatic patients present with problems that relate to bony overgrowth and foraminal stenosis. Hearing loss may be conductive or sensorineural owing to ossicular involvement or cochlear nerve impingement. Facial nerve function may be weak and spastic as a result of internal auditory canal narrowing. Other cranial nerve neuropathies may result from progressive stenosis of neural foramina.

Pathogenesis

The osteopetroses result from osteoclast dysfunction. Remodeled bone is faulty. Histologically, regions of endochondral ossification contain abnormal calcified cartilage. The osteopetrotic bone is immature, thick, dense, and brittle. This appearance gives rise to the names *chalk* or *marble bone disease.*

Clinical Findings

A. SYMPTOMS AND SIGNS

In osteopetrosis congenita, findings that result from foraminal stenosis include optic atrophy, hearing loss, and facial palsy. Hearing loss tends to be conductive and is the result of ossicular infiltration by osteopetrotic bone and exostoses. In adult-type osteopetrosis, patients suffer multiple cranial nerve palsies involving cranial nerves I, II, III, V, and VII. Facial nerve paralysis can be recurrent and results from narrowing of the internal auditory, and labyrinthine and vertical fallopian canals. Conductive or mixed hearing loss is also due to ossicular chain involvement. Sensorineural hearing loss may arise from otic capsule and internal auditory canal infiltration by osteopetrotic bone.

B. IMAGING STUDIES

Temporal bone CT findings in **osteopetrosis congenita** are notable for a small middle ear cavity with normal ossicles, obliteration of the mastoid antrum, and normal-appearing otic capsule.

Temporal bone CT findings in **osteopetrosis tarda** are remarkable for a diffusely chalky, thickened cranial vault. Stenosis of neural foramina, encroachment of pneumatic spaces, infiltration of ossicles, and involvement of the otic capsule are other findings.

Treatment & Prognosis

There is no effective medical therapy for the osteopetroses, so limited surgical intervention may be indicated to decompress cranial canals and foramina. Of note, conductive hearing loss resulting from osteopetroses may be caused by either direct bony ossicular infiltration or epitympanic fixation. Treatment of conductive hearing loss by ossiculoplasty may be technically difficult because of dense middle ear bony disease and footplate abnormalities. Nonsurgical therapy with hearing aid rehabilitation should be considered before surgical intervention. It may be necessary to perform surgery to enlarge the external auditory canal to accommodate a hearing aid. Surgical decompression of the acoustic nerve for stabilization of sensorineural hearing loss is unproven.

Facial nerve dysfunction generally presents with acute and recurrent episodes of facial palsy. Presurgical planning with a fine-resolution temporal bone CT scan can delineate stenotic sites for decompression.

PAGET DISEASE

ESSENTIALS OF DIAGNOSIS

- *External auditory canal stenosis.*
- *Mixed hearing loss.*
- *Facial nerve dysfunction.*
- *Radiographic "cotton wool" appearing lesions.*

General Considerations

Paget disease, or **osteitis deformans,** is a disorder of excessive bone remodeling, primarily of the axial skeleton. Most cases are sporadic, but up to 15% are inherited in an autosomal pattern. The disease tends to occur after the fifth decade. The diagnosis is often made during evaluation for skeletal pain or incidentally on routine radiography.

Pathogenesis

The evidence for a possible viral etiology for Paget disease is based on findings of an immunoregulatory defect in chromosome 6 in association with viral inclusions in osteoclasts. The histologic pattern in Paget disease is one of alternating waves of osteoclastic and osteoblastic activity. Bone remodeling activity results in haphazard bony resorption followed by deposition of structurally weakened, demineralized cancellous bone. The early phase of the disease is dominated by bone resorption, which is seen as lytic lesions. The marrow space subsequently fills with fibrovascular tissue, which later undergoes sclerosis. Multifocal areas of lysis and sclerosis within the temporal bone and cranial base are seen.

Temporal bone findings in Paget disease are notable for a tortuous external auditory canal, constriction of the middle ear cleft, bony changes of the ossicular chain, and demineralization of the otic capsule. Narrowing of the internal auditory canal can also cause acoustic-vestibular-facial dysfunction.

Clinical Findings

A. SYMPTOMS AND SIGNS

Patients with Paget disease of the temporal bone present with tinnitus, vertigo, and hearing impairment. The pattern of hearing loss is mixed. The conductive component is most pronounced in the lower frequencies, whereas the sensorineural component most commonly involves the higher frequencies. Other cranial neuropathies due to foraminal stenosis are hemifacial spasm, trigeminal neuralgia, and optic atrophy.

B. IMAGING STUDIES

Plain film x-rays of the skull may be diagnostic in Paget disease. The "cotton wool" appearance (coexistence of osteolysis and sclerosis) is almost pathopneumonic. The only other diagnostic consideration is the pagetoid variant of fibrous dysplasia. In approximately 10% of cases, Paget disease may present as a sharply delineated osteolytic skull lesion, *osteoporosis circumscripta cranii.* The CT appearance of the temporal bone reflects varying degrees of bone remodeling activity. There are two radiographic patterns: mosaic and translucent. In the **mosaic pattern,** diffuse areas of radiolucency adjacent to foci of irregular sclerosis are seen. In the **translucent variant,** the appearance is homogeneous, "washed out," and blurred. The otic capsule may lack its usual sharply demarcated boundary and may be accompanied by an overall diffuse demineraliza-

tion of the petrous pyramid. The internal and external auditory canals and middle ear cleft may appear stenotic.

Treatment

A. NONSURGICAL MEASURES

Treatment of symptomatic Paget disease (bone pain, neuropathies, and cardiovascular stress) with calcitonin and bisphosphonates has been shown to induce biochemical and clinical improvement. Decremental levels of alkaline phosphatase and urinary hydroxyproline are seen in association with clinical improvement. Radiographic evaluation may document the arrest of bony lesions.

B. SURGICAL MEASURES

Surgical therapy for hearing loss and cranial neuropathy in Paget disease should be considered only as the last resort. Surgery for conductive hearing loss in Paget disease has not been satisfactory. Modern hearing devices are excellent alternatives to middle ear exploration and should be encouraged. Persistent symptomatic internal auditory canal stenosis with sensorineural hearing loss and facial nerve dysfunction following medical therapy may be an indication for surgical decompression.

OSTEOGENESIS IMPERFECTA

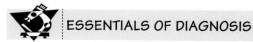 ESSENTIALS OF DIAGNOSIS

- Fragile bones.
- Blue sclera.
- Conductive and sensorineural hearing loss.

General Considerations

Osteogenesis imperfecta carries the hallmark of fragile bones susceptible to easy fracture. Osteogenesis imperfecta has two major variants: congenita and tarda. The **congenita variant** is lethal. The newborn suffers from severe and life-threatening fractures sustained in utero and in the peripartum period. The **tarda variant** has a broad range of clinical outcomes that span the range from mild to lethal disease. Inheritance of the tarda variant is through either autosomal dominant or recessive transmission. The classic triad of blue sclera, multiple fractures, and early hearing loss is inherited through an autosomal dominant pattern of transmission.

Pathogenesis

The histopathology of osteogenesis imperfecta is marked by the deposition of osteopenic immature bony tissue that is weak and fragile. There is an increase in osteocytes in both woven and lamellar bone, and a relative reduction of matrix substance. The bone turnover rate is high. Conflicting theories have been proposed to explain the pathogenesis of this disease. Some advocate the hypothesis of osteoblast dysfunction that is responsible for immature bone deposition; others advocate the hypothesis of increased osteoclast activity. Still others implicate abnormal cell signaling due to defects of the extracellular matrix. Clinically, the regulatory defect in bone turnover results in pathologic fractures and hearing loss.

Clinical Findings

A. Symptoms and Signs

Osteogenesis imperfecta tarda is a systemic disease and thus affects multiple organ systems, producing a broad array of clinical manifestations. Some of these conditions are dentinogenesis imperfecta, blue sclerae, loose joints, mitral valve prolapse, easy bruising, and growth deficiency. The hearing loss pattern may be conductive, sensorineural, or mixed. The onset of hearing loss is between the second and third decades. Hearing loss in osteogenesis imperfecta tarda can be audiometrically indistinguishable from otosclerosis. However, osteogenesis imperfecta has an earlier onset of hearing impairment and a higher incidence of sensorineural loss compared with otosclerosis. Footplate fixation in osteogenesis imperfecta tarda can arise either from an otospongiosis-like focus, as seen in early otosclerosis, or diffuse changes within the otic capsule.

Several operative findings during stapedectomy differentiate osteogenesis imperfecta from otosclerosis. The canal wall skin is thin and fragile, and the scutum is brittle. Crural fractures are not uncommon, and there is excessive bleeding. The sensorineural component of the hearing loss in osteogenesis imperfecta is poorly understood but may involve microfractures of the otic capsule and encroachment of the bony labyrinth by dysplastic bone. Facial nerve dysfunction is a rare complication of osteogenesis imperfecta.

B. Imaging Studies

Temporal bone CT findings in osteogenesis imperfecta have substantial overlap with those found in otosclerosis. Both entities may have fenestral and retrofenestral findings. In fenestral disease, CT scanning shows an excrescent mass at the level of the promontory. In retrofenestral disease, the cochlea may be demineralized, with or without sclerosis. The "double ring" sign refers to the hypodense band that spirals along the cochlea. Extensive endochondral demineralization of the otic capsule is evident in severe cochlear otosclerosis. However, diffuse resorptive changes in vast areas of the otic capsule are more often seen in osteogenesis imperfecta. The findings of extensive facial nerve canal involvement and severe proliferative otic capsule dysplasia differentiate osteogenesis imperfecta tarda from cochlear otosclerosis.

Treatment & Prognosis

The primary otologic symptom in osteogenesis imperfecta is conductive hearing loss that occurs between the second and third decades. The benefit of medical therapy with calcitonin, sodium fluoride, and vitamin D is unclear. Surgical intervention with stapedectomy to improve conductive hearing loss in osteogenesis imperfecta tarda is technically more demanding than in otosclerosis. There is a greater tendency for bleeding and difficult footplate mobilization. Despite these challenges, stapes surgery in osteogenesis imperfecta has favorable short- and long-term results. Alternately, patients may choose to improve hearing with an amplification device.

In the rare event of facial nerve dysfunction, CT imaging is useful to evaluate the fallopian canal. Sites obstructed by dysplastic bone can be delineated for surgical decompression.

Aharinejad S, Grossschmidt K, Streicher J et al. Auditory ossicle abnormalities and hearing loss in the toothless mutation in the rat and their improvement after treatment with colony-stimulating factor 1. *J Bone Miner Res*. 1999;14:415. [PMID: 10027906] (Describes the effects of treating mutant rats with CSF-1 on hearing and temporal bone pathology.)

Albright F, Butler MA, Hampton AO et al. Syndrome characterized by osteitis fibrosa disseminata, areas of pigmentation and endocrine dysfunction with precocious puberty in females. *N Engl J Med*. 1937;216:727. (Seminal article describing McCune Albright syndrome.)

Bartynski WS, Barnes PD, Wallman JK. Cranial CT of autosomal-recessive osteopetrosis. *Am J Neuroradiol*. 1989;10:543. [PMID: 2501985] (Radiographic, clinical review of 8 patients with autosomal recessive osteopetrosis.)

Benecke JE. Facial nerve dysfunction in osteopetrosis. *Laryngoscope*. 1993;103:494. [PMID: 8483364] (Review of the literature regarding facial nerve outcome in osteopetrosis.)

Bergstrom LV. Osteogenesis imperfecta: otologic and maxillofacial aspects. *Laryngoscope*. 1977;87(Suppl 6):1. [PMID: 330992] (Review article of patient clinical manifestations of osteogenesis imperfecta in the temporal bone and maxillofacial region.)

Bollerslev J, Grontved A, Andersen PE Jr. Autosomal dominant osteopetrosis: an otoneurologic investigation of the two radiological types. *Laryngoscope*. 1988;98:411. [PMID: 3352441] (Clinical findings correlated in a retrospective fashion with radiographic findings of 14 patients with autosomal dominant osteopetrosis.)

Collins DH, Winn JM. Focal Paget's disease of the skull (osteoporosis circumscripta). *J Pathol*. 1955;69:1. (Seminal article describing the pathologic features of osteogenesis.)

d'Archambeau O, Parizel PM, Koekelkoren E et al. CT diagnosis and differential diagnosis of otodystrophic lesions of the temporal bone. *Europ J Radiol*. 1990;11:22. [PMID: 2397727] (Retrospective review of 55 patients and their CT scans in order to assess the diagnostic and differential value of high-resolution CT scanning in the evaluation of temporal bone dysplasia.)

Dort JC, Pollak A, Fisch U. The fallopian canal and facial nerve in sclerosteosis of the temporal bone: a histopathologic study. *Am J Otol.* 1990;11(5):320. [PMID: 2240173] (Study looking at detailed measures of the fallopian canal and facial nerve, correlating cross-sectional areas with facial nerve function.)

Freeman DA. Southwestern internal medicine conference: Paget's disease of bone. *Am J Med Sci.* 1988;295(2):144. [PMID: 3278610] (Review of Paget disease.)

Garretsen JTM, Cremers WRJ. Ear surgery in osteogenesis imperfecta. *Arch Otolaryngol.* 1990;116:317. [PMID: 2306350] (Presentation of pre- and postoperative hearing results after stapes surgery in osteogenesis imperfecta.)

Hamersma H. Osteopetrosis (marble bone disease) of the temporal bone. *Laryngoscope.* 1970;80:1518. [PMID: 4991443] (Review article of osteopetrosis involving the temporal bone.)

Khetarpal U, Schuknecht HF. In search of pathologic correlates for hearing loss and vertigo in Paget's disease: a clinical and histopathologic study of 26 temporal bones. *Ann Otol Rhinol Laryngol.* 1990;99(Suppl 145):1. [PMID: 2106820] (Histopathologic review of 26 patients to determine the etiology of conductive hearing loss.)

Lustig LR, Holliday MJ, McCarthy EF, Nager GT. Fibrous dysplasia involving the skull base and temporal bone. *Arch Otolaryngol.* 2001;127:1239. [PMID: 11587606] (Retrospective review of the clinical presentation of 21 patients with histopathologically confirmed fibrous dysplasia.)

McCune DJ, Bruch H. Osteodystrophia fibrosa: report of a case in which the condition was combined with precocious puberty, pathologic pigmentation of the skin, and hyperthyroidism, with review of the literature. *Am J Dis Child.* 1937;54:806. (Seminal article describing McCune Albright syndrome.)

Milroy CM, Michaels L. Temporal bone pathology of adult-type osteopetrosis. *Arch Otolaryngol.* 1990;116:79. [PMID: 2294946] (Case presentation of the pathologic features in a patient with adult osteopetrosis.)

Papadakis CE, Skoulakis CE, Prokopakis EP et al. Fibrous dysplasia of the temporal bone: report of a case and a review of its characteristics. *Ear Nose Throat J.* 2000;79:52. [PMID: 10665192] (Case presentation and review of clinical features of fibrous dysplasia.)

Pedersen U. Osteogenesis imperfecta: clinical features, hearing loss and stapedectomy. *Acta Oto-Laryngologica.* 1985;Suppl 415:1. [PMID: 3859176] (Comparison of stapes surgery in osteogenesis imperfecta.)

Reid IR, Miller P, Lyles K et al. Comparison of a single infusion of zoledronic acid with risedronate for Paget's disease. *N Engl J Med.* 2005;353:898. [PMID: 16135834] (Recent double-blinded clinical trial of single infusion versus 60 days of oral intake.)

Silence DO, Senn A, Danks DM. Genetic heterogeneity in osteogenesis imperfecta. *J Med Genet.* 1979;16:101. [PMID: 458828] (Epidemiologic and genetic study of osteogenesis imperfecta in Australia.)

Neoplasms of the Temporal Bone & Skull Base

65

John S. Oghalai, MD

The skull base includes the frontal bone, the sphenoid bone, the temporal bone, and the occipital bone. Tumors arising within the skull base are rare and usually cause few symptoms until they grow to a size in which they begin to affect cranial nerves. Occasionally, an asymptomatic tumor may be diagnosed when a middle ear mass is noted during routine otoscopic examination of the ear. Unfortunately, it is all too common for patients to have complaints of imbalance, unilateral pulsatile tinnitus, mild asymmetric hearing loss, vague headache, facial twitching or facial numbness, as well as to have the diagnosis of a skull base tumor delayed because of an incomplete work-up. By far, the majority of skull base tumors are benign and can be successfully managed with surgical resection by an otolaryngologist specialized in neurotology and skull base surgery. A magnetic resonance imaging (MRI) scan of the brain, skull base, or both, with and without gadolinium contrast, is extremely sensitive at diagnosing these rare tumors with little risk to the patient. Table 65–1 lists the various skull base neoplasms and their imaging characteristics.

Tumors of the temporal bone and skull base tend to arise in one of three locations: (1) the mastoid or middle ear, (2) the jugular foramen, or (3) the petroclival junction or petrous apex. Tumors of the cerebellopontine angle and Meckel cave are not considered in this chapter (see Chapter 61, Nonacoustic Lesions of the Cerebellopontine Angle). Surgical approaches to these three areas are numerous, and the nomenclature is confusing. To remove a lesion of the middle ear or mastoid, a mastoidectomy through a postauricular incision or a middle ear exploration through the ear canal is usually adequate. Tumors of the jugular foramen require a postauricular incision that extends down into the upper neck. A mastoidectomy is performed along with skeletonization of the facial nerve, the sigmoid sinus, and the jugular bulb. One classic approach to the jugular foramen is the Fisch Type A approach (Figure 65–1). This involves dissecting the facial nerve out of its bony canal and rerouting it anteriorly. Permanent facial paresis or synkinesis can occur. Closure of the ear canal is also part of the Fisch Type A approach, which leaves the patient with a maxi-

mal conductive hearing loss. However, newer approaches are available that may permit adequate exposure of the jugular foramen without requiring facial nerve rerouting and closure of the ear canal. Finally, tumors of the petroclival junction and petrous apex require either a middle fossa-transpetrous approach with removal of the petrous apex bone (Kawase triangle, Figure 65–2) or a combined subtemporal-retrolabyrinthine approach (Figure 65–3). The Fisch Type B and C approaches can also be used to access the petroclival junction and can be extended all the way to the nasopharynx. Surgical strategies are chosen by the skull base surgeon based on approaching the tumor with enough exposure to perform a complete and safe resection while minimizing neurologic morbidity.

PARAGANGLIOMAS

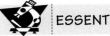 **ESSENTIALS OF DIAGNOSIS**

- *Pulsatile tinnitus.*
- *Reddish-blue middle ear mass.*

General Considerations

Paragangliomas (or glomus tumors) are tumors of paraganglionic tissue, which originally derive from the migration of neural crest cells during fetal development. These tissue rests are distributed predominantly throughout the middle ear, the jugular foramen, the vagus nerve, and the carotid body, but are also found in the upper mediastinum and the retroperitoneum. These cell clusters are innervated by the parasympathetic nervous system and function as chemoreceptors for circulatory regulation.

The most common paraganglioma is the **carotid body tumor.** A well-known, but rare, paraganglioma is the **pheochromocytoma.** Within the temporal bone, there are two main types of paraganglioma: **glomus tympanicum** and **glomus jugulare.** Glomus tympanicum tumors arise within the middle ear, from paraganglionic

Table 65–1. Radiographic appearance of skull base neoplasms.

Neoplasm	Most Common Site of Origin in Skull Base	CT	T1-Weighted MRI	T2-Weighted MRI	Contrast Enhancement
Paraganglioma	Jugular foramen and middle ear	Bone destruction	Intermediate, with flow voids	High, with flow voids	Strongly
Facial nerve schwannoma	Geniculate ganglion	Smooth remodeling and dilation of the surrounding bone of the facial canal	Intermediate	Intermediate	Strongly; follows the course of the facial nerve
Geniculate hemangioma	Geniculate ganglion	Erosion of surrounding bone with bony spicules within tumor	Intermediate	High	Strongly
Leukemia, lymphoma, and plasmacytoma	Petrous apex	Lytic lesion	Low	Intermediate	Moderately
Langerhans cell histiocytosis	Mastoid	Irregular bone destruction; may have other skull lesions as well	Intermediate	High	Moderately
Chondrosarcoma	Petroclival junction	Bone destruction, but can produce calcium matrix in 50% of tumors	Intermediate	High	Moderately or mixed
Chordoma	Clivus	Bone destruction, but can have bone remnants within it	Intermediate, with some areas of low signal representing mucus	High	Moderately or mixed
Meningioma	Posterior face of temporal bone	Surrounding hyperostosis and intratumoral calcification	Intermediate	Intermediate	Strongly; characteristic dural tail
Intralabyrinthine schwannoma	Within the inner ear	Mass within labyrinth; no bone erosion	Low	Intermediate	Strongly
Schwannoma of jugular foramen	Jugular foramen and middle ear	Soft tissue mass posterior to jugular bulb; mild, smooth bone erosion	Low	Intermediate	Strongly
Rhabdomyosarcoma	Anywhere, predominant tumor of children	Bone destruction	Intermediate	High	Strongly
Osteosarcoma	Anywhere	Either lytic osteoblastic or osteolytic; may have concentric rings of calcium	Intermediate	High	Strongly
Fibrosarcoma	Anywhere	Bone destruction	Intermediate	High	Strongly
Adenoma	Middle ear	Middle ear soft tissue mass; no bone erosion	Low	Intermediate	Strongly
Endolymphatic sac tumor	Posterior face of temporal bone	Bone destruction and erosion of otic capsule	Mixed, due to localized areas of mucus	Mixed	Strongly
Carcinoma	Middle ear	Bone destruction	Intermediate	Intermediate	Strongly
Metastatic disease	Petrous apex and internal auditory canal	Lytic lesion	Intermediate	High	Strongly

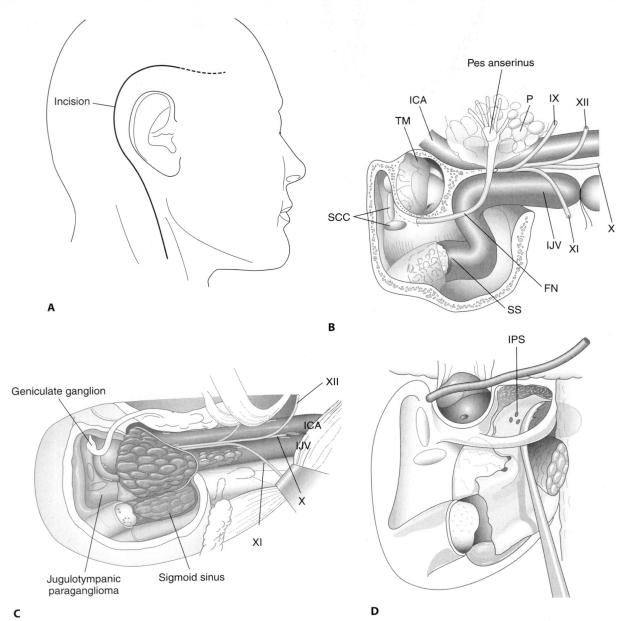

Figure 65–1. Surgical resection of a large jugulotympanic paraganglioma (Fisch Type A approach). **(A)** The incision runs from above the ear down into the upper neck. **(B)** The external auditory canal is oversewn and the pinna reflected anteriorly, exposing the facial nerve, middle ear, parotid gland, internal carotid artery, and internal jugular vein. **(C)** The facial nerve is rerouted out of its bony canal and transposed anteriorly. **(D)** The sigmoid sinus is occluded superiorly and the internal jugular vein is ligated inferiorly; the tumor is then removed from the jugular foramen. Although the classic Fisch Type A approach involves closure of the external auditory canal and rerouting of the facial nerve, these procedures are not often required to resect even large jugular foramen tumors as shown in this example. ICA, internal carotid artery; TM, tympanic membrane; SCC, semicircular canals; P, parotid gland; SS, sigmoid sinus; FN, facial nerve; IJV, internal jugular vein. Roman numerals indicate cranial nerves; IPS, inferior petrosal sinus. *(continued)*

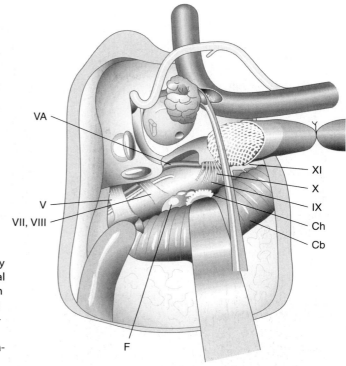

Figure 65–1 (continued). **(E)** If necessary, any remaining tumor is removed off of the internal carotid artery or cerebellopontine angle. Fisch Type B and C approaches (not shown) are not used to approach the jugular foramen, but instead are used to approach tumors of the infratemporal fossa, petroclival junction, and nasopharynx. VA, vertical artery; CH, choroid plexus; CB, cerebellum.

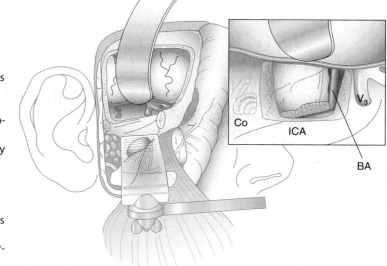

Figure 65–2. Middle fossa-transpetrous approach for resection of petrous apex tumors. These tumors can grow to involve the petroclival junction, around foramen lacerum, and extend posteriorly into the ventral brainstem and superiorly into the temporal lobe. They can be approached by a middle fossa craniotomy with drill-out of the anterior petrous apex (Kawase triangle). Good visualization of the petroclival junction, as well as the anterior brainstem, is obtained by this approach. Co, cochlea; BA, basilar artery; ICA, internal carotid artery.

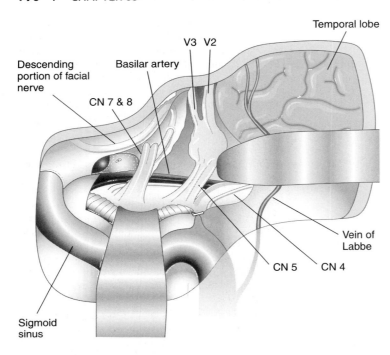

Figure 65–3. Combined subtemporal-retrolabyrinthine approach for resection of tumors of the petroclival junction. This involves opening both the posterior and middle cranial fossa dura, with division of the tentorium. Excellent exposure of the entire brainstem from the posterior circle of Willis to the jugular foramen is obtained.

cell rests associated with branches of cranial nerves IX and X (the glossopharyngeal and vagus nerves, respectively) that run over the promontory. Together these nerves are called the tympanic plexus, which consists of the Jacobsen nerve (a branch of CN IX) and the Arnold nerve (a branch of CN X). Glomus jugulare tumors arise within the jugular foramen from cell rests associated with cranial nerves IX, X, and XI.

Pathogenesis

Paragangliomas are most common in white populations. They typically occur in the fourth or fifth decades of life, although they can be identified at any age. Paragangliomas are slow-growing tumors, and metastases are extremely rare. They grow by spreading along the paths of least resistance. Within the skull base, they tend to extend through fissures and foramina, vascular channels, and air cell tract lines. Paragangliomas also demonstrate locally aggressive behavior with bone destruction and the invasion of soft tissue. They can extend from the temporal bone down into the upper neck.

Approximately 1% of paragangliomas display functionally significant catecholamine secretion similar to a pheochromocytoma. Pathologically, the chief cell is the cell of origin of the tumor and contains acetylcholine, catecholamines, and serotonin. Classic findings are clusters of chief cells, termed *Zellballen*, with a rich vascular plexus throughout the entire tumor. Indeed, these tumors are highly vascular and may bleed substantially during surgical excision.

The overall incidence of multiple lesions is about 10% in sporadic tumors. There is a 1–2% incidence of bilateral glomus jugulare tumors and a 7% incidence of an associated carotid body tumor. Paragangliomas can be based on germline mutations and can be hereditary. Mutations in the mitochondrial complex II genes *SDHB, SDHC,* and *SDHD* cause hereditary paragangliomas. In addition, another form of the disease has an autosomal dominant mode of transmission, and the causative genetic defect has been localized to two separate loci: 11q13.1 and 11q22-23. Patients with hereditary disease display a much higher incidence of synchronous paraganglioma, approximately 25–35%.

Paragangliomas are also associated with phakomatoses (neurologic diseases with cutaneous manifestations). These include von Recklinghausen neurofibromatosis, Sturge-Weber syndrome, tuberous sclerosis, and von Hippel-Lindau disease. In addition, they can be associated with multiple endocrine neoplasia (MEN) Type I syndrome.

Classification

There are two main classification schemes for paragangliomas of the temporal bone: Fisch and Glasscock-Jackson.

A. FISCH CLASSIFICATION

The Fisch classification includes four main categories: (1) Type A (tumors limited to the middle ear), (2) Type B (tumors limited to the tympanomastoid area), (3) Type

C (tumors extending into the petrous apex), and (4) Type D (tumors with intracranial extension).

B. GLASSCOCK-JACKSON CLASSIFICATION

The classification scheme of Glasscock and Jackson differentiates between glomus tympanicum and glomus jugulare tumors.

1. Glomus tympanicum neoplasms—For glomus tympanicum neoplasms, this staging system includes (1) Type I (small masses limited to the promontory of the middle ear), (2) Type II (tumors filling the middle ear space), (3) Type III (tumors filling the middle ear and mastoid), and (4) Type IV (tumors extending into the external auditory canal or around the internal carotid artery).

2. Glomus jugulare neoplasms—For glomus jugulare tumors, this staging system includes (1) Type I (small tumors involving the jugular bulb, the middle ear, and the mastoid); (2) Type II (tumors extending under the internal auditory canal); (3) Type III (tumors extending into the petrous apex); and (4) Type IV (tumors extending beyond the petrous apex into the clivus or infratemporal fossa).

Clinical Findings

A. SYMPTOMS AND SIGNS

The two most common presenting symptoms of a patient with a paraganglioma of the temporal bone are conductive hearing loss and pulsatile tinnitus. Patients may also complain of aural pain, facial nerve weakness, and a neck mass. The patient should be questioned as to symptoms of sympathetic discharge, which may represent a functionally secreting tumor, such as tachycardia, arrhythmias, flushing, or labile hypertension. Moreover, the patient should be queried about any symptoms of dysphagia or hoarseness, which may represent palsy of cranial nerves IX or X.

Physical examination demonstrates a reddish-bluish mass behind the eardrum. An aural polyp may be noted. There are two clinical signs associated with paraganglioma that can be identified during microscopic exam of the tympanic membrane: (1) **Brown sign** is the cessation of tumor pulsation and tumor blanching with positive pressure using the pneumatic otoscope; and (2) **Aquino sign** is the blanching of the mass with manual compression of the ipsilateral carotid artery. A complete examination of the cranial nerves is indicated, with particular attention to cranial nerves VII (the facial nerve), VIII (the vestibulocochlear nerve), IX (the glossopharyngeal nerve), X (the vagus nerve), XI (the accessory nerve), and XII (the hypoglossal nerve).

B. LABORATORY FINDINGS

Patients with a suspected paraganglioma can be screened for a catecholamine secretion by collecting a patient's urine for 24 hours and determining the vanillylmandelic acid (VMA) and metanephrine levels. An audiogram will reveal conductive hearing loss if the middle ear space is invaded with tumor. If the inner ear is invaded, a sensorineural hearing loss will be found. Impedance audiometry will reveal a flat tympanogram if a middle ear mass is present and touches the eardrum. Occasionally, vascular pulsations may be noted on the tympanogram.

C. IMAGING STUDIES

The importance of imaging paraganglioma of the skull base cannot be underestimated (Figure 65–4). Imaging is critical to delineate the extent of these tumors precisely. The first thing to determine is whether the jugular foramen is involved with the tumor. A glomus tympanicum is limited to the promontory and the mastoid though a glomus jugulare begins in the jugular foramen and extends superiorly into the middle ear and mastoid. In addition, the studies should be reviewed with careful attention to the middle ear, jugular foramen, and carotid bifurcation to look for a synchronous tumor.

1. Computed tomography (CT) scanning—CT scanning is useful to visualize the bony structures of the temporal bone. Of key importance is to evaluate the bone above the jugular bulb, the jugular plate. If the tumor is a glomus jugulare tumor that has extended into the middle ear cavity, this bone will be eroded. In contrast, if the tumor is a glomus tympanicum tumor, the bone surrounding the jugular bulb is usually intact. Inner ear or facial nerve involvement may also be noted. There may be a semicircular canal fistula or the tumor may be in close proximity to the fallopian canal, particularly along the vertical segment. The tumor may extend anterior to the internal auditory canal or along the petrous portion of the internal carotid artery. These findings may affect the planned surgical approach.

2. MRI scanning—MRI studies are useful to identify whether there is intracranial extension of the tumor. MRI gives excellent soft tissue contrast resolution and permits delineation of the tumor from the brainstem, the cerebellum, and the cranial nerves. The tumor has intermediate signal intensity on T1-weighted MRI and high intensity on T2-weighted MRI. Both may demonstrate a speckled pattern within the tumor, termed a "salt and pepper" pattern. This pattern is due to flow voids from the large number of intratumoral blood vessels. The tumor enhances strongly with gadolinium contrast.

3. Magnetic resonance angiography and venography—Magnetic resonance angiography (MRA) can be used to evaluate for compression of the internal carotid artery. Magnetic resonance venography (MRV) is useful to assess collateral circulation within the dural sinuses of the skull, since blood flow within the sigmoid sinus is often blocked by the tumor.

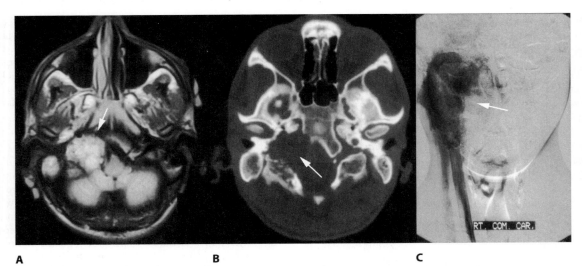

A   **B**   **C**

Figure 65–4. Jugulotympanic paraganglioma. **(A)** Axial view, T1-weighted image MRI with gadolinium contrast demonstrates a large enhancing mass in the right jugular bulb extending intracranially into the cerebellopontine angle (arrow). **(B)** Computed tomography at the same level shows significant bone destruction of the temporal bone and clivus (arrow). **(C)** Coronal-view angiogram demonstrates the highly vascular tumor extending from the skull base inferiorly into the upper neck. This mass was embolized prior to surgical excision.

4. Angiography—Angiography of glomus jugulare tumors is usually done 1 or 2 days before surgical excision. This permits definitive diagnosis of the tumor by visualizing the tumor blush characteristic of such highly vascular tumors. In addition, the feeding vessels can be identified and embolized to reduce blood loss during surgery. The typical feeding vessels for a glomus jugulare tumor are the ascending pharyngeal artery and the stylomastoid branch of the occipital artery. Glomus tympanicum tumors typically do not need to be embolized preoperatively because of their small size and easy accessibility.

Differential Diagnosis

The differential diagnosis of a patient with a middle ear mass includes otitis media, cholesterol granuloma, other types of middle ear neoplasms—including middle ear adenoma or carcinoma—a vascular anomaly such as a high-riding dehiscent jugular bulb, an aberrant carotid artery, or a persistent stapedial artery. Other temporal bone neoplasms that might involve the middle ear space include meningiomas, schwannomas or neuromas, adenomas, or endolymphatic sac tumors.

Complications

A. HEARING LOSS

Progressive conductive hearing loss usually is the presenting symptom of patients with a temporal bone paraganglioma. This may occur directly if the tumor contacts the ossicular chain or indirectly if the tumor blocks the eustachian tube, producing a serous middle ear effusion. Sensorineural hearing loss is uncommon but can occur if the tumor erodes the dense otic capsule bone and invades the inner ear. Alternately, the tumor may extend intradurally and affect cranial nerve VIII in the cerebellopontine angle and internal auditory canal.

B. FACIAL NERVE PALSY

Paragangliomas of the temporal bone may cause facial nerve palsy (21%) by invading the nerve within the temporal bone. Usually, this occurs along the vertical portion of the nerve within the mastoid. Even if nerve function is unaffected, most glomus jugulare tumors grow to wrap around the facial nerve and erode its bony canal in this location. A microsurgical dissection of a dehiscent nerve surrounded by tumor is the norm and can be quite challenging. (A dehiscent nerve is one in which the bony canal surrounding the nerve has been eroded.)

C. JUGULAR FORAMEN SYNDROME

If the jugular foramen is involved with the paraganglioma, the insidious onset of neuropathy of the lower cranial nerves (IX, X, and XI) ensues as they are slowly encroached upon by the tumor. Symptoms include dysphagia and aspiration, as the sensation to the pharynx (CN IX) and the larynx (CN X) is diminished. Also, hoarseness may be noted owing to vocal cord paralysis (CN X). It should be noted that rather than an isolated recurrent laryngeal nerve injury that causes vocal cord paralysis (such as with a Pancoast tumor), the jugular foramen syndrome includes a high vagal nerve injury. This is much more severe because the combination of a lack of sensation to the upper larynx and vocal cord paralysis puts these patients at extremely high risk of aspiration. The paralysis of cranial nerve XI can be noted as weakness and atrophy of the sternocleidomastoid and trapezius muscles.

D. HYPOGLOSSAL NERVE PARALYSIS

The hypoglossal nerve exits the skull base through the hypoglossal foramen in the occipital bone, anteroinferior to the jugular foramen. Large paragangliomas that extend inferiorly may affect the hypoglossal nerve. The patient may complain of worsening articulation, and the physical exam will demonstrate ipsilateral tongue atrophy, muscular fasciculations, and deviation to the affected side with protrusion.

E. HORNER SYNDROME

The sympathetic nerves to the head run from the superior cervical ganglion up along the internal carotid artery into the skull base. Paragangliomas that envelop the petrous portion of the internal carotid artery may cause an ipsilateral Horner syndrome with ptosis, miosis, and ipsilateral facial flushing and sweating.

F. OTHER COMPLICATIONS

Large paragangliomas can affect other neurologic functions, depending on the tumor extension. Intradural tumors can grow within the cerebellopontine angle, producing cerebellar dysfunction and imbalance, brainstem compression, and even obstructive hydrocephalus. Tumors that grow superiorly or medially can affect other cranial nerves, causing diplopia (CN IV or VI), facial numbness or pain (CN V), or dry eye (the greater superficial petrosal branch of CN VII).

Treatment

A. NONSURGICAL MEASURES

1. Observation—Observation with no treatment is reasonable in patients with minimal symptoms, particularly if they are older. Because glomus tumors are slow growing, serial MRI scans can be obtained, reserving surgery or radiation therapy for obvious tumor growth. This approach is less acceptable for younger patients in whom the tumor would be expected to grow substantially during their life span.

2. Radiation—The role of radiation therapy in the management of paragangliomas is controversial. Radia-

tion is thought to reduce the growth rate of these tumors; however, it does not eliminate viable tumor cells within the mass. Tumors have been known to recur even more than a decade after radiation therapy. Radiation therapy for paragangliomas of the temporal bone can be useful as a treatment for elderly patients with symptomatic tumors or for patients who are unwilling to undergo a surgical resection. Postoperative stereotactic radiation therapy may be used for patients in whom total tumor removal could not be achieved.

B. SURGICAL MEASURES

Microsurgical total tumor removal is the treatment of choice for most patients. Patients with functionally secreting tumors need to be alpha-blocked with phentolamine before and during surgical resection to prevent life-threatening hypertension as the alpha-adrenergic hormones are released with tumor manipulation.

The surgical approach for resection of paragangliomas of the temporal bone depends on the tumor extent. For a glomus tympanicum tumor that is limited to the middle ear cavity, a simple middle ear exploration through the ear canal may be all that is indicated. After raising the tympanic membrane, the tumor can be visualized on the promontory. It may then be cauterized with a bipolar cautery and removed. If the tumor is larger and extends into the mastoid air cells, a tympanomastoidectomy with an extended facial recess approach may be required. This is a standard mastoidectomy via a postauricular incision with sacrifice of the chorda tympani nerve to allow exposure of the middle ear and hypotympanum from the mastoid. A tumor extending medially to the facial nerve (the retrofacial air cells) can be resected after exposing the facial nerve along its vertical segment to prevent injury to it.

For glomus jugulare tumors, a larger surgical approach is required. One very important aspect during the removal of these tumors is delineation and preservation of the facial nerve. Unfortunately, the vertical segment of the facial nerve lies in the middle of the operative field, and the tumor is usually based directly behind it, wrapping around it. A tympanomastoid approach with an extended facial recess and complete skeletonization of the facial nerve to the stylomastoid foramen typically provides adequate exposure. If possible, the preservation of a thin layer of bone surrounding the facial nerve circumferentially is ideal to minimize risk to the facial nerve (the fallopian bridge technique). It is also important to extend the skin incision into the neck and identify the internal carotid artery and internal jugular vein. The sternocleidomastoid and digastric muscles are separated from the mastoid tip so that the great vessels can be followed up to the skull base. These vessels need to be controlled both proximally and distally to the tumor in case a great vessel rupture occurs.

The most important part of the surgery is resection of the jugular bulb. Superiorly, the sigmoid sinus is occluded in the mastoid cavity, inferior to the junction of the transverse sinus and sigmoid sinus because the vein of Labbé enters at that location. Occlusion of the vein of Labbé may cause venous infarction of the temporal lobe since it is the only vein draining this territory. Inferiorly, the internal jugular vein is divided and ligated in the neck. Next, the jugular bulb (the lateral wall of the sigmoid sinus and the tumor filling the sinus) is dissected from the posterior fossa dura and cranial nerves IX, X, and XI. There is usually substantial bleeding from the entry point of the inferior petrosal sinus to the jugular bulb during this process. It is important to quickly remove this tumor and pack this area with an absorbable knitted fabric (eg, Surgicel) to control the bleeding. After tumor removal, the mastoid cavity is often packed with fat harvested from the abdominal wall and closed in layers.

Large glomus jugulare tumors, which extend anteriorly along the internal carotid artery, typically require a larger infratemporal fossa surgical approach (Fisch Type A, see Figure 65–1). This approach involves following the facial nerve from the geniculate ganglion to the pes anserinus, lifting it out of the bony canal, and transposing it anteriorly to displace it out of the surgical field. The jugular spine, the bone between the internal jugular vein and the internal carotid artery as they enter the skull base, can then be fully delineated and removed. This permits dissection of the tumor from the internal carotid artery into the petrous apex. If needed, tumor dissection can extend from the jugular foramen all the way to the nasopharynx. If the tumor extends intracranially, this portion of the tumor should be removed after the vascular base of the tumor around the great vessels has been controlled. This reduces potentially massive intracranial hemorrhage. Large tumors require complete exenteration of the middle ear cavity, packing of the eustachian tube, and closure of the external auditory canal to form a blind pouch. If the tumor is extensive, it is possible that some type of soft tissue reconstructive flap may be needed to reconstruct the defect, such as a pedicled temporalis muscle flap.

Prognosis

Paragangliomas have a slow but relentless growth pattern. For most patients, the treatment of choice is a complete microsurgical removal to prevent worsening morbidity from tumor progression. Observation with no treatment can be performed if the patient is elderly and has only minimal symptoms. The use of radiation therapy is limited to elderly patients with symptomatic tumors, hopefully slowing the growth rate of an already slow-growing tumor. The main question, however, is whether this tumor will cause serious morbidity or mor-

tality in the patient's remaining years. In the end, the treatment of paragangliomas needs to be individualized based on the patient, the disease, and the physician.

The most common complications from surgical excision are those related to cranial neuropathy. These include paresis or palsy of the jugular foramen nerves (CN IX, X, and XI) with resultant hoarseness, dysphagia, and aspiration. These complications may be temporary or permanent. In either case, patients can usually regain the ability to eat within the first few weeks after surgery with swallowing therapy. Facial nerve palsy also can occur during tumor removal, although if the facial nerve is anatomically intact at the end of surgery, a good return of function is expected. As with any skull base surgery, meningitis or cerebrospinal fluid (CSF) leak may occur. There can be significant amounts of blood loss during the resection of these tumors because of their highly vascular nature. Preoperative embolization is quite helpful in reducing the amount of blood loss.

Jackson CG, McGrew BM, Forest JA, Netterville JL, Hampf CF, Glasscock ME III. Lateral skull base surgery for glomus tumors: long-term control. *Otol Neurotol.* 2001;22:377. [PMID: 11347643] (Surgical control rates for paragangliomas.)

Oghalai JS, Leung MK, Jackler RK, McDermott MW. Transjugular craniotomy for the management of jugular foramen tumors with intracranial extension. *Otol Neurotol.* 2004;25:570; discussion 579. [PMID: 15241237] (Newer approaches for jugular foramen tumors.)

Weber PC, Patel S. Jugulotympanic paragangliomas. *Otolaryngol Clin North Am.* 2001;34:1231. [PMID: 11728943] (A good review.)

FACIAL NERVE SCHWANNOMAS

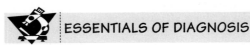 ESSENTIALS OF DIAGNOSIS

- *Facial twitch.*
- *Slowly progressive facial palsy.*
- *Conductive hearing loss.*

General Considerations

Primary tumors of the facial nerve can arise anywhere from the glial-Schwann cell junction in the cerebellopontine angle into the parotid gland. These are very slow-growing tumors and tend to spread longitudinally along the course of the facial nerve within the temporal bone (the fallopian canal). These tumors are histologically similar to vestibular schwannomas (acoustic neuromas) except for the fact that they rise along a different cranial nerve.

The diagnosis of a facial nerve schwannoma is frequently delayed because of the slow rate of tumor growth and symptom development. Patients with Bell's palsy in whom facial nerve function was not of acute onset should be evaluated for a facial nerve schwannoma. Also, patients with facial palsy that does not begin to demonstrate the return of function within 6–9 months of onset should be evaluated for a facial nerve schwannoma.

Clinical Findings

A. SYMPTOMS AND SIGNS

The clinical findings depend on the precise location of the tumor. For facial nerve schwannomas that begin in the cerebellopontine angle or internal auditory canal, the most common clinical findings are sensorineural hearing loss, tinnitus, vestibular dysfunction, and balance. These findings are precisely the same symptomatology as those of a patient with an acoustic neuroma. Patients with facial nerve schwannomas within the fallopian canal present with facial nerve palsy and twitch. They can also present with conductive hearing loss if the mass impinges upon the middle ear ossicles. Extratemporal facial nerve schwannomas typically present as an asymptomatic firm mass in the parotid gland.

For all locations, a common patient history is a slow onset of facial nerve palsy over 3–6 months, which has not improved even after several years. Usually, facial spasm is noted before the onset of facial paralysis. Occasionally, a patient with a facial nerve schwannoma presents with facial palsy of rapid onset (over 1–2 days). These patients are diagnosed with idiopathic Bell's palsy and treated with corticosteroids. Although steroids may reduce tumor edema and initially lead to an improvement in facial nerve function, the facial nerve palsy will return over the next few weeks as the effects wear off.

B. IMAGING STUDIES

1. CT scanning and MRI—CT scanning is quite useful in identifying the extent of bony erosion and dilatation of the fallopian canal. In addition, it delineates whether the tumor mass impinges upon the ossicles. An MRI scan with gadolinium contrast is superior for defining the extent of the tumor within the cerebellopontine angle and the parotid gland (Figure 65–5). The tumor has an intermediate signal intensity on both T1- and T2-weighted MRI.

It can be difficult to differentiate between an acoustic neuroma and a facial nerve schwannoma within the internal auditory canal. However, facial nerve schwannomas typically follow the course of the facial nerve. They extend into the temporal bone, involving the geniculate ganglion and horizontal portion of the facial

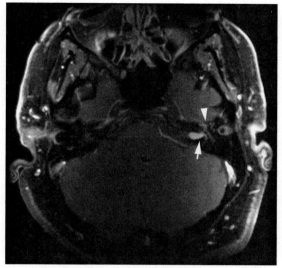

Figure 65–5. Facial nerve schwannoma. Axial view, T1-weighted image MRI with gadolinium contrast demonstrates an enhancing tumor of the left internal auditory canal (arrow) that extends anteriorly to the geniculate ganglion (arrowhead).

nerve within the middle ear. In contrast, acoustic neuromas stop at the fundus, which is the distal portion of the internal auditory canal (IAC).

2. Audiometry—Audiometry often demonstrates conductive hearing loss. The ipsilateral acoustic reflex may have elevated thresholds or show abnormal decay functions.

Differential Diagnosis

The differential diagnosis of a facial nerve schwannoma in the cerebellopontine angle and IAC includes vestibular schwannoma, meningioma, and epidermoid cyst. If the tumor involves the geniculate ganglion or the intratemporal facial nerve, the differential diagnosis includes cholesteatoma, paraganglioma, and geniculate hemangioma. If a parotid mass is palpable, all types of benign and malignant parotid tumors are within the differential diagnosis. For any patient with unilateral peripheral facial palsy, both idiopathic Bell's palsy and Ramsey-Hunt syndrome should be included in the differential diagnoses.

Treatment

A. NONSURGICAL MEASURES

These tumors are extremely slow growing and typically cause slowly progressive facial nerve palsy. Observation is the treatment of choice until the facial nerve palsy is substantial (House-Brackmann Grade 4 or greater) or symptoms of brainstem compression occur.

B. SURGICAL MEASURES

Because surgical excision requires resection of the involved segment of the nerve and grafting of the facial nerve, a significant postoperative facial nerve deficit is to be expected. After nerve grafting or hypoglossal-facial nerve transfer has been performed, the best facial nerve function that can be expected is a House-Brackmann Grade 3. The surgical approach depends on the precise location of the tumor. If the tumor is limited to the IAC and cerebellopontine angle, a retrosigmoidal or middle cranial fossa approach can be used to try to preserve hearing. Typically, the middle fossa approach allows better exposure of the facial nerve as it lies on the superior aspect of the nerves within the IAC. If hearing has already been lost, a translabyrinthine approach allows the best exposure of the complete length of the facial nerve. If the facial nerve schwannoma is limited to the middle ear or mastoid, a postauricular tympanomastoidectomy approach can be used. Although this approach does not allow exposure of the IAC, complete exposure from the geniculate ganglion to the parotid gland can be obtained.

Tumor removal involves transecting the facial nerve on either side of the schwannoma. If only a small segment of the nerve is involved, the nerve may be mobilized out of its canal and repaired primarily. Otherwise, a nerve graft either from the great auricular nerve or the sural nerve can be grafted between the segments. If the proximal portion of the facial nerve is involved at the brainstem, nerve grafting may be impossible and a hypoglossal-facial nerve transposition can be performed.

Prognosis

After the initial diagnosis, close follow-up is warranted with a serial MRI, CT scan, or both to determine whether there is evidence of tumor growth. As long as symptoms are stable, these tumors can be followed. If surgical excision is required, routine eye care is needed until facial nerve function returns. This may require the use of artificial tears and Lacri-Lube (a nighttime eye lubricant), a protective eye shield, or the placement of a gold weight in the upper eyelid. Patients may also have conductive or sensorineural hearing loss that needs to be managed accordingly.

Fenton JE, Chin RY, Tonkin JP, Fagan PA. Transtemporal facial nerve schwannoma without facial nerve paralysis. *J Laryngol Otol.* 2001;115:559. [PMID: 11485588] (Surgical excision of facial nerve tumors.)

Liu R, Fagan P. Facial nerve schwannoma: surgical excision versus conservative management. *Ann Otol Rhinol Laryngol.* 2001;110:1025. [PMID: 11713912] (The management of facial nerve tumors.)

GENICULATE HEMANGIOMAS

General Considerations

Hemangiomas are benign tumors of blood vessels. They are the most common tumor of infancy and typically resolve spontaneously by the time the child is 5 to 6 years old. Within the temporal bone, hemangiomas have a predilection for the geniculate ganglion of the facial nerve. These are different from typical hemangiomas in that they are not associated with pediatric patients. They are usually identified in middle-aged adults.

Pathogenesis

Geniculate hemangiomas arise directly from the geniculate ganglion. The bony floor of the middle cranial fossa is dehiscent over the tumor in nearly all cases. The tumor can extend superiorly into the middle cranial fossa but typically remains extradural. It can also track distally along the distal portion of the facial nerve but does not extend beyond the horizontal segment. Geniculate hemangiomas usually do not extend proximally into the IAC; however, hemangiomas can arise primarily within the internal auditory canal, which similarly do not extend to the geniculate ganglion.

Clinical Findings

A. SYMPTOMS AND SIGNS

The most common presenting symptom of geniculate hemangiomas is slowly progressive facial paralysis. Rarely, a patient may present with a rapid onset of facial paralysis. Although a patient may have a geniculate hemangioma without facial paralysis, it would be unusual to diagnose this lesion without this symptom. Facial paralysis may simulate Bell's palsy (idiopathic facial paralysis), with improvement in facial function with steroid treatment; however, the facial palsy recurs as the effect of the steroids wears off.

Facial twitch and spasm can be identified in patients with tumors compressing the facial nerve and have been reported in patients with geniculate hemangiomas. Hearing loss is typically conductive owing to impingement of the tumor on the ossicular mass in the middle ear. These tumors usually do not erode the otic capsule and do not affect the IAC; therefore, sensorineural hearing loss is unusual. Patients may complain of symptoms related to compression of the greater superficial nerve, including either epiphora or dry eye. On physical exam, the patient may present with a red mass behind the eardrum and the Weber and Rinne tuning fork tests suggest a conductive hearing loss in that ear.

B. IMAGING STUDIES

CT scans demonstrate a soft tissue density in the area of the geniculate ganglion with bony dehiscence and ero-

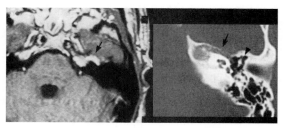

A　　　　　　**B**

Figure 65–6. Geniculate hemangioma. **(A)** Axial view, T1-weighted image MRI with gadolinium contrast demonstrates an enhancing lesion in the vicinity of the geniculate ganglion (arrow). **(B)** CT scan of the temporal bone demonstrates an expansile lesion with moderate bone erosion (arrow). There are characteristic calcium flakes within the tumor. The malleus and incus are also identified as a landmark (arrowhead).

sion of the floor of the middle cranial fossa around the geniculate ganglion (Figure 65–6). Classically, there may be intratumoral calcifications or bone spicules within the tumor, which are diagnostic for a hemangioma. However, the absence of calcium within the tumor does not rule out a hemangioma. MRI is useful in delineating the intracranial extent of the tumor. It enhances intensely with gadolinium contrast. On T1-weighted images without contrast, the tumor has the same density as brain tissue; on T2-weighted images, the tumor is bright.

Differential Diagnosis

The differential diagnosis of a geniculate lesion includes facial nerve schwannomas, meningioma, metastases, cholesteatomas, cholesterol granulomas, and mucoceles.

Treatment

A. Nonsurgical Measures

These lesions demonstrate slow but progressive growth. Observation can be considered in an older or debilitated patient in whom surgical risks are felt to be too great.

B. Surgical Measures

Surgical excision is the treatment of choice for most patients with these tumors since they clearly grow and cause worsening symptoms. Although they are next to the facial nerve, they usually do not infiltrate the nerve nor do they extend intradurally. Surgery often permits complete tumor resection with minimal impact on the facial nerve function. However, large tumors can affect final facial

nerve outcomes. The best surgical strategy is via a middle cranial fossa approach, with care to identify the interface between the tumor and the dura during the initial elevation of the dura off the floor of the middle cranial fossa. The tumor can usually be delicately microdissected from the geniculate ganglion with facial nerve preservation.

Prognosis

Surgical excision is curative. There have been no recurrence rates reported.

Isaacson B, Piccirillo E, Agarwal M, Rohit, Khrais T, Sanna M. Management of temporal bone hemangiomas. *Ann Otol Rhinol Laryngol.* 2004;113:431. [PMID: 15224824] (Facial nerve results after surgical tumor resection.)

Telian SA, McKeever PE, Arts HA. Hemangiomas of the geniculate ganglion. *Otol Neurotol.* 2005;26:796. [PMID: 16015187] (Hemangiomas infiltrate the facial nerve.)

MALIGNANT HEMATOLOGIC DISORDERS

1. Leukemia

Leukemia is the production of an abnormally high number of white blood cells that become deposited in various organs and sites within the body. The temporal bone is one site that occasionally becomes infiltrated, typically within the marrow of the petrous apex. Involvement of the middle ear cleft and mastoid can also occur; however, it is unusual for leukemic infiltrates to involve the inner ear or the facial nerve. Patients with leukemia are immunosuppressed and are highly prone to developing acute otitis media. Hemorrhage into the middle ear can also occur. Up to 32% of patients with leukemia have otologic symptoms, usually due to eustachian tube dysfunction with resultant middle ear effusion and conductive hearing loss. Obstruction of the eustachian tube can occur along its length or at its opening to the nasopharynx at the adenoid bed. A solid tumor known as a granulocytic sarcoma or chloroma is occasionally noted with myelogenous leukemia. This is a localized concentration of neoplastic granulocytic cells that begins within the marrow of the petrous apex.

CT scanning demonstrates a lytic lesion, and MRI shows the mass to have low-signal intensity on T1-weighted images and intermediate intensity on T2-weighted images. It enhances moderately with contrast. The treatment for leukemic infiltrates, granulocytic sarcoma, or both is based on systemic chemotherapy; there is no need for surgical treatment of this disease. Occasionally, a myringotomy is useful to drain fluid out of the middle ear cleft and for culture of the middle ear effusion if infection is suspected. Very rarely, a mastoidectomy is required if coalescent mastoiditis has developed or for biopsy purposes.

2. Lymphoma

Lymphoma can infiltrate the marrow spaces of the temporal bone, typically within the petrous apex. Like patients with leukemia, these patients can have eustachian tube dysfunction or hemorrhage into the middle ear with resultant middle ear effusion and conductive hearing loss. It is unusual to see destruction of the inner ear or facial nerve in this group of patients. The treatment of the disease is systemic chemotherapy and radiation therapy.

3. Plasmacytoma

The head and neck are the most common sites of an extramedullary plasmacytoma (ie, plasmacytoma arising anywhere outside of the bone marrow). Lesions usually involve the Waldeyer ring, which includes the tonsils, adenoids, and lymphoid tissue along the base of tongue. Very rarely, extramedullary plasmacytomas may involve the temporal bone, usually within the middle ear and mastoid air cells. Patients with this lesion present with eustachian tube dysfunction, middle ear effusion, and conductive hearing loss. Occasionally, a middle ear mass is identified. Surgery may be required to perform a biopsy, but once the diagnosis has been made, it is important to search for disseminated disease suggestive of multiple myeloma (found in 31% of patients with extramedullary plasmacytoma). This includes staging CT scans and a bone marrow biopsy.

The treatment for a solitary extramedullary plasmacytoma is based on radiation therapy alone. Debulking surgery is not generally recommended; however, limited resection with preservation of the facial nerve and inner ear can be performed during the biopsy. It is not recommended to perform a radical resection because this is not thought to improve outcomes. The 5-year survival rate is 69% for patients with isolated extramedullary plasmacytomas of the head and neck. If disseminated plasmacytoma or multiple myeloma is identified, chemotherapy is usually recommended in combination with radiation therapy.

Chiang SK, Canalis RF, Ishiyama A, Eversole LR, Becker DP. Plasmacytoma of the temporal bone. *Am J Otolaryngol.* 1998;19: 267. [PMID: 9692637] (Review article.)

Lewis WB, Patel U, Roberts JK, Palis J, Teot L. Angiocentric T-cell lymphoma of the temporal bone. *Otolaryngol Head Neck Surg.* 2002;126:85. [PMID: 11821775] (Case report.)

LANGERHANS CELL HISTIOCYTOSIS

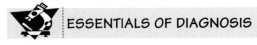

ESSENTIALS OF DIAGNOSIS

- *Chronic otitis media, otorrhea, and an aural polyp in a child.*

General Considerations

Langerhans cell histiocytosis is a proliferation of cells that arise from the bone marrow and are found circulating within the blood and lymph nodes and at junctional areas between the body and the outside environment (eg, along epithelial and endothelial surfaces). The role of normal histiocyte function is to present antigens to both T cells and B cells to initiate an immune response.

Other terms for Langerhans cell histiocytosis include histiocytosis X, eosinophilic granuloma, Hand-Schüller-Christian disease, and Letterer-Siwe disease. All of these diseases have now been categorized as Langerhans cell histiocytosis, and the latter terms are no longer used.

Langerhans cell histiocytosis is typically a disease of children, although it can occur at any age. There are three standard presentations. Localized Langerhans cell histiocytosis (Group 1) often occurs in children between the ages of 5 and 9 and presents as a single bony lesion. Multifocal Langerhans cell histiocytosis (Group 2) typically occurs in children between the ages of 2 and 5 and presents with two or more osseous, cutaneous, or soft tissue lesions with or without endocrine abnormalities. Disseminated Langerhans cell histiocytosis (Group 3) is found throughout the entire body in association with vital organ dysfunction. These patients are under 2 years of age.

Pathogenesis

The cause of Langerhans cell histiocytosis is unclear. Current theories suggest that it may represent an immune dysfunction that is either primary or secondary to an external stimulus, such as an infection. In addition, it may represent a low-grade type of lymphoma. Langerhans cells appear as mononuclear cells under light microscopy. With electron microscopy, Langerhans cells display the characteristic Birbeck granule or X-body. This is a rod-shaped structure that contains a central striated line and often expands at one end to form a shape similar to a tennis racket.

Clinical Findings

A. SYMPTOMS AND SIGNS

The most common presenting symptoms of Langerhans cell histiocytosis include a swelling of the skull (45%), cervical adenopathy (25%), cephalic rash (20%), and otorrhea (20%). Within the temporal bone, the disease often masquerades as otitis media, mastoiditis, and otorrhea that fail to resolve with antibiotic therapy. Conductive hearing loss is often noted, and an aural polyp may be realized during the physical exam. Indeed, Langerhans cell histiocytosis should be considered in all

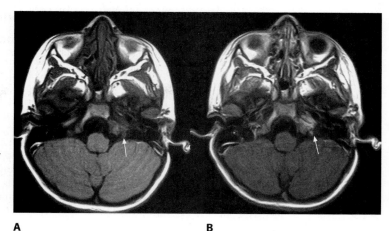

Figure 65–7. Langerhans cell histiocytosis. Axial views, T1-weighted MRI without (**A**) and with (**B**) gadolinium contrast demonstrate a subtle, mildly enhancing lesion in the petrous apex of the temporal bone and lateral clivus (arrow). There is no bony destruction.

A   **B**

children with aural polyps and chronic otitis media. Facial nerve paralysis, vertigo, dysequilibrium, tinnitus, and sensorineural hearing loss are rare.

Patients with disseminated Langerhans cell histiocytosis are quite sick and present with failure to thrive, fever, and extensive systemic involvement. There may also be cervical lymphadenopathy and cutaneous manifestations. These patients may have anemia and bleeding diatheses if the hematopoietic system is involved. Involvement of the central nervous system manifests as diabetes insipidus (polyuria and polydipsia), as well as other aspects of pituitary dysfunction such as growth hormone deficiency, hypothyroidism, and diminished sex hormone function.

B. IMAGING STUDIES

Plain radiographs of the skull often reveal multiple lytic skull lesions. CT scanning reveals a soft tissue mass with diffuse irregular bone destruction. The lesions have intermediate intensity on T1-weighted imaging and high intensity on T2-weighted MRI (Figure 65–7). They enhance moderately with gadolinium contrast. One should always look for other central nervous system lesions of Langerhans cell histiocytosis, especially in the pituitary stalk. Often, patients present with diabetes insipidus because of this second lesion. A bone scan can also be useful in identifying any other sites of involvement throughout the body.

Differential Diagnosis

Langerhans cell histiocytosis mimics many disorders. Chronic otitis media, aural polyps, cholesteatoma, external otitis, and coalescent mastoiditis are common inflammatory diseases with similar presenting symptoms. Other tumors of the temporal bone, including rhabdomyosarcoma, chondrosarcoma, adenocarcinoma, Ewing sarcoma,

osteosarcoma, and metastasis, also mimic Langerhans cell histiocytosis. Lymphoma, leukemia, and plasmacytoma are uncommon lesions of the temporal bone that may also simulate this disorder as well.

Treatment

A. NONSURGICAL MEASURES

1. Radiation therapy—Low-dose radiation therapy may be used if adequate curettage is not feasible for localized or multifocal Langerhans cell histiocytosis and is commonly used in patients with disseminated Langerhans cell histiocytosis.

2. Chemotherapy—Patients with disseminated Langerhans cell histiocytosis require both chemotherapy and radiation. The most common chemotherapeutic regimen is a combination of corticosteroids, vincristine or vinblastine, and methotrexate. Response rates vary widely and depend on the presence or absence of organ dysfunction.

B. SURGICAL MEASURES

The surgical management of Langerhans cell histiocytosis involves diagnostic biopsy and curettage. Conservative curettage is indicated, and there is no need for radical resection of the lesion. In particular, the inner ear, the ossicles, and the facial nerve should be carefully preserved. Surgical treatment is usually all that is required for patients with localized or multifocal disease.

Prognosis

Patients with localized disease can be treated equally well with either curettage or low-dose radiation therapy; their survival rate is 95–100%. Patients with multifocal disease also have a good survival rate, ranging from 65% to 100%. Patients with disseminated disease are treated with a combination of radiation therapy and chemotherapy. Their survival rate is quite poor and varies from 0% to 75%.

Cochrane LA, Prince M, Clarke K. Langerhans' cell histiocytosis in the paediatric population: presentation and treatment of head and neck manifestations. *J Otolaryngol.* 2003;32:33. [PMID: 12779259].

Marioni G, De Filippis C, Stramare R, Carli M, Staffieri A. Langerhans cell histiocytosis: temporal bone involvement. *J Laryngol Otol.* 2001;115:839. [PMID: 11668004] (Review article.)

OTHER RARE NEOPLASMS

1. Chondrosarcoma

General Considerations

Chondrosarcomas are thought to arise from cartilage rests left within the skull base after endochondral ossification during embryogenesis. Although theoretically these tumors can occur anywhere within the temporal bone, usually they are found at the petroclival junction around the foramen lacerum. They are very slow-growing tumors. Pathologically, they are usually well or moderately-differentiated tumors, although poorly differentiated tumors have been reported.

Clinical Findings

Clinically, patients may present with pulsatile tinnitus, hearing loss, headaches, diplopia, facial numbness, and dysphagia, depending on the tumor location. Radiographic findings usually demonstrate an expansile mass at the petroclival junction with bony erosion on CT. There may be small areas of calcification within the tumor, referred to as a "popcorn" pattern. The tumor has intermediate intensity on T1-weighted MRI and high intensity on T2-weighted MRI. The lesion also enhances heterogeneously with gadolinium contrast, although some tumors are quite avascular and may demonstrate only minimal enhancement throughout. The differential diagnosis includes chordoma, osteosarcoma, fibrosarcoma, meningioma, and paraganglioma.

Treatment & Prognosis

The mainstay of therapy is surgical excision. Microsurgical total tumor removal can usually be achieved via the middle fossa-transpetrous approach with removal of the bone of the petrous apex medial to the cochlea (Kawase triangle) to expose the petroclival junction (see Figure 65–2). Alternately, an infratemporal fossa approach (Fisch Type B or C) or a combined subtemporal-retrosigmoidal approach (see Figure 65–3) may be used. Postoperative radiation therapy appears to improve patient prognosis. The 5-year survival rate is 40% to 90%.

2. Chordoma

General Considerations

Chordomas arise from remnant cells of the primitive notochord, an embryonic structure important during the embryologic development of the central nervous system, spinal cord, and vertebral bodies. Pathologically, chordomas are gelatinous tumors filled with vacuolated stellate cells in a background of glycoprotein matrix. Within the skull base, the predominant site where chordomas originate is the midline clivus. As the tumor grows and erodes the surrounding bone, it may extend anteriorly into the sphenoid sinus and nasopharynx, laterally into the cavernous sinus and temporal bone, and posteriorly to compress the brainstem. It is uncommon for chordomas to extend intradurally.

Clinical Findings

Presenting symptoms most commonly include headache and diplopia (palsy of CN III, IV, or VI), although any cranial nerve can be affected, depending on tumor extension. CT scanning reveals an expansile lesion of the midclivus with bone destruction. MRI demonstrates the tumor to be multilobular and to have intermediate signal intensity on T1-weighted images and high intensity on T2-weighted images. There is strong contrast enhancement with gadolinium, although this may be heterogeneous if there are cystic areas within the tumor filled with mucin. The differential diagnosis includes chondrosarcoma, osteosarcoma, fibrosarcoma, meningioma, and paraganglioma.

Treatment

Microsurgical total tumor removal is the goal of therapy; however, this is difficult because of the location of the tumor and the proximity of vital vascular structures (eg, internal carotid arteries, the circle of Willis, and the cavernous sinus) and neurologic structures (eg, CN II, III, IV, V, VI, the brainstem, and the pituitary gland). If the tumor is only in the midline and is extradural, an anterior approach is used. This may be performed through two routes: (1) by traversing the sinuses and resecting the tumor through an opening in the posterior wall of the sphenoid sinus or nasopharynx, or (2) via a transoral approach and tumor resection through the posterior pharyngeal wall. CSF leak through contaminated oral or nasal passageways can be a serious complication of these anterior approaches. If the tumor extends laterally or intradurally, a lateral approach should be used. Lateral approaches include an infratemporal fossa approach (Fisch Type B or C), a middle fossa-transpetrous approach with removal of the anterior petrous apex (Kawase triangle) (see Figure 65–2), or a combined subtemporal-retrolabyrinthine approach (see Figure 65–3).

Prognosis

Postoperative radiation therapy may play a role in reducing recurrence, although data are lacking. Although metastases are distinctly uncommon, the natural history of this disease is local recurrence with eventual mortality. The 5-year survival rate ranges widely from 35% to 85%, depending on the amount of tumor removal achieved at surgery.

3. Meningioma

General Considerations

Meningiomas arise from arachnoidal cap cells associated with arachnoid villi. Within the posterior cranial fossa, these tumors can be found along the dura anywhere from the sigmoid sinus (posteriorly) to the cavernous sinus (anteriorly). Similar to schwannomas, meningiomas are usually sporadic, but they are also associated with neurofibromatosis Type II. Although most meningiomas are benign, 5% have malignant cell characteristics as well as a tendency for early and aggressive recurrence. Meningiomas usually grow slowly by expanding into the cerebellopontine angle or along the Meckel cave (around the gasserian ganglion). However, any posterior fossa meningioma also has the potential to invade the temporal bone.

Clinical Findings

A. SYMPTOMS AND SIGNS

Patients with meningiomas may present with hearing loss from tumor expansion into the IAC, the inner ear (sensorineural loss), or the middle ear (conductive loss). Jugular foramen syndrome, which includes dysphagia, vocal cord paralysis, and shoulder weakness, may be present if the tumor infiltrates cranial nerves IX, X, and XI of the jugular foramen.

B. IMAGING STUDIES

On CT scan, meningiomas demonstrate hyperostosis of the adjacent bone and calcification within the tumor on CT scan. The tumors have intermediate intensity on both T1- and T2-weighted MRI. They enhance strongly with contrast and show a characteristic "dural tail," with enhancement of the dura bordering the tumor mass because of its infiltration within the tumor; this finding is a key diagnostic difference between meningioma and schwannoma. Flow voids may be noted on larger tumors, and occasionally angiography with embolization is useful as a preoperative measure to reduce blood loss during a planned surgery.

Treatment

The treatment of meningiomas includes observation with serial MRI, stereotactic radiation, and surgery. In a younger patient with a larger tumor, surgery is usually recommended, whereas in an older patient with minimal symptoms, observation or radiation should be considered. Surgical resection depends on the tumor location but often requires a retrosigmoidal or combined subtemporal-retrolabyrinthine approach (see Figure 65–3). Although the complete resection of these infiltrative tumors is nearly impossible, a good subtotal resection, sparing vital neurovascular structures, is adequate. If the tumor recurs, further resection or radiation therapy can be performed.

4. Intralabyrinthine Schwannoma

General Considerations

In general, vestibular schwannomas are usually found within the IAC. However, they can arise anywhere Schwann cells are present, which extends from the oligodendrogliocyte-Schwann cell junction (the Obersteiner-Redlich zone) near the porus acousticus to the hair cells of the inner ear.

Clinical Findings

A. SYMPTOMS AND SIGNS

Patients with a vestibular schwannoma arising within the inner ear labyrinth have symptomatology similar to those with a vestibular schwannoma arising within the IAC. Vague imbalance, unilateral tinnitus, and asymmetric hearing loss are the common presenting symptoms.

B. IMAGING STUDIES

Imaging features include an enhancing mass within the inner ear on gadolinium contrast T1-weighted MRI, which simulates acute labyrinthitis. However, the absence of fluid density within the inner ear on T2-weighted MRI is what differentiates these two processes. Of note, the bone of the otic capsule is usually not expanded by the tumor. Indeed, these tumors continue to grow by slowly filling the entire labyrinth before bone erosion occurs.

Treatment

If the only symptom is mild sensorineural hearing loss, the treatment is usually observation. Surgical resection requires labyrinthectomy and results in profound hearing loss in the affected ear. If chronic dysequilibrium develops, surgical excision by a transcochlear approach (through both the vestibular labyrinth and the cochlea) is warranted.

5. Schwannomas of the Jugular Foramen, Jacobson Nerve, & Arnold Nerve

General Considerations

Besides seventh and eighth cranial nerve schwannomas, schwannomas can also arise from other nerves that pass through the temporal bone. Cranial nerves IX, X, and XI run from the brainstem through the jugular foramen and down into the neck. These nerves are located medial to the jugular vein at the skull base. Jacobson nerve is a branch of cranial nerve IX that runs along the promontory of the middle ear, supplying sensation and parasympathetic fibers to the parotid gland. Arnold nerve is a branch of cranial nerve X that carries fibers that supply sensory innervation to the ear canal.

Clinical Findings

Patients with a jugular foramen schwannoma present with dysphagia, hoarseness due to vocal cord paralysis, and shoulder weakness. A middle ear mass may also be noted. Patients with a schwannoma of Jacobson or Arnold nerves present with conductive hearing loss and have a bulging, white middle ear mass on otoscopy. Like all schwannomas, these tumors are smooth and gently erode the surrounding bone. They enhance on gadolinium contrast MRI.

Treatment

Treatment is surgical resection. Schwannomas of the lower cranial nerves require a transtemporal approach to the jugular foramen, like the Fisch Type A approach (see Figure 65–2A) or transjugular craniotomy, although often the facial nerve does not require rerouting and the ear canal does not need to be closed off, preserving hearing.

6. Rhabdomyosarcoma

General Considerations

Rhabdomyosarcoma is the most common soft tissue sarcoma in children, accounting for 5–15% of all childhood cancers. The average age at presentation is 4.4 years.

Clinical Findings

A. SYMPTOMS AND SIGNS

Rhabdomyosarcoma involving the temporal bone presents as chronic otitis media recalcitrant to antibiotic therapy. Otorrhea, earache, and an aural polyp are commonly noted. This disease process is highly aggressive. Local destruction of surrounding bone can produce either conductive or sensorineural hearing loss. Facial nerve paralysis can manifest if the mastoid or middle ear is involved with tumor. If the petrous apex is involved, facial numbness, diplopia, or both can be exhibited owing to involvement of cranial nerves V and VI. Extension of tumor to the internal auditory canal and cerebellopontine angle can also develop.

B. IMAGING STUDIES

CT scanning demonstrates an enhancing soft tissue mass with bony destruction. MRI shows an intermedi-

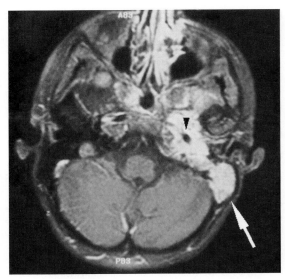

Figure 65–8. Rhabdomyosarcoma. Axial view, T1-weighted image MRI with gadolinium contrast demonstrates a large enhancing tumor involving the entire temporal bone (arrow) and surrounding the internal carotid artery (arrowhead).

ate-intensity mass on T1-weighted imaging and a high-intensity mass on T2-weighted images (Figure 65–8). The lesion enhances with gadolinium contrast.

Treatment & Prognosis

Initially, a biopsy of the temporal bone mass must be performed, which may require a mastoidectomy through a postauricular incision if no aural polyp is available to biopsy. Treatment is based upon chemotherapy and external beam radiation therapy. There are five histologic subtypes of rhabdomyosarcoma: (1) pleomorphic (5%), (2) alveolar (20%), (3) embryonal (55%), (4) botryoid (5%), and (5) mixed. The botryoid and pleomorphic subtypes have a favorable prognosis, the embryonal subtype has an intermediate prognosis, and the alveolar and mixed subtypes have an unfavorable prognosis. The prognosis is also worsened if distant metastases have developed.

7. Osteosarcoma

Osteosarcoma is extremely rare within the temporal bone. It presents as a rapid, painful swelling of the bone and is most often found in patients between the ages of 10 and 30. Imaging characteristics depend on the amount of osteoblastic and osteolytic activity of the tumor. An enhancing soft tissue mass may be present. If the tumor has osteoblastic components, concentric rings are usually seen, termed "onion skinning." The treatment is surgical resection followed by chemotherapy and radiation therapy. Patients have a 5-year survival rate of 9%.

8. Fibrosarcoma

More than half of all fibrosarcomas are diagnosed within the first year of life, with less than 2% occurring in the head and neck. This tumor may appear as a soft tissue tumor within the temporal bone with local bony destruction. Treatment is surgical resection. Often, preoperative chemotherapy can be attempted to reduce the tumor mass, permitting a more conservative resection. The prognosis is good, with 5-year survival rates of 84–92%.

9. Hemangiopericytoma

Hemangiopericytoma is a malignant vascular neoplasm arising from the contractile cells around blood vessels, the "pericytes of Zimmerman." These mesenchymal tumors arise within the musculoskeletal system and rarely may arise within the middle ear cleft. Pathologically, sheets of spindle-shaped tumor cells with numerous vascular channels are noted. Treatment is based upon complete surgical resection, with consideration of postoperative radiation. Metastases occur in about 50% of cases, predominantly to the lung, bones, and liver.

10. Adenoma

Middle ear adenomas are rare tumors that arise from the middle ear mucosa. Patients with these neoplasms present with conductive hearing loss because the mass compresses the ossicular chain. Examination reveals a middle ear mass that enhances on gadolinium contrast MRI. An aural polyp may also be noted. The differential diagnosis includes glomus tympanicum tumors and schwannomas of the facial, Jacobson, or Arnold nerve. Treatment is middle ear exploration and resection. These are benign tumors with minimal propensity for malignant degeneration.

11. Endolymphatic Sac Neoplasms (Papillary Adenocarcinoma)

General Considerations

Endolymphatic sac tumors are extremely uncommon and are most often identified in young patients with von Hippel-Lindau disease, an autosomal dominant disease with multiple central nervous system and retinal hemangioblastomas, renal cell carcinoma, pancreatic cysts, and islet cell tumors. Von Hippel-Lindau disease is caused by germline mutations of the tumor suppressor gene located on chromosome 3p25. Isolated endolymphatic sac tumors can occur as well. Tumors arise from the cuboi-

dal epithelium of the endolymphatic sac and are low-grade adenocarcinomas, with both papillary and cystic areas. They are highly vascular. The hallmark of these tumors is that they invade the inner ear and infiltrate bone, including the otic capsule.

Clinical Findings

A. Symptoms and Signs

The aggressive, infiltrative behavior of these tumors leads to the primary symptoms of sensorineural hearing loss, pulsatile tinnitus, imbalance, and facial nerve paralysis. Physical examination may demonstrate a reddish-purple middle ear mass on otoscopy that originates from the mastoid.

B. Imaging Studies

CT and MRI demonstrate an enhancing mass based in the posterior cranial fossa with significant erosion of the posterior face of the temporal bone and the otic capsule (Figure 65–9). The signal intensity on T1- and T2-weighted images without contrast is heterogeneous because of areas of mucin collection with variable protein and fluid content.

Treatment

Treatment is complete surgical excision, usually via a transcochlear approach with obliteration of the middle ear and mastoid and with closure of the external auditory canal. The dura of the posterior and possibly the middle cranial fossa also need to be resected. If the disease extends intradurally, this also needs to be removed. Close follow-up of these patients is indicated, reserving the use of radiation therapy for unresectable, recurrent disease.

12. Carcinoma

Carcinoma arising primarily within the temporal bone is rare. However, the mucosa of the middle ear may dedifferentiate into carcinoma, including squamous cell carcinoma and adenocarcinoma. Patients with squamous cell carcinoma originating from the middle ear have a high likelihood of having had a long history of chronic otitis media, suggesting that squamous metaplasia with subsequent chronic inflammation may underlie the etiology of the tumor. More commonly, patients have squamous cell carcinoma that originated from the skin of the ear canal and has grown medial to the tympanic membrane, invading the temporal bone. These tumors present in middle-aged adults as a painful, chronically draining ear. An aural polyp or external auditory canal lesion may be noted. These patients are usually treated with a temporal bone resection, parotidectomy, and neck dissection. A free flap or regional myocutaneous flap may be needed to

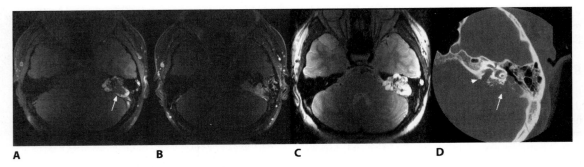

Figure 65–9. Endolymphatic sac tumor. Axial views. **(A)** T1-weighted MRI demonstrates an infiltrative tumor of the posterior temporal bone (arrow) with some areas of low intensity (representing tumor) and some areas of high intensity (representing proteinaceous fluid). **(B)** The addition of gadolinium contrasts makes the entire tumor of high signal intensity. **(C)** T2-weighted MRI demonstrates high signal intensity. **(D)** CT scan of the temporal bone demonstrates significant bony destruction of both the mastoid air cells and the otic capsule bone (arrow). The internal auditory canal (arrowhead) is infiltrated with tumor.

close a soft tissue defect. Postoperative radiation therapy is usually given.

13. Metastatic Disease

General Considerations

The most common primary sites of malignant growth that spreads to the temporal bone are the breasts (25%), the lungs (11%), the kidneys (9%), the stomach (6%), the bronchus (6%), and the prostate (6%). The most common route of metastasis to the temporal bone is via hematogenous spread. The most common site of disease metastatic to the temporal bone is the petrous apex (33%), and the second most common is the internal auditory canal (16%).

Clinical Findings

A. SYMPTOMS AND SIGNS

Growth of the lesion may interfere with eustachian tube function, producing middle ear effusion and conductive hearing loss. The facial nerve and inner ear may become infiltrated as well. The most common symptoms of metastasis to the temporal bone are hearing loss (60%), facial paralysis (50%), and vertigo (30%). Commonly, these symptoms are overshadowed by other systemic symptoms because temporal bone metastases occur late in the disease process. Meningeal carcinomatosis can also occur, producing headache, altered mental status, and cranial neuropathy. Concurrent brain metastasis can be found in 26% of patients.

B. IMAGING STUDIES

CT scanning usually reveals an osteolytic lesion, although breast and prostate metastatic lesions may demonstrate new bone growth consistent with osteoblastic activity. MRI reveals an intermediate signal intensity on T1-weighted images and a high signal intensity on T2-weighted images. The lesion enhances brightly with gadolinium contrast. A bone scan can be quite useful in making the diagnosis of metastasis.

Treatment & Prognosis

Treatment for temporal bone metastasis is directed toward palliative care. The prognosis for these patients is universally poor. External-beam radiation therapy or radiation therapy can be offered to the patient with symptomatic temporal bone metastasis.

Colli B, Al-Mefty O. Chordomas of the craniocervical junction: follow-up review and prognostic factors. *J Neurosurg.* 2001;95:933. [PMID: 11765837] (Review of the management of chordomas.)

Oghalai JS, Buxbaum JL, Jackler RK, McDermott MW. Skull base chondrosarcoma originating from the petroclival junction. *Otol Neurotol.* 2005;26:1052. [PMID: 16151358] (Review of chondrosarcoma.)

Oghalai JS, Jackler RK. Anatomy of the combined retrolabyrinthine-middle fossa craniotomy. *Neurosurg Focus.* 2003;14:e8. [PMID: 15669793] (Surgical approach for petro-clival lesions.)

Neurotologic Skull Base Surgery

66

Robert K. Jackler, MD

Although in widespread use, the term "skull base surgery" is somewhat of a misnomer. Only a minority of such procedures are undertaken to expose lesions actually located primarily within the skull base. Most procedures are conducted to expose deep-seated intracranial lesions situated either adjacent to the brainstem (eg, midbrain, pons, or medulla) or beneath the cerebral cortex. Previously, many such tumors were approached via simple openings in the calvaria, which require vigorous and often injurious degrees of brain retraction.

The fundamental principle in transbasal craniotomy is removal of the skull base bone to minimize the need for brain retraction. Although current techniques represent a major enhancement in our ability to control inaccessible tumors while minimizing morbidity, they are not panaceas. For example, experience has shown that these procedures are far more suitable for benign lesions (eg, meningiomas, schwannomas, and paragangliomas) and even for low-grade malignant growths (eg, chordomas and chondrosarcomas) than for high-grade malignant lesions (eg, squamous cell carcinoma, adenocystic carcinoma, and soft tissue sarcomas). Currently, more emphasis is placed on the preservation of function, especially cranial nerves, than on the necessity for radical resection in every case. The value of neurophysiologic nerve monitoring for motor nerves within the surgical field has become well established. In the developmental years of skull base surgery, two-stage procedures were common. More recently, single-stage procedures have become preferred in most centers, even for tumors with sizable intra- and extracranial components, as well as those involving multiple cranial fossae. Computerized imaging modalities provide localizing information that guides the surgeon around vital structures and helps to enable thorough tumor removal.

Jung HW, Yoo H, Paek SH, Choi KS. Long-term outcome and growth rate of subtotally resected petroclival meningiomas: experience with 38 cases. *Neurosurgery.* 2000;46(3):567. [PMID: 10719852]

Kurtsoy A, Menku A, Tucer B, Oktem IS, Akdemir H. Neuronavigation in skull base tumors. *Min Invas Neurosurg.* 2005;48(1):7. [PMID: 15747210]

APPROACHES TO CRANIAL BASE LESIONS

TEMPORAL BONE

Temporal bone resection is a fairly radical operation conducted for malignant disease, particularly squamous cell carcinoma originating in the external auditory canal. Some other indications include adenomatous tumors, such as the aggressive papillary adenocarcinoma of the endolymphatic sac and those arising in salivary tissue (eg, adenocystic carcinoma). In most cases, the lateral portion of the temporal bone housing the ear canal is removed en bloc (Figure 66–1). The posterior margin consists of the dural lining of the petrous pyramid, which is exposed via mastoidectomy. The anterior margin often includes some or all of the parotid gland and, at times, the mandibular condyle and the temporomandibular joint (Figure 66–2).

Most surgeons remove more deeply involved regions (eg, the cochlea, semicircular canal, and internal auditory canal) piecemeal, using a high-speed drill as resection en bloc risks injury to the internal carotid artery. In advanced lesions, the resection can be carried medially to the internal carotid artery, but its resection is seldom justified. After resection of the condyle, exenteration of the pterygoid muscles, including the third division of the trigeminal nerve to the level of the pterygoid plates, may be accomplished in deeply penetrating lesions. As a general rule, if the facial nerve works preoperatively, a diligent effort should be made to preserve it, although this is not always feasible and engraftment may be needed.

Reconstruction of the defect needs to anticipate the need for radiation therapy. Leaving an open cavity increases the risk of osteoradionecrosis. For this reason, the external auditory meatus is typically sewn shut. A rotation flap of temporalis muscle is often desirable to reinforce the closure with well-vascularized tissue. Regional (eg, pectoralis or trapezius) or even free (rectus abdominis) flaps may be needed for closure in cases where auriculectomy has been required.

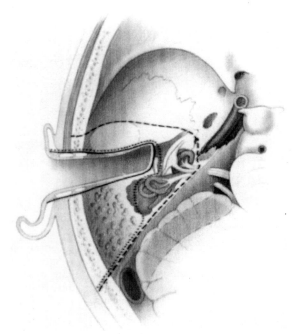

Figure 66–1. The degrees of temporal bone resection. The solid lines demarcate the so-called sleeve resection of the soft tissue of the canal. This is an insufficient approach to malignant tumors of the region. The dotted lines depict subtotal temporal bone resection. The dashed lines illustrate total temporal bone resection. (Reprinted with permission of Jackler RK.)

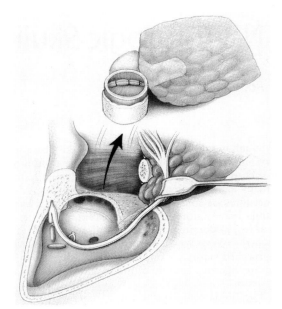

Figure 66–2. Temporal bone resection with a specimen, en bloc, including the external auditory canal, the mandibular condyle, and a portion of the parotid gland. (Reprinted with permission of Jackler RK.)

Jackler RK, Driscoll C. *Tumors of the Ear and Temporal Bone.* Philadelphia: Lippincott Williams & Wilkins, 2000.

Nyrop M, Grontved A. Cancer of the external auditory canal. *Arch Otolaryngol Head Neck Surg.* 2002;128(7):834. [PMID: 12117346]

PETROUS APEX, PETROCLIVAL JUNCTION, & FORAMEN LACERUM

1. Petrous Apicotomy

The majority of procedures conducted for disease in the petrous apex involves creation of a narrow drainage pathway that circumnavigates the inner ear. Such procedures, which are usually carried out to drain petrositis or cholesterol granulomas, are best termed petrous apicotomy (Figure 66–3). In the subcochlear route, a channel is excavated along the floor of the external auditory canal and the hypotympanum, which traverses the narrow window between the cochlea, the carotid genu, and the dome of the jugular bulb.

An alternate pathway is the infralabyrinthine approach, conducted between the posterior semicircular canal and the jugular bulb, immediately behind the descending portion of the facial nerve. However, because most apical cysts

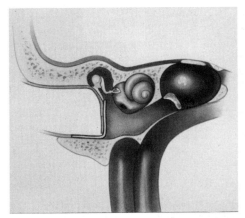

Figure 66–3. Petrous apicotomy is a narrow drainage opening created circumventing the inner ear to drain an apical fluid collection (cholesterol granuloma or infection). (Reprinted with permission of Jackler RK.)

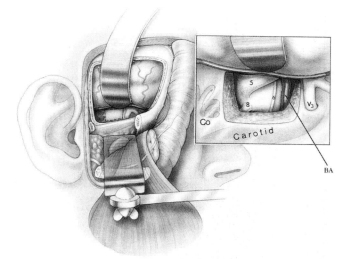

Figure 66–4. Petrous apicectomy is the surgical resection of the petrous apex and is carried out through a subtemporal exposure of the ventral surface of the petrous pyramid. Note the transapical view of the superior aspect of the cerebellopontine angle. Downward displacement of the zygomatic arch is optional. BA, basilar artery; Co, cochlear. (Reprinted with permission of Jackler RK.)

are located anteriorly medial to the cochlea, the infralabyrinthine route is deeper, more difficult, and creates a less adequate drainage portal.

Brackmann DE, Toh EH. Surgical management of petrous apex cholesterol granulomas. *Otol Neurotol.* 2002;23(4):529. [PMID: 12170157]

Jacob CE, Rupa V. Infralabyrinthine approach to the petrous apex. *Clin Anat.* 2005;18(6):423. [PMID: 1601561]

Telischi FF, Luntz M, Whiteman ML. Supracochlear approach to the petrous apex: case report and anatomic study. *Am J Otol.* 1999;20(4):500. [PMID: 10431893]

2. Petrous Apicectomy

Petrous apicectomy, the formal removal of the petrous apex, is conducted for neoplasms of the apex and petroclival junction. It is conducted via a low subtemporal craniotomy, which exposes the anterior face of the petrous pyramid (Figure 66–4). Anatomically, the resection is limited inferiorly by the horizontal portion of the internal carotid artery, laterally by the cochlea and internal auditory canal, and medially by Meckel cave and the trigeminal nerve. Exposing the infratemporal fossa beneath the internal carotid artery requires downfracture and subsequent repair of the zygomatic arch. The characteristic tumor of this region is the chondrosarcoma of the petroclival junction, which arises in the cartilaginous section of the foramen lacerum (Figure 66–5). Although it is not often necessary, apicectomy is sometimes used for the resection of cholesterol granulomas that have proven recalcitrant to drainage procedures.

Oghalai JS, Buxbaum JL, Jackler RK, McDermott MW. Skull base chondrosarcoma originating from the petroclival junction. *Otol Neurotol.* 2005;26(5):1052. [PMID: 16151358]

CLIVUS

The clivus is not a bone in and of itself, but is rather a region composed of the dorsal part of the sphenoid bone and the portion of the occipital bone located anterior to the foramen magnum. The clivus, which, in Latin, means *slope*, spans from the posterior clinoid to the anterior margin of the foramen magnum. Adjacent to its dorsal surface is the entire brainstem and the vertebrobasilar system. The subject of clival tumors falls into two categories: (1) intrinsic tumors (especially chordo-

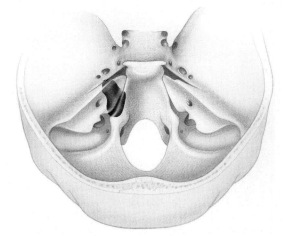

Figure 66–5. Chondrosarcoma of the petroclival junction arising from the cartilage of foramen lacerum. (Reprinted with permission of Jackler RK.)

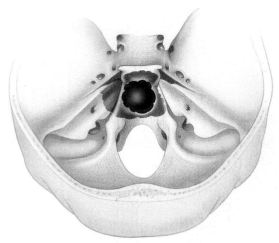

Figure 66–6. Chordoma of the clivus with intracranial involvement due to breaching of the dorsal clival surface. (Reprinted with permission of Jackler RK.)

mas) and (2) meningiomas arising from the dural lining of its dorsal surface.

Chordomas arise from notochordal remnants in the midline of the skull base (Figure 66–6). Initially, they grow to fill the clival marrow compartment but later erode its cortical plate to spread intradurally. This brings them into contact with the brainstem, which may be compressed posteriorly. Intrinsic clival lesions, which remain extradural, are approached anteriorly via either a **transsphenoethmoidal** or **transoral approach.** The transsphenoethmoidal approach is well suited for lesions of the mid- and upper clivus, whereas the transoral approach is preferred when lower clival and craniovertebral junction exposure is needed. Recently, endoscopic techniques are increasingly used in surgery of clival tumors.

Enepekides DJ, Donald PJ. Transoral approaches to the clivus and nasopharynx. *Otolaryngol Clin N Am.* 2001;34(6):1105. [PMID: 11728936]

Solares CA, Fakhri S, Batra PS, Lee J, Lanza DC. Transnasal endoscopic resection of lesions of the clivus: a preliminary report. *Laryngoscope.* 2005;115(11):1917. [PMID: 16319599]

JUGULAR FORAMEN

The jugular foramen is traversed by the jugular vein and the three lower cranial nerves (CN IX, the glossopharyngeal nerve; CN X, the vagus nerve; and CN XI, the accessory nerve). The vertical segment of the facial nerve lies immediately lateral to the jugular foramen, presenting one of the classic challenges in cranial base surgery. The dome of the jugular bulb approaches the hypotympanic portion of the middle ear. Three tumor types predominate in tumors of this region: (1) glomus jugulare tumors, (2) meningiomas, and (3) lower cranial nerve schwannomas. These may remain confined to the cranial base, but most often possess a component in the upper neck, posterior cranial fossa, or both (Figure 66–7).

The jugular foramen approach begins control of the great vessels in the upper neck (Figure 66–8). Exposure of the foramen itself commences with a mastoidectomy and decompression of the bony covering of the sigmoid sinus. After skeletonization of the descending fallopian canal, the lateral aspect of the jugular foramen is exposed. Tumor resection commences after connecting the skull base and neck dissection followed by proximal and distal occlusion of the jugular vein (Figure 66–9).

Traditionally, many surgeons rerouted the facial nerve anterior to obtain unobstructed access to the jugular foramen. However, this frequently leads to transient palsy, which does not always recover to normal. More recently, a **fallopian bridge** technique has gained popularity. In this procedure, the facial nerve remains in situ, and microdissection is carried out around it (Figure 66–10). Some surgeons use facial

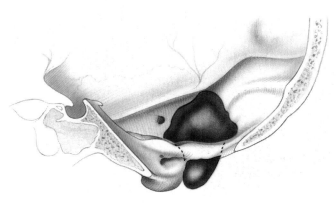

Figure 66–7. Jugular foramen tumor with intracranial, foraminal, and extracranial component. (Reprinted with permission of Jackler RK.)

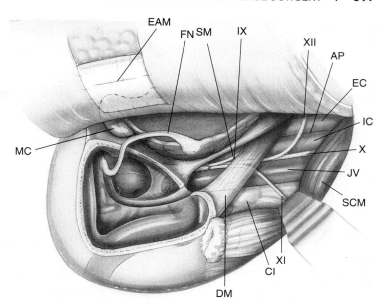

Figure 66–8. Surgical exposure of the jugular foramen region after mastoidectomy, anterior rerouting of the facial nerve, and upper neck dissection. MC, mandibular condyle; EAM, closed external auditory meatus; FN, facial nerve; SM, styloid muscle; IX, glossopharyngeal nerve; DM, digastric muscle; C1, the transverse process of C1; XI, accessory nerve; XII, hypoglossal nerve; AP, ascending pharyngeal artery; EC, external carotid artery; IC, internal carotid artery; X, vagus nerve; JV, jugular vein; SCM, sternocleidomastoid muscle. (Reprinted with permission of Jackler RK.)

nerve rerouting selectively when encasement of the carotid artery necessitates obtaining augmented anterior exposure.

Meningiomas and glomus tumors both have a proclivity for growing proximally into the sigmoid sinus and distally into the jugular view. Meningiomas and schwannomas are also more likely to involve the neural plane containing cranial nerves IX–XI, although these structures may certainly become involved with larger paragangliomas as well. To reduce blood loss and facilitate orderly microdissection, preoperative embolization is usually conducted. Tumor removal is conducted piecemeal, with resection of involved segments of the sigmoid-jugular system (typically occluded from disease) as required. Although preservation of the stout cranial nerves in the neck is usually readily accomplished, the multiple fine neural branches of the jugular foramen region can be a challenge to preserve when infiltrated by tumor. In such cases, meticulous microdissection, guided by neurophysiologic monitoring, can sometimes be rewarded by preservation of part or all of the lower nerve branches.

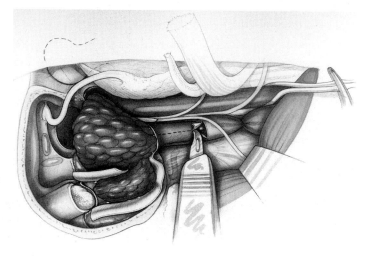

Figure 66–9. Large glomus jugulare tumor with retrograde spread into the sigmoid sinus and distal involvement of the lumen of the jugular vein. The hypotympanum is extensively eroded. (Reprinted with permission of Jackler RK.)

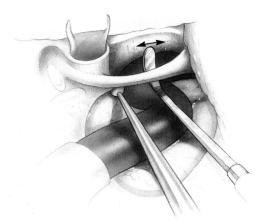

Figure 66–10. Fallopian bridge approach to the jugular foramen, leaving the descending facial nerve in situ. (Reprinted with permission of Jackler RK.)

The removal of jugular foramen tumors can often be accomplished with preservation of the auditory apparatus. Resection of the middle ear and ear canal with closure of the meatus is necessary under two circumstances: (1) extensive destruction of the ear canal and (2) substantial involvement of the carotid genu (Figure 66–11). Intradural penetration of jugular foramen tumors will be discussed with transjugular craniotomy.

Gilbert ME, Shelton C, McDonald A et al. Meningioma of the jugular foramen: glomus jugulare mimic and surgical challenge. *Laryngoscope.* 2004;114(1):25. [PMID: 14709990]

Jackson CG. Glomus tympanicum and glomus jugulare tumors. *Otolaryngol Clin North Am.* 2001;34(5):941. [PMID: 11557448]

Pensak ML, Jackler RK. Removal of jugular foramen tumors: the fallopian bridge technique. *Otolaryngol Head Neck Surg.* 1997; 117(6):586. [PMID: 9419083]

Tekdemir I, Tuccar E, Aslan A, Elhan A, Ersoy M, Deda H. Comprehensive microsurgical anatomy of the jugular foramen and review of terminology. *J Clin Neurosci.* 2001;8(4):351. [PMID: 11437579]

Wilson MA, Hillman TA, Wiggins RH, Shelton C. Jugular foramen schwannomas: diagnosis, management, and outcomes. *Laryngoscope.* 2005;115(8):1486. [PMID: 16094130]

INFRATEMPORAL FOSSA

The infratemporal fossa is not a well-demarcated anatomic compartment but is rather the region of the upper neck that lies beneath the temporal bone and the sphenoid wing. Within it are the jugular vein, the carotid artery, the styloid process, the third division of the trigeminal nerve, the eustachian tube, the pterygoid muscles and their associated bony plates, and a rather impressive venous plexus. Laterally, the infratemporal fossa is defended by the mandible (condyle and ramus) and the zygomatic arch. Medially, it is bounded by the nasopharynx and the lateral wall of the sphenoid sinus. As previously mentioned, jugular foramen tumors often involve the superficial portion of the infratemporal fossa in proximity to the great vessels. Tumors involving the deeper regions include trigeminal schwannomas in the vicinity of the foramen ovale and penetrating malignant neoplasms such as those from the deep lobe of the parotid gland and ear. The most common tumor involving the deep aspect of the infratemporal fossa is nasopharyngeal carcinoma.

Lesions involving the lateral portion of the infratemporal fossa, such as glomus jugulare tumors, are approached via a postauricular incision and include some degree of temporal bone surgery. More anteriorly situated lesions are approached preauricularly, often with access gained through downfracture of the zygomatic arch and either downward displacement or resection of the condyle. When necessitated by penetration of the skull base, the exposure can be combined with middle fossa craniotomy. Resection of the glenoid fossa and division of V3 is needed to expose Meckel cave and the cavernous sinus from this perspective. A reasonably functional pseudoarthrosis usu-

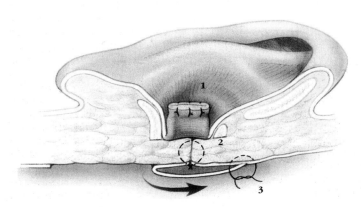

Figure 66–11. Ear canal closure is carried out with a meticulous three-layer technique to withstand cerebrospinal fluid pressure, if necessary. 1, everted canal skin; 2, subcutaneous tissue; 3, periosteum. (Reprinted with permission of Jackler RK.)

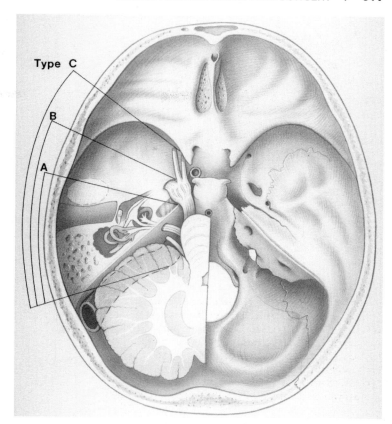

Figure 66–12. Infratemporal fossa approaches types A, B, and C (after Fisch). (Reprinted with permission of Jackler RK.)

ally forms after resection of the glenoid. In one commonly used system of nomenclature, the various depths of infratemporal fossa dissection are referred to as approaches A, B, and C (Figures 66–12 and 66–13).

■ TRANSBASAL APPROACHES TO INTRACRANIAL NEOPLASMS

INTERNAL AUDITORY CANAL & CEREBELLOPONTINE ANGLE

Surgery of tumors of the internal auditory canal (IAC) and cerebellopontine angle (CPA) is a central issue to neurotology. Some of the complex issues in this involved subject are considered, in greater depth, in the chapter that discusses vestibular schwannomas (see Chapter 56, Vestibular Disorders). A decision among the three approaches in widespread use (translabyrinthine, retrosigmoidal, and middle fossa) depends on a number of variables such as size, shape, anatomic location, and pathologic type of tumor, as well as status of hearing (Figure 66–14).

1. Retrosigmoidal Approach

The retrosigmoidal approach is a classic means of exposing the CPA (Figures 66–15, 66–16, and 66–17). It provides wide access to the CPA from the tentorium to the foramen magnum. Although not relevant in vestibular schwannoma surgery, the retrosigmoidal approach provides enhanced access to the inferior region of the CPA when compared with the translabyrinthine approach. The opening is created by removing the calvaria immediately behind the sigmoid and below the transverse sinus. Retraction of the cerebellar hemisphere brings the CPA into view. Access to the IAC is obtained by drilling off its posterior bony lip. Approximately the medial two thirds of the IAC can be exposed without violating a portion of the inner ear. Thus, when the fundus of the canal is involved, direct exposure of the deepest portion of the tumor in the IAC precludes an attempt at hearing conservation. The primary disadvantage of the retrosigmoidal approach is a higher incidence of persistent headache

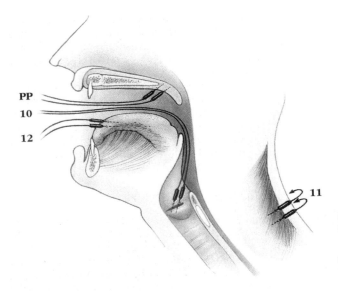

Figure 66–13. Neurophysiologic monitoring of the lower cranial nerves in jugular foramen surgery. 10, vagus nerve; 11, accessory nerve; 12, hypoglossal nerve; PP, pharyngeal plexus. (Reprinted with permission of Jackler RK.)

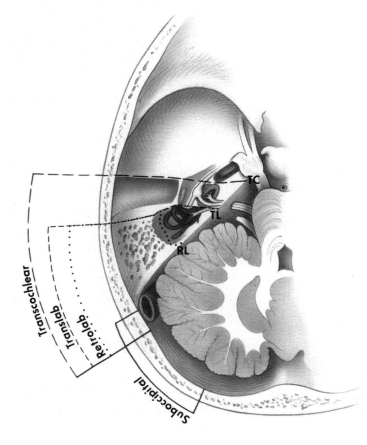

Figure 66–14. Overview of posterior fossa approaches to the cerebellopontine angle: retrosigmoidal, retrolabyrinthine, translabyrinthine, and transcochlear. (Reprinted with permission of Jackler RK.)

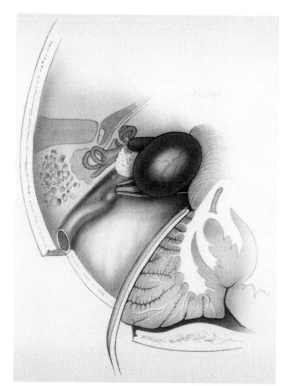

Figure 66–15. Overview of the retrosigmoidal approach from an axial perspective. Note the removal of the posterior lip of the internal auditory canal. (Reprinted with permission of Jackler RK.)

when compared with the translabyrinthine or middle fossa approaches. Although still used routinely as a hearing conservation method in many centers, comparison data show that the middle fossa approach appears to be more successful in this regard, at least for tumors with modest-sized components within the CPA.

2. Translabyrinthine Approach

The translabyrinthine approach provides direct exposure of the CPA through the petrous pyramid, the shortest route from the surface (Figures 66–18 and 66–19). When properly performed, it provides excellent exposure of the lateral aspect of the pons and upper medulla. Exposure of the CPA is bounded superiorly by the tentorium cerebelli and inferiorly by the limitation imposed by the sigmoid sinus and jugular bulb. Because the opening provided by petrosectomy alone is fairly narrow, the exposure is augmented by removing the bone overlying the sigmoid sinus and a variable degree of retrosigmoidal posterior fossa dura (depending on the amount of posterior fossa expo-

sure required). After mastoidectomy and decompression of the sigmoid sinus, removal of the semicircular canals brings into view the bone surrounding the IAC. Excavations around the IAC place it into high relief so that it is fully accessible for microsurgical dissection.

The translabyrinthine approach is primarily used for vestibular schwannomas, although it has some role in posterior fossa meningioma surgery as well. Since a portion of the inner ear is removed during the craniotomy, in most centers, this approach is used either for CPA tumors associated with poor hearing or for patients in whom hearing preservation is not a realistic option.

3. Middle Fossa Approach

The middle fossa approach provides exposure to the IAC from above and limited access to the CPA (Figure 66–20). Most centers do not use this approach for tumors exceeding approximately 1.5 cm in CPA diameter. After removal of an approximately 3.0-cm by 3.0-cm plate of calvaria above the ear, the temporal lobe is elevated extradurally off the petrous floor. With the exposure maintained through a specially designed retractor, the bone is removed from the superior aspect of the IAC. Wide excavation of the petrous apex and the region of the porus acusticus provides limited access to the CPA from above. The primary advantage of the middle fossa approach is its superior ability to preserve hearing. The primary disadvantage is the inconvenient location of the facial nerve on the superior surface of the tumor that must be manipulated to a greater degree and thus has a higher rate of temporary postoperative dysfunction.

Baumann I, Polligkeit J, Blumenstock G, Mauz PS, Zalaman IM, Maassen MM. Quality of life after unilateral acoustic neuroma surgery via middle cranial fossa approach. *Acta Otolaryngol.* 2005;125(6):585. [PMID: 16076706]

Ciric I, Zhao JC, Rosenblatt S, Wiet R, O'Shaughnessy B. Suboccipital retrosigmoid approach for removal of vestibular schwannomas: facial nerve function and hearing preservation. *Neurosurgery.* 2005;56(3):560; discussion 560. [PMID: 15730582]

Day JD, Chen DA, Arriaga M. Translabyrinthine approach for acoustic neuroma. *Neurosurgery.* 2004;54(2):391. [PMID: 14744286]

Sharp MC, MacFarlane R, Hardy DG, Jones SE, Baguley DM, Moffat DA. Team working to improve outcome in vestibular schwannoma surgery. *Br J Neurosurg.* 2005;19(2):122. [PMID: 16120514]

INTRACRANIAL ASPECTS OF THE JUGULAR FORAMEN

Meningiomas, schwannomas, and paragangliomas frequently extend intracranially. Meningiomas and schwannomas originate in the intracranial compartment, whereas glomus tumors spread posteriorly from their

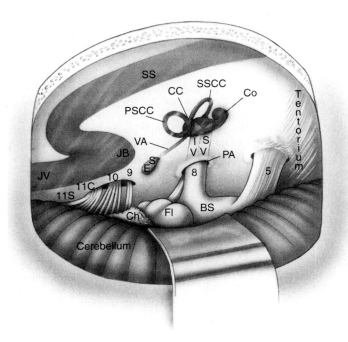

Figure 66–16. Operative view of the cerebellopontine angle via the retrosigmoidal approach. JV, jugular vein; JB, jugular bulb; 11S, spinal root of accessory nerve; 11C, cranial root of accessory nerve; 10, vagus nerve; 9, glossopharyngeal nerve; ES, endolymphatic sac; VA, vestibular aqueduct; PSCC, posterior semicircular canal; CC, common crus; SSCC, superior semicircular canal; Co, cochlea; IV, inferior vestibular nerve; SV, superior vestibular nerve; PA, porus acusticus; Ch, choroids plexus; Fl, flocculus; BS, brainstem; 7, facial nerve; 8, audiovestibular nerve; 5, trigeminal nerve. (Reprinted with permission of Jackler RK.)

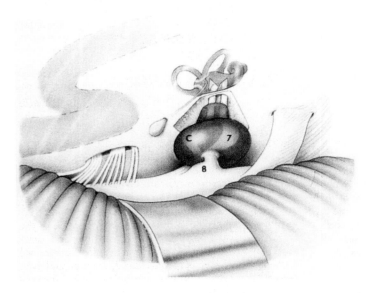

Figure 66–17. Retrosigmoidal approach to a small vestibular schwannoma that extends only partly down the internal auditory canal. Note that the inner ear overlies the lateral one third of the internal auditory canal. C, cochlear nerve; 7, facial nerve; 8, audiovestibular nerve. (Reprinted with permission of Jackler RK.)

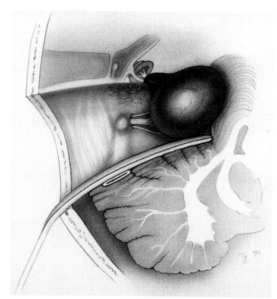

Figure 66–18. Overview of the translabyrinthine approach from an axial perspective. Note that the craniotomy extends from the posterior edge of the external auditory canal to a distance behind the sigmoid sinus, which is posteriorly displaced. (Reprinted with permission of Jackler RK.)

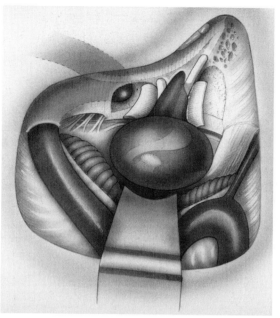

Figure 66–19. Translabyrinthine approach to a medium-sized vestibular schwannoma. Note the deviation and splaying of the facial nerve on the anterior surface of the tumor. (Reprinted with permission of Jackler RK.)

skull base component via either the neural portion of the foramen or by penetrating the posterior surface of the jugular bulb or sigmoid sinus. In the past, these tumors were commonly approached with a multistage procedure in which the skull base and neck component were removed separately from the intracranial portion. The current trend is toward a single-stage removal via a **transjugular craniotomy.** This procedure involves the creation of a posterior fossa craniotomy through resection of the sigmoid sinus and jugular bulb, both of which have usually been occluded by tumor growth (Figures 66–21 and 66–22). This maneuver provides direct visualization of the intracranial aspect of the jugular foramen, including the lower nerve roots emanating from the lateral aspect of the medulla.

Some tumors, especially meningiomas, but occasionally lower cranial nerve schwannomas as well, are largely intracranial with little or no foraminal involvement. In such cases, a retrosigmoidal approach is appropriate. It is possible, from this perspective, to drill open the introitus of the intracranial aspect of the jugular foramen from above.

George B, Tran PB. Surgical resection of jugulare foramen tumors by juxtacondylar approach without facial nerve transposition. *Acta Neurochir.* 2000;142(6):613. [PMID: 10949434]

Oghalai JS, Leung MK, Jackler RK, McDermott MW. Transjugular craniotomy for the management of jugular foramen tumors with intracranial extension. *Otol Neurotol.* 2004;25(4):570; discussion 579. [PMID: 15241237]

THE VENTRAL SURFACE OF THE BRAINSTEM

1. Transcochlear Approach

In the past, lesions situated anterior to the brainstem were considered to be unresectable. Typical tumors of the region include clival meningiomas and chordomas that had broken through the posterior surface of the clivus to become intradural. **Radical petrosectomy,** also known as the transcochlear approach, is one method used to expose this inaccessible region (Figure 66–23). This procedure entails complete rerouting of the facial nerve, which results in a complete paralysis that recovers only partially and with synkinesis; sacrifice of the entire inner ear; closure of the external auditory meatus and eustachian tube; and skeletonization of the intrapetrous carotid artery. After removal of the apical petrous bone, petroclival junction, and even the lateral aspect of the clivus, an excellent view of the ventral surface of the pons and upper medulla is obtained with minimal brain retraction. Although this method affords

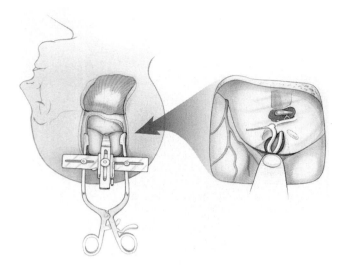

Figure 66–20. Middle fossa approach to the internal auditory canal and cerebellopontine angle. (Reprinted with permission of Jackler RK.)

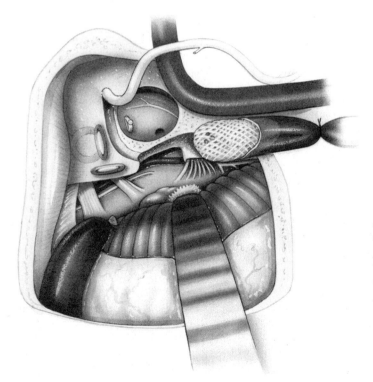

Figure 66–21. Transjugular craniotomy is conducted through resection of the sigmoid-jugular system (usually occluded preoperatively by tumor growth). This affords an excellent view of the intracranial aspect of the jugular foramen nerves as well as the lateral aspect of the pons and upper medulla. Note that although the facial nerve is rerouted in this illustration, this is not necessary in most cases. (Reprinted with permission of Jackler RK.)

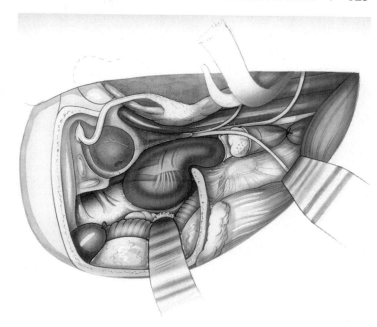

Figure 66–22. A jugular foramen schwannoma as visualized through a transjugular craniotomy. (Reprinted with permission of Jackler RK.)

excellent exposure, it is associated with high morbidity, including ipsilateral deafness and permanent facial nerve dysfunction. In recent years, this aggressive technique has become increasingly supplanted by the so-called combined approach craniotomies.

2. Retrolabyrinthine-Subtemporal Approach

In the combined retrolabyrinthine-subtemporal approach (also called simply the **petrosal approach**), a limited presigmoid petrosectomy is combined with a subtemporal opening (Figures 66–24 and 66–25). The two fossae are connected by division of the tentorium. This affords a wide exposure of the lateral aspect of the midbrain, pons, and medulla. This versatile approach has become the heavily used option in modern neurotology for a wide range of tumors in and around the brainstem. Although exposure is limited in the inferior reaches of the CPA by the sigmoid sinus and jugular bulb, superiorly it readily exposes the cavernous sinus. A partial (retrolabyrinthine) petrosectomy is usually chosen as this approach allows for hearing preservation. In lesions predominantly involving the anterior midline, a greater degree of petrosectomy (eg, translabyrinthine or even transcochlear) may be needed. During a combined-approach craniotomy, care must be taken in elevation and retraction of the posterior temporal lobe to avoid injury to the vein of Labbé. Injury to this bridging vein may result in a venous infarct of the temporal-parietal cortex.

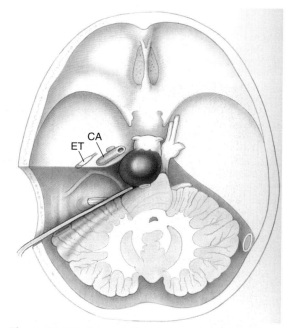

Figure 66–23. Transcochlear approach to a prepontine tumor. The anterior limits are the eustachian tube (ET), which has been obliterated with bone wax and the carotid artery (CA). Note that the facial nerve has been rerouted. (Reprinted with permission of Jackler RK.)

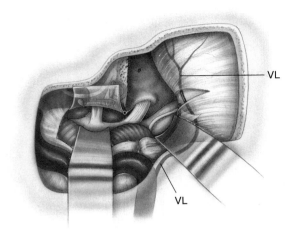

Figure 66–24. Combined retrolabyrinthine-subtemporal craniotomy with access to the lateral aspect of the pons and midbrain. Note the preservation of the semicircular canals and endolymphatic sac. The posterior and middle cranial fossae have been made confluent by division of the tentorium. The vein of Labbé (VL) is noted on the temporal lobe and joining the transverse sinus. (Reprinted with permission of Jackler RK.)

Abdel Aziz KM, Sanan A, van Loveren HR, Tew JM Jr, Keller JT, Pensak ML. Petroclival meningiomas: predictive parameters for transpetrosal approaches. *Neurosurgery*. 2000;47(1):139. [PMID: 10917357]

Angeli SI, de la Cruz A, Hitselberger W. The transcochlear approach revisited. *Otol Neurotol*. 2001;22(5):690. [PMID: 11568681]

Bambakidis NC, Gonzalez LF et al. Combined skull base approaches to the posterior fossa. *Neurosurg Focus*. 2005;19:1. [PMID: 16122215]

Horgan MA, Anderson GJ, Kellogg JX, et al. Classification and quantification of the petrosal approach to the petroclival region. *J Neurosurg*. 2000;93(1):108. [PMID: 10883912]

Magliulo G. Modified retrolabyrinthine approach with partial labyrinthectomy: anatomic study. *Otolaryngol Head Neck Surg*. 2001;124(3):287. [PMID: 11240993]

Mortini P, Mandelli C, Franzin A, Giugni E, Giovanelli M. Surgical excision of clival tumors via the enlarged transcochlear approach: indications and results. *J Neurosurg Sci*. 2001;45(3):127. [PMID: 11731737]

MECKEL CAVE

Meckel cave, also known as the cavum trigeminale, overlies the petroclival junction. Traversing it is the semilunar ganglion of the fifth cranial nerve (the trigeminal nerve). In close relationship anteromedially is the cavernous sinus. Posteriorly, its mouth opens into the superior aspect of the CPA. The oculomotor nerves IV and VI are in the immediate vicinity of the roof of Meckel cave. Because of the

rich representation of arachnoid granulations in this region, meningiomas are especially prevalent. The second most common lesion is trigeminal schwannoma.

The optimal surgical exposure of Meckel cave depends upon whether the tumor is dominantly in the middle fossa, posterior fossa, or bilobed (Figure 66–26A–C). Middle fossa lesions are approached via a subtemporal craniotomy. Posterior fossa lesions are exposed via a standard retrosigmoidal approach, modified, when necessary, by drilling open the posterior aspect of Meckel cave. In current practice, a bilobed lesion with substantial components in both posterior and middle cranial fossae is addressed by a single opening that connects both fossa (retrolabyrinthine-subtemporal).

Al-Mefty O, Ayoubi S, Gaber E. Trigeminal schwannomas: removal of dumbbell-shaped tumors through the expanded Meckel's cave and outcomes of cranial nerve function. *J Neurosurg*. 2002;96(3):453. [PMID: 11883829]

Danner C, Cueva RA. Extended middle fossa approach to the petroclival junction and anterior cerebellopontine angle. *Otol Neurotol*. 2004;25(5):762. [PMID: 15354008]

Samii M, Tatagiba M, Carvalho GA. Retrosigmoidal intradural suprameatal approach to Meckel's cave and the middle fossa: surgical technique and outcome. *J Neurosurg*. 2000;92(2):235. [PMID: 10659009]

FORAMEN MAGNUM & CRANIOVERTEBRAL JUNCTION

The exposure of posterior lesions of foramen magnum presents relatively little challenge. Extradural lesions located ventral to the craniovertebral junction are usually approached transorally (eg, lower clival chordoma or odontoid displacement upward). Intradural lesions in this ventral location, such as meningiomas, require a

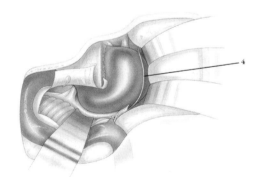

Figure 66–25. Combined retrolabyrinthine-subtemporal craniotomy for a meningioma with substantial components in both the middle and posterior cranial fossae. Note the trochlear nerve (4) on the superior surface of the tumor. (Reprinted with permission of Jackler RK.)

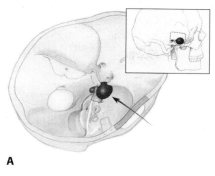

A

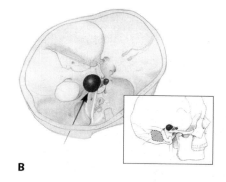

B

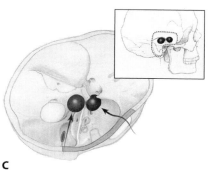

C

Figure 66–26. Surgery for tumors of Meckel cave. **(A)** Middle fossa predominant lesions are approached subtemporally. **(B)** Posterior fossa predominant lesions are approached retrosigmoidally. **(C)** Bilobed lesions are exposed via a combined craniotomy. (Reprinted with permission of Jackler RK.)

sterile approach from a lateral perspective. The **far lateral (transcondylar) approach** has been devised for just such cases (Figure 66–27; see also Figure 66–26). After a retrosigmoidal craniotomy and removal of the posterior ring of the foramen magnum, the posterior margin of the jugular foramen is skeletonized. Working beneath the jugular foramen, the cerebellum is elevated extradurally while a variable portion of the occipital condyle is removed. Usually, adequate exposure is obtained following the removal of approximately half of the condyle. Additional condylar resection may lead to instability that requires the insertion of hardware for stabilization. Resection of the tumor ventral to the medulla and upper spinal cord is carried out between the lower cranial nerve roots and the upper spinal roots.

Wanebo JE, Chicoine MR. Quantitative analysis of the transcondylar approach to the foramen magnum. *Neurosurgery.* 2001;49 (4):934. [PMID: 11564256]

Suhardja A, Agur AM, Cusimano MD. Anatomical basis of approaches to foramen magnum and lower clival meningiomas: comparison of retrosigmoid and transcondylar approaches. *Neurosurg Focus.* 200315;14(6):9. [PMID: 15669794]

VERTEBROBASILAR LESIONS

Neurotologic cranial base approaches have a role in the exposure of aneurysms of the posterior circulation. The **subtemporal transapical approach,** similar to that used for an apical petrosectomy (noted previously), was initially devised as a means of both exposing basilar tip aneurysms and establishing proximal control of the intrapetrous carotid (see Figure 66–4). Through the window created in the petrous apex, access is provided to the upper basilar artery. The transcochlear approach is capable of providing access for midbasilar artery aneurysms. Similarly, the transcondylar approach has use in approaching vascular lesions in the region of the vertebrobasilar junction.

Gonzalez LF, Amin-Hanjani S et al. Skull base approaches to the basilar artery. *Neurosurg Focus.* 2002;19:1. [PMID: 16122212]

Ng PY, Yeo TT. Petrosal approach for a large right posterior cerebral artery (P2) aneurysm. *J Clin Neurosci.* 2000;7(5):445. [PMID: 10942668]

MENINGOCELES & ENCEPHALOCELES

Defects in the dura of the roof of the petrous pyramid may occur spontaneously or following trauma or may arise as a consequence of long-standing elevated intracranial pressure. The thin bone of the tegmen overlying the mastoid or middle ear is most frequently breached. The petroclival junction is a site where congenital meningoceles may occur. Postsurgical defects after mastoid surgery commonly involve the herniation of brain tissue (encephalo-

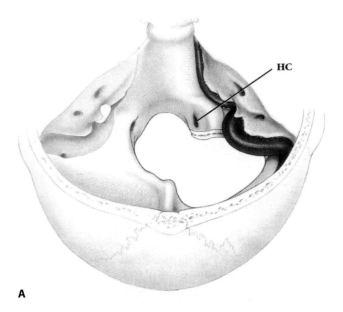

A

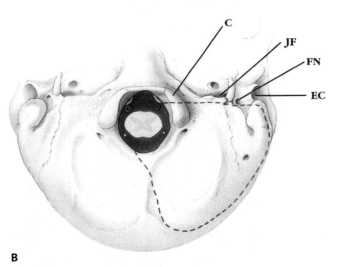

B

Figure 66–27. Bone removed via the far lateral (transcondylar) approach to the foramen magnum as seen from above **(A)** and below **(B)**. HC, hypoglossal canal; C, condyle; JF, jugular foramen; FN, facial nerve; EC, ear canal. (Reprinted with permission of Jackler RK.)

celes). The operative approach to such defects is generally from above, with repair of the temporal floor defect with fascia and, when a substantial defect exists, reinforcement with a plate of bone (Figures 66–28 and 66–29). In extensive lateral defects, the temporalis muscle may be rotated to augment the repair (Figure 66–30).

Mayeno JK, Korol HW, Nutik SL. Spontaneous meningoencephalic herniation of the temporal bone: case series with recommended treatment. *Otolaryngol Head Neck Surg.* 2004;130(4):486. [PMID: 15100650]

■ RECONSTRUCTION OF THE CRANIAL BASE

CLOSURE OF DEFECTS

Free adipose tissue, usually harvested from the anterior abdominal wall or iliac crest region, is the mainstay of skull base defect obliteration. Local rotation flaps, such

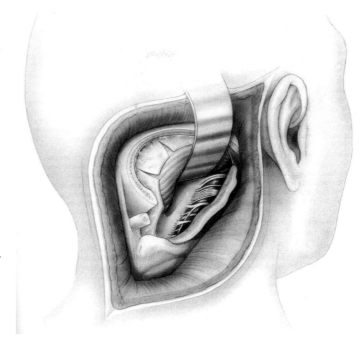

Figure 66–28. Surgical view of the far lateral approach to a ventrally situated meningioma in the foramen magnum region. Note that tumor resection must be conducted through a veil of lower cranial nerves. (Reprinted with permission of Jackler RK.)

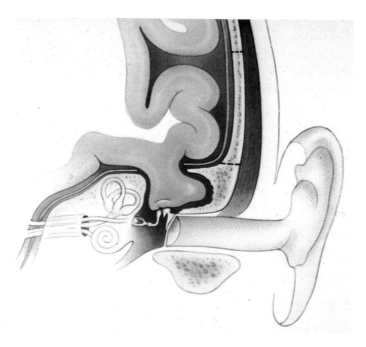

Figure 66–29. Encephalocele of the tegmen tympani. (Reprinted with permission of Jackler RK.)

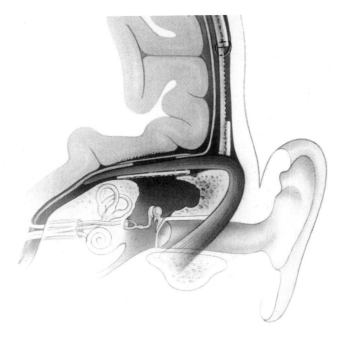

Figure 66–30. Multilayer repair of a large tegmen defect with fascia (intradural), bone (spanning the skull base defect), and inward rotation of the temporalis muscle. (Reprinted with permission of Jackler RK.)

as those fashioned using the temporalis muscle or pericranium, are useful supplements for minor soft tissue deficits. More substantial deficits require the use of either regional rotation flaps, such as the pectoralis major or trapezius myocutaneous flaps, or microvascular free flaps, such as the rectus abdominis.

CEREBROSPINAL FLUID RHINORRHEA & OTORRHEA

Aside from cranial nerve neuropathy, cerebrospinal fluid (CSF) leakage is the most prevalent morbidity in cranial base surgery. These surgeries frequently violate pneumatic tracts that ultimately connect to the middle ear and, from there, via the eustachian tube to the nasopharynx. Methods in common use to discourage CSF leak include packing the craniotomy defect with adipose tissue and sealing transected cell tracts with bone wax or other obliterative material. Despite diligent efforts at preventing this complication, CSF rhinorrhea occurs in about 10% of CPA surgeries, regardless of operative technique used, and an even higher percentage of more major skull base resections. Jugular

foramen tumors that possess both intracranial and upper neck components are particularly prone to formation of large pseudomeningoceles. This risk can be minimized by avoiding both the opening of unnecessary tissue planes and multilayer closure of the neck tissues. Meticulous hemostasis is important to avoid the need for a cervical drain.

One reason for this persistent incidence is the frequency of transient postoperative CSF hypertension brought about by the impaired resorptive function of arachnoid granulations. Management of CSF leakage includes fluid restriction, medication to reduce CSF production (eg, acetazolamide [Diamox] at 250 mg qid), and CSF diversion via a lumbar subarachnoid drain. Although most CSF leaks halt with such conservative management, a small percentage of skull base surgeries require secondary operative intervention. The most common remedial procedure is obliteration of the eustachian tube.

Becker SS, Jackler RK, Pitts LP. Cerebrospinal fluid leak after acoustic neuroma surgery: a comparison of the translabyrinthine, middle fossa, and retrosigmoidal approaches. *Otol Neurotol.* 2003;24:107. [PMID: 12544038]

SECTION XV
Facial Nerve

Anatomy, Physiology, & Testing of the Facial Nerve

Lawrence R. Lustig, MD, & John K. Niparko, MD

67

■ FACIAL NERVE ANATOMY

The facial nerve is involved in numerous pathologic conditions affecting the temporal bone, ranging from congenital anomalies to degenerative disorders and from infectious to neoplastic conditions. In each instance, a solid understanding of its complex anatomy and physiology is crucial to the physician's ability to both diagnose and treat disorders of the facial nerve with an awareness of future prognosis.

EMBRYOLOGY

Intratemporal Development

The facial nerve (Figure 67–1; Table 67–1) first develops near the end of the first month of gestation, when the acousticofacial primordium, giving rise to both the facial and acoustic nerves, develops adjacent to the primordial inner ear, the otic placode. Anlagen of the geniculate ganglion appear early in the second month of gestation. Adjacent to the developing geniculate ganglion, the acousticofacial primordium differentiates into a caudal trunk, becoming the main trunk of the facial nerve, and a rostral trunk, eventually developing into the chorda tympani nerve. The complex, tortuous course of these two nerves is explained by their separate origin and subsequent intersection. During the sixth week of gestation, the motor division of the facial nerve establishes its position in the middle ear between the membranous laby-

rinth (an otic placode structure) and the developing stapes (a second arch structure). During this time, the chorda tympani nerve becomes associated with the trigeminal nerve, which carries the chorda tympani on its way to the tongue via the lingual nerve. The greater superficial petrosal nerve, which carries preganglionic parasympathetic fibers toward the pterygopalatine ganglion, also develops during this time period.

Anatomic relationships of the facial nerve are established by the end of the second gestational month. In subsequent development, the nerve elongates as the temporal bone grows, while the fallopian canal, the bony canal that transmits the facial nerve through the temporal bone, begins to form. Although the fallopian canal begins its development in the fifth gestational month, it is not complete until several years after birth. Incomplete development of the fallopian canal is responsible for the natural dehiscences identified in temporal bone specimens, and may contribute to facial palsies associated with otitis media.

Extratemporal Development

During the sixth gestational week through the end of the second gestational month, all five divisions of the extratemporal nerve—the temporal, zygomatic, buccal, mandibular, and cervical branches—are present. During the third month, the parotid bud enlarges and engulfs the facial nerve. The facial muscles (Figure 67–2), developing independently, are formed at 7–8 weeks' gestation and must be innervated by the distal

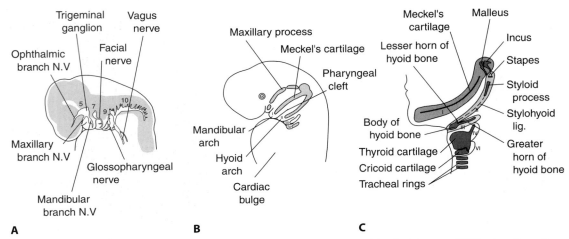

Figure 67–1. A schematic illustration demonstrating the embryology of the facial nerve. **(A)** The location of the primitive facial nerve in the developing embryo is shown in relation to other important nerves in the head and neck. **(B)** The location of the second branchial arch, giving rise to the main trunk of the facial nerve is shown in relation to the other branchial arches. **(C)** Other derivatives of the second branchial arch are shown and help explain the complex innervation pattern of the facial nerve. (Reproduced with permission from Sadler TW. *Langman's Medical Embryology,* 5th ed. Baltimore: Williams & Wilkins, 1985.)

facial nerve branches or else the muscle will degenerate, although this critical time period before degeneration is not currently known. By the end of the third gestational month, a majority of the facial musculature is identifiable and functional.

Postnatal Development

At birth, the facial nerve is located just beneath the skin near the mastoid tip as it emerges from the temporal bone, and is vulnerable to the postauricular inci-

Table 67–1. Facial nerve development.

Gestational Month	Development
1	Acousticofacial (AF) primordium gives rise to both the facial and acoustic nerves
2	Geniculate ganglion develops
	Caudal trunk of AF primordium develops into main trunk of facial nerve (FN)
	Rostral trunk of AF primordium develops into chorda tympani nerve
	Motor division of FN establishes position between labyrinth and stapes
	Chorda tympani nerve becomes associated with trigeminal nerve
	Greater superficial petrosal nerve develops
	5 extratemporal branches develop
	Facial muscles develop independently
3	FN elongates
	Fallopian canal develops, continuing through birth
	Parotid bud engulfs extratemporal FN
	Facial musculature is identifiable and functional
4–Birth	FN elongates
	Fallopian canal continues to develop
Postnatal	FN axon myelination, continuing through age 4 years
	Lateral location of extratemporal facial nerve gradually medializes under developing mastoid tip

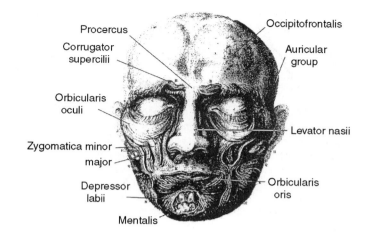

Figure 67–2. An adaptation of Sir Charles Bell's classic illustration of the muscles of facial expression, with the muscles labeled. (Reproduced from Bell C. *Essays on the Anatomy of Facial Expression,* 2nd ed. Murray, 1824.)

sion in a young child. As the mastoid tip forms and elongates during childhood however, the facial nerve assumes its more medial and protected position. Individual axons of the facial nerve also undergo myelination until the age of 4 years, an important consideration during electrical testing of the nerve during this time period.

CENTRAL NEURONAL PATHWAYS

Supranuclear Pathways

The primary somatomotor cortex of the facial nerve, controlling the complex motor function of the face, is located in the precentral gyrus, corresponding to Brodmann areas 4, 6, and 8 (Figure 67–3). Neural projec-

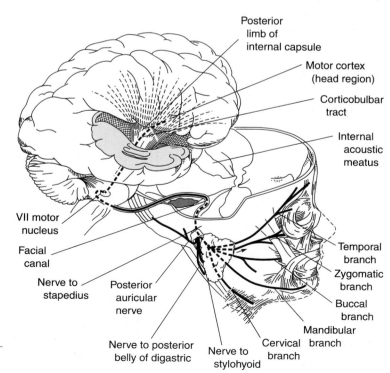

Figure 67–3. A schematic illustration of the complete pathway of the motor division of the facial nerve. (Reproduced, with permission, from Wilson-Pauwels L, Akesson EJ, Stewart PA. *Cranial Nerves: Anatomy and Clinical Comments.* Toronto: B.C. Decker, 1988.)

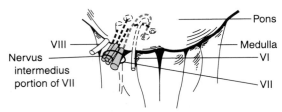

Figure 67–4. The anatomy of the facial nerve (CN VII), cochlear nerve, and vestibular nerve (CN VII), as they exit the brainstem at the level of the pontomedullary junction. (Reproduced, with permission, from Wilson-Pauwels L, Akesson EJ, Stewart PA. *Cranial Nerves: Anatomy and Clinical Comments.* Toronto: B.C. Decker, 1988.)

tions from this area making up the corticobulbar tract descend through the internal capsule and then through the pyramidal tracts within the basal pons. In the caudal pons, most of the facial nerve fibers cross the midbrain to reach the contralateral facial nucleus. A small number of facial nerve fibers innervate the ipsilateral facial nucleus, a majority of which are destined for the temporal branch of the nerve. This innervation pattern explains why central nervous system lesions spare the forehead muscle, since they receive input from both cerebral cortices, whereas peripheral lesions involve all branches of the facial nerve.

In addition to these voluntary neural projections to the facial nerve, there is also an extrapyramidal cortical input to the facial nucleus from the hypothalamus, the globus pallidus, and the frontal lobe, all of which control involuntary facial expression associated with emotion. Additional projections to the facial nuclei from the visual system are involved in the blink reflex. Projections from the trigeminal nerve and nuclei contribute to the corneal reflex, whereas those from the auditory nuclei help the eye close involuntarily in response to loud noises.

Facial Nucleus & Brainstem

The efferent projections from the facial motor nucleus emerge dorsomedially to form a compact bundle that loops over the caudal end of the abducens nucleus beneath the facial colliculus or internal genu (or turn). The neurons then pass between the facial nerve nucleus and the trigeminal spinal nucleus, emerging from the brainstem at the pontomedullary junction (Figure 67–4).

Nervus Intermedius

The nervus intermedius, or Wrisberg's nerve, mediates taste, cutaneous sensation of the external ear, proprioception, lacrimation, and salivation. The nervus intermedius exits the brainstem adjacent to the motor branch of the facial nerve (Table 67–2; Figure 67–5).

Table 67–2. Subdivisions and functions of the facial nerve.

Facial Nerve Subdivision	Function
Branchial motor	Muscles of facial expression Posterior belly of digastric muscle Stylohyoid muscle Stapedius muscle
Visceral motor	Salivation—lacrimal, submandibular, and sublingual Nasal mucosa or mucous membrane
General sensory	Sensory to auricular concha External auditory canal Tympanic membrane
Special sensory	Chorda tympani nerve—taste to anterior two-thirds of the tongue

The nerve commonly clings to the adjacent cochleovestibular nerve complex rather than the facial nerve and crosses back to the seventh nerve as it approaches the internal auditory meatus.

General visceral efferent fibers of the nervus intermedius are preganglionic parasympathetic neurons that innervate the lacrimal, submandibular, sublingual, and minor salivary glands. The cell bodies of these nerves arise in the superior salivatory nucleus and join the facial nerve after it has passed the abducens nucleus. They travel together until reaching the geniculate ganglion in the temporal bone. At this point, the greater superficial petrosal nerve branches off, composed of neurons destined for the pterygopalatine ganglion. The greater superficial petrosal nerve ultimately innervates the lacrimal, minor salivary, and mucosal glands of the palate and nose. Remaining fibers form part of the chorda tympani nerve, proceed to the submandibular ganglion, and eventually proceed to the submandibular and sublingual salivary glands.

The special visceral afferent fibers, which also form a portion of the chorda tympani nerve, receive input from the taste buds of the anterior two thirds of the tongue, as well as the hard and soft palates (Figure 67–6). These sensory afferents for taste have their cell bodies in the geniculate ganglion and will eventually synapse in the medulla, in the nucleus solitarius.

The general sensory afferent neurons of the nervus intermedius are responsible for cutaneous sensory information from the external ear canal and postauricular region. These cutaneous sensory fibers enter the spinal

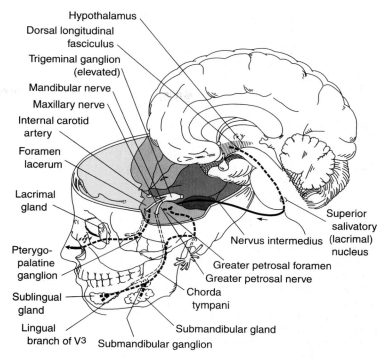

Figure 67–5. The anatomy of the visceral motor portion of the facial nerve, making up the *nervus intermedius,* or Wrisberg nerve. The preganglionic, parasympathetic portions of this nerve have cell bodies located in the abducens nucleus. From there they travel toward the geniculate ganglion in the temporal bone, located at the first genu of the facial nerve on the floor of the middle cranial fossa. Fibers from this nerve are destined to innervate the lacrimal gland, the minor salivary glands, and the mucosal glands of the palate and nose. (Reproduced, with permission, from Wilson-Pauwels L, Akesson EJ, Stewart PA. *Cranial Nerves: Anatomy and Clinical Comments.* Toronto: B.C. Decker, 1988.)

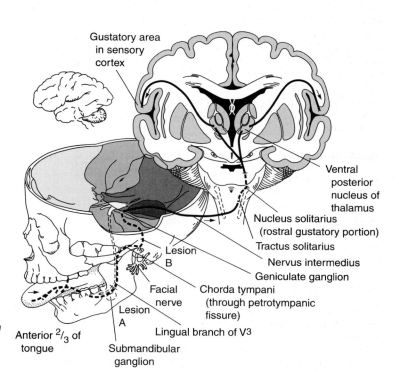

Figure 67–6. The anatomy of the special sensory component of the facial nerve, comprising the chorda tympani nerve. (Reproduced, with permission, from Wilson-Pauwels L, Akesson EJ, Stewart PA. *Cranial Nerves: Anatomy and Clinical Comments.* Toronto: B.C. Decker, 1988.)

trigeminal tracts without synapsing in the geniculate ganglion.

Cerebellopontine Angle

The facial nerve leaves the brainstem at the pontomedullary junction (see Figure 67–4), where it lies in close approximation to the vestibulocochlear nerve. This intimate relationship takes on critical importance when lesions such as a vestibular schwannoma arise in the region of the cerebellopontine angle, a common location for central nervous system tumors. In this location, the facial nerve is placed in jeopardy both during the growth of the tumor and during attempted surgical resection in this area.

During its lateral course through the cerebellopontine angle and internal auditory canal, the relative positions of the facial and cochleovestibular nerves change by rotating 90°. In the cerebellopontine angle, the facial nerve is covered with pia, is bathed in cerebrospinal fluid, and is devoid of epineurium, leaving it susceptible to manipulation trauma during intracranial surgery.

INTRATEMPORAL NERVE PATHWAYS

After traversing the cerebellopontine angle, the facial nerve enters the temporal bone along the posterior face of the petrous bone. Within the temporal bone, the facial nerve successively passes through four regions before its exit out of the stylomastoid foramen: (1) the internal auditory canal, (2) the labyrinthine segment, (3) the intratympanic segment, and (4) the descending segment (Figures 67–7, 67–8, and 67–9). From the lateral end of the internal auditory canal to its exit out the stylomastoid foramen, the nerve travels approximately 3 cm within the fallopian canal.

Internal Auditory Canal

The facial nerve enters the temporal bone along the posterior face of the petrous bone, piercing the internal auditory meatus. At the lateral end of the internal auditory canal (IAC), the traverse crest divides the IAC into superior and inferior portions. The superior portion is in turn further divided by the smaller and more laterally located vertical crest or "Bill's bar." At this lateral portion of the IAC, the anatomy is most consistent: The superior portion is occupied by the facial nerve anteriorly and the superior vestibular nerve posteriorly (see Figure 67–8). Within the IAC, the dural covering of the facial nerve is transformed to epineurium.

Labyrinthine Segment

At the lateral portion of the IAC, the facial nerve pierces the meatal foramen to enter the labyrinthine segment. The labyrinthine segment is notable in that it is the narrowest portion of the fallopian canal,

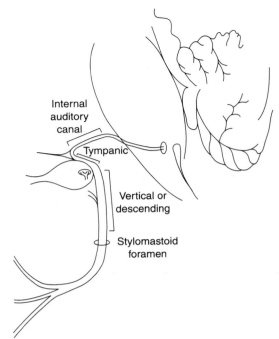

Figure 67–7. The intratemporal divisions of the facial nerve. After passing through the internal auditory meatus on the posterior face of the petrous temporal bone, the nerve enters its canalicular segment, within the internal auditory canal. It then becomes the labyrinthine segment, as it traverses between the cochlea and the vestibular labyrinth. After making its first genu (bend) at the geniculate ganglion, it becomes the tympanic segment, coursing through the middle ear space, just superior to the oval window. It then makes its second major genu at the level of the horizontal semicircular canal, and becomes the vertical or descending segment. After passing through the stylomastoid foramen, it becomes extracranial.

where it averages < 0.7 mm in diameter, occupies the canal to the greatest proportional extent, and is lined by a fibrous annular ligament. As a result, it is believed that infections or inflammations causing edema of the facial nerve within this region can lead to temporary or permanent paralysis of the nerve, such as in Bell palsy.

The geniculate ganglion is considered the end of the labyrinthine segment of the nerve and lies just superior to the nerve. Arising from the geniculate ganglion is the greater superficial petrosal nerve, containing preganglionic parasympathetic fibers destined for the lacrimal gland, as well as for the nasal and palatine mucosal glands. The nerve also contains some minor taste neurons that supply the posterior palate.

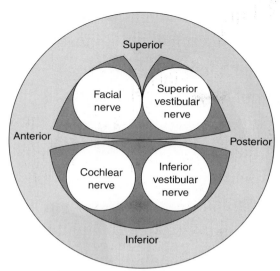

Figure 67–8. A stylized representation of the anatomy of the lateral aspect of the internal auditory canal. The facial nerve lies at the most anterior and superior location at th is level.

Tympanic Segment

At the geniculate ganglion, the facial nerve makes its first genu and becomes the tympanic segment of the facial nerve, so called because it travels within the middle ear space. This portion of the nerve is approximately 10 mm long. Landmarks for the nerve at this location include the cochleariform process, which gives rise to the tensor tympani muscle, and the "cog," a small bony prominence projecting from the roof of the epitympanum. The facial nerve then travels posteriorly, just superior to the oval window and stapes. The nerve then curves inferiorly at its second genu, just posterior to the oval window, pyramidal process, and stapedial tendon, and anterior to the horizontal semicircular canal. It is this portion of the nerve that is most susceptible to injury during surgery because processes such as cholesteatoma frequently erode the bone covering the facial nerve in this region, leaving it precariously exposed.

In addition to bony dehiscence from pathology, natural fallopian canal dehiscences have also been described in cadaver specimens, a majority of which occurred in the tympanic segment. In more than 80% of cases, the dehiscences involved the portions of the canal adjacent to the oval window.

Vertical, Descending, or Mastoid Segment

After the second genu, the nerve traverses the synonymously named vertical, descending, or mastoid segment

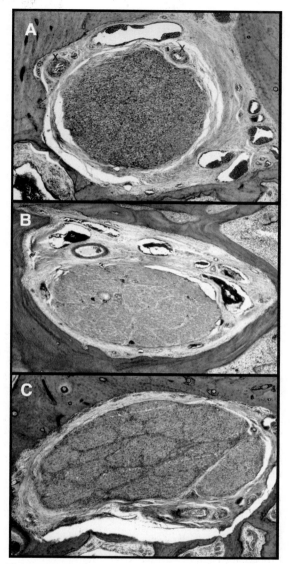

Figure 67–9. Histologic cross sections of the facial nerve at three points along its course within the temporal bone. Proximally within the temporal bone at the level of the internal auditory canal **(A),** the individual nerve fascicles are not defined, and nerve elements appear homogeneous. **(B)** As the nerve proceeds through the tympanic segment and **(C)** at the level of the stylomastoid foramen, individual nerve fascicles becomes increasingly defined.

en route to the stylomastoid foramen. As the facial nerve descends inferiorly in this portion, it gradually assumes a more lateral position. Important branches of the nerve in this segment include the nerve to the stapedius muscle and the chorda tympani nerve. As it arises from the facial nerve, the chorda tympani nerve makes an approximately 30° angle and delineates a triangular space known as the "facial recess," an important surgical route of entry into the middle ear space.

In its most inferior portion, the facial nerve takes on a close proximity to the digastric ridge and muscle, where the nerve is consistently medial and anterior to these structures. On exiting the stylomastoid foramen, the nerve becomes encased in the thick fibrous tissue of the cranial base periosteum and digastric muscle.

Although the facial nerve most commonly descends in its vertical segment as a single nerve, bifurcations, trifurcations, and hypoplasia of the facial nerve have been found within the mastoid segment. In addition, the chorda tympani nerve has been noted to arise from the facial nerve anywhere from the stylomastoid foramen to the geniculate ganglion.

PERIPHERAL FACIAL NERVE ANATOMY

The facial nerve exits the skull base through the stylomastoid foramen, between the mastoid tip laterally and the styloid process medially (Figure 67–10). At the stylomastoid foramen, the facial nerve passes into the parotid gland, typically as a single large trunk. The nerve then divides within the parotid gland into its temporofacial and cervicofacial branches. Rarely, this division can occur within the temporal bone and exit the stylomastoid foramen as separate branches.

Within the parotid gland, the nerve can assume numerous configurations, with frequent anastomoses between branches. However, generally five main branches of the nerve can be identified: (1) the temporal, (2) the zygomatic, (3) the buccal, (4) the mandibular, and (5) the cervical. The temporal branch innervates the frontalis muscle, which allows for the voluntary raising of eyebrows. The zygomatic branch innervates the orbicularis oculi muscle and is critical for proper eye closure. The buccal nerve innervates the buccinator and orbicularis oris, allowing for proper mouth closure and cheek musc le activity. The mandibular branch innervates the platysma. The posterior auricular nerve, arising just after the exit of the facial nerve from the stylomastoid foramen, sends branches to the occipitalis muscle posteriorly on the skull.

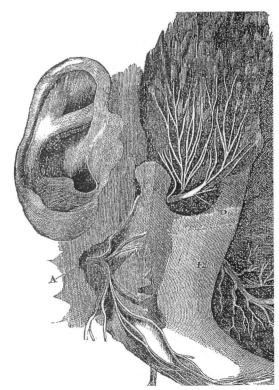

Figure 67–10. A portion of an illustration from Sir Charles Bell, demonstrating the exit of the facial nerve from the stylomastoid foramen. (Reproduced from Bell C. *The Nervous System of the Human Body.* Longman, 1830. Plate VII.)

Fowler E. Variations in the temporal bone course of the facial nerve. *Laryngoscope.* 1961;91:937.

Gasser RF. The development of the facial nerve in man. *Ann Otol Rhinol Laryngol.* 1967;76:37. [PMID: 6020340] (A classic manuscript on the embryologic development of the facial nerve.)

Gasser RF. The development of the facial nerve muscles in man. *Am J Anat.* 1967;120:357. [PMID: 5447369] (A classic manuscript on the development of the muscles of facial expression.)

Gasser RF. The early development of the parotid gland around the facial nerve and its branches in man. *Anat Rec.* 1970;167:63. [PMID: 5447369] (A classic manuscript on the development of the parotid gland in relation to the facial nerve.)

Gasser RF, May M. Embryonic development of the facial nerve. In: May M, ed. *The Facial Nerve.* New York: Thieme, Inc., 1987:3.

Ge XX, Spector GJ. Labyrinthine segment and geniculate ganglion of facial nerve in fetal and adult human temporal bones. *Ann Otol Rhinol Laryngol Suppl.* 1981;90(4 Pt 2):1. [PMID: 6792965] (A classic study of the intratemporal portion of the facial nerve.)

Nager GT, Proctor B. Anatomic variations and anomalies involving the facial canal. *Otolaryngol Clin North Am.* 1991;24:531.

Baxter A. Dehiscence of the fallopian canal: an anatomical study. *J Laryngol Otol.* 1971;85:587. [PMID: 5581361] (An anatomic study describing naturally occurring dehiscences of the facial nerve.)

Courbille J. The nucleus of the facial nerve: the relation between cellular groups and peripheral branches of the nerve. *Brain.* 1966;1:338. [PMID: 5961910] (A classic study of the anatomy of the facial nerve nucleus.)

[PMID: 1762775] (A classic, comprehensive study of the anatomy of the facial canal.)

Proctor B, Nager GT. The facial canal: normal anatomy, variations and anomalies. II. Anatomical variations and anomalies involving the facial canal. *Ann Otol Rhinol Laryngol Suppl.* 1982;97:45. [PMID: 6814329] (A classic study of the anatomy of the facial canal.)

Rhoton AL Jr, Kobayashi S, Hollinshead WH. Nervus intermedius. *J Neurosurg.* 1968;29:609. [PMID: 5708034] (A classic study of the anatomy of the nervus intermedius.)

Sherwood CC. Comparative anatomy of the facial motor nucleus in mammals, with an analysis of neuron numbers in primates. *Anat Rec A Discov Mol Cell Evol Biol.* 2005;287(1):1067. [PMID: 16200649] (A contemporary study of the central motor pathways of the facial nerve.)

Toth M, Moser G, Patonay L, Olah I. Development of the anterior chordal canal. *Ann Anat.* 2006;188(1):7. [PMID: 16447906] (A contemporary study of the chorda tympani nerve pathway.)

Vidic B, Wozniak W. The communicating branch of the facial nerve to the lesser petrosal nerve in human fetuses and newborns. *Arch Anat Histol Embryol.* 1969;52(5):369. [PMID: 4926584] (A classic anatomic study of the communicating branch of the facial nerve.)

■ FACIAL NERVE PHYSIOLOGY

ANATOMIC CONSIDERATIONS

The facial nerve trunk consists of approximately 10,000 nerve fibers, approximately 7000 of which are myelinated motor fibers. The facial nerve sheath consists of several layers. The endoneurium, closely adherent to the layer of Schwann cells of the axons, surrounds each nerve fiber. The perineurium, which is the intermediate layer surrounding groups of fascicles, provides tensile strength to the nerve and is believed to represent the primary barrier to the spread of infection. The outermost layer of the nerve is the epineurium. This outer layer contains the vasa nervorum, which provides the blood supply to the nerve.

CLASSIFICATION OF FACIAL NERVE DEGENERATION

If the facial nerve is injured, various degrees of injury may result. The most widely used model of clinical-pathologic classification of nerve injury is the classification originally proposed by Sunderland (Figure 67–11):

(1) **First-degree injuries,** also referred to as **neuro-praxia**, are characterized by the blockage of axoplasm flow within the axon. Although an action potential cannot be propagated across the lesion site, a stimulus applied distal to the lesion will con-

duct normally to produce an evoked response.

(2) **Second-degree injuries** entail axonal and myelin disruption distal to the injury site as a result of the progression of a first-degree injury. Such injuries eliminate the propagation of an externally applied stimulus as wallerian degeneration of the axon ensues.

(3) **Third-degree injuries** involve complete disruption of the axon, including its surrounding myelin and endoneurium.

(4) **Fourth-degree injuries** entail the complete disruption of the perineurium.

(5) **Fifth-degree injuries** entail the disruption of the epineurium.

(6) **Sixth-degree injuries,** a proposed addition to the Sunderland classification by later authors, takes into account the observed patterns of blunt and penetrating injuries of the nerve. These injuries are characterized by normal function through some fascicles and varying degrees of injury (first-degree through fifth-degree injuries), differentially involving fascicles across the nerve trunk.

Central to Sunderland's classification is the notion that axonal recovery depends on the integrity of the connective tissue elements of the nerve trunk. This model predicts a high likelihood for the complete recovery of peripheral innervation when endoneurial tubules remain intact to support reinnervation, as is the case with first- and second-degree injuries. In contrast, disruption of the endoneurium—a third-degree injury or worse in this model—increases the likelihood of irreversible axonal injury and aberrant patterns of regeneration.

An example of abnormal neural regrowth is "crocodile tears," or increased lacrimation associated with eating. It occurs when efferent fibers normally targeted to travel with the chorda tympani nerve to the submandibular and sublingual glands are misdirected through the greater superficial petrosal nerve to the lacrimal gland. This results in parasympathetic innervation of the lacrimal gland as well as the normal target, the salivary glands.

Moran LB, Graeber MB. The facial nerve axotomy model. *Brain Res Brain Res Rev.* 2004;44(2-3):154. [PMID: 15003391] (Contemporary, scientific study of facial nerve injury and repair.)

Myckatyn TM, Mackinnon SE. The surgical management of facial nerve injury. *Clin Plast Surg.* 2003;30(2):307. [PMID: 12737358] (Review of the management of injuries to the facial nerve based on clinical presentation.)

Sunderland S, Cossar DF. The structure of the facial nerve. *Anat Rec.* 1953;116(2):147. [PMID: 13065751] (A classic study of the structure of the facial nerve that helped lead to Sunderland's classification of facial nerve injury.)

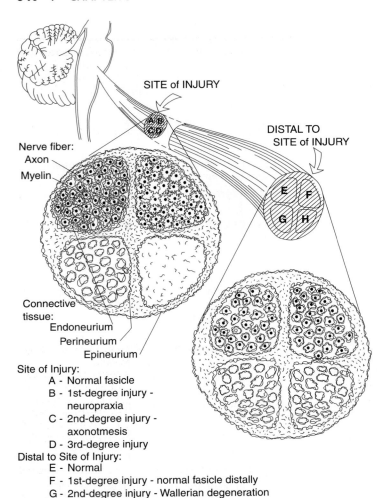

SITE of INJURY

DISTAL TO
SITE of INJURY

Nerve fiber:
Axon
Myelin

Connective
tissue:
Endoneurium
Perineurium
Epineurium

Site of Injury:
A - Normal fasicle
B - 1st-degree injury - neuropraxia
C - 2nd-degree injury - axonotmesis
D - 3rd-degree injury
Distal to Site of Injury:
E - Normal
F - 1st-degree injury - normal fasicle distally
G - 2nd-degree injury - Wallerian degeneration has produced axonal loss distally
H - 3rd-degree injury

Figure 67–11. A model of graded neural injury that details clinical-pathologic classifications. Microanatomic changes in cranial nerve injury are demonstrated in cross-section. The potential for appropriate axonal regeneration across the site of injury is dictated principally by the status of connective tissue elements.

■ FACIAL NERVE TESTING

The impaired transmission of neural impulses can result from physiologic blockage (in the absence of nerve fiber degeneration) and axonal discontinuity with wallerian degeneration. Because the clinical presentation of a facial paralysis does not distinguish between simple conduction block and axonal disruption, investigators have explored an array of testing procedures designed to define the extent of nerve injury (Table 67–3).

In an initial evaluation of patients with acute facial paralysis, the clinician should aim to determine the prognosis for recovery as well as the cause of the paraly-

sis. Early determination of the prognosis for recovery may permit intervention both to minimize nerve injury and to optimize regeneration.

TOPOGNOSTIC TESTING

Topognostic test batteries are intended to determine the level of facial nerve injury by testing peripheral facial nerve function. The underlying hypothesis is that injury to the facial nerve at a particular location will affect all branches proximal to the lesion, yet leave distal branches with normal function. For example, if tearing is diminished (Schirmer test), the lesion is assumed to be proximal to the point at which the greater superficial petrosal nerve branches from the geniculate ganglion. Additional testing includes immittance testing (abnor-

Table 67–3. Tests of facial nerve function.

Test	Measure	Advantages	Disadvantages
Minimal excitability test	The lowest stimulus intensity that consistently excites all branches on the uninvolved side	Portability Patient comfort Easy to perform	Subjective Relies on visual detection
Maximal excitability test	Compares response on involved vs. uninvolved side of face	Portability Patient comfort Easy to perform	Subjective Relies on visual detection
Electroneuronography and evoked electromyograph (EMG)	Assesses the facial motor response to a supramaximal stimulus Records the compound muscle action potential Reflects % motor fibers of the facial nerve that have undergone degeneration < 90% denervation prognosticates excellent recovery Repeated every other day to detect ongoing degeneration beyond the 90% critical level	Useful early in the course of facial paralysis Some measures useful in predicting the ultimate level of spontaneous recovery	Patient discomfort
Electromyography	Measures postsynaptic membrane potentials Motor unit potentials in five muscle groups in the first 3 days after onset of palsy associated with good outcome in > 90% of patients	Precision characterization of motor units	Possible pitfalls with early testing Sparse residual motor units that suggest a favorable outcome may be evident despite severe injury to large portions of fibers that are at risk for degeneration
Antidromic conduction	F wave represents activity in facial muscles generated by antidromically activated motor neurons In Bell palsy, F wave seen only after recovery begun	Can provide direct and immediate assessment of facial nerve function	Limited dynamic range and prognostic value Primarily animal testing, research
Magnetic simulation	Electromagnetic coil to produce neural activation	Intensity of the stimulus is minimally attenuated by intervening tissue	Limited clinical utility Difficult to interpret results
Trigeminofacial reflex	EMG recording of the blink reflex Compares responses between the affected and normal sides Abolished R1 reflex associated with little chance of recovery in the first 2 months after onset of paralysis	Easy to perform	May be limited by small response amplitude

mal stapedial muscle function reflecting nerve impairment above the stapedial motor branch), and salivary secretion and taste testing (chorda tympani nerve function). Although attractive in theory, topognostic modalities have often provided inconsistent information on the level of neural injury, since lesions of the nerve can affect the motor, sensory, and autonomic portions of the nerve differently.

For example, the Schirmer tear test has been shown to have an accuracy rate of only 60% using intraoperative electrical stimulation to specify the site of nerve conduction block in Bell palsy. However, the Schirmer test does have great practical value in assessing tear production and the need for adjunctive measures for eye care.

ELECTROPHYSIOLOGIC TESTING

The interpretation and validity of electrophysiologic testing of an acute facial palsy rests on two tenets with regard to nerve fiber function:

(1) Segmentally demyelinated fibers maintain the capacity to propagate a stimulus, albeit at a higher threshold, than that of normal fibers. Anatomically intact fibers will therefore continue to propagate an applied stimulus, whereas those that have become disrupted and subsequently degenerated will not.

(2) By estimating the proportion of degenerated motor fibers, a clinician may distinguish palsies that will fail to recover spontaneously and will produce long-term sequelae.

Ideally, electrophysiologic testing provides an index of the severity of injury to the nerve trunk by reflecting the proportion of motor fibers that have progressed beyond a first-degree injury. Correlation of the ultimate level of recovery with early electrophysiologic findings determines the prognostic value of the test in identifying the subset of facial palsy patients who will not obtain satisfactory, spontaneous recovery.

Electrophysiologic tests can only indirectly assess the severity of injury to the intratemporal facial nerve; because this portion of the nerves lies entirely within the temporal bone, electrical stimulation proximal to the site of conduction blockade is possible only when the nerve is activated intracranially. For this reason, clinical tests of facial nerve function rely on measures of nerve stimulation distal to the stylomastoid foramen. Even in the presence of severe neural injury, conduction distal to a lesion continues until its axoplasm is consumed and wallerian degeneration ensues. This process requires 48–72 hours to progress from intratemporal to extratemporal segments, thereby rendering electrical stimulation tests falsely normal during this period. Routine electrophysiologic tests therefore fail to detect nerve conduction as it occurs, thereby delaying the differentiation of neuropraxia from degeneration.

Nerve Excitability Testing

Minimal excitability testing with the Hilger nerve stimulator has provided a readily accessible method of facial nerve assessment. The test is indexed according to the thresholds for visually detectable activity generated by

surface stimulation of a facial nerve branch. The test reflects elevated thresholds for neuromuscular stimulation produced by axonal disruption and degeneration. The lowest stimulus intensity that consistently excites all branches on the uninvolved side establishes the normal threshold. A 2.0–3.5 mA difference between the uninvolved and involved sides is considered abnormal and suggests impending denervation. Additional advantages of the test include the portability of the equipment and less patient discomfort compared with other tests (such as the maximal stimulation test).

A disadvantage of the test is the subjective nature of the measured response, relying on the visual detection of a limited number of facial muscles. In addition, current threshold levels for peripheral branches are likely to selectively activate large nerve fibers with lower thresholds and those fibers closer to the stimulating electrode, thereby excluding an unknown proportion of motor fibers from the assessment.

Dumitru D, Walsh NE, Porter LD. Electrophysiologic evaluation of the facial nerve in Bell's palsy. A review. *Am J Phys Med Rehabil.* 1988;67(4):137. [PMID: 3041998] (Comprehensive review of electrophysiologic facial nerve testing that is still timely.)

Gantz BJ, Gmur A, Fisch U. Intraoperative evoked electromyography in Bell's palsy. *Am J Otolaryngol.* 1982;3(4):273. [PMID: 7149140] (The technique of intraoperative evoked electromyography is described in detail. The limited extent of the blocked motor fibers suggests that segmental, rather than total, intratemporal decompression is needed in Bell palsy.)

Gates GA. Nerve excitability testing: technical pitfalls and threshold norms using absolute values. *Laryngoscope.* 1993;103(4 Pt 1):379. [PMID: 8459745] (Practical review of nerve excitability testing.)

Ikeda M, Abiko Y, Kukimoto N, Omori H, Nakazato H, Ikeda K. Clinical factors that influence the prognosis of facial nerve paralysis and the magnitudes of influence. *Laryngoscope.* 2005;115(5):855. [PMID: 15867653] (Contemporary study evaluating the factors resulting in facial nerve recovery outcomes using clinical and electrophysiologic testing.)

Lewis BI, Adour KK, Kahn JM, Lewis AJ. Hilger facial nerve stimulator: a 25-year update. *Laryngoscope.* 1991;101(1 Pt 1):71. [PMID: 1984555] (Review of the impact of the Hilger nerve stimulator on facial nerve assessment.)

Maximal Stimulation Test

A test of maximal electrical stimulation can be used to determine whether nerve degeneration has developed in the course of an acute facial paralysis. It involves a transcutaneous electrical impulse designed to saturate the nerve with current, activating all functioning fibers. The response on the involved side is characterized as being (1) equal to the contralateral side, (2) minimally diminished (50% of normal), (3) markedly diminished (< 25% of normal), or (4) absent.

When the response is markedly diminished or absent within the first 2 weeks of the clinical paralysis, it has been found that there is a 75% chance of incomplete facial nerve recovery. When the response completely disappeared within the first 10 days, recovery was typically incomplete and significant sequelae ensued. Conversely, if responses were symmetric during the first 10 days of a clinical paralysis, complete return was found in more than 90% of patients tested. The use of supramaximal stimulation provides sensitivity and consistency in testing when used early in the course of an acute facial paralysis. However, the interpretation of the maximal stimulation test relies on a subjective evaluation of the visually graded evoked response.

Gates GA. Nerve excitability testing: technical pitfalls and threshold norms using absolute values. *Laryngoscope.* 1993;103(4 Pt 1):379. [PMID: 8459745] (Practical review of nerve excitability testing.)

Ikeda M, Abiko Y, Kukimoto N, Omori H, Nakazato H, Ikeda K. Clinical factors that influence the prognosis of facial nerve paralysis and the magnitudes of influence. *Laryngoscope.* 2005; 115(5):855. [PMID: 15867653] (Contemporary study evaluating the factors resulting in facial nerve recovery outcomes using clinical and electrophysiologic testing.)

May M. Nerve excitability test in facial palsy: limitations in its use based on a study of 130 case. *Laryngoscope.* 1972;82:2122. [PMID: 5081746] (This study describes the usefulness and drawbacks of the facial nerve excitability test based on the author's personal experience.)

May M, Blumenthal F, Klein S. Acute Bell's palsy: prognostic value of evoked electromyography, max stimulation and other electrical tests. *Am J Otol.* 1983;5:107. [PMID: 6881304] (Evoked electromyography and maximal stimulation tests were the most accurate electrical tests for predicting the course of acute facial paralysis when performed serially within the first 10 days after onset.)

Evoked Electromyography & Electroneuronography

Similar to the maximal stimulation test, evoked electromyography (EEMG) or electroneuronography (ENoG) assesses the facial motor response to a supramaximal stimulus. In contrast to maximal stimulation testing, the EEMG technique records the compound muscle action potential (CMAP) with surface electrodes placed in the nasolabial fold. The CMAP can be graphically displayed for quantitative analysis and printed for the medical record (Figure 67–12). Waveform responses are analyzed to compare peak-to-peak amplitudes between normal and involved sides.

Patients with incomplete paralyses due to Bell palsy invariably recover function to normal or near-normal levels and do not require EEMG evaluation. The reappearance of facial movement within 3–4 weeks after onset also predicts an excellent prognosis for functional recovery. EMG sampling of motor activity to detect visually imperceptible facial function is advised.

When assessed within a critical time window, reductions in the amplitude of the EEMG response of the affected side are considered to reflect the percentage of

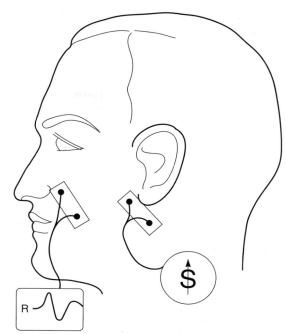

Figure 67–12. Placement of recording and stimulating electrodes for facial EEMG recordings. The compound muscle action potential is reflected in the biphasic electromyographic response.

motor fibers of the facial nerve that have undergone degeneration. Facial EEMG is most reliable during the initial phase of accelerated denervation when reliable results can be obtained (ie, in the first 2–3 weeks after the onset of a paralysis due to Bell palsy or herpes zoster oticus). When neuropraxic fibers become "de-blocked" either in the recovery phase or later as axons regenerate peripherally, stimulated nerve fibers discharge asynchronously. Because regenerated fibers do not discharge in synchrony, the response is disorganized and consequently diminished. This phenomenon imposes a time constraint on the reliability of EEMG testing that must be considered in interpreting the test results.

ENoG is most useful early in the course of facial paralysis. More than 50% of patients with complete paralysis who exhibit a ≥ 90% reduction in CMAP amplitude have less than a satisfactory, spontaneous return of facial function. When results demonstrate < 90% denervation (> 10% in CMAP amplitude relative to the normal side), excellent recovery has been uniformly observed.

It is recommended that EEMG testing should be repeated on an every-other-day basis to detect ongoing degeneration beyond the 90% critical level. The time span of reduced electrical excitability (ie, the velocity of denervation as demonstrated by repeated testing) and the degree of degradation of the CMAP response (ie, the nadir of the response) are most useful in predicting the ultimate level of spontaneous recovery. The earlier the EEMG response drops to ≤ 10% of normal, the worse the prognosis is. Some surgeons have advocated a decompression of the facial nerve proximal to the geniculate ganglion if the 90% level is reached, although this decompression must be performed within 2 weeks of the onset of the facial palsy.

Chung WH, Lee JC, Cho Do Y, Won EY, Cho YS, Hong SH. Waveform reliability with different recording electrode placement in facial electroneuronography. *J Laryngol Otol.* 2004;118(6):421. [PMID: 15285858] (Examining four parameters of facial nerve electroneuronography, the authors found that with the electrode placed on the nasal ala, the threshold was significantly lower, thus concluding that placement of the recording electrode on the nasal ala is the preferred method.)

Coker NJ. Facial electroneuronography: analysis of techniques and correlation with degenerating motoneurons. *Laryngoscope.* 1992;102:747. [PMID: 9226049] (Comprehensive review of electroneuronography.)

Fisch U. Maximal nerve excitability testing vs electroneuronography. *Arch Otolaryngol.* 1980;106:352.

Fisch U. Surgery for Bell's palsy. *Arch Otolaryngol.* 1981;107:1. [PMID: 6246866] (This study shows that the advantage of electroneuronography vs maximal nerve excitability test (NET) is the quantitative analysis of the number of degenerated fibers and the assessment of an accurate degeneration profile in Bell palsy.)

Gantz BJ, Rubinstein JT, Gidley P, Woodworth GG. Surgical management of Bell's palsy. *Laryngoscope.* 1999;109(8):1177. [PMID: 10443817] (The study showed that electroneurography in with voluntary EMG successfully predicts that surgical decompression within 2 weeks of onset medial to the geniculate ganglion significantly improves the chances of normal or near-normal return of facial function in the group that otherwise has a high probability of a poor result.)

May M, Blumenthal F, Klein S. Acute Bell's palsy: prognostic value of evoked electromyography, max stimulation and other electrical tests. *Am J Otol.* 1983;5:107. [PMID: 6881304] (Evoked electromyography and maximal stimulation tests were the most accurate electrical tests for predicting the course of acute facial paralysis when performed serially within the first 10 days after onset.)

Sillman JS, Niparko JK, Lee SS, Kileny PR. Prognostic value of evoked and standard electromyography in acute facial paralysis. *Otolaryngol Head Neck Surg.* 1992;107:377. [PMID: 1408222] (The findings from this study support previous reports of the prognostic value of evoked electromyography in idiopathic facial paralysis, but suggest that this test may have less predictive value in the evaluation of facial paralysis as a result of trauma.)

Thomander L, Stalberg E. Electroneurography in the prognostication of Bell's palsy. *Acta Otolaryngol.* 1981;92:221. [PMID: 7324892] (Using electroneurography, the prognosis for recovery for the individual patient can be judged with relatively high accuracy on day 4 [70%].)

Electromyography

The electromyographic (EMG) response reflects postsynaptic membrane potentials that may be either initiated at the neuromuscular junction with voluntary activation or generated spontaneously across the muscle membrane. These potentials are easily recorded with either bare-tip (monopolar) or concentric (coaxial) needle electrodes.

Voluntarily and spontaneously generated facial motor responses can help to characterize the condition of motor units with precision. However, the results obtained with testing in any single field should be buttressed with testing in adjacent fields. Motor unit potentials in four of five muscle groups in the first 3 days after the onset of an acute facial paralysis is associated with a satisfactory outcome in more than 90% of patients. Motor units in two of three muscle groups predicted a satisfactory outcome in 87% of patients. When motor units were either limited to one muscle group or abolished, satisfactory recovery was found in only 11% of cases.

Although these findings suggest a role for early EMG testing in prognosticating functional recovery, others have noted potential pitfalls of early EMG testing that may mislead the examiner. Sparse residual motor units that suggest a favorable outcome may be evident despite severe injury to large portions of fibers that are at risk for degeneration. The clinical evidence of this was noted as an unsatisfactory recovery despite voluntary motor potentials in 38% of Bell palsy patients. These observations suggest that EMG assessment should be performed within at least two muscle groups to more accurately assess the degree of denervation.

Early in the course of an acute facial paralysis, preserved facial motor activity may escape clinical inspection and yet provide prognostic information when combined with other testing modalities. For example, subclinical motor activity that is still detectable by the EMG may complement the use of evoked electromyography in the early phase of a clinical paralysis. EMG monitoring is of limited use in detecting early degeneration, since electrical evidence of nerve degeneration is absent in the first 10 days of the paralysis. Ten to fourteen days after the onset of a clinical paralysis, EMG recordings reflect the dynamic resting membrane potentials of postsynaptic elements. In this phase, muscle membrane, deprived of "trophic" substances that are normally transported through the axon, undergoes changes that destabilize the resting potential. These changes produce spontaneous depolarizations reflected in the EMG as fibrillation potentials. Such changes are interpreted as indicative of persistent denervation.

Substantial axonal loss and impaired reinnervation yield fibrillation potentials as long as postsynaptic membranes remain electrically active. With persistent denervation, EMG recordings are silent and the short burst of discharges normally found on needle insertion is absent. Conversely, successful reinnervation generates high-frequency polyphasic potentials that increase in amplitude and duration and replace fibrillation potentials. In rare cases of protracted paralysis due to Bell palsy, longitudinal EMG evaluations detect persistent nerve degeneration or reinnervation.

Bozorg Grayeli A, Kalamarides M, Fraysse B et al. Comparison between intraoperative observations and electromyographic monitoring data for facial nerve outcome after vestibular schwannoma surgery. *Acta Otolaryngol.* 2005;125(10):1069. [PMID: 16298788] (A four-channel facial EMG device was shown to be an excellent indicator of good immediate facial function outcome during vestibular schwannoma surgery.)

Cronin GW, Steenerson RL. The effectiveness of neuromuscular facial retraining combined with electromyography in facial paralysis rehabilitation. *Otolaryngol Head Neck Surg.* 2003; 128(4):534. [PMID: 12707657] (This study demonstrates that neuromuscular facial retraining exercises and electromyography are effective for improving facial movements in patients with recovering facial nerve paralysis.)

Dumitru D, Walsh NE, Porter LD. Electrophysiologic evaluation of the facial nerve in Bell's palsy: a review. *Am J Phys Med Rehabil.* 1988;67(4):137. [PMID: 3041998] (Comprehensive review of electrophysiologic facial nerve testing that is still timely.)

Gordon AA, Friedberg MD. Current status of testing for seventh nerve lesions. *Otolaryngol Clin North Am.* 1978;11:301. [PMID: 3041998] (Electromyography may assist in prognosticating a functional return, determining neural conduction across the site of injury and following reinnervation in the recovery period.)

Granger C. Prognosis in Bell's palsy. *Arch Phys Med Rehabil.* 1976; 57:33. [PMID: 1247374] (Using clinical and electromyographic methods, it should be possible to forecast recovery within 3 days after onset to preselect patients in need of any proposed curative treatment program designed to salvage the facial nerve.)

May M, Blumenthal F, Klein S. Acute Bell's palsy: prognostic value of evoked electromyography, max stimulation and other electrical tests. *Am J Otol.* 1983;5:107. [PMID: 6881304] (Evoked electromyography and maximal stimulation tests were the most accurate electrical tests for predicting the course of acute facial paralysis when performed serially within the first 10 days after onset.)

Sillman JS, Niparko JK, Lee SS, Kileny PR. Prognostic value of evoked and standard electromyography in acute facial paralysis. *Otolaryngol Head Neck Surg.* 1992;107:377. [PMID: 1408222] (The findings from this study support previous reports of the prognostic value of evoked electromyography in idiopathic facial paralysis, but suggest that this test may have less predictive value in the evaluation of facial paralysis as a result of trauma.)

Facial Nerve Assessment with Central Activation

The previously described electrodiagnostic tests indirectly assess the severity of injury to the intratemporal segment of the facial nerve. Investigators have explored alternate testing procedures in which the facial nerve is activated central to the presumed site of involvement within the temporal bone.

A. ANTIDROMIC CONDUCTION

Testing via antidromic (retrograde) conduction provides an alternative to electrodiagnostic testing of peripheral fibers that, at least theoretically, can provide a direct and immediate assessment of facial nerve function. Antidro-

mic conduction of electrical activity in the facial nerve can be measured with near- and far-field techniques in animals (Figure 67–13) and clinically with middle ear recording electrodes. It has been demonstrated that the far-field response to antidromic stimulation represented composite activity along the facial pathway and did not appear to reflect stimulation of the facial nerve at a specific site along the intracranial segment.

The F wave represents activity in facial muscles generated by antidromically activated motor neurons and contains no reflex components. For electrodiagnostic purposes, F waves evoked by electrical stimulation may be recorded with intramuscular needle electrodes. This response has a long latency and is normally small in amplitude, thereby limiting its dynamic range and prognostic value. In patients with Bell palsy, electrical stimulation of the nerve reliably produces F-wave responses only after recovery has begun.

B. MAGNETIC STIMULATION

Transcranial magnetic stimulation uses an electromagnetic coil to produce neural activation. This method of neural activation is unique in that the intensity of the stimulus is minimally attenuated by intervening tissue. This feature enables central activation via a transcranial application of induced current. Animal studies have demonstrated that transcranial magnetic stimulation can be used to activate the facial nerve centrally, although the precise site of stimulation is difficult to determine. Observations suggest that the evoked response is likely due to excitation of the facial nerve intratemporally or intracranially rather than via cortical or brainstem excitation.

Clinical experience with electromagnetic stimulation in pathologic states, including Bell palsy, is in keeping with observations that localize the lesion intratemporally. In 11 patients with recent onset of Bell palsy, none demonstrated evoked CMAPs with magnetic stimulation. The lack of response is attributed to the elevation in threshold associated with segmental demyelination and the inability of the current generated by the electromagnetic field to reach the threshold.

Further refinement in the application and interpretation of transcranial magnetic stimulation for prognosticating facial nerve lesions awaits further understanding of the actual site of activation. The development of coils that facilitate a more focused current offers the possibility of site-specific stimulation of the central facial motor tract and intracranial segment of the facial nerve—sites proximal to the typical sites of nerve injury for most acute facial paralyses.

C. TRIGEMINOFACIAL REFLEX

The blink reflex can be tested clinically to assess the efferent arc contributed by cranial nerve VII. Electromyographic recording of the trigeminofacial reflex

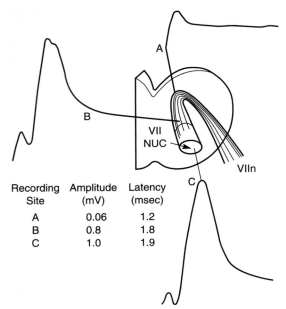

Recording Site	Amplitude (mV)	Latency (msec)
A	0.06	1.2
B	0.8	1.8
C	1.0	1.9

Figure 67–13. Topographic representation of mean amplitude and latency of evoked neural potentials from **(A)** the facial genu, **(B)** the dorsal region to the facial nucleus, and **(C)** the nucleus in experimental rodent preparation. Stimulus intensity = 0.4 mA; duration = 100 μs; N = 100 stimuli for each trial. (Reproduced, with permission, from Niparko JK, Kartush JM, Bledsoe SC, Graham MD. Antidromically evoked facial nerve response. *Am J Otolaryngol.* 1985;6:353.)

provides a quantitative assessment of facial nerve conduction via activation of the facial nucleus centrally. This technique records action potentials reflexively generated in the orbicularis oculi muscle in response to an electrical stimulus applied to the supraorbital area (V1 branch). Responses between the affected and normal sides are compared to provide quantitative assessment of the reflex, thereby providing a measure of the functional integrity of the facial nerve. Trigeminofacial reflex testing of acute facial paralysis may be limited by small response amplitudes.

An abolished R1 trigeminofacial reflex response is associated with little chance of recovery in the first 2 months after onset of paralysis. Preserved, early R1 responses predicted return to normal facial nerve function within the first month. The performance of this test in selecting those patients with an absent R1 response who have a poor long-term prognosis is yet to be evaluated.

Hallett M, Cohen LG. Magnetism: a new method for stimulation of nerve and brain. *JAMA.* 1989;262:538. (Describes the use of magnetic stimulation as a means of activating cortical regions of the brain.)

Kartush JM, Bouchard KB, Graham MD, Linstrom C. Magnetic stimulation of the facial nerve. *Am J Otol.* 1989;10:14. [PMID: 2719085] (Normal volunteers and one patient with acute facial paralysis were studied with both magnetic and electric stimulation of the facial nerve.)

Kartush JM, Garcia P, Telian SA. The source of far-field antidromic facial nerve potentials. *Am J Otolaryngol.* 1987;8:199. [PMID: 3631416] (This study identifies the generator sites of the far-field antidromic facial nerve response in dogs and shows that complete transection of the facial nerve at the CPA has little effect on the responses.)

Kimura J. *Electrodiagnosis in Diseases of Nerve and Muscle: Principles and Practice.* Philadelphia: FA Davis, 1983.

Maccabee PJ, Amassian VE, Cracco RQ, Cracco JB, Anziska BJ. Intracranial stimulation of the facial nerve in humans with the magnetic coil. *Electroencephalogr Clin Neurophysiol.* 1988;70:350. [PMID: 2458243] (This noninvasive technique may be useful in evaluating patients with peripheral facial nerve disorders, including Bell palsy.)

Nakatani H, Iwai M, Takeda T, Hamada M, Kakigi A, Nakahira M. Waveform changes in antidromic facial nerve responses in patients with Bell's palsy. *Ann Otol Rhinol Laryngol.* 2002; 111(2):128. [PMID: 11860064] (This study demonstrates that monophasic or flat waves with a low facial score strongly suggest nerve degeneration and that antidromic facial nerve response is recommended as a method of diagnosing paralysis and monitoring the progression of intratemporal facial nerve damage during its early stages.)

Niparko JK, Kartush JM, Bledsoe SC, Graham MD. Antidromically evoked facial nerve response. *Am J Otolaryngol.* 1985;6:353. [PMID: 4073377] (Results of antidromic conduction testing suggest that the recorded potentials measured represent antidromic activation of the facial nerve, further suggesting that antidromic testing may provide a useful means of assessing proximal facial nerve function in pathologic states.)

Nowak DA, Linder S, Topka H. Diagnostic relevance of transcranial magnetic and electric stimulation of the facial nerve in the management of facial palsy. *Clin Neurophysiol.* 2005;116(9):2051. [PMID: 16024292] (The authors demonstrate that transcranial magnetic stimulation in the early diagnosis of Bell palsy is less specific than previously thought, although transcranial magnetic stimulation may be capable of localizing the site of lesion within the fallopian canal.)

Sawney BB, Kayan A. A study of the F wave from the facial muscles. *Electromyography.* 1970;3:287. [PMID: 5509973]

Schriefer TN, Mills KR, Murray NMF, Hess CW. Evaluation of proximal facial nerve conduction by transcranial magnetic stimulation. *J Neurol Neurosurg Psych.* 1988;51:60. [PMID: 3351531] (A magnetic stimulator was used for direct transcutaneous stimulation of the intracranial portion of the facial nerve in patients with a variety of facial nerve pathologies.)

Stennert E, Frentup KP, Limberg CH. Modern recording technique of the trigeminofacial reflexes. In: Fisch U, ed. *Facial Nerve Surgery.* Birmingham, AL: Aesculapius, 1977.

Wigand ME, Bumm P, Berg M. Recordings of antidromic nerve action potentials in the facial nerve. In: Fisch U, ed. *Facial Nerve Surgery.* Birmingham, AL: Aesculapius, 1977:101.

Zealar D, Kurago Z. Facial nerve recording from the eardrum. *Otolaryngol Head Neck Surg.* 1985;93:474. [PMID: 3931021] (Noninvasive technique described for recording from the facial nerve within the fallopian canal using electrodes placed on the eardrum.)

Disorders of the Facial Nerve

68

Lawrence R. Lustig, MD, & John K. Niparko, MD

Facial nerve dysfunction can dramatically affect a patient's quality of life. The human face is a focal point for expression and interpersonal communication whereas facial motor movement contributes to eye protection, speech articulation, chewing, and swallowing. Thus, the patient with a facial palsy suffers not only the functional consequences of impaired facial motion, but also the psychological impact of a skewed facial appearance.

ACUTE FACIAL PALSIES

 ESSENTIALS OF DIAGNOSIS

BELL'S PALSY

- *Acute onset, with unilateral paresis or paralysis of the face in a pattern consistent with peripheral nerve dysfunction (all branches affected).*
- *Rapid onset and evolution (< 48 hours).*
- *Facial palsy may be associated with acute neuropathies affecting other cranial nerves (particularly cranial nerves V–X).*

HERPES ZOSTER OTICUS (RAMSAY HUNT SYNDROME)

- *Acute peripheral facial palsy associated with otalgia and varicella-like cutaneous lesions that involve the external ear, skin of the ear canal, or the soft palate.*
- *Involvement often extends to cranial nerves V, IX, and X, and cervical branches that have anastomotic communications with the facial nerve.*
- *Differentiated from Bell's palsy by characteristic cutaneous ulcers and a higher incidence of hearing loss or balance dysfunction.*

General Considerations

There are a large variety of disorders that may be associated with unilateral facial palsies (Table 68–1). Bilateral facial palsy is much less common and occurs in less than 2% of patients presenting with an acute facial palsy (Table 68–2). Bilateral involvement typically reflects a systemic disorder with multiple manifestations. Because of their overlapping clinical presentation and treatment paradigms, Bell's palsy and herpes zoster oticus (also known as Ramsay Hunt syndrome) are considered together.

1. Bell's Palsy

No identifiable cause is present for approximately 60–70% of cases of acute facial palsy. The clinical diagnosis of Bell's palsy is appropriately applied in such cases. Bell's palsy manifests as an acute, unilateral paresis or paralysis of the face in a pattern consistent with peripheral nerve dysfunction (Figure 68–1). The onset and evolution are rapid—typically less than 48 hours. Other cranial nerves, particularly the trigeminal, abducens, facial, vestibulocochlear, glossopharyngeal, and vagus nerves, may manifest deficits.

There may also be subtle but frequent associated dysfunction of cranial nerves V, VIII, IX, and X in association with Bell's palsy. Pain or numbness affecting the ear, mid-face, and tongue, as well as taste disturbances, are common. These observations suggest that the facial weakness seen in Bell's palsy is the inflammatory facial-motor component of a wider cranial polyneuropathy.

Recurrent Bell's palsy, both ipsilateral and contralateral, occurs in up to 12% of patients. Recurrences are more likely in patients with a family history of Bell's palsy, and the incidence of diabetes mellitus in recurrent Bell's palsy patients is 2.5 times that noted in nonrecurrent cases. Immunodeficiency is also associated with recurrences. As noted below, any recurrence warrants a complete workup for another etiology.

2. Herpes Zoster Oticus

Herpes zoster oticus (Ramsay Hunt syndrome) is a syndrome of acute peripheral facial palsy associated with otalgia and varicella-like cutaneous lesions. It accounts for approximately 10–15% of acute facial palsy cases. The pathognomonic lesions may involve the external ear, particularly the meatal and preauricular skin, the skin of

Table 68–1. Differential diagnoses of facial paralysis.

Birth
  Molding
  Forceps delivery
  Myotonic dystrophy
  Möebius syndrome (facial diplegia associated with other cranial nerve deficits)

Trauma
  Cortical injuries
  Basilar skull fractures
  Brainstem injuries
  Penetrating injury to middle ear
  Facial injuries
  Altitude paralysis (barotrauma)
  Scuba diving (barotrauma)

Neurologic
  Opercular syndrome (cortical lesion in facial motor area)
  Millard-Gubler syndrome (abducens palsy with contralateral hemiplegia due to lesion in base of pons involving corticospinal tract)

Infection
  Malignant otitis externa
  Acute or chronic otitis media
  Cholesteatoma (acquired and congenital)
  Mastoiditis
  Meningitis
  Parotitis
  Chickenpox
  Herpes zoster oticus (Ramsay Hunt syndrome)
  Encephalitis
  Poliomyelitis (type I)
  Mumps
  Mononucleosis
  Leprosy
  HIV and AIDS
  Influenza
  Coxsackie virus
  Malaria
  Syphilis
  Scleroma
  Tuberculosis
  Botulism
  Mucormycosis
  Lyme disease

Genetic and Metabolic
  Diabetes mellitus
  Hyperthyroidism
  Pregnancy
  Hypertension
  Alcoholic neuropathy
  Bulbopontine paralysis
  Oculopharyngeal muscular dystrophy

Vascular
  Anomalous sigmoid sinus
  Benign intracranial hypertension
  Intratemporal aneurysm of internal carotid artery
  Embolization for epistaxis (external carotid artery branches)

Neoplastic
  Acoustic neuroma
  Glomus jugulare tumor
  Leukemia
  Meningioma
  Hemangioblastoma
  Hemangioma
  Pontine glioma
  Sarcoma
  Hydradenoma (external canal)
  Facial nerve neuroma
  Teratoma
  Fibrous dysplasia
  von Recklinghausen disease
  Carcinomatous encephalitis (Bannworth syndrome)
  Cholesterol granuloma
  Carcinoma (invasive or metastatic, from breast, kidney, lung, stomach, larynx, prostate, thyroid)

Toxic
  Thalidomide (Miehlke syndrome: cranial nerves VI and VII with atretic external ears)
  Tetanus
  Diphtheria
  Carbon monoxide
  Lead intoxication

Iatrogenic
  Mandibular block anesthesia
  Antitetanus serum
  Vaccine treatment for rabies
  Otologic, neurotologic, skull base, and parotid surgery iontophoresis (local anesthesia)
  Embolization

Idiopathic
  Familial Bell's palsy
  Melkersson-Rosenthal syndrome (recurrent facial palsy, furrowed tongue, faciolabial edema)
  Hereditary hypertrophic neuropathy (Charcot-Marie-Tooth disease, Dejerine-Scottas disease)
  Autoimmune syndromes of temporal arteritis, periarteritis nodosa, and other vasculitides
  Thrombotic thrombocytopenic purpura
  Landry-Guillain-Barré syndrome (ascending paralysis)
  Multiple sclerosis
  Myasthenia gravis
  Sarcoidosis (Heerfordt syndrome, uveoparotid fever)
  Wegener granulomatosis
  Eosinophilic granuloma
  Amyloidosis
  Hyperostoses (Paget disease, osteopetrosis)
  Kawasaki disease (infantile acute febrile mucocutaneous lymph node syndrome)

Reproduced, with permission, from May M: Differential diagnosis by history, physical findings, and laboratory results. In: May M, ed. *The Facial Nerve.* New York: Thieme-Stratton; 1986.

Table 68–2. Etiologies associated with bilateral facial palsies (may be simultaneous or delayed).

Bell palsy
Diabetes mellitus
Sarcoidosis (Heerfordt syndrome)
Periarteritis nodosa
Guillain-Barré syndrome
Myasthenia gravis
Basilar skull fracture
Bulbar palsies
Porphyrias
Leukemia
Myotonic dystrophia
Meningitis
Möbius syndrome
Botulism
Infectious mononucleosis
Leprosy
Malaria
Poliomyelitis
Lyme disease
Syphilis
Postvaccination neuropathy
Isoniazid
Osteopetrosis

the ear canal, or the soft palate (Figure 68–2). Hearing loss, dysacusis, and vertigo reflect extension of the infection to involve the eighth cranial nerve. Involvement often extends to other cranial nerves (V, IX, and X) and cervical branches (2, 3, and 4) that have anastomotic communications with the facial nerve. Herpes zoster oticus is therefore differentiated from Bell's palsy by the characteristic cutaneous changes and a higher incidence of hearing and balance dysfunction and other cranial neuropathies.

Pathogenesis

Studies of the intratemporal facial nerve suggest that Bell's palsy and herpes zoster oticus result from impaired facial nerve conduction within the temporal bone. In the labyrinthine segment of the fallopian canal, the facial nerve occupies more than 80% of the cross-sectional area of the surrounding facial canal between the meatal foramen and the geniculate fossa (in contrast to less than 75% in the tympanic and vertical segments of the canal) (Figure 68–3). Because the narrow diameter of the meatal foramen (Figure 68–3A) and the presence of a circumferential band of periosteum that virtually seals the entry site and constricts the nerve at this location (Figure 68–4), the meatal foramen appears to constitute a pressure transition zone or "physiologic bottleneck" in the presence of neural

edema. The ratio of the cross-sectional areas of the nerve to the meatal foramen is significantly smaller in pediatric temporal bones relative to those of adults, perhaps explaining the low incidence of Bell's palsy in pediatric populations.

In patients with near-total degeneration undergoing facial nerve decompression for Bell's paralysis, electrical stimulation demonstrated a transition in responsiveness in the (decompressed) region of the meatal foramen. Sequential stimulation in a distal-to-proximal direction from the second genu to the meatal foramen consistently revealed substantially diminished responses proximal to the meatal foramen. These observations strongly implicate the meatal foramen as the primary pathophysiologic site in Bell's palsy.

Most postmortem studies from patients with Bell's palsy demonstrate that diffuse involvement of the facial nerve in its intratemporal course was typical. Evidence of an inflammatory neuritis suggesting a viral etiology is frequently evident, though not uniformly observed. One study in a patient who died 13 days after the onset of Bell's palsy demonstrated intraneural inflammatory changes with leukocytic infiltration and demyelinization in the proximal intratemporal portion of the nerve, consistent with a viral infection. Other studies have demonstrated intraneural vascular congestion and hemorrhage in the labyrinthine segment of the nerve. The likelihood of the meatal foramen also being the critical site for nerve injury in herpes zoster oticus is supported by neuropathologic findings demonstrating a sharp demarcation between the degenerated nerve distal to and normal nerve proximal to the meatal foramen. It is also possible that several pathologic events may be sequential and synergistic in manifesting a clinical facial palsy, and the disease may represent a spectrum of entities with varied pathogeneses. Although inflammation and ischemia likely dominate early processes in Bell's palsy, neural blockade and degeneration, as well as subsequent fibroblastic response, probably manifest later in the sequence. Given the confinement of the nerve trunk within the meatal foramen, it is likely that compression at this site is a critical if not determinative event in the genesis of Bell's palsy and is triggered by one or a combination of the above etiologies. Histopathologic findings suggest that the facial palsy component of herpes zoster oticus is manifested by a similar process of entrapment, with typically a higher risk of irreversible degeneration of nerve fibers.

Eicher SA, Coker NJ, Alford BR, Igarashi M, Smith RJH. A comparative study of the fallopian canal at the meatal foramen and labyrinthine segment in young children and adults. *Arch Otolaryngol Head Neck Surg.* 1990;116:1030. [PMID: 2383386] (This report, documenting the differences in facial nerve palsy between children and adults, suggests that the facial nerve is not as tightly contained at the meatal foramen in children and

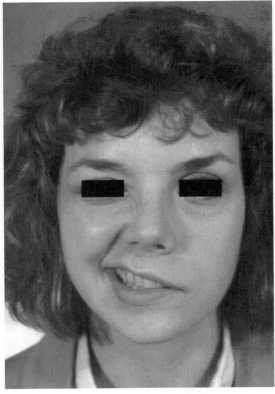
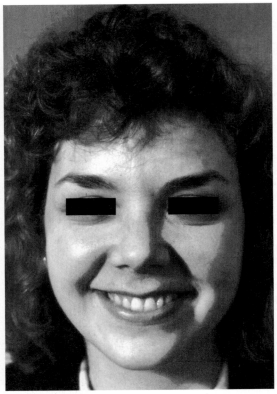

A

B

Figure 68–1. **(A)** Prototypic case of Bell's palsy. This 28-year-old woman experienced the onset of an acute, left-sided paralysis of the face over a 24-hour period, in a pattern consistent with peripheral nerve dysfunction. Treatment consisted of oral steroid dosing at pharmacologic doses for 10 days, followed by a 2-week taper. **(B)** Full recovery of facial motor function 2 months after onset.

provides a possible explanation for the relative infrequency of Bell's palsy in this age group.)

Fisch U, Esslen E. Total intratemporal exposure of the facial nerve: pathologic findings in Bell's palsy. *Arch Otolaryngol.* 1972;95:335. [PMID: 5018255] (This classic report highlights the intraoperative and pathologic findings of the facial nerve during intratemporal decompression of the nerve.)

Fowler EP. The pathologic findings in case of facial paralysis. *Trans Am Acad Ophthalmol Otolaryngol.* 1963;67:187. (This classic study evaluates the pathophysiology of facial paresis in a case of facial palsy.)

Gantz B, Gmur A, Fisch U. Intraoperative evoked electromyography in Bell's palsy. *Am J Otolaryngol.* 1982;3:273. [PMID: 7149140] (In this report, the technique of intraoperative evoked electromyography is described in detail.)

Jackson CG, Hyams VJ, Johnson GD, Poe DS. Pathologic findings in the labyrinthine segment of the facial nerve in a case of facial paralysis. *Ann Otol Rhinol Laryngol.* 1990;99:327. [PMID: 2337309] (The histopathologic findings for a patient with acute facial paralysis caused by herpes zoster oticus

who obtained no return of active facial function after 1 year are presented in this manuscript and are consistent with observations that the lesion producing Bell's palsy and herpes zoster oticus usually is situated at the meatal foramen.)

Liston SL, Kleid MS. Histopathology of Bell's palsy. *Laryngoscope.* 1989;99:23. [PMID: 2642582] (The histopathology of the facial nerve 1 week after the onset of Bell's palsy is reported.)

McKeever P, Proctor B, Proud G. Cranial nerve lesions in Bell's palsy. *Otolaryngol Head Neck Surg.* 1987;97:326. [PMID: 3118317] (This report documents all associated cranial nerve deficits in patients who present with Bell's palsy.)

Niparko JK, Kileny PR, Kemink JL, Lee SH, Graham MD. Neurophysiologic intraoperative monitoring: II. Facial nerve function. *Am J Otol.* 1989;10:55. [PMID: 2655465] (This report outlines the use of facial nerve monitoring in neurotologic surgery.)

Proctor B, Corgill DA, Proud G. The pathology of Bell's palsy. *Trans Am Acad Ophthalmol Otolaryngol.* 1976;82:70. [PMID: 969098] (This classic study examines the pathophysiology of Bell's palsy.)

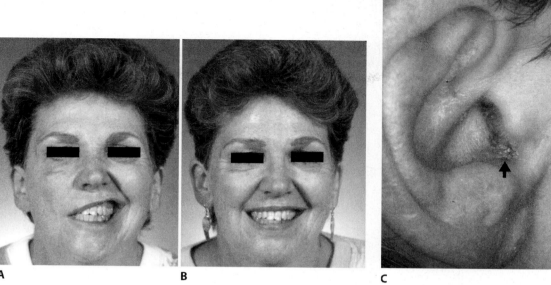

A **B** **C**

Figure 68–2. **(A)** Prototypic case of herpes zoster oticus. This 53-year-old woman experienced the onset of a right-sided facial paralysis with marked right-sided otalgia and throat pain. She presented 3 days after the onset of her symptoms and demonstrated minimal facial motor activity on evoked electromyography. Treatment consisted of oral steroid dosing at pharmacologic doses for 10 days, followed by a 2-week taper, and acyclovir given intravenously for 1 week. **(B)** Full recovery of facial motor function 4 months after onset. **(C)** Skin lesion of the right external meatus in the same patient with oticus in the crusting phase at the time of presentation.

Proctor B, Nager GT. The facial canal: normal anatomy variations and anomalies. *Ann Otol Rhinol Laryngol.* 1982;97:33. [PMID: 6814328] (This classic study provides a detailed descriptive anatomy with emphasis on the relations of the facial canal to adjacent structures, including the variations in the course of the facial canal.)

Wakisaka H, Hato N, Honda N et al. Demyelination associated with HSV-1-induced facial paralysis. *Exp Neurol.* 2002;178(1):68. [PMID: 12460609] (An experimental model of facial paralysis in mice demonstrates that facial nerve paralysis in this model is caused mainly by facial nerve demyelination in the descending segment).

Etiology

A. VIRAL NEURITIS

There is significant resemblance between Bell's palsy and other viral neuropathies. Poliomyelitis, mumps, Epstein-Barr virus, and rubella infections can include progressive neural dysfunction, often with subtotal regeneration as is often observed with Bell's palsy and herpes zoster oticus. There are multiple lines of evidence for a viral etiology in Bell's palsy based on clinical observations and experimental models reported over the past 20 years. Rabbit facial nerve trunks inoculated with herpes simplex virus (HSV)

demonstrate facial motor dysfunction that progressed to paralysis within the first week after inoculation. HSV Type I has been identified in isolates of the HSV from the nasopharynx of patients during the acute phase of Bell's palsy. A higher incidence of HSV antibodies has been identified in patients with Bell's palsy compared with gender- and age-matched controls. HSV has a well-known predilection for sensory neurons and can exist in a latent phase in sensory cell bodies of the ganglion. The facial nerve contains sensory neurons with cell bodies located in the geniculate ganglion, and it is believed that infection of the facial nerve, such as a geniculate ganglionitis, underlies Bell's palsy.

The presence of the HSV has been detected in epineurial biopsies from a patient undergoing facial nerve decompression for Bell's palsy. Lastly, ultrastructural studies of autopsy material from asymptomatic patients have demonstrated herpes simplex viral particles in sensory ganglia of regional cranial nerves, most notably the trigeminal ganglion. Thus, the preponderance of evidence highly suggests, but does not conclusively prove, that HSV is the cause of Bell's palsy.

The role of the varicella-zoster virus (VZV) as etiologic in herpes zoster oticus is supported strongly by the charac-

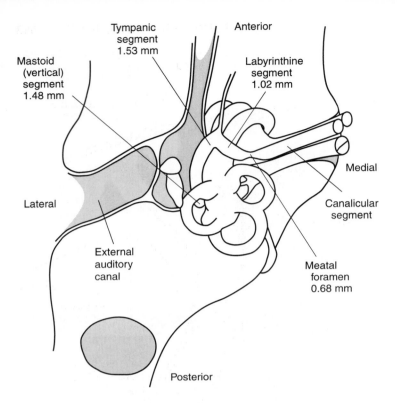

A

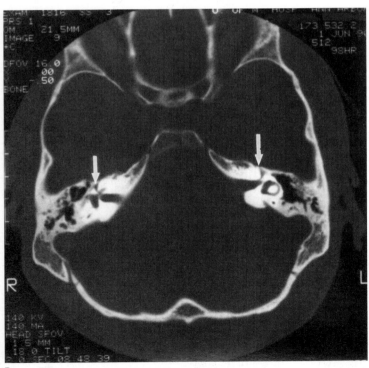

B

Figure 68–3. **(A)** Caliber of the (intratemporal) facial canal from the meatal foramen to the mastoid segment. **(B)** CT scan of temporal bones revealing the fallopian canal caliber for the labyrinthine segment proximal to the geniculate ganglion (white arrows).

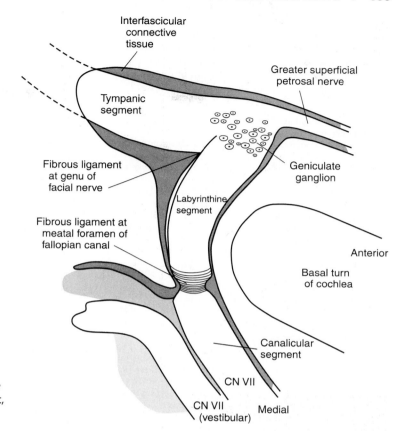

Figure 68–4. Surgical anatomy of the meatal foramen, labyrinthine segment, and geniculate fossa.

teristic varicelliform rash. This rash assumes a dermatologic distribution in a pattern that mimics the distribution of afferent fibers of the facial nerve. Serologic confirmation of VZV infection is often, but not always, possible. Histologic studies indicate facial dysfunction with herpes zoster oticus to be the result of an entrapment neuropathy, with more pronounced nerve fiber degeneration than that typically found in histopathologic studies of Bell's palsy.

The HSV and VZV are both DNA viruses of the herpes virus group and differ subtly in their ultrastructural features. Although differences in biologic behavior suggest that neuritides resulting from these viruses should manifest clinically distinguishable differences in their presentation, infections from HSV and VZV may mimic one another. Furthermore, HSV, mumps, and cytomegalovirus infections may produce a clinical picture resembling herpes zoster oticus, whereas varicella-zoster neuritis may occur in the absence of a rash, occasionally making a clear distinction between these clinical entities difficult.

B. ALTERNATIVE ETIOLOGIC THEORIES

Two other causes of Bell's palsy that have been proposed include ischemic insult and immunologic injury.

Theories advocating ischemic insult as a cause argue that impaired neural conduction follows small-vessel ischemia. The facial nerve derives its blood supply from an extrinsic, circumneural vessel network derived from the labyrinthine middle meningeal and the stylomastoid arteries. The circumneural system in turn connects to an intrinsic vascular supply of small-vessel tributaries within the perineurial compartment. The pathologic process is thought to involve this intrinsic system of vessels: Pressure elevations within the intraneural compartments produces venous stasis, stagnation of capillary flow, and a cycle of additional edema and an elevation in intraneural pressure. Circulatory sludging and, ultimately, tissue damage through acidosis and anoxia ensue. In this theory, the mechanism by which the cascade of primary ischemia is initiated remains unclear.

An alternate theory proposes that immunologic injury may be a potential cofactor in Bell's palsy. Studies demonstrating neuropathologic findings of segmental demyelination accompanied by lymphocytic infiltration of the perineurium support this etiology. Autoimmune mechanisms of nerve injury have also been suggested. Immunoassay methods have been used to detect acute-phase antibodies within the chorda tympani nerve from three of seven patients with Bell's palsy. Immune complexes found in the chorda tympani nerve fibers were characteristic of viral-antibody (Type III) immunologic reaction, suggesting an immune injury triggered by the presence of viral antigens.

Adour KK, Byl FM, Hilsinger RL, Kahn ZM, Sheldon MI. The true nature of Bell's palsy: analysis of 1000 consecutive patients. *Laryngoscope.* 1978;88:787. (This classic manuscript suggests that Bell's palsy be termed "idiopathic facial paralysis" and that it should be recognized as an acute benign cranial polyneuritis.)

Bance M, Rutka J. Speculation into the etiologic role of viruses in the development of Bell's palsy and disorders of inner ear dysfunction. *J Otolaryngol.* 1990;19:46. [PMID: 2179576] (Discussion of a case history of a patient who initially presented with an idiopathic facial palsy that years later developed into a spectrum of vestibular dysfunction associated with herpes zoster.)

Djupseland G, Berdal P, Johannsen TA et al. Virus infection as a cause of acute peripheral facial palsy. *Acta Otolaryngol.* 1976;102:403. [PMID: 938319] (This study examines the relationship between acute facial palsy and evidence of varicella-zoster infection and also demonstrates that an inflammatory reaction preceded or coincided with the facial palsy in all patients.)

Furuta Y, Ohtani F, Kawabata H, Fukuda S, Bergstrom T. High prevalence of varicella-zoster virus reactivation in herpes simplex virus-seronegative patients with acute peripheral facial palsy. *Clin Infect Dis.* 2000;30(3):529. [PMID: 10722439] (This study demonstrates that varicella-zoster virus is one of the major etiologic agents of clinically diagnosed Bell's palsy and that viral reactivation causes acute facial paralysis in most patients who lack antibodies to herpes simplex virus.)

Giannoni E, Corbacelli A. Aspects immunofluoroscopiques de la corde du tympan sur de sujets atteints de paralysie de Bell. *Rev Laryngol Otol Rhinol.* 1977;98:31. [PMID: 323952] (This report examines the pathology of the chorda tympani nerve in patients with Bell's palsy.)

Jackson CG. Facial nerve paralysis: diagnosis and treatment of lower motor neuron facial nerve lesions and facial paralysis. American Academy of Otolaryngology-Head & Neck Surgery Foundation, Washington, DC; 1986.

Kuhweide R, Van de Steene V, Vlaminck S, Casselman JW. Ramsay Hunt syndrome: pathophysiology of cochleovestibular symptoms. *J Laryngol Otol.* 2002;116(10):844. Review. [PMID: 12437843] (This study argues that the cochleovestibular symptoms in Ramsay Hunt syndrome may result from varicella-zoster virus transmission across the nerves inside the internal auditory canal and that prompt treatment with an antiviral-corticosteroid combination might be justified in any acute nonhydropic cochleovestibular syndrome.)

Linder T, Bossart W, Bodmer D. Bell's palsy and herpes simplex virus: fact or mystery? *Otol Neurotol.* 2005;26(1):109. [PMID: 15699730] (This study used polymerase chain reaction to detect herpes virus (HSV) and varicella-zoster virus in patients with acute facial paralysis and concluded that HSV genomic DNA within the sensory ganglion along the facial nerve does not explain the direct association with Bell's palsy.)

Mair IW, Flugsrud LB. Peripheral facial palsy and herpes zoster infection. *J Laryngol Otol.* 1976;90:373. [PMID: 178812] (This classic paper evaluates 133 consecutive cases of peripheral facial palsy and provides evidence for simultaneous infection with the varicella-zoster virus in nine patients [6–8%].)

Njoo FL, Wertheim-van Dillen P, Devriese PP. Serology in facial paralysis caused by clinically presumed herpes zoster infection. *Arch Otorhinolaryngol.* 1988;245:230. [PMID: 2845904] (Retrospective study examines the relationship between facial palsy and varicella-zoster virus infection.)

Ohtani F, Furuta Y, Aizawa H, Fukuda S. Varicella-zoster virus load and cochleovestibular symptoms in Ramsay Hunt syndrome. *Ann Otol Rhinol Laryngol.* 2006;115(3):233. [PMID: 16572614] (This study shows that several different patterns in the development of eighth cranial nerve dysfunction are caused by progression of neuritis or labyrinthitis following varicella-zoster virus reactivation.)

Peitersen E. The natural history of Bell's palsy. *Am J Otol.* 1982;4:107. [PMID: 7148998] (This classic study describes the spontaneous course of idiopathic facial palsy without treatment of any kind and included 1011 patients seen over a 15-year period.)

Pitts DB, Adour KK, Hilsinger RL. Recurrent Bell's palsy: analysis of 140 patients. *Laryngoscope.* 1988;98(5):535. [PMID: 3362016] (This report documents the clinical presentation, treatment, and outcome in a group of 140 patients with recurrent Bell's palsy and outlines a new classification system for ease of computer analysis and a simplified discussion of recurrent facial paralysis.)

Robillard PRB, Hilsinger RL, Adour KK. Ramsay Hunt facial paralysis: clinical analysis of 185 patients. *Otolaryngol Head Neck Surg.* 1986;95:292. [PMID: 3108776] (This prospective study evaluating 185 patients with Ramsay Hunt syndrome found that the facial palsy of Ramsay Hunt syndrome was more severe, caused late neural denervation, and had a less favorable recovery profile than Bell [herpes simplex] facial palsy.)

Tovi F, Sidi J, Haikin H, Sarov B, Sarov I. Viral infection and acute peripheral facial palsy: a study with herpes simplex and varicella zoster viruses. *Isr J Med Sci.* 1980;16:576. [PMID: 6252119] (The role of herpes simplex virus and varicella-zoster virus in acute peripheral facial palsy was evaluated according to clinical symptomatology and serologic findings in a series of 70 patients seen over a 1-year period, suggesting a relationship between herpes simplex and varicella-zoster.)

Vahlne A, Edstrom S, Arstila P et al. Bell's palsy and herpes simplex virus. *Arch Otolaryngol.* 1981;107:79. [PMID: 6258547] (The possible association of some viral infections with the onset of Bell's palsy was examined in a study of 142 patients.)

Incidence & Risk Factors

A wide spectrum of health care providers manage cases of acute facial palsy; an assessment of the true incidence of Bell's palsy is therefore complicated by this wide distribution of specialists. Nonetheless, this disorder is recognized as one of the most common neuropathies and appears to be universal in its occurrence. The incidence is approximately 15–40 per 100,000 individuals in the general population.

Age and gender influence the likelihood of contracting Bell's palsy; it is uncommon in patients under the age of 10 years but thereafter increases in incidence with age. Females in their teens and 20s carry a predilection for the disorder. Among middle-aged adults, there is a nearly equal distribution by gender with a slight male predominance in older age groups. Epidemiologic surveys indicate a seasonal variation in incidence in some geographic regions.

The risk posed by diabetes mellitus in developing Bell's palsy remains undetermined, although most studies suggest a heightened susceptibility. Several authors have demonstrated a correlation between pregnancy and acute facial palsy, particularly during the third trimester and with the presence of preeclampsia.

Immunodeficiency may also entail a heightened risk for acute facial palsy. Cranial neuropathies, including facial palsy, are observed with human immunodeficiency virus (HIV) infection, often in association with a symmetrical polyneuropathy. Facial dysfunction in this setting may also reflect either susceptibility to other infectious agents or the development of lymphoma. Facial palsy in association with HIV may occur in a clinical course characteristic of Bell's palsy or herpes zoster oticus. Neuropathies may appear at any stage of HIV infection: early after initial infection, as part of the chronic illness characterized by the acquired immunodeficiency syndrome (AIDS), or with AIDS-related meningitis. Case series suggest that facial palsy in the setting of HIV infection not associated with neoplasm demonstrates patterns of spontaneous recovery that are not unlike those of the general population.

Facial palsy associated with the conditions noted above is not necessarily diagnostic of Bell's palsy. Patients should be evaluated as completely as those who do not carry these risk factors, with the notable caveat of considering the risk and benefit of radiologic studies in pregnancy.

Clinical Findings

A. PATIENT EVALUATION

The diagnosis of Bell's palsy is one of exclusion. Facial motor disturbance should be characterized as Bell's palsy only after the exclusion of traumatic, neoplastic, infectious, metabolic, and congenital etiologies. Strict attention to the evaluation, particularly the history and otoscopic and neurologic findings, often differentiates an acute facial palsy of another origin from a true case of Bell's palsy.

On the clinical examination, the severity of the facial nerve weakness should be recorded by one of the standard facial nerve grading schemes. In particular, one should assess for the ability to close the eyelid, because this has the greatest functional significance. Vesicles within the auricle or external auditory canal may reveal the diagnosis of herpes zoster oticus. Pain or numbness affecting the ear, midface, and tongue, as well as taste disturbances, are common. Other cranial nerve deficits should also be noted.

B. LABORATORY FINDINGS

Blood and cerebrospinal fluid (CSF) studies only rarely differentiate a facial palsy and are largely unwarranted for most cases of Bell's palsy. For atypical cases though, one should consider Lyme titers and a search for a paraneoplastic syndrome.

C. IMAGING STUDIES

Routine radiologic evaluation is generally not recommended for most cases of acute facial palsy, particularly when the clinical course matches that of Bell's palsy or herpes zoster oticus. However, if the patient's recovery is incomplete over 3 months' time, the palsy becomes recurrent, or associated cranial nerve deficits develop, then scans are warranted. Magnetic resonance imaging (MRI) scanning with dye enhancement should include the brain, the skull base, and the temporal bone to rule out a lesion along the entire course of the facial nerve. High-resolution computed tomography (CT) scanning may be useful to define the bony detail in the course of the facial nerve within the fallopian (facial) canal.

Treatment

A. PRETREATMENT ASSESSMENT

Both pharmacologic and surgical treatments are designed to reduce the likelihood of residual facial dysfunction in susceptible patients with acute facial palsies. Prior reports have documented the reasons underlying the difficulty in assessing the efficacy of steroids and other therapeutic modalities for Bell's palsy. Evaluation of the response is complicated by the potential for spontaneous remission for most acute palsies. Impediments such as the fragmentation of care of facial palsy patients as well as the difficulty in obtaining early assessment and maintaining strict experimental conditions have thwarted systematic, definitive studies.

To assess the response to treatment, patients with facial palsy should be initially stratified using clinical and electrophysiologic criteria (see Chapter 67, Anatomy, Physiology, & Testing of the Facial Nerve). The assessment of the ultimate outcome requires sensitive and objective measures and a classification system that is universally accepted. As with any study of treatment effect, inconclusive or negative results may reflect insensitive measures of outcome.

A variety of facial nerve classification schemes have been proposed. The difficulty, of course, lies in translating facial impairment into a classification that is continuous and enables precise comparisons of functional recovery. Presently, the House-Brackmann grading system has been adopted by the American Academy of Otolaryngology-Head and Neck Surgery and has found the greatest acceptance among otolaryngologists in the United States (Table 68–3).

Table 68–3. The House-Brackmann facial nerve grading scale.

Grade	Function
I	Normal
II	Normal tone and symmetry at rest Slight weakness on close inspection Good to moderate movement of forehead Complete eye closure with minimum effort Slight asymmetry of mouth with movement
III	Normal tone and symmetry at rest Obvious but not disfiguring facial asymmetry Synkinesis may be noticeable but not severe, ± hemifacial spasm or contracture Slight to moderate forehead motion Complete eye closure with effort Slight weakness of mouth with maximum effort
IV	Normal tone and symmetry at rest Asymmetry is disfiguring or results in obvious facial weakness No perceptible forehead movement Incomplete eye closure Asymmetrical motion of mouth with maximum effort
V	Asymmetrical facial appearance at rest Slight, barely noticeable movement No forehead movement Incomplete eye closure Slight movement of mouth with effort
VI	No facial function perceptible

Reproduced, with permission, from House JW, Brackmann DE. Facial nerve grading system. *Otolaryngol Head Neck Surg.* 1985;93:146.

B. Non-Surgical Measures

1. Steroid therapy—Most early studies of the value of steroids in treating Bell's palsy were based on comparisons of treated patients with retrospective controls. Although double-blinded, randomized, controlled clinical trials have demonstrated a significantly higher rate of complete functional recovery in glucocorticoid-treated patients compared with the control group in most studies, the lack of randomization and concurrent controls and the dose of glucocorticoid used have not completely resolved the question.

Prospective, randomized trials have suggested, though not with statistical significance, that using larger doses of steroids with dextran and pentoxifylline demonstrated improved rates of recovery in the treated groups. Other double-blinded trials have demonstrated beneficial effects of glucocorticoid therapy as long as therapy was initiated early in the course of the palsy.

Oral prednisone has been used extensively to treat patients with Bell's palsy and herpes zoster oticus. Proof of efficacy is, however, controversial. Several series have compared the use of oral steroids with either no treatment or placebo; some have purported to show benefit in reducing residual weakness or aberrant regeneration and others suggest no benefit.

Meta-analytic reviews of steroids in the treatment of Bell's palsy suggest that they may have the following effects: (1) reducing the risk of denervation if initiated early on, (2) preventing or lessening synkinesis, (3) preventing progression of incomplete to complete paralysis, (4) hastening recovery, and (5) preventing autonomic synkinesis (crocodile tearing). However, no single investigation has yet been conducted with adequate size and experimental design to conclusively prove or disprove the effectiveness of steroids. However, in light of the low risk of side effects and minimal costs involved, prednisone is commonly started at the initial visit—even in patients with partial palsy—on the chance that a complete palsy might evolve within a few days. The initiation of steroid therapy during the first 24 hours of symptoms might confer a higher likelihood of recovery. In patients with Ramsay Hunt syndrome, higher rates of full recovery have been noted by some studies for patients receiving intravenous therapy.

a. Glucocorticoid steroids—Glucocorticoid steroids exert an inhibitory effect on virtually every phase of the inflammatory response and thus have assumed an important role in treating a vast range of inflammatory and immune-mediated disorders. The precise mechanism by which steroids exert beneficial effects is incompletely defined in many of the conditions for which they are prescribed. The pharmacologic effects of steroids make them attractive agents for ameliorating symptoms associated with the acute phases of Bell's palsy and herpes zoster oticus and, theoretically, for improving the likelihood of full recovery. In addition to their anti-inflammatory properties, the glucocorticoid steroids also exert a facilitatory action on the neuromuscular junction. These combined effects may contribute to the recovery of neuromusculature function in disorders such as inflammatory polyradiculoneuropathies (the Landry-Guillain-Barré syndrome), the pathology of which is marked by inflammatory, segmental demyelinization.

The desired goal of glucocorticoid therapy for acute facial paralysis is to induce effective anti-inflammatory control. To provide such control, the inflammatory process should be countered with consistent, pharmacologic levels of an anti-inflammatory agent, beginning as soon as possible. Once the inflammatory process is checked and the stimulus for inflammation removed, therapy can be discontinued. However, abrupt withdrawal may be followed by a rebound of disease activity. To prevent reacceleration of the inflammatory process, a tapered withdrawal of the daily glucocorticoid dose over 10–14 days is recommended.

Based on the theoretical active phase of the herpes simplex and varicella-zoster viruses (3 and 14 days, respectively), the following strategy for steroid treatment of Bell's palsy and herpes zoster oticus has been proposed: oral prednisone (1 mg/kg/d) divided into 3 doses per day for 7–10 days. The daily dose should then be tapered to zero over the following 10 days. Theoretically, this dosing regimen maximizes anti-inflammatory activity while minimizing side effects and is consistent with anti-inflammatory schedules that are effective in controlling acute hypersensitivity as well as autoimmune and other inflammatory disorders.

When administered intravenously, methylprednisolone is prescribed at 1 g/d administered intravenously as either a single dose or in 3 divided doses for 3–7 days, followed by an oral prednisone taper.

b. Side effects of steroid therapy—Side effects that are likely to be manifest during short-term steroid treatment include hyperglycemic action. Given the high incidence of glucose intolerance in some series of acute facial palsy patients, steroids should be initially prescribed with caution. Other acute side effects include CNS changes such as psychotic breaks, fluid and electrolyte disturbances, acne, increased intraocular pressure, and gastrointestinal irritation. Corticosteroids are category C drugs in pregnant patients.

An adverse effect of glucocorticoid administration that deserves special consideration is a heightened susceptibility to infection. Glucocorticoids should be used with caution in patients with existing gastrointestinal infections and in cases of latent tuberculosis. The effects of glucocorticoids on cellular and humoral components of inflammation may lessen host immunity to bacterial, viral, and fungal infections. Latent infections may become reactivated and spread. Moreover, suppression of the inflammatory response may conceal symptoms and signs of infection.

Although effects on host resistance have been demonstrated in experimental trials, typical daily doses of glucocorticoids (1 mg/kg/d of prednisone or its equivalent) given for 2 weeks or less are only rarely associated with an increased susceptibility to infection. The risk of steroid-induced dissemination of viruses presents a particular concern in treating acute facial palsies of viral origin. The risk of virus dissemination is significant with steroid therapy beyond 1 month and in immunosuppressed patients. Otherwise, clinical experience suggests that the risk of this complication is minimal and that steroids can ameliorate postherpetic neuralgia.

2. Antiviral therapy—Antiviral therapy represents a newer adjunct in treating acute facial palsy of viral origin. Based on its spectrum of activity and low toxicity, acyclovir, a synthetic purine nucleoside analogue, has found clinical use in treating herpes zoster oticus. In cell culture, acyclovir inhibits the herpes simplex Types I and II, varicella-zoster, and Epstein-Barr viruses and cytomegalovirus.

Indications for the use of acyclovir include herpes simplex viral infections in genital herpes, immunocompromised patients, herpes simplex encephalitis, and varicella-zoster infections in immunocompromised patients. Early reports suggest that acyclovir may mitigate neurologic deficits produced by herpes zoster oticus.

a. Intravenous antiviral agents—Intravenous acyclovir (10 mg/kg every 8 hours for 7 days) produced substantially greater functional return in patients treated within the first 72 hours after the onset of paralysis. Moreover, preliminary reports have demonstrated early recovery of facial nerve function and reversal of sensorineural hearing loss associated with herpes zoster oticus in response to the drug early on, though these are nonrandomized trials. Given the high incidence of nerve degeneration associated with this disorder, these results appear promising. The efficacy of acyclovir in treating herpes zoster oticus and its potential role in treating Bell's palsy are currently under evaluation.

b. Oral antiviral agents—Oral antiviral agents are significantly less costly and more convenient than intravenous agents. An exception to the general preference for oral antiviral agents exists in immunocompromised patients with severe or widespread herpes zoster oticus. Newer antiviral drugs, including valacyclovir, famciclovir, and penciclovir, are better absorbed after oral administration than acyclovir and have increasingly been used in treating Ramsay Hunt syndrome. However, these drugs are more expensive than acyclovir. Valacyclovir may be superior to acyclovir in limiting zoster pain.

Acyclovir has also been used for the treatment of Bell's palsy. When compared with patients who received oral prednisone alone, some studies have identified a higher recovery rate as well as reduced rates of synkinesis in Bell's palsy patients given oral acyclovir plus prednisone. Conflicting studies have found little benefit from adding oral acyclovir to prednisone in Bell's palsy.

Synthesizing the myriad clinical trials on the topic, one can say that oral acyclovir appears reasonably indicated in all cases of herpes zoster oticus. Although proof of efficacy is limited in Bell's palsy, low risks and costs associated with acyclovir suggest that it may be reasonable to include its use in patients with complete facial paralysis. Acyclovir is prescribed at 400 mg or 800 mg 5 times daily and administered orally for 7–10 days in Bell's palsy. Alternately, acyclovir may be prescribed at 300–1000 mg (5–10 mg/kg) three times daily administered intravenously. Higher acyclovir doses (ie, 4000 mg per day orally) are recommended for patients suffering from herpes zoster oticus. Intravenous dosing is often indicated for immunocompromised individuals with severe infection. The main side effects of antiviral agents are nausea, malaise, injection site reactions, and mild renal insufficiency. Acyclovir is a category B drug in pregnant patients.

3. Physical therapy

a. Electrical stimulation—Transcutaneous electrical (galvanic) stimulation of the facial muscles has been used in an effort to maintain membrane conductivity and reduce muscle atrophy. It has also been used to potentially limit residua such as persistent paresis in patients with long-standing facial palsy. There exist few compelling, comparative trials to support this practice, although interest in this measure persists. Electrical stimulation may also improve function in chronic facial palsy. Patients left with partial deficits often benefit from physical therapy. Electromyographic and mirror feedback has been used to facilitate muscle reeducation to assist in the recovery of symmetric facial tone and expression.

b. Eye care—The cornea is vulnerable to drying and foreign body irritation in acute facial palsy due to orbicularis oculi dysfunction. Corneal desiccation and abrasion can result from incidental contact, particularly during sleep and can progress to cataract formation. Measures that confer corneal protection are recommended. Examination of the cornea by slit-lamp biomicroscopy and either fluorescein or rose Bengal staining provides the most sensitive measure for the early detection of corneal compromise. For mild facial paresis, therapy is generally not needed, unless dysfunction of cranial nerve V is present because the combination of a facial weakness and dysesthesia dramatically increases the risk of corneal exposure and ulceration. For moderate to severe deficits, a corneal moistening regimen should consist of a moisture chamber, artificial tears during the daytime, and ocular ointments at night. Sunglasses or other protective eyewear should be worn to protect the eyes in the outdoors. The lower eyelid can be gently elevated with adhesive tape running obliquely from the lower lid to the orbital rim, temporarily improving lid closure.

In longer-standing cases of facial palsy, lubrication and occlusion are insufficient to protect the cornea. Implanting a gold weight in the upper lip, which induces ptosis, and reducing the exposed area of cornea may augment lid suturing. This procedure is often augmented by elevating the lower lid via a lateral canthopexy, in which the tarsal ligament is suspended to the periorbital periosteum. Joining the upper and lower lid margins laterally (tarsorrhaphy) may be performed to narrow the palpebral fissure. The standard procedure calls for suturing a margin of upper and lower lid together from the lateral canthus inward. The width of the tarsorrhaphy is adjusted to optimize the degree of lid closure. If neural recovery ensues, the tarsorrhaphy can be reversed.

C. Surgical Measures

Mounting anatomic and electrophysiologic evidence of a specific anatomic lesion site in Bell's palsy has guided the choice of procedures for surgical intervention. These approaches now focus on decompressing the meatal foramen and adjacent labyrinthine segment of the nerve for cases thought to have a poor prognosis for complete recovery with medical treatment alone.

1. Nerve decompression—Surgical approaches to treating acute facial palsy are based on the premise that axonal ischemia can be reduced by the decompression of nerve segments presumed to be inflamed and entrapped. Facial nerve decompression, aimed at alleviating Bell's palsy and herpes zoster oticus, has been variably embraced for more than 70 years. The role of surgery has evolved in concert with developments in electrophysiologic testing and techniques of enhanced surgical exposure of the facial nerve.

a. Preoperative considerations—Evoked electromyography (EEMG) may be used to help stratify patients who might benefit from facial nerve decompression. Surgical treatment is offered when evoked response amplitudes are 10% (or less) of the normal side. This criterion is based on the observation that approximately one half of patients who progressed to a nadir of 95–100% degeneration within 2 weeks of the onset of the paralysis demonstrated a permanent, unsatisfactory recovery of facial function. Furthermore, most patients who reach a 90% level of degeneration progressed beyond 94% degeneration in the EEMG profile. Therefore, the proposal that immediate surgical decompression be performed as soon as the 90% level of degeneration has been reached entailed unnecessary surgery in, at most, 10% of patients. All patients who underwent decompression when degeneration reached 90% demonstrated a satisfactory return of facial movement. The 90% rate of satisfactory outcome with surgery compared favorably with the 50% chance of satisfactory return noted in patients who were not operated on and who were matched by EEMG profile. Surgery performed on eight patients in the third week after onset of the palsy, when degeneration exceeded 90%, did not significantly improve the return of facial function. However, two patients in this group demonstrated an exceptional return of facial movement after decompression. These observations suggest that studies of more patients with delayed degeneration are needed before the role of surgical decompression can be assessed definitively in this subset of patients.

b. Transmastoid approach—Both transmastoid and middle fossa approaches have been described, although transmastoid approaches are thought to provide limited

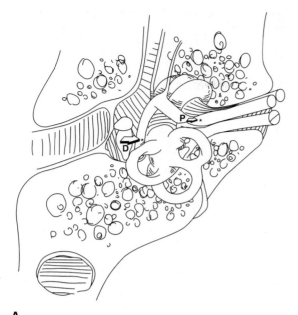

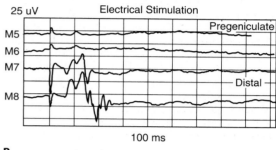

Figure 68–5. **(A)** Schematic of the approach to the intracanalicular and labyrinthine segments of the facial nerve via a middle cranial fossa. P, Pregeniculate (proximal) site of stimulation. D, Distal site of stimulation at the tympanic segment of the facial nerve. **(B)** Electrically evoked responses obtained after decompression of the meatal foramen in a patient with Bell's paralysis and > 90% reduction on preoperative EEMG. Responses of reduced amplitude to pregeniculate stimulation suggest the lesion is in the labyrinthine segment of the facial nerve. (A: Adapted, with permission, from Fisch U, Esslen E. Total intratemporal exposure of the facial nerve: Pathologic findings in Bell palsy. *Arch Otolaryngol.* 1972;95:335; B: Adapted, with permission, from Gantz B, Gmur A, Fisch U. Intraoperative electromyography in Bell's palsy. *Am J Otolaryngol.* 1982;3:273.)

exposure of the meatal foramen owing to the interposed labyrinth. The transmastoid approach to the geniculate ganglion and the labyrinthine segment obviates a craniotomy, but requires removal of the incus in poorly pneumatized bones to facilitate exposure of the facial nerve proximal to the cochleariform process. Some studies have shown that facial nerve decompression using the transmastoid approach improved recovery in patients whose maximal nerve stimulation responses were reduced by 75% or more. However, long-term follow-up of these patients failed to evidence significant benefit from this procedure as compared to the spontaneous recovery rate found in other studies.

c. **Middle cranial fossa approach**—The middle cranial fossa approach to the meatal, labyrinthine, and geniculate segments of the nerve facilitates direct decompression with small though significant risk to the labyrinth (Figure 68–5A). Permanent ipsilateral auditory and vestibular loss, meningitis, and subarachnoid hemorrhage are potential complications of facial nerve

decompression via a middle cranial fossa approach. This approach also permits direct stimulation of the facial nerve proximal to the meatal foramen, enabling verification of the site of impairment if a complete loss of response to electrical stimulation has not yet occurred. Intraoperative stimulus trials typically reveal severely decreased to absent responses proximal to the foramen. However, stimulation distal to the foramen typically evokes potentials of substantially greater amplification (Figure 68–5B).

2. **Nerve grafting**—Facial motor reinnervation may be accomplished by grafting a section of normal peripheral nerve over a damaged area, or bringing fibers from the intact facial nerve across the midline to innervate the paralyzed side, or by direct anastomosis of the ipsilateral hypoglossal nerve with the peripheral facial nerve. Nerve grafting may be augmented by muscle transfer procedures, since atrophy of facial muscles may render the muscle fibers less amenable to reinnervation. A wide variety of

reconstructive procedures, including rhytidectomy, blepharoplasty, brow lift, and facial slings, can improve resting tone and symmetry.

Aberrant regeneration may give rise to inappropriate patterns of reinnervation wherein specific muscle groups receive excessive neural inputs. Spasm and synkinesis with facial nerve recovery often produce undesired eye closure (Figure 68–6). This form of aberrant facial nerve regeneration can often be managed with subcutaneous or intramuscular botulinum toxin injections. Botulinum toxin, which induces temporary paresis in targeted muscles for up to 6 months, can reduce disability with tonic contractions, hemifacial spasm, and synkinesis. Side effects of botulinum toxin are rare and typically reveal severely decreased to absent responses proximal to the foramen. However, stimulation distal to the foramen typically evokes potentials of substantially greater amplification.

Prognosis

Most series that have assessed surgical decompression of the facial nerve in Bell's palsy have been small and retrospective and have targeted subjects most likely to suffer residual deficits (ie, patients with complete palsies and severe reductions in neural conductivity as demonstrated by electrophysiologic testing). Results that have used the middle fossa approach have included multicenter, prospective data, although subjects were nonrandomized. In these studies, patients recovered completely or with slight residual deficits in 91% of the surgical group, but in only 42% of a similar, medically treated group, suggesting a benefit of decompression using this surgical approach. Because of the difficult nature of designing such a controlled trial, the precise role of facial nerve decompression in the management of Bell's palsy and herpes zoster oticus remains unclear at present.

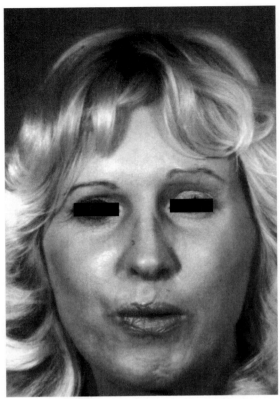

Figure 68–6. 38-year-old woman 1 year after recovery from Bell's paralysis with synkinetic closure of left eye with lip movement.

Adour KK, Byl FM, Hilsinger RL, Kahn ZM, Sheldon MI. The true nature of Bell's palsy: analysis of 1000 consecutive patients. *Laryngoscope.* 1978;88:787. [PMID: 642672] (This classic study of 1502 patients with Bell's palsy led to the conclusion that Bell's palsy is an acute benign cranial polyneuritis probably caused by reactivation of the herpes simplex virus and that the dysfunction of the motor cranial nerves [V, VII, X] may represent inflammation and demyelination rather than ischemic compression.)

Adour KK, Diamond C. Decompression of the facial nerve in Bell's palsy: a historical review. *Otolaryngol Head Neck Surg.* 1982;90: 453. [PMID: 6817276] (This article reviews, in chronologic order, the history and present status of facial nerve decompression in the surgical management of patients with Bell's palsy.)

Adour KK, Ruboyianes JM, Von Doersten PG et al. Bell's palsy treatment with acyclovir and prednisone compared with prednisone alone: a double-blind, randomized, controlled trial. *Ann Otol Rhinol Laryngol.* 1996;105(5):371. [PMID: 8651631] (This double-blind study compared the final outcome of 99 patients with Bell's palsy treated with either acyclovir-prednisone or placebo-prednisone, and demonstrated

that the outcome in acyclovir-prednisone-treated patients was superior to that in placebo-prednisone-treated patients.)

Allen D, Dunn L. Acyclovir or valacyclovir for Bell's palsy (idiopathic facial paralysis). *Cochrane Database Syst Rev.* 2004;(3):CD001869. [PMID: 15266457] (This meta-analysis of the use of antiviral medications for Bell's palsy suggests that more data are needed from a large multicenter randomized, controlled, and blinded study with at least 12 months' follow-up before a definitive recommendation can be made regarding the effect of acyclovir or valacyclovir on Bell's palsy.)

Brach JS, Van Swearingen JM. Physical therapy for facial paralysis: a tailored treatment approach. *Phys Ther.* 1999;79(4):397. [PMID: 10201545] (This case report describes a classification system used to guide treatment and to monitor recovery of an individual with facial paralysis and describes how the use of this classification system may help simplify the rehabilitation process.)

Brown J. Bell's palsy: a five-year review of 174 consecutive cases; an attempted double-blind study. *Laryngoscope.* 1982;92:1369. [PMID: 6757616] (This paper examines 174 consecutive cases of Bell's palsy that were clinically divided into a group with incomplete facial palsy and a group with complete facial palsy, outlining the prognosis in each group.)

Claman H. Glucocorticosteroids II: the clinical responses. *Hosp Pract.* 1983;18(7):143. [PMID: 6407967] (This paper reviews the use and treatment responses of the class of glucocorticosteroid medications.)

Fauci A, Dale D, Balow J. Glucocorticosteroid therapy: mechanisms of action and clinical considerations. *Ann Intern Med.* 1976;84:304. [PMID: 769625] (This review outlines the mechanisms of action of steroids and their use in various clinical scenarios.)

Fisch U. Surgery for Bell's palsy. *Arch Otolaryngol.* 1981;107:1. [PMID: 7469872] (This electroneuronographic study of the spontaneous course of Bell's palsy shows that the chance of a satisfactory spontaneous return of facial function is reduced by 50% when 95% or more maximal degeneration is reached within two weeks of onset.)

Fisch U, Esslen E. Total intratemporal exposure of the facial nerve: pathologic findings in Bell's palsy. *Arch Otolaryngol.* 1972; 95:335. [PMID: 5018255] (This report highlights the intraoperative and pathologic findings of the facial nerve during intratemporal decompression of the nerve.)

Gantz B, Rubinstein J, Gidley P, Woodworth G. Surgical management of Bell's palsy. *Laryngoscope.* 1999;109(8):1177. [PMID: 10443817] (This prospective study examines surgical decompression of the facial nerve in a population of patients with Bell's palsy who exhibit the electrophysiologic features associated with poor outcomes.)

House JW. Facial nerve grading systems. *Laryngoscope.* 1983;93:1056. [PMID: 3921901] (This classic study outlines the basis of the House-Brackmann facial nerve grading scale, the most widely used facial grading scale used.)

House JW, Brackmann DE. Facial nerve grading system. *Otolaryngol Head Neck Surg.* 1985;93:146. [PMID: 3921901] (This classic study outlines the basis of the House-Brackmann facial nerve grading scale, the most widely used facial grading scale used.)

Kartush J, Linstrom C, McCann P, Graham M. Early gold weight eyelid implantation for facial paralysis. *Otolaryngol Head Neck Surg.* 1990;103(6):1016. [PMID: 2126116] (This study evaluates the use of the gold weight for facial reanimation in patients with facial palsy.)

Keczkes K, Basheer AM. Do corticosteroids prevent postherpetic neuralgia? *Br J Dermatol.* 1980;102:551. [PMID: 7387900] (This study evaluates 20 patients who received prednisolone for the treatment of postherpetic neuralgia, compared with 20 patients who received carbamazepine.)

Kinishi M, Hosomi H, Amatsu M, Tani M, Koike K. Conservative treatment of Ramsay Hunt syndrome. *Jibiinkoka Gakkai Kaiho.* 1992;95(1):65. [PMID: 1709354] (This study evaluates the use of a "steroid-dextran" in 172 cases of Bell's palsy.)

Laskawi R, Damenz W, Roggenkamper P, Baetz A. Botulinum toxin treatment in patients with facial synkinesis. *Eur Arch Otorhinolaryngol Suppl.* 1994;S195:9. [PMID: 10774349] (This study outlines the treatment rationale and technique of botulinum [Botox] toxin to treat facial synkinesis.)

May M. Total facial nerve exploration: transmastoid, extralabyrinthine, and subtemporal. *Laryngoscope.* 1979;89:906. [PMID: 312987] (This paper describes a transmastoid operation that provides exposure of the labyrinthine segment of the facial nerve without performance of a craniotomy.)

May M, Klein SR, Taylor FH. Idiopathic (Bell's) facial palsy: natural history defies steroid or surgical treatment. *Laryngoscope.* 1985;95:406. [PMID: 3982183] (The results from this and prior studies indicate transmastoid facial nerve surgery is not recommended to treat Bell's palsy because no benefits have been identified that outweigh the risks of surgery.)

Morrow M. Bell's palsy and herpes zoster oticus. Current treatment options. *Neurology.* 2000;2(5):407. [PMID: 11096766] (This report outlines the author's approach to treating patients with Bell's palsy and herpes zoster oticus, including the use of oral prednisone in those patients with complete facial palsy and no contraindications to their use, and the use of antivirals [acyclovir].)

Peitersen E. The natural history of Bell's palsy. *Am J Otol.* 1982; 4:107. [PMID: 7148998] (This classic study describes the spontaneous course of idiopathic facial palsy without treatment of any kind and included 1011 patients seen over a 15-year period.)

Ramos Macias A, de Miguel Martinez I, Martin Sanchez AM, Gomez Gonzalez JL, Martin Galan A. The incorporation of acyclovir into the treatment of peripheral paralysis: a study of 45 cases. *Acta Otorrinolaringol Esp.* 1992;43(2):117. [PMID: 1605959] (The relation between use of acyclovir and facial nerve palsy prognosis was studied, but found no added benefit in patients treated with acyclovir compared with steroids.)

Salinas RA, Alvarez G, Ferreira J. Corticosteroids for Bell's palsy (idiopathic facial paralysis). 2004;18(4):CD001942. [PMID: 15495021] (This recent meta-analysis of randomized controlled trials did not show significant benefit from treating Bell's palsy with corticosteroids. More randomized controlled trials with a greater number of patients are needed to determine reliably whether there is real benefit (or harm) from corticosteroid therapy in patients with Bell's palsy.)

Stankiewicz J. Steroids and idiopathic facial paralysis. *Otolaryngol Head Neck Surg.* 1983;91:672. [PMID: 6320082] (This article reviews 92 papers that study steroids used for facial paralysis.)

Targan R, Alon G, Kay S. Effect of long-term electrical stimulation on motor recovery and improvement of clinical residuals in patients with unresolved facial nerve palsy. *Otolaryngol Head Neck Surg.* 2000;122(2):246. [PMID: 10652399] (This study investigated the efficacy of a pulsatile electrical current to shorten neuromuscular conduction latencies and minimize clinical residuals in patients with chronic facial nerve damage caused by Bell's palsy or acoustic neuroma excision.)

Tyring SK, Beutner KR, Tucker BA, Anderson WC, Crooks R. Antiviral therapy for herpes zoster: randomized, controlled clinical trial of valacyclovir and famciclovir therapy in immunocompetent patients 50 years and older. *Arch Fam Med.* 2000;9(9):863. [PMID: 11031393] (This randomized study compares the efficacy and safety of valacyclovir hydrochloride and famciclovir for the treatment of herpes zoster.)

Wolf S, Wagner J, Davidson S et al. Treatment of Bell's palsy with prednisone: a prospective randomized study. *Neurology.* 1978;28:158. [PMID: 340980] (Two hundred thirty-nine patients with Bell's palsy were randomly distributed into prednisone-treated and control groups and studied.)

Wood M, Shukla S, Fiddian A, Crooks R. Treatment of acute herpes zoster: effect of early (less than 48 hours) versus late (48- to 72-hour) therapy. [PMID: 9852981] (Acyclovir significantly shortened the time to complete resolution of zoster-associated pain compared with placebo—and valacyclovir was superior to acyclovir in this regard—even when therapy was delayed up to 72 hours after the onset of rash.)

Yanagihara N, Honda N, Hato N, Murakami S. Edematous swelling of the facial nerve in Bell's palsy. *Acta Otolaryngol.* 2000;120:667. [PMID: 11039881] (Considering the etiology and the analysis of edematous swelling, the authors propose that the course of Bell's palsy be differentiated into an acute phase [the first 3 weeks after onset], a subacute phase [from 4th–9th weeks] and a chronic phase [after 10th week].)

OTHER FACIAL NERVE DISORDERS

Next to Bell's palsy, the most common causes of acute, peripheral facial paralysis are trauma, herpes zoster oticus, bacterial infection, perinatal factors, and neoplastic involvement of the nerve. An acute facial palsy due to trauma or infection often presents with characteristic findings that readily point to a diagnosis. In contrast, differentiating neoplastic involvement of the facial nerve from Bell's palsy frequently poses a dilemma. Several other disorders (described below) should be considered in the clinical evaluation of an acute facial palsy. It must always be remembered that Bell's palsy is a diagnosis of exclusion, and one should therefore consider the following disorders in the context of the presenting symptoms and signs of the patient.

1. Facial Nerve Neoplasms

A variety of neoplasms may induce a facial palsy, which is occasionally acute in onset (Table 68–1 and Figure 68–7). It is estimated that there is an incidence of sudden facial palsy in 27% of patients found to have neoplastic involvement of the nerve—a surprisingly high incidence given the slow growth and encapsulation of most tumors responsible for the palsy.

Although patients with Bell's palsy may present with a variety of associated symptoms, atypical presentations

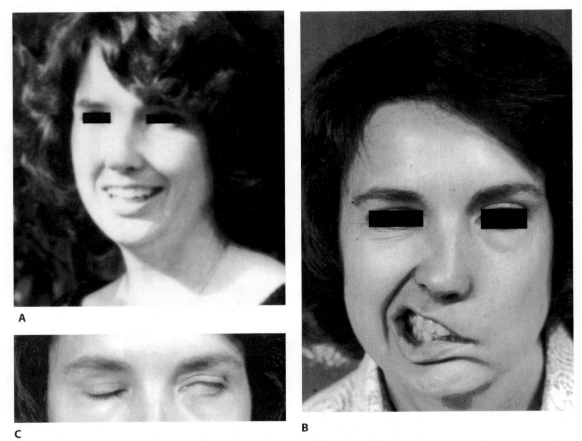

Figure 68–7. **(A)** A 42-year-old woman before onset of facial dysfunction. **(B)** Left facial paralysis of 1-year's duration mistakenly attributed to Bell's palsy. Severe facial skewing due to complete loss of facial motor tone is apparent. **(C)** The severity of the patient's facial nerve dysfunction allows for only passive closure of the left eye. *(Continued)*

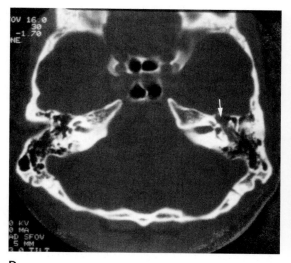

D

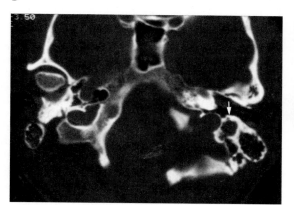

E

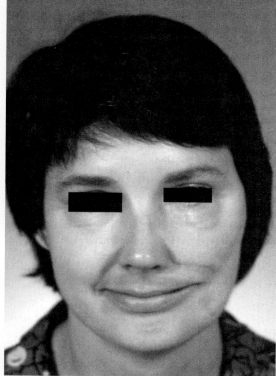

G

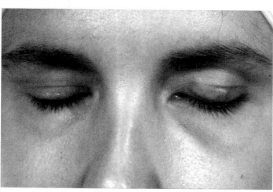

F

Figure 68–7(Cont'd). **(D)** CT scan of temporal bones demonstrating facial nerve neuroma involving the tympanic segment (arrow). **(E)** CT scan of temporal bones revealing expansion of fallopian canal within the mastoid segment that is filled with soft-tissue density. **(F)** After resection of facial schwannoma from meatal foramen to stylomastoid foramen, a sural nerve graft was placed. Reinnervation did not occur, requiring lower lid acanthopelyx and (gold) weighting of upper eyelid to achieve eye closure. **(G)** Early postoperative view after left temporalis transposition to achieve lower facial soft tissue support.

warrant consideration of other causes, particularly neoplasms. A facial palsy produced by a neoplasm may differ only subtly from Bell's palsy. There are characteristic historical and clinical features that suggest that a neoplasm is responsible for a facial palsy: (1) progression of a facial palsy over 3 weeks or longer; (2) no return of facial function within 3–6 months of the onset of paralysis; (3) failure to resolve an incomplete paresis within 2 months; (4) facial hyperkinesia, particularly hemifacial spasm, antecedent to the palsy; (5) associated dysfunction of regional cranial nerves; (6) prolonged otalgia or facial pain; (7) a mass in the middle ear, external ear canal, digastric region, or parotid gland; and (8) recurrent ipsilateral palsy.

Although Bell's palsy may recur, a recurrent palsy indicates the need for an exhaustive tumor search with radiologic evaluation. When the diagnosis of a neoplasm is delayed or missed, the neoplasm carries the potential consequences of extension into the labyrinth and cranial fossae. Extension into the cerebellopontine angle diminishes the opportunity for effective reanimation with direct neural anastomosis, underscoring both the need for vigilance in cases of atypical facial palsy and the importance of early diagnosis.

Facial nerve hemangiomas may also present with facial palsy. A classic presentation of a patient with a facial nerve hemangioma is one of recurrent and progressively more severe episodes of unilateral facial palsy. Treatment involves surgical excision, often at the expense of residual facial nerve function.

Angeli SI, Brackmann DE. Is surgical excision of facial nerve schwannomas always indicated? *Otolaryngol Head Neck Surg.* 1997;117 (6):S144. [PMID: 9419130] (This article outlines the indications for surgical excision of facial nerve schwannomas.)

Isaacson B, Telian SA, McKeever PE, Arts HA. Hemangiomas of the geniculate ganglion. *Otol Neurotol.* 2005;26(4):796. [PMID: 16015187] (Review of the presentation and clinical course of six patients with hemangiomas of the geniculate ganglion.)

Jackson CG, Glasscock ME, Hughes GB, Sismanis A. Facial paralysis of neoplastic origin: diagnosis and management. *Laryngoscope.* 1980;90:1581. [PMID: 6999266] (This classic article outlines the basis for differentiating facial palsy with a neoplastic origin from that with an idiopathic origin [ie, Bell's palsy].)

Liu R, Fagan P. Facial nerve schwannoma: surgical excision versus conservative management. *Ann Otol Rhinol Laryngol.* 2001;110 (11):1025. [PMID: 11713912] (This study compares a series of 22 patients with facial nerve schwannoma, of whom 12 underwent definitive excision and 10 were managed more conservatively.)

Perez R, Chen JM, Nedzelski JM. Intratemporal facial nerve schwannoma: a management dilemma. *Otol Neurotol.* 2005;26(1):121. [PMID: 15699732] (This report outlines the clinical management of 24 patients with facial nerve schwannomas).

Salib RJ, Tziambazis E, McDermott AL, Chavda SV, Irving RM. The crucial role of imaging in detection of facial nerve hemangiomas. *J Laryngol Otol.* 2001;115(6):510. [PMID: 11429083] (This report supports the assertion that the definitive diagnosis

of a facial nerve tumor rests exclusively with high-resolution imaging of the temporal bone using enhanced MRI and thin-sectioned CT scanning.)

Wiggins RH 3rd, Harnsberger HR, Salzman KL, Shelton C, Kertesz TR, Glastonbury CM. The many faces of facial nerve schwannoma. *AJNR Am J Neuroradiol.* 2006;27(3):694. [PMID: 16552018] (This paper reviews the clinical presentation and radiographic appearance of 24 patients with facial nerve schwannomas.)

2. Melkersson-Rosenthal Syndrome

General Considerations

Melkersson-Rosenthal syndrome (MRS) is a granulomatous neuromucocutaneus systemic disorder characterized by a variable course that includes unilateral facial palsy, episodic or progressive facial edema, and lingua plicata (scrotal or fissured tongue). The syndrome is usually sporadic in occurrence, although familial occurrence has been described.

Pathogenesis

Patients with MRS demonstrate orofacial granulomatosis, including oral lesions with noncaseating granulomas, features often associated with Crohn's disease, sarcoidosis, focal dental sepsis, and food or contact allergies. Recent studies have shown a possible link with mycobacterial infection. The syndrome may also reflect a more generalized autonomic dysfunction that manifests as vasomotor instability rather than a purely inflammatory condition. Further support for this assertion comes from the association of MRS with migraine headaches and megacolon.

Clinical Findings

Patients may variably present with several symptoms that mark the syndrome. Lingua plicata is most likely to occur early in life, whereas facial edema generally occurs after the initial episode of facial weakness (Figures 68–8 and 68–9). Facial dysfunction may be heralded by the onset of a facial swelling, but more typically precedes the swelling by months or years.

Episodes of facial paresis or paralysis typically begin in childhood or adolescence. Edema of the lips and palatal mucosa produces a ruddy appearance. Swelling often extends to the cheeks, eyelids, nose, and chin and may be dramatic. Progressive disfigurement can result from recurrent facial swelling. Facial weakness assumes a peripheral distribution and can be differentiated from Bell's palsy only when other manifestations of the syndrome are apparent or noted on the history. Although a relapsing course is usual, good to excellent recovery is typical. However, cases of progressive dysfunction have been described.

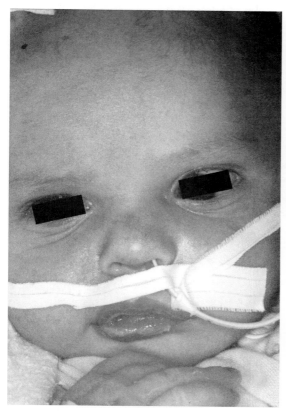 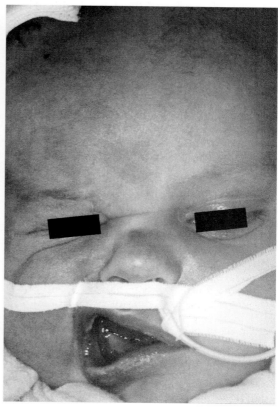

A   **B**

Figure 68–8. Facial paralysis in newborns and young infants can be difficult to detect at rest owing to high facial tone in these age groups. Right facial paralysis in a neonate with medulloblastoma of the caudal brainstem is shown. A right esotropia indicates a right abducens paralysis combined with right facial nerve paralysis. **(A)** Face at rest. **(B)** An asymmetric crying facies.

Treatment

The treatment of facial palsy associated with MRS is empiric. Anti-inflammatory (steroid) therapy has been used with mixed success. Antibiotics, antihistamines (tetracycline derivatives), sulfasalazine (an aspirin-like compound), and clofazimine (used to treat leprosy) have all been used with varying degrees of success. Reports of surgical decompression of the meatal and labyrinthine segments suggest a benefit in preventing further recurrence of the palsy.

Apaydin R, Bahadir S, Kaklikkaya N, Bilen N, Bayramgurler D. Possible role of *Mycobacterium tuberculosis* complex in Melkersson-Rosenthal syndrome demonstrated with Gen-Probe amplified *Mycobacterium tuberculosis* direct test. *Australas J Dermatol.* 2004;45(2):94. Erratum in: *Australas J Dermatol.* 2005;46(3):209. [PMID: 15068454] (This report demon-strates a possible link between *Mycobacterium* and Melkersson-Rosenthal syndrome.)

Dutt SN, Mirza S, Irving RM, Donaldson I. Total decompression of facial nerve for Melkersson-Rosenthal syndrome. *J Laryngol Otol.* 2000;114(11):870. [PMID: 11144840] (This study describes a successful case of a surgical decompression of the facial nerve in a 27-year-old woman with Melkersson-Rosenthal syndrome and reviews the literature pertaining to facial nerve decompression for this syndrome.)

Glickman LT, Gruss JS, Birt BD, Kohli-Dang N. The surgical management of Melkersson-Rosenthal syndrome. *Plast Reconstr Surg.* 1992;89(5):815. [PMID: 1561252] (This article reports on 14 patients with Melkersson-Rosenthal syndrome and provides an algorithm that guides the surgeon with regard to both the medical and surgical treatment of the patient with this syndrome.)

Graham MD, Kemink JL. Total facial nerve decompression in recurrent facial paralysis and Melkersson-Rosenthal syndrome: a preliminary report. *Am J Otol.* 1986;7(1):34. [PMID: 3946579]

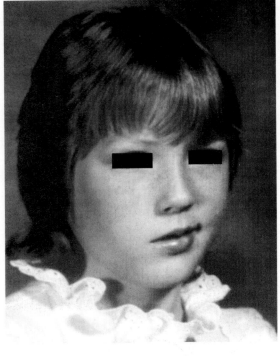

A

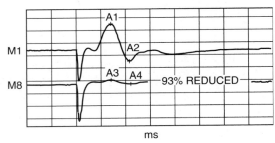

B

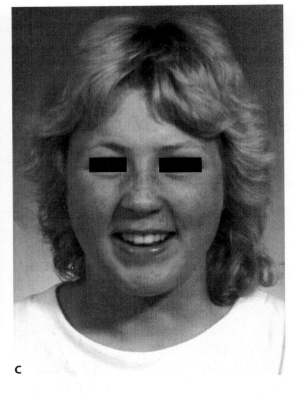

C

Figure 68–9. **(A)** An 8-year-old girl during the initial episode of right facial paralysis associated with lower facial and lip swelling. This patient experienced three subsequent episodes of right facial paralysis with swelling on a yearly basis. **(B)** At age 12, evoked electromyography demonstrated poor responsiveness on the right side in association with an episode of paralysis. Facial nerve decompression via a middle cranial fossa approach was performed. No subsequent episodes of facial palsy have been noted over the ensuing 5 years. **(C)** Patient at age 13 years. *(Continued)*

(This preliminary report describes two patients—one with unilateral Melkersson-Rosenthal syndrome and the other with a bilateral recurrent idiopathic facial paralysis—who were treated with combined transmastoid and middle cranial fossa total facial nerve exposure, decompression, and slitting of the fibrous nerve sheath.)

Gerressen M, Ghassemi A, Stockbrink G, Riediger D, Zadeh MD. Melkersson-Rosenthal syndrome: case report of a 30-year misdiagnosis. *J Oral Maxillofac Surg.* 2005;63(7):1035. [PMID: 16003636] (Report of a case and review of the literature of patients with Melkersson-Rosenthal syndrome.)

Pigozzi B, Fortina AB, Peserico A. Successful treatment of Melkersson-Rosenthal syndrome with lymecycline. *Eur J Dermatol.* 2004;14(3):166. [PMID: 15246942] (This report documents the successful treatment of a patient with Melkersson-Rosenthal syndrome with the tetracycline-like drug lymecycline.)

Sciubba JJ, Said-Al-Naief N. Orofacial granulomatosis: presentation, pathology and management of 13 cases. *J Oral Pathol Med.* 2003;32(10):576. [PMID: 14632932] (A large series of patients with Melkersson-Rosenthal syndrome.)

3. Lyme Disease

General Considerations

Lyme disease is a multisystem infection induced by the tick-borne strain of the *Borrelia burgdorferi* spirochete. The occurrence of acute facial palsy in association with

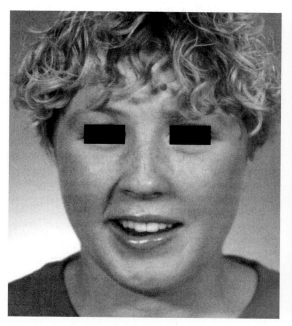

D

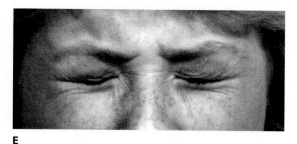

E

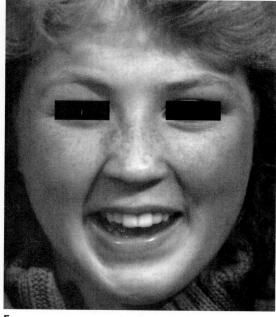

F

Figure 68–9 (Cont'd). (D) Patient at age 15 years. **(E and F)** Patient at age 17 revealing full facial movement, with some synkinetic eye closure with lip movement.

Lyme disease is well recognized. Unilateral or bilateral facial palsy may occur in up to 11% of patients with Lyme disease. The ratio of unilateral to bilateral involvement is 3:1.

Clinical Findings

A. SYMPTOMS AND SIGNS

Although most patients with facial palsy associated with Lyme disease note an antecedent rash adjacent to the site of a tick bite, others do not; the palsy may be the presenting sign of the illness. The interval between the onset of the rash and facial palsy is less than 2 months. Facial palsy may occur in association with other neurologic deficits produced by meningoencephalitis and radiculoneuritis.

After a tick bite and a 1- to 4-week incubation period, skin lesions develop in approximately 50% of infected individuals in association with flu-like symptoms. Less than half of patients suspected to have Lyme disease can recall a previous tick bite. Within weeks to months after the initial infection, constitutional, neurologic, and cardiac manifestations, including ipsilateral or bilateral facial palsy, may appear. Arthritic symptoms typically follow.

B. LABORATORY FINDINGS

If Lyme disease is suspected, diagnostic testing should include serologic testing with ELISA (**E**nzyme-**L**inked **I**mmuno**s**orbent **A**ssay) to search for IgG and IgM antibodies. By some reports, serologic evidence of Lyme disease has been found in up to 20% of patients diagnosed with Bell's palsy.

Treatment

Early antibiotic treatment is thought to enhance symptomatic improvement and prevent long-term sequelae. A 3-week course of tetracycline, doxycycline, or amoxicillin (for adults) or penicillin (for children) is recommended, with erythromycin administered as an alternative choice. Success in over 90% of patients has been reported with this treatment. Adequate antibiosis provides high rates of recovery of facial function with a generally good prognosis for facial nerve recovery. Residual dysfunction was more likely in patients with bilateral involvement.

Bagger-Sjoback D, Remahl S, Ericsson M. Long-term outcome of facial palsy in neuroborreliosis. *Otol Neurotol.* 2005;26(4):790. [PMID: 16015186] (This study shows that not all children with neuroborreliosis-related facial palsy recover with 100% normal function.)

Burgdorfer W, Barbour AG, Hayes S, Benach J, Grunwaldt E, David J. Lyme disease: a tickborne spirochetosis? *Science.* 1982;216:1317. [PMID: 7043737] (This classic paper is the first that links the newly discovered spirochete in the etiology of Lyme disease.)

Clark JR, Carlson RD, Pachner AR, Sasaki CT, Steere AC. Facial paralysis in Lyme disease. *Laryngoscope.* 1985;95(11):1341. [PMID: 4058212] (This paper reviews the clinical course, distinguishing features, and outcome of 124 patients with facial palsies. The authors believe that antibiotics should be given to patients with this facial palsy to treat any other concurrent manifestations of the illness and to prevent subsequent complications.)

Jonsson L, Stiernstedt G, Thomander L. Tick-borne *Borrelia* infection in patients with Bell's palsy. *Arch Otolaryngol Head Neck Surg.* 1987;113:303. [PMID: 3814376] (This classic study evaluates 94 patients diagnosed as having Bell's palsy for evidence of Lyme disease infection.)

Kalish RA, Kaplan RF, Taylor E, Jones-Woodward L, Workman K, Steere AC. Evaluation of study patients with Lyme disease: 10–20-year follow-up. *J Infect Dis.* 2001;183(3):453. [PMID: 11133377] (This classic article describes the long-term impact of Lyme disease in 84 patients from the Lyme, Connecticut, region who had erythema migrans, facial palsy, or Lyme arthritis 20 years previously.)

Peltomaa M, McHugh G, Steere AC. The VlsE (IR6) peptide ELISA in the serodiagnosis of Lyme facial paralysis. *Otol Neurotol.* 2004;25(5):838. [PMID: 15354020] (This study demonstrates the usefulness of ELISA in the diagnosis of Lyme disease–associated facial paralysis.)

Skogman BH, Croner S, Odkvist L. Acute facial palsy in children—a 2-year follow-up study with focus on Lyme neuroborreliosis. *Int J Pediatr Otorhinolaryngol.* 2003;67(6):597. [PMID: 12745151] (This study is a long-term examination of children with facial palsy from Lyme neuroborreliosis, demonstrating that one fifth of children with an acute facial palsy get a permanent dysfunction of the facial nerve. Other neurologic symptoms or health problems do not accompany the sequelae of the facial palsy.)

Taylor RS, Simpson IN. Review of treatment options for Lyme borreliosis. *J Chemother.* 2005;17(Suppl 2):3. [PMID: 16315580] (This review outlines contemporary treatment algorithms for patients with Lyme borreliosis.)

4. Acute Otitis Media & Mastoiditis

Clinical Findings

If the history or physical examination suggests evidence of prior or existing otitis media or if there is a history of otologic surgery, an otogenic etiology for a facial palsy should be suspected (Figure 68–10). Concomitant symptoms of hearing loss, otorrhea, and vestibular symptoms are highly suggestive of an otogenic etiology. Facial palsy due to acute suppurative otitis media (ASOM) is typically seen in children who appear toxic and manifest otoscopic findings of middle ear empyema. The palsy is often progressive over a 2- to 3-day interval. In such cases, there is often a history of recent episodes of otitis media that have been partially treated. In cases of prolonged palsy, radiographic evaluation of the temporal bone may rarely disclose coalescence of infection in the mastoid. Facial palsy associated with ASOM is generally the result of toxic neuritis and can be adequately treated with wide myringotomy and systemic antibiotics.

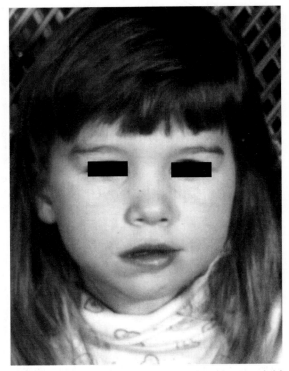

Figure 68–10. Unsuspected right facial palsy in a child who was found 2 weeks later to have a complete facial paralysis in association with right-sided otitis media, underscoring the subtle nature of facial paralysis in young children.

Treatment

Cortical mastoidectomy is required when antibiotics and myringotomy fail to render the patient afebrile after 24 hours or when facial paralysis persists beyond 1 week. The surgical objective is to drain the empyema; extended nerve decompression is unnecessary except in cases of prolonged dysfunction.

Agrawal S, Husein M, MacRae D. Complications of otitis media: an evolving state. *J Otolaryngol.* 2005;34(Suppl 1):S33. [PMID: 16089238] (This review discusses the intracranial and extracranial complications of acute and chronic otitis media, including the clinical presentation, work-up, and management of the individual complications such as facial paralysis.)

Gaio E, Marioni G, de Filippis C, Tregnaghi A, Caltran S, Staffieri A. Facial nerve paralysis secondary to acute otitis media in infants and children. *J Paediatr Child Health.* 2004;40(8):483. [PMID: 15265194] (This study reviews the authors' experience with facial nerve paralysis secondary to otitis media and outlines the indications for surgical intervention.)

Goldstein NA, Casselbrant ML, Bluestone CD, Kurs-Lasky M. Intratemporal complications of acute otitis media in infants and children. *Otolaryngol Head Neck Surg.* 1998;119(5):444. [PMID: 9807067] (This review of 100 children with an intratemporal complication of acute otitis media includes 22 children who presented with facial paralysis; complete in 5 [22.7%] and incomplete in 17 [77.3%].)

Kvestad E, Kvaerner KJ, Mair IW. Otologic facial palsy: etiology, onset, and symptom duration. *Ann Otol Rhinol Laryngol.* 2002;111(7 Pt 1):598. [PMID: 12126015] (This 10-year retrospective review showed that facial palsy was a complication of acute otitis media in 56%, of acute mastoiditis in 17%, of secretory otitis media in 17%, and of chronic otitis media in 11%; total remission was achieved in all patients.)

5. Chronic Otitis Media

Chronic suppurative otitis media (CSOM), manifesting mucosal inflammation or cholesteatoma, may produce an associated facial palsy (Figure 68–11; also see Figure 68–10). Facial nerve dysfunction associated with CSOM reflects a toxic neuritis, external compression, or intraneural compression from edema or abscess.

Facial palsy associated with this disorder should be addressed surgically as soon as possible. Surgical removal of irreversible disease in the middle ear and mastoid, as well as decompression of the involved segment of the nerve without slitting the sheath, is advised. Long-standing paralysis (but less than 2 years in duration) requires sectioning of attenuated tympanic or mastoid segments of the nerve followed by grafting.

Agrawal S, Husein M, MacRae D. Complications of otitis media: an evolving state. *J Otolaryngol.* 2005;34(Suppl 1):S33. [PMID: 16089238] (This review discusses the intracranial and extracranial complications of acute and chronic otitis media, including the clinical presentation, work-up, and management of the individual complications such as facial paralysis.)

Ikeda M, Nakazato H, Onoda K, Hirai R, Kida A. Facial nerve paralysis caused by middle ear cholesteatoma and effects of surgical intervention. *Acta Otolaryngol.* 2006;126(1):95. [PMID: 16308261] (This study demonstrates that in patients with advanced and facial paralysis, the outcome of facial paralysis was good; however, poor outcomes were observed in patients with petrosal cholesteatoma and in those who underwent surgical decompression more than 2 months after the onset of paralysis.)

Omran A, De Denato G, Piccirillo E, Leone O, Sanna M. Petrous bone cholesteatoma: management and outcomes. *Laryngoscope.* 2006;116(4):619. [PMID: 16585869] (This review of 94 patients with petrous cholesteatoma demonstrates the high incidence of facial nerve palsy in this presentation.)

Osma U, Cureoglu S, Hosoglu S. The complications of chronic otitis media: report of 93 cases. *J Laryngol Otol.* 2000;114(2):97. [PMID: 10748823] (The aim of this study was to investigate the incidence, mortality, and morbidity of complications due to chronic otitis media in 93 patients.)

Yetiser S, Tosun F, Kazkayasi M. Facial nerve paralysis due to chronic otitis media. *Otol Neurotol.* 2002;23(4):580. [PMID: 12170164] (This study demonstrated that a middle ear cholesteatoma was present in the majority of patients with facial paralysis caused by chronic otitis media.)

6. Necrotizing (Malignant) Otitis Externa
Clinical Findings

Infection by *Pseudomonas aeruginosa* is the primary offending agent in necrotizing infection of the external auditory canal and temporal bone. These infections are observed in patients with diabetes mellitus or in others who are immunocompromised. Patients typically present with symptoms of otorrhea and progressive, disabling otalgia. The pathognomonic signs are otoscopic evidence of ear canal inflammation or a breech of the external canal skin at the bony-cartilaginous junction. The breech is filled with granulation tissue. Facial palsy is ominous and reflects skull base extension of the osteomyelitic process along vascular channels. The diagnosis is based on the clinical presentation in association with radioisotope gallium and technetium scanning that demonstrates osteomyelitis of the temporal bone.

Treatment

Treatment of necrotizing otitis externa requires aggressive management with intravenously administered antipseudomonal antibiotics, which should be maintained for 8–12 weeks to facilitate sequestration of the infection. Oral fluoroquinolones (ciprofloxacin) are also becoming increasingly popular for treatment of malignant otitis externa after an initial treatment with intravenous antibiotics for early disease. Aggressive debridement of granulation tissue within the ear canal is key to promoting the replacement of necrotic bone with viable tissue. Because necrotizing otitis externa is associated with extensive ischemia of the skull base, the operative

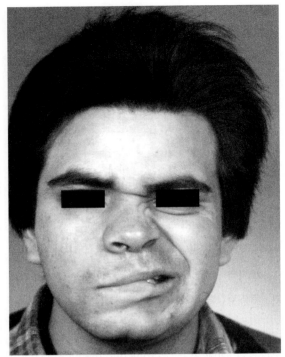

Figure 68–11. Chronic suppurative otitis media manifesting as an associated facial palsy.

debridement of the tympanic bone, the mastoid, and the skull base is indicated only when medical treatment fails to produce improvement. Radioisotope scanning can be helpful while following the progress of the infection and helps to determine the length of the course of intravenous therapy that is required. Hyperbaric oxygen has also been used as an adjuvant therapy in some cases with success, although recent meta-analyses have failed to find it significantly adds to the rate of cure.

Benecke JE Jr. Management of osteomyelitis of the skull base. *Laryngoscope.* 1989;99(12):1220. [PMID: 2601534] (This classic paper reviews 13 patients with skull base osteomyelitis treated over a 4-year period and describes a now commonly used method of staging and monitoring this malady using gallium and technetium scanning techniques.)

Chandler JR. Malignant otitis externa. *Laryngoscope.* 1968;78:1257. [PMID: 4970362] (This classic article describes the clinical presentation and treatment of malignant external otitis.)

Phillips JS, Jones SE. Hyperbaric oxygen as an adjuvant treatment for malignant otitis externa. *Cochrane Database Syst Rev.* 2005;2:CD004617. [PMID: 15846724] (This meta-analysis shows no added benefit of hyperbaric oxygen therapy for malignant otitis externa).

Rubin Grandis J, Branstetter BF 4th, Yu VL. The changing face of malignant (necrotizing) external otitis: clinical, radiological, and anatomic correlations. *Lancet Infect Dis.* 2004;4(1):34.

[PMID: 14720566] (This review outlines contemporary management of malignant otitis externa.)

Sreepada GS, Kwartler JA. Skull base osteomyelitis secondary to malignant otitis externa. *Curr Opin Otolaryngol Head Neck Surg.* 2003;11(5):316. [PMID: 14502060] (This review summarizes the diagnosis and treatment of patients with skull base osteomyelitis.)

Weber PC, Seabold JE, Graham SM, Hoffmann HH, Simonson TM, Thompson BH. Evaluation of temporal and facial osteomyelitis by simultaneous In-WBC/Tc-99m-MDP bone SPECT scintigraphy and computed tomography scan. *Otolaryngol Head Neck Surg.* 1995;113(1):36. [PMID: 7603719] (The results from this study suggest that dual In-WBC/Tc-99m MDP bone SPECT scintigraphy provides an accurate imaging modality for diagnosis and follow-up of temporal and facial osteomyelitis when existing clinical or postoperative bone changes make it difficult to detect active osteomyelitis by CT scan.)

7. Childhood Facial Palsy

General Considerations

The evaluation of a facial palsy in a child should be guided by the fact that although Bell's palsy is the most common cause of childhood facial palsies, it accounts for a substantially smaller proportion of palsies relative to adults. For instance, a clinically or radiographically identified etiology can be found in 20% of adult palsies initially diagnosed as Bell's palsy; this incidence may reach as high as 72% in childhood palsies. Patients under the age of 18 years with facial palsy are most likely to have an etiology of Bell's palsy (42%), trauma (21%), infection (13%), congenital causes (8%), and neoplasms (2%).

Clinical Findings

The onset of facial palsy in childhood is frequently obscured by the excellent tone of aponeurotic tissues and skin and, therefore, the excellent static suspension of central and lower portions of the face. Consequently, childhood facial nerve disorders are often referred to as "asymmetric crying facies" (see Figure 68–8).

Treatment

The treatment for childhood facial palsies generally follows that for adults, with the appropriate adjustment in medication strength and dosing schedules.

Carr MM, Ross DA, Zuker RM. Cranial nerve defects in congenital facial palsy. *J Otolaryngol.* 1997;26(2):80. [PMID: 9106081] (This paper evaluates the cranial nerve defects in 29 children with congenital facial palsy presenting for reanimation.)

Evans AK, Licameli G, Brietzke S, Whittemore K, Kenna M. Pediatric facial nerve paralysis: patients, management and outcomes. *Int J Pediatr Otorhinolaryngol.* 2005;69(11):1521. Epub 2005 June 27. [PMID: 15985298] (This retrospective review of 35 cases of facial palsy in children demonstrated that infectious causes were the most likely etiology, followed by trauma, iatrogenic, congenital, Bell/idiopathic, relapsing, and neoplastic.)

Gaio E, Marioni G, de Filippis C, Tregnaghi A, Caltran S, Staffieri A. Facial nerve paralysis secondary to acute otitis media in infants and children. *J Paediatr Child Health.* 2004;40(8):483. [PMID: 15265194] (This series and review of the literature demonstrate that facial paralysis is an uncommon complication of otitis media and recommends antibiotic therapy and myringotomy as first-line interventions, with surgery reserved for cases of acute or coalescent mastoiditis, suppurative complications, and lack of clinical regression.)

May M, Fria RJ, Blumenthal F et al. Facial paralysis in children: differential diagnosis. *Otolaryngol Head Neck Surg.* 1981;89:841. [PMID: 6799919] (The differential diagnosis in 170 patients with facial paralysis between birth and 18 years of age is reviewed in this classic article, and symptoms and signs associated with each diagnosis are presented.)

Saito H, Takeda T, Kishimoto S. Neonatal facial nerve defect. *Acta Otolaryngol Suppl.* 1994;510:77. [PMID: 8128879] (This important study reports on the findings from 42 temporal bones with facial nerve, and includes 9 temporal bones in which the facial nerve disappeared midway through the course of the temporal bone.)

Singhi P, Jain V. Bell's palsy in children. *Semin Pediatr Neurol.* 2003;10(4):289. [PMID: 14992461] (This review outlines the presentation and management of Bell's palsy in children.)

8. Perinatal Facial Palsy

Traumatic Perinatal Facial Palsy

Intrauterine trauma to the facial nerve may occur as a consequence of compression from the maternal sacrum. Prolonged labor and forceps delivery may produce facial nerve trauma. The extratemporal facial nerve is at risk because the absence of an overlying mastoid tip places the vertical segment of the nerve at risk for injury. A traumatic cause of the facial nerve dysfunction is suggested by hemotympanum, periauricular ecchymosis, and the progressive decline of facial nerve responsiveness to an applied stimulus.

The assessment of perinatal facial nerve dysfunction relies heavily on electrodiagnosis. Electromyographic evidence of preserved or declining neuromuscular activity is most diagnostic. In the absence of such activity, muscle biopsy may be required to determine whether a congenital palsy exists.

A review of the etiologic basis for facial palsy in 95 newborns indicated that a traumatic etiology was suspected in 74 cases (78%), as suggested by signs of periauricular injury or electrical testing (evoked and spontaneous electromyography). There was excellent recovery in 41 of 45 children with perinatal trauma. Occasional cases of poor recovery, however, suggest the need for a radiographic and electrodiagnostic evaluation to detect an unfavorable prognosis for spontaneous recovery. In such cases, surgical exploration and decompression of the nerve may be critical for effective reanimation.

May M, Fria RJ, Blumenthal F et al. Facial paralysis in children: differential diagnosis. *Otolaryngol Head Neck Surg.* 1981;89: 841. [PMID: 6799919] (The differential diagnosis in 170 patients with facial paralysis between birth and 18 years of age is reviewed in this classic article, and symptoms and signs associated with each diagnosis are presented.)

Renault F. Facial electromyography in newborn and young infants with congenital facial weakness. *Dev Med Child Neurol.* 2001;43(6):421. [PMID: 11409833] (This study highlights the importance of electrophysiologic measures for diagnosing and treating children with facial paralysis.)

Sapin SO, Miller AA, Bass HN. Neonatal asymmetric crying facies: a new look at an old problem. *Clin Pediatr (Phila).* 2005;44 (2):109. [PMID: 15735828] (This article describes asymmetric facies as a means of diagnosing newborn facial paralysis and describes the use of ultrasound to aid in diagnosis.)

Congenital Perinatal Facial Palsy

Newborn facial palsy unrelated to trauma accounts for a smaller proportion of cases than does traumatic facial palsy. Both syndromic and nonsyndromic forms of congenital facial palsy occur. The palsy may be complete or incomplete, unilateral or bilateral, and isolated to particular branches. Associated craniofacial malformations, often those involving first and second branchial arch derivatives, are common. Microtia and facial clefts are most frequently noted. Palsies isolated to a single branch, particularly the marginal mandibularis, indicate the need for a cardiac evaluation in light of a high rate of concurrent cardiac conductive and anatomic anomalies.

Otologic, electrodiagnostic, and radiologic evaluations are performed, as necessary, to determine the etiology. A congenital neuromuscular etiology is suggested by a concomitant defect (or defects) involving other cranial nerves and the absence of evidence of electrical responsiveness to evoked and spontaneous electromyographic evaluation.

The Möbius syndrome encompasses a wide spectrum of anomalies due to dysgenesis at the level of the brainstem with resultant neuromuscular deficits peripherally. The bilateral absence of facial and abducens nerve function, as well as other cranial neuropathies, may occur. The auditory brainstem response is often abnormal and is a helpful adjunct in diagnosis.

The prognosis for effective facial animation with congenital facial palsies is poor. However, resting tone may provide adequate eye coverage and oral competence even into adulthood. Facial motor rehabilitative procedures and reconstructive procedures to effect better symmetry may be indicated later in life.

Abramson DL, Cohen MM Jr, Mulliken JB. Möbius syndrome: classification and grading system. *Plast Reconstr Surg.* 1998; 102(4):961. [PMID: 9734409] (This paper retrospectively analyzes 27 patients with Möbius syndrome using a newly developed grading system termed the CLUFT, which permits categorization and comparison of patients with Möbius for phenotypic and management outcome studies.)

Jemec B, Grobbelaar AO, Harrison DH. The abnormal nucleus as a cause of congenital facial palsy. *Arch Dis Child.* 2000;83(3):256. [PMID: 10952650] (This study documents that developmental abnormalities of the facial nucleus itself constitute an important, and previously ignored, cause of monosymptomatic unilateral congenital facial palsy.)

Saito H, Takeda T, Kishimoto S. Neonatal facial nerve defect. *Acta Otolaryngol Suppl.* 1994;510:77. [PMID: 8128879] (This study reports on the pathologic findings in temporal bones with congenital anomalies of the facial nerve. Some of the nerve fibers suggested regeneration after necrotic lesions induced during the perinatal period.)

Sudarshan A, Goldie WD. The spectrum of congenital facial diplegia (Möbius syndrome). *Pediatr Neurol.* 1985;1(3):180. [PMID: 3880403] (This manuscript reviews Möbius syndrome, congenital facial diplegia with associated anomalies, and includes six cases that manifest a very broad spectrum of associated neurologic anomalies.)

Toelle SP, Boltshauser E. Long-term outcome in children with congenital unilateral facial nerve palsy. *Neuropediatrics.* 2001;32(3):130. [PMID: 11521208] (This study follows the long-term outcome of 12 children with congenital unilateral facial nerve palsies and note a poor long-term functional prognosis.)

Verzijl HT, van der Zwaag B, Lammens M, ten Donkelaar HJ, Padberg GW. The neuropathology of hereditary congenital facial palsy vs Möbius syndrome. *Neurology.* 2005;64(4):649. [PMID: 15728286] (This study demonstrates that neuropathologic findings confirm clinical observations that hereditary congenital facial palsy and Möbius syndrome are two different entities with a different pathogenesis.)

SECTION XVI
Implants

Implantable Middle Ear Hearing Devices

69

Kenneth C. Y. Yu, MD, & Steven W. Cheung, MD

◼ GENERAL CONSIDERATIONS OF IMPLANTABLE MIDDLE EAR HEARING DEVICES

SOCIETAL FACTORS

Hearing loss is a common disability among adults. In the aging population, 25% of individuals between age 65 and 74, and 50% of individuals age 75 and older have hearing problems. Overall, approximately 14.4 million adults in the United States have moderate to severe sensorineural hearing loss. For this group, acoustic amplification (a conventional hearing aid) is an important rehabilitative strategy that often restores hearing to a serviceable level.

Despite the potential benefits of acoustic amplification, many hearing-impaired patients do not accept hearing aids. Some common complaints about hearing aids include feedback annoyance, ear canal discomfort, stigma of wearing an external appliance, and psychological rejection. It is estimated that only 20% of individuals within the United States who may benefit from a hearing aid own one. Only half of those who own a hearing aid use their device on a long-term basis.

ADVANTAGES OF IMPLANTABLE MIDDLE EAR HEARING DEVICES

The search for alternatives to conventional hearing aids motivated the development of implantable hearing devices that deliver sound energy more directly to middle ear structures. This design eliminates many of the disadvantages of conventional hearing aids. Implantable hearing devices endeavor to deliver more natural sound quality, increase gains across the frequency spectrum, reduce feedback, improve comfort and cosmesis, and eliminate ear canal occlusion.

IMPLANTATION-RELATED RISKS

Risks associated with middle ear device implant surgery include sensorineural hearing loss, ossicular chain disruption, facial nerve injury, external canal laceration, and cerebral spinal fluid (CSF) leak. Beyond surgical risks, other considerations associated with implantable hearing devices are higher costs compared with conventional hearing aids, incompatibility with magnetic resonance imaging (MRI), and uncertain need for future explantation (ie, device removal) and reimplantation. Nevertheless, emerging technologies in implantable middle ear hearing devices (IMEHD) are very exciting for both patients and care providers.

HEARING DEVICE COMPONENTS

An IMEHD is a device that converts acoustic energy to mechanical energy and delivers it to a vibratory structure in the middle ear. The basic components of an IMEHD consist of an **acoustic signal detector** (receptor), a **transmission link,** and an **actuator** that vibrates the ossicular chain (effector). The two basic transducer types used to drive the ossicular chain are electromagnetic and piezoelectric systems. **Electromagnetic fields** generated by induction coils can put magnets into oscillatory motion. **Piezo-**

electric transducers are generally ceramic materials that vibrate in response to applied electrical energy. The general design of an IMEHD consists of separate receptor and effector limbs. For semi-implantable devices, the receptor limb is an external, removable component that houses the microphone, the speech processor, and the power supply. It is held in a stable position relative to the fixed internal component across the scalp interface by using a centering magnet. Acoustic information is transferred from the external receptor component to the internal effector system through radiofrequency coupling. For totally implantable devices, the receptor and effector limbs are completely internalized; there is no external component. Transcutaneous technologies are used to power and replenish energy to the internal batteries. The effector limb of implantable hearing devices differs in the location of ossicular chain stimulation. The sites of contact are the incus head, body, and lenticular process, and the stapes superstructure.

ACOUSTIC, IMAGING, AND OTHER DEVICE CONSIDERATIONS

Acoustic considerations for IMEHDs relate to increased stiffness and mass loading of the ossicular chain, which may result in a deepening of the existing hearing loss. Because middle ear mechanics may be impacted by all IMEHDs, normal middle ear function is a strict criterion in selecting patients for implantation. Ossicular chain stiffness is increased when there is rigid coupling between the device and the ossicles. Mass loading is increased when an effector component is attached to the incus or the stapes.

Currently, none of the IMEHDs is compatible with MRI. Unforeseen clinical problems in the future might warrant device explantation for diagnostic and therapeutic interventions. Once an IMEHD is implanted, electrocautery cannot be used in surgical procedures because electrical discharges might damage the device. Electromagnetic interference from other environmental sources might possibly interact with IMEHDs in unknown ways. Device-related uncertainties include lifespan of IMEHDs, output protection safeguards to prevent noise-induced hearing loss, hermitic seal dependability to reduce device failure rates, ease of upgrade from a semi- to a fully implantable model, and performance capacity to accommodate progressive hearing loss.

■ SPECIFIC IMPLANTABLE MIDDLE EAR HEARING DEVICES

The semi-implantable Vibrant Soundbridge (Med-El, Innsbruck, Austria) and totally implantable Envoy (Envoy Medical, Minneapolis, MN) devices are featured in this section to provide examples of innovative IMEHD technologies. The Vibrant Soundbridge was FDA approved for distribution in the U.S. market under Symphonix (San Jose, CA) corporation, but its availability under Med-El, which acquired Vibrant Soundbridge from Symphonix in 2003, has been on hold in the United States because FDA approval for the Med-El manufacturing facility is under review. The Vibrant Soundbridge is available in Europe. The Envoy is an investigational device undergoing clinical trials in the United States and Germany.

VIBRANT SOUNDBRIDGE

The Vibrant Soundbridge is a semi-implantable device that uses an electromagnetic effector to drive the ossicular chain. The external component is the Audio Processor, and the internal component is the surgically implanted Vibrating Ossicular Prosthesis. The Audio Processor houses the microphone, the speech processor, and the battery. The Vibrating Ossicular Prosthesis (Figure 69–1) contains the radiofrequency link, the demodulator, and the ossicular stimulator—the floating mass transducer—which is attached to the incus lenticular process with a titanium clip. The floating mass transducer is an electromagnetic effector with a magnet housed within an induction coil.

Implantation & Candidate Criteria

The surgical procedure consists of a mastoidectomy with a facial recess approach to place the floating mass transducer onto the lenticular process. After a 2-month period of healing, the device is activated. The speech processor delivers electronically controlled currents to drive the floating mass transducer into vibratory motion. Candidates for implantation are adults (≥ 18 years) with a moderate to severe sensorineural hearing loss and speech discrimination scores > 50%.

Testing

For the Vibrant Soundbridge Phase III FDA study, statistically significant improvements in average functional gain on the order of 10–15 dB across the frequency spectrum was reported. Mass loading of the incus did not adversely affect hearing in a clinically significant manner. Subjects reported improved satisfaction and performance; they preferred the Vibrant Soundbridge to a heterogeneous group of conventional hearing aids. Occlusion and feedback were virtually eliminated. Of note, aided speech recognition was comparable between the Vibrant Soundbridge and conventional hearing aids.

Safety

The trial also demonstrated acceptable safety. Most patients did not have a significant change in residual

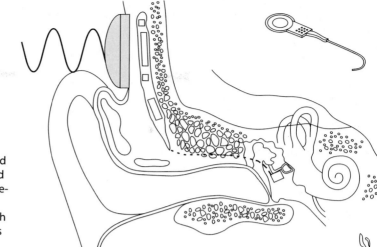

Figure 69–1. The Symphonix Vibrant Soundbridge Semi-Implantable Device. The external Audio Processor receives and processes sounds. Signals are transmitted to the internal Vibrating Ossicular Prosthesis (inset, right) via radiofrequency coupling. The floating mass transducer, which is attached to the incus lenticular process with a titanium clip, vibrates the stapes.

hearing (ie, change in pure-tone average < 10 dB). However, a small percentage of patients (4% or 2 of 53 patients) experienced a 12–18 dB decrease in residual hearing. Other adverse effects have been reported during the U.S. trial. There were six device failures; these devices were successfully reimplanted after the manufacturer revised the product. One subject had a disconnection of his floating mass transducer; the device was successfully reimplanted.

ENVOY

The Envoy is a totally implantable hearing device that uses piezoelectric transducers. The Envoy device is undergoing a Phase II FDA trial. A major design challenge of totally implantable hearing devices is the management of mechanical and acoustic feedback. By necessity, receptor (sensor) and effector (driver) limbs of the system are in close proximity. At high output levels by the effector limb, feedback may occur because the sensor detects the output signal. This results in feedback oscillation. The Envoy system addresses this difficult problem by segregating the receptor and effector limbs through controlled ossicular discontinuity.

Implantation & Candidate Criteria

The surgical procedure is a mastoidectomy with a facial recess approach to vaporize the distal 2–3 mm of the incus lenticular process with a laser (Figure 69–2). Bone cement is used to stabilize the sensor and driver to the mastoid and to affix the device tips to the incus body and stapes capitulum. When incoming sounds vibrate the native drum, the incus head is set in motion. The sensor tip, which is firmly attached to the incus head, deflects the piezoelectric transducer. Electrical signals are gener-

ated and transmitted to the speech processor. Outflow electrical signals from the processor guide the movements of the driver tip, which is transmitted to the stapes. Candidates for Envoy device implantation are adults (≥ 18 years) with a mild to severe sensorineural hearing loss and speech discrimination scores > 60%.

Phase I Testing and Safety Data

For the Envoy Phase I FDA study in 7 patients, 5 of 7 perceived benefit over their best-fit hearing aid at the 2-month activation period. Two of the 5 patients who ultimately experienced benefit required revision surgery after initial implantation because immediate benefit was insufficient. In the original cohort of 7 patients, 3 were explanted owing to infection or patient request. Functional gain with the Envoy was similar to hearing aids. Cochlear reserve in study patients appeared to be preserved following Envoy implantation, whereas air conduction thresholds for frequencies greater than 1 kHz were increased by 10–20 dB at 12 months after implantation. Device modifications were implemented prior to Phase II clinical trial, which is currently under way.

Chen DA, Backous DD, Arriaga MA et al. Phase 1 clinical trial results of the envoy system: a totally implantable middle ear device for sensorineural hearing loss. *Otolaryngol Head Neck Surg.* 2004;131(6):904. [PMID: 15577788] (Phase I clinical study results in 7 patients.)

Fisch U, Cremers CW, Lenarz T et al. Clinical experience with the Vibrant Soundbridge implant device. *Otol Neurotol.* 2001;22(6):962. [PMID: 11698826] (Multicenter clinical study demonstrating successful implantation and fitting of the Vibrant Soundbridge.)

Fraysse B, Laveille JP, Schmerber S et al. A multicenter study of the Vibrant Soundbridge middle ear implant: early clinical results

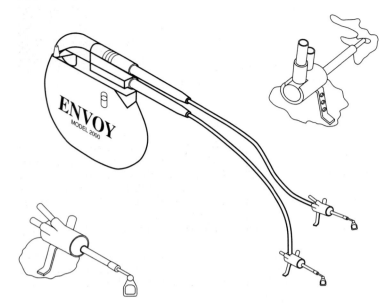

Figure 69–2. The Envoy Totally Implantable Device. Sensor and driver limbs connect to the processor with detachable pins. The sensor is affixed to the incus body with bone cement. Note that the distal incus lenticular process is shortened to segregate sensor and driver vibrations (inset, upper right). The driver is also attached to the stapes capitulum with bone cement (inset, lower left). (Reproduced with permission of Envoy Medical Corporation, St. Paul, MN.)

and experience. *Otol Neurotol.* 2001;22(6):952. [PMID: 11698825] (Study showing the Vibrant Soundbridge procedure is generally a safe procedure.)

Ko WH, Zhu WL, Kane M, Maniglia AJ. Engineering principles applied to implantable otologic devices. *Otolaryngol Clin North Am.* 2001;34(2):299. [PMID: 11382572] (Summary of engineering principles of possible actuators and sensors for totally implantable middle ear and cochlear hearing devices.)

Luetje CM, Brackman D, Balkany TJ et al. Phase III clinical trial results with the Vibrant Soundbridge implantable middle ear hearing device: a prospective controlled multicenter study. *Otolaryngol Head Neck Surg.* 2002;126(2):97. [PMID: 11870337] (Phase III study demonstrating safety and efficacy of the Vibrant Soundbridge system.)

WEB SITES

http://www.envoymedical.com/Envoy_device.htm (This website provides information on their product.)

Cochlear Implants

70

Michael B. Gluth, MD, Colin L.W. Driscoll, MD, & Anil K. Lalwani, MD

An absence or disturbance of cochlear hair cells causes most cases of deafness. This defect in normal cochlear function—specifically, in the transduction of a mechanical acoustic signal into auditory nerve synaptic activity—represents a broken link in the sometimes delicate chain that constitutes the human sense of hearing. Cochlear implants afford an artificial means to bypass this disrupted link and thereby allow the transmission of acoustic information through the central auditory pathway via direct electric stimulation of auditory nerve fibers. Most deaf individuals maintain an adequate surplus of viable auditory nerve fibers to permit this intervention.

Although current technologic and scientific boundaries preclude the artificial transduction of sound by using the exact native cochlear patterns of synaptic activity at the level of each individual residual auditory nerve fiber, knowledge of these native patterns has aided the development of cochlear implants by allowing the processing of speech into novel synthetic electronic codes that contain the key features of spoken sound. By using these codes to systematically regulate the firing of intracochlear electrodes, it is possible to convey the timing, frequency, and intensity of sound. Cochlear implants have progressively evolved with increasing complexity and elegance from an experimental concept to a proven tool used in the management of patients with sensorineural hearing loss. Worldwide, the number of implants is rapidly increasing. As with many other technology-driven medical treatment modalities, recent innovations in microcircuitry and computer science are continuing to drive the performance profiles of cochlear implants to new heights.

◼ COCHLEAR IMPLANT SYSTEMS

HARDWARE

Currently, three separate corporations manufacture multichannel implant systems that are commercially available and approved by the FDA for use in both adults and children. The approximate cost for implant systems is $25,000, with an additional cost of approximately $20,000–25,000 for the surgical procedure and other associated costs. Nevertheless, multiple studies have demonstrated that the cost-utility of cochlear implantation is excellent and that it compares well with other common medical interventions such as coronary angioplasty.

All modern implant systems function by the use of the same basic components, including a microphone, a speech processor, and an implanted receiver-stimulator (Figure 70–1).

Microphone & Receiver-Stimulator

Sound is first detected by a microphone (usually worn on the ear) and converted into an analog electrical signal. This signal is then sent to an external processor where, according to one of a number of different processing strategies, it is transformed into an electronic code. This code, usually a digital signal at this point, is transmitted via radiofrequency through the skin by a transmitting coil that is held externally over the receiver-stimulator by a magnet. Ultimately, this code is translated by the receiver-stimulator into rapid electrical impulses distributed to electrodes on a coil implanted within the cochlea (Figure 70–2).

Speech Processor

Newer innovations directed at discreteness and convenience have led to a new generation of speech processors that may be worn ear-level (behind-the-ear [BTE] processors). Processors worn on the belt like a pager are still preferred for very young children as well as some adults (Figures 70–3 through 70–6). In addition, entirely implantable devices are presently under development.

SPEECH PROCESSING

The literature uses the term *speech processing,* but this component may be more aptly termed **sound processing,** because the manipulations are not limited to speech only. In fact, a greater focus is now on enhanc-

877

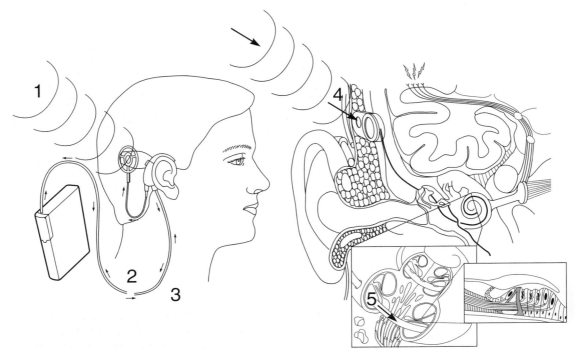

Figure 70–1. Schematic depiction of how cochlear implant systems operate. 1. Sound is detected by an external microphone. 2. This signal is directed to an external sound processor. 3. Once processed, a digital electronic code is sent by a transmitting coil situated over the receiver-stimulator via radiofrequency through the skin. 4. The receiver-stimulator delivers electronic impulses to electrodes on a coil located within the cochlea according to whichever strategy is being used by the processor. 5. Electrodes electrically stimulate spiral ganglion cells and auditory nerve axons.

ing the quality of all sound and specifically an effort to improve music appreciation. No matter what processing strategy is used, part of this process must include both amplification (ie, gain control) and compression. Since the deaf ear responds to electrical stimulation with a dynamic response in the range of 10–25 dB, processing must compress the signal to fit within this narrow range. How to best convert sound into an electrical signal is being actively investigated.

Electrical Stimulation Strategies

A. MULTICHANNEL STRATEGIES

Some of the earliest multichannel strategies, known as analog filter bank strategies (**continuous analog,** or CA), channel speech through multiple frequency-dependent filters and deliver distinct outputs of sinusoidal analog signals directly to separate electrodes. Other so-called feature extraction strategies (F0, F1 and F0, F1, F2) work by rapidly drawing out frequency-based details that are considered to be the most essential in speech recognition; these include both fundamental fre-

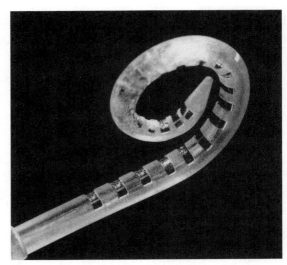

Figure 70–2. The Nucleus Contour Advance curled electrode array. (Image courtesy of the Cochlear Corporation, Sydney, Australia.)

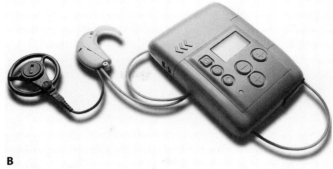

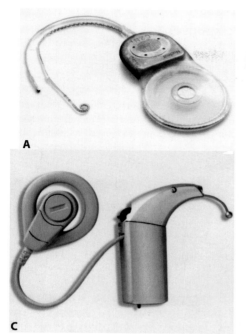

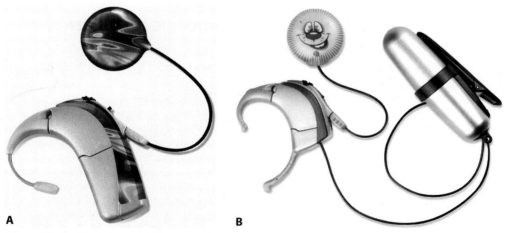

Figure 70–3. The Nucleus Contour System. **(A)** Nucleus 24 Contour Advance cochlear implant. **(B)** Sprint body-worn speech processor. **(C)** ESPrit 3G BTE speech processor. (Image courtesy of the Cochlear Corporation, Sydney, Australia.)

Figure 70–4. The Advanced Bionics Implant System. **(A)** HiRes™ Auria™ speech processor. **(B)** HiRes™ Auria™ with separate PowerPac designed primarily for small children who have difficulty wearing full behind-the-ear processors.

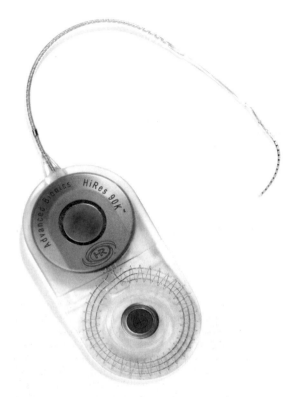

Figure 70–5. The Advanced Bionics HiResolution™ 90K implant with removable magnet and titanium case.

quency and vowel formants. Disbursement of this key information is accomplished through pulsatile signals having rates synchronous to the fundamental frequency and a tonotopic order that is derived from formants.

B. PULSATILE STIMULATION

Modern adaptations of direct analog strategies have sought to overcome the problem of channel interaction or "spillover" that readily occurs when adjacent electrodes are simultaneously stimulated with continuous analog signals. The result of such efforts has led to the development of a strategy, **continuous interleaved sampling,** or CIS, which delivers very rapid noncontinuous pulsatile stimulation over multiple filtered channels.

C. SPECTRAL ANALYSIS

In addition, newer high-rate spectral analysis strategies, **SPEAK** (**Sp**ectral **P**eak) and **ACE** (**A**dvanced **C**ombination **E**ncoders), for example, determine 6–10 spectral maxima for each input signal. Other newer approaches, such as "n-of-m" strategies (n = filters, m = channels), are constantly undergoing innovation and refinement with the

goal of combining the theoretical advantages of each type of system while incorporating ever-progressing new technologies.

Neural Responses

In speech processing, consideration is given to the incoming acoustic signal; in addition, actual neural responses (**neural response telemetry,** NRT; **neural response imaging,** NRI; or auditory nerve response telemetry, ART) to stimulation may be measured and accounted for in the formulation of a neural stimulation scheme. By measuring evoked action potentials from specific electrodes, it is possible to predict the needed amplitudes for each channel of the speech processor.

Cheng AK, Rubin HR, Powe NR, Mellon NK, Francis HS, Niparko JK. Cost-utility analysis of the cochlear implant in children. *JAMA.* 2000;284:850. [PMID: 10938174] (Cost-utility in children is favorable.)

Cheng AK, Niparko JK. Cost-utility of the cochlear implant in adults: a meta-analysis. *Arch Otol Head Neck Surg.* 1999; 125:1214. [PMID: 10555692] (Cost-utility of cochlear implantation in adults shown to be in line with many other common medical and surgical modalities.)

■ SELECTION & EVALUATION OF PATIENTS

AUDIOLOGIC ASSESSMENT

Candidacy for cochlear implantation relies heavily upon the audiologic evaluation. Although the audiometric criteria continue to change, the goal remains the same—identify those patients in whom the implant is likely to provide better hearing. Because of device improvements, the ability to hear with an implant has dramatically improved over time. Therefore, the accepted audiometric criteria for implantation have expanded to include patients with more residual hearing.

In adults, candidacy is based on sentence recognition test scores (eg, **Hearing-in-Noise Test,** or HINT) with properly fitted hearing aids. Scores of 60% or less are generally needed to establish candidacy.

In children undergoing an evaluation for cochlear implantation, it is first necessary to establish a hearing threshold. A hearing aid trial can then be initiated and speech and language development assessed. Even children with a profound hearing loss undergo a hearing aid trial. Input is elicited from audiologists, parents, teachers, and speech and language pathologists. The cochlear implant team then assimilates the information and a determination is made regarding the child's progress with amplification. If the audiograms indicate poor hearing levels and there is

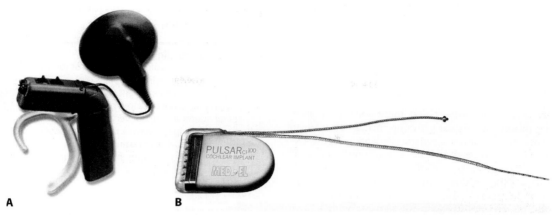

Figure 70–6. The Med El System. **(A)** TEMPO + BTE speech processor and **(B)** PULSAR implant. (Image courtesy of the Med-El Corporation, Innsbruck, Austria.)

a limited progression in language skills, the child is a candidate for implantation.

OTOLOGIC ASSESSMENT

A thorough otologic history and physical examination are obtained as part of the preimplantation assessment and include an investigation into the etiology of the hearing loss. (For a thorough discussion of the evaluation of sensorineural hearing loss [SNHL] in adults and children, which is beyond the scope of this chapter, see Chapter 52, Sensorineural Hearing Loss.)

Assessment of Pediatric Patients

In pediatric patients, it is important to ascertain whether there is a history of recurrent ear infections, pressure equalization (PE) tube placement, or other otologic surgeries. Patients with acute otitis media should be both treated with appropriate conventional antibiotics and demonstrated to be clear of infection before proceeding with surgery. For patients with a chronic middle ear effusion or recurrent acute otitis media, myringotomy with PE tube placement may be considered. Cochlear implants can coexist with PE tubes, although, ideally, patients would have an intact tympanic membrane at the time of surgery. Because children can be implant recipients at a very young age, there is a high likelihood of undergoing an episode of otitis media after implantation. These infections should be treated promptly and with broad-spectrum antibiotics. Curiously, it has been documented that an ear with a cochlear implant is less likely to develop otitis media than the contralateral ear, probably due to the fact that a mastoidectomy is performed as a part of the implantation.

Cochlear Patency

When deafness is a result of meningitis, special attention is required preoperatively to account for the possibility of cochlear ossification. If a patient has lost hearing as a result of meningitis, cochlear patency can be evaluated with either computed tomography (CT) scanning or magnetic resonance imaging (MRI). CT scanning should generally demonstrate cochlear ossification; however, obliteration due to fibrosis and the presence of soft tissue can be best assessed with a T2-weighted MRI. When the cochlea appears to be actively undergoing obliteration, the surgeon may wish to implant quickly—assuming that hearing is not expected to be recovered.

Tympanic Membrane

For adult implant recipients, an intact tympanic membrane is preferred. Accordingly, those patients with a tympanic membrane perforation, a chronic draining ear, or cholesteatoma often require other surgical procedures before implantation. For patients with long-dormant chronic ear disease and a modified radical cavity, it is not uncommon to combine cochlear implantation, closure of the ear canal, and obliteration of the mastoid cavity and middle ear into a single surgical procedure. Patients with active chronic ear disease processes, however, are better served with initial conventional otologic surgery with cochlear implantation delayed until the ear is stable.

Vestibular Evaluation

A vestibular evaluation, including at least electronystagmography (ENG), should be obtained if there is suspicion of a unilateral or bilateral vestibular hypofunction. Although the risk of losing balance function in the ear being implanted is low, if function was lost and the contralateral ear already lacked function, the resulting balance problems can be devastating, particularly in elderly adults.

Other Otologic Conditions

Other otologic conditions that merit special attention in the process of surgical planning include otosclerosis and congenital cochlear dysplasia. Patients with otosclerosis are likely to be at a higher risk of unwanted facial nerve stimulation because of coexistent demineralization of the surrounding bone. If the patient has previously undergone a stapes procedure, the prosthesis can usually be left undisturbed. For patients with known cochlear dysplasia, unusual surgical anatomy and a higher incidence of cerebrospinal fluid leak should be anticipated. Preoperative imaging is invaluable in avoiding complications.

RADIOLOGIC ASSESSMENT

Radiologic assessment for cochlear implantation typically consists of fine-cut CT scanning and/or MRI of the temporal bone. CT is preferred to delineate the detailed bony anatomy of the labyrinth, which may include evidence of cochlear ossification, abnormal facial nerve course, or congenital abnormalities. In patients in whom soft tissue detail is required, as in a patient with an elevated suspicion of central pathology or when cochlear patency is in question, MRI with and without gadolinium plus high-resolution T2-weighted images may prove to be valuable. The modification of MRI pulse sequences, such as fast-spin echo (FSE), and the development of new coils are leading to continuously improving resolution of the inner ear and internal auditory canal. Specifically, MRI can now allow reliable imaging of the internal auditory canal contents and afford confirmation of the presence of an auditory nerve. The Michel deformity (ie, congenital cochlear agenesis) and an absence of the auditory nerve, which may be present with the narrow internal auditory canal malformation or in the setting of auditory neuropathy, are the two absolute contraindications to cochlear implantation that may be found on radiologic assessment.

CANDIDACY

General Considerations

In addition to meeting audiometric and medical criteria, the basic evaluation of cochlear implant candidates involves analyzing multiple other factors (Table 70–1). The goals of the evaluation are (1) to determine whether the patient is likely to benefit from the implant; (2) to

Table 70–1. General criteria for cochlear implant candidacy.

Prelingual and Postlingual Children
Bilateral severe-to-profound hearing loss (only profound hearing loss in children < 2 years old)
Lack of auditory development with a proper binaural hearing aid trial as documented by objective testing or a parental questionnaire (for very young children)
Properly aided open-set work recognition scores < 20–30% in children capable of testing
Suitable auditory developmental education plan
Lack of medical contraindication

Postlingual Adults
18 years of age
Bilateral severe to profound hearing loss
Properly aided sentence (HINT) recognition scores < 40%
Lack of medical contraindication, with cochlea and auditory nerve present

Prelingual Adults
18 years of age
Bilateral profound deafness
Minimal benefit from properly fitted hearing aid
Lack of medical contraindication, with cochlea and auditory nerve present

establish realistic expectations concerning the outcome; and (3) to assess the needs and expectations of the patient, the patient's family, or both. Not all patients who meet audiometric and medical criteria should be given an implant. There must be grounded expectations as well as a firm commitment to follow through with the necessary postimplantation rehabilitation and programming. Furthermore, in many parts of the world, financial limitations preclude providing implants to all qualifying individuals.

Clearly, some patients are "better" candidates than others in that the positive impact of the implant on their lives is more dramatic. For example, an adult whose deafness is prelingual and who communicates with sign language may be made able to hear some environmental sounds; yet the device would not likely help the person to secure a different job or change his or her mode of communication. Conversely, a child led to develop near-normal speech and language abilities would live a very different life than would have been realized without implantation. Ultimately, it is hoped that patients use the device long term. Patients most likely to become nonusers are postlingual teens and adults.

Patients with Other Disorders

A unique group of individuals requiring careful consideration are those with hearing loss and other developmental and cognitive deficits. Historically, children with cerebral palsy or children with other conditions in addition to hearing loss were denied implantation. It is now clear, however, that many of these patients are very good candidates. In fact, if a hearing disability can be reduced with a cochlear implant, other disabilities (eg, a learning disability) may become less pronounced or more manageable. In contrast, in a child with very severe developmental issues and a poor prognosis for cognitive development, a cochlear implant may simply be another burden.

Timing of Implantation

The timing of implantation is very important. Earlier implantation in children generally yields more favorable results. In engaging this pursuit, complex questions arise with regard to how early children should undergo cochlear implantation in order to optimize eventual developmental outcomes. Although the answers to all these questions have yet to be definitively answered, success in progressively younger patient populations is driving the age of implant recipients lower. Early implantation essentially limits how far behind the child is in language development. Likewise, adults do better with a shorter duration of deafness. Excellent results can be obtained in older children and adults with long-term deafness, but expectations for the outcome should be modified. Current devices are FDA approved for implantation in children 12 months and older, with no upper age restrictions. Furthermore, it has been shown that outcomes in adults over age 65 are no better or no worse than those in young adults.

Of particular note, when the decision to proceed with cochlear implantation in prelingual deaf children is made, it is essential that the child subsequently undergo education in an oral-based environment. The more the child works with and depends on the implant, the better the eventual outcome.

IMPLANT SELECTION

All three currently available devices are excellent, and rarely are there strong reasons to prefer one to another. The outcomes seem to be similar regardless of the device, thereby indicating that patient factors are more important than the device variations. There are a few clinical situations that may make the physician favor one device over another. For example, a device with MRI compatibility or a removable magnet may be the best type to implant in a patient who will need future MRI scans. Some companies have multiple electrode configurations that are useful in an obliterated or malformed cochlea. Lastly, multiple family members or friends may have implants, and being able to share experiences and tips is facilitated if the devices are the same.

■ SURGICAL CONSIDERATIONS & GENERAL TECHNIQUES

SURGERY

Implant Location

Surgery is performed under a general anesthetic without muscle relaxation to allow for facial nerve monitoring. The device location is marked out with the use of templates. It is important to place the internal device far enough posteriorly so that the processor that is placed behind the ear does not lie against it and render the underlying skin at risk. In an effort to avoid the complications associated with a skin flap breakdown, it is imperative to plan the skin incision in order to provide adequate exposure while both preserving tissue viability and avoiding the placement of a suture line directly over implanted hardware. The location of prior incisions should be taken into account. Most surgeons use a postauricular incision that may be extended slightly more superiorly than what might be typically used in a routine ear surgery. The smaller devices in use can be placed through a 3–4 cm cosmetically acceptable incision. In children, the scar is less likely to widen with head growth if it is located only in the postauricular area and does not extend up into the scalp. Due diligence should be rendered in manipulating the tissues of the skin flap to assure minimal trauma.

Mastoidectomy & Cochleostomy

After the initial incision, the periosteum is elevated from the mastoid and a mastoidectomy is performed. The facial recess is opened to gain access to the middle ear—specifically to the promontory, the round window niche, and the stapes (Figure 70–7). The chorda tympani nerve is preserved and the incus buttress can be left in place or removed as needed. A cochleostomy is then made approximately 1 mm anteroinferior to the round window niche. The actual size of the cochleostomy needed may differ depending on the specific device being implanted.

According to the shape and size of the particular device chosen, a well may be drilled posterior to the mastoid cavity in the cortex to harbor the receiver-stimulator package. In children, this dissection is often carried down to the dura so that the device can be recessed. This better protects the device from trauma and is more cosmetically appealing. In adults, because of thicker bone, the device can be adequately recessed by removing bone to the inner table of the skull. The device can be placed in a tight subperiosteal pocket or secured by various means such as permanent suture or

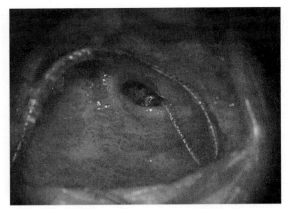

Figure 70–7. The basal turn of the cochlea is approached via drilling out the facial recess. The coiled electrode array is inserted into a cochleostomy that is fashioned 1 mm anterior and inferior to the round window.

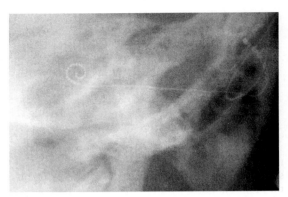

Figure 70–8. Postoperative x-ray image of a cochlear implant. Note the spiral coil within the cochlea.

overlying mesh. After the device is seated, the electrode array is gently inserted into the scala tympani. Following successful insertion, small pieces of fascia or periosteum are used to carefully plug the cochleostomy.

Hearing Preservation

When a patient with residual hearing (usually in the low tones) undergoes implantation, various strategies may be used to preserve or use this hearing after implantation. Namely, a shortened "hybrid" electrode that does not extend into and disturb the apical cochlear neural elements may be considered. When full-length electrode insertion is planned, "soft surgery" approaches to implantation aimed at preservation of natural hearing may be used. When hearing is preserved, a cochlear implant and a hearing aid in the same ear may be of some benefit.

Intraoperative Electrical Tests

Depending on the device and the availability of audiology support, intraoperative electrical tests can be performed to confirm the proper functioning of the device. Evoked potential and stapedial reflexes can be measured, which may be particularly helpful in programming with young children. Finally, if cochlear nerve action potentials can be recorded and a stapedial reflex elicited, the surgeon can be quite confident the device is indeed in the cochlea. After wound closure, a Stenver's view x-ray can be obtained for further confirmation of the device location and for reference in the case of future trauma or device migration (Figure 70–8). Patients may be discharged from the hospital on the same day, or they may spend one night in the hospital.

SPECIAL CIRCUMSTANCES

Cochlear Ossification

When cochlear ossification is encountered, various approaches may be used to ultimately attain satisfactory electrode placement. Often the obliteration involves only the first few millimeters of the basal turn, which can be removed with a drill or other small instruments. In these cases, the device can then be fully inserted. A preoperative MRI can usually predict this situation. For more extensive disease, other options exist, such as partial electrode insertion, insertion into the scala vestibuli, or other more elaborate drill-out approaches. Split electrodes (ie, two distinct electrodes) have been designed so that one electrode can be partially inserted in the scala tympani and the second can be inserted in the scala vestibuli or further along the scala tympani.

Cochlear Malformation

Cochlear malformations provide another surgical challenge. Everything from finding the cavity to inserting and stabilizing the electrode may be problematic. Fortunately, specifically designed electrodes are available to facilitate implantation. A CSF leak should be anticipated and may require plugging the eustachian tube and packing the middle ear.

Bilateral Implantation

The benefits of bilateral cochlear implantation have more recently been studied. Specifically, improvements in sound localization and speech understanding have been noted. Bilateral implantation can be staged months apart or undertaken safely in one setting When a second implant is placed, monopolar cautery must be avoided.

INITIAL STIMULATION & DEVICE PROGRAMMING

After the patient has healed from surgery, usually in 1–4 weeks, the device hardware is fully engaged and programmed. The initial programming is often done over 2–3 days. There are a myriad of variables that can be adjusted to improve the sound quality. After the first day, most adults report that speech sounds like static or voices sound either like "Donald Duck" or sound metallic in character. Amazingly, without any changes to the device, over the next 24 hours the sound quality improves. The brain somehow manages to adapt to the signal. This learning by the brain occurs mostly within the first 3–6 months, after which the rate of improvement in sound quality slows. Most adults have programming sessions 4–6 times in the first year, then annually or as needed.

Children (particularly infants) are more difficult to program because of the lack of a consistent feedback response regarding volume and clarity. Objective intraoperative measurements are helpful in estimating hearing thresholds and comfort levels. It is obviously very important to not provide too much gain. Children are seen more frequently for programming. Programming is critical to the success of the device, and experienced audiologists are able to achieve better outcomes than less experienced audiologists.

INTRAOPERATIVE & POSTOPERATIVE COMPLICATIONS

Cochlear implantation requires a surgical procedure under general anesthesia and therefore carries some risk. In particular, risks such as those encountered when removing a cholesteatoma or performing any surgery for chronic ear pathology do exist, including wound infection, facial nerve injury, taste disturbance, tinnitus, and balance problems. Overall, the complication rate of cochlear implantation has been reported as being 5–10%.

Wound Infection

A postoperative wound infection can usually be adequately treated with local wound care and antibiotics, but because of the presence of an indwelling foreign body, explantation of the device is occasionally required. Wound or skin breakdown can occur with an acute infection or may be related to excessive pressure of the magnet over the implant. It is important for patients to monitor the condition of the skin between the magnet and the implant device; the magnet strength can be adjusted to account for skin thickness.

Facial Nerve Injury

Facial nerve injury has been reported as well, which may not be surprising because of the wide array of aber-rant anatomy potentially encountered in this unique patient population. The anticipation of an abnormal nerve location and the use of intraoperative facial nerve monitoring should result in very few cases of temporary or permanent nerve injury.

Tinnitus

Patients need to understand that the residual hearing in the ear with the implant is likely to be lost and that a hearing aid will be of no benefit. Cochlear trauma from device insertion not only results in a loss of hearing, but it also may lead to or exacerbate tinnitus. When encountered in this setting, tinnitus typically lessens in time and often markedly improves after device programming.

Vestibular Dysfunction

Breaching the confines of the inner ear may also result in vestibular dysfunction with temporary balance problems; however, permanent balance difficulty has, in rare cases, been reported as well. Accordingly, if the patient is at all suspected of having contralateral vestibular dysfunction, a preoperative ENG should be considered.

Electronic Malfunction

Although the implanted device has no moving parts to wear out, there are still instances of electronic malfunction or failure due to trauma. Mechanically spoiled devices can usually be replaced with good results.

Risk of Meningitis

The risk of meningitis in implant recipients is being scrutinized. Patients with inner ear malformations have a higher risk of meningitis pre- and postoperatively unrelated to the cochlear implantation. The role of the electrode design and its impact on the risk of meningitis is under investigation. It is prudent for adult and pediatric implant recipients to receive the available pneumococcal vaccine; moreover, children should be vaccinated against *Haemophilus*.

ASSESSMENT OF OUTCOMES

Subjective Measurements

Cochlear implantation, not long ago viewed as experimental, is now a proven treatment for sensorineural hearing loss in properly selected patients. Adult implant recipients with positive outcomes have seen benefits as far-reaching as a restored capability to communicate on the telephone (attained by roughly 60% of adult recipients) and the ability to converse without the necessity of lip-reading. More modest outcomes have included the improved reception of environmental sounds and augmented lip-reading capabilities. Other selected benefits that have been described include the treatment of tinnitus, the improvement of preimplantation depression, and a perceived overall improvement in the quality of life (reported to be as high as 96% of recipients in one report).

Rarely in medicine is there a procedure that has such a profoundly positive impact on the quality of life. Successful cochlear implantation is extremely rewarding for implant team members and patients alike. Yet, it is essential to stress that the outcomes seen with cochlear implantation vary widely both within given patient populations and among differing groups. Multiple factors have been shown to have a bearing on the degree of benefit obtained from implantation (Table 70–2). Although these factors are helpful in anticipating performance levels, additional unaccounted-for dynamics, which are difficult to gauge and recognize, do exist and account for about 50% of the variance in performance.

Objective Measurements

A. OPEN-SET SENTENCE AND WORD RECOGNITION SCORES

More specific objective measures in postlingual deafened adults following implantation include an evaluation of both open-set sentence and word recognition scores. Various reports have documented open-set sentence recognition scores of 60–70% and word recognition scores of 30–50%. Note that patient variability, evolving inclusion criteria, and ever-changing technologic innovations render the objective analysis between various implant systems and processing strategies quite difficult.

B. MEASUREMENTS FOR PEDIATRIC PATIENTS

In children, results seem to have greater variability and are more difficult to measure.

1. Mainstream schooling—A common goal (and one that has been frequently attained) for implant recipients in the very young pediatric population is to achieve communication abilities sufficient to allow enrollment in mainstream schooling by the second grade. In fact, an especially high number of children who have received an implant before age 3 have been known to eventually achieve age-appropriate speech recognition and production, with the most frequent success coming in the subset of patients who are younger than 18 months when they receive the implant.

2. Word understanding—The objective markers of pediatric outcomes in postlingual deafened children (the minority of deaf children) include word understanding test scores 3 years after implantation that are documented to reach as high as 100%. The prelingual

Table 70–2. Factors generally associated with better outcomes in cochlear implantation (listed in random order).

Adults and Children
  Shorter duration of deafness
  Better preoperative word or sentence recognition (or both)
  Lip-reading ability
  Higher intelligence quotient (IQ)
  Better preoperative residual hearing
  Optimized implant technology and processing strategy
  Cause of deafness (eg, meningitis associated with poor outcomes)
  Intact, nonossified cochlea
Additional Factors in Children
  Younger age at implantation
  Motivated family assistance
  Oral preoperative education
  Oral education rehabilitation program as opposed to *total communication*

deafened child, who represents the majority of pediatric deaf patients, has shown to make slower and more variable improvements over a longer time span, including reported progress at up to 8 years after implantation. As previously alluded to, evidence seems to indicate that these children do better if implantation is undertaken before age 8 with the best outcomes usually obtained in children less than 3–4 years old.

Chmiel R, Sutton L, Jenkins H. Quality of life in children with cochlear implants. *Ann Otol Rhinol Laryngol.* 2000;185(Suppl):103. [PMID: 11140975] (Quality of life gauged to be significantly better in children with cochlear implants.)

Franz DC. Pediatric performance with the Med-El Combi 40+ cochlear implant system. *Ann Otol Rhinol Laryngol.* 2002;189 (Suppl):66. [PMID: 12018352] (Good outcomes in children with the Med-El Combi 40+.)

Geers A, Brenner C, Nicholas J, Uchanski R, Tye-Murray N, Tobey E. Rehabilitation factors contributing to implant benefit in children. *Ann Otol Rhinol Laryngol.* 2002;189(Suppl):127. [PMID: 12018339] (Children and family nonverbal IQ, implant characteristics, and educational variables each account for variability in the outcomes in pediatric implantation.)

Geers AE, Nicholas J, Tye-Murray N et al. Effects of communication mode on skills of long-term cochlear implant users. *Ann Otol Rhinol Laryngol.* 2000;185(Suppl):89. [PMID: 11141021] (Results in children using an oral-auditory communication mode are superior to total communication.)

Hammes DM, Novak MA, Rotz LA, Willis M, Edmondson DM, Thomas JF. Early identification and cochlear implantation: critical factors for spoken language development. *Ann Otol Rhinol Laryngol.* 2002;189(Suppl):74. [PMID: 12018355] (Infants implanted at 18 months and younger shown to develop age-appropriate speech.)

Kirk KI, Miyamoto RT, Lento CL, Ying E, O'Neill T, Fears B. Effects of age at implantation in young children. *Ann Otol Rhi-*

nol Laryngol. 2002;189(Suppl):69. [PMID: 12018353] (Rate of language development significantly faster in recipients under age 3; also, development with an oral-auditory communication mode is faster than total communication.)

Labadie RF, Carrasco VN, Gilmer CH, Pillsbury HC III. Cochlear implant performance in senior citizens. *Otol Head Neck Surg.* 2000;123:419. [PMID: 11020178] (Equally good outcomes with cochlear implants seen in both young and older adults with Clarion device.)

Osberger MJ, Kalberer A, Zimmerman-Phillips S, Barker MJ, Geier L. Speech perception results in children using the Clarion multistrategy cochlear implant. *Ann Otol Rhinol Laryngol.* 2000;185(Suppl):75. [PMID: 11892207] (Good outcomes in children with the Clarion device.)

Staller S, Parkinson A, Arcaroli J, Arndt P. Pediatric outcomes with the Nucleus 24 Contour: North American clinical trial. *Ann Otol Rhinol Laryngol.* 2002;189(Suppl):56. [PMID: 12018350] (Good outcomes in children with the Nucleus 24 Contour device.)

SECTION XVII
Facial Plastic & Reconstructive Surgery

Scar Revision 71

Nathan Monhian, MD, & Anil Shah, MD

General Considerations

With advances in the knowledge of wound healing, as well as the development of better materials and techniques, many options have become available in the treatment of patients with unsightly scars. Nevertheless, no technique has been devised to allow total and permanent removal or effacement of scars. Patients should be counseled to understand that the goal of scar revision is to replace one scar for another to improve the appearance and the acceptability of the scar.

The wound healing process is divided into three stages. In the **inflammatory phase,** the release of inflammatory mediators results in migration of fibroblasts into the wound. During the **proliferative phase,** an extracellular matrix is formed that comprises proteoglycans, fibronectin, hyaluronic acid, and collagen secreted by fibroblasts. Angiogenesis and re-epithelialization of the wound also occur during the proliferative phase. Collagen and the extracellular matrix mature in the **remodeling phase,** and the wound contracts. Wound strength reaches 20% of its preinjury strength at 3 weeks. The ultimate tensile strength of the wound is 70–80% of that of the uninjured skin.

Pathogenesis

A. GENETIC FACTORS

Genetic factors contributing to poor scar formation are likely to be present in patients with Fitzpatrick skin Types III and above. Darker skins tend to form postinflammatory hyperpigmentation and are more likely to form keloids or hypertrophic scars. Younger skin has more tensile strength, which can lead to widening of

the scar, whereas older skin tends to scar better because of a lesser amount of tension on the wound.

B. IATROGENIC CAUSES

Iatrogenic causes of poor scar formation include excessive soft tissue trauma while handling the skin, failure to reapproximate and evert the wound edges properly, and closure under excessive tension. Failure to evert the wound edges at the time of closure leads to formation of a depressed scar. Lack of deep support of the wound can lead to excessive tension on wound edges, resulting in a widened scar. Sutures from facial wounds should be removed after 5–7 days. Removing sutures too early or too late may lead to a wide scar or unsightly tracking, respectively. Early treatment with steroids or isotretinoin (Accutane) can adversely affect wound healing. It is recommended that elective surgery, especially on the face, be delayed for at least 12–18 months after completing a course of isotretinoin.

C. HYPERTROPHIC SCAR, KELOIDS, AND WIDENED SCARS

Hypertrophic scars are self-limited scars, which hypertrophy within the limits of the wound but above the skin level. Hypertrophic scars are more common than keloids and occur without race predilection and in any age group. Initially, these scars are red, raised, pruritic, and occasionally painful, but they tend to flatten over time. They appear worse at 2 weeks to 2 months after wound closure. In general, hypertrophic scars are more responsive to steroid injections than are keloids.

Keloid scars can be distinguished from hypertrophic scars by spreading beyond the original wound. Keloids have a distinct race predilection to darker skins and occur most often in patients 10–30 years old. In contrast to hypertrophic scars, keloid scars remain raised, red, pruritic, and occasionally painful rather than regressing at a few months.

Widened scars are typically flat and depressed and do not have an erythematous or pruritic phase. They occur without race or age tendency and occur most frequently on the body. Wound color typically improves to match the uninjured skin with time.

Histologically, the collagen in both keloids and hypertrophic scars is organized in discrete nodules, frequently obliterating the rete pegs in the papillary dermis of the lesions. While collagen in normal dermis is arranged in discrete fascicles separated by considerable interstitial space, collagen nodules in keloids and in hypertrophic scars appear avascular and unidirectional and are aligned in a highly stressed configuration. Collagen synthesis is greater in keloids than hypertrophic scars. Collagen synthesis is three times greater in keloids than hypertrophic scars and 20 times greater in normal scars. Disagreement exists about whether hypertrophic scars can be differentiated from keloids using light microscopy. Blackburn and Cosman described eosinophilic refractile hyaline collagen fibers, an increase in mucinous ground substance, and a lack of fibroblasts in keloids. Scanning electron microscopy findings clearly demonstrate the randomly organized sheets of collagen with no obvious relationship to the skin surface in keloid scar formation.

Clinical Findings

Skin is anisotropic and nonlinear and has time-dependent properties. The term **anisotropic** indicates that the mechanical properties of skin vary with direction. The **relaxed skin tension lines** (RSTLs) are the lines of minimal tension of the skin; incisions parallel with these lines are under the least possible tension while healing. Perpendicular to the RSTLs are the lines of maximal extensibility. A fusiform excision parallel with the RSTLs and closed in the direction of the lines of maximal extensibility heals under minimal closing tension and results in the best scar.

Complications

Complications of scar revision vary according to the method used. These include local infection, graft or flap necrosis, and further scarring after the revision. Viral reactivation of the herpes zoster virus is a potential complication after dermabrasion or laser resurfacing. Laser resurfacing can also cause postinflammatory hyperpigmentation, which may last several months. Resurfacing methods that go beyond the deep reticular dermis can cause further scarring instead of improving a scar.

Treatment

A. Nonsurgical Measures

1. Intralesional agents—For many years, corticosteroid injection has been established in the reduction of hypertrophic scars and keloids. Common preparations include triamcinolone acetonide (Kenalog) and triamcinolone diacetate (Aristocort). Steroids decrease fibroblast proliferation, reduce blood vessel formation, and interfere with fibrosis by inhibiting extracellular matrix protein gene expression (downregulates pro-α_1 collagen gene). By decreasing the production of collagen, a smaller scar is created. Doses ranging from 5 mg/mL to 40 mg/mL are injected at 3- to 6-week intervals. Typically, multiple injections are required to obtain the desired benefit. Complications of steroid injection include atrophy of the subcutaneous layer, granuloma formation, pigmentary changes, and development of telangiectasias.

New intralesional treatments have included the use of antimitotic agents such as bleomycin and 5-fluorouracil (5-FU). Small doses of these drugs may be injected into hypertrophic scar tissue with good results. Intralesional injections of 5-FU in combination with triamcinolone acetonide plus concomitant use of a pulsed-dye laser have had good results. Injections can be performed as frequently as three times per week. Injections of bleomycin into a keloid using a multipuncture technique have also shown some promise in scar flattening and preventing recurrence. Antimitotic medications should not be administered to pregnant women.

2. Soft tissue fillers—Atrophic and depressed scars may also be treated with injectable fillers in an attempt to provide bulk in areas of tissue deficiency. The most commonly used agents include bovine collagen (Zyderm, Zyplast), pooled human collagen (micronized AlloDerm or Cymetra, CosmoDerm, CosmoPlast), hyaluronic acid (Hylaform, Restylane), hydroxyapatite (Radiesse), autologous dermis, and fat. These biologically derived materials provide temporary correction (2–12 months). Synthetic materials such as expanded polytetrafluoroethylene (e-PTFE, GoreTex, SoftForm, or Ultrasoft) may also be used to provide a filling effect in depressed areas. Injectable Fibrel and silicone are no longer in widespread use.

3. Silicone sheeting, hydration, and compression—Silicone has been used with relative success in the management of hypertrophic scars, although its mechanism of action is not clearly understood. Although it was initially hypothesized to work through pressure over the scar tissue, the efficacy of silicone has been demonstrated even in nonpressure dressings. It appears that hydration, or rather the ability of silicone to prevent wound desiccation, is a contributing mechanism. Hydration inhibits the in vitro production of collagen and glycosaminoglycans by fibroblasts. Silicone sheeting can be worn daily for as long as 12–24 hours daily, although its application is somewhat cumbersome. An alternative to silicone sheeting, silicone gel can be applied to the scar. Both silicone gel and silicone sheeting have shown positive results in the reduction of scar size and erythema.

Continuous pressure at 80 mm Hg provided by tight-fitting dressings has been shown to prevent and modify scar formation. The potential mechanisms of action are local tissue hypoxia and reduction of the intralesional population of mast cells, which may affect fibroblast growth.

4. Pulsed-dye laser—The pulsed-dye 585-nm-wavelength laser can be effective in reducing scar erythema by reducing neovascularization. Several treatments are usually required using a low to moderate fluence (5.0–7.0 J/cm^2) with no overlap. Hypertrophic scars may also shrink with this treatment as a result of a reduction in the number and activity of fibroblasts.

5. Dermabrasion—Raised, depressed, or hyperpigmented scars may benefit from superficial abrasion of the skin, which blends the scar with its surrounding tissue by changing the texture, color, and depth of the scar. The technique of resurfacing depends on the nature of the deformity. The goal of this technique is to even out any uneven surfaces. The depth of the dermabrasion depends on the depth of the scar. However, dermabrasion should not go beyond the reticular dermis; otherwise, greater scarring or hypopigmentation will result.

6. Laser resurfacing—Laser resurfacing has replaced mechanical dermabrasion in many practices. One advantage of laser resurfacing over mechanical dermabrasion is that the depth of penetration is easier to control. Another advantage is that there is no aerosolization of skin and blood, thereby lowering the risk of viral transmission. The thermal damage that results from laser resurfacing is advantageous in that it produces collagen contracture of 20–60%. However, the postoperative period of laser resurfacing is marked by prolonged erythema. The most common lasers in use for resurfacing are the high-energy pulsed CO_2 laser, which produces photothermal injury, and the erbium:YAG laser, which results in photomechanical injury to the skin. Combining different laser modalities, such as the pulsed-dye and CO_2 lasers, may provide an added advantage in scar improvement.

7. Camouflage—Many patients who seek scar revisions may not be able to camouflage the scar or have minimal knowledge of available camouflage techniques. Makeup, hair, and accessories can sometimes offer excellent coverage of the scar. Newer makeup materials and techniques allow for better and more complete coverage of unsightly defects. Opaque cosmetics with a slightly low tone, which disguises the erythema of scars, generally provide better results.

B. Preoperative Considerations

1. Patient expectations—As with any cosmetic procedure, the patient's motivations and expectations for seeking corrective surgery should be carefully considered. In general, well-informed patients with realistic expectations have better overall outcomes. A patient should understand that scar revision is a process to improve the appearance of the scar by adjusting, repositioning, or narrowing the scar and that complete elimination of the scar is impossible at this point. However, the physician should be sensitive to the fact that the scar may represent a traumatic experience to the patient. If the revision does not meet the patient's expectations, the patient may suffer additional trauma. Occasionally, psychological counseling should be recommended in conjunction with scar revision.

2. Timing of scar revision—Scars in the inflammatory phase are prone to hypertrophy. The initial scar can be expected to change due to collagen remodeling and collagen fiber reorientation. Although collagen remodeling continues for 1–3 years, most significant changes occur in the first 4–6 months, and an average of 6 months' delay before revision is reasonable. Nevertheless, in clinical situations, where skin edges are grossly misaligned or the scar lies in an unfavorable direction, scar revision may prove beneficial as early as 2 months.

3. Scar analysis—Before embarking on a revision, the primary scar, and its desired location when revised, should be carefully analyzed. Scars can be classified according to their location, etiology, size, shape, contour, and color. Cosmetically favorable scars are similar in color to the surrounding tissue. They are also fine, flat, and well positioned in the face. Scars that are located in the periphery of the face, at a transition line between two cosmetic subunits, or directly in the midline are less conspicuous. The lack of one or more of these qualities results in an unsightly scar. Noticeable scars are wide, raised, or depressed, or are often hyperpigmented or hypopigmented compared with the adjacent skin. They may cut across different subunits or lie in an unfavorable direction. A scar contracture in sensitive areas—for example, at the vermilion or the eyelid—can distort adjacent structures and create cosmetic or functional deformities.

C. Surgical Measures

Appropriate scar management begins at the time of injury. Good surgical technique is essential for normal wound healing. Crushing the skin edges, tying sutures too tightly, and cauterizing too excessively may result in local tissue inflammation, necrosis, and poor scarring. Adequate wound humidity and coverage are also important for minimizing scar formation. Studies suggest that epithelial cells migrate more readily with adequate surface moisture. If the wound is kept moist, particularly with an occlusive dressing, migration proceeds more directly and efficiently. Local tissue ischemia caused by infection, hematoma, foreign bodies, anemia, or poor surgical technique may slow wound healing. In addition, local wound infection prolongs wound healing. Bacteria delay normal healing phases by directly damaging cells of wound repair by prolonging the inflammatory phase as well as competing for oxygen and nutrients within the tissue. Surgical excision of hypertrophic scars or keloids may lead to recurrence rates of 45–100%.

1. Primary excision and straight-line closure—The most common technique in the revision of scars 2 cm or shorter is primary excision and linear closure. Typically with this procedure, a small margin of normal skin in the periphery of the scar is excised with the scar in a fusiform fashion, and the defect is closed in a linear fashion. The optimal length-to-width ratio to prevent standing cone deformities while maintaining the minimum length of the new scar is 3:1. The wound edges should be undermined to reduce the tension on the closure line. The defect is then closed in two layers, with subdermal absorbable sutures to minimize tension and fine monofilament sutures, such as 5.0 or 6.0 nylon or polypropylene, for the superficial layer. Wound eversion should be meticulously achieved.

With large scars, where total excision of the scar is not practical, serial excisions of the central portion of the scar with advancement of the peripheral tissue can be useful. A minimum period of 6 weeks should be allowed between each two excisions.

Small and pitted or depressed scars, such as deep acne scars, can be revised by punch excision and primary closure with wound eversion. As an alternative, small, full-thickness skin grafts can be placed into the defects and secured in position with sutures, bolstering techniques, or both.

2. W-Plasty—The W-plasty is a series of connected, triangular advancement flaps mirrored along the length of the scar. A W-plasty, unlike a Z-plasty, incorporates shorter limbs and does not result in an overall change in the length of the scar. Unfavorable scars that are short and located in forgiving locations, such as the forehead or cheeks, scars that lie perpendicular to RSTLs, pretrichial scars, and scars over curved surfaces such as the inferior mandibular border are particularly good indications of W-plasty. This procedure can make the scar less conspicuous by making it irregular and thus more difficult for the observing eye to track. It also disrupts wound contracture with its irregular pattern.

In designing a W-plasty, dots representing the apices of the triangles are placed 3–5 mm from the scar edge. These dots should be spaced 5–6 mm apart, and each

limb of the triangle should be 3–5 mm in length. The angle of the apex of each triangle should be determined by its relationship to the RSTLs, making one of the limbs of the triangle parallel with these lines. The ends of the W-plasty should be less than 30° to avoid standing cone deformities. Alternately, an M-plasty can be used at the ends to prevent extending the excision. The scar is excised, the adjacent tissue is undermined, and the wound is closed with a two-layer closure. Horizontal mattress sutures can be used to enhance wound eversion.

3. Geometric broken-line closure—Geometric broken-line closure (GBLC) differs from W-plasty in that, instead of using a series of triangles, it includes other alternating geometric shapes, such as squares and semicircles, along with triangles (Figure 71–1). Scars that respond well to GBLC are those that are relatively long and 45° or greater from RSTLs. Scars that are perpendicular to these lines have the best cosmetic result using GBLC. GBLC is slightly more challenging than W-plasty, but the principles and techniques are otherwise identical.

4. Z-Plasty—The Z-plasty consists of two transposition-advancement flaps designed to accomplish three goals: (1) change scar direction, (2) interrupt scar linearity, and (3) lengthen scar contracture (Figure 71–2). Z-pasty is particularly beneficial if it can reorient a scar with RSTLs or in a natural junction between facial

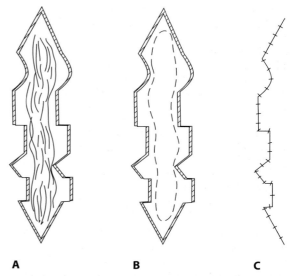

A   **B**   **C**

Figure 71–1. Geometric broken-line closure. **(A)** Random geometric patterns in mirror images are marked around the scar. **(B)** The scar is excised. **(C)** Wound edges are advanced and closed with appropriate sutures.

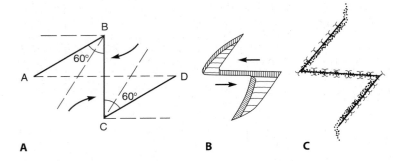

A   **B**   **C**   ***Figure 71–2.*** 60° Z-plasty.

esthetic units. Similarly, with this technique, a long scar can be broken up into several smaller components to allow better camouflage (Figure 71–3). Finally, scars that cause distortion of facial features due to scar contracture are good candidates for revision using Z-plasty.

A main advantage of Z-plasty over other techniques, such as W-plasty, is that usually no additional normal skin needs to be removed. A properly planned Z-plasty results in minimal distortion of surrounding structures. Moreover, it can counter the forces of scar contracture, thus correcting webbed or contracted scars that distort anatomic landmarks.

Precise preoperative planning of this technique is an essential requirement for its success. In its classic description, Z-plasty consists of one central and two peripheral limbs in the shape of a Z, such that two triangular flaps of equal size are created. All three limbs are of equal length, and the central limb consists of the scar that is to be lengthened and realigned. The orientation of the final scar can be determined by the direction in which the lateral limbs are placed and by varying the angles of the lateral limbs in relation to the central limb. The most commonly used angles are 30°, 45°, and 60°, which produce lengthening of the scar of 25%, 50%, and 75%, respectively. For long scars for which a single Z-plasty may produce long, linear scars, multiple Z-plasties can be used along the scar.

In performing this technique, the scar is excised along the central limb and the peripheral limbs are incised. The two triangular flaps and the surrounding tissue are mobilized, and the flaps are transposed and advanced. After meticulous hemostasis, the flaps are closed using tension-reducing techniques and eversion. A passive drain with pressure dressing may be necessary to reduce the dead space and the chance of fluid accumulation under the flaps.

5. Skin grafts—Full-thickness skin grafts can be used in a variety of ways in scar revision. Scars can be simply excised and grafted with a full-thickness graft. Skin grafts can also be used to fill skin defects after punch excision of deep or depressed scars. Contracted scars in the lower eyelid that lead to ectropion often require

replacement of the anterior lamellar defect using a full-thickness graft. Defects in the upper eyelid causing lag ophthalmus can be repaired in a similar fashion using skin grafts.

6. Flaps—Flaps can be beneficial in a variety of ways in scar revision. In general, they can be used when the best option in scar revision is complete excision of the scar and reconstruction of the defect with a local flap. For example, a small scar of the nasal tip may be excised and repaired using a bilobed flap, just as one might repair a defect after ablation of a malignant growth in the same area. (For a more comprehensive discussion of local flaps, see Chapter 76, Local & Regional Flaps in Head & Neck Reconstruction.)

Prognosis

Most scars may be improved using a variety of scar revision techniques. Essentials of wound care are as important after the revision to achieve optimal outcomes. However, a scar may require several revision procedures

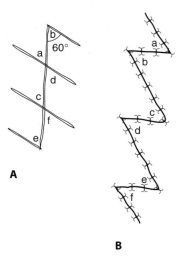

A   **B**

Figure 71–3. Multiple Z-plasties at 45°.

before an outcome acceptable to the patient is achieved. The need for multiple procedures should be clearly discussed with the patient.

Blackburn WR, Cosman B. Histologic basis of keloid and hypertrophic scar differentiation. Clinicopathologic correlation. *Arch Pathol.* 1966;82(1):65. [PMID: 5938452] (An early comparative study of hypertrophic scars and keloids.)

Brown SA, Coimbra M, Coberly D et al. Oral nutritional supplementation accelerates skin wound healing: a randomized, placebo-controlled, double-arm, crossover study. *Plast Reconstr Surg* 2004;114:237. [PMID: 15220599] (This clinical trial suggests that InflammEnz, an oral nutritional supplement, modulates the wound-healing process and suggests that many patients with minor soft-tissue wounds may benefit from treatment.)

Chen MA, Davidson TM. Scar management: prevention and treatment strategies. *Curr Opin Otolaryngol Head Neck Surg.* 2005;13(4):242. ((Discussion of the basic science mechanism underlying aberrant wound healing, as well as the strategies for prevention and management of keloids and hypertrophic scars.)

Clark JM, Wang TD. Local flaps in scar revision. *Facial Plast Surg.* 2001;17(4):295. [PMID: 11735064] (Reviews common techniques used in reconstruction of facial defects and scars and provides several cases in which these techniques were successfully used.)

Cohen IK, McCoy BJ, Mohanakumar T, Diegelmann RF. Immunoglobulin, complement, and histocompatibility antigen studies in keloid patients. *Plast Reconstr Surg.* 1979;63(5):689. [PMID: 432336] (This study suggests that a localized immune response is involved in keloid pathogenesis, one that is not related to either the HLA-A or B histocompatibility loci.)

Ehrlich HP, Desmouliere A, Diegelmann RF et al. Morphological and immunochemical differences between keloid and hypertrophic scar. *Am J Pathol.* 1994;145(1):105. [PMID: 8030742] (An extensive, comparative study of hypertrophic scars and keloids, suggesting that several morphologic and immunohistochemical differences exist between hypertrophic scar and keloid that are useful for the biological and pathologic characterization of the two lesions.)

Lee KK, Mehrany K, Swanson NA. Surgical revision. *Dermatol Clin.* 2005;23:141. (Provides an excellent summary of surgical techniques for scar prevention and updates on scar revision strategies including dermabrasion, laser resurfacing, intralesional steroids, excision, and geometric closures.)

Liu W, Wang DR, Cao YL. TGF-β: a fibrotic factor in wound scarring and a potential target for anti-scarring gene therapy. *Curr Gene Ther.* 2004;4:123. (Provides an update on the role of TGF-β in scar formation and basic science gene therapy study.)

Panin G, Strumia R, Ursini F. Topical α-tocopherol acetate in the bulk phase: eight years of experience in skin treatment. *Ann N Y Acad Sci.* 2004;1031:443. (Provides a useful review of topical vitamin E usefulness in wound healing.)

Rodgers BJ, Williams EF, Hove CR. W-plasty and geometric broken line closure. *Facial Plast Surg.* 2001;17(4):239. [PMID: 11735056] (W-plasty provides a regularly irregular scar, and geometric broken-line closure provides an irregularly irregular scar. Both methods divert the attention of the eye by producing a nonlinear scar pattern.)

Rhytidectomy, Browlifts, & Midface Lifts

72

Anil R. Shah, MD, Eugene J. Kim, MD, & Corey S. Maas, MD

PATHOGENESIS OF FACIAL AGING

Facial aging generally consists of intrinsic and extrinsic processes. Intrinsically, the most extensive changes occur in the dermis, especially in its upper third. The total amount of ground substance, predominantly made of glycosaminoglycans and proteoglycans, diminishes. In addition, elastic fibers, which maintain the wavy pattern of collagen bundles, become thin and fragmented with time, beginning at age 30. Finally, the ratio of type I to type III collagen diminishes over time, along with a general reduction in the total amount of collagen.

Extrinsically, one of the main factors in facial aging is from actinic damage. In a process called elastosis, collagen is degraded and elastin is increased. The dermis becomes thickened and poorly organized. Fine-skin wrinkling from sun-damaged epidermis also occurs. Along with fat atrophy in the subcutaneous tissue, there is a general redistribution of tissue due to gravitational effects. The sagging of tissue leads to the loss of the cervicomental angle and mandibular definition. All these factors contribute to the aging face.

ANATOMY

Superficial Musculoaponeurotic System

Anatomic studies have shown the superficial musculoaponeurotic system (SMAS) to be a distinct layer that is just superficial to and closely applied to the parotid fascia (Figure 72–1). Generally, sensory nerves lie superficial and facial nerve fibers lie deep to the SMAS. Superiorly, the SMAS is contiguous with the temporoparietal fascia. Anteriorly, insertion occurs at the lateral border of the zygomaticus muscle and to the dermis of the upper lip. Thus, the posterior traction of the SMAS actually deepens the nasolabial fold. The SMAS is also in continuity with the orbicularis oculi muscle in the lower eyelid. Inferiorly, there is continuity with the platysma over the body of the mandible and extension in the neck.

Platysma

The platysma is a broad, thin muscle innervated by the cervical branch of the facial nerve. It has been shown to have different configurations in terms of midline decussation. This has implications in the aging face in that platysmal bands can form along with the pseudoherniation of fat. This results in the "turkey gobbler" look and the loss of the cervicomental angle, which contributes to an aged appearance.

Facial Nerve

The facial nerve (cranial nerve VII) gives mimetic function through innervation of the facial musculature. Divisions include the frontal, zygomatic, buccal, mandibular, and cervical branches (Figure 72–2). Crossover innervation occurs up to 70% in the zygomatic and buccal branches and only up to 15% in the frontal and mandibular branches. The frontal branch runs within the temporoparietal fascia and lies just superficial to the superficial layer of the deep temporal fascia. It generally crosses the zygoma approximately 4 cm lateral to the lateral canthus. The zygomatic and buccal branches are deep to the SMAS but become more superficial as they course anteriorly. The marginal branch has a varying course but generally extends up to 1 cm below the inferior edge of the mandible.

Greater Auricular Nerve

The greater auricular nerve provides sensation to the inferior lobule and the upper neck and is a branch of the cervical plexus. The skin and SMAS lie just superficial to the nerve. The nerve has an intimate association with the sternocleidomastoid muscle and has been shown to cross the muscle at its midpoint, approximately 6 cm below the external auditory canal.

PATIENT SELECTION

The appropriate selection of patients has critical importance in ensuring a desirable outcome. Patients need to understand the goals and limitations of rhytidectomy. They should be motivated and willing to participate in other associated changes that support longevity, such as improved diet, smoking cessation, and sun protection. An ideal patient is a healthy, motivated individual aged

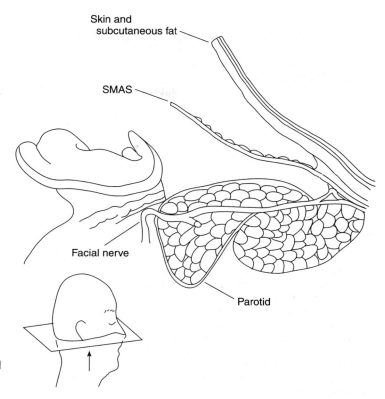

Skin and
subcutaneous fat

SMAS

Facial nerve

Parotid

Figure 72–1. The superficial musculoaponeurotic system (SMAS) is a distinct
layer between the parotid gland, skin, and
subcutaneous fat.

40 to 60 whose skin has some elasticity without severe solar damage, and who is an appropriate weight. The major concern should be of ptotic skin and muscle.

Patients often inquire as to the amount of time their facelifts will last. They should be made aware that rhytidectomy does not stop the aging process but rather gives them a more youthful appearance from which they will continue to age. This process is dictated by their individual genetic predisposition and somewhat by their environment. Multiple consultations may be necessary and should be encouraged if there seem to be any hidden motivations or confusion about the goals of the procedure. Cooperation by patients is critical in their postoperative recovery, and it behooves the surgeon to devote equal effort to the selection process as much as to the operation itself.

PATIENT HISTORY & PHYSICAL EXAMINATION

Preparation for surgery should include a complete history and physical examination. Any history of bleeding problems should alert the physician that a hematologic workup may be necessary. This has obvious implications with regard to a postoperative risk of hematoma. The appropriate control of any medical problems, espe-

cially hypertension, should be assured. Patients should cease smoking and stop the use of nonsteroidal anti-inflammatory drugs (NSAIDs) approximately 2 weeks before and after surgery.

At the time of the preoperative visit, the procedure should be reviewed, informed consent obtained, and any final questions answered. Preoperative photographs are mandatory and are taken in the standard lateral, oblique, and frontal views.

PREOPERATIVE PREPARATION & ANESTHESIA

In the preoperative area, the patient's hair is carefully combed along planned incision lines and rubber bands are applied as twist ties. By twisting the hair in the area of the planned incision sites, hair loss is minimized.

Some surgeons perform rhytidectomy using local anesthesia with sedation. However, general anesthesia is preferred by many others to maximize patient comfort. It also allows the surgeon to concentrate on the operative field and not have his or her attention distracted by monitoring the patient's vital signs and status. A smooth extubation should be a high priority to decrease the risk of hematoma.

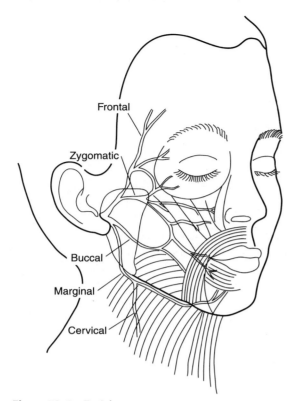

Figure 72–2. Facial nerve anatomy.

After the induction of general anesthesia, an endotracheal tube is fixed in the midline, taking care not to distort the facial anatomy. The first side is infiltrated with 1% lidocaine with 1:100,000 epinephrine along the skin incisions and widely across the planned area of elevation. Adequate local anesthetic is critical in minimizing bleeding during skin flap elevation through the vasoconstrictive effects of epinephrine. The contralateral side is injected while completing the first side to maximize hemostasis and minimize toxicity. Prior to the administration of anesthesia, care should be taken to calculate the maximal dose, which is based on body weight.

SURGICAL TECHNIQUES

Incisions

The placement of incisions is important and influenced by several factors. The principal goals are to minimize hair loss, hairline adjustments, visible scars, and changes in normal anatomic structures. In general, incisions should be placed post-tragal in women and pre-tragal in men. Pre-tragal incisions avoid the need to redrape hair-bearing skin onto the tragus. As the incision is carried superiorly past

the helical root, careful attention should be made to preserving the temporal hair tuft and preventing alopecia in this area. If the temporal area requires lifting, the incision is curved anterosuperiorly into the hair-bearing scalp. If alopecia is a concern, the incision is brought more anteriorly in a pretrichial or "trichophytic" fashion to preserve the patient's hairline (Figure 72–3). The incision is also made irregularly to help camouflage the scar.

The posterior incision is preferably brought into the hair. The alternative to bringing the posterior incision along the hairline can result in visible scar tissue from scar widening. The postauricular incision is brought within 1–2 cm of the sulcus, with a 90° posterior turn into the hair above the external auditory canal. It extends approximately 6–8 cm posteriorly, with a 45° downturn at the end. This helps prevent a standing cutaneous deformity during flap advancement.

Subcutaneous Rhytidectomy

Subcutaneous flap techniques have an extremely low risk of facial nerve injury and remain in common use. The flap is elevated with facelift scissors just superficial to the SMAS using a combination of traction and countertraction (Figure 72–4). Elevation of the flap into the neck

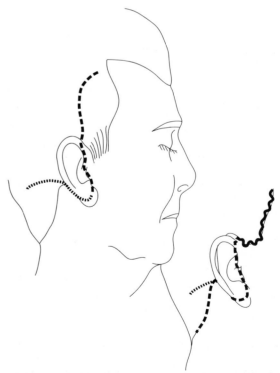

Figure 72–3. Possible incisions in rhytidectomy.

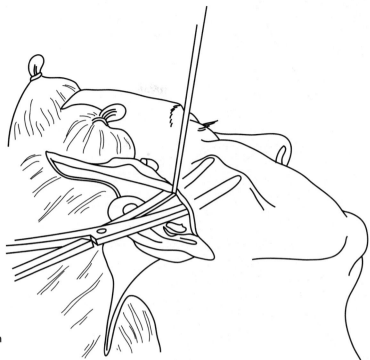

Figure 72–4. Elevation of the skin flap in the subcutaneous plane.

extends to the middle third of the neck. Undermining in the neck is carried anteriorly to the midline, and the physician should always be mindful of staying superficial and using blunt dissection. Care must be taken in dissection around the sternocleidomastoid to avoid injury to the greater auricular nerve and the external jugular vein. The extent of the anterior dissection depends on the individual patient. Once the anterior border of the parotid gland is reached, the risk of facial nerve injury increases. Superiorly, dissection is carried in a plane superficial to the temporalis fascia, which allows the protection of the frontal facial nerve branch.

In general, skin flap length is dictated by the surgeon's experience and the individual patient. The risks of hematoma, skin flap ischemia, and facial nerve injury obviously increase in longer skin flaps. In patients who may be at risk for skin flap ischemia (ie, smokers), a shorter skin flap may be desirable. Meticulous hemostasis of the skin flap is made with bipolar electrocautery to prevent facial nerve injury. The use of a lighted retractor can help in visualizing bleeding sites, especially with longer skin flaps.

SUB-SMAS RHYTIDECTOMY

Techniques that address the SMAS-platysma complex have been shown to have more favorable long-term results compared with skin flap elevation alone. There are many described methods of dealing with the SMAS. Suture plication or the infolding of the SMAS allows for the placement of tension without the need to incise the SMAS, which places the facial nerve at a slightly greater risk of injury. However, the elevation of a SMAS flap may allow for a superior result with a skilled surgeon. The SMAS is incised in the preauricular and neck regions and elevated using blunt dissection. The limits of the flap are just below the zygomatic arch superiorly, the anterior border of the parotid gland anteriorly, and the angle of the mandible inferiorly (Figure 72–5). Facial nerve fibers may be visible and extreme care is taken to preserve them. After the excision of excess tissue, a nonabsorbable suture is used to suspend this flap in a posterosuperior direction to the mastoid periosteum and temporal fascia (Figure 72–6).

Deep-Plane & Composite Rhytidectomy

Deep-plane rhytidectomy attempts to address aging changes in the melolabial fold and malar area. According to advocates of this procedure, these areas are not directly addressed with simple SMAS-platysma suspension techniques. Composite rhytidectomy essentially extends the deep plane by including the orbicularis oculi muscle in the dissection. Essentially, a composite flap is created,

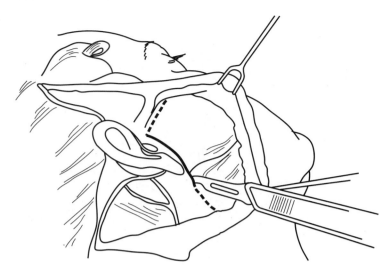

Figure 72–5. Incision of the SMAS.

which is preplatysmal in the neck, suborbicularis oculi in the malar regions, and sub-SMAS anterior to the cheek fat pad. Anteriorly, the investing fascia is released from the zygomaticus major muscle. The composite flap is then suspended in one unit (Figure 72–7). The added risk in this dissection relates to the facial nerve. More specifically, the zygomatic branch and facial nerve branches innervating the orbicularis oculi muscle are at risk of injury. With experience and a detailed anatomic knowledge of the facial nerve branches in this area, the surgeon may achieve an improved result with this technique.

Closure & Drains

The direction of suspension for the skin flap is posterior and superior. Making the majority of the closure tension free is critical. The points of maximal tension are in the temporal and occipital regions and key sutures are placed to suspend the skin flap. Following suspension, excess skin is trimmed so that the skin edges are reapproximated in a tension-free manner. This is especially important at the lobule to prevent the "pixie ear" deformity that occurs when this area is placed under undue tension. This problem can be avoided by incising the skin flap so that the lobule rests in a neutral position without tension directed inferiorly.

The pretragal area is carefully defatted, and a subcutaneous anchoring suture is placed to recreate the normal concave contour of this area. The preauricular and postauricular skin up to the hair-bearing skin is closed with interrupted or running sutures. The hair-bearing skin is closed with surgical clips. All wound edges are everted to minimize visible scarring.

Closed-suction drainage is placed through a separate stab incision in the hair-bearing skin. No studies show that drains actually help prevent hematomas. However, drains allow for the removal of residual fluid and help to keep the skin flap adherent to the underlying tissue. The use of tissue sealants that use fibrin, thrombin, or platelet-rich gel (or any combination of these substances) may obviate the need for drains.

POSTOPERATIVE CARE

The wounds are cleaned and antibiotic ointment is placed on the incisions. Bulky dressings are placed immediately after the procedure and help in keeping pressure

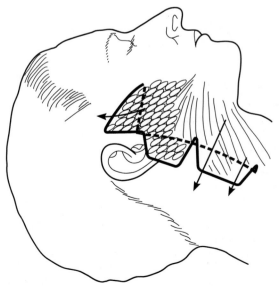

Figure 72–6. Suspension of the SMAS superiorly and posteriorly.

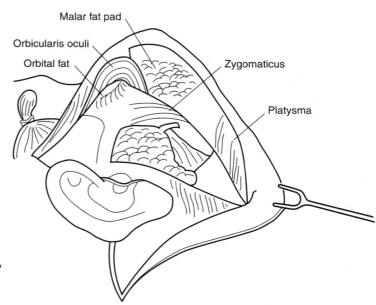

Figure 72–7. Composite rhytidectomy with dissection of the orbicularis oculi and zygomaticus muscles.

on the skin flap. The head of the bed is kept elevated, and patients are placed on limited bedrest. Blood pressure control with the patient's normal medication, along with the control of pain and nausea, are extremely important in the immediate postoperative period. Unilateral pain or pain unresponsive to medication needs an immediate evaluation for the possibility of a hematoma. The drains and bulky dressings are removed on the first postoperative day. Elastic bandages or a light dressing are subsequently placed for comfort and support.

Incisions are cleaned with half-strength hydrogen peroxide, and an antibiotic ointment is placed to keep the wounds moist and to encourage wound healing. Suture removal occurs on postoperative day 5 or 7, and surgical clips are removed on day 10. Patients are reassured that postoperative edema and ecchymosis will resolve.

COMPLICATIONS

Nerve Injury

The most commonly injured nerve in rhytidectomy is the greater auricular nerve, with a 6% rate of injury. The nerve is intimately associated with the sternocleidomastoid muscle and the overlying skin, and can be easily injured during skin flap elevation. If transected, the nerve is reapproximated with fine suture.

Facial nerve injury is relatively rare and has been reported to be 2.6% with subcutaneous techniques and up to 4.3% in sub-SMAS techniques. The buccal branch of the facial nerve is the most commonly injured in rhytidectomy. However, because of overlapping innerva-

tion in the upper lip, it is the least noticed. Because of the minimal overlap, the marginal and frontal branches are at the greatest risk for permanent and obvious paralysis.

Hematoma

Hematoma is the most common complication of rhytidectomy and has an occurrence rate of 1–8%. Men are twice as prone to developing hematoma secondary to the increased vascularity in the hair-bearing skin of the face. Hematoma is a worrisome complication because of the risk of epidermolysis and skin slough. Symptoms and signs of hematoma include an abrupt increase in pain, swelling, and ecchymosis, which are especially concerning if they are unilateral. Rapidly expanding hematomas necessitate a return to the operating room and the control of bleeding points. With prompt management, significant sequelae can usually be avoided. When hematomas are delayed or small, they can be managed with needle aspiration and pressure dressings. The incidence of hematoma can be minimized with careful intraoperative hemostasis, blood pressure control, and the cessation of NSAIDs.

Additional Complications

Other complications of rhytidectomy include scarring, a "pixie ear" deformity, an elevated temporal hairline, and skin slough. These can be prevented by careful incision placement and minimizing tension on the suture line. Infection is a relatively rare complication of rhytidectomy and is treated with antibiotic therapy.

Baker D. Rhytidectomy with lateral SMASectomy. *Facial Plast Surg.* 2000;16(3):209. [PMID: 11802569] (Review of the SMAS excision technique.)

Baker DC, Conley J. Avoiding facial nerve injuries in rhytidectomy. Anatomical variations and pitfalls. *Plast Reconstr Surg.* 1979;64(6):781. [PMID: 515227] (A classic review of facial nerve anatomy in the context of rhytidectomy.)

Brennan HG, Toft KM, Dunham BP, Goode RL, Koch RJ. Prevention and correction of temporal hair loss in rhytidectomy. *Plast Reconstr Surg.* 1999;104(7):2219. [PMID: 11149791] (Review of decision making in approaching the temporal hair tuft.)

Grover R, Jones BM, Waterhouse N. The prevention of haematoma following rhytidectomy: a review of 1078 consecutive facelifts. *Br J Plast Surg.* 2001;54(6):481. [PMID: 11513508] (Retrospective analysis of the risk factors for hematoma.)

Hamra ST. The deep-plane rhytidectomy. *Plast Reconstr Surg.* 1990;86(1):53. [PMID: 2359803] (Classic article first describing the deep-plane rhytidectomy.)

Hamra ST. Composite rhytidectomy. *Plast Reconstr Surg.* 1992; 90(1):1. [PMID: 1615067] (Classic article first describing the composite rhytidectomy.)

Kamer FM. One hundred consecutive deep plane face-lifts. *Arch Otolaryngol Head Neck Surg.* 1996;122(1):17. [PMID: 8554742] (Prospective study of the deep-plane rhytidectomy.)

Kamer FM, Frankel AS. SMAS rhytidectomy versus deep plane rhytidectomy: an objective comparison. *Plast Reconstr Surg.* 1998;102(3):878. [PMID: 9727459] (Retrospective review that favors the deep-plane rhytidectomy.)

Larrabee WF Jr, Henderson JL. Face lift: the anatomic basis for a safe, long-lasting procedure. *Facial Plast Surg.* 2000;16 (3):239. [PMID: 11802572] (Anatomic review and its implications in successful rhytidectomy.)

McCollough EG, Perkins SW, Langsdon PR. SMAS suspension rhytidectomy: rationale and long-term experience. *Arch Otolaryngol Head Neck Surg.* 1989;115(2):228. [PMID: 2643976] (A substantial retrospective review of the SMAS technique by an expert on rhytidectomy.)

Mitz V, Peyronie M. The superficial musculo-aponeurotic system (SMAS) in the parotid and cheek area. *Plast Reconstr Surg.* 1976;58(1):80. [PMID: 935283] (The classic article first describing the SMAS anatomically.)

Perkins SW, Williams JD, Macdonald K, Robinson EB. Prevention of seromas and hematomas after face-lift surgery with the use of postoperative vacuum drains. *Arch Otolaryngol Head Neck Surg.* 1997;123(7):743. [PMID: 9236595] (Retrospective review showing the effectiveness of drains in decreasing seroma and hematoma formation.)

Sherris DA, Larrabee WF Jr. Anatomic considerations in rhytidectomy. *Facial Plast Surg.* 1996;12(3):215. [PMID: 9243990] (Review article of relevant anatomy.)

BROWLIFT

Endoscopic Browlift

The endoscopic browlift is currently the most commonly performed procedure for rejuvenation of the brow. The ideal candidate is a female patient with a normal or low hairline, thin skin, and a flat forehead. The endoscopic browlift can be performed in either a subgaleal or subperiosteal plane. Releasing the periosteum of the arcus marginalis and the orbital ligament adequately mobilizes the brow and helps achieve a long-term result. The method of fixation of the brow varies with polylactic resorbable screws or bone tunnels. Some surgeons have achieved long-term brow elevation without the need for fixation. The endoscopic forehead lift has the advantage of minimal incision length and less risk of paresthesias.

Coronal Browlift/Tricophytic Browlift/Pretrichial Browlift

In a coronal browlift, the surgeon makes an incision within the hair-bearing scalp. The procedure leads to elevation of the hairline. The plane of dissection is in the subgaleal plane allowing access to the frontalis, corrugator, and procerus muscles. Coronal browlifting is contraindicated in patients with high hairlines or with male pattern baldness. In addition, paresthesias are common after this technique owing to resection of the deep branch of the supraorbital nerve.

In the trichophytic browlift, an incision is made within the fine hair of the anterior hairline. A reverse bevel allows for hair growth through the incision. A pretrichial variant places the scar in front of the hairline. Both approaches are effective in patients with high hairlines.

Midforehead Browlift/Direct Browlift

A midforehead browlift is made with an incision in a horizontal furrow in the forehead. A direct browlift is made by directly excising skin above a patient's brow. Typical candidates for both procedures include bald men with prominent forehead wrinkles and patients with a highly asymmetric brow (facial paralysis patients). Forehead wrinkles and corrugator hyperactivity are not addressed with this technique.

MIDFACE LIFT

Midface lifts are techniques designed to specifically address the malar fat pad. A variety of approaches can be used including temporal (via an endoscope) with or without buccal release, and transconjunctival. A suture or polylactic acid device engages the malar fat pad and lifts it in a posterior superior direction, effacing the nasolabial fold. The suture is then fixed to deep temporal fascia. If a transconjunctival approach is used, fixation can occur by drilling a polylactic acid screw within the anterior face of the maxilla. When the nasolabial fold is lifted superiorly, excess skin bunches along the lower lash line. Typically, the excess skin is resected in a conservative fashion.

Patients who are candidates are generally younger patients who have isolated aging in the midface without prominent jowls or signs of aging present in the neck.

Complications

The most common complications of forehead lifting are residual brow asymmetry, hematoma, paresthesias, and temporary paresis of the temporal branch of the facial nerve. Permanent paralysis of the temporal branch is rare. Poor scarring can result with excessive tension on surgical wounds or cauterization of hair follicles. Alopecia can be minimized with limited cautery and atraumatic tissue handling.

Midface lift patients may experience prolonged swelling due to disruption of lymphatics of the midface. Eye shape may change to appear cat-like, but this usually resolves with time. Preservation of a cuff of periosteum along the lateral orbit minimizes this complication. Excessive skin excision may lead to ectropion, especially if the midface returns to its preoperative level.

Cook TA, Brownrigg PJ, Wang TD, Quatela VC. The versatile midforehead browlift. *Arch Otolaryngol Head Neck Surg.* 1989;115(2):163.

Knize DM. A study of the supraorbital nerve. *Plast Reconstr Surg.* 1995;96(3):564.

Schmidt BL, Pogrel MA, Hakim-Faal Z. The course of the temporal branch of the facial nerve in the periorbital region. *J Oral Maxillofac Surg.* 2001;59(2):178.

Sykes JM. Surgical rejuvenation of the brow and forehead. *Facial Plast Surg.* 1999;15(3):183.

Trinei FA, Januszkiewicz J, Nahai F. The sentinel vein: an important reference point for surgery in the temporal region. *Plast Reconstr Surg.* 1998;101(1):27.

Blepharoplasty

Eugene J. Kim, MD, Minas Constantinides, MD, & Corey S. Maas, MD

ANATOMY

Eyelid Surface

Eyelid skin is the thinnest in the body with relatively sparse subcutaneous fat. This allows free movement of the lid in closure and blinking. The upper eyelid skin is thinner than the skin in the lower lid. The skin itself has many fine hairs as well as sebaceous and sweat glands. Healing occurs quickly in this area and scarring is usually minute.

The lid crease of the upper eyelid is formed by the insertion of the levator aponeurosis fibers into the skin and the orbicularis oculi muscle. It is approximately 8–12 mm superior to the lash line and lies just at the level of the upper edge of the tarsal plate. Medially and laterally, the crease is closer to the lid margin and has an arc shape across the lid. The Asian eye usually lacks this crease owing to the lower insertion of the levator aponeurosis on the tarsus, often with interposed fat.

The lid fold describes the tissue above the lid crease and may extend throughout the length of the upper lid or it may be more localized. Excess tissue may develop in the aging face and sag over the lid crease, sometimes obscuring vision. A combination of excess skin, hypertrophied orbicularis oculi muscle, and herniated fat can be responsible for this blepharochalasis. Often, the overhang is exacerbated by the concomitant descent of the lateral eyebrow with aging.

Orbicularis Oculi Muscle

The orbicularis oculi muscle provides the main mimetic function to the eyelid. It receives its innervation from the temporal and zygomatic branches of the facial nerve. The muscle is elliptical and divided into three bands (the pretarsal, preseptal, and preorbital), which attach to the bony orbit at the medial and lateral canthal tendons. The muscle can become hypertrophied over time and result in a full appearance of the eyelids.

Orbital Fat

Orbital fat cushions the globe and its associated structures, and its anterior limit is the orbital septum. In the upper eyelid, the fat separates the levator aponeurosis posteriorly and the orbital septum anteriorly. Here it is divided into two fat compartments: central and medial. In the lower lid, there are three fat compartments: lateral, central, and medial (Figure 73–1).

LEVATOR PALPEBRAE SUPERIORIS MUSCLE

The levator muscle acts to elevate the upper eyelid and has its origin in the periorbita posteriorly. The muscle runs above the superior rectus and fans out anteriorly to become the levator aponeurosis. Insertion occurs at the level of the tarsus, as previously described, forming the lid crease (Figure 73–2). Its innervation is by cranial nerve III (the oculomotor nerve).

Tarsal Plate

The tarsi are composed of fibrous tissue and provide the general shape and firmness to the eyelids. The upper and lower tarsi measure approximately 10 mm and 5 mm in height, respectively. Many meibomian glands are present in both tarsi and open into the ciliary margin.

Conjunctiva

This mucous membrane is attached to the tarsal plate and covers the tarsus and Müller muscle. Because of its firm tarsal attachment, the conjunctiva does not have to be sutured after incision. The gray line marks the border between the conjunctiva and skin. Histologically, there is columnar epithelium posteriorly and stratified squamous epithelium anteriorly. This landmark is frequently used in eyelid surgery.

PREOPERATIVE ASSESSMENT

A thorough history and physical examination, especially an ophthalmologic history, should be performed on every patient. Important historical points include a recent change in vision, significant differences in visual acuity between the eyes, any history of trauma or previous eyelid or facial surgery, and the presence of cheek implants. Dry eye syndrome can be particularly troublesome postoperatively, and the history is often the best way to elicit it. Sensitivity to wind outdoors, excessive burning or tearing, or a

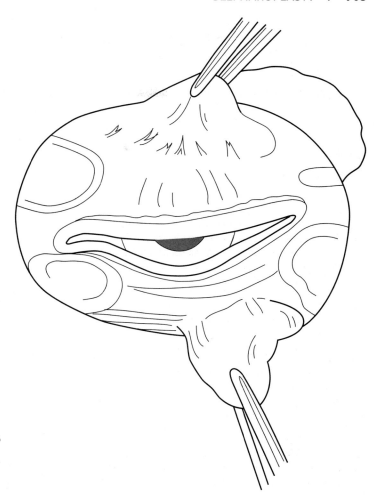

Figure 73–1. The orbital fat is divided into the upper medial and central compartments, and the lower medial, central, and lateral compartments.

history of a corneal abrasion are important clues. Schirmer testing will help screen patients who are prone to dry eye syndrome. Any significant visual problem is best fully documented by an ophthalmologist preoperatively.

On the examination, the snap test allows for the determination of the laxity of the lower lid skin. The lower lid is pulled away from the globe and its snap back to the normal position is observed. If the lid is slow to snap back, lower lid laxity is a concern and the patient may be at risk for postoperative ectropion. A full-thickness shortening of the horizontal lid can help prevent this complication at the time of blepharoplasty.

Close attention to any degree of scleral show should be made; scleral show occurs when the lid margin does not reach the cornea. However, more subtle lateral rounding of the lower lid can also be a warning sign of marginal lid strength. Eyelid-tightening procedures, in particular when a skin-muscle approach is used, are essential in these patients to prevent ectropion. Asymmetries should be documented and discussed with the patient. Patients with proptosis are poor candidates for blepharoplasty because of the risk of lagophthalmos and ectropion. In addition, blepharoplasty in patients found to have dry eye should be done very conservatively.

Aspirin should be discontinued at least 2 weeks before and after surgery to decrease the risk of bleeding. Preoperative photography is mandatory and involves the frontal view with eyes open, closed, and in upward gaze; a lateral view should also be taken. These photographs are reviewed with the patient and realistic goals and limitations are discussed.

ANESTHESIA

Local anesthesia with or without intravenous sedation is usually perfectly adequate for blepharoplasty. Injection

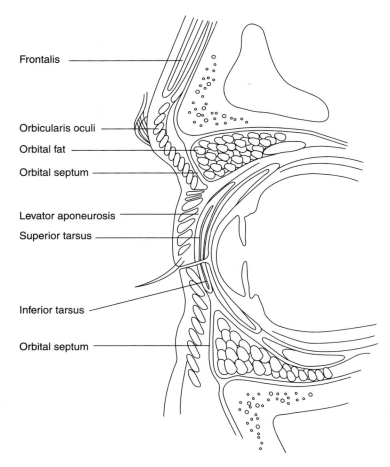

Frontalis

Orbicularis oculi

Orbital fat

Orbital septum

Levator aponeurosis

Superior tarsus

Inferior tarsus

Orbital septum

Figure 73–2. Coronal view of the orbit and its structures.

with 1% lidocaine with 1:100,000 epinephrine is made in the surgical field just underneath the skin surface and superficial to the orbital septum.

UPPER BLEPHAROPLASTY

The skin incision in upper blepharoplasty should follow the natural lid crease. This is measured approximately 8–12 mm above the ciliary margin along the upper edge of the tarsal plate. Laterally, the incision is carried toward the orbital rim and curves slightly superiorly. The exact extent is determined by the amount of excess tissue in that area. Medially, the incision extends to an area above the level of the medial canthus and never onto the nasal skin.

The superior skin incision is determined by the amount of skin to be excised. One method to determine this is by grasping the excess skin with forceps. Another method involves incising the lid crease only and then redraping the lid skin downward. This allows just enough skin to be excised. A simple elliptical skin

excision may also need to be modified both laterally and medially by a Z-plasty or M-plasty closure.

The orbicularis oculi can be addressed following the skin excision or excised with the skin flap (Figure 73–3). Some surgeons advocate the excision of muscle varying from 2 mm in width to a width just 2 mm short of the skin excision. Regardless, care should be taken when tenting the muscle as the septum and levator can be accidentally cut. Hemostasis is obtained with the use of bipolar electrocautery.

Fat excision addresses the process of herniation. The orbital septum is carefully opened above the insertion of the levator aponeurosis. Gentle pressure on the globe can help identify the location of the relevant fat compartments prior to incision. The central and medial fat pads herniate with globe pressure. They are excised anterior to the septum and meticulous attention is made to hemostasis (Figure 73–4). The central compartment may appear darker in color than the medial compartment. Care should be taken to avoid excessive resection of fat because it can create a hollowed-eye look.

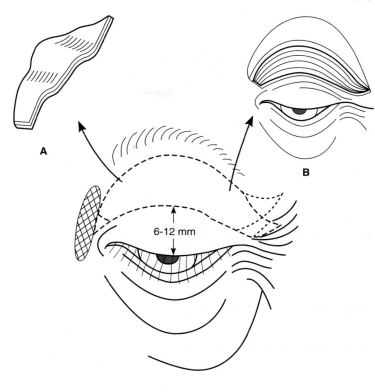

Figure 73–3. The extent of excision in upper blepharoplasty is demonstrated by the dotted line. **(A)** Skin and muscle are excised as one unit. **(B)** Skin is elevated first, followed by muscle excision.

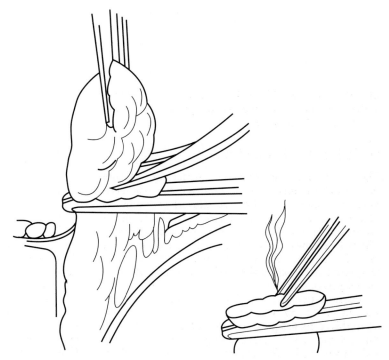

Figure 73–4. Orbital fat is delivered and then carefully excised with the use of cautery.

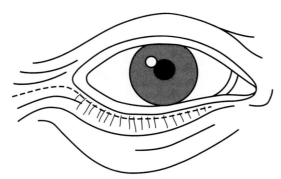

Figure 73–5. Lower blepharoplasty incision.

The incision is then closed initially via the principle of halves using a 6-0 nylon suture. It is completed with a 6-0 fast-absorbing gut suture in a running fashion.

LOWER BLEPHAROPLASTY

Lower blepharoplasty can be approached via several techniques, including a skin flap, a skin-muscle flap, and a transconjunctival technique.

Skin Flap

The use of the skin flap technique is most appropriate in patients who have a significant excess of loose skin but evidence of good orbicularis oculi muscle tone. A subciliary incision is made just inferior to the lash line. Medially, it extends to the punctum and laterally to the canthus with a slight curve inferiorly (Figure 73–5). The plane of dissection is between the skin and the orbicularis muscle down to the level of the orbital rim. Gentle globe pressure then allows localization of areas of fat herniation. The muscle and septum are incised and the fat delivered and excised from all three compartments. Meticulous hemostasis is achieved. The skin flap is then retracted superiorly and laterally. A thin strip of hypertrophied orbicularis muscle may need excision at this point, followed by closure of the muscle edges. Finally, the skin flap is trimmed underneath the lid margin, taking exquisite care not to place any tension on this area. The patient must open his or her mouth and look upward to ensure that excessive skin is not removed (Figure 73–6). A combination of interrupted and running sutures can then be used to close the incision.

Skin-Muscle Flap

The skin-muscle flap is developed in a plane between the orbital septum and the orbicularis muscle and is easier to develop than the skin flap. The incision is made as in the skin flap approach, and dissection is carried through the orbicularis muscle and directed inferiorly toward the orbital rim. From there, the fat excision proceeds in the same fashion as with the skin flap. Excess skin and muscle are also trimmed in the same manner.

Transconjunctival Blepharoplasty

Transconjunctival blepharoplasty does not directly address the lid skin but, rather, only the orbital fat. However, advocates of this approach argue that the main problem is fat herniation rather than excess skin. By remaining postseptal, the orbital septum and muscle are left intact, which decreases the chance of lid retraction. In addition, external scarring is avoided. However, some surgeons believe that this approach is more likely to result in inadequate fat removal secondary to more limited exposure.

In performing a transconjunctival blepharoplasty, the conjunctiva is first anesthetized with topical tetracaine, followed by a direct injection of lidocaine with epinephrine. The globe is protected with a shield during the procedure. The technique itself uses an incision in the lower sulcus of the conjunctiva near the orbital rim (Figure 73–7). This can be made with electrocautery, and the fat is encountered after the lower eyelid retractors are incised. Gentle pressure delivers the fat, and it is excised and cauterized in the usual fashion

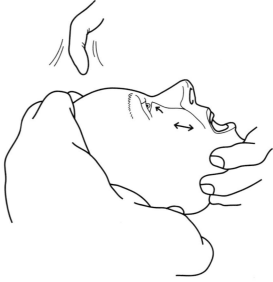

Figure 73–6. An open mouth and upward gaze allows for the precise excision of lower lid skin.

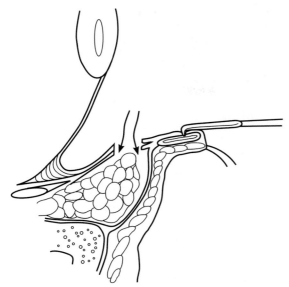

Figure 73–7. Transconjunctival incision below the lower tarsus.

(Figure 73–8). As stated before, the incision does not need to be sutured closed secondary to the tight adherence of the conjunctiva to the tarsal plate. If there is some mild redundant skin, some surgeons advocate the use of a CO_2 laser to tighten the skin in conjunction with the transconjunctival blepharoplasty. The "pinch" technique, in which excess skin is pinched up with a forcep and sharply excised with a sharp scissor, is also effective. Other resurfacing techniques including chemical peels can be performed after recovery is complete.

Fat Transposition Lower Blepharoplasty

One limitation of standard blepharoplasty techniques is their poor ability to improve the hollow created between the prolapsed lower eyelid fat and the infraorbital rim. This hollow anatomically correlates with the arcuate line, where the orbital septum merges with the periosteum of the face of the maxilla. Classic blepharoplasties are excellent at removing excess fat. However, when fat is removed in youth, the eye can become cadaverically hollow with age without sufficient fat volume. Fat preservation techniques, in which fat is transposed rather than removed, address this esthetic concern.

Fat transposition blepharoplasty is performed either using a skin-muscle or transconjunctival approach. The orbital septum is cut at the arcuate line, and orbital fat is freed of attachments while preserving its blood supply. This pedicled fat is then transposed over the orbital rim, resulting in a smooth, full, youthful eyelid. The fat may either be sutured into its new position to the maxillary periosteum (skin-muscle approach), to the overlying skin (transconjunctival approach), or simply allowed

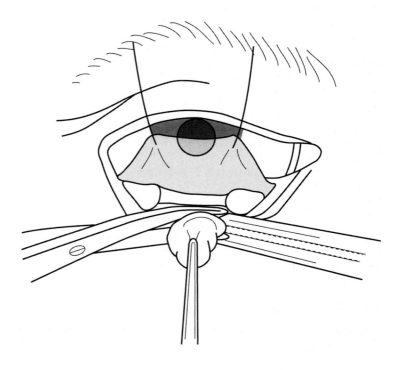

Figure 73–8. The excision of orbital fat in the transconjunctival approach.

to lie in the space created as long as the pedicle has been dissected adequately and there is no tension to retract the fat back into the orbit (transconjunctival approach).

POSTOPERATIVE CARE

Antibiotic ointment is applied to the incisions. Ice packs or cool compresses are applied to decrease edema and ecchymosis. Pressure dressings are not necessary because they hinder the ability to assess the presence of bleeding or vision changes. Pain is usually minimal and many patients may require no medication at all. Instructions are given to return immediately if there is an onset of pain, bleeding, or visual disturbance. Patients are again reminded to refrain from aspirin or nonsteroidal anti-inflammatory drug use. Sutures are removed in 3 or 4 days.

COMPLICATIONS

Loss of Vision

Isolated visual loss is the most serious complication of blepharoplasty and is fortunately a rare occurrence, with a reported rate of 0.04%. In the absence of intraorbital hemorrhage, the exact mechanism is unclear.

Retrobulbar hemorrhage is a surgical emergency. This increases the intraocular pressure and causes an ischemic optic neuropathy, the occlusion of the central retinal artery, or both. The onset of bleeding may often be related to postoperative vomiting or coughing. Clinically, the patient has a rapid onset of pain and proptosis with associated eyelid ecchymosis. Return to the operating room is mandated with clot evacuation and control of any bleeding sites. Lateral canthotomy may also be necessary for immediate decompression. With a visual loss, the intravenous administration of mannitol and steroids is recommended to decrease intraocular pressure. A consultation with an ophthalmologist should also be made.

Lower Eyelid Malposition & Ectropion

Lower eyelid malposition is the most common complication of lower blepharoplasty. It occurs after excessive skin removal or other weakening maneuver on the lower lid. Mild malposition preferentially occurs laterally, resulting in inferior bowing of the lateral lid, called "rounding." More severe cases result in scleral show, and the most severe is ectropion, in which the palpebral conjunctiva no longer touches the bulbar conjunctiva and is visible as the eyelid separates completely from the globe. It usually requires surgical correction either with horizontal lid shortening, muscle suspension, or full-thickness skin grafting.

Milia

The development of milia is the most common complication of upper blepharoplasty. These arise from trapped epithelium within the epidermis, often at the suture line. This problem can easily be addressed by "unroofing" the lesions with a needle in the office.

Lagophthalmos

In the initial postoperative period, lagophthalmos is present in many patients secondary to lid edema. It may be permanent in patients with excessive skin resection or scarring. If lubrication, massage, and taping of the lid fail to correct the problem, surgical correction is necessary with a full-thickness skin graft.

Additional Complications

Some other complications of blepharoplasty are scleral show, lid asymmetry, ptosis, corneal injury, and dry eye. The incidence of all these complications can be minimized with careful surgical attention, a preoperative screening, and a detailed anatomic knowledge.

Becker DG, Kim S, Kallman JE. Aesthetic implications of surgical anatomy in blepharoplasty. *Facial Plast Surg*. 1999;15(3):165. [PMID: 11816079] (Review of orbital anatomy with attention to pathologic changes.)

Castanares S. Anatomy for a blepharoplasty. *Plast Reconstr Surg*. 1974;53(5):587. [PMID: 4821211] (Classic anatomic description of orbital anatomy.)

Castro E, Foster JA. Upper lid blepharoplasty. *Facial Plast Surg*. 1999;15(3):173. [PMID: 11816080] (A comprehensive review of indications and techniques in upper-lid blepharoplasty.)

Gausas RE. Complications of blepharoplasty. *Facial Plast Surg*. 1999;15(3):243. [PMID: 11816087] (A good review and summary of complications and their management.)

Jacono AA, Moskowitz B. Transconjunctival versus transcutaneous approach in upper and lower blepharoplasty. *Facial Plast Surg*. 2001;17(1):21. [PMID: 11518974] (Comparison of these techniques and also adjunctive procedures with the transconjunctival approach.)

Jelks GW, Jelks EB. Preoperative evaluation of the blepharoplasty patient. Bypassing the pitfalls. *Clin Plast Surg*. 1993;20(2):213. [PMID: 8485931] (Classic article by one of the masters of preoperative assessment.)

Kikkawa DO, Kim JW. Asian blepharoplasty. *Int Ophthalmol Clin*. 1997;37(3):193. [PMID: 9279651] (Review of techniques and anatomy unique to the Asian patient.)

Mahaffey PJ, Wallace AF. Blindness following cosmetic blepharoplasty—a review. *Br J Plast Surg*. 1986;39(2):213. [PMID: 3516289] (Review of this devastating complication and the appropriate management of the underlying causes.)

McKinney P, Byun M. The value of tear film breakup and Schirmer's tests in preoperative blepharoplasty evaluation. *Plast Reconstr Surg*. 1999;104(2):566. [PMID: 10654706] (Emphasizes the role of other preoperative tests over Schirmer testing.)

Perkins SW, Dyer WK 2nd, Simo F. Transconjunctival approach to lower eyelid blepharoplasty. Experience, indications, and technique in 300 patients. *Arch Otolaryngol Head Neck Surg.* 1994;120(2):172. [PMID: 8297575] (A substantial retrospective review of this approach with attention to technique.)

Triana RJ Jr, Larrabee WF Jr. Lower eyelid blepharoplasty: the aging eyelid. *Facial Plast Surg.* 1999;15(3):203. [PMID: 11816083] (Discussion of the aging changes in the lower lid and techniques to address them.)

Wolfort FG, Vaughan TE, Wolfort SF, Nevarre DR. Retrobulbar hematoma and blepharoplasty. *Plast Reconstr Surg.* 1999; 104(7):2154. [PMID: 11149784] (An excellent review of the pathogenesis of retrobulbar hematoma and a management algorithm.)

Zarem HA, Resnick JI. Operative technique for transconjunctival lower blepharoplasty. *Clin Plast Surg.* 1992;19(2):351. [PMID: 1576780] (A classic paper describing the modern technique for transconjunctival blepharoplasty.)

Rhinoplasty

Alexander L. Ramirez, MD, Corey S. Maas, MD, & Minas Constantinides, MD

 ESSENTIALS OF DIAGNOSIS

- *Length, projection, and rotation of the nose are three parameters essential to preoperative planning.*
- *Lower lateral cartilage strength and its attachments to the caudal septum and upper lateral cartilage are the three major tip support structures.*
- *The tripod principle may be used to determine what maneuvers intraoperatively will result in the desired tip position postoperatively.*
- *Photographic documentation must be consistent to enable analysis of the postoperative result.*
- *Approaches in rhinoplasty may be open or closed, depending on the complexity of the surgery and surgeon preferences.*

ANATOMY

The nasal skeleton can be divided into thirds (Figure 74–1): (1) the upper compartment (bony vault), (2) the middle compartment (upper cartilaginous vault), and (3) the lower compartment (lower cartilaginous vault). The upper third is bone; the lower two thirds are cartilage.

Bony Vault

The bony vault is made up of the nasal bones and the nasal processes of the maxilla. They join to form a convex bony arch that provides stability to the nose. The nasal bones are widest at the nasofrontal suture, become narrowest at the nasofrontal groove, and then become wide again at the rhinion. The dorsal border of the septum fuses with the caudal end of the nasal bones so that the septum acts like a rigid and fixed beam on which the cartilaginous structures are suspended.

The nasion refers to the nasofrontal suture, where the nasal bones fuse with the frontal process. The rhinion is where the caudal border of the nasal bones meets the upper lateral cartilages. The upper lateral cartilages are not only juxtaposed to the nasal bones here, but there is actual overlap among them. This area is referred to as the "keystone" or "K" area. There is up to 11 mm of overlap in the midline.

Unlike the nasion and rhinion, which correspond to exact anatomic landmarks, the radix or the root of the nose refers to a general location. On frontal view, the radix is formed as the space between two gently curving continuous lines from the superior orbital rims to the lateral nasal walls (Figure 74–2). On profile, it is the lowest portion of the nasal dorsum, correlating to the nasofrontal groove or angle (Figure 74–3).

Upper Cartilaginous Vault

The upper cartilaginous vault comprises the upper lateral cartilages. The cephalic border is relatively immobile because of the fusion of the upper lateral cartilages to the fixed quadrangular cartilage of the septum and the overlap with bone at the keystone area. Laterally, the upper lateral cartilages are fused to the pyriform aperture by dense fibroareolar tissue and are attached to the alar cartilages caudally. The caudal edge of the upper lateral cartilage curves in the same direction as the overlapping cephalic edge of the alar cartilage, creating the scroll. In many ways, the bony pyramid and the upper lateral cartilage act as a single osseocartilaginous unit.

In contrast, the caudal border of the upper lateral cartilage is mobile. The thickened caudal border of the upper lateral cartilage acts as the internal nasal valve and moves with the respiratory cycle in a paradoxical fashion. With inspiration, the respiratory muscles create negative pressure within the entire upper respiratory tract. This causes the internal nasal valve to narrow and increases air resistance and modifies currents to maximize exposure to nasal mucosa. At the same time in the lower cartilaginous vault, the nostrils flare, increasing the diameter of the external nasal valve.

Lower Cartilaginous Vault

The lower lateral cartilages or alar cartilages are responsible for the support and configuration of lower third of the nose. The lower third is mobile and animate. The alar car-

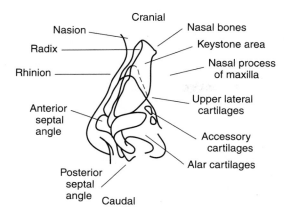

Figure 74–1. Nasal skeleton.

tilages are almost free floating, only loosely connected by fibroareolar and muscular attachments to the septum. They are connected laterally to the sesamoid (accessory) cartilages, the pyriform aperture, and to the upper lateral cartilages. The alar cartilages are divided into three continuous segments called crura (Figure 74–4).

The medial crura form the shape of the columella and the nostril medially. They run along the caudal septum to the apex of the nostril and diverge anteriorly. The most posterior portion, called the medial crural footplates, extends toward but not to the nasal spine. These footplates are short, face outward, and flare variably later-

ally. They do, however, tightly sandwich the caudal septum, a relationship that is important for tip support.

The intermediate or middle crura form the bridge between the medial and lateral crura. The point at which the medial crura diverge is most commonly considered the start of the intermediate crura. This bend in the alar cartilage is called the point of divergence or the medial genu. The angle created between the intermediate crura is defined as the angle of divergence and typically measures 50° to 60°. Angles greater than this tend to create a boxy or bifid nasal tip.

The apex of the alar cartilages is called the dome, lateral genu, or tip-defining point. This is the area where the intermediate crura merge with the lateral crura. The domes are connected to the anterior septal angle by dense connective tissue called the interdomal ligament. The lateral crura then extend laterally but do not parallel the entire rim of the nostril. Initially, the lateral crura follow the curvature of the nostril to the apex of the nostril opening, but then they turn obliquely superior and laterally to the pyriform aperture. While paralleling the alar margins, the lateral crura are outwardly convex, but as they curve superiorly, they flatten. It is the soft tissue of the lobules that create the shape of the nostrils—not the alar cartilages.

The three major factors in nasal tip support all relate to the alar cartilages. They include (1) the integrity and strength of the alar cartilage itself, (2) its attachment to the caudal septum, and (3) its attach-

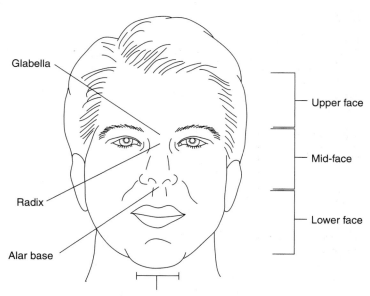

Figure 74–2. Facial proportions (frontal view).

Alar base width = intercanthal distance

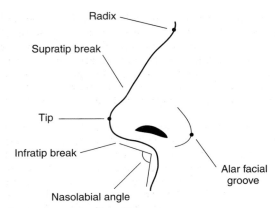

Figure 74–3. Nasal profile.

ment to the upper lateral cartilage. Overzealous resection of alar cartilage can lead to many pitfalls, including the loss of tip support, vestibular stenosis, and alar retraction secondary to scar contracture. The lower third of the nose is also called the tip-lobule complex or the base of the nose.

FACIAL EVALUATION

The concept of facial aesthetics and beauty is highly subjective. However, an understanding of aesthetic facial proportions serves as a guide when evaluating patients. It helps with interpreting surgical goals and concerns, and it improves the surgeon's ability to correct deformities. These evaluative aspects are not consistent for all patients, but are an approximation of ideals.

Frontal View

In the frontal view, the face may be divided into thirds, using the glabella and the base of the alae as points of division (see Figure 74–2). The base of the nose should be equal in width to the intercanthal distance. In the basal view, the alar base should approximate an isosceles triangle (see Figure 74–4). The distance from the base of the ala to the apex of the nostril should be two thirds of the distance from the base of the ala to the tip of the nose. The beginning of the flare of the medial crural footplates should divide the alar bases into equal halves.

The brow-tip esthetic line is a useful concept in evaluating how well a nose approaches the esthetic ideal. A gently sweeping line from medial eyebrow to nasal tip should be elegant, unbroken by deviations, and symmetric from side to side. Deviations of the upper third, middle third, or lower third of the nose disrupt the brow-tip esthetic and signal deformities that may require correction.

Profile View

In the profile view, the length of the nose is defined as the point from the radix to the tip (see Figure 74–3). It should be approximately two thirds of the midfacial height. The radix's horizontal height should approach the level of the upper eyelashes in women and may be somewhat lower in men. The anterior projection of the radix can dramatically affect the overall length of the nose. A deep radix can create the illusion of a dorsal hump or make a small hump look much larger. Ideally, the nasofrontal angle should be between 115° and 130°. A shallow nasofrontal angle in the presence of a dorsal hump may create too straight a line between forehead and dorsum once the hump is removed. An aesthetically pleasing profile has two breaks or bends in the lines that make up the silhouette. First, immediately above the tip, there should be a mild depression called the supratip break. Below the tip, there is another bend called the infratip break or the columellar double break. This break marks the junction between the medial crura and the intermediate crura.

Nasal-Tip Projection

The nasal-tip projection is measured from the alar facial groove to the tip. It is appropriate at 50–60% of the nasal length. If it is greater than this value, then the nose is overprojected. If it is less than this value, it is underprojected. These estimations are helpful in the clinical setting because one can easily be fooled by a cursory examination of the face. A nose may appear overprojected when the chin is retrognathic, or it may appear underprojected when there is a large dorsal hump. On profile, the columella should parallel the long axis of the nostril; the nasolabial angle should be 90–95° in men and 90–110° in women. If the

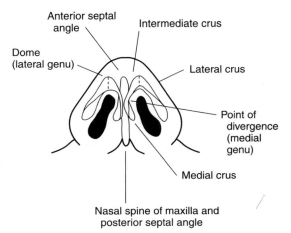

Figure 74–4. Nasal base and alar cartilages.

angle is greater than expected, then the tip is overrotated or vice versa (caudally rotated). However, a prominent nasal spine or caudal septum may create an obtuse nasolabial angle without actually indicating an overrotated tip. Similarly, a deficient premaxilla or posterior septal angle may create an acute nasolabial angle, again without accounting for tip position. Rotation is best judged by looking at the position of the dome with respect to the alar crease, and its relative angle of rotation from the horizontal. However, a prominent nasal spine or caudal septum may create an obtuse nasolabial angle without actually indicating an overrotated tip. Similarly, a deficient premaxilla or posterior septal angle may create an acute nasolabial angle, again without accounting for tip position. Rotation is best judged by looking at the position of the dome with respect to the alar crease, and its relative angle of rotation from the horizontal.

Columellar show, or the distance from the caudal edge of the ala to the cephalic edge of the columella, is ideally between 3 and 4 mm. Excess columellar show may be due to alar retraction, columellar ptosis, or both. In analyzing the amount of show, a line should be drawn on lateral view from the apex to the base of the nostril. If the amount of show is primarily above the line, then alar retraction is the cause of the show. Conversely, if it is below the line, then columellar ptosis is at fault.

The composition of the skin–soft tissue envelope is a critical component of understanding the lower third of the nose. If this layer is thick and sebaceous, it lacks the ability to drape softly over the nasal skeleton. It creates tip definition because of the inherent memory or integrity of skin–soft tissue envelope itself and not from the cartilage. Thick skin may also overburden weakened cartilage, leading to collapse. In contrast, thin skin allows the impressions of the underlying structures to be more prominent.

Byrd HS, Hobar PC. Rhinoplasty: a practical guide for surgical planning. *Plast Reconstr Surg.* 1993;91(4):642. [PMID: 8446718] (Classic article on objective analysis of the face and nose.)

Daniel RK. The nasal tip: anatomy and aesthetics. *Plast Reconstr Surg.* 1992;89(2);216. [PMID: 1732887] (A master of rhinoplasty gives the classic description of the anatomy of the lower lateral cartilages.)

Tardy ME Jr, Dayan S, Hecht D. Preoperative rhinoplasty: evaluation and analysis. *Otolaryngol Clin North Am.* 2002;35(1):1. [PMID: 11781205] (A master of rhinoplasty reviews evaluation and aesthetics.)

Toriumi DM, Mueller RA, Grosch T, Bhattacharyya TK, Larrabee WF Jr. Vascular anatomy of the nose and the external rhinoplasty approach. *Arch Otolaryngol Head Neck Surg.* 1996;122 (1):24. [PMID: 8554743] (Classic article on vascular anatomy and planes of dissections for rhinoplasty.)

Photographic Documentation

Photographs are essential for the evaluation, diagnosis, and surgical planning of every patient. The appearance of the nose is a subtle interplay between concave and convex surfaces, between areas of light and areas of shadow. Poor photography can hide imperfections or conceal deformities from both surgeon and patient. The basic principles of photography apply. All photographs should be performed in a standardized format that allows precise comparison of views before and after surgery.

Photographs should be taken with a solid background, such as medium blue, because this provides contrast but does not obscure facial features. It is important to take pictures at the subject's eye level and to keep the Frankfort horizontal line parallel with the ground. The Frankfort line is an imaginary line from the top of the tragus to the infraorbital rim.

Six views should be obtained because each allows a unique analysis. The frontal view is useful to evaluate the root and base of the nose for any deviations, asymmetries, and curvatures. Bilateral three-quarter views are useful to analyze the alar cartilages and the tip-lobule complex. Bilateral lateral views allow for the evaluation of tip projection and rotation, the length of the nose, and the symmetry of the nostrils and columella. In addition, any disruption of the silhouette of the nose, such as dorsal humps or the absence of supra- or infratip breaks, can be evaluated. Finally, a basal view allows for an evaluation of columellar length, tip projection, base width, nostril notching, deviations, and asymmetries.

Becker DG, Tardy ME Jr. Standardized photography in facial plastic surgery: pearls and pitfalls. *Facial Plastic Surg.* 1999;15(2):93. [PMID: 11816129] (Review of techniques, equipment, and pitfalls.)

ANESTHESIA

Indications

The choice for general anesthesia versus local anesthesia with monitored anesthesia care is largely a decision based on a discussion with the patient, the surgeon's personal experience, and the anesthesia staff. Regardless of choice, local anesthesia should be administered to improve surgical hemostasis, to aid in patient analgesia, and to aid in atraumatic dissection by infiltration into favorable and appropriate tissue planes. The injection should be in the supraperichondrial or subcutaneous musculoaponeurotic plane because this aids in evaluating the skin–soft tissue envelope in the appropriate plane. Overzealous injection should be avoided because this leads to a distortion of anatomy. Regional field blocks of the supratrochlear, infraorbital, and nasopalatine nerves also can improve patient analgesia (in the case of local anesthesia with intravenous sedation) and hemostasis.

Preoperative Considerations

Anesthesia for rhinoplasty begins with topical decongestion with topical phenylephrine (eg, Neo-Synephrine), oxymetazoline, or cocaine at least 15 minutes before surgery to achieve adequate nasal vasoconstriction. Four milliliters of 4% cocaine (160 mg) is below the toxic dose of 3 mg/kg in most adult patients.

Liao BS, Hilsinger RL Jr, Rasgon BM, Matsuoka K, Ardour KK. A preliminary study of cocaine absorption from the nasal mucosa. *Laryngoscope.* 1999;109(1):98. [PMID: 9917048] (Objective analysis of systemic absorption of cocaine through the nasal mucosa.)

Intraoperative Considerations

A 1:100,000 mixture of 1% lidocaine with epinephrine is then injected using a control syringe with a 1.5-inch 27-gauge needle. Each side of the nasal septum is injected, beginning posteriorly and inferiorly. These injections blanch and elevate the mucoperichondrium. Next, the lateral nasal walls should be injected via an intercartilaginous approach, staying close to the nasal bones and injecting as the needle is withdrawn. There is essentially no injection along the dorsum.

The pyriform aperture and the infraorbital foramen are infiltrated. The needle is then inserted through the vestibule toward the alar-facial groove to inject the angular artery. An injection is also placed at the base of the columella toward the nasal spine to control the columellar branch of the facial artery. The tip is finally injected via the vestibule, anterior to the alar cartilage and into the dome, with placement confirmed by blanching. Typically, only 10 mL of a local anesthetic is necessary to inject these sites.

SURGICAL TECHNIQUES

The decision to proceed with an external (open) or endonasal (closed) approach is based on the surgeon's preference and experience.

Endonasal Approach

The endonasal or closed approach includes multiple routes of access (Figure 74–5). The cartilage-delivery method is an example of a closed approach that combines multiple endonasal incisions. In this approach, intercartilaginous incisions are combined with marginal incisions to allow for either externalization or delivery of the lateral crura. This allows for an enhanced visualization of the cartilage, an improved ability to manipulate the domes under direct vision, and better postoperative symmetry. Other examples of closed approaches to the tip include the transcartilaginous approach and the retrograde approach. In the transcartilaginous approach, a predetermined amount of lateral

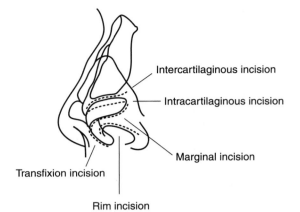

Figure 74–5. Incisions for endonasal approaches.

crus is incised through the vestibular mucosa directly and removed. In the retrograde approach, no marginal incision is made. The lateral crural excision is performed after a retrograde dissection from the intercartilaginous incision. The major benefits of the closed approaches are less dissection leading to less edema and faster healing, and the absence of a transcolumellar incision. The endonasal approach is used by many surgeons primarily when nasal tip morphology is normal. The major benefit is less dissection, leading to faster healing.

External Approach

The external or open approach involves bilateral marginal incisions that are connected in the midline by a transcolumellar skin incision, usually in the shape of an inverted "V." The main difference between an open and closed approach is that the open approach allows exposure of the tip-lobule complex without disturbing intercrural or alar-septal attachments. It also allows for better binocular visualization, both for teaching and studying deformed anatomy. In addition, the open approach allows for a more precise control of bleeding by electrocautery and a more precise correction of deformities. The disadvantage is the skin incision on the columella and the degloving of the nose, which may be associated with more postoperative edema.

Tip-Lobule Complex

Alteration and molding of the alar cartilage must be done with precision to avoid visible deformities. The combination of a well-structured and stable nasal skeleton with a conforming skin–soft tissue envelope produces an aesthetically pleasing tip-lobule complex.

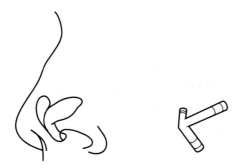

Figure 74–6. Altar "tripod".

When the skin–soft tissue envelope is thick, reducing tip projection is usually contraindicated. Thick skin does not contract well to an underprojected cartilage framework and worsens tip definition. Rather than deprojecting tip cartilages or weakening them by aggressive cephalic trims, definition can be improved only by increasing alar cartilage projection so the underlying framework pushes up into the thick overlying skin envelope. Frequently, tip grafts are required for optimal tip definition in these patients, although other techniques that increase projection can also be effective.

Jack Anderson, who was largely responsible for popularizing the open approach, taught that the alar cartilages can be seen as a tripod (Figure 74–6). The conjoined medial crura form the medial "leg" and each lateral crus forms the other two "legs." The modification of any leg leads to tip rotation. For example, if the conjoined medial crura lose support or are shortened, the tip rotates caudally. If both lateral crura are symmetrically shortened, either posteriorly or in mid-span, cephalic rotation occurs. The resection of one lateral crus leads to nasal-tip deviation toward that side. It is important to note that the shape of a weakened alar cartilage may also be modified by the contraction of scar tissue during the healing process or by the formation of bossae or knuckles over time. Overresection must be avoided to maintain stable alar cartilages, which allows for an accurate prediction of the surgical outcome.

A poorly defined and underprojected tip is well addressed with rhinoplasty. A columellar strut is often used, especially when using the open approach. Made from septal cartilage, it adds stability to the medial crura, allows for enhanced tip definition and projection, and prevents tip ptosis. The strut is placed in a pocket between the medial crura and extends just beyond the medial crura footplate. It should not rest on the nasal spine because this may cause clicking if it moves over the bone. When the caudal septum is long, care should be taken to shorten it before strut placement to prevent excess columellar show results. In addition, tip grafts or dome-binding sutures may be used to improve tip projection and definition.

A bulbous tip is another common problem. It is caused by convex, long, and poorly defined lateral crura that are rounded because of an obtuse angle at the dome. To address this, cephalic trim is used to reduce the curvature of the lateral crura and to create a flat profile. At least 7 mm of remaining crura are needed to ensure sufficient stability and strength. The excision of a triangle of cartilage just lateral to the domes is then used to reduce rounding from the obtuse angle. Staying lateral to the apex of the dome maintains the defining point of an unchanged tip, and the resection of a superior-based triangle allows cephalic rotation and narrowing of the dome. Care should be taken that such excision does not result in increased alar retraction. Suture reconstitution of the lateral crura is important because it maintains the strength of the nasal skeleton.

Nasal Valves

The most common cause of acquired incompetence of the internal or external nasal valves is rhinoplasty. Internal valvular incompetence is seen when the angle between the caudal edge of the upper lateral cartilage and the septum is less than the norm of 15°, creating a static obstruction. Some obstruction can be dynamic, with underlying weakness of the internal or external nasal valve evident only with inspiration. A spreader graft, placed between the dorsal septum and the upper lateral cartilage, is used to widen the angle and improve problems with the internal nasal valve, improving both static and dynamic obstruction at this level.

External valve incompetence is caused by excessive resection and weakening of the lateral crura of the alar cartilage, either congenital or acquired from excessive resection of the lateral crura. Repair is most commonly performed by placement of either a batten graft (overlying the lateral crus or stabilizing a deficient area) or an alar strut graft (underlying the lateral crus and straightening it) to strengthen the cartilage and prevent collapse. Repair is most commonly by placement of either a lateral graft that spans the crura or a batten graft to strengthen the cartilage and prevent collapse.

Alar retraction is most often caused by poor support of the alar margin resulting from aggressive alar cartilage excisions. It may also be caused by lateral crura that lie too cephalad. It may be corrected by placing a graft in a pocket along the alar rim (rim graft), by repositioning a cephalically oriented lateral crus more caudally, or, in severe cases, by using a composite ear cartilage-skin graft to increase vestibular length.

Nasal Dorsum

Skin thickness changes along the length of the nasal dorsum. It is thick over the nasion, thinnest at the rhinion, and thick again in the supratip area. This is essen-

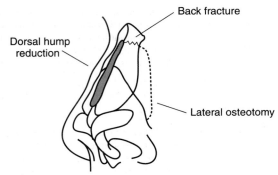

Figure 74–7. Dorsal hump and osteotomy.

tial to note because a straight dorsal profile of the bone and cartilage would not lead to an aesthetic profile; instead, it would lead to a concavity along the dorsum where the skin is thin. Therefore, it is important to preserve a slight convexity near the rhinion to account for the anatomy of the skin–soft tissue envelope.

Dorsal humps are usually more cartilaginous than bony in origin. They may be removed sharply or by rasping and often are combined with lateral osteotomies to prevent an open roof deformity (Figure 74–7). Hump removal is successful only if soft tissue, cartilage, or bone has been removed sufficiently to allow the lateral walls to fall medially to close the roof. Two errors leading to a flat dorsum despite osteotomies are uncorrected high septal deformities and insufficient resection in the keystone area of the upper lateral cartilages.

Lateral osteotomies are typically done intranasally, using a stab incision above the inferior turbinate to gain access to the pyriform aperture. The lateral osteotomy is started 1–2 mm above the base of the pyriform aperture and then follows a low to high trajectory along the nasal sidewalls. If the osteotomy is started at the base of the pyriform aperture, this segment of bone, along with the anterior portion of the inferior turbinate, may displace medially and partially block the airway.

The osteotomy cut is kept low, as close to the face as possible, to prevent any palpable step-off along the nasal wall and a "pinched-nose" appearance. Indeed, the lateral osteotomy is mostly an osteotomy of the nasal (ascending) process of the maxilla rather than of the nasal bone. Only as the osteotomy proceeds cephalically does it include the nasal bone. At the cranial end of the nasal bone, from the osteotomy line to the dorsum, the back-fracture is usually performed digitally or occurs spontaneously with medial rotation and pressure of the osteotomy (see Figure 74–7). The back fracture is usually at the nasofrontal groove, the thin portion of the nasal bone. If the osteotomy enters the thicker bone of the nasofrontal angle, a rocker deformity may result. In this situation,

manual medial pressure to realign the displaced cephalic thick bone would cause lateral displacement of the caudal bone.

Medial and lateral osteotomies are used to completely mobilize the bony skeleton to change its position, width, and appearance. A medial osteotomy, if needed, may be done through the incision used for either a closed or open rhinoplasty.

POSTOPERATIVE CARE

The surgical dressing is applied immediately after osteotomies to minimize edema. If there is significant bleeding, small precut strips of Telfa packing (a smooth-surfaced, absorbent material) may be placed. A thin coat of benzoin is applied over the nose and precut Steri-strips are applied cautiously over the nose from the root to the supratip area with 1–2 mm of overlap. If tip work has been performed, a sling around the columella is placed lightly enough for support, yet sufficient for adequate venous drainage of the tip.

Patients require reassurance and instruction after rhinoplasty. Postoperative antibiotic use is surgeon's choice. Patients should apply ice to their eyes and cheeks for 2 to 3 days. Patients should refrain from heavy lifting, strenuous activity, and nose blowing. If glasses must be worn, they may be worn over the cast during the first week, and then with supportive tape if they are heavy. Sneezing should be performed with an open mouth. In addition, patients should refrain from smoking and taking aspirin or ibuprofen for at least 2 weeks. Finally, nasal saline irrigation and half-strength hydrogen peroxide on a cotton applicator should be used to minimize crusting in the nasal passage and around the vestibule.

COMPLICATIONS

Complications after rhinoplasty are common. The most common complication is a dissatisfied patient due to nasal irregularities or asymmetries, or new or persistent nasal obstruction. Most credible studies cite revision rates after primary rhinoplasty of up to 25%. Fortunately, severe complications are rare after rhinoplasty. The most common early complication is epistaxis. The risk of infection is minimal in the absence of hematoma because of the excellent blood supply to the nose. Other rare complications include septal hematoma, septal abscess, septal perforation, suture granuloma, anosmia, and anesthesia-related complications.

Rhinoplasty is among the most challenging surgeries that the otolaryngologist will perform. Many years of experience are typically needed before a consistently excellent result is achieved. This challenge drives the rhinoplasty surgeon to constantly analyze his or her own technique and results, reaching for an illusive ideal that may eventually satisfy both surgeon and patient.

Constantian MB. Elaboration of an alternative, segmental, cartilage-sparing tip graft technique: experience in 405 cases. *Plast Reconstr Surg.* 1999;103(1):237. [PMID: 9915189] (Discusses a large group of patients who receive tip augmentation from an endonasal approach.)

Foda HM, Kridel RW. Lateral crural steal and lateral crural overlay: an objective evaluation. *Arch Otolaryngol Head Neck Surg.* 1999;125(12):1365. [PMID: 10604416] (Two techniques for the nasal tip are evaluated and clinical guidelines are discussed.)

Guyuron B. Dynamics in rhinoplasty. *Plast Reconstr Surg.* 2000; 105(6);2257. [PMID: 10839427] (Review of how alterations of the nasal appearance can be unexpected and achieved by subtle surgical modifications.)

Guyuron B. Nasal osteotomy and airway changes. *Plast Reconstr Surg.* 1998;102(3):856. [PMID: 9727456] (Objective study on the effects of osteotomies on the nasal airway.)

Harshbarger RJ, Sullivan PK. Lateral nasal osteotomies: implications of bony thickness on fracture patterns. *Ann Plast Surg.* 1999;42(4):365. [PMID: 10213395] (Anatomic study revealing specifics of osteotomy patterns.)

Harshbarger RJ, Sullivan PK. The optimal medial osteotomy: a study of nasal bone thickness and fracture patterns. *Plast Reconstr Surg.* 2001;108(7):2114. [PMID: 11743413] (Anatomic study revealing insights to osteotomy.)

Schlosser RJ, Park SS. Surgery for the dysfunctional nasal valve. Cadaveric analysis and clinical outcomes. *Arch Facial Plast Surg.* 1999;1(2):105. [PMID: 10937087] (Objective evaluation of nasal obstruction from nasal valve dysfunction and deviated septum.)

Sheen JH. Rhinoplasty: personal evolution and milestones. *Plast Reconstr Surg.* 2000;105(5):1820. [PMID: 10809116] (A father of rhinoplasty reviews his pearls from a distinguished career.)

Sheen JH. Closed versus open rhinoplasty—and the debate goes on. *Plast Reconstr Surg.* 1997;99(3):859. [PMID: 9047208] (The classic debate argued from a father of rhinoplasty and strong believer in the closed approach.)

Toriumi DM, Josen J, Weinberger M, Tardy ME Jr. Use of alar batten grafts for correction of nasal valve collapse. *Arch Otolaryngol Head Neck Surg.* 1997;123(8):802. [PMID: 9260543] (Two masters of rhinoplasty with an excellent long-term study on the treatment of nasal valve dysfunction.)

Hair Restoration

Min S. Ahn, MD

■ BIOLOGIC ROLE & SOCIAL RELEVANCE OF HUMAN HAIR

The presence of human scalp hair has important biologic and psychosocial roles for the individual. Biologic functions include providing protection from potentially harmful environmental elements, such as wind and cold temperatures, and dispersing hair follicle products, such as pheromones in nonverbal human interaction. The absence of scalp hair often has a more profound effect since both the individual's appearance and other people's reaction to that person are adversely affected. Whereas only 8% of nonbalding men state that losing hair would concern them, 50% of men with mild hair loss and 75% of men with moderate to severe hair loss express concern over the loss of hair. Men with hair loss feel older and less physically and sexually attractive than nonbalding men. People's impressions of those with hair loss are often unflattering and critical. With the advent of effective medical therapies and refined surgical techniques, a multibillion-dollar hair restoration treatment industry has emerged.

The physician can provide the first step in the therapeutic treatment of the individual with hair loss. The physician may be the only person who can broach the topic of hair loss with the patient without appearing judgmental or grossly inappropriate. With a basic understanding of normal hair physiology and the most common causes of hair loss, the physician from any subspecialty can provide effective care for those with hair loss. More specifically, after recognizing the presence of hair loss in the patient and making the appropriate diagnosis (male pattern baldness or alopecia areata, etc.), one can initiate further workup, if necessary, and discuss medical and surgical treatment options for the patient. The impact of such help on the individual with hair loss can be profoundly positive.

Sinclair R. Male pattern androgenetic alopecia. *BMJ.* 1998;317:865. [PMID: 9748188] (Pathogenesis and treatment of male pattern androgenetic alopecia.)

■ ANATOMY & GROWTH CYCLE OF HAIR FOLLICLES

There are approximately 5 million hair follicles covering the body, 100,000 of which cover the scalp. An individual who does not suffer from androgenetic alopecia (AGA) normally loses 50–150 scalp hairs per day. After birth, no additional follicles arise, although the size of follicles and hair can change with age. A reduction of the total number of follicles occurs only with scarring or skin loss. Androgenetic alopecia, in fact, does not involve a loss of follicles, but an androgen-mediated alteration of their anatomy that causes hair loss.

Hair follicles vary in size and shape, but all have the same basic anatomy. Matrix cells of the hair bulb are rapidly proliferating, producing the hair shaft and its cortex. Melanocytes produce pigment of the hair shaft. Matrix cells proliferate and migrate upward into a shape determined by the inner root sheath. The dimensions and curvature of the inner root sheath determine the diameter and shape of the hair. The dermal papilla resides at the base of the follicle and controls the number of matrix cells. The dermal papilla and the follicular epithelium interact to induce the cyclic and repeating pattern of normal hair growth. Epithelium stem cells of the outer root sheath bulge migrate from the follicle to repopulate the epithelium after injury such as that which occurs in laser resurfacing. The outer root sheath also contains Langerhans and Merkel cells, respectively, serving important immunologic and neurosensory functions.

Each follicle proceeds through three stages throughout the life of the follicle: (1) **anagen** (growth), (2) **catagen** (involution), and (3) **telogen** (resting). After the telogen stage, hair is shed and the follicle reenters the growth phase. Follicles of different parts of the body have differing lengths of time spent in the anagen stage. The amount of time spent in the anagen stage is directly proportional to the length of hair. For example, scalp follicles typically are in the growth phase for 2–8 years and produce long hairs, whereas eyebrow follicles spend 2–3 months in the anagen stage and produce shorter hairs.

Ninety percent of scalp hairs are in the anagen stage at any given moment. Androgens and various growth factors affect the length of time spent in the anagen stage.

During the catagen stage, the follicle involutes with apoptosis of the follicular keratinocytes and melanocytes. The telogen phase of scalp hair lasts 2–4 months, after which the follicle reenters the anagen stage. If a higher percentage of hair follicles are in the telogen stage, more shedding of hair results. Typically, 2–10% of scalp follicles are in the telogen stage. Androgens and certain drugs increase that percentage, thereby causing a further loss of scalp hair.

Paus R, Cotsarelis G. The biology of hair follicles. *N Engl J Med.* 1999;341:491. [PMID: 10441606] (Brief review of hair follicle biology and pathology.)

■ TYPES OF HAIR LOSS

Causes of hair loss affecting both men and women include those that are reversible and those that are irreversible. Reversible causes of hair loss involve an interruption in the natural hair follicle growth cycle. The most common types of reversible alopecia include androgenetic alopecia (eg, male pattern baldness and female pattern hair loss), alopecia areata, and telogen and anagen effluvium. Although androgenetic alopecia is technically reversible because it represents an interruption in the hair follicle growth cycle, no treatment exists that permanently reverses the process. The most common irreversible types of hair loss include those resulting from scars, trauma, surgery, and burns.

REVERSIBLE CAUSES OF HAIR LOSS

1. Androgenetic Alopecia

ESSENTIALS OF DIAGNOSIS

- *Hereditary thinning of scalp hair in genetically susceptible men and women.*
- *Androgen (dihydrotestosterone [DHT]) mediated.*
- *Occurs in both men and women.*

General Considerations

Androgenetic alopecia is the most common cause of hair loss and occurs in genetically susceptible individuals. Hair loss in both affected men and women typically begins between the ages of 12 and 40 and is variable in its rate of progression. Thirty percent of 30-year-old men and 50% of 50-year-old men suffer from male pattern baldness. White men are four times more likely than African-American men to suffer from this type of hair loss.

Pathogenesis

Circulating testosterone is converted peripherally to DHT by 5α-reductase. Two isoforms of 5α-reductase exist, Types 1 and 2. DHT promotes beard, chest, and axillary hair growth. When DHT binds to the androgen receptor on susceptible hair follicles of the scalp, the DHT-receptor complex effects a shortening of the anagen stage of the hair growth cycle and a lengthening of the telogen stage. This results in progressively shorter, finer, de-pigmented hairs.

Prevention

As of yet no preventive measures can be initiated in susceptible individuals. Further progression of hair loss can be delayed with drug therapy.

Clinical Findings

Androgenetic alopecia in men starts with bitemporal hairline recession followed by thinning of the vertex. Further thinning of the vertex results in a bald patch that may enlarge and combine with the progressively receding frontal hairline. This eventually results in a narrow rim of hair of the lower parietal and occipital regions.

Female AGA occurs in approximately 10% of women. Such female hair loss shows a different pattern in which a diffuse thinning of the frontal or parietal scalp occurs. A rim of hair along the frontal hairline is typically retained. The resulting hair loss, though as common in women as in men, is less evident and can be camouflaged with effective hair styling. Affected women typically have normal menses, pregnancies, and general endocrine function. An extensive hormonal evaluation is indicated only in the case of irregular menses, a history of infertility, hirsutism, severe acne, or virilization.

Differential Diagnosis

Androgenetic alopecia has a distinct pattern in both men and women, rendering its diagnosis relatively easy. Other reversible causes of hair loss, such as alopecia areata and certain conditions that induce a telogen effluvium, should be ruled out.

Complications

Complications of alopecia center on the psychosocial impact on the individual as alluded to above.

Treatment

In considering treatment options for androgenetic alopecia, the clinician must communicate to the patient that no medical or surgical means exist that either restore all of the hair that has been lost or achieve the density of hair that existed before the onset of hair loss. Hair weaves and pieces offer a less than natural-appearing option for coverage. Both medical and surgical modalities are available for both men and women. Medical and surgical treatments of hair loss are not mutually exclusive and, in fact, are often used in combination. Individuals undergoing hair restoration surgery will start medical therapy to maintain the existing hairs and therefore limit the amount of additional coverage needed through surgical techniques.

Drug therapy is able to prevent further thinning of existing hair and can restore some of the coverage that has been lost. There are two options for drug therapy currently approved by the FDA: minoxidil (Rogaine) and finasteride (Propecia). The therapeutic effect of both drugs requires the continued use of the medication. With cessation of the treatment, susceptible hair follicles, including those with hair that has been restored, restart the progressive thinning according to the individual's pattern of hair loss. Surgical therapy ultimately achieves an overall scalp density less than that of normal hair. Given its limitations, the goal of surgical restoration is to achieve a well-groomed, presentable appearance with acceptable coverage of the bald scalp.

A. NONSURGICAL MEASURES

1. Minoxidil—Minoxidil is a cream that is available in both 2% and 5% solutions. Both preparations have the effect of prolonging the anagen stage, thus enlarging miniaturized follicles. The 2% topical solution was approved in 1988 for men with androgenetic alopecia. Approval was based on significantly increased hair counts in 2294 men with mild to moderate vertex thinning who participated in a 12-month controlled trial with placebo. The FDA approved a 5% topical solution in 1997 for over-the-counter use. The 5% solution is more effective than the 2% solution in increasing hair counts. Both are applied to the dry scalp twice a day to maintain efficacy. Cessation of the drug results in a shedding of the hair.

Minoxidil is FDA approved for female androgenetic alopecia in both the 2% and 5% solutions. Minoxidil was originally developed as an antihypertensive medication, a result of its potassium-mediated vasodilatory effects. The mechanism of hair restoration is unknown. Adverse effects of minoxidil center on irritation of the scalp and occur in 7% of patients using the 2% solution.

2. Finasteride—Finasteride prevents the conversion of testosterone to DHT by competitively inhibiting the activity of Type 2 5α-reductase. As such, it has beneficial effects on benign prostatic hypertrophy. Individuals with

Type 2 5α-reductase deficiency never experience androgenetic alopecia. Daily treatment of men with AGA with finasteride (1 mg) results in increased hair weight, converts more hair into the anagen growth phase, and reverses miniaturization of scalp hair. The FDA approved the use of once-daily 1-mg tablets of finasteride for the treatment of androgenetic alopecia in men. This was based on three randomized double-blind placebo-controlled trials in which a total of 1879 men experienced increased hair counts at the vertex and frontal regions compared with the placebo group after 1 year. After 2 years, 67% of the men had increased scalp coverage. Finasteride results in a 60% reduction in serum and scalp DHT levels, has no affinity for androgen receptors, and has no androgenetic or steroidal effects. Daily finasteride therapy in men with AGA starting 4 weeks before and continuing until 48 weeks after hair transplantation increases hair density compared with the placebo group as a result of retaining hairs otherwise susceptible to androgen-mediated hair loss. Adverse effects related to sexual dysfunction occur slightly more commonly than with placebo and are largely reversible; 1.8% of men experience decreased libido, 1.3% suffer from erectile dysfunction, and 1.2% experience ejaculatory dysfunction. Such adverse effects typically resolve with continued use. Finasteride is contraindicated in women who may become pregnant or are pregnant because of the potential for 5α-reductase inhibitors to inhibit the virilization of the genitalia of male fetuses.

B. SURGICAL MEASURES

Surgical therapy of androgenetic alopecia relies on the redistribution of follicles that have not been affected by the process of androgenetic alopecia to cover areas of hair loss. The donor hairs that provide the source of hair to be distributed can be transferred in the form of hair flaps, or more commonly as free grafts. The most common surgical technique currently employed involves hair grafting because of its low morbidity, reliable results, and acceptable effect.

Jose Juri described the original flap used for baldness in 1975. He discussed a twice-delayed parieto-occipital flap of hair-bearing scalp that was rotated to restore the frontal hairline and midscalp region. Sheldon Kabaker introduced this technique to North America in 1978 after observing Juri perform the surgery in Argentina. He discussed the technique in detail with further refinements. Other surgical techniques have been described including scalp reduction procedures that remove non–hair-bearing scalp with or without tissue expansion.

Because of relatively higher rates of morbidity, as well as the limited potential for a natural-appearing result, all of these surgical procedures have been supplanted by mini-micro grafting and follicular-unit hair transplantation techniques. Modern hair-grafting methods have been refined from the original use of large grafts, causing a "pluggy" or "doll's head" result into current techniques that provide for a natural appearance.

With regard to terminology, **micrografts** refer to 1–2 hair grafts and **minigrafts** represent 3–6 hair grafts. **Follicular-unit grafts** refer to naturally occurring entities that include 1–4 hairs. Hair grows naturally from the scalp as single hairs or groups of 2–4 hairs. These groupings represent follicular units that contain single hairs or 2–4 hairs. Headington was the first to describe the follicular unit in 1954 as containing 1–4 terminal hairs, 1 vellum hair, sebaceous lobules, and other appendages. Robert Limmer in 1988 was the first to perform follicular unit transplantation (FUT) during which grafts of follicular units containing 1–4 hairs are individually harvested under stereomicroscopic dissection. The method of FUT has evolved to the point where commonly 1000–2000 follicular-unit grafts are harvested and transplanted into recipient site slits during a single session. The majority of grafts become immediately viable, commonly enter a telogen stage of shedding, and ultimately show growth of transplanted hair in approximately 6–12 months. Such hair is permanent and will proceed through the natural hair cycle without being susceptible to the process of AGA.

Often, more than one session is required to achieve adequate coverage. Whereas normal donor site hair has a density of approximately 100 follicular units per square centimeter, transplanted hair has a density of 10–40 follicular units per square centimeter. The result, therefore, is not a high level of density but an adequate amount of coverage that provides a natural, albeit thinning, appearance. Grafting techniques for female androgenetic alopecia, in which the hair loss involves a diffuse thinning, is often less effective because of the limitations on resulting hair density. Adverse effects of FUT are infrequent and are limited to donor site morbidity (widening of the scar, wound infection) or improper recipient site design resulting in a cosmetically unacceptable result.

Bernstein RM. In support of follicular unit transplantation. *Dermatol Surg.* 2000;26:160. [PMID: 10691949] (Follicular unit transplantation method is discussed in detail.)

Bernstein M, Rassman WR, Seager D et al. Standardizing the classification and description of follicular unit transplantation and mini-micrografting techniques. *Dermatol Surg.* 1998;24:957. [PMID: 9754083] (Multiple authors providing guidelines for nomenclature and classification of techniques.)

Juri J. Use of parietooccipital flaps in the surgical treatment of baldness. *Plast Reconstr Surg.* 1975;55:456. [PMID: 1090958] (Classic article describing the Juri flap.)

Kabaker SS. Juri flap procedure for the treatment of baldness: two-year experience. *Arch Otolaryngol.* 1979;105:509. [PMID: 383056] (Classic description of modification of the Juri flap.)

Price VH. Treatment of hair loss. *N Engl J Med.* 1999;341:964. [PMID: 10498493] (Medical treatment of various types of hair loss.)

Rittmaster RS. Finasteride. *N Engl J Med.* 1994;330:120. [PMID: 7505051] (Biologic effects and clinical use of finasteride.)

Sinclair R. Male pattern androgenetic alopecia. *BMJ.* 1998;317:865. [PMID: 9748188] (Pathogenesis and treatment of male pattern androgenetic alopecia.)

Swerdloff I, Kabaker S. The state of the art: donor site harvest, graft yield estimation, and recipient site preparation for follicular-unit hair transplantation. *Arch Facial Plast Surg.* 1999;1:49. [PMID: 10937077] (State-of-the-art technique by leading hair restoration surgeons.)

Unger WP. The history of hair transplantation. *Dermatol Surg.* 2000;26:181. [PMID: 10759790] (Hair transplantation history.)

2. Alopecia Areata

 ESSENTIALS OF DIAGNOSIS

- *Wide range of severity from small, round, patchy areas of baldness of the scalp and body to total loss of hair of the scalp (alopecia totalis) and body (alopecia universalis).*
- *Occurs in both men and women.*
- *More commonly affects children and young adults.*
- *Affected individuals are typically otherwise healthy.*

General Considerations

Alopecia areata affects approximately 2% of the U.S. population. The process is typically self-limited and commonly results in spontaneous remission. Persistent cases can be treated medically with good success.

Pathogenesis

Alopecia areata is thought to be an autoimmune process based on the presence of activated CD4 and CD8 lymphocytes around follicles in the anagen stage of the growth cycle.

Prevention

No preventive measures exist, although further progression of alopecia areata can be halted with medical therapy.

Clinical Findings

Alopecia areata typically manifests as patchy, round, smooth areas of balding scalp. Hairs at the periphery of the patch are often easily dislodged. The eyebrows, beard, and eyelashes can be affected. Alopecia totalis and alopecia universalis refer to more extensive forms of the disease that involve the entire scalp, as well as the scalp and body, respectively. Although most often the patient is otherwise healthy, atopy, vitiligo, Hashimoto thyroiditis, pernicious anemia, and Addison disease are occasionally associated. Serum thyroid-stimulating hormone levels should therefore be measured in affected children.

Complications

Complications of alopecia areata are limited to an adverse psychosocial impact on the individual.

Treatment

Treatment options include intralesional and systemic steroids, topical 5% minoxidil, topical immunotherapy, and anthralin. Limited cases respond better to treatment than larger areas of hair loss. Most commonly, triamcinolone (10 mg/mL) is injected into the area at intervals of 4–6 weeks until regrowth occurs. The choice of treatment depends on the age of the individual and the extent of hair loss.

Other reversible causes of hair loss involve a **telogen effluvium**, in which the majority of hairs become transiently shifted to the telogen stage and are subsequently shed. This may be precipitated by fever, the latter stages of pregnancy, the stress of surgery, iron deficiency, malnutrition states, and certain drugs, such as thallium, vitamin A, oral contraceptive pills, and propranolol. Most commonly, the process is temporary and requires no treatment. Antineoplastic drugs and radiation therapy induce an **anagen effluvium** in which the rapidly proliferating bulb matrix cells are specifically affected.

Price VH. Treatment of hair loss. *N Engl J Med*. 1999;341:964. [PMID: 10498493] (Medical treatment of various types of hair loss.)

IRREVERSIBLE CAUSES OF HAIR LOSS

The loss of hair follicles from scarring is complete and irreversible. Scalp trauma, surgical trauma, burns, and inflammatory states such as lichen planopilaris and discoid lupus erythematosus all result in scarring and permanent loss of the hair follicle. With such loss, the only treatment options are hair weaves, hair-bearing flaps, or hair-grafting sessions. Scarring of the hair-bearing scalp near improperly placed or poorly healed facelift incisions is very effectively treated with follicular-unit grafting techniques.

Nordstrom RE, Greco M, Vitagliano T. Correction of sideburn defects after facelift operations. *Aesthetic Plast Surg*. 2000;24:429. [PMID: 11246431] (Useful technique for correction of facelift scars in hair-bearing regions.)

Paus R, Cotsarelis G. The biology of hair follicles. *N Engl J Med*. 1999;341(7):491. [PMID: 10441606] (Brief review of hair follicle biology and pathology.)

Local & Regional Flaps in Head & Neck Reconstruction

76

Nathan Monhian, MD, & Jeffrey Wise, MD

Local facial flaps are most often used in reconstruction of defects left after excision of skin tumors and represent the method of choice for repair of most facial defects that are too large for primary closure. Although skin grafts should be considered in reconstructing defects, local flaps are better suited for poorly vascularized recipient beds and frequently offer a better skin color match. Local flaps are the method of choice for repair of most facial defects that are too large for primary closure. This chapter reviews the commonly used flaps in facial reconstruction with an emphasis on their indications in particular circumstances. A review of regional flaps in head and neck reconstruction is also presented. Detailed information on skin tumors and their differential diagnosis is provided in corresponding chapters.

CLASSIFICATION

Method of Flap Movement

Local flaps can be classified by method of movement into pivotal, advancement, or hinged flaps (Table 76–1).

A. Pivotal Flaps

Pivotal flaps rotate around a pivotal point and form one standing cutaneous deformity. Pivotal flaps may in turn be divided into transposition, rotation, and interpolated flaps. **Transposition flaps** have a linear axis with their base adjacent to the defect. In transposition, a lifting of the flap occurs, usually across a normal bridge of tissue. **Rotation flaps** are curvilinear in shape, with one border of the defect being the leading border of the flap. Although transposition and rotation flaps are both pivotal flaps, they differ in that the axis of a transposition flap is linear, whereas the axis of a rotation flap is curvilinear. An **interpolated flap** has a linear axis and its base is removed from the defect site. This flap requires either detachment of the pedicle as a separate procedure or burying of the pedicle under a bridge of skin at the time of reconstruction.

B. Advancement Flaps

Advancement flaps are flaps with sliding movement in one vector of movement. In an advancement flap, one border of the defect is the leading border of the flap. Advancement flaps have two standing cutaneous deformities. These flaps can be further divided into single pedicle, bipedicle, or subcutaneous pedicle flaps.

C. Hinged Flaps

Hinged flaps move like a page of a book in a swinging movement. They can be raised as subcutaneous flaps to fill a tissue defect in an adjacent site.

Flap Blood Supply

Flaps may also be classified according to their blood supply. The most commonly discussed are random and axial flaps.

A. Random Flaps

Random flaps are created by dissecting in the level of the subcutaneous fat. In so doing, the flap base derives its blood supply from perforating musculocutaneous vessels that lie in the deep subdermal and muscular plane. Perfusion at the free portion of the flap is derived from communication between the superficial papillary dermal plexus and the deeper subdermal plexus. Most advancement and rotation flaps fall into this category. An example of a random flap is the **rhombic flap.** For most random flaps, a length-to-width ratio of 1:1 is safe; however, in the face, this ratio can be extended to 2:1 or even greater without significant risk of flap loss or skin necrosis.

B. Axial Flaps

In contrast to a random flap, an axial flap is based on a named vessel, which supplies the majority of the flap. Axial flaps have a subcutaneous artery extending along the linear axis of the flap. The blood supply of the most distal portion of an axial flap is often random. An example of an axial flap is the **paramedian forehead flap,** which is based on the supratrochlear artery and vein.

Table 76–1. Local flaps classified by tissue movement.

Pivotal Flaps
Rotation
Transposition
Interpolation
Advancement Flaps
Single pedicle
Bipedicle
Y-V
Hinged Flap

Principles of Aesthetic Subunits and Wound Dynamics

Understanding the concept of aesthetic regions and the borders defining them is important in the design and performance of flap surgery. The face is divided into several aesthetic regions and each region may be divided into several units. These are natural anatomic areas, which must be respected. When possible, the flap should be designed in the same aesthetic unit as the defect. Incisions are best hidden when they are placed in aesthetic borders. When a defect involves two or more aesthetic units, it is often best to reconstruct each portion of the defect separately. Therefore, each subunit may be reconstructed with a separate local flap. This places the scars along the borders of aesthetic units and prevents the obliteration of important boundary lines between the units.

In planning a reconstruction, especially for nasal defects, it may be beneficial to enlarge a defect to include an entire aesthetic region or unit and then reconstruct the entire unit with a flap.

The **relaxed skin tension lines** (RSTLs) are the lines of minimal tension of the skin. Perpendicular to the RSTLs are the **lines of maximal extensibility** (LME). Incisions parallel with RSTLs heal with less wound closure tension than incisions placed perpendicular to RSTLs. Whenever possible, it is preferable to design the excision of skin lesions in such a manner that the necessary skin incisions are parallel with RSTLs. Likewise, when designing cutaneous flaps, it is prudent to orient the flap so that the linear axis of the flap is parallel with RSTLs.

ROTATION FLAPS

Rotation flaps are pivotal flaps with a curvilinear shape. They rotate around a pivotal point near the defect (Figure 76–1). Rotation flaps are most appropriate for triangular-shaped defects. A curvilinear incision is made immediately adjacent to the defect. The standing cutaneous deformity that is formed can be excised as a Burrow triangle to facilitate wound closure. By combining rotation and advancement tissue movement and using the principle of halving (ie, dividing the length of the closure into equal halves until the entire defect is closed), the defect may often be closed without the need for excision of a Burrow triangle. The vector of greatest tension is from the pivotal point to the most distal point along the curvilinear incision. This flap usually has a random blood supply, but depending on the location of the base of the flap, it may acquire an axial pattern.

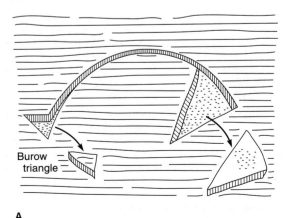

A

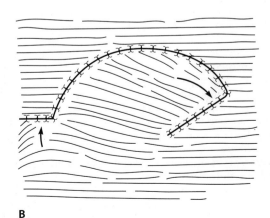

B

Figure 76–1. Rotation flap. **(A)** The flap is rotated and advanced into the defect. **(B)** Burrow triangle is removed to eliminate a standing cutaneous deformity at the base of the flap (small arrow).

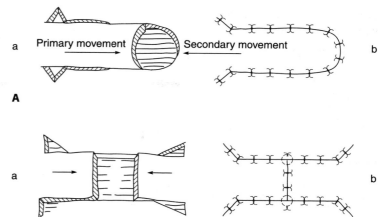

Figure 76–2. **(A)** Single-pedicle flap and **(B)** bilateral advancement flap.

The rotation flap is ideal for medium to large defects of the cheek, neck, and scalp. It is not useful in nasal reconstruction because of the lengthy incision required to achieve the proper tissue movement and the need to undermine and advance the pivotal point. One advantage of a rotation flap is its viability in an irradiated area or in patients with poor vascularity due to smoking or diabetes.

ADVANCEMENT FLAPS

1. Simple Linear Closure

A simple linear closure involves the undermining and movement of opposite wound margins toward each other and is the most basic of advancement flaps. Studies using animal models have demonstrated that undermining in the subcutaneous plane 2 to 4 cm provides benefit by decreasing wound tension. However, undermining tissue for distances greater than 6 cm does not alleviate wound tension and may actually increase flap tension. The classic rectangular-shaped advancement flap is created by parallel incisions extending from the border of the defect and involves a sliding movement of tissue into the defect. The incision lines can be placed into appropriate RSTLs or cosmetic boundary lines, when possible. Two standing cutaneous deformities are created at the corners of the flap and can be corrected by excising Burrow triangles. Occasionally, a simple halving technique allows closure without the need to excise normal skin in the forms of Burrow triangles. Advancement flaps may be designed unilaterally (the so-called U-plasty) or bilaterally (H-plasty or T-plasty) (Figure 76–2). In designing these flaps, it is best not to exceed a 3:1 ratio of flap-to-defect length. The wound closure tension is maximal along the leading border of the flap. Advancement flaps are particularly useful in the forehead, lip, and eyelid areas, where it is necessary to avoid any tension in a superior or inferior direction, thus avoiding distortion of important anatomical structures.

2. Cheek Advancement Flaps

Cheek advancement flaps have the advantage of relative mobility and elasticity of the soft tissue of the cheek area. They are useful in reconstruction of medium to large defects of the medial cheek, near the nasal-facial sulcus. The standing cutaneous deformities are excised superiorly at the junction of the cheek and lower eyelid and inferiorly along the melolabial fold.

3. V to Y Island Advancement Flaps

The V to Y island advancement flap works especially well for medium-sized defects of the medial cheek, the nasal sidewall, or the upper lip near the alar base. It involves the isolation of a segment of skin as an island dependent on the deep perforating vessels in the subcutaneous tissue. As the flap is advanced, the donor wound defect is closed primarily, creating a Y configuration at the wound closure. Undermining is performed at the periphery of the flap. Deep tissues remain attached to the center of the flap and provide the vascular supply to the flap. This flap has the potential for developing a pincushion-like or "trapdoor" deformity, but this is usually self-limited and is minimized by proper undermining in the periphery of the defect.

TRANSPOSITION FLAPS

Transposition flaps are pivotal flaps with their base immediately adjacent to the defect. They are usually designed so that the borders of the flap are at some distance from the defect to be repaired.

1. S Flaps

When designing an S flap, a transposition flap 30–40% of the size of the defect is created slightly longer and narrower (as narrow as one half) than the defect. The wound is closed in an S-shaped configuration. The note flap allows a circular defect to be closed with a triangular flap. A tangent is drawn on the side of the circular defect parallel with the RSTLs. This tangent is extended approximately 1.5 times the diameter of the defect. At the end of the tangent, a 50–60° flap is designed with a length approximately equal to the diameter of the defect. The flap is transposed into the defect, and the distal tip of the flap is usually trimmed. This flap is useful in the cheek, lip, and nasal areas. The small standing cutaneous deformity that develops may require correction by excision of a Burrow triangle.

Larger defects may be reconstructed by the use of multiple transposition flaps. The major disadvantages of these flaps include the risk of necrosis and the development of a trapdoor deformity. Poor design of the flap, poor handling of the tissue, and impaired skin vascularity because of smoking or diabetes increase the risk of flap loss or necrosis. A trapdoor deformity may occur a few weeks after transfer. The flap appears bulky, protruding from the surrounding skin and having the appearance of a pincushion. The predisposing factors to this deformity include round defects, curvilinear flaps, inadequate undermining of the periphery of the defect, and interpolated flaps (circumferential scars). This deformity usually resolves with time. Resolution can be assisted by intralesional Kenalog (ie, triamcinolone acetonide) injections every 6–8 weeks. If the deformity is not resolved after 6–8 months, a scar revision with thinning of the flap or multiple Z-plasties of the scar can correct the deformity.

2. Rhombic Flaps

A variant of the transposition flap is the rhombic flap (Figure 76–3). The movement of a rhombic flap is by a combination of pivotal movement and advancement and is commonly used for repair of defects of the cheek and temple area. The classic rhombic flap, as described by Limberg, reconstructs a rhombic defect (an equilateral parallelogram) with opposing angles of 60° and 120°. Once the rhombus defect has been created with all sides equal, by definition, the short diagonal is directly extended. This creates the first side of the flap and is extended to a distance equal to one of the sides. The second side of the flap is drawn parallel with one of the sides of the defect.

The Webster 30° flap is a modification of the classic Limberg flap (Figure 76–4). A flap with a 30° acute

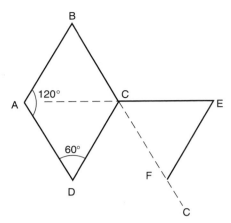

Figure 76–3. Classic rhombic flap.

angle is designed and transposed. This flap has the advantage of minimizing the standing cutaneous deformities and dissipating wound closure tension more evenly along the border of the flap. Performing an M-plasty at the corner of the rhombic defect can reduce the large amount of tissue that must be excised to correct the resulting standing cutaneous deformity.

3. Bilobe Flaps

The bilobe flap is a double transposition flap. The primary flap is used to repair the cutaneous defect and a

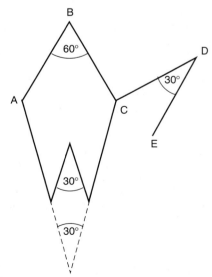

Figure 76–4. Webster 30° flap. This flap is more appropriate for longer, oval defects.

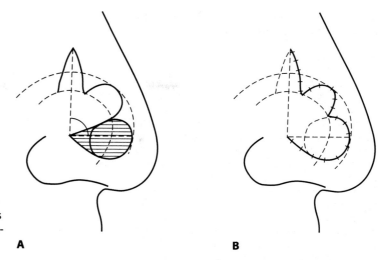

A   **B**

Figure 76–5. Modification of the bilobe flap, resulting in a 90° rotation, minimizes standing cutaneous deformities and trapdoor deformities.

secondary flap is used to repair the primary flap donor site. The secondary flap donor site is then closed primarily (Figure 76–5).

The original design of the bilobe flap required that the angle of tissue transfer be 90° between each lobe, for a total transposition of 180°. The wide angles have the disadvantage of maximizing standing cutaneous deformities and the likelihood of developing trapdoor deformities of both primary and secondary flaps. Zitelli's modification of the bilobe flap requires a 45° angle of transfer between each lobe, thus limiting the total transposition to 90–110°. With this modified approach, standing cutaneous deformities are minimized and a trapdoor deformity is avoided.

The bilobe flap is best suited for use in repairing 1-cm cutaneous defects of the nasal tip. The upper limit in the size of nasal defects that can be easily repaired with a bilobe flap is approximately 1.5 cm. With minimal wound closure tension on the primary flap, there is limited or no distortion when the flap is used to repair defects located near the alar rim. The use of adjacent skin provides excellent color and texture match for reconstruction. The base of the flap is usually located laterally, and the nasalis muscle is included in the substance of the flap, thus providing excellent vascularity to the flap with little risk of necrosis. The bilobe flap is also useful for reconstruction of cheek defects, away from the central part of the face. Because of the curvilinear design of the flap, the scars do not fall in wrinkle lines. However, this may be outweighed by good tissue mobility, a lack of wound tension, and minimal distortion of anatomic landmarks.

4. Melolabial Flaps

The melolabial fold adjacent to the nose and lips provides abundant skin with excellent color match for nasal and perinasal reconstruction. The cheek skin in this region has an extensive blood supply from perforating branches of the facial artery and is drained by facial and angular veins. Because of this rich blood supply, the melolabial flaps may be based superiorly or inferiorly with little risk of flap necrosis. The donor site is closed primarily, and the closure line is usually well hidden in the melolabial sulcus. The pedicle of the flap is divided after 3–4 weeks, at which time flap thinning and contouring may also be performed.

5. Midforehead Flaps

Midforehead flaps were first described in the Indian medical treatise, the *Sushruta Samita,* in approximately 700 BC. Median and paramedian forehead flaps are interpolated axial flaps, supplied primarily by the supratrochlear artery and secondarily by the dorsal nasal (angular) artery and the supraorbital artery. In the absence of the supratrochlear artery, the median and paramedian forehead flaps can still be harvested based on the dorsal nasal artery. The supratrochlear artery exits the superior medial orbit approximately 1.7–2.2 cm lateral to the midline, corresponding to the location of the medial portion of the eyebrow. It continues its course vertically in a paramedian position approximately 2 cm lateral to the midline. At the level of the eyebrow, the supratrochlear artery passes through the orbicularis and frontalis muscles and continues superiorly in the superficial subcutaneous tissue. Therefore, the flap can be thinned and contoured for better aesthetic results by removing the fascia and frontalis muscle without concern for compromise of the flap vasculature.

Midforehead flaps are used primarily for the reconstruction of larger defects of the nose or nasal tip, where the defect is too large or too deep to close with full-thickness skin grafts, composite auricular grafts, or adjacent tissue flaps, such as the bilobe or melolabial flaps. In general, nasal defects larger than 2.5 cm in length along the horizontal transverse plane are best closed with a midforehead flap. Nasal defects with exposed bone or cartilage deficient of periosteum or perichondrium, or wounds in irradiated fields, are ideally reconstructed by this well-vascularized flap.

The major disadvantages of the midforehead flap are a vertical forehead scar, the potential for transferring hair, and the need for a second operation to divide the pedicle. It is important to counsel the patient preoperatively regarding the deformity caused by the flap during the interval between flap transfer and pedicle division.

6. Z-Plasty

Z-plasty is a transposition flap of two identical triangles. This technique is used primarily to lengthen a scar in an effort to treat scar contractures. In addition, Z-plasty can reorient the position of a scar so that it lies parallel with RSTLs.

In the design of a Z-plasty, limbs are drawn at angles ranging from 30° to 90° from the central scar. With an increase in angle size, the degree of lengthening of a scar predictably increases. A 30° angle produces a 25% increase in scar length, a 45° angle produces a 50% increase in scar length, and so on (Table 76–2). The optimal angle for Z-plasty appears to be from 45° to 60°. Angles less than 45° tend not to achieve significant lengthening and result in thin flaps. Alternatively, angles that exceed 60° produce significant tension on the wound and prevent successful transposition of the triangular flaps. The use of multiple Z-plasties reduces lateral tension and more evenly distributes the tension across the entire wound. In addition, multiple Z-plasties, in contrast to a single Z-plasty, often produce better cosmesis, particularly in the head and neck region.

Demir Z, Velidedeoglu H, Celebioglu S. V-Y-S plasty for scalp defects. *Plast Reconstr Surg.* 2003;112(4):1054. [PMID: 12973223] (Presentation of a V-Y advancement/rotation flap for reconstruction of large scalp defects.)

Jellinek, Nathaniel J. Local flaps in head and neck reconstruction. *J Am Acad Dermatol.* 2005;52(4):740. [ISSN 0190-9622] (Re-

Table 76–2. The relationship of size and limb length in Z-plasty.

Angle Size	Length Increase
30°	25%
45°	50%
60°	75%
75°	100%
90°	120%

Table 76–3. Regional flaps and their primary blood supply.

Flap	Blood Supply
Deltopectoral fasciocutaneous flap	Internal mammary artery (first four perforators)
Pectoralis major myocutaneous flap	Thoracoacromial artery
Trapezius myocutaneous flap	Occipital artery
Sternocleidomastoid muscle flap	Superior thyroid, transverse cervical occipital arteries

view of several flaps and their applications in head and neck reconstruction.)

Sedwick JD, Graham V, Tolan CJ, Sykes JM, Terkonda RP. The full-thickness forehead flap for complex nasal defects: a preliminary study. *Otolaryngol Head Neck Surg.* 2005;132(3):381. [PMID: 15746847] (Reports a new technique using a bivalved, full-thickness paramedian forehead flap in which the skin and subcutaneous tissue are separated from the frontalis muscle and pericranium.)

REGIONAL FLAPS

Defects that are too extensive to repair with local, random flaps can frequently be repaired with regional flaps. Four such flaps, the deltopectoral, pectoralis major, trapezius, and sternocleidomastoid muscle flaps are described herein. The primary blood supply of each flap is outlined in Table 76–3.

1. Deltopectoral Flaps

This fasciocutaneous flap is based on the first four perforators of the internal mammary artery with the second and third perforators serving as the primary contributors. The second is the larger of the two. The use of this flap in an undelayed fashion requires the continuity of the second perforator. To prevent injury to the perforators, flap elevation should remain lateral to a vertical line approximately 2 cm from the sternal border. The vessels provide an axial blood supply to the proximal two thirds of the flap; the remaining third is random in distribution. The elevation of this flap below the pectoralis fascia protects the subdermal network of vasculature for the random distribution. The donor site of the deltopectoral flap requires a skin graft for a shoulder defect. Primary closure can be completely or partially accomplished for a resulting donor defect of the chest.

2. Pectoralis Major Myocutaneous Flaps

The pectoralis major flap has been the workhorse flap in head and neck reconstruction. It can be elevated as a myofascial or myocutaneous flap. The primary blood supply to this flap is from the pectoral branch of the thoracoacromial artery, a branch of the subclavian. A secondary contributor that occasionally can be left intact is the lateral thoracic artery. This artery is usually ligated if the flap is to be extended farther superiorly, and the humeral attachment of the muscle is divided for mobilization. The skin paddle elevated with the flap is based on the deep perforating vessels. The flap is delivered to the neck under a tunnel created by elevating the skin overlying the remaining pectoralis muscle. The harvest site on the chest is closed primarily. The flap can successfully be used to reconstruct defects as superior as the lateral temporal bone.

3. Trapezius Myocutaneous Flaps

The trapezius myocutaneous flap can be elevated with an inferior pedicle based on the transverse cervical artery. The superiorly based trapezius flap is a nape of neck flap with the trapezius muscle beneath it. The ipsilateral occipital artery and posterior scalp vessels, in conjunction with the trapezius muscle branches of the vertebral artery superiorly, contribute to the blood supply of this flap. This flap can be used to resurface defects of the neck, ear, parotid, and posterior cheek. The bulk of the flap can fill defects created by radical resection. However, this bulk does not lend itself to being tubed or readily used intraorally. The donor site can usually be partially or totally closed primarily.

4. Sternocleidomastoid Myocutaneous Flaps

The sternocleidomastoid flap was initially used for intraoral reconstruction. This flap has been designed with an inferior or superior base. The inferior base allows for anterior floor of mouth reconstruction but cannot be used to reconstruct defects above the mandible. The superiorly based flap is supplied by the occipital artery. If the flap is not dissected to the superior one third, the superior thyroid artery supplies the flap as well. The superiorly based flap can be transposed in an arc from the malar eminence to the melolabial fold, buccal area, or lateral and anterior floor of the mouth.

Hamaker RC, Singer MI. Regional flaps in head and neck reconstruction. *Otolaryngol Clin North Am.* 1982;15(1):99. [PMID: 7099655] (Pectoralis major flap has a wide range of applications in head and neck construction. Deltopectoral flap, a fasciocutaneous flap, has limited application and is used in lower neck reconstruction. Trapezius flap is a bulky flap useful for reconstruction of the neck, ear, parotid gland, and posterior cheek defects.)

COMPLICATIONS OF LOCAL FLAPS

When performing surgical procedures, complications are inevitable. A thorough understanding of prevention and management of complications is as important as learning how to perform any surgical procedure.

Ischemia & Necrosis

Apart from fearsome complications, such as a cardiovascular or neurologic event or the death of the patient, the next most serious complications in flap surgery are ischemia and necrosis. A number of events may compromise the blood supply to a flap. The most critical factor is excessive tension on wound edges. Insufficient undermining of the flap or distention of the flap secondary to hematoma or edema can add to the tension at the wound edges. The type of flap also determines the tension at the distal edge. Transposition flaps generate less distal wound tension than rotation or advancement flaps. An inappropriately high length-to-width ratio of the flap increases the risk of necrosis at the tip of the flap. The risk of necrosis is greatly increased with smoking. Cigarette smoke affects the cutaneous blood supply by at least two interrelated mechanisms: (1) nicotine in cigarette smoke is a potent vasoconstrictor, and (2) carbon monoxide can cause tissue hypoxemia by competing with oxygen for hemoglobin-binding sites. If the patient can stop smoking for 2 days before and 7 days after surgery, flap reconstruction is much less hazardous.

Wound Infection

Fortunately, wound infection of head and neck reconstruction using local cutaneous flaps is uncommon. Aseptic surgical practice, proper surgical technique, and the rich blood supply of the region reduce the risk of infection. However, when infection does occur, it can have devastating effects on the local flap. Necrosis of all or part of the flap may ensue. The flap may dehisce or the final scar may widen or thicken. Infection can impair wound healing by lengthening the inflammatory phase of the healing process. The role of perioperative antibiotics to prevent wound infection remains controversial.

Bleeding & Clotting

Bleeding and clotting are destructive to flap viability. A significant collection of blood under the flap as well as the undermined area can create several problems, including necrosis, subdermal fibrosis with trapdoor deformity, and suboptimal scarring. Toxic mediators, especially hemoglobin-derived oxygen free radicals, interfere with flap circulation. The space-occupying hematoma may increase tension on the closure line. Separation of the flap from the wound bed may interfere with normal cohesion and normal wound healing. Blood in the wound acts as an excellent culture medium for bacteria and thus increases the risk of wound infection.

Wound Dehiscence

Wound dehiscence or separation is often secondary to another major complication: infection, hematoma, or a full-thickness necrosis. Minor wound separations may occur from direct trauma or as a result of dynamic movement of the flap in the perioral or periocular areas. In addition, the lack of buried dermal sutures or early suture removal may lead to wound separation. Uncom-

plicated, clean separations from trauma or early suture removal may be resutured within 24 hours, without the need for debridement. Complicated separations secondary to infection, hematoma, or necrosis that have been present for longer than 24 hours are best left to heal by secondary intention, usually followed by scar revision.

Vural E, Key JM. Complications, salvage, and enhancement of local flaps in facial reconstruction. *Otolaryngol Clin North Am.* 2001;34(4):739. [PMID: 11511473] (Discussion of various complications in flap surgery, as well as methods of prevention and management.)

Microvascular Reconstruction

77

Jeannie Hye-Joon Chung, MD, & Daniel G. Deschler, MD, FACS

Microvascular free-tissue transfer is a reconstructive technique in which tissue units are separated from their native blood supply and moved from one part of the body to a new location. The donor tissue has an identifiable artery and vein that are reanastomosed to recipient vessels, thus reestablishing blood flow. The potential for sensory reinnervation also exists through the reanastomosis of cutaneous nerves.

The basic goal of head and neck reconstruction is to replace soft tissue and bony defects with similar tissue, restoring function and optimizing cosmesis. Refinements in free-tissue transfer over the last two decades have revolutionized reconstruction of head and neck defects resulting from trauma, congenital anomalies, and ablative procedures for neoplastic processes. Free-tissue units are custom-designed for defects to provide characteristics similar to those of the original tissue. This versatility allows free flaps to serve multiple purposes, such as lining oropharyngeal defects and providing soft tissue support for maxillary defects. Free flaps offer other advantages because they do not have the anatomic constraints of pedicled flaps; they can be completed in a single stage, allow a simultaneous two-team approach, and have allowed ablative surgeons to expand their resection boundaries.

PREOPERATIVE CONSIDERATIONS & PLANNING

Important considerations in patient selection for free-flap reconstruction include age, comorbidities, and functional needs. Older patients are more likely to have comorbid factors that may increase their risk of exposure to prolonged anesthesia, affect wound healing, and decrease their tolerance for donor site morbidity. Some patients may not need the additional functional advantages gained from free-flap reconstruction. The risks and benefits of free-flap reconstruction must be considered for each individual patient.

Preoperative planning and communication with the anesthesia, nursing, and other involved surgical teams facilitate an efficient and well-executed surgical procedure. The tissue defect, functional needs of the patient, or both must be anticipated so that the optimal free flap is selected. Factors to be considered are tissue character-istics, the length of pedicle, color match, soft tissue bulkiness, and the functional disability of the donor site. Communication about the patient's intraoperative position and the preservation of adequate donor vessels for anastomosis should also be relayed with the appropriate teams.

Technical Considerations

Although careful preoperative planning, patient selection, and flap design are important factors in free-tissue transfers, a meticulous microvascular technique is essential for the successful insetting and revascularization of tissue units. Critical to the execution of microvascular techniques are proper instruments, an operating microscope, and the expertise of microvascular surgeons who are trained in the techniques of vessel selection, handling, and preparation.

A. Vessel Preparation

As a rule, vessel handling should be minimal to decrease the risk of trauma or injury. Vessels should be handled by the adventitia because direct contact with the intima may cause spasm, endothelial damage, and thrombosis, all with the potential of compromising blood flow to and from the transferred tissue. Vessels in the vascular pedicle are skeletonized, freeing the arteries from the veins within the vascular pedicle. Atraumatic vascular clamps are then placed. The vessels are transected and irrigated intermittently with dilute heparinized saline solution to prevent thrombosis. Finally, the excess adventitia is removed from the vessels to expose the media; adventitia trapped in the lumen at the suture line may initiate clot formation.

B. Microvascular Anastomosis

After both donor and recipient vessels are prepared, arterial anastomosis is followed by venous anastomosis. End-to-end anastomosis is the most commonly used technique, using appropriately sized monofilament sutures (8-0, 9-0, or 10-0). The end-to-side technique is used when there is a significant size mismatch between vessels (> 3:1) or when the internal jugular vein is the recipient vessel. Tension should not exist at the suture line and vessels should be sutured to lie without twists or kinks.

FASCIAL & FASCIOCUTANEOUS FREE-TISSUE FLAPS

Fascial and fasciocutaneous free-tissue flaps are commonly used flaps in head and neck reconstruction. They are characterized by thin, pliable fascia or skin without the bulk of pedicled myocutaneous flaps. Furthermore, they have the potential for crude sensation through the reanastomosis of an accompanying cutaneous nerve to nerves at the recipient site. They are primarily used for complex intraoral, pharyngeal, and cutaneous defects of the head and neck.

1. Radial Forearm Free-Tissue Flaps

The free-tissue flap of the radial forearm is based on the radial artery and cephalic vein. The skin is supplied by fasciocutaneous vessels in the intermuscular septum.

The main advantages of the radial forearm flap are its thin and pliable tissue characteristics. This flap is an excellent choice to reconstruct oral cavity and oropharyngeal defects without limiting mobility of the tongue or remaining structures. Furthermore, this tissue can be tubed for pharyngeal, laryngeal, and esophageal defects. Crude sensation may be achieved through the reanastomosis of the lateral and medial antebrachial cutaneous nerves to nerves at the recipient site.

Possible ischemic injury to the hand is the main disadvantage to this flap. Preoperatively, the Allen test is performed to verify collateral flow to the hand from the ulnar artery via the palmar arch. Other potential drawbacks include tendon exposure, dysesthesia, motor dysfunction of the hand, and cosmetic results at the donor site from coverage with a split-thickness skin graft (Figure 77–1).

2. Lateral Arm Free-Tissue Flaps

The fasciocutaneous flap of the lateral arm is supplied by the posterior branches of the radial collateral vessels from the profunda brachii artery. This flap has both a superficial and a deep venous system, the cephalic vein and paired venae comitantes, respectively. The perforators travel to the skin via the lateral intermuscular septum.

The advantages of this flap include a pliable skin paddle, the potential for sensory innervation through the posterior cutaneous nerve, and a donor site that can be closed primarily with minimal functional impairment. The disadvantages of this flap include smaller-caliber vessels and the variability of subcutaneous fat, which depends on the patient's body habitus.

3. Fasciocutaneous Flaps of the Lateral Thigh

The fasciocutaneous flap of the lateral thigh receives its blood supply from the cutaneous perforators of the profunda femoris artery, with the dominating third perforator. Venous drainage occurs through paired venae comitantes that accompany branches from the third perforator. The lateral femoral cutaneous nerve may also provide some sensation to the skin paddle.

The advantage of this flap is the availability of a sizable amount of pliable skin. The long axis of the skin paddle is designed over the intermuscular septum between the long head of the biceps femoris and the vastus lateralis muscles. This flap has been used after laryngopharyngectomy, and the ample subcutaneous tissue is useful in total glossectomy and skull base defects.

Donor site morbidity is minimal but may include wound dehiscence and compartment syndrome. Another disadvantage is the potential anatomic variation of the vascular bundle.

The anterior lateral thigh flap was initially described at the time of the lateral thigh flap, but it did not gain widespread acceptance and popularity until recently. This flap is similar to the lateral thigh flap in tissue characteristics, yet in a more favorable position for simultaneous harvest, since the approach is to the anterior thigh. The anterior lateral thigh flap is based on a septocutaneous or septomyocutaneous perforator off of the circumflex femoral artery and vein. The vascular pedicle travels between the rectus femoris and vastus lateralis muscles until giving off perforating branches that supply the cutaneous segment. This perforator is situated within a 3-cm circle located midway between the anterior iliac crest and the lateral patella.

Advantages of the flap include the minimal donor site morbidity, since primary closure is usually achievable and minimal muscular loss is required. Disadvan-

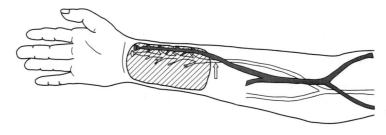

Figure 77–1. Radial forearm free-tissue flap (hatched lines) based on the radial artery (open arrow) and cephalic vein.

tages include the somewhat short vascular pedicle, requirement for delicate perforator dissection, and the somewhat small vessel diameter. The clinical uses of this flap are similar to those of the lateral thigh free flap.

Lueg EA. The anterolateral thigh flap: radial forearm's "big brother" for extensive soft tissue head and neck defects. *Arch Otolaryngol Head Neck Surg.* 2004;130(7):813.

Wei FC, Jain V, Celik N, Chen HC, Chuang DC, Lin CH. Have we found an ideal soft-tissue flap? An experience with 672 anterolateral thigh flaps. *Plast Reconstr Surg.* 2002;109(7):2219; discussion 2227. (An outstanding review with the single greatest experience with this flap.)

4. Scapular Fasciocutaneous Flaps

The scapular fasciocutaneous flap is based on the circumflex scapular artery and vein and may be harvested either as a fasciocutaneous or an osseocutaneous flap (see Osseomyocutaneous Free-Tissue Flaps in the following text). The circumflex scapular artery originates from the subscapular artery and terminates into the transverse and descending branches, which may be used to supply two separate skin islands—the scapular and parascapular flaps, respectively. Two skin flaps supplied by a single vascular pedicle offer an excellent choice when both intraoral and external coverage are needed. The scapular region provides a large amount of tissue (14–21 cm) useful for larger defects, large-caliber vessels, and an acceptable color match to facial skin.

The major drawback of this flap is the lateral decubitus position of the patient during flap harvest, which limits a simultaneous two-team approach. Furthermore, no potential for sensory reinnervation exists. Although the donor site can be closed primarily with minimal morbidity, patients need to wear a sling and undergo physical therapy for a short period of time postoperatively.

5. Temporoparietal Fascial Flaps

The temporoparietal fascial flap derives its blood supply from the superficial temporal artery and vein. The temporoparietal fascia is thin, pliable, and well vascularized, allowing it to mold into complex facial defects and drape over skeletal frameworks such as the ear. This flap also has the unique property of providing a viscous gliding surface that is excellent for tendon excursion. Moreover, it is an excellent choice for reconstruction of dorsal hand and foot defects with exposed tendon and bone. The temporoparietal fascial flap is most often used as a pedicled flap. As a free flap, it can be used for orbital reconstruction and a nasal lining in the setting of total nasal reconstruction; it has recently been described for laryngeal reconstruction after partial laryngectomy.

The disadvantages of this flap include a donor-site scar, potential alopecia along the region of flap elevation, and a small-caliber vessel (Table 77–1).

Azizzadeh B, Yafai S, Rawnsley JD et al. Radial forearm free flap pharyngoesophageal reconstruction. *Laryngoscope.* 2001;111 (5):807. [PMID: 11359159] (Evaluates wound healing, speech, and swallowing outcomes.)

Cheney ML, Varvares MA, Nadol JB Jr. The temporoparietal fascial flap in head and neck reconstruction. *Arch Otolaryngol Head Neck Surg.* 1993;119(6):618. [PMID: 8388696] (Techniques, advantages, and applications are described.)

Hayden RE, Deschler DG. Lateral thigh free flap for head and neck reconstruction. *Laryngoscope.* 1999;109(9):1490. [PMID: 10499060] (Describes favorable outcomes in the largest case series.)

Ninkovic M, Harpf C, Schwabegger AH, Rumer-Moser A, Ninkovic M. The lateral arm flap. *Clin Plast Surg.* 2001;28(2): 367. [PMID: 11400830] (Describes the anatomy, surgical approach, advantages, and disadvantages of the lateral arm flap.)

Urken ML, Bridger AG, Zur KB, Genden EM. The scapular osteofasciocutaneous flap: a 12-year experience. *Arch Otolaryngol Head Neck Surg.* 2001;127(7):862. [PMID: 11448364] (Describes favorable outcomes for patients with large surface area defects, those with preexisting gait disturbances, and older patients.)

OSSEOMYOCUTANEOUS FREE-TISSUE FLAPS

A variety of composite flaps, comprising both soft tissue and bone, are available for mandibular, maxillary, and palatal defects. Because each flap has advantages and limitations, the surgeon needs to consider the soft tissue characteristics, the length of bone stock and vascular pedicle, and the suitability for osseointegration (ie, the placement of dental implants) of each flap.

The bony components of these composite flaps are vascularized by the periosteum, which in turn receives perforators from the main pedicle. The bone is plated to the viable remaining native bone, allowing primary bone healing. These free-tissue techniques, which include a bone segment, offer advantages over traditional techniques, which use reconstruction plates and myocutaneous pedicled flaps. Free-tissue techniques also provide an advantage to the high rates of plate extrusion and wound breakdown associated with traditional techniques.

1. Scapular Osseomyocutaneous Flaps

As described previously, the circumflex scapular artery divides into the transverse and descending branches. The transverse branch of the scapular circumflex artery travels approximately 2 cm below and parallel with the scapular spine whereas the descending branch parallels the lateral border of the scapula. Approximately 10–14 cm of bone can be harvested from the lateral scapular border, which is suitable for osseointegration. The advantages and disadvantages are sim-

Table 77–1. Anatomy, advantages, and disadvantages of various fasciocutaneous flaps.

Type of Flap	Neurovascular Pedicle	Advantages	Disadvantages
Radial forearm	Radial artery Cephalic vein Lateral and medial antebrachial nerves	Thin, pliable Potential sensation	Possible ischemia, tendon exposure, motor dysfunction, and unfavorable cosmesis at donor site
Lateral arm	Radial collateral vessels from the profunda brachii artery Cephalic vein and paired venae comitantes Posterior cutaneous nerve	Thin, pliable Potential sensation Donor site can be closed primarily	Smaller-caliber vessels Variability of subcutaneous fat
Lateral thigh	Perforators off the profunda femoris artery (with dominant third perforator) Paired venae comitantes Lateral femoral cutaneous nerve	Sizable amount of pliable skin Excess subcutaneous tissue useful for large defects	Possible wound dehiscence and compartment syndrome Anatomic variability of vascular bundle
Scapula	Circumflex scapular artery and vein	Large amount of tissue Possibility of two skin islands Large-caliber vessels Acceptable color match with facial skin	Patient lies in lateral, decubitus position No potential for sensory reinnervation
Temporoparietal fascia	Superficial temporal artery and vein	Thin, pliable Rich, vascular capillary network Gliding surface	Donor site scar Potential alopecia

ilar to the scapular fasciocutaneous flap described earlier (Figure 77–2).

2. Osseomyocutaneous Flaps of the Iliac Crest

The iliac crest composite flap is based on the deep circumflex iliac artery and vein, which arise from the external iliac system. Perforators from the deep circumflex iliac artery supply the skin overlying the iliac crest and the ascending branch of this artery forms an arcade on the undersurface of the internal oblique muscle.

Although up to 16 cm of bone stock can be harvested from the iliac crest, this flap was limited by the lack of maneuverability of the soft tissue component. The iliac crest flap was modified to include the internal oblique muscle. An osseomyocutaneous flap of the internal oblique-iliac crest offers increased flexibility of the soft tissue components as well as decreased bulk, making it a more versatile flap for oromandibular reconstruction. The iliac crest also provides a hardy bone stock suitable for osseointegrated implants.

The drawbacks of this flap are a short vascular pedicle, bulky skin island, and morbidity at the donor site. The donor site has an increased risk of abdominal hernias, even with the use of mesh, and gait abnormality.

3. Fibular Osseomyocutaneous Flaps

The fibular composite flap is based on the peroneal artery and vein. Perforators from the posterior intermuscular septum supply the thin overlying skin; sensation to the flap may be restored through the lateral sural cutaneous nerve. This flap offers the longest length of available revascularized bone (24 cm), allowing near-total oromandibular reconstruction. Although the height of the fibular bone stock is shorter than the iliac crest, it can still support osseointegrated implants.

Preoperatively, angiography or magnetic resonance angiography (MRA) is recommended to verify the collateral vascular supply to the foot. Approximately 6–8 cm of fibular bone should be left proximally to prevent injury to the common peroneal nerve and distally to prevent destabilization of the ankle.

Although the skin island is thin and pliable, it is somewhat limited by its linear orientation to the bone. However, technical modifications have made the skin harvest dependable. The donor site can usually be closed primarily, but a skin graft may be required. Functional mobility of the leg is expected postoperatively.

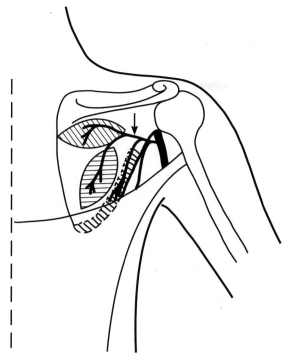

Figure 77–2. Scapular fasciocutaneous flap based on the circumflex scapular artery (arrow), which may include bone from the lateral border of the scapular (shaded region).

4. Osseocutaneous Flaps of the Radial Forearm

The fasciocutaneous flap of the radial forearm, described in the previous section, may also be harvested as a composite flap. The length of radius that may be harvested is limited to 10–12 cm in length and to 40% of the diameter to prevent donor site complications. The use of this flap has been limited by the risk of pathologic fracture and short bone stock available (Table 77–2).

Genden EM, Wallace D, Buchbinder D, Okay D, Urken ML. Iliac crest internal oblique osteomusculocutaneous free flap reconstruction of the postablative palatomaxillary defect. *Arch Otolaryngol Head Neck Surg.* 2001;127(7):854. [PMID: 11448363] (Describes favorable results for competent oral rehabilitation without the need for a prosthetic obturator.)

Shpitzer T, Neligan PC, Gullane PJ et al. Oromandibular reconstruction with the fibular free flap: analysis of 50 consecutive flaps. *Arch Otolaryngol Head Neck Surg.* 1997;123(9):939. [PMID: 9305243] (Describes favorable functional and cosmetic results.)

Urken ML, Bridger AG, Zur KB, Genden EM. The scapular osteofasciocutaneous flap: a 12-year experience. *Arch Otolaryngol Head Neck Surg.* 2001;127(7):862. [PMID: 11448364] (Describes favorable outcomes for patients with large surface area defects, with preexisting gait disturbances, and older patients.)

Werle AH, Tsue TT, Toby EB, Girod DA. Osseocutaneous radial forearm free flap: its use without significant donor site morbidity. *Otolaryngol Head Neck Surg.* 2000;123(6):711. [PMID: 11112963] (Internal fixation reduces the incidence of donor radius fractures while preserving excellent function.)

Table 77–2. Anatomy, advantages, and disadvantages of various osseocutaneous flaps.

Type of Flap	Neurovascular Pedicle	Length of Bone Stock	Advantages	Disadvantages
Scapula	Circumflex scapular artery and vein	Up to 10–14 cm	Large amount of tissue Possibility of two skin islands Large-caliber vessels Acceptable color match with facial skin Suitable for osseointegration	Patient lies in lateral, decubitus position No potential for sensory reinnervation
Iliac crest	Deep circumflex iliac artery and vein	Up to 16 cm	Flexible soft tissue component Suitable for osseointegration	Short vascular pedicle Bulky skin island Risk of abdominal hernia
Fibula	Peroneal artery and vein	Up to 24 cm	Offers greatest length of bone for possible near-total mandibular reconstruction	Little maneuverability of soft tissue around bone May need skin graft to cover donor site
Radius	Radial artery Cephalic vein Lateral and medial antebrachial nerves	Up to 10–12 cm	Thin, pliable Potential sensation	Possible pathologic fracture Short bone stock

MYOGENOUS & MYOCUTANEOUS FREE-TISSUE FLAPS

Before the advances in microvascular techniques, pedicled myocutaneous flaps were the standard of care for head and neck reconstruction. Pedicle flaps still play an important role, but free-tissue myogenous and myocutaneous flaps offer greater versatility with fewer limitations. The following flaps may be harvested as muscle only or with skin and adipose tissue.

1. Myogenous & Myocutaneous Flaps of the Rectus Abdominis Muscle

Although the rectus abdominis muscle has a dual blood supply from the inferior and superior epigastric arteries, the harvested free-tissue flap is based on the larger-caliber inferior epigastric system. These vessels arise from the external iliac vessels.

This flap is used primarily for its significant muscle and soft tissue bulk, long vascular pedicle, and reliability. It is an excellent choice for large maxillary and skull base defects.

The main donor site morbidity is a potential ventral hernia, with the most susceptible region below the arcuate line. To decrease the risk of tissue and viscera herniation, the anterior rectus sheath below the arcuate line must be meticulously closed; mesh may be used as an adjunct to strengthen the abdominal wall (Figure 77–3).

2. Myocutaneous Flaps of the Latissimus Dorsi Muscle

The latissimus dorsi muscle receives its blood supply from the thoracodorsal artery and vein with innervation from the thoracodorsal nerve. It is potentially the largest flap used in head and neck reconstruction.

An advantage of this flap is the versatility in the amount of muscle that is harvested, ranging from a small amount of muscle under the skin paddle to the entire muscle. Other advantages include its long pedicle length (9 cm), large-caliber vessels, and the ability to design a bilobed flap based on the medial and lateral branches of the thoracodorsal artery. This flap is used for glossectomy, the skull base, and large cervical cutaneous defects. Muscle only may be harvested and used with skin grafting for large scalp defects.

Disadvantages to this flap are the potential for seroma formation and wound dehiscence at the donor site. The lateral decubitus position of the patient, needed for flap harvest, limits the simultaneous two-team approach (Figure 77–4).

3. Myogenous & Myocutaneous Flaps of the Gracilis Muscle

The dominant vascular supply to the gracilis muscle is the adductor artery, which arises from the profunda

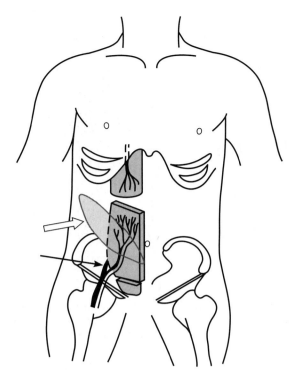

Figure 77–3. Rectus abdominis muscle and overlying skin paddle (dark arrow) supplied by the inferior epigastric vascular pedicle (open arrow).

femoris. Venous drainage occurs via accompanying venae comitantes. Motor innervation to the gracilis is supplied by the obturator nerve, which divides into fascicles to different portions of the muscle.

The gracilis muscle is a medial rotator and superficial adductor of the medial thigh whose primary role in head and neck reconstruction is for facial reanimation. The main advantages of the gracilis flap for facial reanimation are the fascicular neuroanatomy of the obturator nerve, the long vascular pedicle (up to 6 cm), and the ability to allow a simultaneous two-team harvest. Donor morbidity is minimal (Table 77–3).

Browne JD, Burke AJ. Benefits of routine maxillectomy and orbital reconstruction with the rectus abdominis free flap. *Otolaryngol Head Neck Surg.* 1999;121(3):203. [PMID: 10471858] (Describes the functional benefits and acceptable cosmesis.)

Papadopoulos ON, Gamatsi IE. Use of the latissimus dorsi flap in head and neck reconstructive microsurgery. *Microsurgery.* 1994;15(7):492. [PMID: 7968480] (Describes the benefits for wide defects of the head and neck.)

Shindo M. Facial reanimation with microneurovascular free flaps. *Facial Plast Surg.* 2000;16(4):357. [PMID: 11460302] (Describes the excellent functional and aesthetic results of free-flap reconstruction for facial reanimation.)

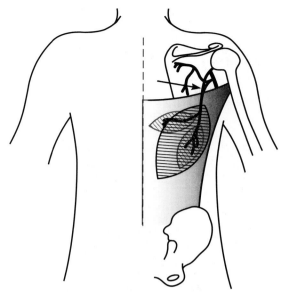

Figure 77–4. Latissimus dorsi flap based on the thoracodorsal artery (arrow); it is shown here as a single large skin paddle (horizontal lines) or as two separate paddles (vertical lines).

ENTERIC FREE-TISSUE FLAPS

The jejunal enteric free-tissue flap was the first example of head and neck free flap reconstruction in humans (1959). The unique aspect of jejunal and omental-gastroomental tissue in head and neck reconstruction is the availability of a mucosal surface that may be used to reconstruct the aerodigestive tract. Both jejunum and gastroomentum flaps may be used as a tubed flap or mucosal patch.

1. Jejunal Enteric Free-Tissue Flaps

The jejunal enteric free-tissue flap is based on arborizing vessels from the superior mesenteric artery and vein. The antimesenteric border of this flap may be filleted, exposing a mucosal surface and providing a pliable and secretory flap for pharyngeal and oral cavity reconstruction. This tubular flap has been used extensively for pharyngoesophageal defects and the diameter of the jejunum makes it appropriate for this purpose.

The disadvantages of this flap include its fragile vessels, poor tolerance to ischemia, and the risks associated with the laparotomy required for harvest: bowel adhesions, obstruction, and wound dehiscence (Figure 77–5).

2. Omental & Gastroomental Free-Tissue Flaps

The omental flap derives its vascular supply from the right and left gastroepiploic vessels. This flap includes the double layer of peritoneum that hangs off the greater curvature of the stomach. A segment of the greater curvature is included in the gastroomental flap.

Because of its excellent blood supply, the omentum has a wide variety of uses in the head and neck, including reconstruction of the skull base and large scalp defects, carotid coverage, the management of wounds with osteomyelitis and osteoradionecrosis, and facial contouring. The gastroomental tissue includes gastric mucosa, which provides potential secretions useful for oropharyngeal defects.

Donor site morbidity includes potential intra-abdominal complications such as a gastric leak and gastric outlet syndrome.

Genden EM, Kaufman MR, Katz B, Vine A, Urken ML. Tubed gastroomental free flap for pharyngoesophageal reconstruc-

Table 77–3. Anatomy, advantages, and disadvantages of myogenous and myocutaneous flaps.

Type of Flap	Neurovascular Pedicle	Advantages	Disadvantages
Rectus abdominus	Inferior epigastric artery and vein	Significant soft tissue bulk Long vascular pedicle	Potential ventral hernia, especially below arcuate line
Latissimus dorsi	Thoracodorsal artery and vein Thoracodorsal nerve	Large amount of available muscle Long vascular pedicle Large-caliber vessels Two soft tissue islands possible	Possible wound dehiscence and seroma formation Patient lies in lateral, decubitus postion for harvest
Gracilis	Adductor artery Venae comitantes Obturator nerve	Fascicular neuroanatomy suitable for facial reanimation Minimal donor site morbidity	Minimal

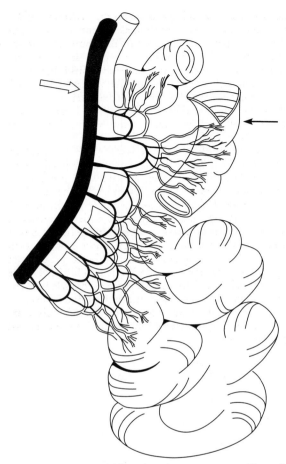

Figure 77–5. Jejunal flap showing a segment of bowel (dark arrow) based on the mesenteric branches of the superior mesenteric artery and vein (open arrow).

Table 77–4. Clinical applications for various microvascular free-tissue flaps.

Type of Flap	Clinical Applications
Fasciocutaneous	
Radial forearm	Oral cavity defects Oropharyngeal and esophageal defects
Lateral arm	Oral cavity and oropharyngeal defects
Lateral thigh	Laryngopharyngectomy, skull base, and total glossectomy defects
Scapula	Intraoral and external defects
Temporoparietal fascia	Dorsal hand and foot defects Auricular defects, nasal defects Laryngeal reconstruction Complex facial defects
Osseomyocutaneous	
Scapula	Maxillary and mandibular defects
Iliac crest	Maxillary and mandibular defects
Fibula	Maxillary and mandibular defects Near-total mandibular defects
Radial forearm	Mandible, orbit
Myogenous-Myocutaneous	
Rectus abdominis	Large maxillary and skull base defects
Latissimus dorsi	Skull base, glossectomy, and large cervical cutaneous defects
Gracilis	Facial reanimation
Enteric	
Jejunum	Pharyngeal, esophageal defects Can be filleted for oral cavity; pharyngeal defects
Omentum	Skull base , large scalp defects Coverage for wounds with osteomyelitis and osteoradionecrosis Carotid coverage Facial contouring
Gastro-omentum	Oropharyngeal defects Cervical, esophageal defects

tion. *Arch Otolaryngol Head Neck Surg.* 2001;127(7):847. [PMID: 11448362] (Describes the benefits for patients previously treated with multimodality therapy.)

Theile DR, Robinson DW, Theile DE, Coman WB. Free jejunal interposition reconstruction after pharyngolaryngectomy: 201 consecutive cases. *Head Neck.* 1995;17(2):83. [PMID: 7558817] (Describes a large series with excellent swallowing outcome and low morbidity.)

POSTOPERATIVE CARE

Once the microvascular unit has been successfully transplanted and vessels have been reanastomosed, the viability of the flap depends on the maintenance of arterial and venous flow. Factors that may reduce vascular flow, such as external compression from hematoma and edema, hypotension, and vessel spasm, need to be minimized (Table 77–4).

Postoperative Monitoring

The dreaded complication of microvascular reconstruction is flap loss from vascular compromise. Early detection may mean the difference between flap salvage and flap failure, with most surgeons favoring the frequent monitoring of flap viability for the first 48–72 hours. Venous congestion usually precedes arterial insufficiency owing to a low-flow system with an increased risk of thrombus formation. The most commonly used monitoring techniques are clinical assessment and Doppler ultrasound flowmeter.

Clinical evidence of venous congestion includes a purplish, turgid flap with rapid capillary refill (less than 1 second). Arterial insufficiency manifests with a pale, cold flap with prolonged capillary refill (> 3–4 seconds). Pinprick of the cutaneous portion of the flap with an 18-gauge needle is also an excellent means of assessing the quality of blood flow to and from the flap. A congested flap rapidly bleeds dark blood, whereas a flap with arterial insufficiency may not bleed at all or may bleed bright blood after a significant delay (> 4 seconds).

The Doppler ultrasound flowmeter is also a convenient tool to assess vascular flow. The quality of the Doppler signal can give evidence of the velocity of blood flow. Other monitoring methods, such as temperature probes, oxygen tension measurement, and color-flow Doppler, have been used.

Thrombus Prevention

The use of pharmacologic adjuncts to prevent thrombus formation is controversial. However, a variety of agents exist and their use is left to the discretion of the surgeon. Aspirin is an antiplatelet agent that has been used postoperatively to prevent thrombus formation. Heparin can be given as a low-dose intraoperative bolus followed by 5–7 days of intravenous infusion, or as a perioperative, subcutaneous injection of 5000 units twice a day. Dextran has been used for its antithrombin and antifibrin effects. An intraoperative bolus is followed by 5 days of intravenous infusion at 25 mL/h.

Medicinal leeches (*Hirudo medicinalis*) are useful for congested flaps and salvaging areas of marginal viability. Leeches release hirudin, an agent that inhibits the conversion of fibrinogen to fibrin at the bite site. The bite wounds then slowly ooze venous blood for up to 6 hours, relieving venous congestion. Patient hematocrit levels must be monitored to prevent significant blood loss, and an antibiotic, third-generation cephalosporin or ciprofloxacin is given intravenously for prophylaxis against specific gram-negative bacterial infection unique to the leech bite. The leech is removed from its attachment to the tissue after withdrawing approximately 5—10 mL of blood by exposing it to an alcohol swab. Each leech is used only once and disposed of using universal precautions.

Otoplasty

78

Jeffrey B. Wise, MD, Anil R. Shah, MD, & Minas Constantinides, MD

ESSENTIALS OF DIAGNOSIS

- *Prominauris (prominent ears) occurs in approximately 5% of the population.*
- *Knowledge of anatomy, embryology, and normal aesthetic proportions is essential for accurate diagnosis and surgical treatment of auricular deformities.*
- *Conchal prominence and the absence of an antihelical fold represent the most common causes of prominence of the ears.*
- *Although there are hundreds of techniques to correct auricular prominence, the most common are suture techniques for conchal setback (technique of Furnas) and for creation of an antihelical fold (technique of Mustarde).*
- *Otoplasty refinement techniques exist for deformities such as large earlobes and excessive helical prominences.*
- *Complication rates from otoplasty range from 7% to 12% and may be subdivided into early, late, and aesthetic/anatomic in etiology.*
- *Auricular hematoma occurs in 1% of otoplasties. Complaints of unilateral pain or tightness within the first 48 hours postoperatively require prompt removal of dressings to examine the wound site for hematoma collection.*

General Considerations

Deformities of the external ear, specifically prominent ear deformities, are relatively common. While posing negligible physiologic consequences, prominent ear deformities can be a source of profound psychological stress on the patient. Dieffenbach is credited with performing the first otoplasty in 1845 through resection of postauricular skin and conchomastoid fixation. Since that time, hundreds of techniques have been reported for correction of the prominent ear. Proper analysis, in combination with

meticulous surgical technique, can optimize form, symmetry, and ultimately patient satisfaction.

ANATOMY & EMBRYOLOGY OF THE AURICLE

The external ear is a composite of cartilage and skin. Important topographic landmarks of the external ear include the circumferential structures of the helix, tragus, and lobule (Figure 78–1). These structures encase a multitude of well-described folds and involutions of the external ear, such as the conchal bowl, which is subdivided into the superior cymba concha and inferior cavum concha by the anterior helical crus. The antihelical fold courses superiorly and anteriorly, dividing into the superior crus and sharper inferior crus. The resulting depression that is formed between the antihelix and the helix is known as the *scaphoid fossa,* and the depression that is formed between the superior and inferior crura of the antihelical fold is known as the *triangular fossa.*

Embryologically, auricular development is first seen in the 5-week embryo and stems from six mesenchymal proliferations, or hillocks, of the first (mandibular) and second (hyoid) branchial arches. These primitive hillocks develop into mature auricular landmarks. Most of these anatomic landmarks are derived from second arch structures (helix, scapha, antihelix, antitragus, lobule), and a less significant contribution is made by first arch components (tragus and helical crus).

The ear consists of six clinically insignificant intrinsic muscles (major and minor helices, tragus, antitragus, transverse, and oblique muscles) and three extrinsic muscles that contribute minor structural support to the ear (anterior auricularis, superior auricularis, and posterior auricularis muscles). The arterial blood supply to the external ear is derived from the superficial temporal, posterior auricular, and occipital arteries. Motor innervation to the external ear, which varies among individuals, is supplied by the facial nerve. Multiple nerves are responsible for sensation to the auricle and include the lesser occipital, greater auricular, auriculotemporal, and Arnold's (CN X) nerves.

Janis JE, Rohrich RJ, Gutowski KA. Otoplasty. *Plast Reconstr Surg.* 2005;115:60e. [PMID: 15793433] (Comprehensive review

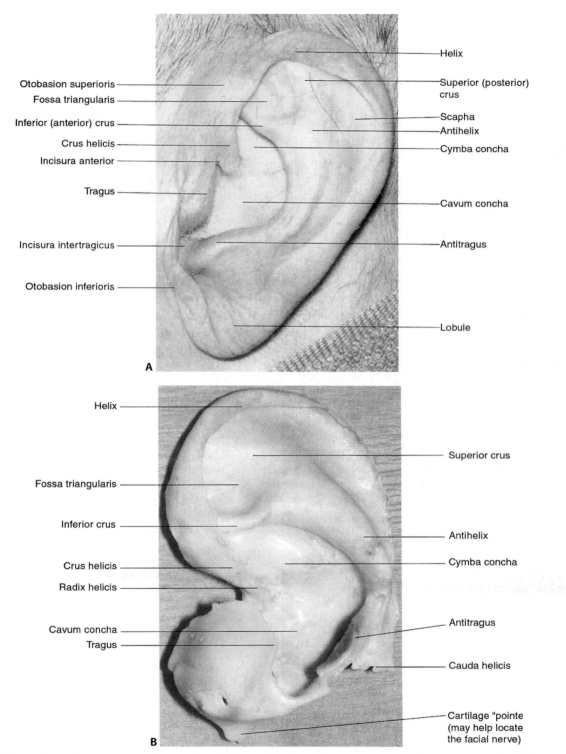

Figure 78–1. External landmarks of auricle with intact skin **(A)** and corresponding cartilaginous landmarks **(B)**. (Reproduced, with permission, from Larrabee WF, Makielski KH, Henderson JL. *Surgical Anatomy of the Face,* 2nd ed. Philadelphia: Lippincott Williams & Wilkins, 2004:171.)

that highlights the history of otoplasty and specific otoplasty techniques based on anatomic deformities.)

Larrabee WF, Makielski KH, Henderson JL. *Surgical Anatomy of the Face,* 2nd ed. Philadelphia: Lippincott Williams & Wilkins, 2004:171–172.

Wise JB. Otoplasty. In: Ruckenstein MJ, ed. *Comprehensive Review of Otolaryngology.* Philadelphia: Saunders, 2004:273.

PROPORTIONS & AESTHETIC CONSIDERATIONS OF THE EXTERNAL EAR

The adult Caucasian ear averages 63.5 mm and 35.5 mm in height and width, respectively. The average height and width of a Caucasian female ear is 59.0 mm and 32.5 mm, respectively. Generally, people of African descent possess ears that are slightly shorter in length, whereas Asians tend to have slightly longer ears. Proportionately, ear width is typically 50–60% of height. In context with the face, the lateral view demonstrates a "line of balance." Specifically, the slope of the ear approximates the nasal dorsum to within 15°, or lies approximately 20° posterior to the vertical plane. The superior aspect of the ear rests at the level of the brow.

In terms of ear protrusion, normal distances from the helix to the mastoid are 10–12 mm in the upper third of the ear, 16–18 mm in the middle third, and 20–22 mm in the lower third. On frontal view, the helix should project 2–5 mm more laterally than the antihelix. Conchal protrusion from the mastoid is typically 12–15 mm. The angle between the superior helix and mastoid in the aesthetically ideal ear is 20–30°. Prominauris, or excessive protruding of the ears, occurs when angles exceed 30–40°.

Campbell AC. Otoplasty. *Facial Plast Surg.* 2005;21:310. [PMID: 16575709] (This article reviews the aesthetic considerations in otoplasty with particular emphasis on otoplasty of the male patient.)

Kelley P, Hollier L, Stal S. Otoplasty: evaluation, technique and review. *J Craniofacial Surg.* 2003;14:643. [PMID: 14501322] (Summarizes evaluation and technique in otoplasty, underscoring the importance of a rational, stepwise evaluation of external ear deformities.)

PREOPERATIVE EVALUATION/TIMING OF SURGICAL CORRECTION

The incidence of excessively prominent ears is about 5%. It is inherited as an autosomal dominant trait with 25% partial penetrance; it most commonly results from two anatomic irregularities, specifically the absence of an antihelical fold and excessive depth or projection of the conchal bowl.

Precise analysis of auricular deformities is paramount to achieving successful outcomes. Surgeons must identify the specific cause of auricular prominence in the formu-

lation of an appropriate surgical plan. Although frequently bilateral, asymmetries in ear protrusion should be noted. As such, standard preoperative photography should be performed, including frontal, full right and left oblique, full right and left lateral, and close-up right and left lateral views.

Although there exist proponents of earlier surgical correction, most authors agree that the ideal age for otoplasty is between 5 and 6 years. Physiologically, the auricle is roughly 90% of adult height by 6 years of age. Psychosocially, correction is undertaken before or soon after a child's entrance to grammar school, where children are subject to peer ridicule. Moreover, by 5 or 6 years, children are able to participate in their own postoperative care (ie, not pulling off bandages or disturbing the wound).

Gosain AK, Kumar A, Huang G. Prominent ears in children younger than 4 years of age: what is the appropriate timing for otoplasty? *Plast Reconstr Surg.* 2004;114:1042. [PMID: 15457011] (This article provides a retrospective analysis of the efficacy of otoplasty in patients younger than 4 years of age.)

TECHNIQUES OF SURGICAL CORRECTION

Over 200 techniques have been described for correction of the prominent ear. Conceptually, they can be subdivided into procedures that address an absent antihelical fold, procedures that reduce excess in the conchal bowl, and those that reduce prominent or enlarged lobules. Most of the latter techniques involve reshaping auricular cartilage, which can be accomplished through a number of cartilage-manipulating techniques such as suturing, scoring, and excision/repositioning, to name a few. Herein, the most commonly used technique for correction of an absent antihelical fold, originally described by Mustarde, is discussed in greater detail. In addition, the Furnas technique for reduction of an excessive conchal bowl is described.

Technique of Mustarde

In 1963, Mustarde first described a technique for creating an antihelical fold by using permanent conchoscaphal mattress sutures. Since that time, many subtle refinements of this technique have been described, but the fundamentals of the procedure remain unchanged.

Pediatric patients most commonly undergo general anesthesia for this procedure, and perioperative broadspectrum antibiotics are administered. The face is prepped into a sterile field such that both ears can be visualized simultaneously. After infiltration with lidocaine 1% with epinephrine 1/100,000, an eccentric fusiform incision is made into the postauricular surface. Typically, more skin is excised from the postauricular surface than from the mastoid, in an effort to camou-

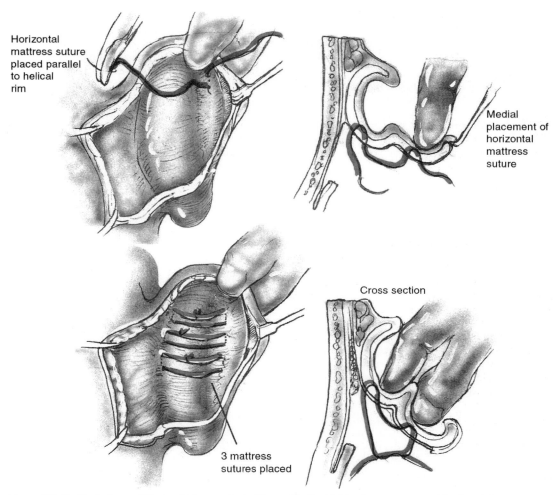

Figure 78–2. Technique of Mustarde for creation of the antihelical fold—three permanent horizontal mattress sutures are placed parallel with the helical rim. Care is taken to place sutures through the anterior perichondrium without violating the anterior skin. (Reproduced, with permission, from Adamson PA, Constantinides MS. Otoplasty. In: Bailey BJ, Calhoun KH, Coffey AR, Neely JG, eds. *Atlas of Head & Neck Surgery—Otolaryngology.* Philadelphia: Lippincott-Raven, 1996:429.)

flage the resultant scar into the postauricular sulcus following setback.

Once the fusiform of skin is excised, the remaining skin of the posterior aspect of the helix, antihelix, and concha is undermined with scissors, leaving perichondrium attached to the auricular cartilage. The extent of antihelical fold creation is determined by pinching the anterior auricle with a thumb and index finger. Alternatively, some surgeons mark cartilaginous landmarks with several ink-dipped fine needles. Permanent horizontal mattress sutures (eg, 4-0 Mersilene [Ethicon, Inc., Somerville, NJ]) are placed into the helical carti-

lage, parallel with the helical rim at the lateral extent of the desired antihelical fold (Figure 78–2). It is critical that sutures are placed through the cartilage and lateral perichondrium but not the lateral helical skin. The first helical suture is placed at the level of the helical root to create the superior crus. The second suture is typically placed just inferior to the junction of the superior and inferior crura. Third and fourth sutures are placed as needed. Some overcorrection is necessary during placement of the most superior suture, because it has been demonstrated that as much as 40% loss of correction at this site may occur within the first postoperative year.

The wound is irrigated with antibiotic solution and closed with resorbable sutures. Antibiotic ointment, along with cotton impregnated in mineral oil, is applied to the new antihelix and postauricular sulcus, and a mastoid dressing is applied.

The dressing is removed on the first postoperative day to check for hematomas, and replaced for 3–4 more days. Subsequently, a head band is worn continuously for 2 weeks and at night for an additional 4–6 weeks.

Technique of Furnas

In 1968, Furnas popularized a technique of conchal setback using permanent conchomastoidal suturing. This procedure is often undertaken in conjunction with techniques to correct an absent antihelical fold, as described above.

The patient is prepped and draped in a manner similar to that described for correction of the antihelical fold. After infiltration of lidocaine 1% with epineph-

rine 1/100,000, a fusiform incision is made in the postauricular region. The width of the incision is estimated by manually pushing the concha toward the mastoid. Care is taken to avoid excessive skin excision, since tension on the wound predisposes to hypertrophic scar formation. Little to no skin excision is required inferior to the level of the antitragus. After excision of skin, soft tissue and postauricular muscle are excised from the postauricular sulcus. Sufficient soft tissue is excised to produce a pocket that will receive the concha during suture placement.

The skin over the helix, antihelix, and concha is undermined with scissors, and permanent horizontal mattress sutures (eg, 4-0 Mersilene [Ethicon, Inc., Somerville, NJ]) are placed at the lateral third of the concha cavum and concha cymba parallel with the natural curve of the auricular cartilage (Figure 78–3). The sutures are thrown through cartilage and lateral perichondrium, but not lateral auricular skin. At least three sutures are placed for adequate setback. The sutures are placed on what was

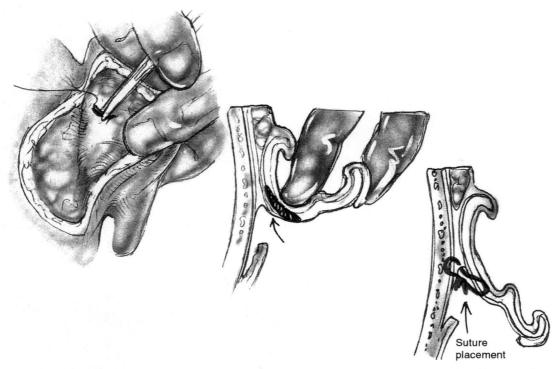

Suture
placement

Figure 78–3. Technique of Furnas for correction of conchal excess. Permanent conchomastoid horizontal mattress sutures are placed at the lateral third of the concha. A full-thickness bite of cartilage and perichondrium is performed, with care taken to avoid suture placement through the anterior skin. In addition, the sutures must pull the ear posteriorly as well as medially to prevent stenosis of the external auditory canal. (Reproduced, with permission, from Adamson PA, Constantinides MS. Otoplasty. In: Bailey BJ, Calhoun KH, Coffey AR, Neely JG, eds. *Atlas of Head & Neck Surgery—Otolaryngology.* Philadelphia: Lippincott-Raven, 1996:429.)

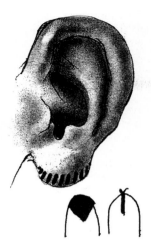

Figure 78–4. Fusiform wedge excision for reduction of large ear lobule. (Reproduced, with permission, from Adamson PA, Constantinides MS. Otoplasty. In: Bailey BJ, Calhoun KH, Coffey AR, Neely JG, eds. *Atlas of Head & Neck Surgery—Otolaryngology*. Philadelphia: Lippincott-Raven, 1996:435.)

the ascending wall of the concha and, when tightened, convert the wall into a longer floor of the concha. For long-term successful conchal reduction, suture bites of mastoid periosteum must be taken. With extremely thick cartilage, as frequently seen in older persons, the cartilage may be weakened by excising small vertical ellipses of cartilage. It is important for the conchomastoidal sutures to allow the concha to be set not only medially but posteriorly. If not, external auditory canal stenosis can result.

The wound is irrigated and closed as after the Mustarde technique. A mastoid dressing is placed, and subsequent postoperative management is the same as that of antihelical fold surgery.

Otoplasty Refinement Techniques

Frequently, small deformities of the auricle are present that can be corrected by subtle surgical refinements. These techniques are applicable to both congenital irregularities and deformities that are detected after more substantial otoplasty correction (ie, conchal setback and correction of absent antihelical fold). Such refinements include correction of the prominent lobule and reduction of helical prominences.

Reduction of a large ear lobule rarely requires general anesthesia in the adult population. A new earlobe size is designed with a marking pen. After infiltration with local anesthesia, a fusiform incision is made anteriorly and posteriorly in a curvilinear fashion, and a V-shaped, wedge excision of lobule excess is performed (Figure 78–4). The skin is closed with permanent suture (eg, 6-0 nylon), with suture removal occurring on the sixth postoperative day.

Helical prominences, such as superior outer helical rim cartilage excess (ie, elf ears, Spock ears) and superior helical fold cartilage excess (ie, lop ear), may be corrected by a variety of helical reduction techniques. After the infiltration of local anesthesia, a fusiform incision is made on the outer helical rim in the case of helical rim excess and under the helical fold in the case of superior helical fold excess (Figure 78–5). After skin elevation, excess cartilage is shaved using a blade. Skin is trimmed as necessary to ensure appropriate draping over the cartilaginous rim. The incision is closed with permanent suture (eg, 6-0 nylon), with suture removal occurring on the sixth postoperative day. No pressure dressing is requ ired.

Figure 78–5. Reduction of helical prominences. (Reproduced, with permission, from Adamson PA, Constantinides MS. Otoplasty. In: Bailey BJ, Calhoun KH, Coffey AR, Neely JG, eds. *Atlas of Head & Neck Surgery—Otolaryngology*. Philadelphia: Lippincott-Raven, 1996:435.)

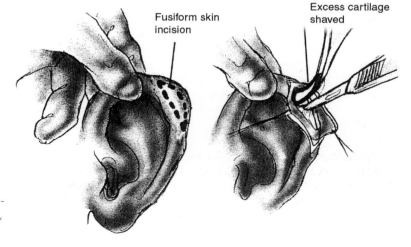

Fusiform skin incision

Excess cartilage shaved

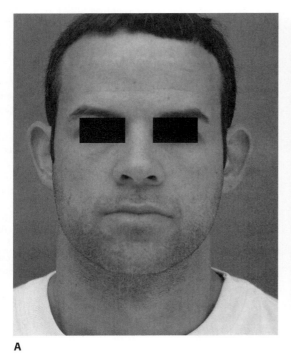

A

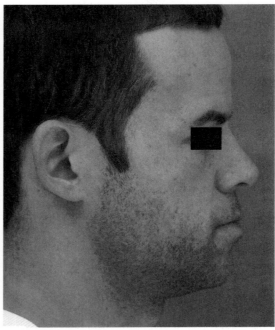

B

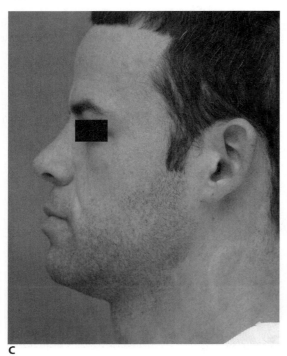

C

Figure 78–6. **(A–C)** Young man with prominauris, specifically conchal excess and an absent antihelical rim. **(D–F)** Patient 4 months postoperative from antihelical fold creation and conchal setback using suture techniques. *(Continued)*

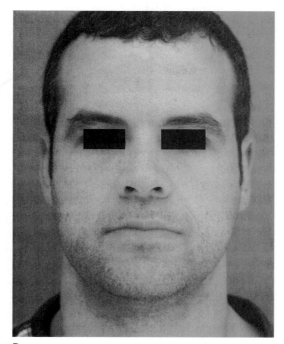

D

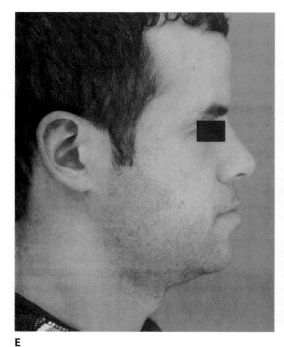

E

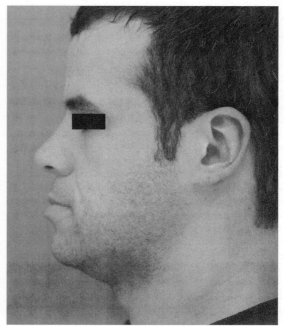

F

Figure 78–6 (Cont'd).

Table 78–1. Otoplasty complications.

Early Complications	Late Complications	Aesthetic/Anatomic Complications
Hematoma	Paresthesia/hypersensitivity	Inadequate correction
Infection	Suture extrusion	Antihelical overcorrection (ie, "hidden helix")
Chondritis	Suture granuloma formation	Telephone ear
Pruritis	Skin necrosis	Reverse telephone ear
	Hypertrophic scar formation	Malposition of the lobule
	Keloid scar formation	Sharp cartilaginous edges
		External auditory canal stenosis (from conchal setback)

From Becker DG, Lai SS, Wise JB, Steiger JD. Analysis in otoplasty. *Facial Plast Surg Clin North Am.* 2006;14:63–71.

Adamson PA, Constantinides MS. Otoplasty. In: Bailey BJ, Calhoun KH, Coffey AR, Neely JG, eds. *Atlas of Head & Neck Surgery—Otolaryngology.* Philadelphia: Lippincott-Raven, 1996: 429.

Furnas DW. Correction of prominent ears with multiple sutures. *Clin Plast Surg.* 1978;5:491. [PMID: 359225] (This article describes the author's suture technique for conchal setback using permanent conchomastoidalsuturing.)

Mustarde JC. The treatment of prominent ears by buried mattress sutures: a ten-year survey. *Plast Reconstr Surg.* 1967;39:382. [PMID: 5336910] (This article reviews the author's otoplasty suture technique for correcting a deficient antihelical fold.)

COMPLICATIONS OF OTOPLASTY

Overall, there is a high satisfaction rate among patients who undergo otoplasty surgery (85%). Complication rates range from 7% to 12%, with unsatisfactory aesthetic outcomes accounting for the majority of complications. Complications arising from otoplasty may be subdivided into early, late, and aesthetic/anatomic in etiology (Table 78–1).

Hematoma formation occurs following approximately 1% of all otoplasty procedures. Studies suggest a slightly higher incidence of hematoma formation in cartilage-cutting procedures compared with cartilage-suturing operations. Symptoms include unilateral or bilateral ear pain, usually within the first 48 hours after surgery. Hematoma formation may lead to perichondritis and the devastating sequelae of cartilage necrosis and ear disfigurement. Therefore, complaints of ear tightness or pain should be taken seriously with prompt removal of bandages and inspection of wounds. Infections after surgery typically manifest on postoperative day 3 or 4. Treatment involves systemic antibiotics, with particular emphasis on coverage for staphylococci, streptococci, and *Pseudomonas aeruginosa.*

Late complications include paresthesias of the ear, particularly to cold temperatures, which typically improve over 4–6 months. In addition, suture otoplasty techniques may result in complications surrounding permanent suture placement, such as suture extrusion and suture granuloma formation. These risks are minimized by meticulous placement of sutures. Hypertrophic scars or keloids may form as the wound heals, and conservative treatment with serial triamcinolone acetonide injections is indicated.

Aesthetic complications result from abnormalities in the relationship of the auricle to the scalp or from distortion of the auricle itself. These often stem from overcorrection or undercorrection of the initial deformity. Often, an unsatisfactory outcome occurs when there is asymmetry between the left and right ear (typically, less than 3 mm difference in the mastoid-helical distance between left and right ear is satisfactory). Classic deformities include the "telephone ear" deformity that results from overcorrection of the middle third of a prominent ear. "Reverse telephone ear" deformity occurs when the midauricle protrudes after overcorrection of the superior pole and lobule. Alternatively, inadequate conchal setback may produce a similar aesthetic deformity. Isolated antihelical overcorrection, or "hidden helix," produces the suboptimal appearance of the helix positioned medial to the antihelix on frontal view. All of the above aesthetic complications can usually be addressed through revision surgery, if desired by the patient.

Becker DG, Lai SS, Wise JB, Steiger JD. Analysis in otoplasty. *Facial Plast Surg Clin North Am.* 2006;14:63. [PMID: 16750764] (This article reviews otoplasty evaluation and provides a thorough description of potential otoplasty complications.

SUMMARY

Protrusion of the ears is a relatively common deformity. Successful surgical correction can relieve both children and adults of the psychosocial distress often associated with these deformities. An understanding of auricular anatomy and aesthetic ideals, plus with accurate analysis and meticulous surgical technique, can yield outcomes that are gratifying to both patient and surgeon (Figure 78–6).

Facial Fillers & Implants

Anil R. Shah, MD, Jeffrey B. Wise, MD, & Minas Constantinides, MD

ESSENTIALS OF DIAGNOSIS

- *Analysis of the type of rhytid, including anatomic location and depth and whether it is static or dynamic.*
- *Knowledge of the longevity of each facial injectable.*
- *Analysis of facial skeletal proportion, occlusion, and preoperative symmetry.*

General Considerations

Facial contouring is a recent trend in facial aesthetic surgery. Facial implants serve to add volume, providing a more appealing shape to a person's face. Facial injectables have reached tremendous popularity due to their safety, "no-down-time" appeal, and economics. Both are discussed to provide background on an exhaustive topic.

FACIAL FILLERS AND INJECTABLES

There are a large variety of facial injectables, each serving a different purpose. A brief summary of the most commonly used facial injectables with a delineation of their advantages and disadvantages will be highlighted.

Botulinum Toxin

Botulinum toxin A (BOTOX® [Allergan, Irvine, CA]) decreases facial lines and wrinkles at sites of skin pleating caused by hyperfunctioning mimetic muscles. Botulinum toxin A is FDA approved for treatment of the glabella. Off-label uses have included periorbital lines (crow's feet), platysmal bands, the forehead, and nasolabial and melolabial lines. Botulinum toxin A is also used for hyperhydrosis of the palms and armpits.

Botulinum toxin A causes paralysis by inhibiting acetylcholine release at the neuromuscular junction. This is accomplished in three steps. First, the toxin binds the nerve. Second, the toxin is internalized into the nerve. Third, the toxin is cleaved by internal proteolytic enzymes, and the degradation by-products interfere with the normal process of vesicle fusion to the plasma membrane. This results in the inhibition of the exocytosis of acetylcholine.

The toxin requires 24–72 hours to take effect, reflecting the time necessary to disrupt the synaptosomal process. In very rare circumstances, some individuals require as many as 5 days for the full effect to be observed. The effects of botulinum toxin last from 2 to 6 months.

The dose of the toxin is measured as 1 standard unit, which is equal to the amount necessary to kill 50% of Swiss-Webster mice injected with that dose. Extrapolating the data from mouse experimentation, Meyer and Eddie estimated that a 104-kg adult male would sustain a lethal dose of botulinum toxin type A at amounts exceeding 3500 units, a dose that far surpasses any dosing regimen in the cosmetic treatment of the aging face.

Botulinum toxin is contraindicated in patients with peripheral motor neuropathic diseases or neuromuscular functional disorders such as Eaton-Lambert syndrome and myasthenia gravis. Similarly, botulinum toxin type A is contraindicated in pregnant patients and those who are lactating, although unintentional administration has not resulted in birth defects or pregnancy issues. Finally, caution should be taken when injecting botulinum toxin type A to those taking aminoglycoside antibiotics or other agents that interfere with neuromuscular transmission, since these agents may potentiate the effects of botulinum toxin both locally and regionally.

Hyaluronic Acid Derivatives

Hyaluronic acid derivatives (Restylane [Medicis Aesthetics, Scottsdale, AZ], Captique [Allergan, Irvine, CA] Juvaderm [Allergan, Irvine, CA]) are glycosaminoglycan biopolymers, similar to the substance found in the intercellular layers of the dermis of the skin, and are very biocompatible. They are used primarily for lip and nasolabial fold augmentation and for fine wrinkles. Some recent uses of hyaluronic acid derivatives include nonsurgical rhinoplasty and volumetric filling in senile earlobe repair. Rare cases of hypersensitivity have been reported, but preinjection skin testing is generally not advocated. Volume enhancement with hyaluronic acid derivatives lasts 4–6 months, with some reports of material lasting for up to 16 months.

Complications are relatively uncommon with hyaluronic acid derivatives. In cases of overaugmentation, hyaluronidase can be used to decrease the amount of dermal filling. Caution should be used when injecting superior to the Frankfort horizontal line. Peter describes a case of retinal artery occlusion through retrograde flow through a peripheral branch of the ophthalmic artery. Skin necrosis is rare (a report of 2 cases of 400,000).

Poly-L-lactic Acid

Poly-L-lactic acid (Sculptra) is a volumetric filler currently FDA approved for treatment of lipoatrophy in HIV patients. Lipoatrophy in HIV is due to a number of factors including reverse transcriptase inhibitors and the disease process itself. Recently, poly-L-lactic acid has been used in an off-label capacity as a non-HIV facial filler. The main complication is nodule formation. This can be avoided by injecting deep to subcutaneous tissues and not in areas of significant muscle motion such as the lips. The duration of augmentation with poly-L-lactic acid is up to 3 years.

Calcium Hydroxylapatite

Calcium hydroxylapatite (Radiance FN, Bioform, Inc, Franksville, WI) is a major mineral constituent of bone. It has an off-label use for soft tissue augmentation in the face, primarily for reduction of nasolabial folds. Calcium hydroxylapatite should be injected subdermally to avoid nodule formation. The true longevity of calcium hydroxylapatite is not known.

Bovine Collagen

Bovine collagen (Zyderm and Zyplast; McGhan Medical Corporation, Fremont, CA) is composed of 95% type I collagen and is most commonly used to augment lips and nasolabial folds. Zyplast is cross-linked with glutaraldehyde (creates a longer-lasting effect) but must be injected into the deep dermis. Zyderm is injected into the superficial dermis. Hypersensitivity reactions occur in about 3% of patients; therefore, skin testing and even secondary skin testing are advocated. Bovine collagen augmentation lasts 2–4 months.

Human-Derived Collagen

Human-derived collagen (Cosmoderm and Cosmoplast, Inamed Corporation, Santa Barbara, CA) is used for the treatment of facial rhytids and lip augmentation. In contrast to bovine-derived collagen, human-derived collagen carries essentially no risk of hypersensitivity reactions,

obviating the necessity for pretreatment skin testing. Typically, injections maintain augmentation similar to that of bovine collagen. Adverse reactions may occur in patients with known allergy to bovine collagen.

Autologous Fat

Fat transplantation has the advantage of being an autologous substance. Fat transplantation is used as a volumetric filler. The concept of loss of facial volume is recent, and surgeons recontour the face, the nasolabial folds, temporal fossa, prejowl sulcus, and perioral and periorbital areas.

Most commonly, fat is harvested from the lateral thigh or abdominal region. Fat is then either strained or centrifuged, and injected into areas requiring volume. Technique in handling fat is crucial in maintaining adipocyte viability. Fat transplantation often requires multiple treatment sessions and has variable degrees of resorption. Fat can be frozen with minimal loss in fat viability and reinjected at a future date.

Disadvantages of fat harvest include donor site morbidity, potential for prolonged facial swelling, and unpredictable resorption. In addition, fat can lead to granulomas that can be treated with triamcinolone injections or direct excision. Advantages of fat transplantation include a potentially permanent, natural facial filler that can serve as an adjunctive or stand-alone procedure.

Butterwick KJ, Bevin AA, Iyer S. Fat transplantation using fresh versus frozen fat: a side-by-side two-hand comparison pilot study. *Dermatol Surg.* 2006;32(5):640. [PMID: 16706758] (This pilot study supports the use of autologous frozen fat or equivalent to improve results regarding longevity and aesthetic appearance versus fresh fat at 1, 3, and 5 months for fat augmentation of aging hands.)

Carruthers J, Fagien S, Matarasso, and the Botox Consensus Group. Consensus recommendations on the use of botulinum toxin type A in facial aesthetics. *Plast Reconstr Surg.* 2004;114(Suppl):1. [PMID: 15507786] (The review of each area encompasses the relevant anatomy, specifics on injection locations and techniques, starting doses (total and per injection point), the influence of other variables, such as gender, and assessment and retreatment issues by a consensus panel on botulinum toxin.)

Castor SA, To WC, Papay FA. Lip augmentation with AlloDerm acellular allogenic dermal graft and fat autograft: a comparison with autologous fat injection alone. *Aesthetic Plast Surg.* 1999;23(3):218. [PMID: 10384022] (Authors concluded that AlloDerm in conjunction with autologous fat injection constitutes a safe, reliable, and lasting method of lip augmentation, providing increased vermilion show compared with that with autologous fat injection alone.)

Coleman SR. Facial recontouring with lipostructure. *Clin Plast Surg.* 1997;24:347. [PMID: 9142473] (Landmark article describing the use of fat transplantation.)

Elson ML. The role of skin testing in the use of collagen injectable materials. *J Dermatol Surg Oncol.* 1989;15(3):301. [PMID:

2783212] (Skin testing can identify those patients with an allergic reaction, compromising approximately 2–3% of all patients.)

Friedman PM, Mafong EA, Kauvar ANB et al. Safety data of injectable nonanimal stabilized hyaluronic acid gel for soft tissue augmentation. *Dermatol Surg.* 2002;28:491. [PMID: 12081677] (According to the reported worldwide adverse events data, hypersensitivity to nonanimal hyaluronic acid gel is the major adverse event and is most likely secondary to impurities of bacterial fermentation.)

Han SK, Shin SH, Kang HJ, Kim WK. Augmentation rhinoplasty using injectable tissue-engineered soft tissue: a pilot study. *Ann Plast Surg.* 2006;56(3):251. [PMID: 16508353] (Description of a novel use of Restylane as a material for augmentation in rhinoplasty.)

Matarasso SL, Herwick R. Hypersensitivity reaction to nonanimal stabilized hyaluronic acid. *J Am Acad Dermatol.* 2006;55(1):128. [PMID: 16781306] (First report of a reaction to NASHA [nonanimal stabilized hyaluronic acid].)

Peter S, Mennel S. Retinal branch artery occlusion following injection of hyaluronic acid (Restylane). *Clin Exp Ophthalmol.* 2006;34(4):363. [PMID: 16764658] (Report of a retinal branch artery occlusion after facial injection of a dermal filler. The superior temporal artery showed occlusion due to a clearly visible long and fragmented embolus suggestive of gel and clearly distinguishable from calcific or cholesterol emboli.)

Sattler G. Long-lasting results with polylactic acid. *J Drugs Dermatol.* 2003;9:422. [PMID: 15303782] (Review article demonstrating benefits of polylactic acid as a facial filler.)

Sklar JA, White SM. Radiance FN. A new soft tissue filler. *Dermatol Surg.* 2004;30:764. [PMID: 15099322] (Retrospective review demonstrating favorable results with Radiance FN.)

Shoshani O, Ullmann Y, Shupak A et al. The role of frozen storage in preserving adipose tissue obtained by suction-assisted lipectomy for repeated fat injection procedures. *Dermatol Surg.* 2001;645. [PMID: 11442616] (Fat obtained by suction-assisted lipectomy may be preserved for future use by freezing.)

Vartanian AJ, Frankel AS, Rubin MG. Injected hyaluronidase reduces Restylane-mediated cutaneous augmentation. *Arch Facial Plast Surg.* 2005;7(4):231. [PMID: 16027343] (Intradermal hyaluronidase injections can be used to reduce dermal augmentation from previously injected Restylane. A small dose of hyaluronidase equivalent to 5–10 U may be injected initially.)

FACIAL IMPLANTS

Preoperative Assessment

The hypoplastic chin is the most common indication for chin augmentation. On frontal view, the face can be divided into thirds, with the lower third spanning from the subnasale to the mentum. Aging results in loss of vertical height of the mandible. On lateral view, a vertical line can be dropped from the lower lip. In females, the chin should be 1–2 mm posterior to this line. In males, the chin should lie at the same level as this line. There are a number of techniques to analyze chin size and projection (Table 79–1).

Patients' occlusion should be assessed preoperatively to ensure that orthognathic treatment is not necessary. Type I occlusion is when the mesial-buccal cusp of the maxillary first molar contacts with the mandibular first molar's buccal groove. Type II occlusion is when the maxillary first molar is anterior to the buccal groove (an overbite), and Type III is when the maxillary molar is posterior (an underbite).

Table 79–1. Chin analysis.

Rish technique	A line perpendicular to the Frankfort horizontal line is projected tangential to the most anterior edge of the lower lip vermilion border. This perpendicular line is the meridian that marks the desired chin projection.
Legan's angle	One line is projected through the glabella and the subnasale, and a second line is projected through the subnasale and the pogonion. The ideal angle created between these two lines is 12° ± 4°.
Merrifield Z-angle	A line is projected through the pogonion and the most anterior point of the upper lip vermilion border. The angle this creates with the Frankfort horizontal line should be 80° ± 5°.
Zero meridian of Gonzales-Ulloa	A line perpendicular to the Frankfort horizontal line projected through the nasion. The pogonion is supposed to be within 5 mm of this line. Retraction of the chin ≥ 1 cm is deemed first-degree retraction, 1–2 cm is second-degree retraction, and > 2 cm is classified as third-degree retraction. Significant is that first- and second-degree retractions are treatable with implants, but third-degree retraction is best treated with maxillofacial surgery.

Table 79–2. Midface analysis.

Hinderer	In a frontal view, draw a line from the lateral commissure of the lip to the lateral canthus of the ipsilateral eye. Another line projects from the tragus to the inferior edge of the nasal ala. The area posterior and superior to the junction of these two projections should be the most prominent area of the malar eminence.
Powell	A vertical line is drawn through the middle of the face, then the segment between the nasion and the nasal tip is bisected by a line that curves gently upward to the tragus on both sides. A line is drawn from the inferior ala to the lateral canthus and another one, parallel with this one, is drawn from the lateral intersection of the curvilinear horizontal line and the line from the oral commissure marks the point where the malar area should be most prominent.

Analysis of the malar and submalar region is much more complex and requires three-dimensional planning. The submalar triangle is the area below the malar eminence and the location of many facial deficiencies. Binder classified patterns of midfacial deformity and the resultant augmentation required. There are a variety of methods of analyzing the midface and its projection (Table 79–2).

Procedure

Chin implantation can take place by an external or intraoral route. The extraoral approach has the advantage of not contaminating the implant through the oral cavity. The intraoral approach prevents an external scar. Implants placed intraorally tend to "ride" high postoperatively, partly because of the difficulty in fixating the implant. The surgeon should be aware of the position of the mental nerve, which emanates from the bone approximately 1 cm above the edge of the mandible and approximately 2.5–3.5 cm from the midline, lying in the vertical plane between the first and second premolar.

Typically, malar and submalar implants are placed by an intraoral route. An incision is made along the upper gingivobuccal sulcus, and an elevator is used to lift the periosteum off the face of the maxilla. The masseteric fibers are released off of the face of the maxilla.

The infraorbital nerve is avoided as it exits the infraorbital foramen 4–7 mm below the inferior orbital rim on a vertical line that descends from the medial limbus of the iris. A tight periosteal pocket is created that is small enough to fit the implant tightly. The implant can be further fixated with a titanium screw, a resorbable suture, or a temporary external suture and bolster.

Complications

Complications of facial implants are rare and include hematoma, infection, nerve paresthesia (transient or permanent), and motor nerve injury. No study has shown a change in infection rates in extraoral versus intraoral approaches.

ePTFE (W.L. Gore & Associates, Flagstaff, AZ) is an expanded, strongly hydrophobic, fibrillated polymer that can be produced in sheets, three-dimensional strands, and suture material. ePTFE has been associated with infection, extrusion, and scarring. It has been used with success in a recent study with only 0.62% of implants requiring removal for infection. ePTFE has the advantage of being soft, with minimal encapsulation and bony resorption. ePTFE is unavailable at this time as a preformed facial implant.

Silicone is a relatively inert substance, which has more encapsulation than ePTFE. Bony resorption increases with overlying muscle action translating to implant mobility. Therefore, the implant should be secured in a tight pocket with either sutures or titanium screws. In addition, subperiosteal placement increases bony resorption. Well-positioned implants with osseous erosion should not be replaced. Silicone implants are easier to place than ePTFE owing to less flexibility at the peripheral portion of the implant and higher resistance to crushing.

Malar and submalar implants can result in injury to sensory nerve (V2) or motor nerve (buccal or temporal branch), albeit a rare event. More commonly, midface implants may result in asymmetry due to preexisting facial skeleton imbalances.

Godin M, Costa L, Romo T, Truswell W, Wang T, Williams E. Gore-Tex chin implants: a review of 324 cases. *Arch Facial Plast Surg.* 2003;5(3):224. [PMID: 12756115] (Description of results with Gore-Tex chin implants: two [0.62%] of the 324 implants became infected and were ultimately removed. No other complications occurred.)

Gonzalez-Ulloa M. Building out the malar prominences as an addition to rhytidectomy. *Plast Reconstr Surg.* 1974;53(3):293. [PMID: 4813762] (Technical article describing use of malar and submalar implants to improve rhytidectomy.)

Hinderer UT. Malar implants to improve facial proportions and aging. In: Stark RB, ed. *Plastic Surgery of the Head and Neck.* New York: Churchill Livingstone, 1987.

Matarasso A, Elias AC, Elias RL. Labial incompetence: a marker for progressive bone resorption in Silastic chin augmentation. *Plast Reconstr Surg.* 1997;98:1007. [PMID: 8911470] (A study of six patients with aesthetically positioned and appropriately sized Silastic implants revealed a correlation between preoperative baseline labial incompetence and mentalis muscle hyperactivity and progressive bony erosion.)

Tobias GW, Binder WJ. The submalar triangle: its anatomy and clinical significance. *Fac Plast Surg Clin North Am.* 1994;2:255. (Describes the submalar triangle and classifies the region to help with selection of appropriate implant.)

Index

Page numbers followed by *t* and *f* indicate tables and figures, respectively. Drugs are listed under their generic names; when a trade name is listed, the entry is cross-referred to the generic name.